230,-

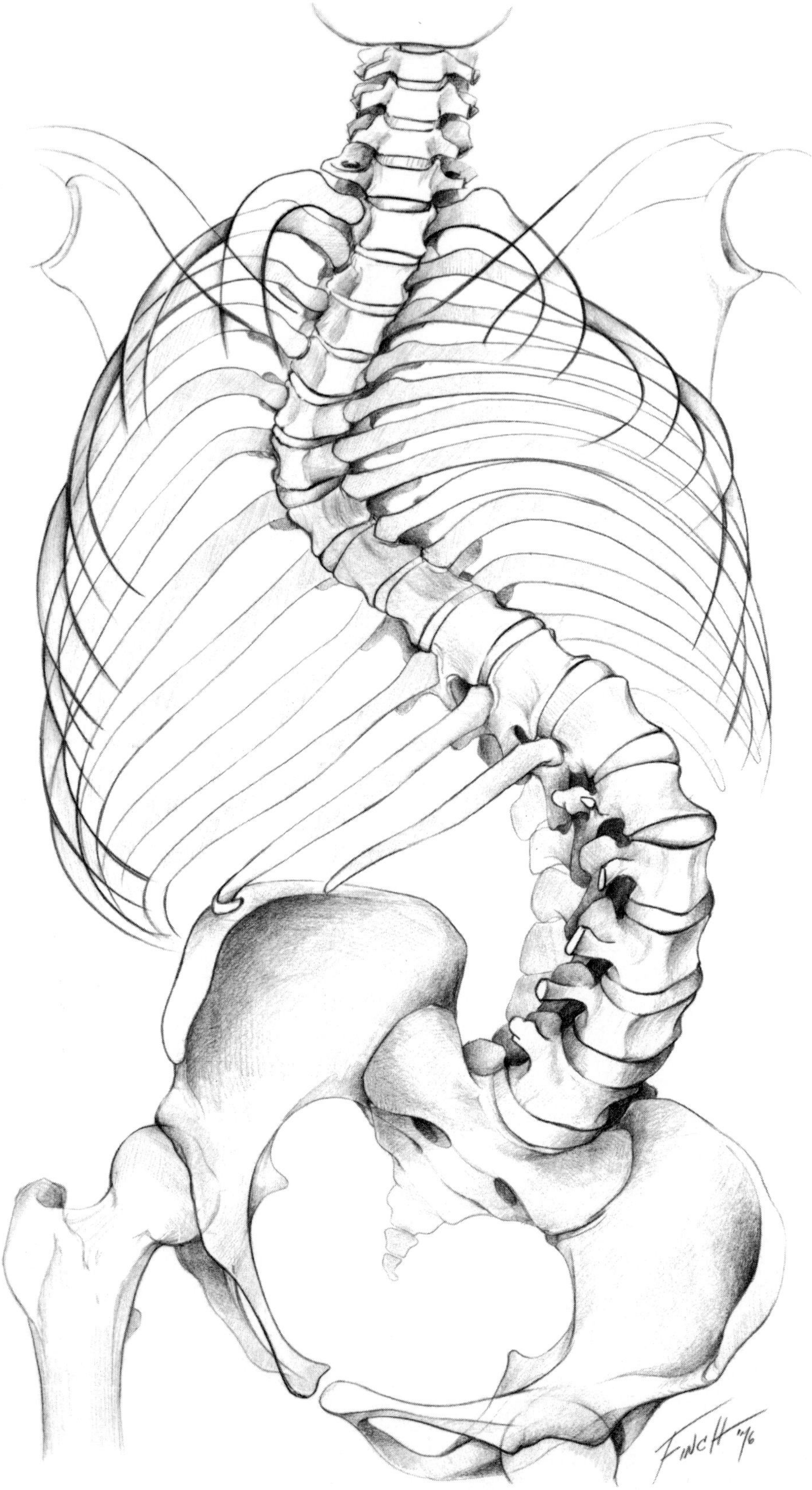
FINCH '96

Moe's Textbook of
SCOLIOSIS
and
Other Spinal Deformities

Second Edition

David S. Bradford, M.D.
Professor, Orthopaedic Surgery
Department of Orthopaedic Surgery, University of Minnesota
Director, Twin Cities Scoliosis Center, Spine Service
Department of Orthopaedic Surgery, University of Minnesota
Attending Staff, Fairview-Riverside Hospital and Twin Cities Scoliosis Center

John E. Lonstein, M.D.
Clinical Associate Professor, Orthopaedic Surgery
Department of Orthopaedic Surgery, University of Minnesota
Attending Staff, Minnesota Spine Center, Fairview-Riverside Hospital
Spine and C. P. Spine Services, Gillette Children's Hospital

John H. Moe, M.D.
Professor Emeritus, Orthopaedic Surgery
Department of Orthopaedic Surgery, University of Minnesota

James W. Ogilvie, M.D.
Assistant Professor, Orthopaedic Surgery
Department of Orthopaedic Surgery, University of Minnesota
Attending Staff, Fairview-Riverside Hospital and Twin Cities Scoliosis Center
Consulting Staff, Shriner's Hospital for Crippled Children

Robert B. Winter, M.D.
Clinical Professor, Orthopaedic Surgery
Department of Orthopaedic Surgery, University of Minnesota
Chief of Spine Service, Gillette Children's Hospital
Attending Staff, Minnesota Spine Center, Fairview-Riverside Hospital

Illustrated by
Martin Finch
Professor and Director, Biomedical Graphic Communications
Health Science Center, University of Minnesota

1987
W.B. Saunders Company
Philadelphia   London   Toronto   Sydney   Tokyo   Hong Kong

W. B. Saunders Company: West Washington Square
Philadelphia, PA 19105

Library of Congress Cataloging-in-Publication Data

Textbook of scoliosis and other spinal deformities.

Moe's textbook of scoliosis and other spinal deformities.

Rev. ed. of: Scoliosis and other spinal deformities. 1978.

Includes index.

1. Spine—Abnormalities.   2. Scoliosis.   I. Moe, John H., 1905–   II. Bradford, David S., 1936–
III. Scoliosis and other spinal deformities.   IV. Title.
[DNLM: 1. Scoliosis.   2. Spinal Diseases.   3. Spine—abnormalities. WE 735 T355]

RD768.T445 1987   617'.375   86-26060

ISBN 0-7216-6428-8

Cover art modified by Sharon Iwanczuk from the drawing of Martin Finch

Listed here are the latest translated editions of this book together with the language of the translation and the publisher.

Italian (*1st Edition*)–Verduci Editore, Rome, Italy.
Spanish (*1st Edition*)–Salvat Editores S.A., Barcelona, Spain.

Editor: W. B. Saunders Staff
Developmental Editor: David Kilmer
Designers: Karen O'Keefe and Patti Maddaloni
Production Manager: Carolyn Naylor
Manuscript Editor: Susan Short
Illustration Coordinator: Lisa Lambert
Page Layout Artist: Patti Maddaloni
Indexer: Erika Shapiro

Moe's Textbook of Scoliosis and Other Spinal Deformities   ISBN   0-7216-6428-8

© 1987 by W. B. Saunders Company. Copyright 1978 by W. B. Saunders Company. Copyright under the Uniform Copyright Convention. Simultaneously published in Canada. All rights reserved. This book is protected by copyright. No part of it may be reproduced, stored in a retrieval system, or transmitted in any form or by any means, electronic, mechanical, photocopying, recording, or otherwise, without written permission from the publisher. Made in the United States of America. Library of Congress catalog card number 86-26060.

Last digit is the print number: 9   8   7   6   5   4   3   2   1

CONTRIBUTORS

BRUCE BEN-DAVID, M.D.
Chairman, Department of Anesthesiology, Fairview Riverside Hospital, Minneapolis, MN.
Anesthesia for Surgery of the Spine

J. ABBOTT BYRD, III, M.D.
John H. Moe Spine Fellow, Twin Cities Scoliosis Center, Department of Orthopaedic Surgery, University of Minnesota, Minneapolis, MN; Assistant Professor of Orthopaedics, Department of Orthopaedic Surgery, West Virginia University, Morgantown, WV.
Idiopathic Scoliosis

KATHRYN A. HALE, M.D.
Clinical Assistant Professor, University of Minnesota; Attending Staff, Abbott-Northwestern Hospital, Fairview Riverside Hospital, Minneapolis, MN.
Pulmonary Function Testing

GLENN S. HALLER, M.D.
Attending Staff, Department of Anesthesiology, Fairview Riverside Hospital, Minneapolis, MN.
Anesthesia for Surgery of the Spine

NIKKI JACKSON JACOBS, M.S., MT(ASCP) SBB
American Red Cross Blood Services, St. Paul Region, Minneapolis, MN.
Bone Transplantation, Bone Banking, and Establishing a Surgical Bone Bank

WILLIAM E. KLINE, M.S., MT(ASCP) SBB
American Red Cross Blood Services, St. Paul Region, Minneapolis, MN.
Bone Transplantation, Bone Banking, and Establishing a Surgical Bone Bank

J. JEFFREY McCULLOUGH, M.D.
Professor, Department of Laboratory Medicine and Pathology, University of Minnesota; Director, Blood Bank, University of Minnesota; Director, American Red Cross Blood Services, St. Paul Region, Minneapolis, MN.
Bone Transplantation, Bone Banking, and Establishing a Surgical Bone Bank

FRED L. RASP, M.D., F.C.C.P.
Clinical Associate Professor of Medicine, University of Minnesota, Minneapolis, MN; Attending Staff, Parkview Memorial Hospital, St. Joseph's Medical Center, Lutheran Hospital, Fort Wayne, IN.
Pulmonary Function Testing

PETER D. TAYLOR, M.D.
Attending Staff, Department of Anesthesiology, Fairview Riverside Hospital, Minneapolis, MN.
Anesthesia for Surgery of the Spine

BRUCE E. van DAM, M.D.
Assistant Professor of Surgery, Uniformed Services University of the Health Sciences, Bethesda, MD; Director of Spine Surgery, Orthopaedic Surgery Service, Walter Reed Army Medical Center, Washington, DC.
Neurofibromatosis

FOREWORD

Eight years have elapsed since the first volume of *Scoliosis and Other Spinal Deformities* was published. The response to our first effort was indeed gratifying. *Scoliosis and Other Spinal Deformities* reached worldwide distribution with 3,000 volumes circulated in English outside North America. However, in the past decade there has been an ever expanding interest in spinal deformities, and development in this field has been explosive. Newer techniques, methodologies, and implant design along with increased knowledge of spinal biomechanics and the natural history of spinal deformity have made our past effort understandably obsolete.

We felt a new and expanded volume on spinal deformities was necessary. In this work we have attempted to present a clear and concise picture of the current state of the art and to provide the reader not only with our experience but also with a composite review and update of data presented and published elsewhere. The book has been expanded to include information on biomechanics, pulmonary function, bone banking, and anesthesia. We feel the reader will find this information useful and relevant. Although we have sought to individualize somewhat our respective contributions, we each have benefited from the critical review of all members of our group and have drawn freely on each other's experience as well as illustrative material when we felt it was desirable.

Finally, in acknowledgment of our respect and gratitude to our teacher, mentor, and friend, Dr. John H. Moe, we have dedicated this volume to him and have retitled our revised effort *Moe's Textbook of Scoliosis and Other Spinal Deformities*. This acknowledgment is but a small token of our appreciation to him for his contributions, leadership, and pivotal role in establishing the Twin Cities Scoliosis Center and the Scoliosis Research Society. As Dr. Paul Harrington so aptly said, "Dr. John H. Moe can truly be considered the father of the modern treatment of scoliosis."

DAVID S. BRADFORD
JOHN E. LONSTEIN
JOHN H. MOE
JAMES W. OGILVIE
ROBERT B. WINTER

ACKNOWLEDGMENTS

Preparing a textbook such as *Moe's Textbook of Scoliosis and Other Spinal Deformities* indeed requires an immense amount of work, not only for the authors but also for their supporting staff. We would be remiss in our responsibility if we did not formally acknowledge those who contributed so tirelessly, in a dedicated and energetic fashion, to facilitate our work in completing this effort.

We would like to formally acknowledge our secretaries and other clerical staff—Ruby Bauer, Jo Borovsky, Pat Ed, Debbie Kline, JoAnn Maier, Bonnie Stephens, and Cindy Warmbo—for their work and effort in typing, retyping, and editing our manuscripts. We would like specifically to acknowledge the dedicated efforts of Ms. Katherine Lindstrom, Administrative Secretary, Twin Cities Scoliosis Center, who was of tremendous help in manuscript preparation, data retrieval, and galley proof editing. Likewise, we benefited from the careful computerization and data retrieval by Ms. Cheryl Noren, who has kept our patient data base up to date and in a useful and retrievable form.

We would also like to thank the photographic departments of the University of Minnesota, Fairview Riverside Hospital, and Gillette Children's Hospital whose staffs spent many hours obtaining the best possible prints from sometimes marginal radiographs in order to have them available for this publication.

Fairview Riverside Hospital	Gillette Children's Hospital
Becky Johnson	Myke Bear
Barbara Szurek	Brian Benish
	Ken Jandle

University of Minnesota Photography Staff of the Biomedical Graphic Communications Department

The orthotics staff at Fairview Riverside Hospital and Gillette Children's Hospital have shown a tireless devotion to their duty in providing our patients with useful and effective orthoses for operative as well as nonoperative treatments, and we appreciate their efforts as well.

Fairview Riverside Hospital	Gillette Children's Hospital
Mary Cantin	Marty Carlson
Merv Larson	Lani Case
Nick McArdell	Paul Lemke
Ted Markgren	Charles Schemitsch
	Paul Swanlund

Finally, to the nursing staff at Fairview Riverside Hospital, Gillette Children's Hospital, and the University of Minnesota Hospital, a special note of acknowledgment is appropriate. New staff members have come, old ones have departed, but the consistency of high quality care has remained, and to this we owe a deep debt of gratitude.

DAVID S. BRADFORD
JOHN E. LONSTEIN
JOHN H. MOE
JAMES W. OGILVIE
ROBERT B. WINTER

CONTENTS

1
HISTORICAL ASPECTS OF SCOLIOSIS... 1
John H. Moe, M.D.

2
BIOMECHANICS.. 7
James W. Ogilvie, M.D.

3
EMBRYOLOGY AND SPINE GROWTH 25
John E. Lonstein, M.D.

4
CLASSIFICATION AND TERMINOLOGY.. 41
Robert B. Winter, M.D.

5
PATIENT EVALUATION 47
John E. Lonstein, M.D.

6
NATURAL HISTORY OF SPINAL DEFORMITY 89
Robert B. Winter, M.D.

7
ORTHOTICS 97
James W. Ogilvie, M.D.

8
TRACTION IN SPINE DEFORMITIES.. 109
James W. Ogilvie, M.D.

9
CAST TECHNIQUES... 119
John E. Lonstein, M.D.

10
TECHNIQUES OF SURGERY... 135
David S. Bradford, M.D.

11
IDIOPATHIC SCOLIOSIS 191
John H. Moe, M.D., and J. Abbott Byrd, III, M.D.

12
CONGENITAL SPINE DEFORMITY 233
Robert B. Winter, M.D.

13
NEUROMUSCULAR SPINAL DEFORMITY 271
David S. Bradford, M.D.

14
MYELOMENINGOCOELE.. 307
Robert B. Winter, M.D.

15
NEUROFIBROMATOSIS.. 329
John H. Moe, M.D., and Bruce E. van Dam, M.D.

16
JUVENILE KYPHOSIS 347
David S. Bradford, M.D.

17
ADULT SCOLIOSIS 369
John E. Lonstein, M.D.

18
SALVAGE AND RECONSTRUCTIVE SURGERY............................... 391
John E. Lonstein, M.D.

19
SPONDYLOLYSIS AND SPONDYLOLISTHESIS............................... 403
David S. Bradford, M.D.

20
DEFORMITIES OF THE THORACIC AND LUMBAR SPINE
SECONDARY TO SPINAL INJURY 435
David S. Bradford, M.D.

21
COMPLICATIONS OF TREATMENT... 465
John E. Lonstein, M.D.

22
MISCELLANEOUS PROBLEMS 491

CONTENTS

Benign and Malignant Tumors of the Spine 491
David S. Bradford, M.D.

Spinal Cord Tumors 505
Robert B. Winter, M.D.

Hysterical (Conversion) Scoliosis 511
Robert B. Winter, M.D.

Post Laminectomy Spine Deformity 513
John E. Lonstein, M.D.

Dwarfs 522
Robert B. Winter, M.D.

Cord Compression 540
John E. Lonstein, M.D.

Spine Deformity Following Radiation 547
James W. Ogilvie, M.D.

Marfan's Syndrome 554
Robert B. Winter, M.D.

Arthrogryposis 561
Robert B. Winter, M.D.

Osteogenesis Imperfecta 562
David S. Bradford, M.D.

Osteomyelitis 568
Robert B. Winter, M.D.

Congenital Heart Disease and Scoliosis 576
Robert B. Winter, M.D.

Scoliosis and Congenital Limb Deficiency 578
Robert B. Winter, M.D.

Thoracic Cage Defects and Contractures with Scoliosis 582
Robert B. Winter, M.D.

Pulmonary Function Testing 585
Kathryn A. Hale, M.D., and Fred L. Rasp, M.D.

Bone Transplantation, Bone Banking, and Establishing a Surgical Bone Bank 592
Nikki Jackson Jacobs, M.S., MT(ASCP) SBB,
William E. Kline, M.S., MT(ASCP) SBB,
and J. Jeffrey McCullough, M.D.

Anesthesia for Surgery of the Spine 607
Bruce Ben-David, M.D., Glen S. Haller, M.D.,
and Peter D. Taylor, M.D.

Ankylosing Spondylitis 628
David S. Bradford, M.D.

Kyphosis in the Elderly 635
David S. Bradford, M.D.

INDEX 639

HISTORICAL ASPECTS OF SCOLIOSIS

John H. Moe, M.D.

Scoliosis is derived from the Greek word meaning curvature. When used in medical literature, it signifies a lateral curvature of the spine. A normal spine has physiological curvatures when viewed from the side, but there is no lateral deviation when viewed anteriorly or posteriorly.

Scoliosis is a spinal deformity that has been recognized since ancient times; it was first described by Hippocrates in "De Articulationes" of the *Corpus Hippocraticum*.[1] One passage states, "There are many varieties of curvatures of the spine even in persons who are in good health, for it takes place from natural conformation and from habit, and the spine is liable to be bent from old age and from pains." The possible relationship between spinal deformity and pulmonary disease was also mentioned. Treatment was recognized to be difficult and ineffectual. The poor prognosis for patients with an early onset of spine deformity was described, but no distinction was made between deformity from infection and true scoliosis. Treatment of spinal deformities was with forcible horizontal traction and underarm and leg distraction in suspension (Fig. 1–1).

Galen (A.D. 131–201) coined the words kyphosis, lordosis and scoliosis.[16] His treatment of spinal deformities followed that of Hippocrates.

From the fifth to the fifteenth centuries, little progress was made in the treatment of spinal deformities. Paul of Aegina (A.D. 625–690) wrote a treatise of "Seven Books," which was an enlightenment in a dark period of time.[40] During the Middle Ages, deformed individuals were objects of scorn and derision; their disfigurements were considered a form of divine punishment. The hunchback or humpback presented an especially grotesque or ugly appearance, which is often depicted in present day horror films. Dwarfs in Egypt were seen as gods or art figures; in the Middle Ages they served as court jesters or counsellors to royalty. The current diagnosis defines dwarfism as a condition in which the affected person has disproportionately short stature accompanied by complications affecting the musculoskeletal system and involving the spine.

Ambroise Paré (1510–1590) considered poor posture to be a probable cause of scoliosis.[39] He first described congenital scoliosis, and he also recognized cord compression as a cause of paraplegia. His treatment of scoliosis adhered closely to the Hippocratic method, but he is given credit for inventing a steel corset made by armorers.

André, who first coined the word orthopedia in 1741, wrote about spine curvatures, calling special attention to postural and sitting habits as a preventative measure and recommending corsets and exercise for methods of treatment.

The "jury mast" for sustained head traction during ambulation was developed by Levacher in 1764.[30] Myotomies, the first surgical technique for correcting scoliosis, were advocated by Guérin in 1839.[20, 21] Volkmann resected protruding rib deformities in 1889.[49] MacClennan performed anterior fusion and epiphyseodesis and reported it in 1922.[32] Royle[44] reported a hemivertebral resection for congenital scoliosis in 1928 following a suggestion made by Codivilla in 1901.[10]

Postural habits continued to be considered the cause of scoliosis throughout the nineteenth century; exercise and body bracing were the recommended treatments. Distrac-

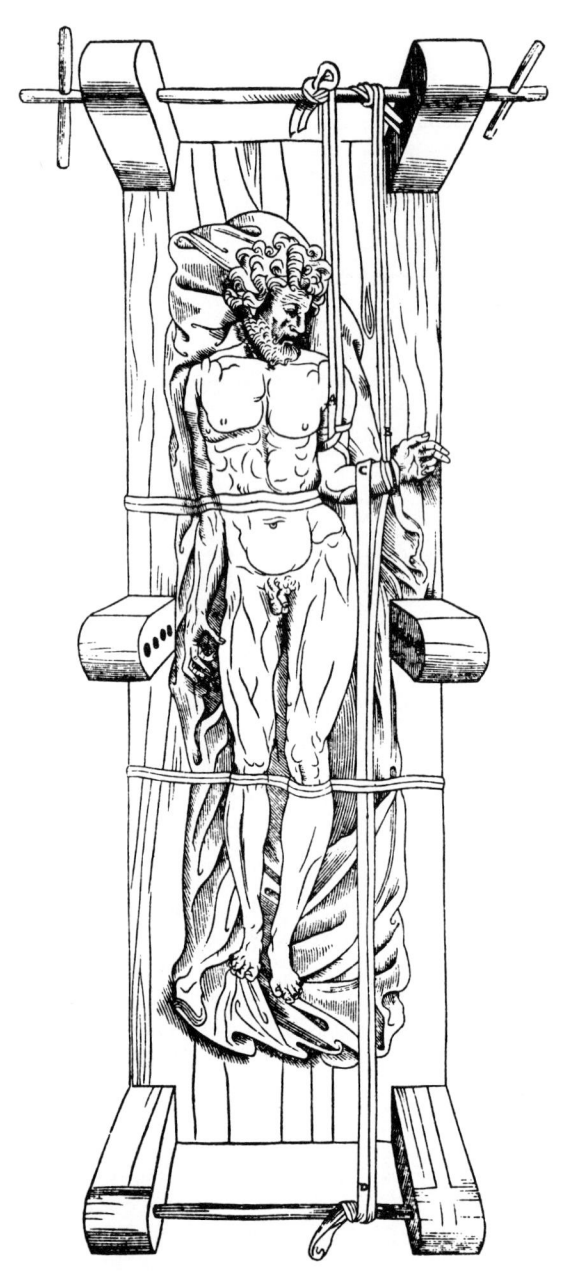

Figure 1–1. The Machine of Hippocrates. It was used in a like manner for torso distraction.

tion in bed or on a frame continued to be used to correct spinal deformities. In 1849, Hare showed startling improvement in his plaster replicas of the patients' torsos (Fig. 1–2).[22] The flagrant dishonesty of these improvements is quite evident.

Ingenious vertical distraction frames with corrective pressure pads appeared under the name of Hoffa[29] and others in Germany, and Louis Sayre[45] applied plaster torso casts in vertical suspension. Bradford and Brackett[8] in 1895 devised a horizontal distraction frame with a "localizer" attachment, very similar to that used by Risser in 1952 (Fig. 1–3).[42, 43]

With the discovery of roentgen rays in 1895 by Wilhelm Konrad Roentgen, professor of physics in Strassburg, Würtzburg, and later in Munich, the etiologic factors involved in scoliosis became increasingly evident. Although Calot[9] performed a fusion for tuberculosis of the spine prior to Hibbs, he abandoned the procedure as unsuccessful.

De Quervain[12] published a description of his method of spine fusion in 1917, but the successful surgical treatment of scoliosis began with Hibbs; he described his method of spine fusion for tuberculosis of the spine in 1911.[26] In this article he suggested its possible use in scoliosis, and in 1914 performed the first fusion for scoliosis. He reported 59 scoliosis fusions in 1924.[27] With Risser and Ferguson he published in 1931 an end result study of 360 fusions for scoliosis.[28] In this same article, the use of the turnbuckle corrective cast was described, to which the name of Risser is commonly ascribed. Hibbs's relatively many failures were mainly because of his inability to recognize fusion defects and to prescribe an adequate period of immobilization after fusion.

Others attempting to correct and fuse scoliotic spines met with a high percentage of failure. During the decade of 1930 to 1940, treatment by fusion fell into disrepute because of the many failures. Steindler's fusion results were so poor that he gave up the idea entirely and again resorted to exercises, bracing, and attempts to establish better compensation and balance.[47]

In 1941, a group of 425 cases of idiopathic scoliosis was studied by a committee of the American Orthopaedic Association.[2] This very dismal report gave the following conclusions: 60 per cent of cases treated by exercise and bracing progressed, and 40 per cent were unchanged. Correction and fusion in 180 cases showed pseudarthroses in 54. Of 214 patients treated by fusion, 29 per cent lost all correction. Of the entire group, 69 per cent had an end result rated poor or fair and 31 per cent good or excellent.

Fusion with cast correction provided fairly good results in the hands of the few orthopaedic surgeons who chose to study the problem thoroughly and pay close attention to meticulous details of cast correction, technique of fusion, and protection of the fusion

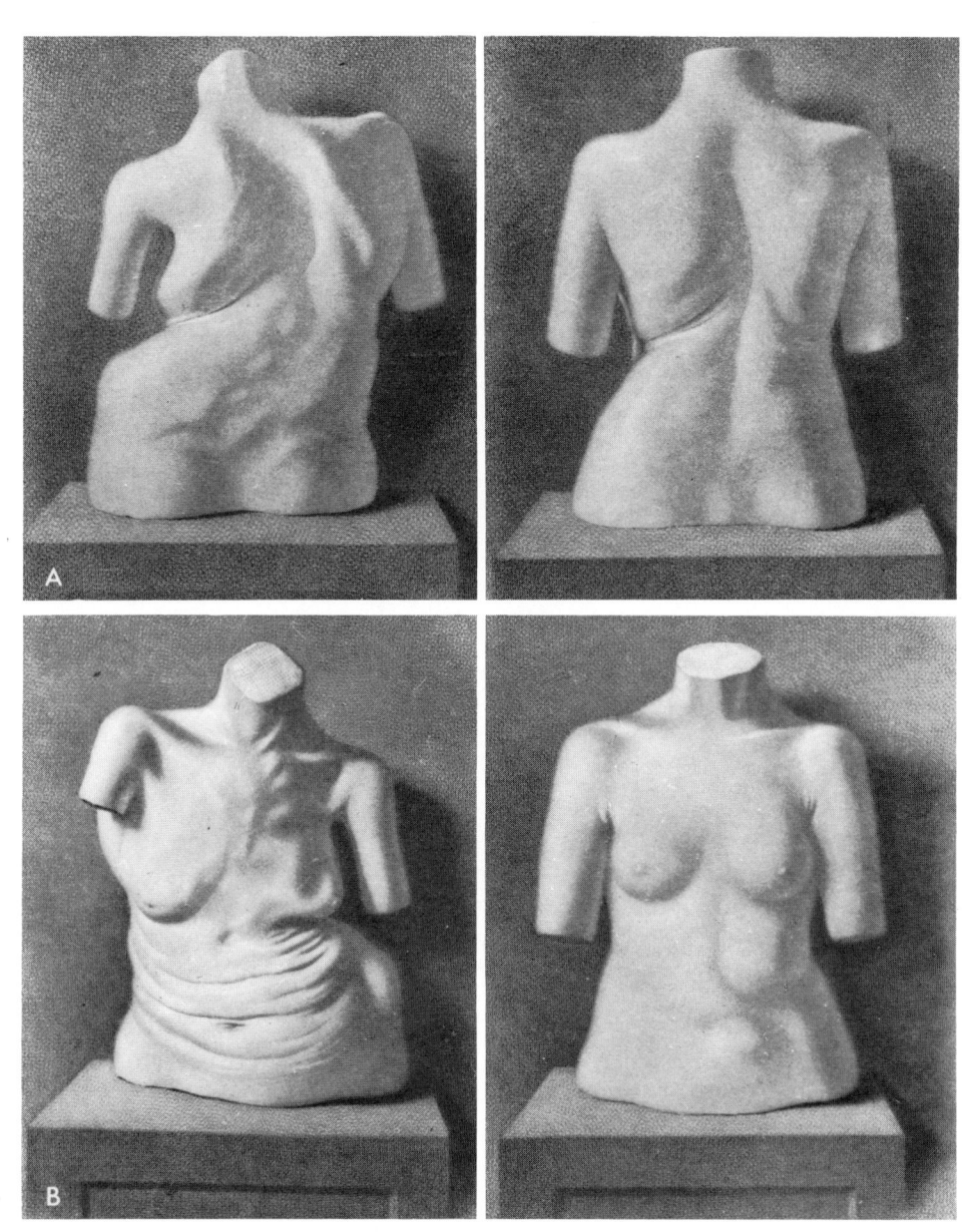

Figure 1–2. "The patient, age 18 years, was treated in lateral recumbency with traction to shoulders and feet, on a specially designed inclined plane of the author's design for 12 months." From "Practical Observations on the Prevention, Causes, and Treatment of Curvatures of the Spine." Samuel Hare, Surgeon, London, 1849.

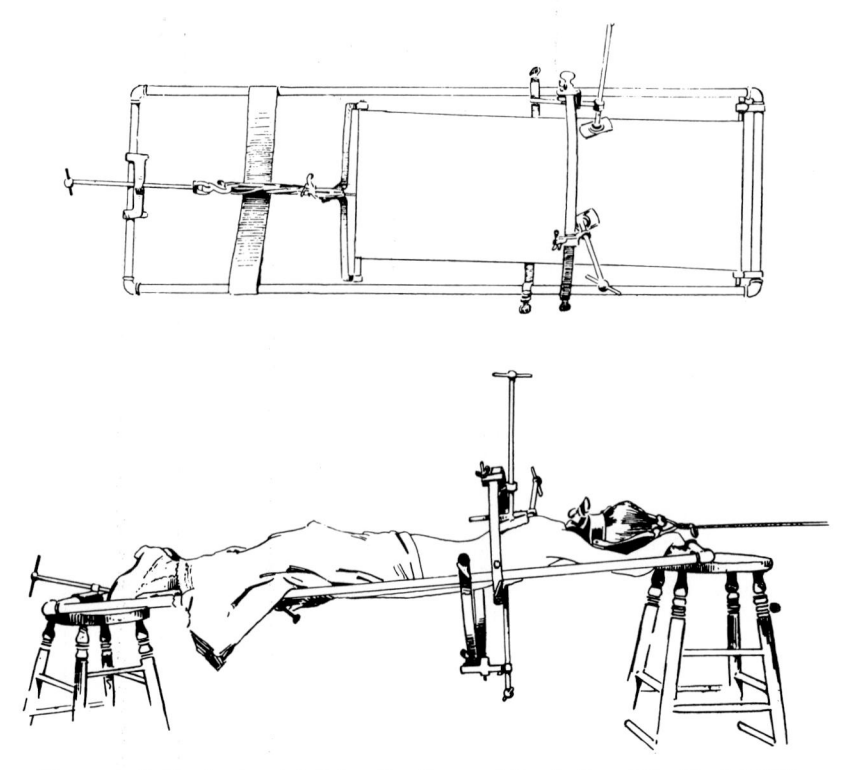

Figure 1–3. The horizontal distraction frame of Brackett and Bradford (1895).

until graft maturation. Through the efforts of these men—Cobb, Risser, and others—surgical treatment of scoliosis slowly began to regain its proper status. In 1946, Blount and Schmidt devised a distraction brace combined with lateral pressure pads. This early Milwaukee brace was at first used only in the operative treatment of scoliosis. Its success in curve correction led to increasing enthusiasm for its improvement, in both fit and construction. Such changes led to greater correction of the curvature and ultimately to use of the appliance as an ambulatory brace in the nonoperative treatment of lesser curves. It has proved successful in a moderate percentage of properly selected patients.[4, 5, 6, 7]

In the past 25 years the surgical management of spinal deformities has undergone tremendous changes. Better techniques of surgical fusion with the addition of copious amounts of bone graft, as proposed by Goldstein[18, 19] and Moe,[35] have withstood the test of time and have now become essential components of any surgical procedure. Advances in the treatment of adults were given great impetus by Stagnara, who contributed so much to scoliosis treatment in France and throughout the world.[46] Internal implants introduced by Harrington[23, 24, 25] added to internal stability of the fused spine and permitted ambulation in a well-fitted cast or brace after surgery without significant loss of correction.[35–38, 48] Anterior spinal implants have been introduced by Dwyer,[14, 15] Zielke,[50] Gardner,[17] Dunn,[13] and many others. Newer concepts and innovative posterior implant designs have been introduced by Resina and Ferriera-Alves,[41] Luque,[31] Marchetti,[33] Moe,[34, 35] and Cotrel and Dubousset,[11] to mention a few. Some have withstood the test of time and others are too new to properly evaluate. The historical development and the current role of these procedures will be addressed in subsequent chapters of this text.

The founding of the Scoliosis Research Society in Minneapolis, Minnesota in 1966 must be considered a landmark in the progress of the operative and nonoperative treatment of scoliosis, providing a forum for dedicated orthopaedic surgeons to present documented data or carefully critique work presented by colleagues. As a result, accelerated development of new and improved techniques and instrumentation has taken place throughout the world. Many of these are included in the following chapters, for the ultimate benefit of those patients with scoliosis and other spinal deformities. Motivation in research and inventiveness in methods of treatment for these medical problems first recognized and described by Hippocrates many centuries ago have never been more intense than in the latter half of this century.

References

1. Adams, F.: The Genuine Works of Hippocrates. New York, William Wood and Company.
2. American Orthopaedic Association Research Committee: End result study of the treatment of idiopathic scoliosis. J. Bone Joint Surg., 23:963, 1941.
3. André, N.: L'orthopaedia, ou l'art de prévenir et de corriger dans les enfants les déformités du corps. Paris, 1741.
4. Blount, W. P.: Scoliosis and the Milwaukee brace. Bull. Hosp. Joint Dis., 19(2):152–165, 1958.
5. Blount, W. P.: Non-operative treatment of scoliosis. A.A.O.S. Symposium on the Spine, St. Louis, C.V. Mosby, pp. 188–195, 1967.
6. Blount, W. P.: Use of the Milwaukee brace. Orthop. Clin. North Am., 3:3–16, 1972.
7. Blount, W. P., and Schmidt, A. C.: The Milwaukee brace in the treatment of scoliosis. Proc. Ann. Acad. Orthop. Surg., J. Bone Joint Surg., 39A:693, 1957.
8. Bradford, G. H., and Brackett, E. G.: Treatment of lateral curvature by means of pressure correction. Boston Med. Surg. J., 128:463, 1895.
9. Calot, F.: L'orthopédie indispensible aux practiciens. Méloine, Paris, 1923.
10. Codivilla, A.: Sulla scoliosi congenita. Arch. di Ortop., 18:65, 1901.
11. Cotrel, Y., and Dubousset, J.: New segmental posterior instrumentation of the spine. Orthop. Trans., 9:118, 1985.
12. De Quervain, L., and Hoessly, H.: Operative immobilization of the spine. Surg. Gynecol. Obstet., 24:428, 1917.
13. Dunn, H. K.: Spinal Instrumentation, Part I: Principles of posterior and anterior instrumentation. Instructional Course Lectures AAOS, Vol. XXXII, St. Louis, C.V. Mosby, pp. 192–209, 1983.
14. Dwyer, A. F., Newton, N. C., Sherwood, A. A.: An anterior approach to scoliosis—a preliminary report. Clin. Orthop., 62:192–202, 1969.
15. Dwyer, A. P., O'Brien, J. P., Seal, P. P., et al.: The late complications after the Dwyer anterior spinal instrumentation for scoliosis. J. Bone Joint Surg., 59B:117, 1977.
16. Galen: De Moto Maerculorum.
17. Gardner, A. D. H.: Four years' experience with an anterior spinal distraction device for the correction of kyphotic deformities and its use as a permanent implant. Orthop. Trans., 7:30, 1983.
18. Goldstein, L. A.: Surgical management of scoliosis. J. Bone Joint Surg., 48A:167–196, 1966.
19. Goldstein, L. A.: Treatment of idiopathic scoliosis by Harrington instrumentation and fusion with fresh autogenous iliac bone grafts. Results in 80 cases. J. Bone Joint Surg., 51A:209–222, 1969.
20. Guérin, J.: Mémoire sur les déviations simulées de l'épine et les moyens. Gaz. Méd. de Paris, 7:241–247, 1839.
21. Guérin, J.: Remarques préliminaires sur le traitement des déviations de l'épine par la section des muscles du dos. Gaz. Méd. de Paris, 10:1–6, 1842.
22. Hare, S.: Practical Observations on the Prevention, Causes and Treatment of Curvatures of the Spine. London, 1849.
23. Harrington, P. R.: Surgical instrumentation for management of scoliosis. J. Bone Joint Surg., 42A:1448, 1960.
24. Harrington, P. R.: Correction and internal fixation by spine instrumentation. J. Bone Joint Surg., 44A:591, 1962.
25. Harrington, P. R.: Technical details in relation to the successful use of instrumentation in scoliosis. Orthop. Clin. North Am. 3:49, 1972.
26. Hibbs, R. A.: An operation for progressive spinal deformities. N.Y. Med. J., 93:1013, 1911.
27. Hibbs, R. A.: A report of fifty-nine cases of scoliosis treated by fusion. J. Bone Joint Surg., 6:3, 1924.
28. Hibbs, R. A., Risser, J. C., Ferguson, A. B.: Scoliosis treated by the fusion operation. An end result study of three hundred and sixty cases. J. Bone Joint Surg., 13:91, 1931.
29. Hoffa, A.: Redression des Buckels nach der Methode von Calot. Dtsch. Med. Wochenschr., 1:3, 1898.
30. Levacher, A. F. T.: Nouveau moyen de prévenir et de guérir la courbure de l'épine. Mém. Acad. R. Chir., 4:596, 1768.
31. Luque, E. R.: Segmental spinal instrumentation for correction of scoliosis. Clin. Orthop., 163:192–198, 1982.
32. MacClennan, A.: Scoliosis. Brit. Med. J., 2:864–866, 1922.
33. Marchetti, P. G., and Valdini, A.: End fusions in the treatment of severe progression or severe scoliosis in childhood or early adolescence. Orthop. Trans. 2:271, 1978.
34. Moe, J. H.: A critical analysis of methods of fusion for scoliosis. J. Bone Joint Surg., 40A:529, 1958.
35. Moe, J. H.: Methods of correction and surgical techniques in scoliosis. Orthop. Clin. North Am., 3(1):17–48, 1972.
36. Moe, J. H., Cummine, J., Winter, R., et al.: Harrington instrumentation without fusion combined with the Milwaukee brace for difficult scoliosis problems in young children. Orthop. Trans., 3:59, 1979.
37. Moe, J. H., Kharrat, K., Winter, R. B., Cummine, J. L.: Harrington instrumentation without fusion plus external orthotic support for the treatment of difficult curvature problems in young children. Clin. Orthop. Rel. Res., 185:35–45, 1984.
38. Moe, J. H., Valuska, J.: Evaluation of treatment of scoliosis by Harrington instrumentation. J. Bone Joint Surg., 48A:1656–1657, 1966.
39. Pare, A.: Collected Works. Trans. Johnson, T. London, 1634.
40. Paul of Aegina: Collected Works. Adams, F. (Trans.) Sydenham Society, London, 1834, et seq.
41. Resina, J., and Ferriera-Alves, A. F.: A technique of correction and internal fixation for scoliosis. J. Bone Joint Surg., 59B:159–165, 1977.

42. Risser, J. C.: The application of body casts for the correction of scoliosis. Am. Acad. Orthop. Surg. Instructional Course Lectures, *12*:255, 1955.
43. Risser, J. C., Lauder, D. H., Norquist, D. M., Craig, W. A.: Three types of body casts. Am. Acad. Orthop. Surg., Instructional Course Lectures, *10*:131, 1953.
44. Royle, N. D.: The operative removal of an accessory vertebra. Med. J. Aust., *1*:467, 1928.
45. Sayre, L. H.: History of treatment of spondylitis and scoliosis by partial suspension and retention by means of plaster of paris bandages. N.Y. Med. J., *11*:12, 1895.
46. Stagnara, P.: Les Déformations du Rachis: Scolioses, Cyphoses, Lordoses. Masson, Paris, 1985.
47. Steindler, A.: Diseases and Deformities of the Spine and Thorax. St. Louis, C.V. Mosby, 1929.
48. Tambornino, J., Armburst, E., Moe, J. H.: Harrington instrumentation in correction of scoliosis. A comparison with cast correction. J. Bone Joint Surg., *44A*:313–321, 1969.
49. Volkmann, R.: Resektion von Rippendtucker bei Scoliose. Berl. Klin. Wehnsehr, 50, 1889.
50. Zielke, K., and Pellin, B.: Neue Instrumente und Implantate zur Erganzung des Harrington Systems. Z. Orthop. Chir., *114*:534–537, 1976.

2
BIOMECHANICS

James W. Ogilvie, M.D.

INTRODUCTION

Spinal biomechanics is a study of directed forces (vectors) that produce equilibrium, motion, and deformity of the vertebral column. An understanding of force application to the spine clarifies the kinematics of normal motion, and the pathogenesis of scoliosis and kyphosis, and it assists in the development of instrumentation and orthoses for the treatment of spine disorders.

Humans possess an axial skeleton uniquely adapted to bipedal ambulation. Sagittal plane contours permit the center of mass for the head and upper torso to remain in line with the vertical axis through the center of mass for the pelvis, therefore a minimum expenditure of energy is required to keep the trunk upright. The upper limbs, thus freed from the task of trunk support, are able to perform other functions associated with a complex society. Various pathologic conditions causing abnormal sagittal plane contour, for example, loss of lumbar lordosis, excessive thoracic kyphosis, or coronal plane deviation of the spine (e.g., scoliosis), may alter balance and coordination, interfere with visceral function, allow premature degeneration of the spinal column, and cause deterioration of neurologic function.

To achieve the balance and mobility required for efficient energy use (ergonomics), humans have a multisegmented bony spinal column. The normal spinal column consists of seven cervical, twelve thoracic, and five lumbar vertebrae connected to fused sacral vertebrae, which are in turn articulated with vestigial coccygeal vertebrae. Normal spinal contour, when viewed in the frontal plane, is straight and when viewed in the lateral plane has physiologic cervical lordosis, thoracic kyphosis, and lumbar lordosis. Stagnara reported that among normal French and Italian adults the thoracic kyphosis averaged 37 degrees while lumbar lordosis averaged −50 degrees, with considerable variation in each range.[105] This study correlates well with studies of Roaf and Rockwell, who stated that normal thoracic kyphosis was 20 to 40 degrees and 35 degrees average, respectively.[90, 91]

HISTORY

Greek artisans literally idolized human form and function. Although movement, grace, and beauty of the human torso have always been appreciated, scholarly investigation of the precise anatomy and function of the vertebral column and its separate elements was first presented by Vesalius in 1543. He noted the variations in facet orientation between lumbar and thoracic vertebrae while describing the apophyseal joints in detail. Necropsy dissections and astute observation of living subjects gave additional data to the Danish anatomist Winslow, and later to Weber in 1827. With the advent of radiographic measurements to document spinal motion, published first by Virchow in 1911, data acquistion on spinal kinesiology proliferated.[109] Ex vivo testing of human spinal elements was first reported by Virgin.[110] Subsequent in vivo measurements utilizing skeletal markers and stereographic radiology have added information with regard to coupled motion, range of motion, instant centers of rotation, and load-deformation curves for the vertebral column.[23, 26, 28, 32, 33, 39, 41, 62, 67, 77, 81, 82]

Finite element analysis subdivides a structure into multiple smaller elements, and the forces acting on each of these individual elements is then studied.[13, 15] Through this simulation it has been possible to understand the internal forces acting on spinal elements such as the bony neural arch and the intervertebral disc.[43]

Mathematical modeling allows simulated stresses to be applied to the computerized spine model and allows the resultant deformation tendencies of the model to be analyzed.[9, 98, 99, 106] Valuable data can be obtained from these methods, but the existing models respond in a linear fashion to stress. Biologic tissues have a nonlinear deformation response to force,[51, 54] and thus the information gained from present mathematical models of the spinal column, while agreeing with empirical data in many instances, has limitations. Boundary conditions and exact knowledge of the nonlinear behavior of spinal soft tissue must be obtained before spinal mathematical modeling lends itself to more diversified use.

ANATOMY

For descriptive purposes, the spine can be divided into anterior and posterior columns. The anterior column consists of the posterior longitudinal ligament, intervertebral disc, vertebral body, and anterior longitudinal ligament. The elements of the posterior column are the pedicles, laminae, transverse processes, spinous process, facet joints, and ligamentous structures, including the facet joint capsule, ligamentum flavum, intertransverse ligaments, interspinous ligaments, and supraspinous ligaments (Fig. 2–1). Each anatomic component of the vertebral column has a function that contributes to the mobility and stability of a motion segment.

The anterior longitudinal ligament attaches to the bony endplate above and below each disc space and is confluent with the anulus fibrosus but can easily be detached from the vertebral body. This ligamentous structure is largest in the thoracic spine but is also structurally significant in the cervical, thoracic, and lumbar areas. It is approximately twice as strong as the posterior longitudinal ligament, which reflects a difference in size rather than a qualitative difference. The tensile strength of the anterior and posterior longitudinal ligaments diminishes with age.[107] Fracture of the neural arch takes place before anterior longitudinal ligamentous rupture when pure extension forces are applied to the spine. Rotation or horizontal shear must be present to tear the ligament.[89] This fact is of considerable importance in correcting kyphotic deformities, since surgical release of the anterior longitudinal ligament is necessary to allow opening of the disc spaces anteriorly.[79] Because shear or rotary subluxation fractures usually result in anterior ligament rupture, care must be taken not to apply excessive force if posterior distraction instrumentation is to be utilized in the acute treatment of such injuries.

Along the posterior aspect of the vertebral body, which is also the anterior border of the spinal canal, lies the posterior longitudinal ligament. It is less substantial than the anterior ligament and is most prominent as it crosses the intervertebral disc. As the ligament extends laterally it thins out, and it also diminishes in substance as it crosses the vertebral body.

Each vertebra except C1 has a cancellous vertebral body. The first cervical vertebra is composed of a bony ring, and the dens of C2 is embryologically the C1 vertebral body. The size and mineral content of each vertebral body increase in a caudal direction, which is a morphologic response to the increasing task of weight-bearing.[14] Pure flexion or compression loads applied to a motion segment result in fracture of the vertebral body endplate and displacement of disc material into the vertebral body rather than herniation of the intervertebral disc into the spinal canal. Roaf noted that when the vertebral body is compressed, the endplate bulges and blood is squeezed out of the cancellous bone before fracture occurs, thus

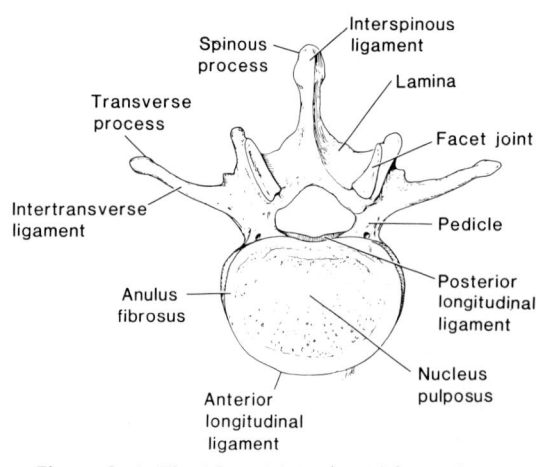

Figure 2–1. The L2 vertebra viewed from above.

performing a shock absorbing function.[89] The vertebral body thus functions as a rigid linkage in the motion segment and a platform for the attachment of the intervertebral disc, muscles, and the anterior and posterior longitudinal ligaments.

From C2 distally each vertebral body is joined to an intervertebral disc.[50] Anatomically, the disc is bordered superiorly and inferiorly by a 1-millimeter thick cartilaginous endplate. Circumferentially, the anulus fibrosus constitutes the outer layer of the intervertebral disc.[39, 117] Peripherally it is composed of 15 to 20 layers of collagenous fibrils obliquely running from one cartilage endplate to the other and crossing at 120 degree angles. On its inner aspect is fibrocartilage, and this portion of the anulus is the major weight-bearing portion of the intervertebral disc complex. In the center is the nucleus pulposus, which contains a loose collagen network with a large amount of hydrophilic proteoglycans. The water content of the nucleus pulposus decreases from a maximum of 70 to 90 per cent as the production of proteoglycans diminishes in the third decade of life. This is manifest as a decrease in the resting tension the nucleus pulposus exerts on the anulus and longitudinal ligaments.[40] Mechanically, the normal intervertebral disc has the diverse functions of allowing motion between adjacent vertebrae and, along with the facet joints and ligamentous restraints, providing stability between adjacent vertebrae.[6, 57] The viscous nucleus pulposus sustains marked changes in pressure, depending on the body position when lifting loads and changing posture.[8, 97] Intradiscal pressures, as measured by Nachemson, were 50 per cent greater in the standing position than in recumbency.[70, 71] Tensile forces on the anulus fibrosus may reach four or five times the applied axial load. Pressure differences inside the nucleus when lifting a 20-kilogram load with knees straight or bent can cause a variation in intradiscal pressure of 100 per cent, with the flexed spine–straight leg lifting posture.[74] The normal intervertebral disc acts as a linkage between two rigid vertebral bodies and transmits the pressure from axial loads evenly to the anulus fibrosus and bony endplates. Acute failure of the intervertebral disc requires compression and torsional load.[2] In general, the facet joints and neural arch protect the disc from large axial rotation. Therefore, torsional loading is not usually a factor in acute disc protrusion if the posterior column restraints are intact. Radial tears in the anulus fibrosus may be produced by chronic fatigue loading of the intervertebral disc, and this mechanism, in conjunction with senescent changes of the disc material, is a factor in the clinical syndrome of herniated nucleus pulposus. In adults, the change in intervertebral disc mechanical properties with age follows no consistent pattern.[75, 101]

A compressive load on the lumbar spine without lordosis results in the disc bearing all of the compression. As lumbar lordosis increases, an increasing load is borne by the facet joints, and the purely compressive load on the disc changes to a combination of compression and shear. The superior articular facet of the subjacent vertebra prevents forward displacement of the posterior element, although the intervertebral disc allows some forward shift of the vertebral body. This creates a tensile load on the pars interarticularis. Lamy and others have shown that tensile loads to failure applied to the neural arch resulted in fractures of the pars interarticularis in about one third of the specimens tested.[55] This report agrees with the observation that those who have sustained loading of the lordotic lumbar spine such as female gymnasts and football interior linemen have an increase in the incidence of spondylolisthesis secondary to spondylolysis.[35]

Situated on the posterior arch are paired diarthrodial articulations called apophyseal or facet joints. Their main function is to restrain the torsional and shear movements of the intervertebral joint, and thus they play a major role in determining the range of motion at that joint.[23, 39, 48] Lumbar facets bear approximately 16 per cent of the axial load in the erect posture.[1] However, in the sitting position they have no compressive load. This correlates well with Nachemson's observation of increased intradiscal pressure in the sitting subject when compared to the standing one.[70] An increase in lumbar lordosis while standing transfers compressive force to the facet joint and thus partially unloads the disc. Intervertebral range of motion is determined for the most part by the orientation of the facet joint. In the thoracic spine, facet joints lie in a coronal plane that is tilted forward, thus permitting flexion-extension and rotation, but restricting lateral bending. Lumbar facets are oriented in the sagittal plane, thereby allowing flexion-extension and lateral bending but limiting torsion. At the thoracolumbar junction, the planar orientation of the joint is midway between coronal and sagittal. Freed from the restraint of the thoracic cage below T10, there is increased rotational movement in the T11 to L1 segments.[65] Excision of one facet allows the remaining facet to rotate and sublux, thereby decreasing contact area. Although the total force transmitted across the remaining facet is diminished, the force per unit area (pressure) is increased.[58] This may accelerate degenerative joint changes in the facet. Putti[84] termed facet asymmetry at the lumbosacral junction trophism, and Brailsford[19] noted its occurrence in 31 per cent of 3,000 asymptomatic lumbar spines. There is, however, a high percentage of facet asymmetry noted in those with symptomatic low back disease, and the facet joint plays an important part in the pathogenesis of low back pain.[18, 101] Badgley, Cyron and Hutton, and Farfan and Sullivan have observed that asymmetrical lumbosacral facet orientation may result in spondylogenic pain.[12, 25, 34] The scientific validation of this opinion has not been established however.

Posterior column ligamentous structures include the facet capsule, ligamentum flavum, interspinous ligament, supraspinous ligament, and intertransverse ligament. Using single-load-to-failure testing, it has been noted that all the posterior ligaments plus at least one component of the anterior column soft tissues must be sacrificed before pathologic motion is recorded in the thoracic spine.[64] Little is known about the chronic effects on disc degeneration when stress loading is done in vivo to a motion segment that has incompetence of only one or two ligamentous elements.

The ligamentum flavum, or yellow ligament, originates from the under side of each lamina caudally from C1 and inserts onto the superior border of the subjacent lamina. Its lateral origins are in the joint capsule attachments. It has the highest percentage of elastin, 65 to 70 per cent, of any structure in the human body.[20] In the resting spine, it is under slight tension and acts as a check rein in flexion.[5, 73, 79] It exerts no function in hyperextension and may even buckle, thus contributing to soft tissue impingement of the spinal canal. Torsion also places the ligamentum flavum under tension, and data suggest that restraint of rotation may also be a significant function.[111]

Each facet joint is encased in fibrous capsule similar to those of other diarthrodial joints. Selective removal of the joint capsule in the laboratory causes no significant decrease in axial load bearing characteristics. Adams has shown that the facet capsule does resist flexion in the lumbar spine, but Posner did not find that instability resulted from facet capsule removal in the lumbar motion segments.[1, 83]

The interspinous and supraspinous ligaments are flexion restraints.[102] They are quadrilateral in shape and thickest in the lumbar spine, where they extend from the ligamentum flavum posteriorly to the lumbosacral fascia. In the thoracic spine they are thin and filamentous. Intertransverse ligaments in the thoracic spine are stout and part of the paraspinous musculature. In the lumbar spine they are poorly developed. They act as passive restraints to lateral bending and rotation.

KINEMATICS

Kinematics deals with motion apart from the influence of mass and force, whereas kinesiology deals with the anatomy and dynamics related to human motion. It is from this knowledge that the pathomechanics of spine deformity is approached. Motion of the spinal column or any of its elements can be separated into six degrees of freedom (Fig. 2–2). Linear motion or translation is a change in position of an object without rotation. The second type of motion, rotation, is motion of an object about an axis or center of rotation. Translation can be along the x, y, or z axis,

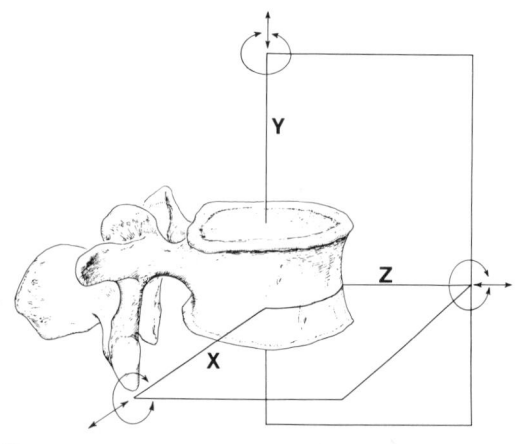

Figure 2–2. Linear motion (translation along the x, y, and z axes) is possible in addition to rotation at each axis, thus allowing six degrees of freedom for vertebral movement.

with three additional possibilities for rotation about those same x, y, and z coordinates. Coupled motion also exists in the human spine. This is defined as motion in one plane linked to concurrent motion in another plane. For instance, lateral motion of the cervical and upper thoracic spine is accompanied by concave rotation of the vertebral body.[78] An understanding of physiologic and pathologic movements of the spinal column is requisite to the understanding of growth and development in the spine, the pathogenesis of spine deformity, and the methods most effective in the treatment of vertebral column disorders.[113]

The movement characteristics of the human spine as listed by Panjabi and others show that torsion and lateral bending are the main functions of the thoracic spine (Fig. 2–3).[80, 113] Considerable variation exists in the observed range of motion present in the lumbar, thoracic, and cervical parts of the spine. These differences are owing to experimental techniques and, while the actual numbers vary, the trends are constant. As the lower thoracic vertebrae gradually change in morphology to that of the lumbar spine and as the stabilizing influence of the thorax is no longer present caudal to T10, more flexion-extension is possible. Lateral bend and flexion-extension are the characteristics of the lumbar motion segments. The orientation of the facet joints, according to the plane in which they are located, dictates the movement possible at a particular motion segment.

Stiffness of the intervertebral joint, which is a measure of resistance to deformation, increases with axial load and decreases with distraction. Although disc height increases, thus increasing flexibility, as one moves caudad in the spinal column vertebral body diameter also increases, thereby decreasing flexibility. Markolf found that these opposing characteristics tend to neutralize each other, thus maintaining relatively constant stiffness for lateral bend, extension, and rotation in the lumbar and thoracic spines.[65] The rib cage, in conjunction with the sternum, provides important stabilizing forces on the tho-

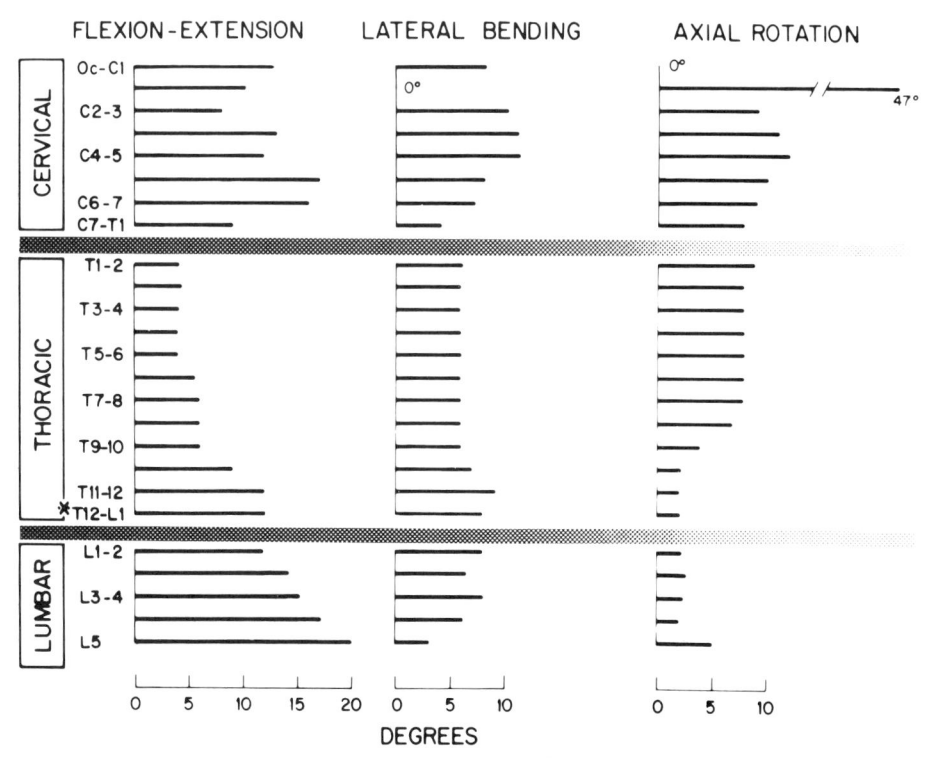

Figure 2–3. This composite graph illustrates the range of motion characteristics in the cervical, thoracic, and lumbar spines. More important than the absolute values are the trends, such as the increasing flexion-extension present in each motion segment as one progresses caudally. (Reprinted with permission from White, A. A., and Panjabi, M. M.: Clinical Biomechanics of the Spine, Philadelphia, J. B. Lippincott, p. 105.)

racic spine.[4] Removal of the sternum negates this stability as does resection of the rib heads or transection of the intercostal muscles.

In contrast to an enarthrodial joint such as the hip, which relies for the most part on its bony components and their orientation for stability, the intervertebral joint is very dependent on soft tissues to maintain proper alignment and stability in its physiologic range of motion. Lucas and Bresler found that an axial load of just 2 kilograms applied to a human spine with intact ligaments, disc, and facet joints but devoid of muscles and bony thorax, caused the column to buckle.[60] This finding illustrates the important principle that the spine itself has very little intrinsic stability. As discussed in the anatomy section, the facets, ligaments, and intervertebral discs continue to determine the range of motion and instant centers of rotation and act as passive restraints at the limits of motion, but they do not provide the stability that results in what we know as normal posture. Although assisted by the stabilizing effect of the thorax, normal posture is an active function, which is both voluntary and a reflex through the righting mechanism.[68]

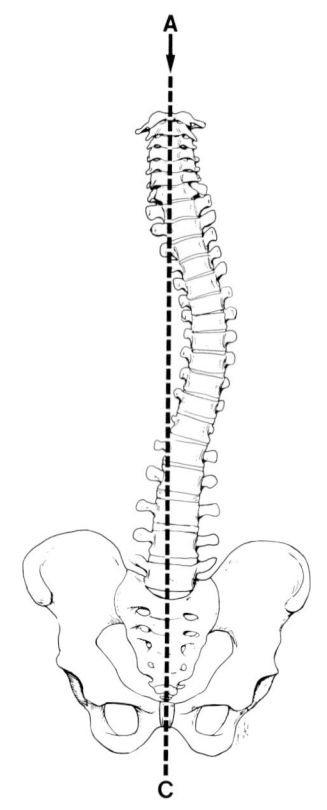

Figure 2–4. The center of body mass (A) is located over the body midline (C) in this compensated scoliosis. Each end of the column, the lumbosacral and craniocervical junctions, must be defined as hinged (able to rotate) or fixed (unable to rotate).

THE MECHANICS OF COLUMN FAILURE

The mechanics of column failure or buckling are increasingly complicated when applied to a biologic system. Euler's mathematical expression assumes that all loads on the column under analysis are vertical and centered over the column. Each end of the column must also be defined as either clamped (unable to rotate) or hinged (free to rotate) (Fig. 2–4). These preconditions to precise mathematical definition may not lend themselves to accurate description when accounting for muscle imbalance, trunk decompensation, pelvic tilt, limb length inequality, neurologic disorders, thoracic cage abnormalities, and intrinsic structural failure such as tumor, trauma, infection, osteopenia, radiation effect, and congenital deformity.

Column failure can be divided into short and long column analysis. Short column stability is defined by the expression $P<YA$, where P is the compressive load, Y is the yield strength of the vertebral element, and A is the cross sectional area of the column. As long as the compressive force remains within the limits set, failure does not occur.

When the compressive load is increased, such as in trauma, or when the strength of the vertebra is diminished from osteopenia or tumor, column failure results.

Most spine deformities can be described as problems in long column stability. For the purposes of this discussion, stability is defined as the tendency of the spinal column to return to normal anatomic configuration when relatively small loads are applied to it. Euler's mathematical expression describing long column stability is $P < K \cdot \frac{EI}{L^2}$.

K is constant, which includes the preconditions defining the degrees of freedom allowed at the ends of the column, EI is the stiffness modulus of the column, and L is the length of the column. Several interesting observations can be made relative to the length of the spinal column in human spine deformity. Idiopathic scoliosis patients are statistically taller, and their individual vertebral bodies are longer than those in nonscoliotic patients.[100, 103, 114, 115] Since the influence of length is inverse and exponential, even small incremental changes in the height of the spinal column may result in a significant shift toward instability. The term EI is a product of the column geometry or area moment of inertia and the column's modulus of elasticity. Slender columns have more tendency to buckle. It has been noted that females have more slender spines than males.[56] In combination, the area moment of inertia and the modulus represent the resistance of the spinal column bone and soft tissue to deform in response to external forces. This is a factor in conditions such as Marfan's syndrome, Ehlers-Danlos syndrome, osteogenesis imperfecta, and other connective tissue disorders associated with spine deformity.

P is the compressive load and is a combination of forces including gravity and muscle forces. Column stability is present as long as P remains within the limits set. When the trunk is decompensated (the occiput is not centered over the sacrum) a bending moment is also added to the compressive force, deforming the spine (Fig. 2–5). Muscle imbalance is the primary deforming force, if gravity and structural abnormalities resulting from trauma, infection, congenital malformations, and intrinsic bone diseases are disregarded. Muscular and neurologic diseases such as poliomyelitis, cerebral palsy, Friedreich's ataxia, cord injury, muscular dystrophy, and others result in diminished or unbalanced muscle tone, often in subtle combinations. Idiopathic scoliosis with its abnormalities in the righting mechanism and asymmetrical distribution of Type I and Type II paraspinal muscle fibers typifies the difficulty in quantifying forces that act to produce spinal column deformity. Euler's mathematical relationship between compressive force and long column stability provides a starting point for critical analysis but it rapidly becomes complicated by the many other parameters to be considered when describing clinical scoliosis. No unified comprehensive mathematical equation has been formulated to accurately describe and predict scoliosis deformity.[96]

In 1905 Lovett observed that lateral bending of the thoracic spine, when accompanied by flexion, was associated with coupled rotation of the vertebral body.[59] Coupled rotation, while still controversial, has been substantiated by White and others.[10, 78] Normally, lateral flexion of the spine is coupled with rotation of the vertebral body into the concavity of the curve. It is more constant in the cervical and upper thoracic spines, becoming less predictable in the lower thoracic and lumbar spines. This physiologic coupled motion is in contrast to thoracic idiopathic scoliosis, which is usually a combination of loss of physiologic kyphosis, convex vertebral body rotation, and lateral bending (Fig. 2–6). The loss of normal kyphosis and vertebral rotation in scoliosis were first described by Adams in 1865.[3] MacLennan, Somerville, and later Roaf have stated that hypokyphosis and rotation are the primary lesions of idiopathic scoliosis, with coronal plane deformity occurring only secondarily.[64, 88, 104] According to Dickson, right thoracic idiopathic scoliosis is preceded by a loss of normal thoracic kyphosis, which can happen during the adolescent growth acceleration.[27] This relative thoracic lordosis decreases vertebral resistance to deforming rotational forces. Theoretically, that deforming torque is provided by the adjacent aortic pulsations on the left ante-

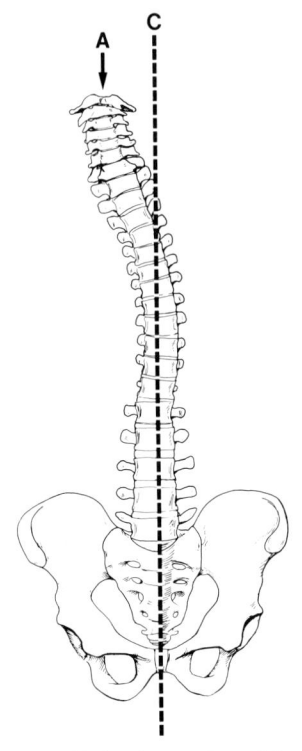

Figure 2–5. A shift in the center of body mass (A) away from the midline (C), as occurs in the decompensated spine, introduces a bending movement. Euler's mathematical expression is only for columns where A and C are concurrent.

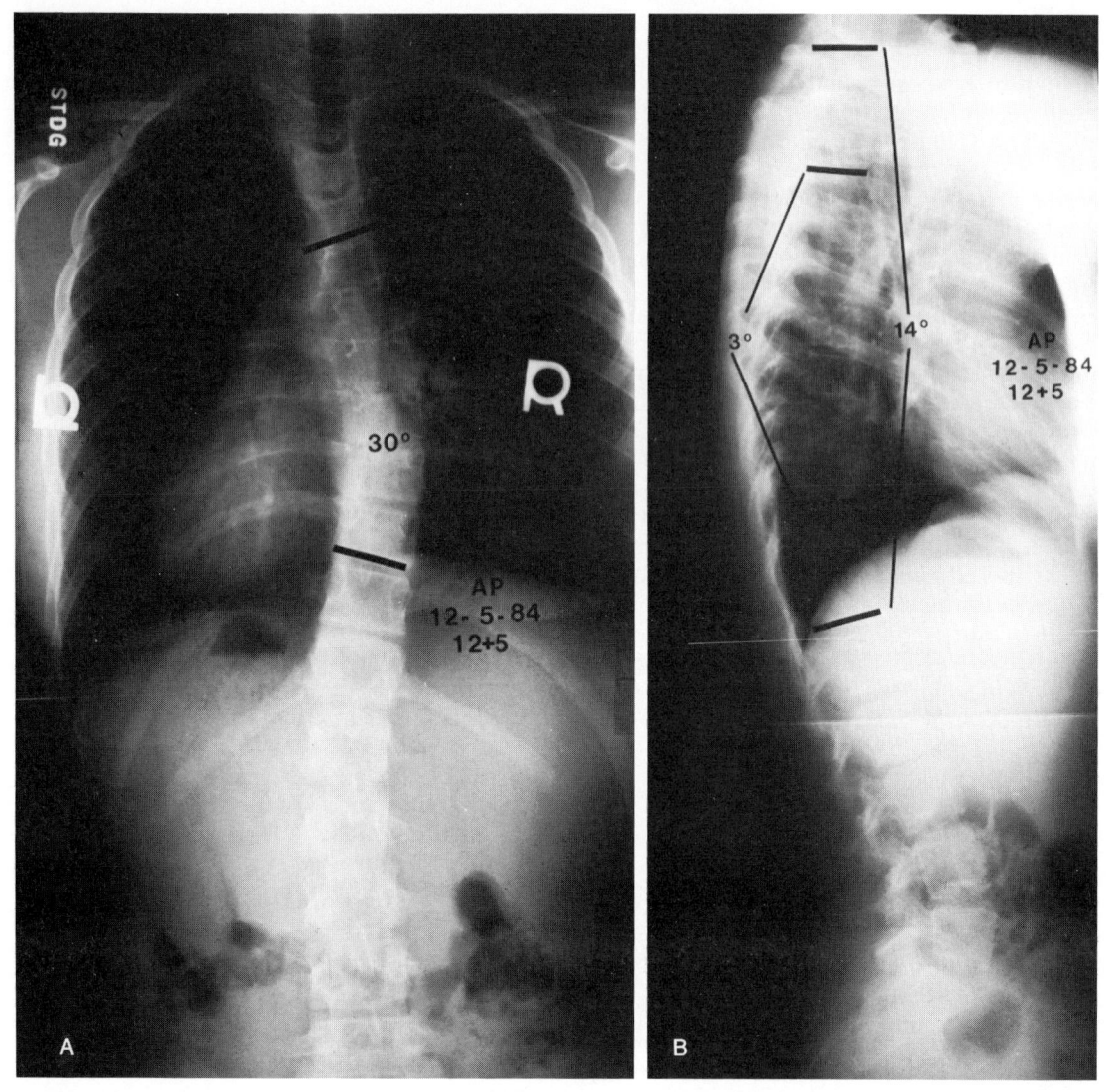

Figure 2–6. *A* and *B*, Radiographs of a 12+5 year old female with idiopathic adolescent scoliosis from T5 through T10. On the lateral view there is a decrease in the normal thoracic kyphosis over those same levels.

rior vertebral border. It should be noted, however, that in patients with dextrocardia and subsequent right-sided vertebral pulsations, there is only a slight increase in left thoracic as opposed to right thoracic scoliosis.[93] This may not be an ideal population for mechanical analysis, since scoliosis is more frequent in cyanotic patients such as those with dextrocardia.[61] As extension becomes fixed, the anterior portion of the vertebral body has relatively less axial load, and in accordance with the Hueter-Volkmann principle, the vertebral body becomes wedged posteriorly. This is analogous but opposite to the anterior wedging observed in Scheuermann's disease. The coronal plane deformity that is observed on frontal radiography is an easily measured but purely secondary result. As the apical vertebra of the scoliosis deformity becomes displaced from the midline of the torso, a stronger contraction of the convex paraspinous musculature is necessary to maintain equilibrium. Reuber and others have suggested that if the righting mechanism cannot supply the asymmetrical force needed to correct or control this small curvature, continued symmetrical paraspinous muscle forces may predispose to curve progression.[86] It is not uncommon for small idiopathic scoliosis curves to spontaneously correct, and this may represent an intrinsic recognition and adaptation of the righting mechanism to an initial purely mechanical curvature. Hormonal and genetically determined growth patterns can be invoked to explain the familial and gender distributions that are clinically observed in adolescent idiopathic scoliosis. Nonstandard vertebral rotation is commonly noted but is rarely associated with clinically significant scoliosis.[11]

Other factors studied in the mechanics of idiopathic scoliosis have suffered from the difficulty in differentiating primary and secondary effects. Unequal distribution of Type I and Type II muscle fibers, asymmetrical paraspinous musculature, and equilibrium dysfunction have been noted but cannot clearly be identified as primary disorders.[35, 36, 47, 53, 87, 94, 116, 118, 120] Asymmetrical intervertebral disc growth and collagen content are secondary phenomena,[22, 38, 49, 52, 108] particularly since Reuber has noted that the disc has a resistance to lateral bend of less than 2 nm. per degree.[86] Lateral forces created by muscular contraction easily exceed 30 to 40 nm. and make disc resistance small by comparison. Once the scoliosis or kyphosis deformity reaches certain proportions, the effect of gravity upon the lever arm created continues to be a major deforming force.[21, 42] The exact pathomechanics of idiopathic scoliosis remain controversial and may represent a spectrum of conditions that are simplistically classified as either progressive or nonprogressive.

THE MECHANICS OF CORRECTION WITH INSTRUMENTATION

Four types of force may be surgically applied to the deformed spinal column to achieve correction: distraction, compression, bending, and torsion (Fig. 2–7). Although others have used distraction devices,[7] Paul Harrington introduced distraction instrumentation as a practical and relatively efficient operative means of improving scoliosis deformities.[45, 66] More than 650 newtons of distraction can be applied to the spine by the Harrington distraction system, using sublaminar hooks on the lumbar and the thoracic vertebrae.[72] The lumbar laminae can sustain

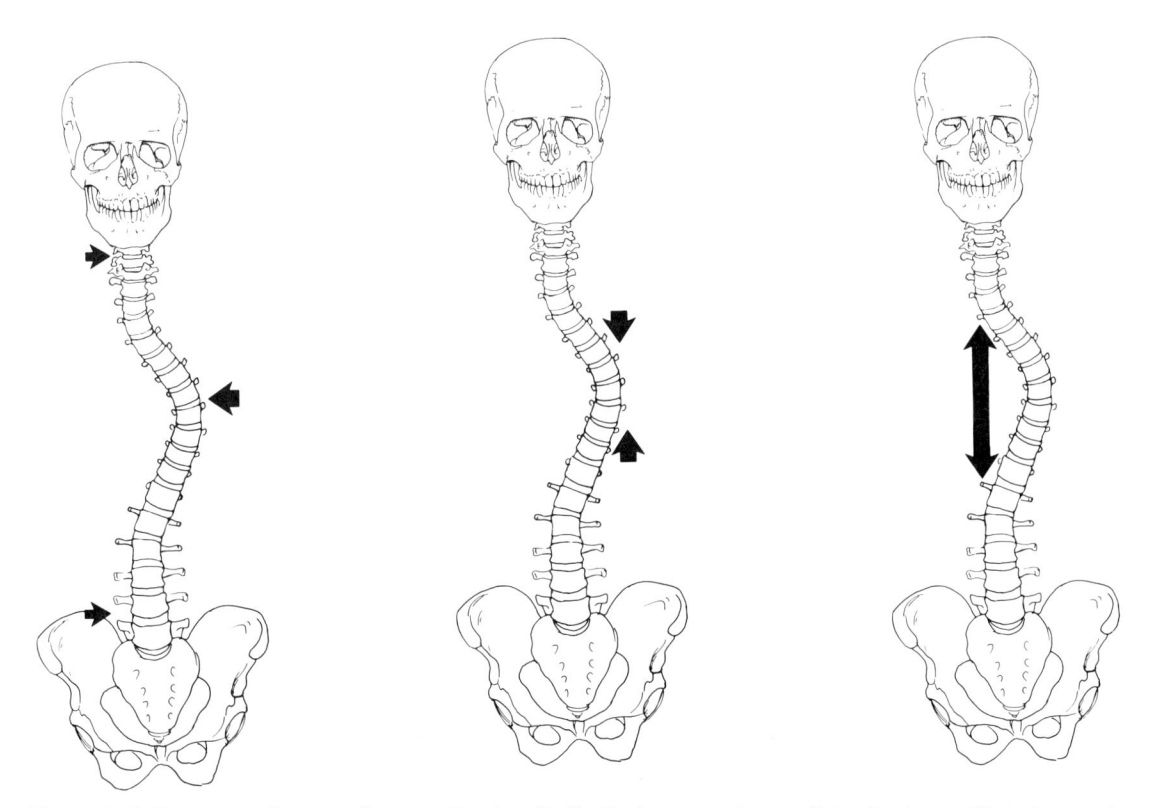

Figure 2–7. Transverse forces or forces acting longitudinally (compression or distraction) can effect changes in spinal contour.

approximately twice the distraction force as the thoracic hook site. Increasing force must be used for incremental curve improvement as the scoliosis decreases in magnitude. In a scoliosis curvature of 90 degrees, 70 per cent of the distractive force is utilized in improving the curvature, whereas in a 45 degree scoliosis curvature, only 35 per cent of the distractive force is directed toward curve improvement.

With distraction alone, it is not possible to control contour in the sagittal plane or to primarily correct rotation. Post-surgical flat back, particularly in the lumbar spine, can result in unfavorable consequences.[29] The center of balance is tilted forward and the patient must flex the knees to stand upright. The addition of multiple hooks to allow more forceful distraction addresses only one shortcoming of the distraction mode. By distributing the upper purchase sites on two or more lamina, rather than one, more distractive force can be applied. This increased ability to apply tensile forces to a small curve increases the potential for traction injury to the spinal cord and its blood supply. Force-limited correction of scoliosis by distraction instrumentation is characterized by structural failure of the lamina or neurologic impairment as the upper limits of force are utilized. Distraction is, in general, a force-limited correction, which is relevant only to correction of uniplanar deformity. It does not allow selective control of rotation or lordosis/kyphosis when applied to the scoliotic spine.

Transverse corrective forces have better efficiency than tensile forces in correcting lateral deformity as the curve diminishes below 53 degrees (Fig. 2–8).[112] While the use of hardware has become increasingly popular, spinal instrumentation is not required to generate these transverse forces. The localizer cast can produce excellent correction of flexible spine deformities. Although originally used by Morscher in 1970,[69] Luque popularized the use of sublaminar wires at multiple levels to provide transverse traction.[63] Others have used the spinous process or transverse process for anchoring the lateral forces,[24, 85] and thus avoided entering the spinal canal. This process distributes corrective forces to multiple laminae, thus reducing the force concentration and the possibility of subsequent laminar failure.[37] Geometry-limited correction is often characteristic of the Luque system. When a Luque rod is pre-bent and then applied to the spine, tightening of the sublaminar wires produces correction. As the laminae are brought into contact with the rod, the predetermined geometry of the rod thus limits further correction. An ideal spinal correction instrument would reach the safe limits of both geometry and force simultaneously as the spine was corrected.

Any force acting at a right angle to the axis of a column creates torque if the force does not pass through the center of the column. All transverse loading devices presently used in surgery apply torsional loads to the spine, which tend to further pathologically rotate

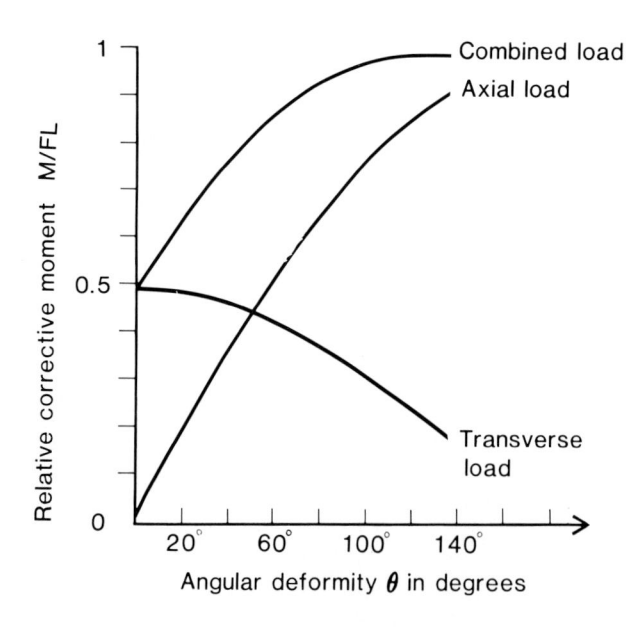

Figure 2–8. Transverse forces are more efficient when correcting curves of small magnitude, whereas axial loads (traction) are more efficient in treating large curves. Parity is reached at approximately 53 degrees. (Adapted with permission from White, A. A., and Panjabi, M. M.: Clinical Biomechanics of the Spine, Philadelphia, J. B. Lippincott, 1978, p. 105.)

the spinal column.[76] The geometry of sublaminar wires fixed to a longitudinal rod in the manner of Luque creates the most favorable vectors. Segmental fixation to a longitudinal rod also provides improved ability to control pathologic lordosis and kyphosis. The Luque system has been clinically demonstrated to be more effective in controlling these sagittal plane deformities than Harrington distraction rods alone. This ability to combine bending moments and to generate torsional forces allows potential control of all six degrees of freedom of the deformed vertebrae. Pure distraction instrumentation can predictably control deformity in only one plane, and the forces generated by any posterior instrumentation now in use have the least ability to correct vertebral rotation.

Compressive forces applied to the convexity of the spine deformity can create significant corrective vectors. When used on the posterior elements of the column, they reduce kyphosis, prevent over-distraction when used in conjunction with a distraction apparatus and provide segmental immobilization of the spine. Their ability to improve scoliosis, however, is not great and their greatest utility is in correcting sagittal plane deformity.[46]

When a convex compression rod is used as the platform for anchoring transverse loading wires to a concave distraction rod, a force is produced that tends to increase malrotation and accentuate hypokyphosis. While very effective in treating kyphotic deformities, compression rods must be used with caution in spines where a decrease is kyphosis is not wanted.

Anterior spinal instrumentation of scoliosis correction was introduced by Dwyer in 1969.[31] Following removal of the intervertebral discs in the area to be instrumented, large cancellous screws are inserted into the vertebral bodies from the convex aspect. These screws are then connected with a flexible cable, which is crimped to the screw heads as tension is applied. This asymmetrical compression across the disc space is an efficient method of scoliosis correction.[95] Technical disadvantages of this apparatus include screw pullout from weak vertebral bodies and the tendency to accentuate kyphus over the instrumented segments. Because the titanium cable does not provide rigid internal fixation, all Dwyer instrumentation must be supplemented with an orthosis until fusion occurs.[44]

Zielke has added a threaded rod in place of the cable for applying compression.[119] This gives both rigidity and the ability to infinitely adjust the tension, features that the Dwyer method lacks. By rotating the Zielke rod with a lordosing bar and by placing the intervertebral bone grafts well anterior to the line of compression, it is possible to dramatically correct rotation and control lordosis. The thin rod and the weakness created by the threading require that patients wear a cast or brace until fusion occurs.

Osteoporosis affects cancellous bone before cortical bone and therefore conditions causing osteopenia result in weakening the vertebral body more than the posterior spinal structures. This can cause pullout of the Dwyer or Zielke screws when tension is applied. Dunn and Bolstad have quantified the failure modes of vertebral body screws.[30] If screw cut out occurs, structural integrity can be restored by removing the screw, injecting liquid methylmethacrylate into the vertebral body, and reinserting the screw. After the methylmethacrylate has hardened, the unit can be treated as a sound structural body.

MECHANICS OF BONE GRAFTING

Although intuitive to most surgeons, there is sound mechanical and biologic reasoning behind the dictum that a spinal fusion mass should lie as close to the weight-bearing lines of the column as possible.

Osseous healing of fractures or arthrodesis masses undergo complex stages of transformation until mature bone is achieved. Further remodelling takes place in accordance with Wolff's axiom, which states that bone responds with changes in architecture according to the stresses applied. Those stresses are either compression/torsion forces in resistance to gravity or compression/torsion forces in resistance to the contractile stress generated by muscles. Bones in general do not increase their strength through remodelling, and they do not heal when subjected to tensile force.

This remodelling concept is brought into focus as the mechanics of bending stress is applied to spinal fusions. When a bending moment is placed on a solid rod, the 60 per cent of the rod's cross sectional area on the concavity of the bend is in compression. The 40 per cent of the rod on the convexity of the

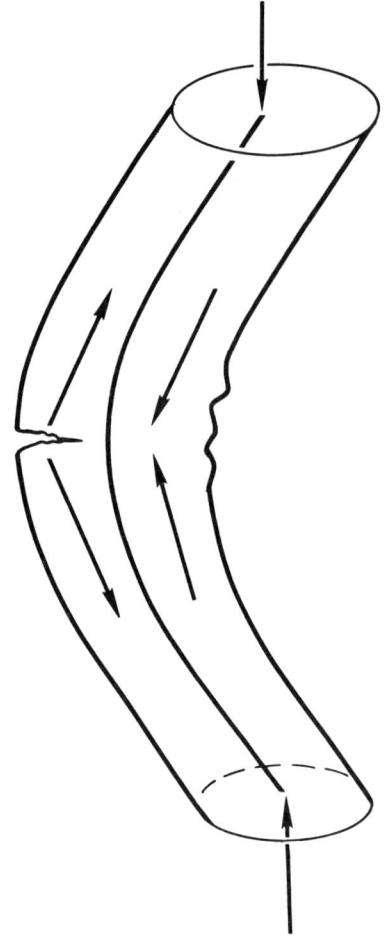

Figure 2–9. The concave 60 per cent of a bent column upper axial load is in compression, whereas the convex 40 per cent is under tension.

bility than can be achieved by posterior fusion alone.[16]

When arthrodesis is performed in Scheuermann's disease, concomitant anterior fusion is also done for two purposes. First stage anterior surgery includes removal of the anterior longitudinal ligament, anulus fibrosus, and nucleus pulposus thus freeing the tether, which prevents correction by extension in the second stage posterior instrumentation and fusion. Anterior discectomy and bone graft also provide a solid anterior column of bone in compression that resists the natural tendency for settling through the disc space and subsequent progression of the kyphosis. Posterior surgery alone in treating Scheuermann's kyphosis has a high incidence of failure because of nonunion and curve progression, an empirical confirmation of the mechanical principles just stated.

If a kyphotic deformity cannot be corrected to less than 50 degrees, it may be necessary to supplement the anterior intervertebral

bend is under tension (Fig. 2–9). Rolander demonstrated this with respect to posterior lumbar spinal fusion in that even solid arthrodesis did not immobilize the disc space. The weight-bearing axis runs through the lumbar discs and the closer a posterior fusion mass is to that weight-bearing line, the less motion is present in the disc space.[92]

This principle regarding the weight-bearing axis has application in scoliosis fusion surgery in which the bone graft is concentrated in the concavity of the deformity. As settling takes place in the postoperative period, the bone graft in the concavity of the deformity comes into compression. This closer approximation of the healing graft fragments promotes osseous union. Arthrodesis of deformities that have a significant kyphotic component often require more sta-

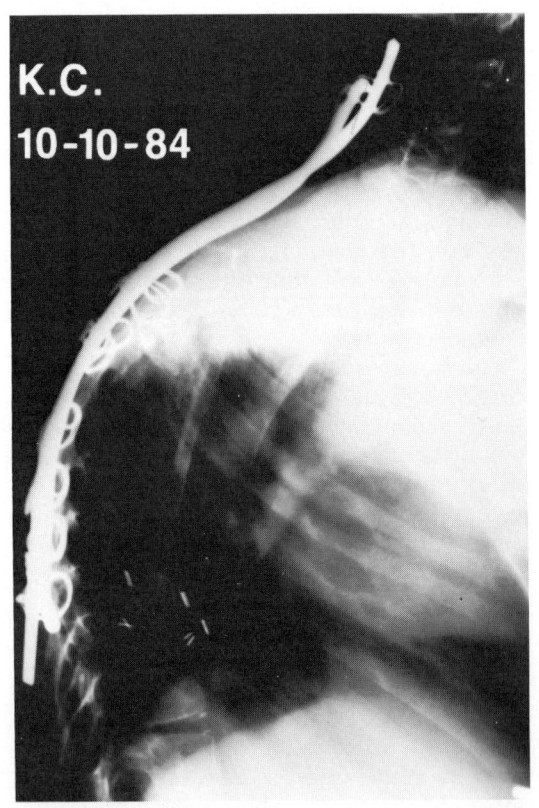

Figure 2–10. This 14 year old male was treated with laminectomy and radiation for a cervicothoracic neuroblastoma. Anterior and posterior fusions have been performed. At 30 months after surgery the T1 to T9 fibular strut has hypertrophied.

body fusion with an anterior strut graft (Fig. 2–10). Placed anteriorly as close to the weight-bearing line as feasible, the bony strut, such as an autogenous fibula or rib, stabilizes the deformity and is eventually incorporated into the fusion. The use of a vascularized pedicle rib can achieve more rapid incorporation, but the rib's geometry may limit the extent of kyphus spanned.[17]

IMPLANT EVALUATION

The mechanical evaluation of spinal implants is a necessary prologue to their clinical employment. Implants have two functions they must fulfill. They must immobilize the segments they span. Immobilization is believed to facilitate healing in fractured long bones and the same principle is applied to spinal fusion. The period of time over which the implant must maintain rigidity varies but usually extends beyond six months, and the continuation of immobilization may be required until the fusion mass matures at two or more years following surgery. Spinal implants are also applied to correct deformity. The ideal implant must generate force vectors that can straighten curves in two planes and correct rotational deformities. After achieving the engineering objectives of correcting spinal deformity and providing prolonged rigidity to the operated segments, the device must be clinically acceptable. It must be reasonably safe to insert, not compromise other body functions, and allow room for biologic healing to achieve bony stability.

When assessing an implant, there are three laboratory evaluations that can be done. No one test is definitive and each gives different information, sometimes incomplete, about an implant's anticipated performance in vivo. The most common method of spinal instrumentation bench testing is the single-load–to-failure stress. In this test mode, force is applied to the implant-spine construct until the failure point of the force-deformation curve is reached. The implant-spine model fails in one of three ways. It can fail outside the instrumented area of the spine; failure can occur at the implant-spine interface; or the implant itself can fail. Although relatively easy to perform, the single-load–to-failure is not the mode usually seen in clinical situations. Information from this test reveals the gross performance of an implant (e.g., When the patient stands up for the first time is it likely that his spine instrumentation will hold?).

Since rigid immobilization is a goal of the ideal implant, the stiffness or spring constant of the device is an important factor. When determining the construct's stiffness, a force-deformation curve is plotted by applying bending, compression, or torsional loads and noting the deflection that results. A flexible spring, for instance, may require great tensile forces before it fails but may have inadequate rigidity to be clinically useful in immobilizing a healing fusion mass.

Cyclical loading is the third method of laboratory testing an implant's structural properties. In this method, the implant is subjected to a given load at a given frequency. The number of cycles necessary to cause implant failure is measured. Although the test's endpoint is the same as the single-load–to-failure test and the failure modes may be the same, several important differences exist. First, mechanical devices may fail at a different location when subjected to cyclical loads than when subjected to a single-load–to-failure stress. Secondly, the variation in frequency of load application can alter the failure pattern. Several different combinations of loads and frequencies may need to be tested before it is possible to predict failure modes that have clinical meaning. Thirdly, spinal implants in vivo have factors influencing them that cannot be duplicated in the laboratory setting. Healing of the spine alters the stress patterns acting on the implant. Failure at the bone-implant interface is influenced by resorption and healing of the fusion. The chemical environment of the metallic implant in vivo may also be a factor in boundary erosion and propagation of cracks. All these factors affect the forces that are encountered in vivo, and few of these can be reproduced in the laboratory. For these reasons, cyclical load tests are of necessity incomplete when used to evaluate an implant's anticipated performance clinically.

The ideal implant will theoretically generate the forces needed to correct or improve a spine deformity. Its engineering design will allow correction along the x, y, and z axis and will also permit rotatory correction where needed. Its mechanical properties will have withstood reasonable laboratory testing to determine its ultimate strength in facing cyclical as well as single loads. The implant's rigidity in stress testing will also be compatible with the goals of spine immobilization until healing occurs. Although no such ideal implant is available, the spine surgeon should have a reasonable expectation that the implant used meets as many of the criteria as possible.

SUMMARY

It is necessary for the surgeon to understand the kinematics of the normal spine, the pathomechanics of spine deformity, and the mechanics of orthotic and spinal instrumentation before initiating a treatment plan.

When surgical planning is done for a spine deformity, the instrumentation in consideration must be capable of safely generating those vectors that will achieve the desired correction and stabilization. Instrumentation must be selected to maintain physiologic lumbar lordosis and thoracic kyphosis in addition to correcting deformities. The instrumentation selected must also be rigid enough to provide immobilization, which is necessary to promote healing of the fusion mass created by scoliosis surgery.

References

1. Adams, M. A., and Hutton, W. C.: The effect of posture on the role of the apophysial joints in resisting intervertebral compressive forces. J. Bone Joint Surg., 62B:358, 1980.
2. Adams, M. A., and Hutton, W. C.: Mechanical factors in the etiology of low back pain. Orthopedics, 5:1461, 1982.
3. Adams, W.: Lectures on the Pathology and Treatment of Lateral and Other Forms of Curvature of the Spine. London, J. Churchill, 1865.
4. Agostini, E., Mognoni, G., Torri, G., and Miserocki, G.: Forces deforming the rib cage. Respir. Physiol., 2:105, 1966.
5. Akerblom, B.: Standing and sitting posture. Thesis, A. B. Nordiski Bokhandeln, Stockholm, 1948.
6. Akeson, W. H., Woo, S. L. Y., Taylor, T. K. F., et al.: Biomechanics and biochemistry of the intervertebral disks: the need for correlation studies. Clin. Orthop., 129:133, 1977.
7. Allen, F. G.: Scoliosis: operative correction of fixed curves. J. Bone Joint Surg., 37B:92, 1955.
8. Andersson, G. B. J., Ortengren, R., and Schultz, A.: Analysis and measurement of the loads on the lumbar spine during work at a table. J. Biomech., 13:513, 1980.
9. Andriacchi, T. P., Schultz, A. B., Belytschko, T. B., and DeWald, R. L.: Milwaukee brace correction of idiopathic scoliosis: a biomechanical analysis and a retrospective study. J. Bone Joint Surg., 58A:806, 1976.
10. Arkin, A. M.: The mechanism of rotation in combination with lateral deviation in the normal spine. J. Bone Joint Surg., 32A:180, 1950.
11. Armstrong, G. W. D., Livermore, N. B., Suzuki, N., and Armstrong, J. G.: Nonstandard vertebral rotation in scoliosis screening patients: its prevalence and relation to the clinical deformity. Spine, 7:50, 1982.
12. Badgley, C.: The articular facets in relation to low back pain and sciatic radiation. J. Bone Joint Surg., 23A:481, 1941.
13. Balasubramanian, K., Ranu, H. S., and King, A. I.: Vertebral response to laminectomy. J. Biomech., 12:813, 1979.
14. Bell, G. H., Dunbar, O., Beck, J. S., and Gibb, A.: Variation in strength of vertebrae with age and their relation to osteoporosis. Calcif. Tissue Res., 1:75, 1967.
15. Belytschko, T., Kulak, R. F., and Schultz, A. B.: Finite element analysis of an intervertebral disc. J. Biomech., 7:277, 1974.
16. Bjerkreim, I., Magnaes, B., and Semb, G.: Surgical treatment of severe angular kyphosis. Acta Orthop. Scand., 53(6):913, 1982.
17. Bradford, D. S.: Anterior vascular bone grafting for the treatment of kyphosis. Spine, 5:318, 1980.
18. Bradley, K. C.: The anatomy of backache. Aust. N.Z. J. Surg., 44:227, 1974.
19. Brailsford, J. F.: Deformities of lumbosacral region of the spine. Brit. J. Surg., 16:562, 1929.
20. Brus, H.: Anastomic des meschen. Band I. Bewegungsapparat. Springer, Berlin, 1921.
21. Bunch, W. H., Patwardhan, A., Vanderby, R., and Knight, G. W.: Stability of scoliotic spines. Orthop. Trans. 8:145, 1984.
22. Bushell, G. R., Ghosh, P., and Taylor, T. F.: Collagen defect in idiopathic scoliosis. Lancet, 2:94, 1978.
23. Cossette, J. W., Farfan, H. F., Robertson, G. H., and Wells, R. V.: The instantaneous center of rotation of the third lumbar intervertebral joint. J. Biomech., 4:149, 1971.
24. Cotrel, V.: Techniques nouvelles dans le traitement de la scoliose idiopathique. Int. Orthop., 1:247, 1968.
25. Cyron, B. M., and Hutton, W. C.: Articular tropism and stability of the lumbar spine. Spine, 5:168, 1980.
26. DeSmet, A. A., Tarlton, M. A., Cook, L. T., et al.: A radiographic method for three-dimensional analysis of spinal configuration. Radiography, 137:343, 1980.
27. Dickson, R. A., Lawton, J. O., Archer, I. A., and Buxt, W. P.: The pathogenesis of idiopathic scoliosis. J. Bone Joint Surg., 66B:8, 1984.
28. Dimnet, J., Fischer, L. P., Gonon, G., and Carret, J. P.: Radiographic studies of lateral flexion in the lumbar spine. J. Biomech., 11:143, 1978.
29. Doherty, J.: Complications of fusion in lumbar scoliosis. J. Bone Joint Surg., 55A:438, 1973.
30. Dunn, H. K., and Bolstad, K. E.: Fixation of Dwyer screws for treatment of scoliosis. J. Bone Joint Surg., 59A:54, 1977.
31. Dwyer, A. F., Newton, N. C., and Sherwood, A. A.: An anterior approach to scoliosis. A preliminary report. Clin. Orthop., 62:192, 1969.
32. Elward, J. F.: Motion in the vertebral column. Read at the Fifth International Congress of Radiology, Chicago, IL, Sept. 13–17, 1937.

33. Evans, G., and Lissner, M. S.: Biomechanical studies of the lumbar spine and pelvis. J. Bone Joint Surg., 41A:278, 1959.
34. Farfan, H. F., and Sullivan, J. D.: The relation of facet orientation to intervertebral disc failure. Can. J. Surg., 10:179, 1967.
35. Ferguson, R. J., McMaster, J. H., and Stanitski, C. L.: Low back pain in college football linemen. J. American Sp. Med., 2:63, 1974.
36. Fidler, M. W., and Jowett, R. L.: Muscle imbalance in the aetiology of scoliosis. J. Bone Joint Surg., 58B:200, 1976.
37. Flatley, T. J.: Application of segmental spinal instrumentation. Orthopedics, 6:441, 1983.
38. Francis, M. J. D., Smith, R., and Sanderson, M. C.: Collagen abnormalities in idiopathic adolescent scoliosis. Calcif. Tissue Res., 22:381, 1977.
39. Frymoyer, J. W., Frymoyer, W. W., Wilder, D. G., and Pope, M. H.: The mechanical and kinematic analysis of the lumbar spine in normal living human subjects in vivo. J. Biomech., 12:165, 1979.
40. Galante, J. O.: Tensile properties of the human lumbar annulus fibrosus. Acta Orthop. Scand. Suppl. 100, 1967.
41. Gregersen, G. G., and Lucas, D. B.: An in vivo study of the axial rotation of the human thoracolumbar spine. J. Bone Joint Surg., 49A:247, 1967.
42. Haderspeck, K., and Schultz, A.: Progression of idiopathic scoliosis: an analysis of muscle actions and body weight influences. Spine, 6:447, 1981.
43. Hakim, N. S., and King, A. I.: A three-dimensional finite element dynamic response analysis of a vertebra with experimental verification. J. Biomech., 12:277, 1979.
44. Hall, J. E., Gray, J., and Allen, N.: Dwyer instrumentation and spinal fusion. A follow-up study. J. Bone Joint Surg., 59A:117, 1977.
45. Harrington, P.: Treatment of scoliosis. J. Bone Joint Surg., 44A:591, 1962.
46. Herndon, W. A., Ellis, R. D., Hall, J. A., and Millis, M. G.: Correction with a transverse loading system in the operative management of scoliosis. Clin. Orthop., 165:168, 1982.
47. Herman, R., and MacEwen, G. D.: Idiopathic scoliosis: Visuovestibular disorder of the CNS. In Zorab, P. A., and Siegler, D. (eds.): Scoliosis 1979. London, Academic Press, p. 61, 1980.
48. Humphry, G. M.: A treatise on the human skeleton. London, MacMillan, 1858.
49. Hunter, R. E., Bradford, D. S., and Oegema, T. R.: Biochemistry of the intervertebral disc in scoliosis. Trans. Orthop. Res. Soc., 4:135, 1978.
50. Jensen, G. M.: Biomechanics of the lumbar intervertebral disk: a review. Phys. Ther., 60:765, 1980.
51. Kazarian, L. E., Kazarian LE: Creep characteristics of the human spinal column. Orthop. Clin. North Am., 6:3, 1975.
52. Keetley, C. B.: On the etiology and essential nature of scoliosis. Ann. Surg., 7:126, 1888.
53. Khosla, S., Tredwell, S. J., Day, B., et al.: An ultrastructural study of multifidus muscle in progressive idiopathic scoliosis. J. Neurol. Sci., 46:13, 1980.
54. Kulak, R. F., Belytschko, T. B., and Schultz, A. B.: Nonlinear behavior of the human interverte-bral disc under axial load. J. Biomech., 9:377, 1976.
55. Lamy, C., Bazergui, A., Kraus, H., and Farfan, H. F.: Strength of the neural arch and the etiology of spondylolysis. Orthop. Clin. North Am., 6:215, 1975.
56. Leong, J. C., Low, W. D., Mok, C. K., et al.: Linear growth in southern Chinese female patients with idiopathic scoliosis. Spine, 7:471, 1982.
57. Lin, H. S., Liu, Y. K., and Adams, K. H.: Mechanical response of the lumbar intervertebral joint under physiological (complex) loading. J. Bone Joint Surg., 60A:41, 1978.
58. Lorenz, M., Patwardhan, A., and Vanderby, R.: Load bearing characteristics of lumbar facets in normal and surgically altered spinal segments. Spine, 8:122, 1983.
59. Lovett, R. W.: The mechanism of the normal spine and its relation to scoliosis. Boston Med. Surg. J., 153:349, 1905.
60. Lucas, D. B., and Bresler, B.: Stability of the ligamentous spine. Biomechanics Laboratory, University of California, San Francisco and Berkeley Technical Report. p. 40, 1961.
61. Luke, M. J., and McDonnell, E. J.: Congenital heart disease and scoliosis. J. Pediatr., 73:725, 1968.
62. Lumsden, R. M., and Morris, J. M.: An in vivo study of axial rotation and immobilization at the lumbosacral joint. J. Bone Joint Surg., 50A:1591, 1968.
63. Luque, E. R., and Cardosa, P.: Segmental correction of scoliosis with rigid internal fixation. Read at the Scoliosis Research Society. Ottawa, 1976.
64. MacLennan, A.: Scoliosis. Brit. Med. J., 2:864, 1922.
65. Markolf, K. L.: Deformation of the thoracolumbar intervertebral joints in response to external loads: a biomechanical study using autopsy material. J. Bone Joint Surg., 54A:511, 1972.
66. Moe, J. H.: Modern concepts of treatment of spinal deformities in children and adults. Clin. Orthop., 150:137, 1980.
67. Morris, J. M., Benner, G., and Lucas, D. B.: An electromyographic study of the intrinsic muscles of the back in man. J. Anat., 96:509, 1962.
68. Morris, J. M., Lucas, D. B., and Bresler, B.: Role of the trunk in stability of the spine. J. Bone Joint Surg., 43A:327, 1961.
69. Morscher, E.: A modification of Harrington operative technique in scoliosis. Proceedings of the 12th Congress of the International Society of Orthopaedic Surgery and Traumatology. Tel Aviv, 1972.
70. Nachemson, A.: The load on lumbar discs in different positions of the body. Clin. Orthop., 45:107, 1966.
71. Nachemson, A., and Elfstrom, G.: Intravital dynamic pressure measurements in lumbar discs: a study of common movements, maneuvers and exercises. Scand. J. Rehabil. Med., Suppl. 1, 1970.
72. Nachemson, A., and Elfstrom, G.: Intravital wireless telemetry of axial forces in Harrington distraction rods in patients with idiopathic scoliosis. J. Bone Joint Surg., 53A:445, 1971.
73. Nachemson, A. L., and Evans, J. H.: Some me-

chanical properties of the third human lumbar interlaminar ligament (ligamentum flavum). J. Biomech., 1:211, 1968.
74. Nachemson, A., and Morris, J. M.: In vivo measurements of intradiscal pressure: discometry, a method for the determination of pressure in the lower lumbar discs. J. Bone Joint Surg., 46A:1077, 1964.
75. Nachemson, A. L., Schultz, A. B., and Berkson, M. H.: Mechanical properties of human lumbar spine motion segments: influences of age, sex, disc level, and degeneration. Spine, 4:1, 1979.
76. Ogilvie, J. W., and Millar, E. A.: Comparison of segmental spinal instrumentation devices in the correction of scoliosis. Spine, 8:416, 1983.
77. Panjabi, M. M.: Experimental determination of spinal motion segment behavior. Orthop. Clin. North Am., 8:169, 1977.
78. Panjabi, M. M., Brand, R. A., and White, A. A.: Mechanical properties of the human thoracic spine. J. Bone Joint Surg., 58A:642, 1976.
79. Panjabi, M. M., Hausfeld, J., and White, A. A.: Experimental determination of thoracic spine stability. Read at the 24th Annual ORS Meeting, Dallas, Texas, Feb. 21–23, 1978.
80. Panjabi, M. M., and White, A. A.: Basic biomechanics of the spine. Neurosurgery, 7:76, 1980.
81. Pearcy, M., Portek, I., and Shepherd, J.: Three-dimensional x-ray analysis of normal movement in the lumbar spine. Spine, 9:294, 1984.
82. Pope, M. H., Wilder, D. G., Matteri, R. E., and Frymoyer, J. W.: Experimental measurement of vertebral motion under load. Orthop. Clin. North Am., 8:155, 1977.
83. Posner, I., White, A. A., Edwards, W. T., and Hayes, W. C.: A biomechanical analysis of the clinical stability of the lumbar and lumbosacral spine. Spine, 7:374, 1982.
84. Putti, V.: On new conceptions in the pathogenesis of sciatic pain. Lancet, 2:53, 1927.
85. Resina, J., and Ferreira-Alues, A. F.: A technique of correction and internal fixation for scoliosis. J. Bone Joint Surg., 59B:159–165, 1977.
86. Reuber, M., Schultz, A., McNeill, T., and Spencer, D.: Trunk muscle myoelectric activities in idiopathic scoliosis. Spine, 8:447, 1983.
87. Riddle, H. F. V., and Roaf, R.: Muscle imbalance in the causation of scoliosis. Lancet, 1:1245, 1955.
88. Roaf, R.: Rotational movements of the spine with special reference to scoliosis. J. Bone Joint Surg., 40B:312, 1958.
89. Roaf, R.: A study of the mechanics of spinal injuries. J. Bone Joint Surg., 42B:810, 1960.
90. Roaf, R.: Vertebral growth and its mechanical control. J. Bone Joint Surg., 42B:40, 1960.
91. Rockwell, H., Evans, F. G., and Pheasant, H. C.: The comparative morphology of the vertebrate spinal column. Its form as related to function. J. Morphol., 63:87, 1938.
92. Rolander, S. D.: Motion of the lumbar spine with special reference to the stabilizing effect of posterior fusion: an experimental study on autopsy specimens. Tryckeri AB Litotyp, Goteborg, 1966.
93. Roth, A., Rosenthal, A., Hall, J. E., and Mizel, M.: Scoliosis and congenital heart disease. Clin. Orth., 93:95, 1973.
94. Sahlstrand, T., and Lidstrom, J.: Equilibrium factors as predictors of the prognosis in adolescent idiopathic scoliosis. Clin. Orthop., 152:232, 1980.
95. Schafer, M. F.: Dwyer instrumentation of the spine. Orthop. Clin. North Am., 9:115, 1978.
96. Schultz, A. B.: A biomechanical view of scoliosis. Spine, 1:162, 1976.
97. Schultz, A. B., and Andersson, G. B. J.: Analysis of loads on the lumbar spine. Spine, 6:76, 1981.
98. Schultz, A. B., Benson, D. R., and Hirsch, C.: Force-deformation properties of human costosternal and costo-vertebral articulations. J. Biomech., 7:311, 1974.
99. Schultz, A. B., Haderspeck, K., and Takashima, S.: Correction of scoliosis by muscle stimulation. Spine, 6:468, 1981.
100. Schultz, A. B., Sorenson, S., and Andersson, G. B. J.: Measurement of spine morphology in children ages 10–16. Spine, 9:70, 1984.
101. Selby, D. C., and Paris, S. V.: Anatomy of facet joints and its clinical correlation with low back pain. Orthop., 3:1097, 1981.
102. Silver, P. H. S.: Direct observation of changes in tension in the supraspinous and interspinous ligaments during flexion and extension of the vertebral column in man. J. Anat., 88:550, 1954.
103. Skogland, L. B., and Miller, J. A. A.: The length and proportions of the thoracolumbar spine in children with idiopathic scoliosis. Acta Orthop. Scand., 52:177, 1981.
104. Somerville, E. A.: Rotational lordosis: the development of the single curve. J. Bone Joint Surg., 34B:421, 1952.
105. Stagnara, P., DeMauroy, J. C., Dran, G., et al.: Reciprocal angulation of vertebral bodies in a sagittal plane: approach to references for the evaluation of kyphosis and lordosis. Spine, 7:335, 1982.
106. Takashima, S. T., Singh, S. P., Haderspeck, K. A., and Schultz, A. B.: A model for semi-quantitative studies of muscle actions. J. Biomech., 12:929, 1979.
107. Tkaczuk, H.: Tensile properties of human lumbar longitudinal ligaments. Acta Orthop. Scand., Suppl. 115, 1968.
108. Trueta, J.: Studies of the Development and Decay of the Human Frame. Philadelphia, W. B. Saunders Co., 1968.
109. Virchow, H.: Einzelbeträge bei der sagittalen Biegung der menschlichen Wirbelsäule. Verh. Anat. Ges., 25:176, 1911.
110. Virgin, W. J.: Experimental investigations into the physical properties of the intervertebral disc. J. Bone Joint Surg., 33B:607, 1951.
111. White, A. A.: Analysis of the mechanics of the thoracic spine in man. Acta Orthop. Scand., 42:482, 1969.
112. White, A. A., and Panjabi, M. M.: Clinical Biomechanics of the Spine. Philadelphia, J. B. Lippincott, p. 105, 1978.
113. White, A. A., and Panjabi, M. M.: The basic kinematics of the human spine: a review of past and current knowledge. Spine, 3:12, 1978.
114. Willner, S.: The proportion of legs to trunk in girls with idiopathic structural scoliosis. Acta Orthop. Scand., 46:84, 1975.
115. Willner, S.: A study of growth in girls with adolescent idiopathic structural scoliosis. Clin. Orthop., 101:129, 1974.
116. Wolfe, E., Robin, G. C., Yarom, R., and Gonen,

B.: Myopathy of deltoids in patients with idiopathic scoliosis. Electromyogr. Clin. Neurophysiol., 22:357, 1982.
117. Wu, H., and Yao, R.: Mechanical behavior of the human annulus fibrosus. J. Biomech., 9:1, 1976.
118. Yettram, A. L., and Jackman, M. J.: Equilibrium analysis for the forces in the human spinal column and its musculature. Spine, 5:402, 1980.
119. Zielke, K., Stundat, R., and Beaujean, F.: Ventrale Derotation spondylodese. Vorlaufiger Ergebnissbericht über 26 operierte Falle. Arch. Orthop. Unfall-Chir., 85:257, 1976.
120. Zuk, T.: The role of spinal and abdominal muscles in the pathogenesis of scoliosis. J. Bone Joint Surg., 44B:102, 1962.

3
EMBRYOLOGY AND SPINE GROWTH

John E. Lonstein, M.D.

Fetal development, and development of all organs, is divided into three stages. The preembryonic period is the first three weeks after fertilization. The second period or the embryonic period lasts from week three to week eight, and during this phase all the organs of the body develop. The embryo starts the second phase as a 1 mm. disc and ends it as an embryo 25 mm. in length, weighing 1 gram and having a definite human appearance. The third phase or the fetal stage extends from eight weeks to term and is characterized by growth, enlargement, and maturation of all structures and organs.

Embryonic age is measured two ways—gestational (ovulation) age and menstrual age. Gestational age is determined from the day of ovulation and is used in the pre-embryonic and embryonic periods. Because of the rapid development in these periods precise staging is difficult when related to age in days. To be more accurate, staging is related to the number of somites present; the first 29 form in the fourth week of development, and the remainder form in the fifth week. The menstrual age, measured from the date of the last menstrual period, is 14 days longer than the gestational age. It is used in discussing development in the fetal period, when knowledge of the exact stage of development is not necessary.

DEVELOPMENT OF THE NOTOCHORD AND NEURAL TUBE[2, 21, 39, 45, 52]

The early stages of development of the neural system, muscular system, and axial skeleton are intimately related to the notochord. This development involves the biologic principle of metamerism, the craniocaudal repetition of anatomically similar segments. This process is well seen in higher invertebrates and in adult fish, and it forms the basic pattern of early vertebrate morphologic development.

In embryonic development, many organs are developing simultaneously, and the development of these structures is often interrelated. For ease of description, the development of the notochord, neural tube, and axial skeleton are described separately, with the understanding that their development occurs together.[7, 8, 15, 16, 20, 27, 29, 34, 38, 40, 49, 51]

After fertilization, the ovum migrates down the fallopian tube into the uterine cavity. During the six to seven days that this occurs, the single-celled ovum divides a number of times to form a solid mass of cells called the morula. The morula becomes a hollow ball, the blastocyst, and at seven days implants in the endometrium. At one side of the blastocyst a cluster of cells develops. This cluster, or embryonic disc, thickens and forms a distinct bilaminar structure. The ectoderm, continuous with the amniotic cavity, is on the dorsal surface, and the endoderm and the yolk sac on the ventral surface (Fig. 3–1*A*).

In the third week of embryonic life, at the future caudal end of the embryonic disc, the midline cells proliferate. This proliferating area is the primitive streak. The proliferating cells push laterally and forward between the ectoderm and endoderm, forming the mesoderm. The embryonic disc is now a trilaminar structure (Fig. 3–1*C*). In the midline just cranial to the primitive streak, an invagination of the ectoderm forms. The proliferating cells form a hollow tube that runs cranially

25

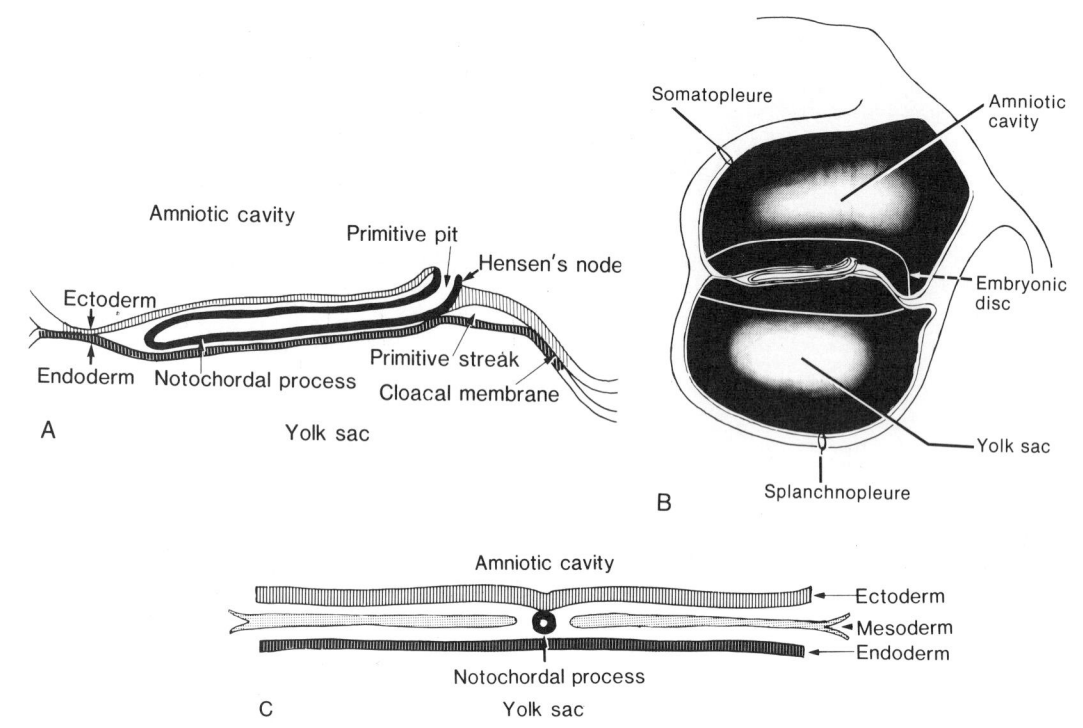

Figure 3–1. Sixteen to seventeen day old embryo in longitudinal section (A and B) and in cross-section (C). The midline notochordal process is forming from the ectoderm at Hensen's node, and the mesoderm from the primitive streak. B, The orientation of the longitudinal section in relation to the yolk sac ventrally and the amniotic cavity dorsally. (Reprinted with permission from Lonstein, J. E.: Spine embryology. In Winter, R. B. (ed.): Congenital Deformities of the Spine, New York, Thieme Stratton, 1983.)

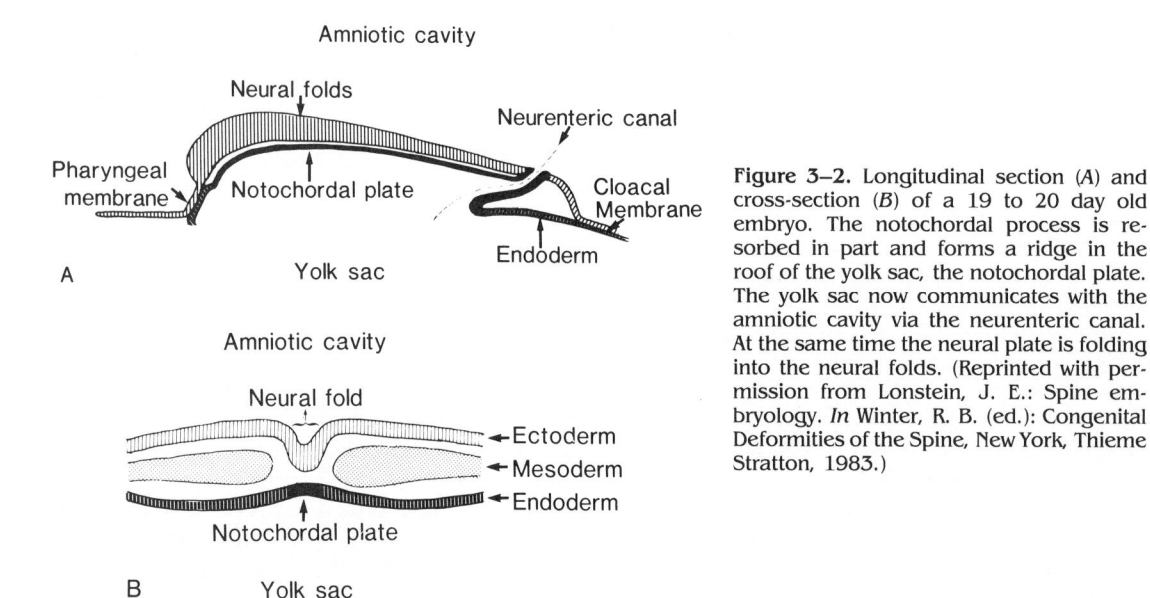

Figure 3–2. Longitudinal section (A) and cross-section (B) of a 19 to 20 day old embryo. The notochordal process is resorbed in part and forms a ridge in the roof of the yolk sac, the notochordal plate. The yolk sac now communicates with the amniotic cavity via the neurenteric canal. At the same time the neural plate is folding into the neural folds. (Reprinted with permission from Lonstein, J. E.: Spine embryology. In Winter, R. B. (ed.): Congenital Deformities of the Spine, New York, Thieme Stratton, 1983.)

Figure 3–3. Longitudinal section (A) and cross-section (B) of a 21 to 22 day old embryo. The definitive notochord is formed, and the endoderm has approximated, forming a continuous layer. The mesoderm laterally shows early differentiation into three areas, the paraxial, intermediate, and lateral plate mesoderm. The neural folds are further developed and are approximating each other. (Reprinted with permission from Lonstein, J. E.: Spine embryology. *In* Winter, R. B. (ed.): Congenital Deformities of the Spine, New York, Thieme Stratton, 1983.)

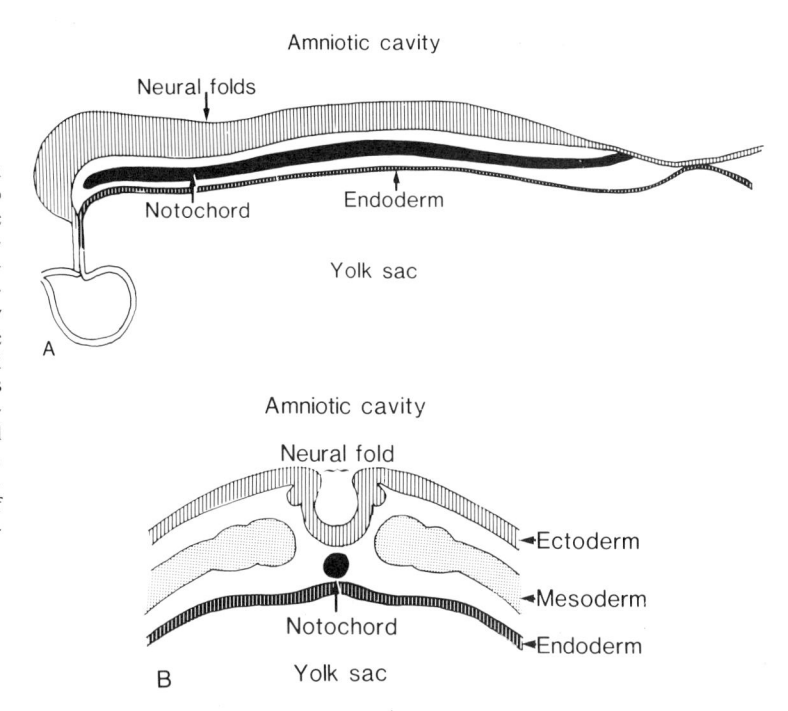

in the midline axis of the embryonic plate between the ectoderm and endoderm. The area of proliferating ectoderm is Hensen's node. The tubular notochordal process formed is in contact with ectoderm and endoderm throughout its length (Fig. 3–1B). The ventral portion of the process and the endoderm with which it is in contact disappear. The dorsal portion of the notochordal process becomes continuous with endoderm and forms a ridge in the "roof" of the yolk sac, the notochordal plate. The cavity of the notochordal process is now part of the yolk sac, and there is communication between the yolk sac and amniotic cavity through the neurenteric canal (Fig. 3–2). The notochordal cells separate from the endoderm, forming a solid notochord that lies in close relationship to the neural plate and neural tube dorsally (Fig. 3–2). The cells of the endoderm reunite, forming a continuous endodermal layer (Fig. 3–3).

During the third week the midline cells of the ectoderm overlying the notochordal process, and later the notochord, enlarge, proliferate, and fold over, forming the neural folds (see Fig. 3–2B). The edges of the neural folds curl over dorsally, separate from the ectoderm, and form the neural tube. The cells at the junction of the neural tube and ectoderm become detached as the tube closes. These cells form two parallel columns of cells, the neural crest, which lie dorsolateral to the neural tube. This column of cells becomes segmented, forming the anlage of the spinal ganglia, which develop opposite developing somites. Other cells of the neural crest detach from the column and form the ganglia of the autonomic nervous system, pigment cells, and Schwann cells.

The closure of the neural tube starts in the middle of the embryo, extending both cranially and caudally. The neural tube is thus open at the two ends, the openings being the neuropores. The rostral neuropore closes between the 18 and 20 somite stage; the caudal neuropore closes at the 25 somite stage, the site of closure being in the lumbar area. The above process is called primary neurulation.

The primitive streak regresses caudally as the embryo grows. Cells migrate from the ectodermal layer as the primitive streak regresses caudally, adding to the mesodermal cells. In the midline the cells extend the existing neural tissue and notochord by continuously adding cells to their caudal ends, the end bud (Fig. 3–4). The extension to the neural tube is initially a solid mass of cells, the medullary cord. Several small lumina appear and coalesce to form a central lumen. This lumen becomes continuous with the central lumen of the neural tube, which has been formed cranially by the neural plate.

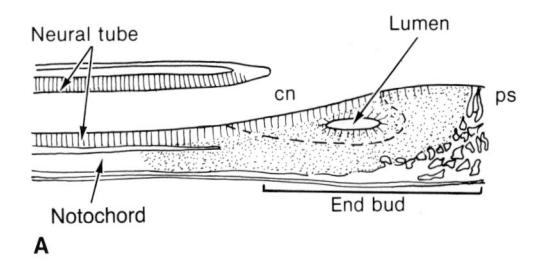

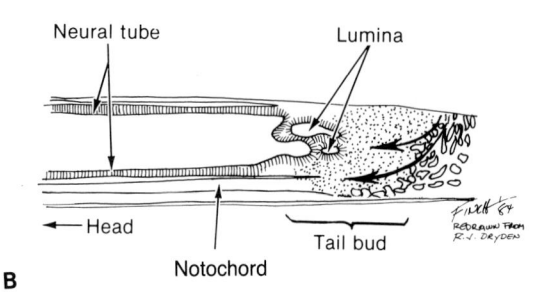

Figure 3–4. Longitudinal section of the development of caudal neural tube and notochord. *A,* The end bud stage is shown. *B,* The tail bud stage is shown. Cells migrate from the primitive streak (*ps*) to the end bud, which is in the area of the caudal neuropore (*cn*). Intercellular lumina coalesce to add to the neural tube (*A*). After closure of the caudal neuropore the process continues in the tail bud (*B*). (Adapted from Dryden, R. J.: Duplication of the spinal cord: a discussion of the possible embryogenesis of diplomyelia. Develop. Med. Child Neurol., 22:234–243, 1980.)

This process of secondary neurulation involves cells of the neural plate dorsally, with contributions from the primitive streak ventrally and caudally; this area is referred to as the transitional zone (Fig. 3–4).

As the active growing area migrates caudally, more cells are received from the primitive streak, forming additional neural and notochordal tissue. When there is no more contribution from the neural plate dorsally, the caudal neuropore having closed, the proliferating center is renamed the tail bud. As in the transitional zone, the initially solid mass of cells becomes progressively canalized by coalescence of the intercellular lumina (Fig. 3–4).[10]

As the aforementioned process is occurring, the embryo is folding laterally because the platelike endoderm is in the initial stage of forming the primitive gut. With the tremendous proliferation dorsally as the neural plate forms and tubulates, the dorsal surface of the embryo lengthens and the embryo folds on itself from end to end.

MESODERMAL DIFFERENTIATION

At the end of the third week the embryo consists of ectoderm dorsally, endoderm ventrally, and mesoderm between these two layers. Mesoderm is absent in the midline where the notochord is situated and cranially and caudally where the ectoderm and endoderm are in intimate contact at the pharyngeal and cloacal membranes. The mesoderm differentiates in two directions, mediolaterally and craniocaudally, simultaneously. The initial sheet of mesoderm proliferates lateral to the notochord, forming two highly cellular parallel tubular structures, the paraxial mesoderm. Further lateral proliferation forms the intermediate mesoderm and the lateral mesoderm; the lateral mesoderm is continuous with the extra-embryonic mesoderm at the edge of the embryo (Fig. 3–5*A*). The lateral plate mesoderm splits into a dorsal and a ventral layer of cells because of the appearance of intercellular clefts, which coalesce. The dorsal layer or somatic mesoderm gives rise to the muscles of the ventrolateral body wall, and the ventral layer forms the splanchnic mesoderm from which the muscular layer of the gut is derived. The intermediate mesoderm differentiates into the urogenital system.

SOMITES

The paraxial mesoderm differentiates in a craniocaudal direction. The mesoderm proliferates and condenses into paired structures, the somites, which form as the spinal ganglia form from the neural crest, the spinal ganglia being situated opposite the medial surface of the somite, giving a one nerve-one somite relationship. Any muscle derived from the somite will retain its innervation, irrespective of how far the muscle migrates (e.g., diaphragm and phrenic nerve). At the same time as the somites are forming, paired vessels arise from the paired longitudinal vessels and are situated between the somites in an intersegmental position (Fig. 3–6*A*).

Somite formation starts near the cranial end of the embryo in the future occipital area and progresses in a craniocaudal direction, closely following the closure of the neural tube. Formation takes 10 days; 29 pairs form in the fourth week and the remainder form early in the fifth week. A total of 42 to 44

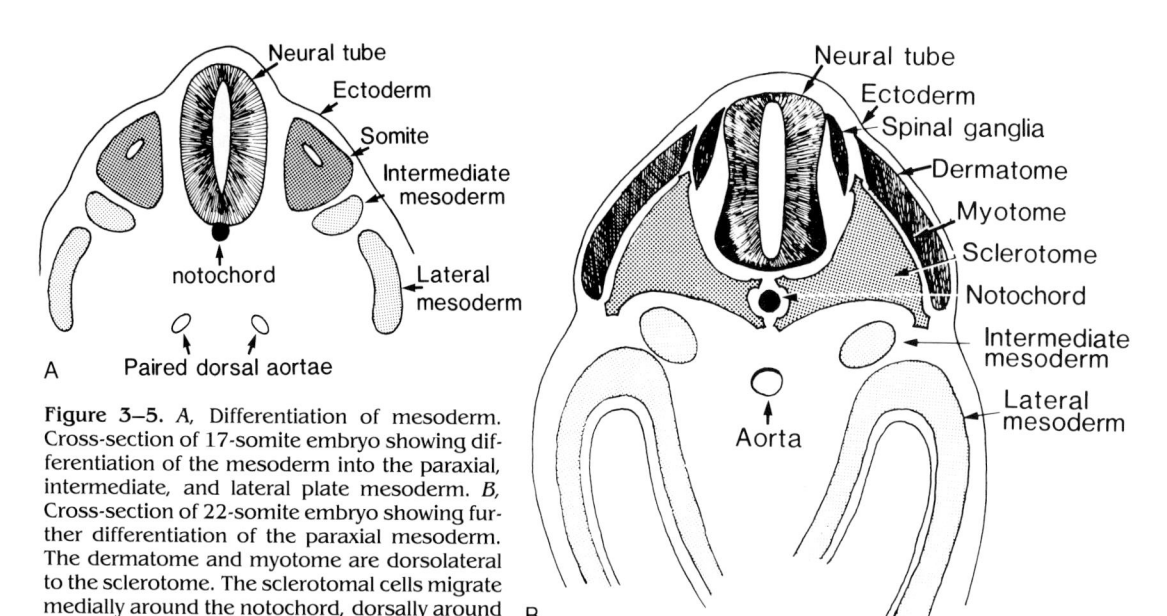

EMBRYOLOGY AND SPINE GROWTH 29

Figure 3–5. *A,* Differentiation of mesoderm. Cross-section of 17-somite embryo showing differentiation of the mesoderm into the paraxial, intermediate, and lateral plate mesoderm. *B,* Cross-section of 22-somite embryo showing further differentiation of the paraxial mesoderm. The dermatome and myotome are dorsolateral to the sclerotome. The sclerotomal cells migrate medially around the notochord, dorsally around the neural tube, and ventrally into the lateral plate body wall mesoderm. (Reprinted with permission from Lonstein, J. E.: Spine embryology. *In* Winter, R. B. (ed.): Congenital Deformities of the Spine, New York, Thieme Stratton, 1983.)

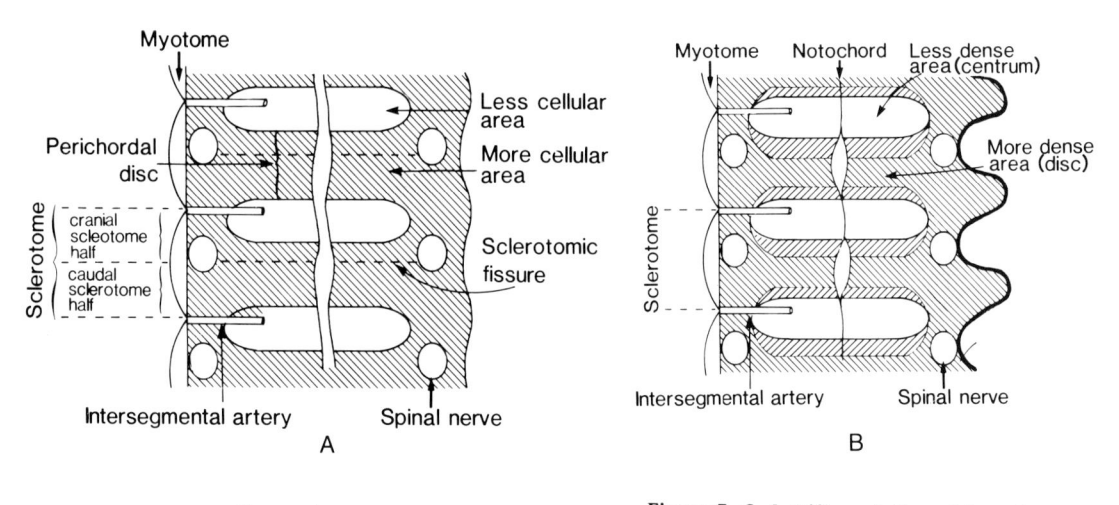

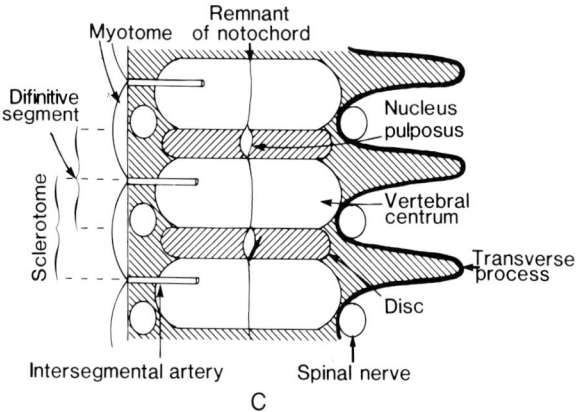

Figure 3–6. *A,* Differentiation of the sclerotome to form the definitive vertebra. The cells around the notochord are initially divided into a more cellular perichordal disc around the sclerotomic fissure and a less cellular area. The sclerotomic fissure divides the sclerotome into cranial and caudal sclerotome halves. *B,* The area on each side of the perichordal disc becomes less cellular and forms part of the vertebral centrum anlage, which enlarges. *C,* The definite centrum and intervertebral disc are formed with resegmentation of the sclerotome. (Reprinted with permission from Lonstein, J. E.: Spine embryology. *In* Winter, R. B. (ed.): Congenital Deformities of the Spine, New York, Thieme Stratton, 1983.)

pairs of somites differentiate—4 occipital, 8 cervical, 12 thoracic, 5 lumbar, 5 sacral, and 8 to 10 coccygeal. The occipital somites form part of the base of the skull and craniocervical articulation. The last five to seven coccygeal somites disappear.

The cells of the somite are initially arranged around a cavity, the myocoele. Cell proliferation occurs, the somite becoming triangular in shape and developing three distinct areas (see Fig. 3–5A). The dorsal cells adjacent to the overlying ectoderm become the dermatome, which gives rise to the skin integuments. The cells medial to the dermatome become spindle-shaped and migrate deep to the dermatome, giving rise to the skeletal muscle of the posterolateral body wall. The cells on the ventral and medial portions of the somite proliferate and migrate toward the notochord and neural tube, forming the sclerotome (see Fig. 3–5B).

SCLEROTOME[2, 4, 5, 46, 55]

The sclerotomal cells stream around the notochord, completely surrounding it and separating it from its intimate relationship with the neural tube. Initially the cells are equally distributed craniocaudally, the separation into somites being marked by the intersegmental vessels. Once the right and left somites fuse across the midline, incorporating the notochord, resegmentation occurs, starting at five to six weeks of development. The mesenchymal cells of the somite form a densely staining cluster of cells, which are aggregated around a cleft or fissue called the sclerotomic fissure of von Ebner. The cells around the notochord now show division into more dense areas, the perichordal discs, which lie around the sclerotomic fissure, and these alternate with less densely cellular areas. The perichordal disc cells lie opposite the developing spinal nerve, and its cells are continuous with the sclerotomal cells that are migrating dorsally and ventrally. These migrations will form the dorsal neural process and the ventrolateral costal element (see Fig. 3–6A).

Initial descriptions of the resegmentation depicted the somite as dividing into a less cellular cranial half and a more cellular caudal half. The work of Sensenig and others has shown that this is not completely accurate.[35, 36] They showed that the densely cellular area, situated around the sclerotomic fissure, was derived from cells from both sclerotome halves, from the cranial two thirds of the caudal sclerotome half and the caudal one third of the cranial sclerotome half (see Fig. 3–6A). The densely cellular perichordal disc forms the majority of the intervertebral disc, while the less cellular area forms the majority of the vertebral centrum.

The less dense area gets larger at the expense of the perichordal disc; as the areas on each side of the perichordal disc become less cellular, they form part of the vertebral centrum anlage (see Fig. 3–6B). This occurs perhaps because of continued migration of cells toward the sclerotomatic fissue area. Resegmentation of the somite has now occurred. The primary segmentation of the paraxial mesoderm is into somites, each somite being related to a spinal nerve and being separated by intersegmental vessels (see Fig. 3–6A). Resegmentation consists of the caudal half of one somite combining with the cranial half of the next somite to form definitive segments. The new segment thus extends from the upper margin of the intervertebral disc down to the lower endplate of the next caudal vertebra (see Fig. 3–6C). The previous segmental nerve lies in a intersegmental position opposite the intervertebral disc while the intersegmental vessel lies over the center of the vertebral centrum (body). The myotomes, which are segmental, associated with a somite now bridge two vertebral segments and thus provide intersegmental motion (see Fig. 3–6C).

The notochord is surrounded by the sclerotomal cells that are migrating to the midline. The cells in the area of the centrum disappear, either because of degeneration or migration to the future disc area. In this area the notochordal cells undergo mucoid degeneration, forming the gelatinous nucleus pulposus. The surrounding cells of the perichordal disc form the anulus fibrosus.

Simultaneous with the medial migration of the cells of the sclerotome, the lateral cells migrate dorsally and ventromedially (see Fig. 3–5B). The dorsal migration also consists of a dense and less dense area. The cells in the denser area are continuous with the perichordal disc and give rise to the neural arches, which migrate dorsally around the neural tube. The arches do not meet in the midline; local cells in the area develop into the neural arches and spinous processes. The two arches (laminae) unite first in the mid-lumbar area, union progressing cranially and

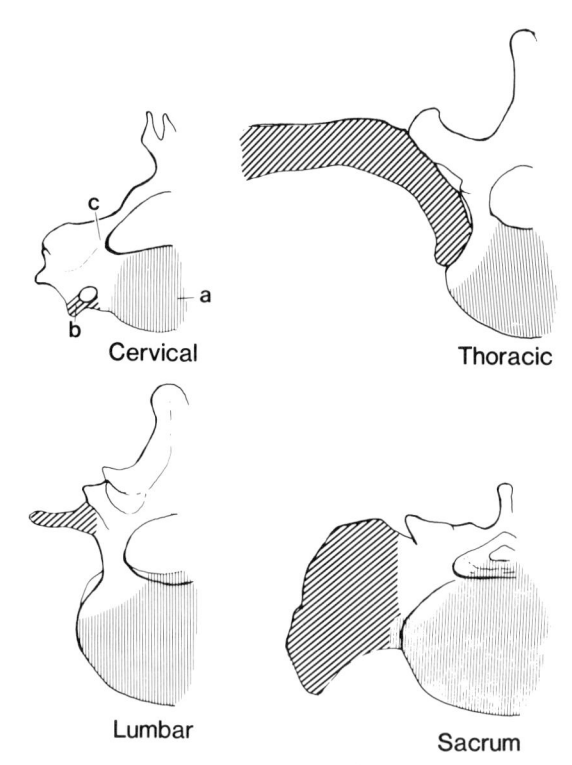

Figure 3–7. Embryonic contributions to the vertebrae in the cervical, thoracic, lumbar, and sacral areas. The centrum contribution is indicated by a, the rib rudiment contribution by b, and the vertebral arch contribution by c. (Reprinted with permission from Lonstein, J. E.: Spine embryology. In Winter, R. B. (ed.): Congenital Deformities of the Spine, New York, Thieme Stratton, 1983.)

caudally. The dorsal migration of the cells of the less dense area is restricted by the large spinal ganglia. A bridge of cells, the future articular processes, connects adjacent neural arches.

The cells migrating ventrally are continuous with the cellular perichordal disc, and migrate into the area between adjacent myotomes. This is the costal process of the vertebra. It forms the rib in the thoracic area; in the other areas of the spine, the costal process contributes different parts of the vertebra (Fig. 3–7).

The development of the occiput, axis, and atlas proceeds in a different manner. The first four somites, the occipital somites, fuse to form the basiocciput in which the rostral extension of the notochord terminates at the hypophyseal fossa. The cranial portion of the first cervical somite combines with the caudal portion of the fourth occipital somite to form the terminal portion of the basiocciput. The intervertebral disc at this level is represented by the apical portion of the dens and the adjacent apical and alar ligaments.

The caudal portion of the first cervical somite and the cranial part of the second cervical somite fuse and form the odontoid process, which is incorporated into the next caudal centrum—the vertebral body of C2. There is a dense band of tissue that extends ventrally around the developing vertebrae called the hypochordal bow. This is best developed at C1, where it gives rise to the anterior arch of the atlas. Caudally it gives rise to the thick portion of the anterior longitudinal ligament that overlies the anterior aspect of each vertebral body.

Chondrification starts at the cervicothoracic level and extends cranially and caudally. Two chondrification centers appear in the vertebral centrum, one on each side of the notochord; these two fuse and form a single chondrification center for the centrum. Two additional centers form on each side. A center appears in the neural arch, and chondrification extends into the transverse and articular processes. The other centers appear in the costal process, just lateral to the junction of centrum and neural arch (Fig. 3–8A). Chondrification extends from these centers, forming a solid cartilage model of the vertebra, with no line of demarcation between body, neural arch, or rib rudiments.

Ossification, except for the atlas, axis, and sacrum, follows a similar pattern, with primary and secondary ossification centers.[3, 28] Each vertebra has three primary and five secondary ossification centers. Ossification of the centrum starts from a single center, starting in the lower thoracic and upper lumbar areas, with ossification extending cranially and caudally, the cranial development being slower. There are two primary ossification centers in the vertebral arches, which appear first in the cervical area. Ossification progresses caudally (Fig. 3–8B) Ossification extends into the spinous, transverse, and articular processes. At birth, a typical vertebra consists of an ossified centrum and two ossified arches that have not fused in the cervical area. An area of cartilage, the neurocentral synchondrosis, lies between the ossified arch and the centrum (Fig. 3–8C) This area is anterior to the junction of body and pedicle, and thus the definitive vertebral body is formed by the centrum and adjacent part of the neural arch. Fusion of the ossified arches

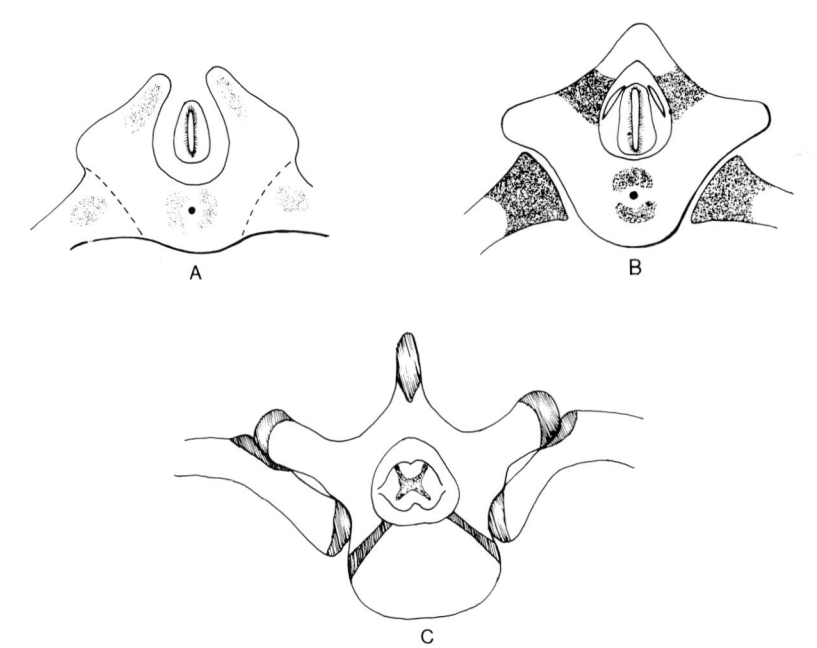

Figure 3–8. Chondification and ossification of a thoracic vertebra. *A,* There are four chondrification centers in the membranous anlage, the ribs being continuous with the vertebra in the cartilaginous stage. There are three primary ossification centers in the vertebra. *B,* The rib is now separate from the vertebra with a primary ossification center in the future head of the rib. *C,* Thoracic vertebra at birth. Note the area of cartilage (neurocentral junction) at the junction of the centrum and the vertebral arch contributions. (Reprinted with permission from Lonstein, J. E.: Spine embryology. *In* Winter, R. B. (ed.): Congenital Deformities of the Spine, New York, Thieme Stratton, 1983.)

and centrum starts in the upper lumbar area and continues cranially and caudally. This process starts in the late fetal period and continues after birth.

Ossification of the centrum leaves two cartilage plates at the superior and inferior margins of the vertebral body. These plates are the growth centers or physes of the vertebra, with typical enchondral ossification occurring. These plates are vascularized by vascular tufts originating in the bony centrum. With growth, a C-shaped ring apophysis develops around the ventral and lateral margins of the centrum disc interface. This ring apophysis anchors the disc to the body and remains cartilaginous until the second decade.

Secondary centers of ossification develop in the ring apophyses at the upper and lower surfaces of the vertebral body. These centers expand in late adolescence, with fusion of the ring apophysis to the adjacent vertebral end plate. In adolescence, in addition, three secondary centers develop in the neural arches—one for the tip of the spinous process and one for each transverse process.

In the thoracic area, a primary center of ossification appears in the cartilage anlage at the future angle of the rib at about the ninth week. Ossification proceeds proximally and distally, the distal end of the rib always remaining cartilaginous. With this ossification (which preceeds ossification of the centrum), a joint is formed between the head of the rib and the vertebra. Secondary centers of ossification in the rib appear in adolescence—two in the tubercle, and one in the head of the rib. In the cervical region, the costal process regresses and forms the anterior half of the foramen for the vertebral artery. In the lumbar area the costal process forms the majority of the transverse process. In both of these areas, the costal process has the potential to form an accessory rib. In the sacrum, the costal process forms the ala (see Fig. 3–7).

ATLAS AND AXIS

The atlas (C1) has two primary and one secondary center of ossification. The two primary centers correspond to the neural arch centers of a typical vertebra. The secondary center develops in the anterior arch; this center is the remnant of the hypochordal bar of lower vertebrates.

The axis (C2) has five primary and two secondary centers of ossification. These are the normal centers for the centrum and neural arches, plus two laterally placed centers for the odontoid, representing the original centrum of C1. These two odontoid centers fuse near the end of gestation; fusion

EMBRYOLOGY AND SPINE GROWTH

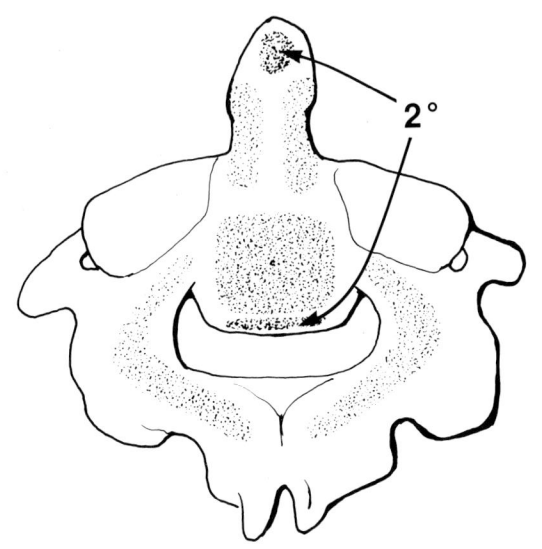

Figure 3–9. Ossification of the axis. There are five primary and two secondary centers of ossification. (Reprinted with permission from Lonstein, J. E.: Spine embryology. In Winter, R. B. (ed.): Congenital Deformities of the Spine, New York, Thieme Stratton, 1983.)

between the odontoid and centrum occurs in the second decade. A secondary ossification center appears in the tip of the odontoid in the second year. In addition an inferior ring apophysis forms as in the other vertebrae in adolescence (Fig. 3–9).

SACRUM

Ossification of the sacrum forms from primary centers in the sacral centra, with rudimentary physeal plates without ring apophyses forming. Each neural arch develops from two centers. In addition three centers develop laterally to produce the sacral alae. Fusion of all these elements starts in adolescence and is only completed in the third decade. The coccygeal vertebrae lack a neural arch, and thus there is only a primary ossification center for each vertebral centrum.

CONTROL OF DIFFERENTIATION[13, 14, 19, 25, 33, 37]

The formation of tissues and organs in the embryo is under local control; it is regulated by interactions among embryonic components. The large body of experimental work has been well summarized by Angevine.[2] Cells cause or induce a change in surrounding cells, controlling their differentiation. This induction, at a cellular level, is based on either a chemical interaction, an electrical charge, or a mechanism as yet undiscovered.

In very early embryonic development the bilaminar disc does not have any cranial or caudal orientation until the notochordal process develops. With the appearance of the notochordal process a longitudinal axis is established, with cranial and caudal differentiation. Once the true notochord forms, it plays an important role in neural tube and vertebral development.

The notochord induces the formation of the neural plate and is involved in folding of the plate and closure into the neural tube. It also appears to induce changes in the neural tube that cause differentiation into the spinal cord. Cranially, where there is no notochord, the neural tube enlarges and forms the brain. It appears that the neural tube causes thickening of the adjacent mesoderm, forming the paraxial mesoderm. Somite formation seems to be under the control of the spinal ganglia as they differentiate from the continuous neural crest.

Sclerotomal development appears to be under the control of the notochord and ventral neural tube. Dorsal migration of sclerotomal cells is related to the dorsal root ganglia, and closure of the neural arches depends on closure of the neural tube.

Recent experimental work of Rivard and others[31, 32, 41] on induction of congenital vertebral anomalies in mouse embryos, has introduced the concept of a notochord-sclerotome inductive complex. It appears from this work that the notochord controls the migration of sclerotomal cells and their further differentiation. Glycosaminoglycans (GAGs) were shown to be very important in the inductive complex. It is still unknown whether GAGs are the causal molecules in this inductive process or only the results, and thus a measure of the process.

When considering the etiology of congenital vertebral anomalies, the time of causation of the anomaly is often controversial. Rivard and coworkers have shown that anomalies occur at the stage of the membranous vertebral anlage. Once the membranous vertebral body is formed, the processes of chondrification and ossification are passive and occur in the cellular model already laid down.[31, 33, 48]

GROWTH OF THE SPINE[57]

A knowledge of spinal growth is essential in treating spinal deformities both nonoperatively and operatively. This includes a knowledge of total body growth, spinal growth, and the pubertal growth spurt.

As shown by Tanner, growth does *not* proceed in a uniform linear pattern.[42, 43, 44] There are two periods of rapid growth, the first from birth to age three and the second at the adolescent growth spurt. The intervening period from age three to the onset of puberty is a period of steady linear growth. Normal growth can be plotted two ways, by height attained or by growth velocity (e.g., cm. growth/year) (Fig. 3–10). The growth spurt of puberty is well seen in these charts.

Total body height is composed of several regions of growth—the head, spine, pelvis, and lower extremities. The head is relatively large at birth and subsequently grows the least. The lower limbs are relatively short at birth and grow the most. The spine is intermediate in growth between the two. An alternate height measurement is sitting height. This includes the head, pelvis, and spine. The head, as stated, grows negligibly, but pelvic height is appreciable. The sitting height chart (Fig. 3–11) has a similar shape to the total height attained chart (see Fig. 3–10A). Pelvic height is 18 to 20 per cent of sitting height. To approximate spine height, sitting heights in Figure 3–11 can be multiplied by .78 in girls and by .85 in boys.[43, 44]

Spine growth alone has been investigated by DiMeglio, who measured spine growth related to three age periods, birth to age five, age five to age ten, and age ten to age sixteen.[9] As most spinal deformities involve the thoracic and lumbar spines, he concentrated on these areas, which he calculated as 48 per cent of sitting height. He divided the growth into the thoracic segment, which accounted for 63 per cent of the T1 to S1 segment growth, and the lumbar spine, which accounted for 37 per cent of the growth. The growth velocities that are derived are shown in Table 3–1, and graphed in Figure 3–12. Although the total thoracic spine grows more than the lumbar spine, the growth per segment from birth to maturity in the thoracic spine is 1.1 cm. compared to 1.6 cm. in the lumbar spine.

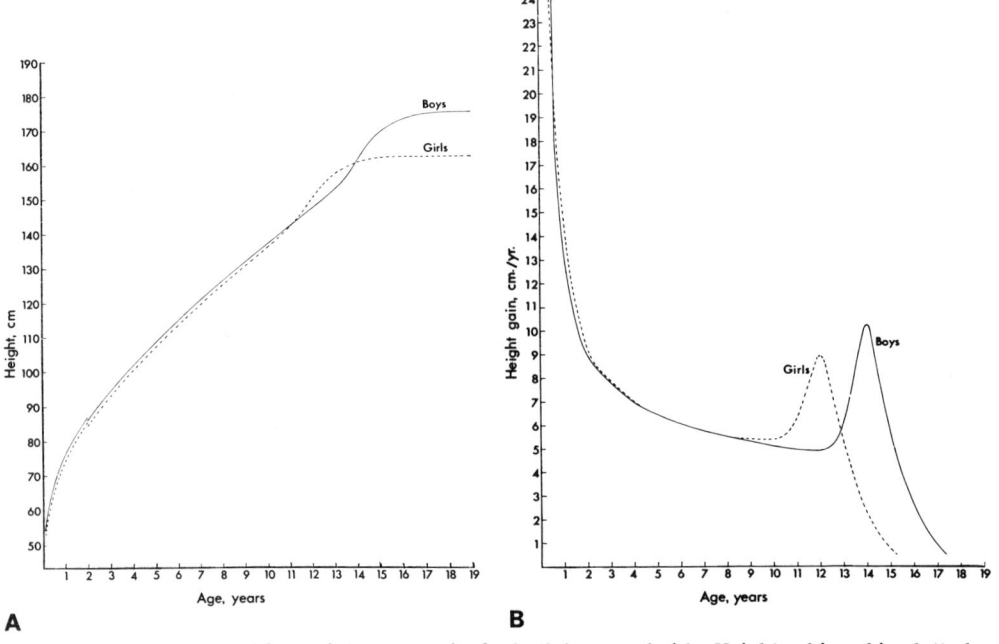

Figure 3–10. *A*, Growth charted from birth to maturity for both boys and girls. Height achieved is plotted against years. *B*, Growth velocity curves. This is the same material as in *A* but charted as growth gain (cm./y.) against years. (Reprinted with permission from Zorab, P. A. (ed.): Scoliosis and Growth. Proceedings of a Third Symposium held at the Institute of Diseases of the Chest, Brompton Hospital, London, on November 13, 1970. London, Churchill Livingstone, 1971.)

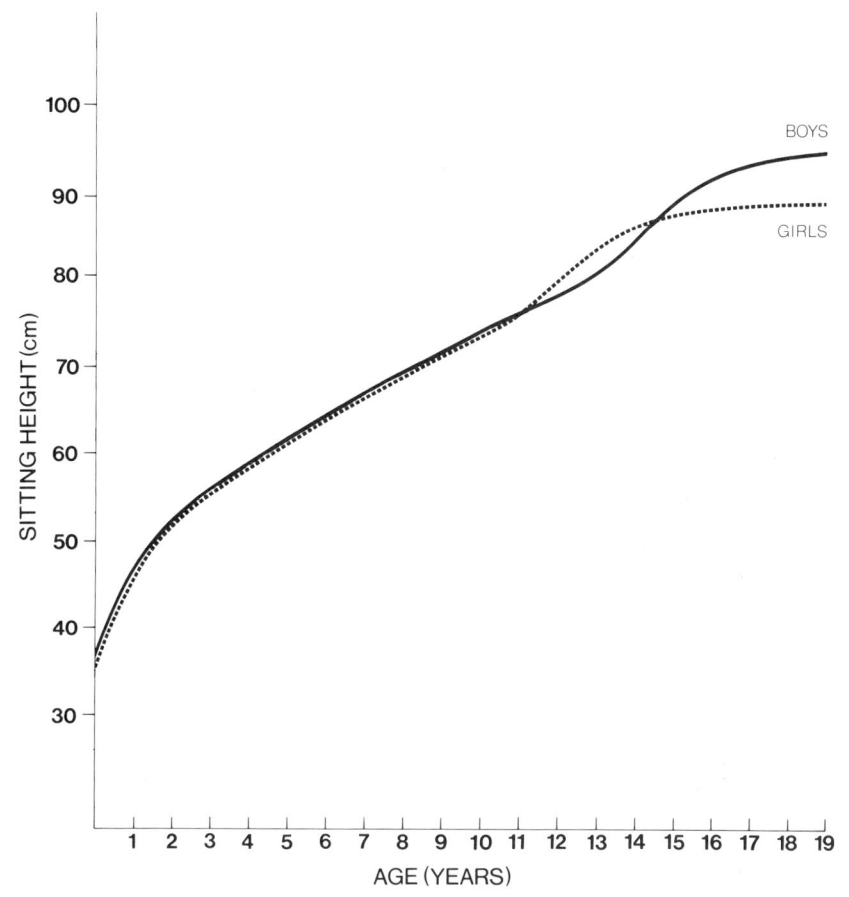

Figure 3–11. Growth charted from birth to maturity for boys and girls. Sitting height achieved is plotted against years.

The pubertal growth spurt is of particular interest. The relationship between scoliosis and growth was well shown by Duval-Beaupère.[11, 12] She studied 560 female scoliosis patients (500 paralytic and 60 idiopathic) with respect to curve increase and growth and compared their growth velocity to 53 normal girls. The curves increased at a steady rate until point P, then acceleration of increase occurred until point R, after which curve increase reached a plateau (Fig. 3–13). What are these points P and R?

Point P coincided with the onset of the growth spurt on the growth velocity graph. In girls this spurt coincides with the start of breast and pubic hair development at a Tanner stage 2 (chronological age 8 to 14 years). The point of maximum growth velocity (peak height velocity) occurs approximately one year later at a mean age of 12, the total growth spurt lasting 2.5 to 3 years. Menarche (and the appearance of axillary hair) occurs two years after the onset of pubic hair development (the onset of the growth spurt) at a mean age of 13 (Fig. 3–14).[6]

In boys the onset of the growth spurt occurs later, at a Tanner stage 3, after the development of pubic hair (chronological age 11 to 16 years). The point of maximum growth velocity occurs at a mean age of 14. Facial hair appearance occurs at the same

TABLE 3–1. Growth Velocity (cm./yr.)*

Spine Segment	Ages		
	Birth–5	*5–10*	*10–16*
T1-S1	2.2	0.9	1.8
T1-T12	1.4	0.6	1.2
L1-S1	0.8	0.3	0.6

*After DiMeglio, A.: Growth of the spine. Unpublished data.

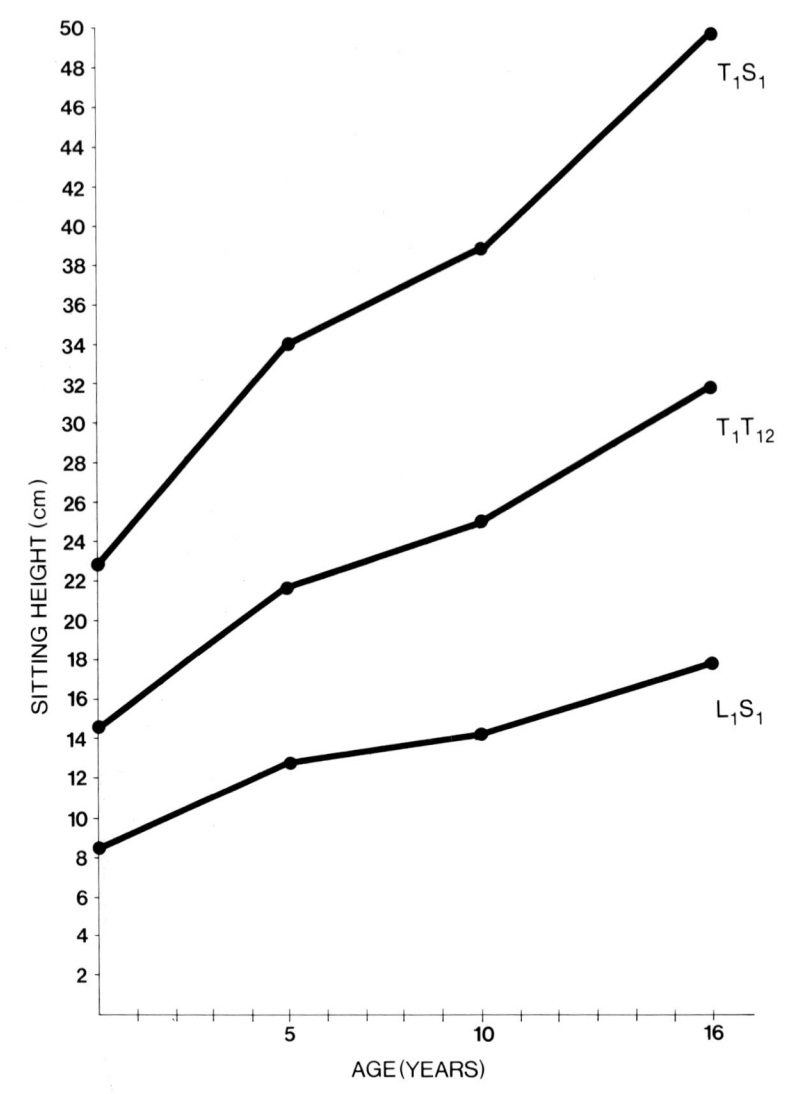

Figure 3–12. Graph showing sitting height increase in the total thoracic and lumbar spines (T1S1) and in the thoracic (T1T12) and lumbar (L1S1) segments. Sitting height is graphed against age. (Adapted from DiMeglio, A.: Growth of the Spine. Unpublished data.)

time as axillary hair, and extension of hair to the chin necessitating shaving occurs with maturity at Tanner stage 5 (Fig. 3–14). It must be remembered that *all* the ages stated above are average values, mainly based on Anglo-Saxon Caucasian or other uniform populations. It has been shown that the height increase in this population has been 10 centimeters from 1880 to 1961.[23] These studies cannot be applied directly to Negro, Oriental, Latin American, or American Indian populations. The maturity landmarks in general hold true for the onset of the growth spurt in these populations.

The point R on Duval-Beaupère's graph (see Fig. 3–13) corresponds to a Risser iliac apophysis sign of 4. Risser divided the ossification of the iliac crest into five grades. Grades 1 to 4 are excursion from 25 per cent to 100 per cent. Excursion usually starts at the anterior superior iliac spine. Grade 5 is fusion of the ossified crest to the ilium. The ossification appears at a mean chronological age of 13.3 to 14.3 years in girls and 14.3 to 15.4 years in boys.[56] The excursion averages 2 years, with a range from 7 months to 3.5 years. As stated, a Risser sign of 4 (complete excursion) correlates with cessation of spinal

EMBRYOLOGY AND SPINE GROWTH

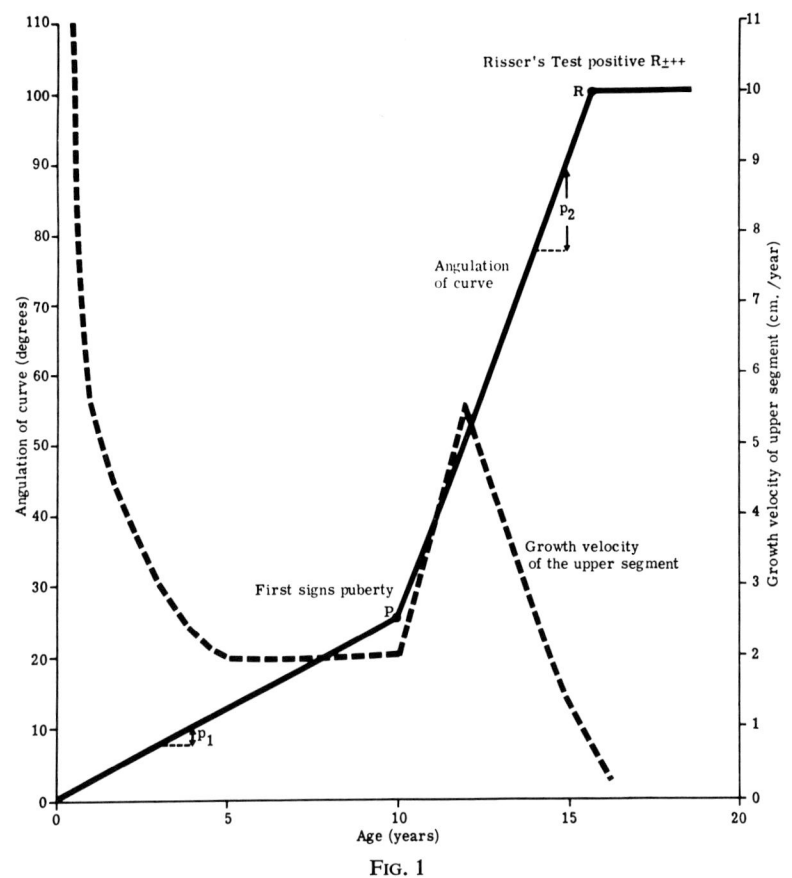

FIG. 1
Longitudinal study of the development of scoliosis compared with growth velocity.
Key: - - - - - - - - 53 Normal girls
——————— 500 Paralytic, 60 Idiopathic scoliotics

Figure 3–13. Growth velocity (*dotted line*) plotted against angulation of the curve in 560 patients followed by Duval-Deaupere. Note that the acceleration of curve increase occurs simultaneously with the accelerated growth. (Reprinted with permission from Zorab, P. A. (ed.): Scoliosis and Growth. Proceedings of a Third Symposium held at the Institute of Diseases of the Chest, Brompton Hospital, London, on November 13, 1970. London, Churchill Livingstone, 1971.)

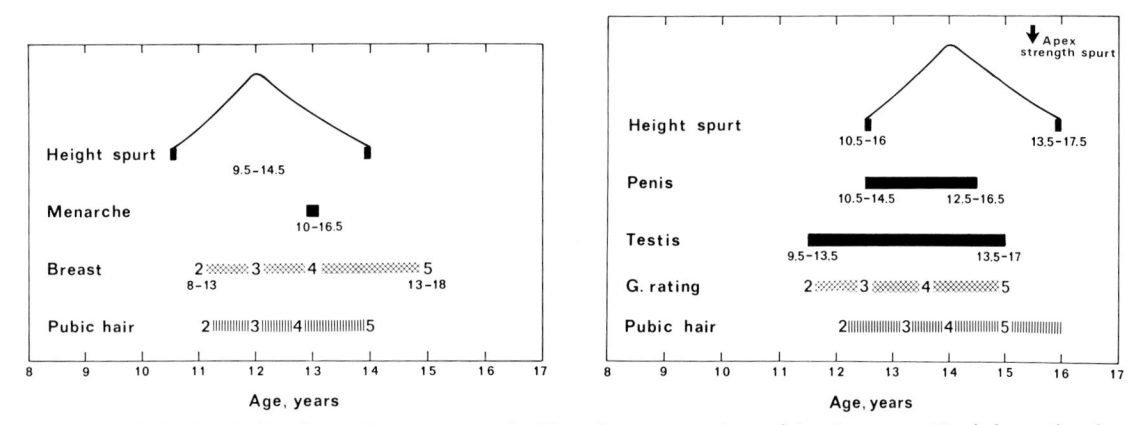

Figure 3–14. Peak velocity of growth as compared with various parameters of development. The information for girls is shown in the left chart; that for boys is in the right chart. (Reprinted with permission from Zorab, P. A. (ed.): Scoliosis and Growth. Proceedings of a Third Symposium held at the Institute of Diseases of the Chest, Brompton Hospital, London, on November 13, 1970. London, Churchill Livingstone, 1971.)

growth and a Risser 5 with cessation of height increase.[48]

The effects of spine fusion on spine growth have been a greatly debated topic for several years. Recently it has been proved that the fused area does not grow longitudinally.[7, 17, 18, 22, 24, 50] The question thus arises: What is the optimal time for a spine fusion in a child with a progressive deformity? It is obvious that there is *no* single best time for fusion.[26] The optimal time varies with the diagnosis and is individualized for each patient, and the factors influencing the decision will be discussed in subsequent chapters. Some general comments are important here.

The total height, as mentioned, is made up of an upper segment (head, spine, and pelvis) and a lower segment (lower extremities). The growth of the legs is linear, and thus they do not participate in the adolescent growth spurt.[1] This makes estimation of leg length relatively easy when planning surgery for leg length inequality.

From charts of sitting and standing heights it is possible to derive a ratio of sitting to standing height. This ratio is about 63 per cent at age 1, 60 per cent at age 2, and 52 per cent in boys and 53 per cent in girls at the end of growth.[30, 53]

Generally speaking, one's total height at the end of growth will be twice the height at age two. Thus an individual at age two who is 80 cm. in height has a sitting height of 48 cm. (60 per cent) and a lower segment of 32 cm. At the end of growth he will be 160 cm. tall, with each segment being 80 cm. Thus the lower segment has grown 48 cm. (80 − 32 cm.) and the sitting segment 32 cm. (80 − 48 cm.), the major height gain being in the lower segment.

An important question is: What is the growth loss due to fusion? This can be calculated as follows for six segments in the individual first discussed who was fused at age 2. At age 2, the six segments account for ⅛ of sitting height. If these six segments are fused at age 2, ⅛ of the amount of growth will be lost. As the sitting height increase is 32 cm., the loss is equal to 5.3 cm. Thus a six segment fusion at age 2 will result in a 5.3 cm. loss of height at the end of growth. Thus the final total height will be 154.7 cm. instead of 160 cm.—a loss of 3.3 per cent. This assumes that the area of the spine would have grown normally and that all areas of the spine grow equally. Usually we are dealing with pathologic spines, which do not have normal growth. Usually the amount of shortening caused by the fusion is less than the amount of shortening that would have been caused by the progressive curve.

An easier method of determining growth loss is possible by using tables for the calculation. Using Tanner tables, the amount of growth remaining can be calculated, as shown in Table 3–2.[43, 44] At the onset of puberty (age 10 in girls, age 12 in boys) 84 per cent of growth is completed. Two years later this figure is approximately 90 per cent. These figures have been represented in a chart showing growth remaining in sitting height for boys and girls (Fig. 3–15).[1] Using this graph and the number of vertebrae to be fused, the height loss from the fusion can be calculated. In the calculation it is approximated that the T1-S1 height is 50 per cent of the sitting height and that the thoracic segment makes up ⅔ of this height, and the lumbar segment the other ⅓. (Percentages are approximated from DiMeglio's statistics.[9])

Winter, using these growth tables calculated a formula for potential shortening caused by a spine fusion.[54] The formula is: cm. of shortening = 0.07 × number of segments fused × number of years of growth remaining. DiMeglio's figures are similar. From age 5 to 10 spine growth averages 0.05 cm./segment/year and after age 10 averages 0.11 cm./segment/year. These average formulae assume that all spinal segments have the same growth, but lumbar segments grow more than thoracic segments. There will be greater stunting if five lumbar vertebrae are fused than if five thoracic vertebrae are fused.

TABLE 3–2. Percentage of Growth Completed*

	Boys		Girls	
Age	Total Height (%)	Sitting Height (%)	Total Height (%)	Sitting Height (%)
2	49	57	53	58
5	62	67	66	70
10	77	80	84	84
12	83	84	92	91
14	90	91	97	97
16	97	97	—	—

*Percentage of total and sitting heights available in boys and girls at different ages. (Adapted from Tanner, J. M., and Whitehouse, R. H.: Clinical longitudinal standards for height, weight, height velocity, weight velocity and stages of puberty. Arch. Dis. Child., 51:170–179, 1976.)

EMBRYOLOGY AND SPINE GROWTH

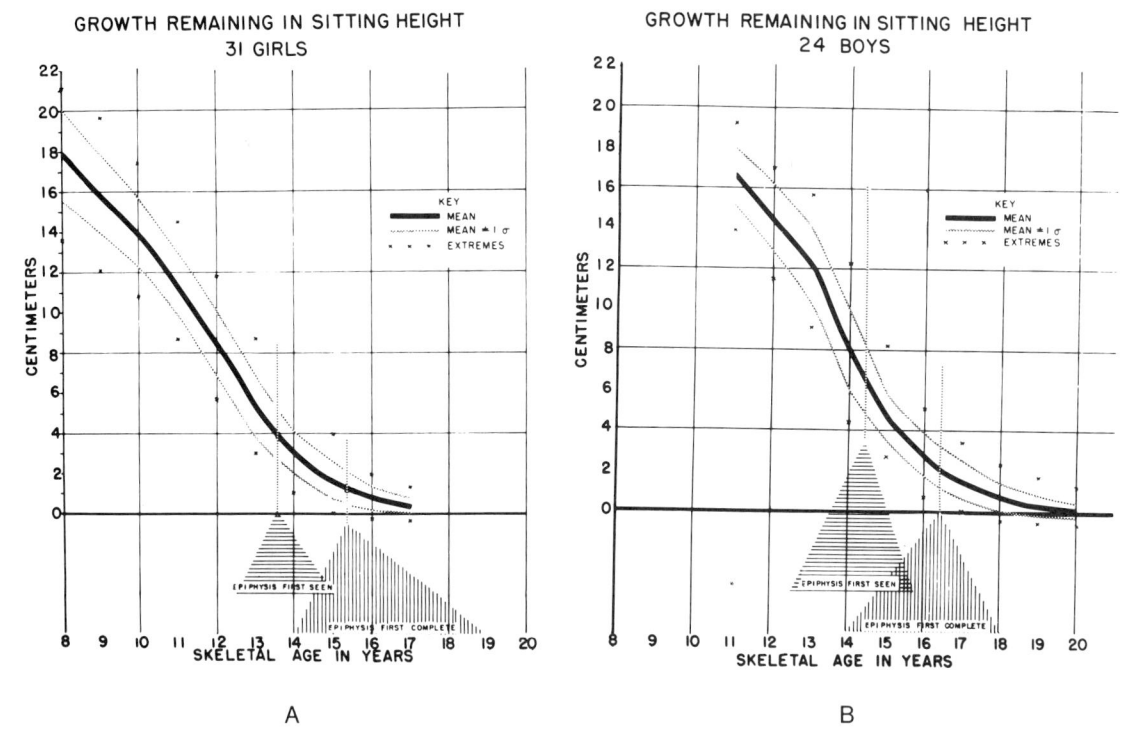

Figure 3–15. Growth remaining in the trunk at consecutive skeletal age levels. The curves indicate averages and ranges for residual growth after attainment of given age in girls (A) and boys (B). Superimposed on the graphs is the skeletal age of appearance and completion of the iliac epiphysis ossification. (Reprinted with permission from Anderson, J., et al.: Growth of the normal trunk in boys and girls during the second decade of life, related to age, maturity, and ossification of the iliac epiphyses. J. Bone Joint Surg., 47A:1561, 1965.)

References

1. Anderson, J., Hwang, S., and Green, W. T.: Growth of the normal trunk in boys and girls during the second decade of life, related to age, maturity, and ossification of the iliac epiphyses. J. Bone Joint Surg., 47A:1554–1564, 1965.
2. Angevine, J. B.: Clinically relevant embryology of the vertebral column and spinal cord. Clin. Neurosurg., 20:95–113, 1973.
3. Bagnali, K. M., Harris, P. F., and Jones, P. R. M.: A radiographic study of the human fetal spine. 2. The sequence of development of ossification centres in the vertebral column. J. Anat., 124:791–802, 1977.
4. Bardeen, C. R.: The development of the thoracic vertebrae in man. Am. J. Anat., 4:163–181, 1905.
5. Bick, M., Copel, J.W., and Spector, S.: Longitudinal growth of the human vertebra. J. Bone Joint Surg., 32A:803–814, 1950.
6. Calvo, J. J.: Observations on the growth of the female adolescent spine and its relation to scoliosis. Clin. Orthop., 10:40, 1957.
7. Crelin, E. S.: Development of the musculoskeletal system. Ciba Clin. Symp., 33:1, 1981.
8. Crowley, L. V.: An Introduction to Clinical Embryology. Chicago, Year Book Medical Publishers, 1974.
9. DiMeglio, A.: Growth of the spine. Unpublished data.
10. Dryden, R. J.: Duplication of the spinal cord: a discussion of the possible embryogenesis of diplomyelia. Develop. Med. Child. Neurol., 22:234–243, 1980.
11. Duval-Beaupère, G.: Les Reperes de maturation dans la surveillance des scoliosis. Rev. Chir. Orthop., 56:56, 1970.
12. Duval-Beaupère, G.: The growth of scoliosis patients. Hypothesis and preliminary study. Acta Orthop. Belg., 38:365–376, 1972.
13. Ehrenhaft, J. L.: Development of the vertebral column as related to certain congenital and pathological changes. Surg. Gynecol. Obstet., 76:282–292, 1943.
14. Fuller, D. J., and Duthie, R. B.: The Timed Appearance of Some Congenital Malformations and Orthopaedic Abnormalities. AAOS Instructional Course Lectures, Vol. 23. St. Louis, C. V. Mosby, pp. 53–61, 1974.
15. Gasser, R. F.: Atlas of Human Embryos. Hagerstown, Md., Harper & Row, 1975.
16. Greenhill, J. P.: Obstetrics. Philadelphia, W. B. Saunders, 1965.
17. Haas, S. L.: Influence of fusion of the spine on growth of the vertebrae. Arch. Surg., 41:607, 1940.
18. Johnson, J. T. H., and Southwick, W. O.: Bone growth after spine fusion. J. Bone Joint Surg., 42A:1396, 1960.
19. Karaharju, E. O.: Deformation of vertebrae in experimental scoliosis. The cause of bone adap-

tation and modeling in scoliosis with reference to the normal growth of the vertebra. Acta Orthop. Scand., Suppl. 105, 1967.
20. LaRocca, H.: Embryology of the musculoskeletal system. In Lovell, W. W., and Winter, R. B. (eds.): Pediatric Orthopaedics. 2nd ed. Philadelphia, J. B. Lippincott, p. 1–24, 1986.
21. Lemire, R. J., Loeser, J. D., Leech, R. W., and Alvord, E. C.: Normal and Abnormal Development of the Human Nervous System. Hagerstown, Md., Harper & Row, 1976.
22. Letts, R. M.., and Bobechko, W. P.: Fusion of the scoliotic spine in young children. Clin. Orthop., 101:136–145, 1974.
23. Meredith, H. V., and Knott, V. B.: Descriptive and comparative study of body size of United States schoolgirls. Growth, 26:283–295, 1962.
24. Moe, J. H., Sundberg, A. B., and Gustilo, R.: A clinical study of spine fusion in the growing child. J. Bone Joint Surg., 46B:784–785, 1964.
25. Nachlas, W., and Borden, J. N.: The cure of experimental scoliosis by directed growth control. J. Bone Joint Surg., 33A:24, 1951.
26. Nordwall, A.: Studies in idiopathic scoliosis. Acta Orthop. Scand., Suppl. 150, 1973.
27. Ogden, J. A.: The development and growth of the musculoskeletal system. In Albright, J. A., and Brand, R. A. (eds.): The Scientific Basis of Orthopaedics. New York, Appleton-Century-Crofts, pp. 41–103, 1979.
28. O'Rahilly, R., and Meyer, D. B.: Roentgenographic investigation of the human skeleton during early fetal life. Am. J. Roentgenol. 76:455–468, 1956.
29. Parke, W. W.: Development of the spine. In Rothman, R. H., and Simeone, F. A. (eds.): The Spine. Philadelphia, W. B. Saunders, pp. 1–18, 1975.
30. Risser, J., Agostini, S., Sampaio, J., and Garibaldi, C.: The sitting-standing height ratio as a method of evaluating early spine fusion in the growing child. Clin. Orthop., 24:7, 1973.
31. Rivard, C. H., LaBelle, P., Simoneau, R., et al.: La kyposie hypoborique moderee, comme inducteur des malformations vertebrales congenitales de l'embryon de souris. Chir. Pediatr., 23:65–67, 1982.
32. Rivard, C. H., Narbaitz, R., and Uithoff, H. K.: Congenital vertebral malformations. Orthop. Rev., 8:135–139, 1979.
33. Roaf, R.: Vertebral growth and its mechanical control. J. Bone Joint Surg., 42B:40, 1960.
34. Schmorl, G., and Junghans, H.: The Human Spine in Health and Disease. New York, Grune and Stratton, 1971.
35. Sensenig, E. C.: The origin of the vertebral column in the deermouse-*Permyseus Maniculatus Rufinus*. Anat. Rec., 86:123–141, 1943.
36. Sensenig, E. C.: Early development of the human vertebral column. Contrib. Embryol., 33:21–42, 1949.
37. Stillwell, D. L.: Structural deformities of vertebrae bone. Adaptation and modeling in experimental scoliosis and kyphosis. J. Bone Joint Surg., 44A:611, 1962.
38. Streeter, G. L.: Developmental horizons in human embryos. Description of age groups XI, 13 to 20 somites and age group XII, 21 to 29 somites. Contrib. Embryol., 30:211–245, 1942.
39. Streeter, G. L.: Factors involved in the formation of the filum terminale. Am. J. Anat., 25:1–11, 1919.
40. Streeter, G. L.: Developmental horizons in human embryos. Description of age groups XIX, XX, XXI, XXII, and XXIII. Contrib. Embryol., 230:167–169, 1942.
41. Tanaka, T., and Uhthoff, H. K.: The pathogenesis of congenital vertebral malformations. Acta Orthop. Scand., 52:413–425, 1981.
42. Tanner, J. M.: Growth at Adolescence, 2nd Ed. London, Blackwell, 1962.
43. Tanner, J. M., and Whitehouse, R. H.: Clinical longitudinal standards for height, weight, height velocity, weight velocity and stages of puberty. Arch. Dis. Child., 51:170–179, 1976.
44. Tanner, J. M., Whitehouse, R. H., and Takaisni, M.: Standards from birth to maturity for height, weight, height velocity and weight velocity: British children, 1965. Arch. Dis. Child., 41:454–471, 613–635, 1966.
45. Taylor, J. R.: Persistence of the notochordal canal in vertebrae. J. Anat., 111:211–217, 1972.
46. Taylor, J. R.: Growth of human intervertebral discs and vertebral bodies. J. Anat., 120:49–68, 1975.
47. Terver, S., Kleinman, R., and Bleck, E. E.: Growth landmarks and the evolution of scoliosis. Develop. Med. Child. Neurol., 22:675–684, 1980.
48. Tsou, P. M.: Embryology of congenital kyphosis. Clin. Orthop., 128:18–25, 1977.
49. Tuchmann-Duplessis, H., David, G., and Haegel, P.: Illustrated Human Embryology, Vol. 1: Embryogenesis. New York, Springer-Verlag, 1972.
50. Veliskakis, K., and Levine, D.: Effects of posterior spine fusion on vertebral growth in dogs. J. Bone Joint Surg., 48A:1367, 1967.
51. Warkany, J.: Congenital Malformations. Chicago, Year Book Medical Publishers, 1971.
52. Williams, L. W.: The later development of the notochord in mammals. Am. J. Anat., 8:251–291, 1908.
53. Willner, S.: The proportion of legs to trunk in girls with idiopathic structural scoliosis. Acta Orthop. Scand., 46:84, 1975.
54. Winter, R. W.: Scoliosis and spinal growth. Orthop. Rev., 6:17–20, 1977.
55. Wyburn, G. M.: Observations on the development of the human vertebral column. J. Anat., 78:94–104, 1944.
56. Zaouss, A. L., and James, J. I. P.: The iliac apophysis and the evolution of curves in scoliosis. J. Bone Joint Surg., 40B:442–453, 1958.
57. Zorab, P. A. (ed.): Scoliosis and Growth. Proceedings of a third symposium held at the Institute of Diseases of the Chest, Brompton Hospital, London, November 13, 1970. London, Churchill Livingstone, 1971.

4

CLASSIFICATION AND TERMINOLOGY

Robert B. Winter, M.D.

INTRODUCTION

In any scientific field, it is important to have a basic language. Without this language, we cannot communicate accurately. In the field of spinal deformity, a standardized language has developed, largely due to the efforts of the Scoliosis Research Society. Throughout this book we shall adhere to this standard terminology, deviating only when absolutely necessary.

CLASSIFICATION

There are three basic types of spine deformity: scoliosis, kyphosis, and lordosis. These may occur singly or in combination. Deformities are also classified according to magnitude, location, direction, and etiology. Thus, a patient may be described as having a "30 degree right thoracic scoliosis due to cerebral palsy." Another patient might be described as having a "110 degree thoracolumbar congenital kyphosis." With such verbal description, an accurate portrayal of the deformity can be communicated.

Classification of spinal deformities by etiology is presented below.

Structural Scoliosis

I. Idiopathic
   A. Infantile (0–3 years)
      1. Resolving
      2. Progressive
   B. Juvenile (3–10 years)
   C. Adolescent (> 10 years)

II. Neuromuscular
   A. Neuropathic
      1. Upper motor neuron
         a. Cerebral palsy
         b. Spinocerebellar degeneration
            i. Friedreich's disease
            ii. Charcot-Marie-Tooth disease
            iii. Roussy-Lévy disease
         c. Syringomyelia
         d. Spinal cord tumor
         e. Spinal cord trauma
         f. Other
      2. Lower motor neuron
         a. Poliomyelitis
         b. Other viral myelitides
         c. Traumatic
         d. Spinal muscular atrophy
            i. Werdnig-Hoffmann
            ii. Kugelberg-Welander
         e. Myelomeningocoele (paralytic)
      3. Dysautonomia (Riley-Day syndrome)
      4. Other
   B. Myopathic
      1. Arthrogryposis
      2. Muscular dystrophy
         a. Duchenne (pseudohypertrophic)
         b. Limb-girdle
         c. Facioscapulohumeral
      3. Fiber type disproportion
      4. Congenital hypotonia
      5. Myotonia dystrophica
      6. Other

III. Congenital
   A. Failure of formation

        1. Wedge vertebra
        2. Hemivertebra
     B. Failure of segmentation
        1. Unilateral (unsegmented bar)
        2. Bilateral
     C. Mixed
  IV. Neurofibromatosis
   V. Mesenchymal disorders
     A. Marfan's syndrome
     B. Ehlers-Danlos syndrome
     C. Others
  VI. Rheumatoid disease
 VII. Trauma
     A. Fracture
     B. Surgical
        1. Post-laminectomy
        2. Post-thoracoplasty
     C. Irradiation
VIII. Extraspinal contractures
     A. Post-empyema
     B. Post-burns
  IX. Osteochondrodystrophies
     A. Diastrophic dwarfism
     B. Mucopolysaccharidoses (e.g., Morquio's syndrome)
     C. Spondyloepiphyseal dysplasia
     D. Multiple epiphyseal dysplasia
     E. Other
   X. Infection of bone
     A. Acute
     B. Chronic
  XI. Metabolic disorders
     A. Rickets
     B. Osteogenesis imperfecta
     C. Homocystinuria
     D. Others
 XII. Related to lumbosacral joint
     A. Spondylolysis and spondylolisthesis
     B. Congenital anomalies of lumbosacral region
XIII. Tumors
     A. Vertebral column
        1. Osteoid osteoma
        2. Histiocytosis X
        3. Other
     B. Spinal cord (see neuromuscular)

Nonstructural Scoliosis

   I. Postural scoliosis
  II. Hysterical scoliosis
 III. Nerve root irritation
     A. Herniation of nucleus pulposus
     B. Tumors
  IV. Inflammatory (e.g., appendicitis)
   V. Related to leg length discrepancy
  VI. Related to contractures about the hip

Kyphosis

   I. Postural
  II. Scheuermann's disease
 III. Congenital
     A. Defect of formation
     B. Defect of segmentation
     C. Mixed
  IV. Neuromuscular
   V. Myelomeningocele
     A. Developmental (late paralytic)
     B. Congenital (present at birth)
  VI. Traumatic
     A. Due to bone and/or ligament damage without cord injury
     B. Due to bone and/or ligament damage with cord injury
 VII. Post-surgical
     A. Post-laminectomy
     B. Following excision of vertebral body
VIII. Post-irradiation
  IX. Metabolic
     A. Osteoporosis
        1. Senile
        2. Juvenile
     B. Osteomalacia
     C. Osteogenesis imperfecta
     D. Other
   X. Skeletal dysplasias
     A. Achondroplasia
     B. Mucopolysaccharidoses
     C. Neurofibromatosis
     D. Other
  XI. Collagen disease
     A. Marie-Strümpell disease
     B. Other
 XII. Tumor
     A. Benign
     B. Malignant
        1. Primary
        2. Metastatic
XIII. Inflammatory

Lordosis

   I. Postural
  II. Congenital
 III. Neuromuscular
  IV. Post-laminectomy
   V. Secondary to hip flexion contracture
  VI. Other

Classification by Anatomic Area

Curvatures are described by the area of the spine in which the *apex* of the curve is located.
  Cervical curve: apex between C1-C6.
  Cervicothoracic curve: apex at C7-T1.
  Thoracic curve: apex between T2-T11.
  Thoracolumbar curve: apex at T12-L1.
  Lumbar curve: apex between L2-L4.
  Lumbosacral curve: apex at L5-S1.

Note: The word dorsal is not used for curve description. Dorsal is the opposite of ventral. All vertebrae have a dorsal aspect (i.e., the laminae and spinous processes).

TERMINOLOGY

The terms listed in the preceding sections and the ones defined in the glossary that follows have been compiled by the terminology committee of the Scoliosis Research Society. This is an ongoing committee, and both the classification and terminology are revised periodically to incorporate advances in knowledge.

A GLOSSARY OF SCOLIOSIS TERMS

Adolescent Scoliosis. Spinal curvature presenting at or about the onset of puberty and before maturity.
Adult Scoliosis. Spinal curvature existing after skeletal maturity.
Angle of Thoracic Inclination. With the trunk flexed 90 degrees at the hips, the angle between the horizontal and a plane across the posterior rib cage at the greatest prominence of a rib hump.
Apical Vertebra. The most rotated vertebra in a curve; the most deviated vertebra from the vertical axis of the patient.
Body Alignment, Balance, Compensation. 1) The alignment of the midpoint of the occiput over the sacrum in the same vertical plane as the shoulders over hips. 2) In roentgenology, when the sum of the angular deviations of the spine in one direction is equal to that in the opposite direction.
Café-au-lait Spots. Light brown irregular areas of skin pigmentation. If sufficient in number and with smooth margins, they suggest neurofibromatosis.
Compensatory Curve. A curve, which can be structural, above or below a major curve that tends to maintain normal body alignment.
Congenital Scoliosis. Scoliosis due to congenitally anomalous vertebral development.
Curve Measurement. Cobb method: Select the upper and lower end vertebrae. Erect perpendiculars to their transverse axes. They intersect to form the angle of the curve. If the vertebral endplates are poorly visualized, a line through the bottom or top of the pedicles may be used.
Double Major Scoliosis. A scoliosis with two structural curves.
Double Thoracic Curves (Scoliosis). Two structural curves within the thoracic spine.
End Vertebra. 1) The most cephalad vertebra of a curve, whose superior surface tilts maximally toward the concavity of the curve. 2) The most caudad vertebra whose inferior surface tilts maximally toward the concavity of the curve.
Fractional Curve. A compensatory curve that is incomplete because it returns to the erect. Its only horizontal vertebra is its caudad or cephalad one.
Full Curve. A curve in which the only horizontal vertebra is at the apex.
Gibbus. A sharply angular kyphos.
Hyperkyphosis. A sagittal alignment of the thoracic spine in which there is more than the normal amount of kyphosis (a kyphos).
Hypokyphosis. A sagittal alignment of the thoracic spine in which there is less than the normal amount of kyphosis, but not so severe as to be truly lordotic.
Hysterical Scoliosis. A nonstructural deformity of the spine that develops as a manifestation of a conversion reaction.
Idiopathic Scoliosis. A structural spinal curvature for which no cause is established.
Iliac Epiphysis, Iliac Apophysis. The epiphysis along the wing of an ilium.
Inclinometer. An instrument used to measure the angle of thoracic inclination or rib hump.
Infantile Scoliosis. Spinal curvature developing during the first three years of life.
Juvenile Scoliosis. Spinal curvature developing between the skeletal age of three years and the onset of puberty.
Kyphos. A change in alignment of a segment of the spine in the sagittal plane that increases the posterior convex angulation; an abnormally increased kyphosis.

Kyphoscoliosis. A spine with scoliosis and a true hyperkyphosis. A rotatory deformity with only *apparent* kyphosis should not be described by this term.

Kyphosing Scoliosis. A scoliosis with marked rotation such that lateral bending of the rotated spine mimics kyphosis.

Lordoscoliosis. A scoliosis associated with an abnormal anterior angulation in the sagittal plane.

Major Curve. Term used to designate the largest structural curve.

Minor Curve. Term used to refer to the smallest curve, which is always more flexible than the major curve.

Nonstructural Curve. A curve that has no structural component and that corrects or overcorrects on recumbent side-bending roentgenograms.

Pelvic Obliquity. Deviation of the pelvis from the horizontal in the frontal plane. Fixed pelvic obliquities can be attributable to contractures either above or below the pelvis.

Primary Curve. The first or earliest of several curves to appear, if identifiable.

Rotational Prominence. In the forward bending position, the thoracic prominence on one side is usually due to vertebral rotation, causing rib prominence. In the lumbar spine, the prominence is usually due to rotation of the lumbar vertebrae.

Skeletal Age, Bone Age. The age obtained by comparing an anteroposterior roentgenogram of the left hand and wrist with the standards of the Gruelich and Pyle Atlas.

Structural Curve. A segment of the spine with a lateral curvature that lacks normal flexibility. Radiographically, it is identified the complete absence of a curve on a supine film or by the failure to demonstrate complete segmental mobility on supine side-bending films.

Vertebral Endplates. The superior and inferior plates of cortical bone of the vertebral body adjacent to the intervertebral disc.

Vertebral Growth Plate. The cartilaginous surface covering the top and bottom of a vertebral body, which is responsible for the linear growth of the vertebra.

Vertebral Ring Apophyses. The most reliable index of vertebral immaturity, seen best in lateral roentgenograms or in the lumbar region in side-bending anteroposterior views.

In the glossary, several terms are used to describe curves. These terms have often been used interchangeably. It seems desirable to comment further at this time in order to avoid confusion for the reader later in this book. The terms causing confusion are: primary curve, secondary curve, compensatory curve, major curve, minor curve, structural curve, and nonstructural curve.

A structural curve is "a segment of the spine with a lateral curvature having lack of normal flexibility. Radiographically, it is identified in supine bending films by the failure to correct." The key phrase here is "lack of normal flexibility." There is a segment or area of the spine that does not have normal mobility. By definition, then, a nonstructural curve has normal flexibility. A good example of a nonstructural curve is that seen in the lumbar spine of a patient with inequality of leg length. When the leg length is corrected by a lift, the curve disappears. In the sitting or supine position, the curve disappears. On bending films, the spine bends equally to the right and left, with no area of fixation. Leg length inequality, even if existing for many years, does not cause a structural curve.

A compensatory curve is "a curve above or below a major curve that tends to maintain normal body alignment. It may be structural or nonstructural." When a patient has a single structural curve, regardless of etiology, there must be a curve above and/or below that structural curve in order to keep the head above the pelvis. At first, the compensatory curve is fully flexible and thus nonstructural. However, over the course of time, because it is constantly present, the tissues develop "fixation" in this curved position, and the compensatory curve becomes structural. Even though it develops structural qualities, it is still a compensatory curve.

The term secondary curve is synonymous with compensatory curve. It is used in conjunction with the term primary curve, which describes the original structural curve of the patient.

A primary curve is "the first or earliest of several curves to appear, if identifiable." Often the patient comes to the physician at the age of 16 with two structural curves, both quite significant, both about equal in magnitude, and both having structural qualities. It can be quite difficult or even impossible to know whether the patient has one primary curve and one secondary curve with highly structural qualities or two primary curves.

CLASSIFICATION AND TERMINOLOGY

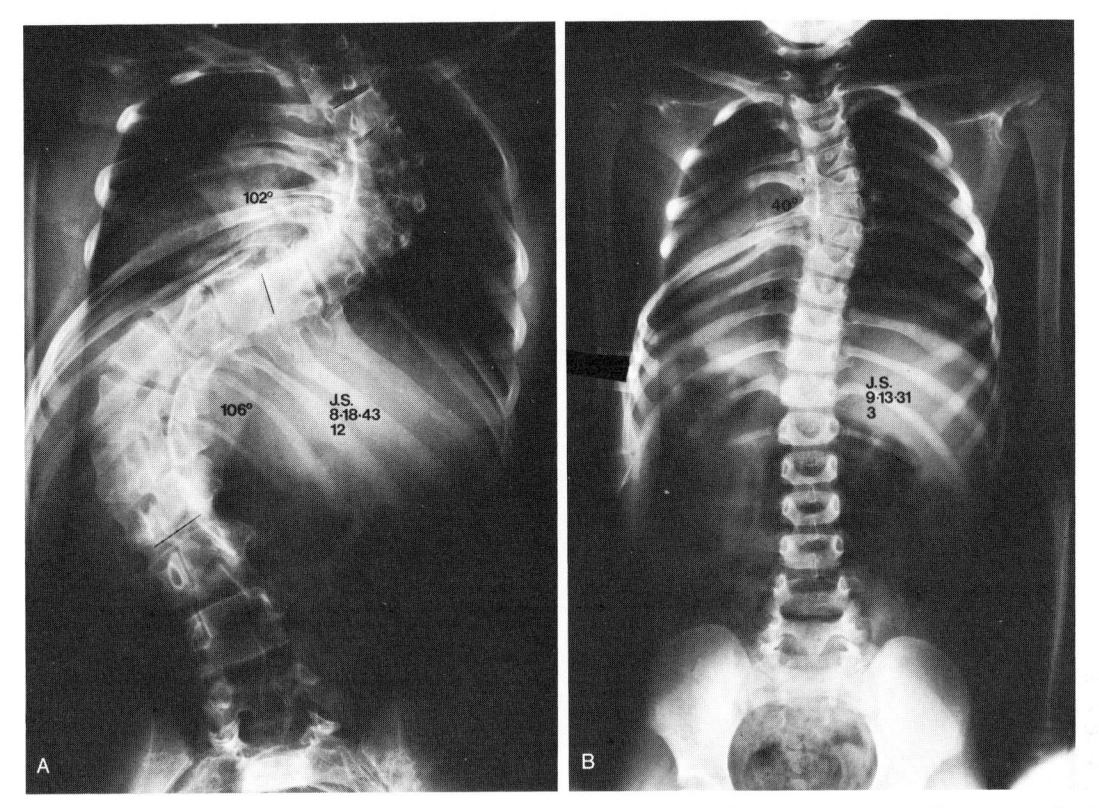

Figure 4–1. *A*, This patient came to us with a double structural curve problem, both curves of large magnitude and quite structural. Is this a *"double primary pattern"*? *B*, Radiographs were found that had been taken 9 years previously at age 3. It was obvious that the thoracic curve was "primary" and the lumbar curve "secondary," but by age 12, the patient had a "double major" curve problem.

Double or even triple primary curves are well-recognized entities.

Because of the frequent impossibility of defining a "primary" curve, many physicians have abandoned that term and use instead the term major curve. A major curve is "the larger curve, always structural," as distinguished from a minor curve, which is "the lesser curve, which may be partially structural or nonstructural."

Thus, the patient presenting with two curves, both large and both structural, might be said to have a "double primary curve pattern" by one physician and a "double major curve pattern" by another. Neither physician is necessarily incorrect.

In this book, we will use the terms primary, compensatory, and major. We will not use the terms secondary or minor. We will use the term primary only when we know for sure that a curve was indeed the first curve. Figure 4–1 shows a patient who came to us with double structural curve problem, both curves of large magnitude and quite structural. Is this a double primary pattern?

When radiographs were found that had been taken nine years previously (at age 3), it was obvious that the thoracic curve was "primary" and the lumbar curve "secondary"; but by age 12, the patient had a "double major" curve problem.

Bibliography

Cobb, J. R.: Outline for the Study of Scoliosis. Instructional Course Lectures, The American Academy of Orthopaedic Surgeons. Ann Arbor, J. W. Edwards, 5:261, 1948.

Goldstein, L. A., and Waugh, T. R.: Classification and terminology of scoliosis, Clin. Orthop., 93:10–22, 1973.

McAlister, W. H., and Shackelford, G. D.: Classification of spinal curvatures. Radiol. Clin. North Am., 13:93–112, 1975.

Terminology Committee, Scoliosis Research Society: A glossary of scoliosis terms. Spine, 1:57–58, 1976.

5

PATIENT EVALUATION

John E. Lonstein, M.D.

When a patient with a spine deformity is first seen by an orthopaedic surgeon, accurate evaluation and documentation of all areas related to the deformity are important. With the aid of a complete history and physical examination, plus appropriate radiographs, the correct diagnosis as to the etiology of the deformity and any co-existing complications of the deformity (e.g., deficient cardiopulmonary function, or neurological symptoms) can be determined. An important part of the evaluation process is the complete and accurate documentation of all findings.

HISTORY[26]

The first part of patient evaluation is a complete history. This includes information regarding the spinal deformity, its effects on the patient, the patient's general condition and health, a family history, and the patient's age and physiologic maturity. The patient's presenting complaint—deformity, pain, neurologic symptoms, cardiopulmonary problems, or functional complications—is important.

Spine Deformity

The examining physician inquires into the onset of the deformity, its progression or subsequent treatment, and the effects of the deformity on the patient. Information as to how the deformity was first noted (i.e., school screening, routine medical physical examination by the family physician, a friend or family member or when fitting clothes) is obtained. Has there been any increase in the size of deformity since it was intially noted? How has this manifested—increased rotational prominence, waistline change, or loss of height in an adult?

Has there been any previous treatment? Was it operative or nonoperative? Was a brace fitted? If so, what kind, and by whom? Was it worn? How long? Full time or part time? How compliant was the patient to the prescribed wearing regimen? If surgery was performed previously, what procedure or procedures were done and by whom? What was the postoperative course and the length of immobilization? When previous treatment has been performed, the physician and hospital records, including operative reports and radiographs, are essential for full patient evaluation.

When pain accompanies the deformity or is the presenting complaint, a full evaluation of the pain is performed. In children and adolescents spinal deformities are not complicated by pain. Thus with pain and a deformity at this age, the same condition is causing both the pain and the deformity (e.g., Scheuermann's disease, spondylolisthesis, and bone or cord tumors). Evaluation must be directed to the etiology of the pain and deformity. Adults, on the other hand, have a high incidence of backpain without the presence of spinal deformity, and, in addition, pain can result from the deformity. Pain without spinal deformity is more common in the lumbosacral area, and pain accompanied by deformity is common in the curve area. The location and radiation of the pain are important. Full details regarding the occurrence of and factors affecting the pain are obtained. Since pain cannot be measured objectively, its effects on the patient are documented. Is the pain increasing? Are analgesics being taken? If so, what analgesic, how much, and how often? How has the pain affected everyday activities, recreational activities, sport? In neuromuscular deformities the effects on the patient's walking, sitting, or performance of everyday functional activities are important.

A history of other complications of the deformity is sought. Is there any history of cardiopulmonary decompensation? Are there any neurologic symptoms? These symptoms could be either associated with the cause of the deformity or a result and complication of the deformity, or they could be entirely separate from the deformity.

General Health

The general health of the patient is evaluated. Have there been any previous illnesses, operations, or injuries? In young children a perinatal and postnatal history is important. This includes the health of the mother during pregnancy, drugs taken during pregnancy, and any problems or complications in the perinatal or postnatal periods. Development milestones during the infantile and juvenile years are documented.

Family History

A family history concerning any other family members with a spinal deformity is obtained. The age of all siblings is documented, and if possible, they are also examined with the forward bending test (see page 50). In familial nueromuscular conditions a family history is important in helping to establish the diagnosis.

Maturity[3, 34, 35]

In adolescence assessment of maturity is important. The important time is the period of rapid growth. Signs of puberty, especially pubic hair development, is important. In girls, onset of pubic hair and breast development occurs just before or at the onset of the rapid growth spurt. In boys, pubic hair development occurs before the onset of the rapid growth spurt. Menarche indicates a point at which the growth is decreasing and occurs approximately 2 to 2½ years later. Axillary hair development starts at this time of decreasing growth velocity in both boys and girls. The above information is used in conjunction with chronological and bone age in decision making.

PHYSICAL EXAMINATION[4, 9]

In the physical examination of the patient three areas are important—the deformity, its etiology, and its complications. The patient should be examined undraped, except for a small pair of underpants (Fig. 5–1A). In females, it is permissible to use an examination gown open at the back, but the chest must be examined at some stage during the evaluation. The overall body habitus and facies are examined. The sitting and standing heights, arm span, and weight are measured and recorded. The general examination will, in some cases, focus subsequent evaluation to definite areas: in dwarfs, examine the cornea for clouding (mucopolysaccharidoses); the palate for high arching (Marfan's syndrome); the ear for deformity (congenital anomalies); and the neck for webbing (Turner's syndrome).

The back is observed. Are there obvious asymmetries in the shoulders, scapulae, waistline, or thoracopelvic relationship (Fig. 5–1A)? Is there an obvious deformity—scoliosis, kyphosis, or lordosis? The balance of the thorax over the pelvis is assessed with the plumbline, a plumb bob being used for this. The plumb bob string is held over the prominent spinous process (vertebra prominens) of C7, and a vertical line obtained with the string and weight. The distance from this vertical to the gluteal cleft is noted and measured in centimeters; the deviation is to the left or right of the gluteal cleft (Fig. 5–1B). When there is a cervical or cervicothoracic component of the scoliosis, the plumbline from the occipital protuberance or inion is also measured and recorded.

The shoulder levels are taken from the acromioclavicular joints, measured either anteriorly or posteriorly. The height of the high shoulder compared to that of the low shoulder is measured and recorded (Fig. 5–2). The trapezius neckline is noted. The pelvic level is evaluated. The iliac crests are difficult to feel and to compare with regard to height. The levels of the anterior superior or posterior superior iliac spines are compared; the difference is approximated in centimeters.

The range of motion of the spine is noted in flexion, extension, and side bending. Side

PATIENT EVALUATION

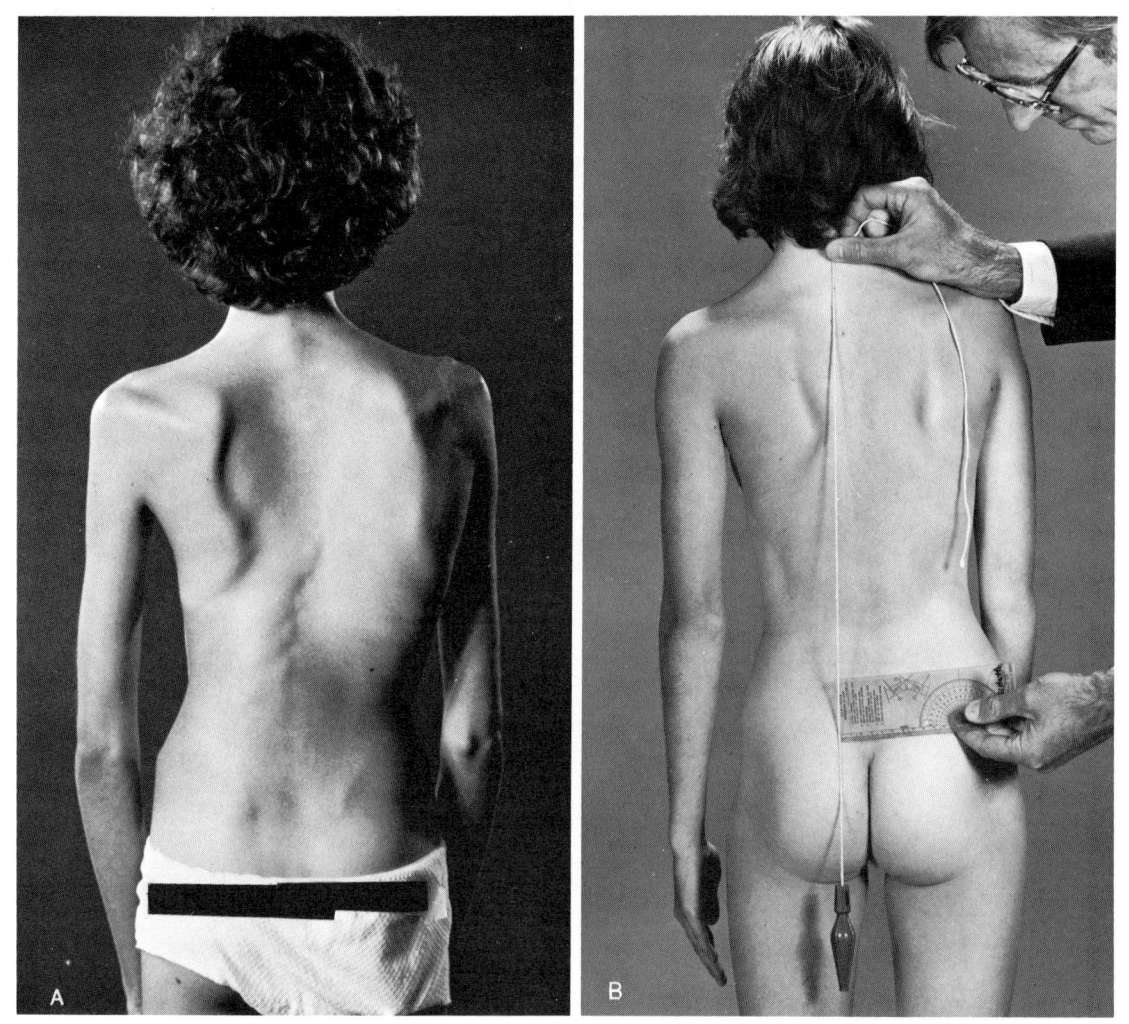

Figure 5–1. *A*, A patient viewed from the back to evaluate the spine deformity. A typical right thoracic curve is shown. The left shoulder is lower, and the right scapula is more prominent. There is a shift of the thorax to the right with a decreased distance between the right arm and the thorax. The left iliac crest appears higher owing to the shift of the thorax to the right and the decrease in the right waistline. *B*, Plumbline dropped from the C7 spinous process (vertebra prominens) measures the decompensation of the upper thorax over the pelvis. The distance from the plumbline to the gluteal cleft is measured in centimeters and is recorded, noting the direction of the deviation (e.g., a 3 centimeter deviation to the left). Where there is a cervical or cervicothoracic curve, the plumb should fall from the occipital protuberance (inion).

Figure 5–2. Measurement of shoulder level using a level. Note the difference in the trapezius neck line and the elevation of the left shoulder with a high left thoracic curve. The level is made horizontal and placed at the level of the acromioclavicular joint on the right. The vertical distance from the level to the high left shoulder is measured in centimeters. An elevation of the left shoulder of 4 centimeters is shown.

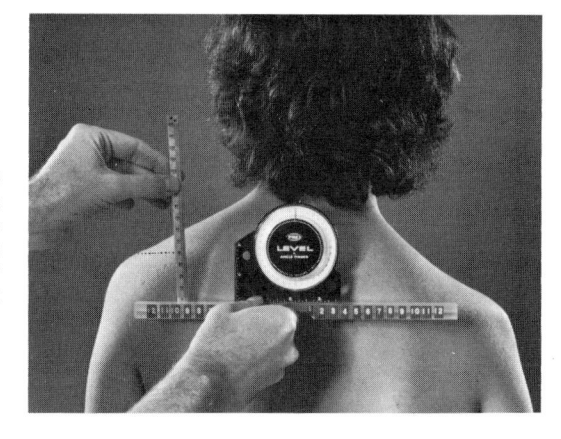

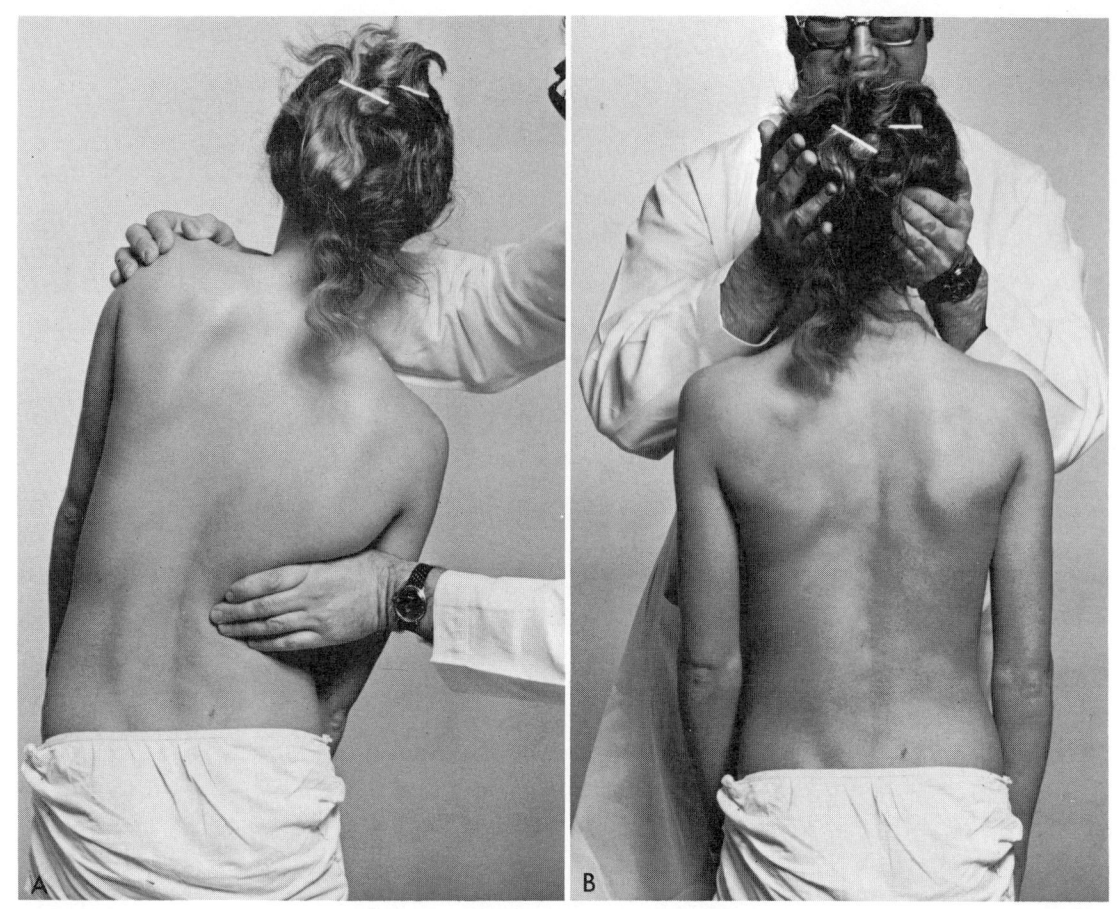

Figure 5–3. Evaluation of spine flexibility. *A*, Side bending to the right aided by the examiner demonstrates the flexibility of the right thoracic curve. *B*, In patients with severe or paralytic deformities, the flexibility is tested by grasping the head in the area of the mastoid processes and lifting the patient.

bending, aided by the examiner, will give an assessment of the flexibility of the scoliosis (Fig. 5–3). In paralytic conditions or in patients with severe deformities a traction evaluation is used. The head is grasped in the area of the mastoid processes, with the patient sitting or standing, and traction is applied by lifting the patient. This demonstrates the flexibility of the curve and whether the thorax compensates over the pelvis in a decompensated curve (Fig. 5–3*B*).

When pain is present, noting the exact location of the pain is essential. This is determined in the standing and prone positions with careful palpation. In addition, restriction of spine motion due to the pain is noted.

The patient is viewed from the side. The sagittal contours of the spine are observed, and areas of increased or decreased sagittal curvature are noted (e.g., areas of hyper- or hypokyphosis or hyper- or hypolordosis).

The patient's posture is also observed. Is there a tilting forward of the trunk? Is the trunk shifted forwards on the pelvis? Is there hip and knee flexion in the relaxed standing posture? Are there subcostal skin folds, indicating a shortened anterior abdominal wall?

The forward bending test is performed. The patient stands with feet together and knees straight and bends forwards at the waist. The arms are dependent with hands together, palms and fingers in opposition (Fig. 5–4*A*). If a knee is flexed, or the hands are not opposed, or the hands are resting on the thighs, the symmetry of the back is impossible to evaluate. The patient is viewed from head on; the examiner compares the sides of the back for symmetry. The two sides, from the upper thoracic to the lumbosacral areas, are compared to see whether one side is higher than the other (Fig. 5–4*B*).

PATIENT EVALUATION 51

Any asymmetry is measured with a spirit level or with a scoliometer. The level is placed over the area or areas of maximum asymmetry (or prominence), with the center of the spirit level placed over the palpable spinous process. The level is made horizontal. The distance from the zero mark (over the palpable spinous process) to the highest point of the prominence is measured. The same distance is taken from the zero mark to the "valley" on the opposite side, and the perpendicular distance of the valley from the spirit level is measured (Fig. 5–4C). Each prominence present is evaluated in a similar manner; the amount of the prominence and its site (high thoracic, thoracic, thoracolumbar, or lumbar) is noted and recorded. The shape of the prominence, e.g., sharp or gentle, is also noted.

During the forward bending test, the man-

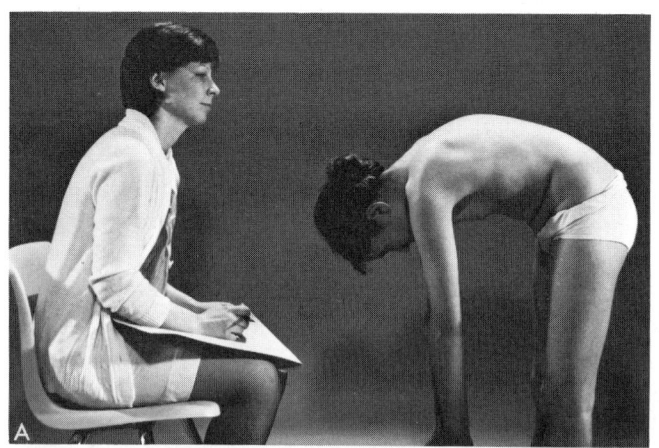

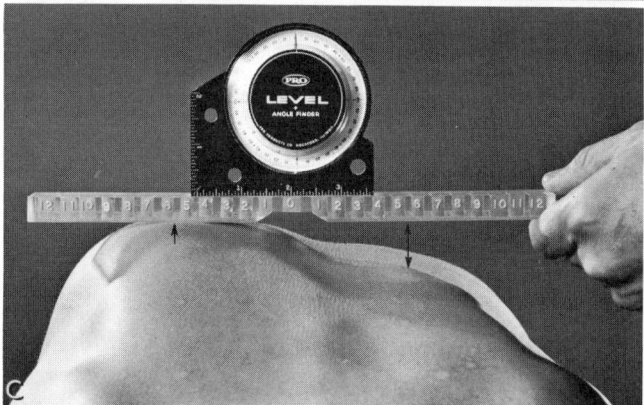

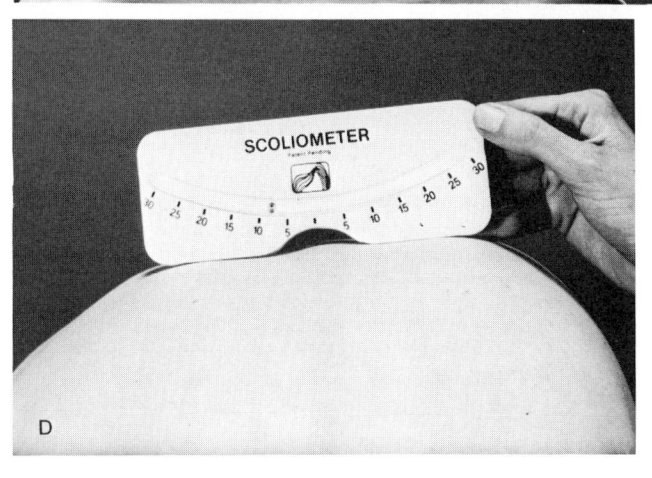

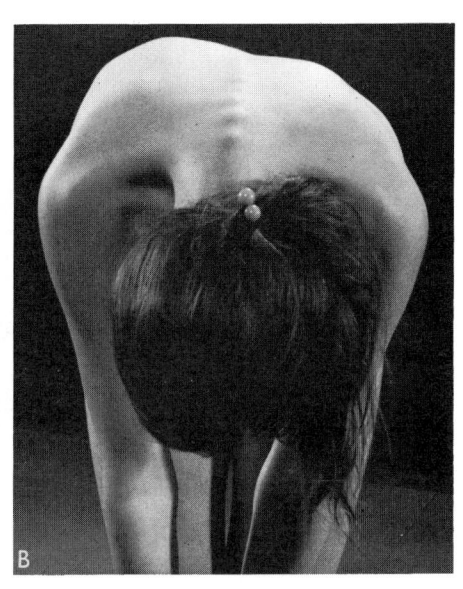

Figure 5–4. Forward bending test. A, The patient stands with feet together, knees straight, and bends at the waist. The arms are dependent and held with fingers and palms opposed. The examiner looks down the back to view the thoracic and lumbar areas. (From Lonstein, J. E., et al.: School screening for early detection of spine deformities. Minn. Med., 59:51, 1976; reprinted with permission.) B, The two sides are compared. Note the presence of a right thoracic prominence. C, Measurement of the prominence. The spirit level is positioned with the zero mark over the palpable spinous process in the area of maximal prominence. The level is made horizontal and the distance to the apex of the deformity (5 to 6 centimeters) noted. The perpendicular distance from the level to the valley is measured at the same distance from the midline. A 2.4 centimeter right thoracic prominence is shown. D, Use of the scoliometer to measure the rotational prominence.

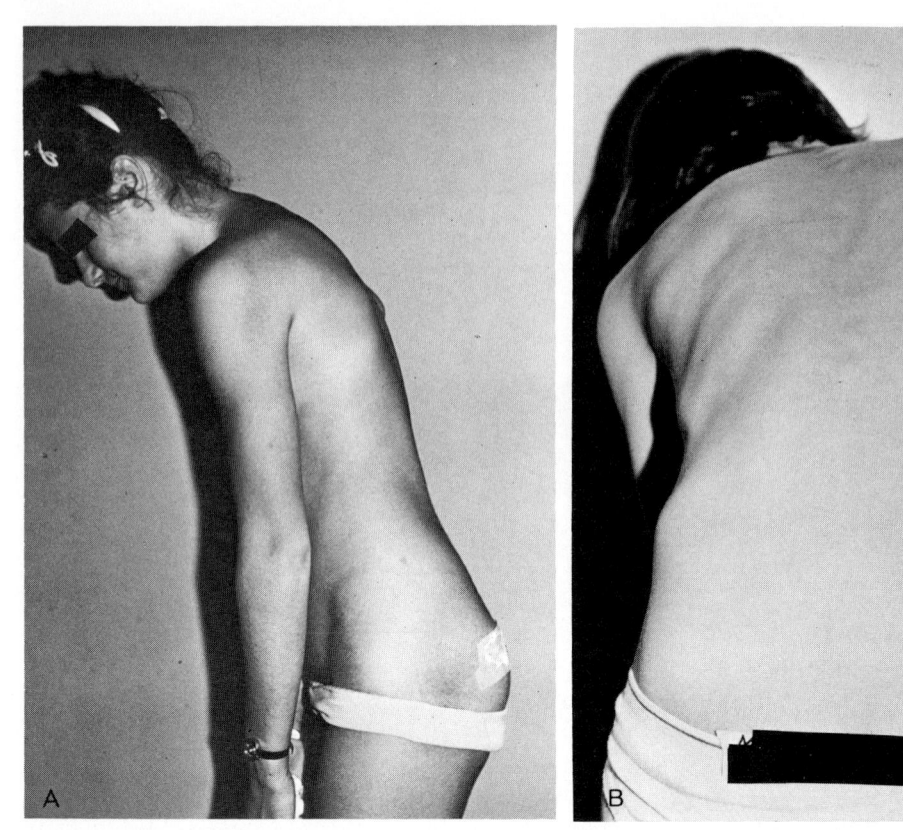

Figure 5–5. *A*, Severe restriction of forward bending due to tight hamstrings is seen in this patient with spondylolisthesis. *B*, A boy with back pain shows marked trunk deviation to the left on forward bending, indicating a "spasm" curve. Further evaluation including CT scan and myelography is indicated to exclude a bone tumor, cord tumor, or ruptured lumbar disc.

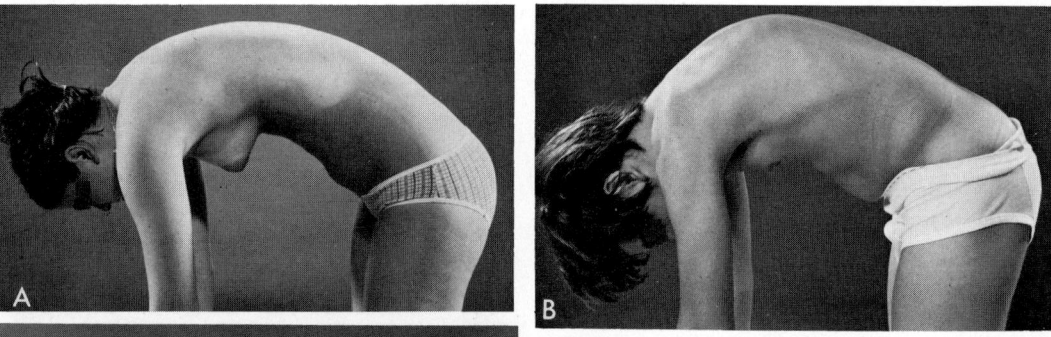

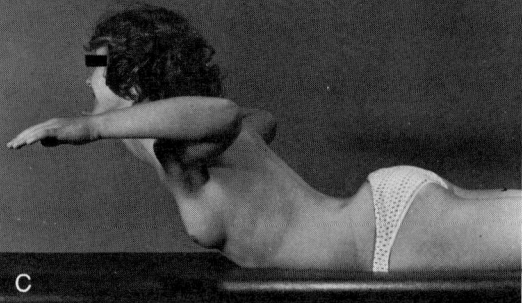

Figure 5–6. *A* and *B*, Side view in forward bending position to view kyphosis. *A*, Normal thoracic roundness is demonstrated with a gentle curve to the whole spine. *B*, An area of increased bending is seen in the thoracic spine, indicating structural changes—Scheuermann's disease, in this example. *C*, Prone hyperextension test to demonstrate the flexibility of hyperkyphosis.

ner in which the patient bends forwards is important. With tight hamstrings or hamstring spasm (in spondylolisthesis) there is an inability to bend forwards (Fig. 5–5). In some cases, the patient bends forwards and consistently deviates to one side. This indicates an irritative lesion (spinal cord tumor, osteoid osteoma, or herniated disc), and in these cases a full neurologic evaluation and appropriate special radiographs are necessary (bone scan, myelogram, CT scan).

With the forward bending test, the back is also viewed from the side. The contour of the back is noted; is it a gentle contour or is there an area of sharp angulation, indicating an area of structural change (Fig. 5–6). The forward bending test also demonstrates the flexibility of lordosis, which is also shown when the patient bends in a knee-chest position. The flexibility of kyphosis is shown clinically by a prone hyperextension evaluation (Fig. 5–6C).

The skin of the back is inspected for hair patches, skin dimples, hyperpigmentation, or midline tumors, which suggest spinal dysraphism. The skin is examined for the presence of café-au-lait hyperpigmentation or subcutaneous nodules, which indicate neurofibromatosis (Fig. 5–7A). In myelodysplasia, the presence of a sac, scars from previous

Figure 5–7. Physical examination. *A*, Skin examination shows numerous café-au-lait areas of pigmentation, indicating neurofibromatosis. *B*, Lumbar hair patch seen in a case of diastematomyelia. In this condition, skin dimples, midline pigmentation, and a lipoma are also seen. *C*, Joint flexibility evaluation using thumb to wrist approximation. A case of extreme flexibility is shown. (Reprinted with permission from Rothman, R. H., and Simeone, F. A.: The Spine, Philadelphia, W. B. Saunders Co.)

Illustration continued on following page

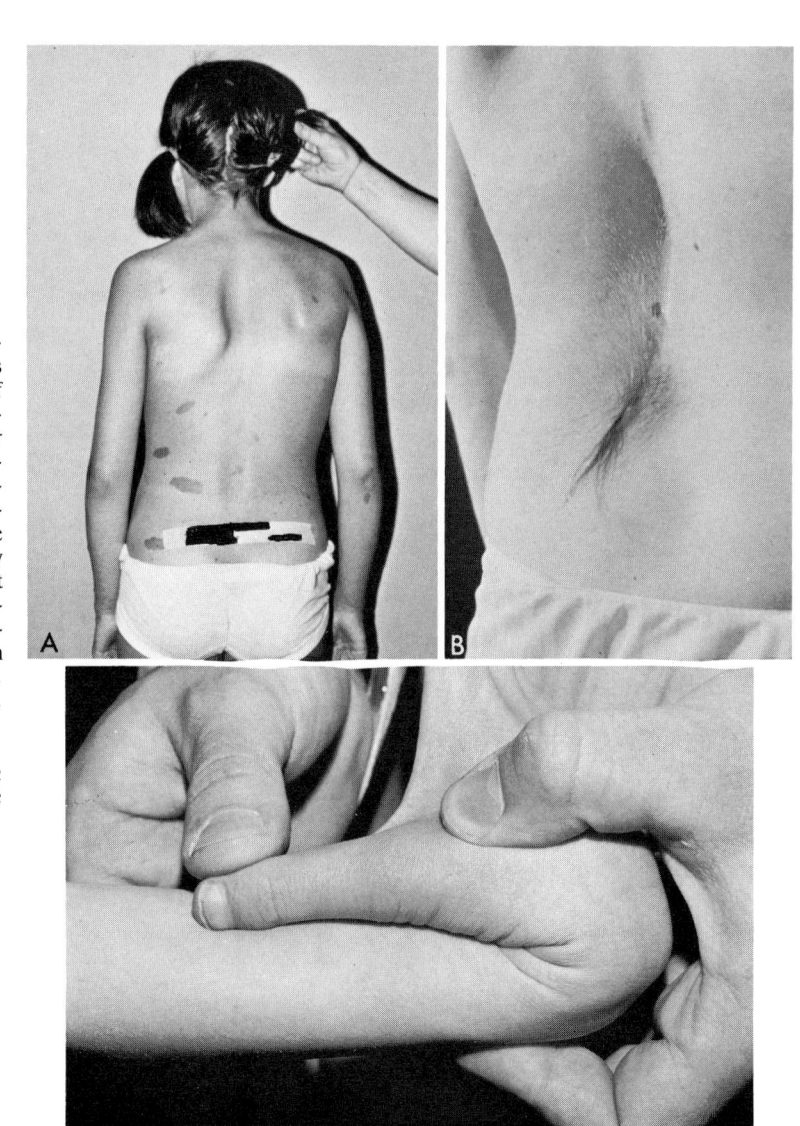

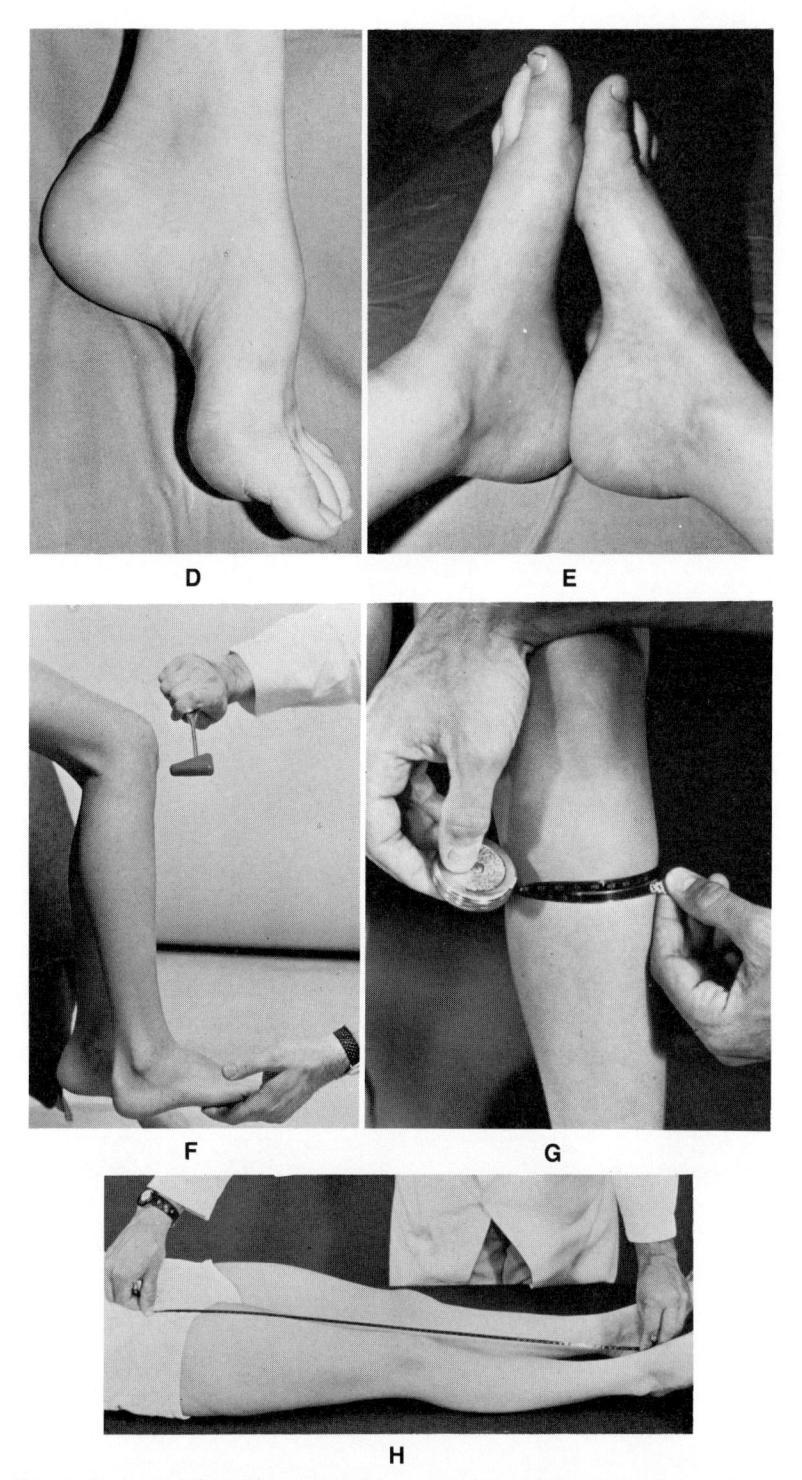

Figure 5–7 *Continued.* *D*, Foot deformities seen with spinal dysraphism. Note the marked cavus. *E*, Marked difference in foot size alerts the examining physician to the possibility of spinal dysraphism. *F*, Neurologic evaluation is mandatory for all patients. *G*, Measurement of thigh and calf circumference to evaluate hypertrophy or wasting. (Reprinted with permission from Rothman and Simeone.) *H*, Leg length accurately measured from the anterior superior iliac spine to the medial malleolus. (Reprinted with permission from Rothman and Simeone.)
Illustration continued on opposite page

PATIENT EVALUATION

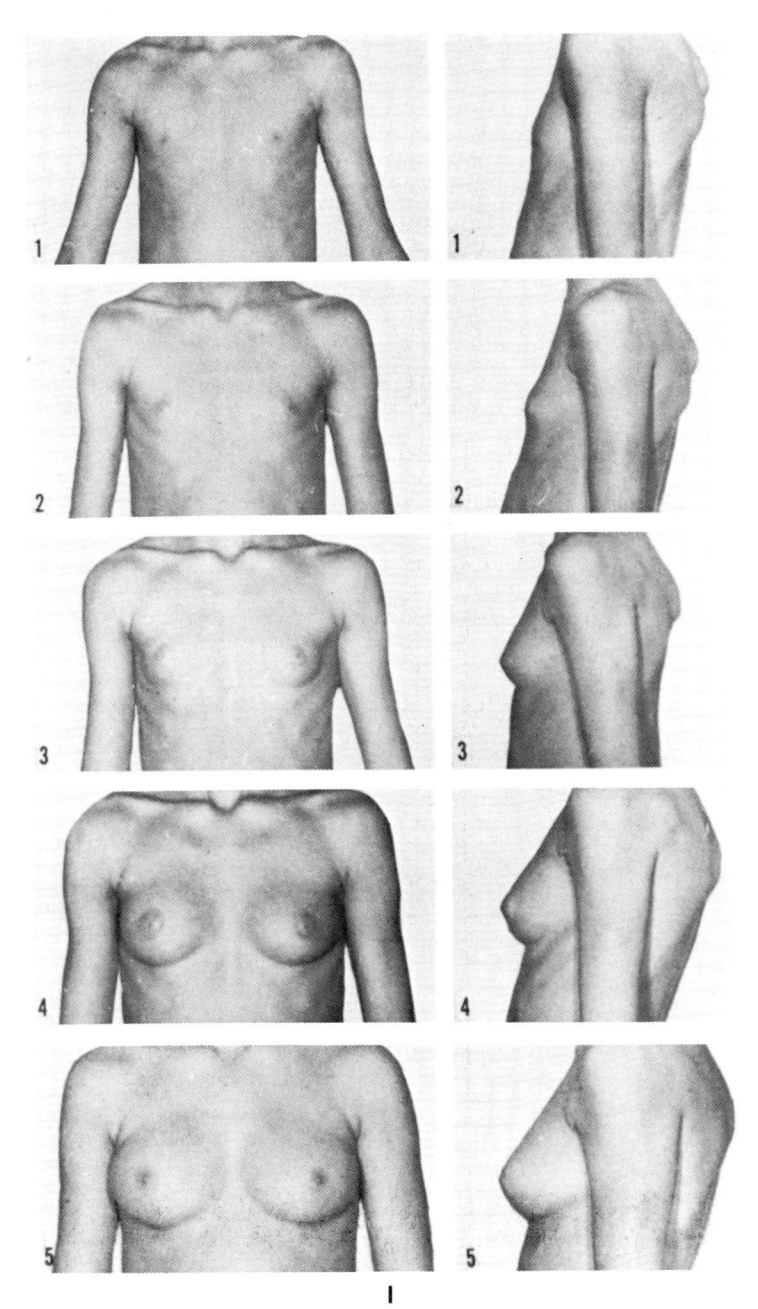

Figure 5–7 *Continued. I,* Standards for breast rating. (Reprinted with permission from Tanner, J. M.: Growth and endocrinology of the adolescent. *In* Gardner, L. (ed.): Endocrine and Genetic Diseases of Childhood and Adolescence, Philadelphia, W. B. Saunders Co., 1975.)

Illustration continued on following page

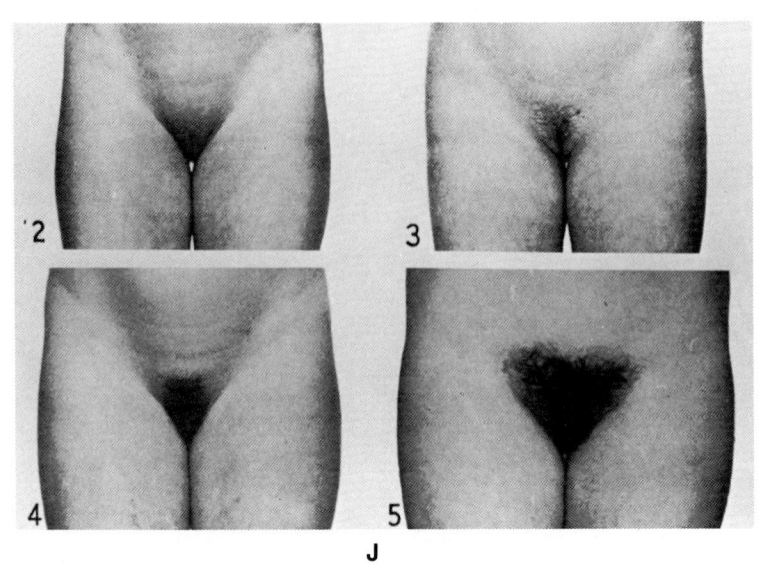

Figure 5–7 *Continued.* J, Standard for pubic hair rating in girls. (Reprinted with permission from Tanner.)

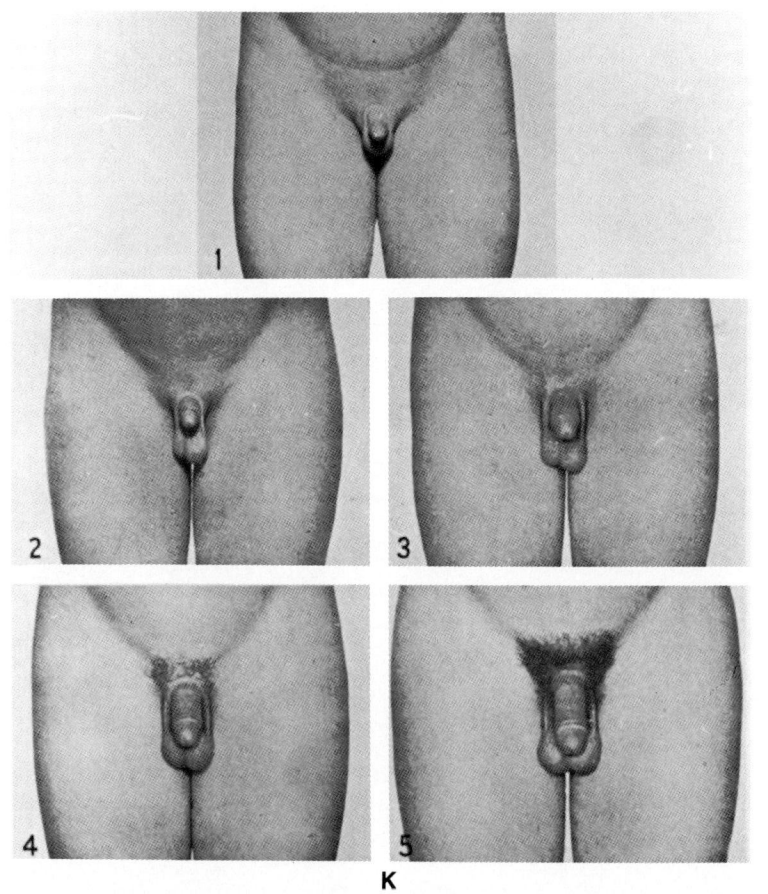

Figure 5–7 *Continued.* K, Standard for genital ratings. (Reprinted with permission from Tanner.)

Illustration continued on opposite page

PATIENT EVALUATION 57

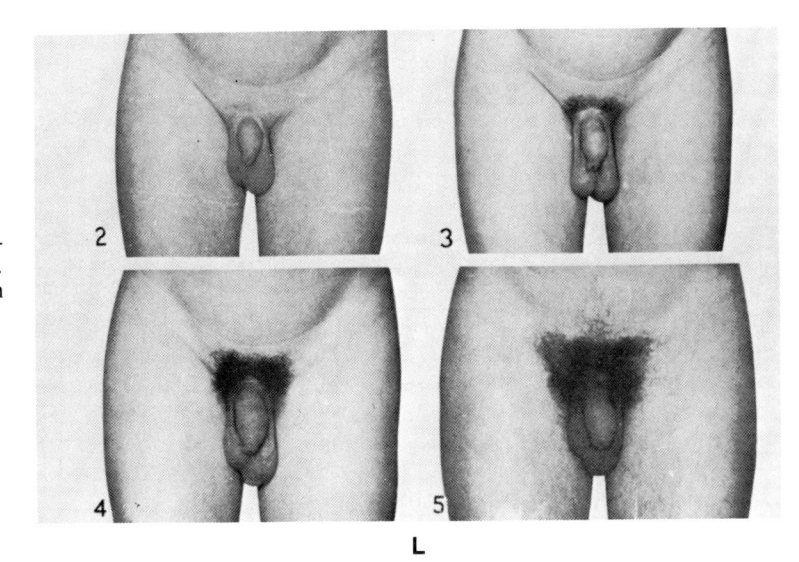

Figure 5–7 *Continued. L*, Standard for pubic hair rating in boys. (Reprinted with permission from Tanner.)

incision closure, and the general nutritional state of the skin of the lumbar area is noted. Any scars from previous surgery (e.g., thoracotomies, spine or abdominal procedures) are noted. The anterior chest is examined for deformity, pectus excavatum or pectus carinatum. There is often an anterior thoracic prominence on the side opposite to the posterior prominence owing to rotation and deformity of the whole thoracic cage.

The child's maturity is assessed. Breast development is assessed in girls, and pubic hair development is assessed in both sexes. Grading is performed using the Tanner System (Table 5–1 and Fig. 5–7*I* to *L*).[34, 35] Joint flexibility is evaluated using thumb-to-wrist

TABLE 5–1. Pubertal Stages in Girls and Boys*

Pubertal Stages in Girls	Pubertal Stages in Boys
Breast Staging	*Genitalia Ratings*
Stage 1. Pre-adolescent; elevation of papilla only.	Stage 1. Pre-adolescent; testes, scrotum and penis are of about the same size and proportion as in early childhood.
Stage 2. Breast bud stage; elevation of breast and papilla as a small mound, enlargement of areola diameter.	Stage 2. Scrotum and testes are enlarged with change in texture of the scrotal skin with slight reddening of the skin.
Stage 3. Further enlargement of breast and areola, with no separation of their contours.	Stage 3. Increase in size of the penis, in length mainly, but also in breadth, with continued growth of the testes and scrotum.
Stage 4. Projection of areola and papilla to form a secondary mound above the level of the breast.	Stage 4. Further enlargement of the testes, scrotum, and penis with development of the glans and darkening of the scrotal skin.
Stage 5. Mature stage; projection of papilla only, due to recession of the areola to the general contour of the breast.	Stage 5. Genitalia adult in size and shape.
Pubic Hair Stages	*Pubic Hair Stages*
Stage 1. Pre-adolescent; no pubic hair.	Stage 1. Pre-adolescent; no pubic hair.
Stage 2. Slight growth of long, slightly pigmented, downy hair, appearing chiefly along the labia.	Stage 2. Slight growth of long, slightly pigmented, downy hair, appearing chiefly at the base of the penis.
Stage 3. Darker, coarser hair that is more curled and spread sparsely over the junction of the pubes.	Stage 3. Darker, coarser hair that is more curled and spread sparsely over the junction of the pubes.
Stage 4. Hair is adult in type with no spread to medial surface of the thigh.	Stage 4. Hair is adult in type with no spread to medial surface of the thigh.
Stage 5. Adult in quantity and quality with no inverse triangle distribution and spread to the medial thighs.	Stage 5. Adult in quantity and quality with no inverse triangle distribution and spread to the medial thighs.

*Reprinted by permission from Tanner, J. M.: Growth and endocrinology of the adolescent. *In* Gardner, L. (ed.): Endocrine and Genetic Diseases of Childhood. Philadelphia, W. B. Saunders Co., p. 14, 1975.

approximation, the hyperflexibility is graded mild, moderate, or extreme (Fig. 5–7C). Joint flexibility can also be assessed using finger hyperextension or knee or elbow recurvatum.

The lower extremities are evaluated for any deformity or contracture. Hip or knee flexion contractures are assessed and measured. Foot size is compared, and any foot deformity is noted (Fig. 5–7D and 7E).

Leg lengths are assessed by measuring the distance between the anterior superior iliac spines and medial malleoli in the supine position (Fig. 5–7H). A brief neurologic examination is performed in all patients (Fig. 5–7F). Muscle tone, strength, and reflexes are evaluated. In patients with neurologic disease, a complete neurologic examination is essential. During the patient examination, an assessment is made of the patient's intelligence and mental status.

SCHOOL SCREENING[32, 48]

The forward bending test is one of the most common tests used in school screening for the early detection of spinal deformities. The school nurse or physical education teacher is instructed in regional workshops in the basics of spinal deformities, their treatment, and the early detection test. With the forward bending test very minor asymmetry can be detected. Once a significant asymmetry has been detected, the child is referred to the family physician. The forward bending test is repeated, and a standing radiograph is taken when necessary. With the diagnosis of scoliosis, the child is referred to an orthopaedic surgeon or a crippled children's clinic for full evaluation and possible treatment.

RADIOGRAPHIC EVALUATION[6, 7, 19, 49, 50]

Radiographs form the basis of patient evaluation during the initial presentation and future therapy. With the aid of the initial radiographs, the determination of the etiology and type of spinal deformity is made. The deformity is evaluated as to type (scoliosis, kyphosis, lordosis), site, magnitude, and flexibility. In addition the patient's maturity is assessed on routine views and with the aid of a bone age radiograph. Occasionally, additional specialized radiographic examinations, including myelography, angiography, laminography, discography, and intravenous pyelography, are necessary.

Correct labeling of each radiograph is essential. All spine films are viewed as if viewing the patient from the back; the right side of the patient is on the right side of the radiograph. All radiographs should be marked with the patient's name, the institution where the films were taken, the date of examination, and the position of the radiograph (e.g., standing, sitting, bending, oblique). In addition, the side (right or left) should be appropriately labeled. Since scoliosis radiographs are viewed opposite to all other radiographs, appropriate adjustment to the labeling is necessary so that all the labeling can be read. It is better to imprint all these markings on the x-ray film radiographically than to write them on later. The markings must be placed on the edge or on a corner of the film so as not to interfere with an evaluation of the spinal deformity (Fig. 5–8).

Routine Radiographic Evaluation of Spinal Deformity

The radiographs necessary for the accurate assessment of a spinal deformity depend on the type of deformity and the treatment plan. In the initial assessment an upright radiograph is all that is necessary to make the diagnosis and to plan treatment. When bracing or surgery is indicated, flexibility views are obtained in addition to special examinations where necessary. With the desire to minimize the radiation exposure to patients, "routines" should not be used; each examination should be tailored to the deformity being evaluated. A radiograph or examination should be ordered only if it is necessary in making a diagnosis or in planning therapy. When ordering a radiograph, the question "How will be information obtained from this examination change my treatment plan?" should be asked. If the information obtained is not necessary in decision making, then the examination need not be ordered.

RADIATION HAZARDS[2, 18, 22, 28, 39, 43]

Any radiograph, as it uses radiation to produce an image, increases the amount of radiation the patient receives. From animal studies and from studies of persons exposed to atomic blasts, it has been determined that

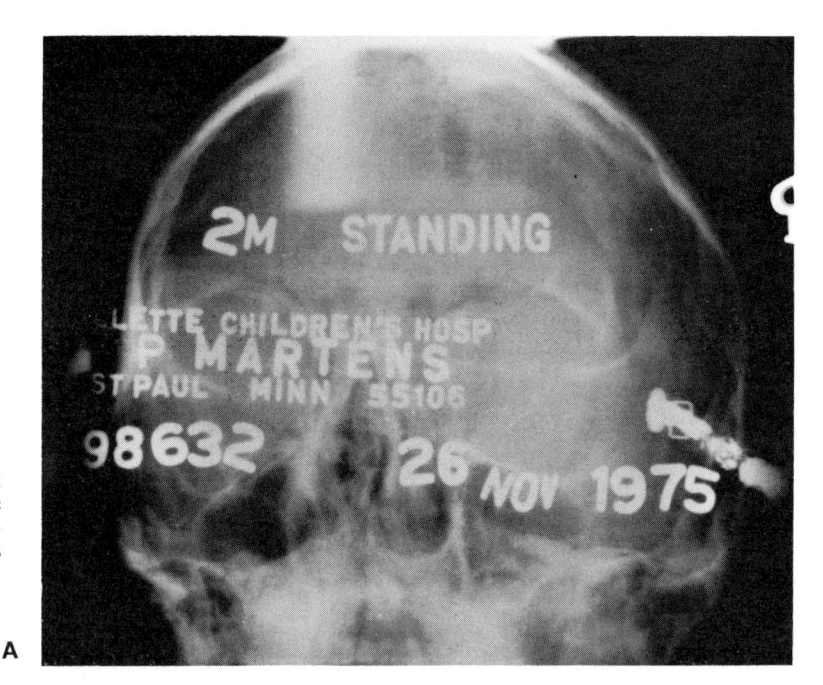

Figure 5–8. *A*, All the required information is imprinted on the film radiographically. *B*, Alternate method of labeling is shown.

the areas of concern are the gonads and organs. Increased gonadal radiation increases the mutation rate; this effect is noncumulative. Experimentally, pregnancy must occur within four to six months of a large dose of gonadal radiation for the effects to occur. Organ irradiation is cumulative, and the most sensitive organs are the breast, bone marrow, and thyroid gland. The breast is the most sensitive and is also very vulnerable in its formative years.

Radiographic technique should therefore minimize radiation and reduce organ dosage as much as possible.[2, 12, 13, 21] The most important reduction is an overall reduction of the number of radiographs taken. Each examination should be tailored to the patient's problem, and repeat examinations should be minimized. The technician, experienced in taking these films, will not have to repeat examinations because of poor quality films.

The x-ray beam should be collimated to only include the body, which reduces scatter and on a lateral view reduces the breast radiation. Antiscatter grids placed between the patient and the cassette require the use of longer exposure (and thus more radiation), but the improvement in quality of the film by reducing scatter overrides this disadvantage. Beam filtration, with the use of filters to give a uniform density to the radiograph, also filters unnecessary radiation (see subsequent section). The use of faster radiographic film reduces the exposure necessary, with an accompanying slight loss of detail. Intensifying screens, for example Quanta rare earth screens, also reduce the exposure by converting the x-ray photons to light, which exposes the film (see Table 5–2).

The gonads are shielded using a gonadal shield (see subsequent section). Breast irradiation can be reduced in a number of ways.

TABLE 5–2. Radiation Doses (in MRAD)*

	No Filter	Filter	Quantum Screen
6 Year Old			
AP	170	55	28
Lat	467	63	21
15 Year Old			
AP	355	150	60
Lat	825	120	40

*X-ray dosages in a 6 year old and a 15 year old with an upright AP or lateral film. Note the reduction of dosage with the use of a filter and further reduction with a Quantum rare earth screen.

With the use of the aforementioned techniques there is a reduction of breast dosage using the anteroposterior position.[18] In this position breast shields (see Fig. 5–10B) or a lead stole can be used.[21] Alternatively, the posteroanterior position which also has been shown to decrease breast dosage, can be used.[2, 13, 39]

UPRIGHT EXAMINATION

Upright sitting or standing radiographs form the basis of the initial evaluation and follow-up. Standing views are taken in patients who are able to stand. Sitting views are used in patients who are unable to stand, including the very young, those with paralysis, and those with weakness of the lower extremities that prevents standing without the aid of support. Routine evaluation of scoliosis used to be in the anteroposterior projection. Because of improved information on radiation dosage and concern regarding dosage to the breast, the standard positioning is now in the posteroanterior projection. A posteroanterior radiograph is used for the evaluation of mild to moderate scoliosis; the lateral view is used with kyphosis or lordosis. To appreciate the spinal deformity in three dimensions both views are necessary.

All upright radiographs are taken at a 6-foot (2-meter) distance. This standarizes the examination and allows a measurement of spinal growth. A 14 × 36 inch (36 × 91 cm.) film is used, allowing complete assessment of the whole spine on a single radiograph. The relationship of the head and thorax to the pelvis can be appreciated on this film. Where this longer film is not available, or in infants and smaller children, a 14 × 17 inch (36 × 43 cm.) film is used. The smaller film is positioned with the lower end of the film

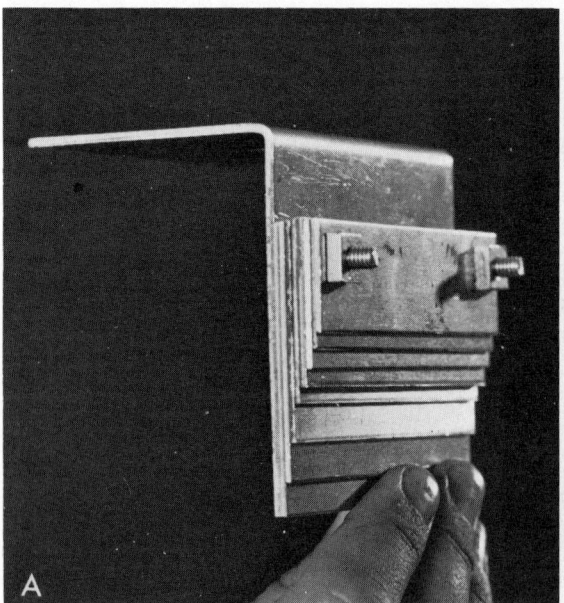

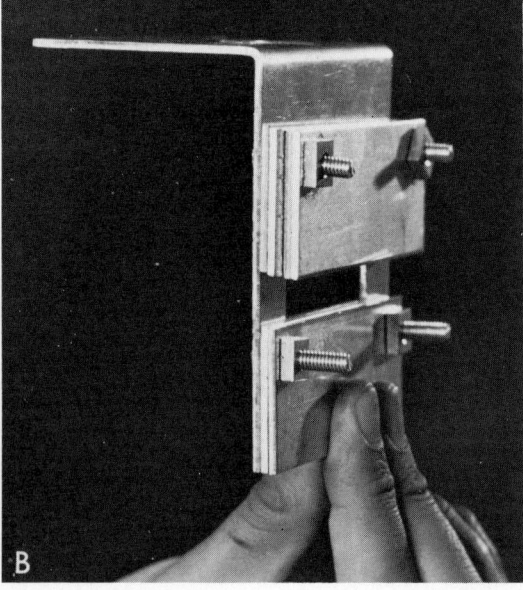

Figure 5–9. The use of aluminum filters screens out a portion of the x-ray beam to give uniform density to the spine on the x-ray film. A, The posteroanterior (anteroposterior) filter consists of 1 mm. thick layers of aluminum, with the thickest portion in the region of the occiput and cervical spines. B, The lateral wedge filter has a thick portion in the region of the occiput and cervical spine. There is no filter in the area of the shoulder, a small filter in the thoracic area, and no filter in the lumbar area.

Illustration continued on opposite page

PATIENT EVALUATION

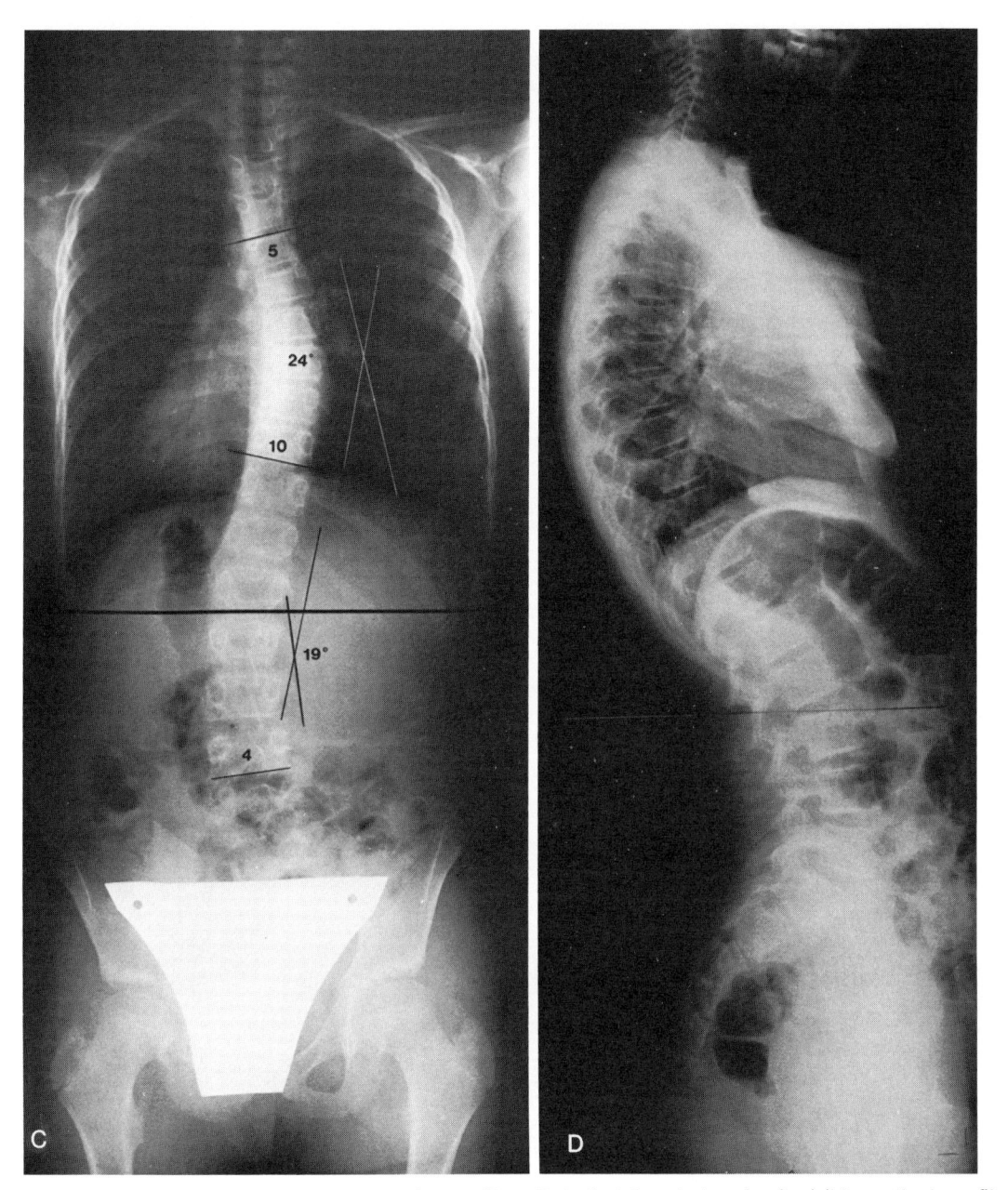

Figure 5–9 *Continued.* C, Radiograph taken with the filter. Note that the whole spine is visible on the long film and that all the vertebrae are well visualized. Note the gonadal shield. D, Radiograph taken with the filter. Note the bone detail of all the vertebrae is seen well.

at the level of the anterior superior iliac spines, which allows all or most of the spine to be viewed on one radiograph. High thoracic or cervical curves are missed using this smaller film.

To help decrease the radiation exposure and to make the radiographic density of the vertebral column on the film uniform, aluminum filters are used to screen out a portion of the radiation beam.[27] The filters are placed on the x-ray tube in the path of the beam. The posteroanterior filter (Fig. 5–9A) has a thicker portion in the area of the occiput and cervical spine, and it gets thinner in the thoracic area, terminating opposite L1. The lateral filter (Fig. 5–9B) also has a thicker portion in the area of the occiput and cervical spine; it has no filter in the area of the shoulders and thoracic spine as a larger amount of radiation is necessary to obtain an adequate radiograph in these areas (Fig. 5–9C and 9D).

In the upright views, the spine is centered in the middle of the bucky, with the appropriate filter being used. The top of the 14 × 35 inch (36 × 91 cm.) cassette is placed at the level of the external auditory meatus. A lead gonadal shield is placed with its top level with the anterior superior iliac spine. The shield is used on all upright examinations except the initial upright films. The patient stands as upright as possible with no rotation present, and with feet together and knees straight (Fig. 5–10). Shoes are not worn unless there is a leg length discrepancy that is corrected with a shoe lift. In patients unable to stand an unsupported sitting view is taken, and because of positioning, this is an anteroposterior view. No hand support is used to stabilize the trunk, thus showing the full effect of gravity on the deformity.

In the lateral projection, a standard position with the arms supported at 90 degrees of flexion is used. The arms are supported on an IV (intravenous) stand, which is raised or lowered to the correct height for each patient (Fig. 5–11). In patients who stand with the aid of support (cane or crutches), unsupported standing or sitting views are necessary to show the true status of the

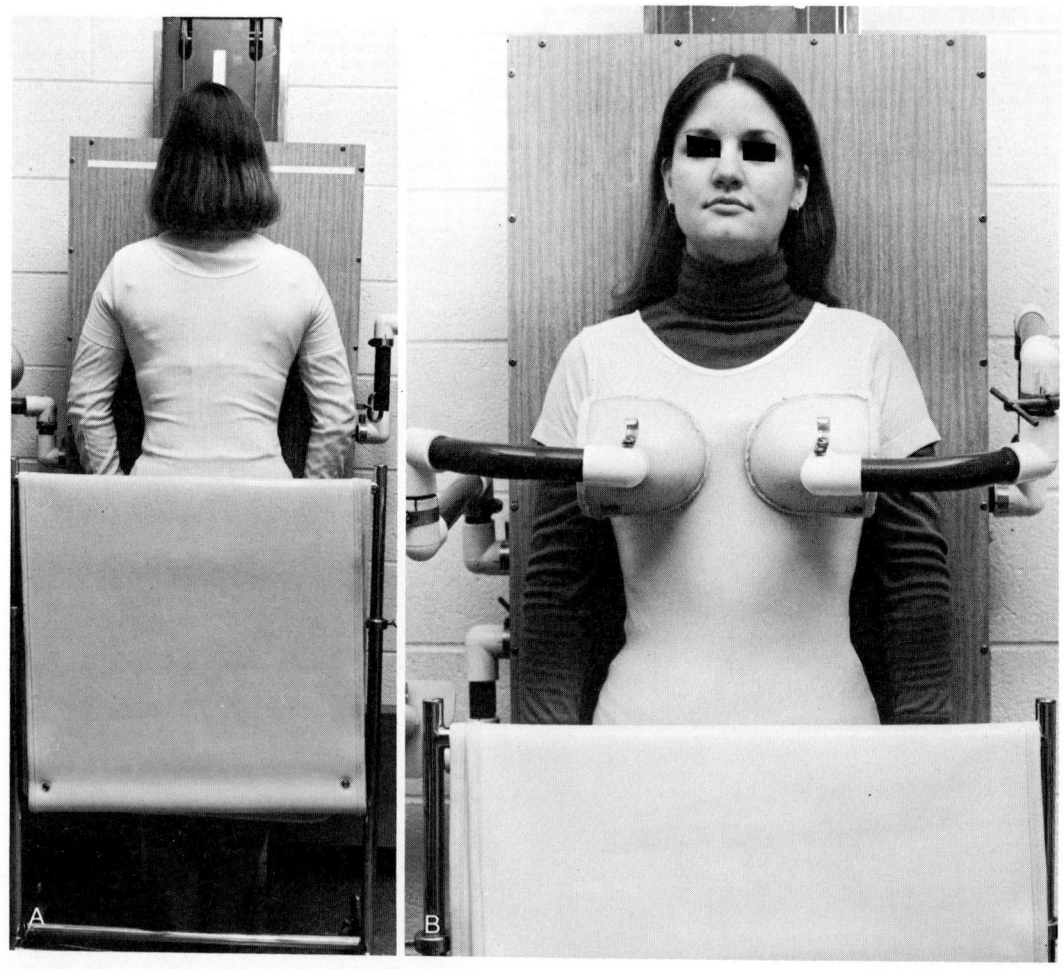

Figure 5–10. A, Position for posteroanterior standing x-ray. The patient stands fully erect with feet together and knees straight. The 14 × 36 inch (36 × 91 cm.) cassette is positioned at the external auditory meatus. Note the gonadal shield positioned at the level of the anterior superior iliac spines; the shield is used in all films except on the initial evaluation. B, Anteroposterior view taken with breast shields; the positioning is the same as in A.

PATIENT EVALUATION

or brace, appropriate adjustments to the exposure are necessary for adequate radiographic evaluation.

SUPINE EVALUATION

Supine radiographs are taken in certain cases to help in the assessment of the spine. In patients unable to sit (the very young or in severely paralyzed patients who are unable to sit) these form the basis of the radiographic evaluation. Supine films are used in the course of treatment to evaluate flexibility with bending or traction and postoperatively in the assessment of the fusion mass. These radiographs are taken on a 14 × 17 inch (36 × 43 cm.) film at a standard 40 inch (102 cm.) distance, without the use of filters. This film, because of the shorter distance, gives better bone detail than the upright view, and is valuable in the assessment of bone detail in congenital anomalies and other lesions.

FLEXIBILITY EVALUATION

Flexibility views consist of active side bending films for scoliosis, a hyperextension film for kyphosis, and flexion film for lordosis. These radiographs are all taken in the supine position and they all involve active muscle power for correction of the deformity. In patients with large deformities or those with neuromuscular scoliosis where there is no active muscle power, a traction film is used to evaluate the flexibility. A "push film" is used by some to assess the spine's flexibility.[31]

Side Bending. After the curves have been identified on the upright radiograph, side bending views are taken to show the flexibility of each curve. The patient is supine with maximum voluntary side bending toward the convexity of each curve. The views are taken supine on a 14 × 17 inch (36 × 43 cm.) film (Fig. 5–12A). For example, for a high left thoracic, right thoracic, left lumbar curve pattern, left side-bending views are taken of the high left thoracic and left lumbar curves and a right side-bending film of the right thoracic curve. Separate exposures are usually necessary for each bending evaluation, except in small children in whom the whole spine is visible on a single radiograph. If obliquity of the lumbosacral area is seen with a fractional lumbosacral curve, a flexibility side-bending evaluation of the lumbo-

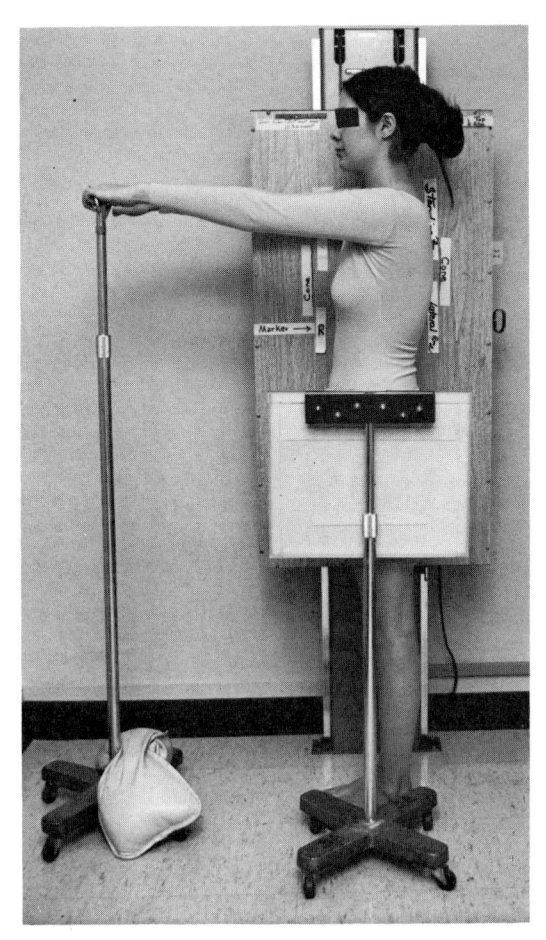

Figure 5–11. Position for lateral standing x-ray. The erect position and cassette placement are the same as in Figure 5–10A. The arms are positioned at shoulder height and are resting on an IV stand, which can be adjusted to the patient's height. Note the gonadal screen positioned with the top at the level of the anterior superior iliac spine. If it is positioned too high, the sacroiliac joint will be obscured. Note the film markers on the cassette holder.

deformity without the suspension effect of the crutches.

As mentioned, on the initial evaluation no gonadal shield is used, allowing an evaluation of the pelvis, hip joints, and proximal femora. The screen is used on all subsequent examinations. The screen found to be most effective and easy to use is a lead screen of appropriate thickness fixed to an IV stand that can be raised and lowered. The shield is positioned over the lower abdomen, with its upper end at the level of the anterior superior iliac spines. This allows the whole spine to be visualized and in addition the iliac crest epiphysis to be assessed. In patients in a cast

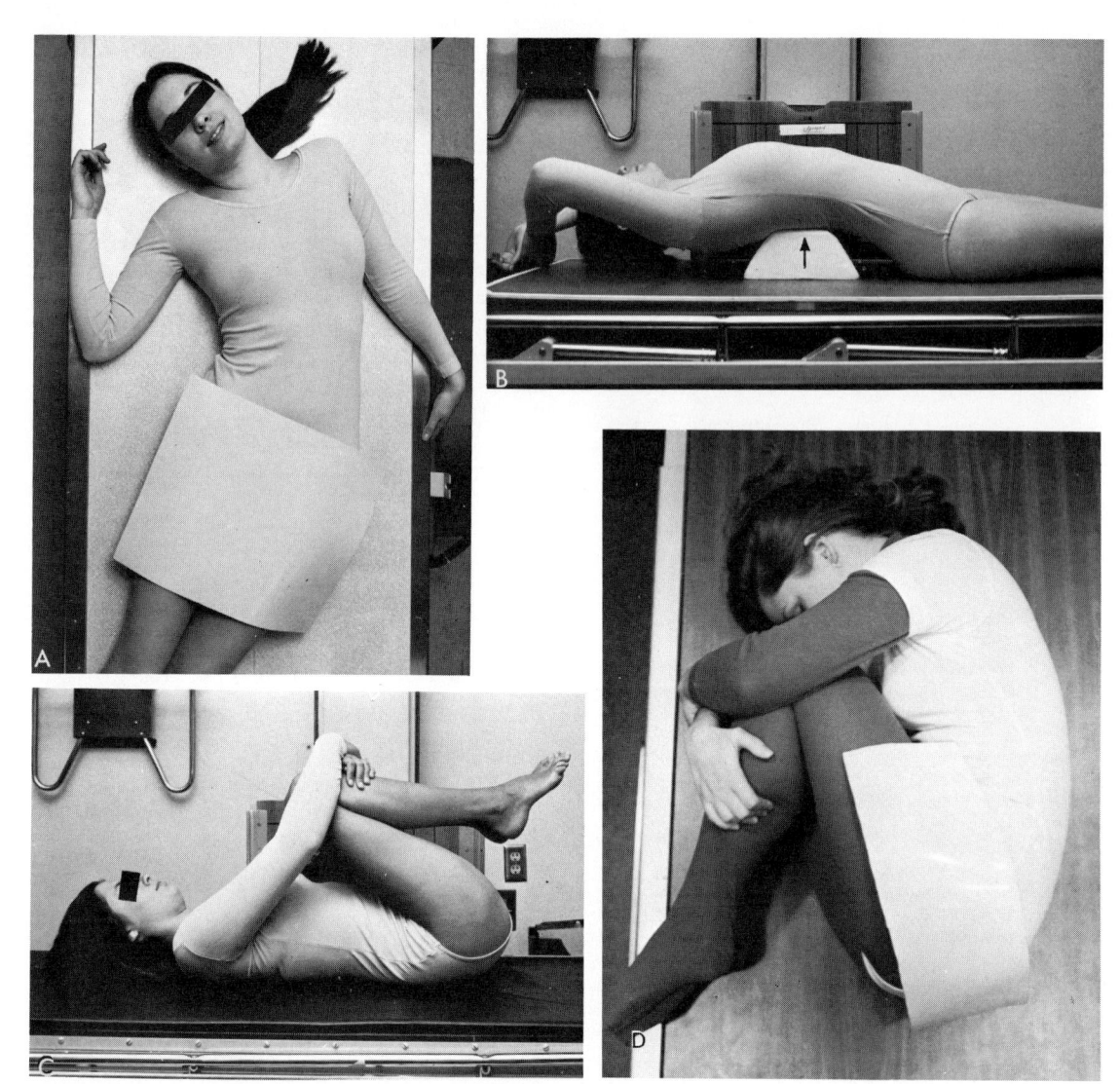

Figure 5–12. Flexibility evaluation. *A*, Supine right side bending position to evaluate the flexibility of a right thoracic curve. The patient bends actively to the right with maximal bending as the exposure is taken. Note the gonadal screen. *B*, Hyperextension position to evaluate the flexibility of kyphosis. The patient lies on a styrofoam block, which is positioned under the apex of the kyphosis. A lead arrow in the block indicates the apex of the hyperextension force on the film. Flexion position for flexibility evaluation of lordosis. Patient is either supine (*C*) or side lying (*D*). The x-ray is taken in maximal flexion with the knees drawn up to the chest (knee-chest position).

sacral area is necessary. Each film has to be marked appropriately to show that the evaluation is supine and marked as RSB for right side bending and LSB for left side bending.

Hyperextension. A hyperextension view is taken to demonstrate the flexibility of kyphosis. With the patient in the forward bending position, the apex of the kyphosis is marked on the skin. The patient is placed supine on a wedge-shaped styrofoam block, which is centered on the kyphosis at the mark on the skin. A lead arrow is placed in the center of the block to show where the maximal corrective force is situated. A cross-table view shows the flexibility of the kyphosis (Fig. 5–12*B*).

Hyperflexion. A hyperflexion view is taken to demonstrate the flexibility of lordosis. As hyperlordosis is usually in the lumbar or thoracolumbar area, flexibility is seen on a lateral radiograph taken in the knee-chest position, with the knees maximally held to the chest and the spine maximally flexed. This view can be taken in the supine position or the side position (Fig. 5–12C and D).

Traction. In neuromuscular disease in which muscle weakness or paralysis prevents active side bending and in large deformities, a traction view will best demonstrate the flexibility of the deformity. A supine anteroposterior radiograph is taken with two technicians applying maximal distraction, one using a disposable head halter for the head, and the other pulling on the legs. Maximal distraction force is applied as the radiograph is taken (Fig. 5–13A). A traction film can also be taken on the Risser-Cotrel casting frame. The patient is positioned with cervical and pelvic traction, with the addition of localizers; the positioning is the same as for the application of a body cast (see Chapter 9). With maximal corrective forces applied, an anteroposterior or lateral view will show correction of the deformity (Fig. 5–13B). In addition, the correction of pelvic obliquity and the balance of the thorax over the pelvis are also shown with this radiograph (Figs. 5–13C and D). A similar view is taken in Europe with the suspension radiograph, where in the upright position the patient is suspended via a head halter as the film is taken.

Evaluation of Maturity

A spot anteroposterior view of the left hand and wrist is taken on patients under 18. This radiograph is compared with the standard views in the Greulich and Pyle Atlas to obtain the skeletal age of the patient, which is compared to the chronological age.[23] In addition the evaluation of the iliac epiphyses and vertebral ring apophysis is important in the adolescent to evaluate spine growth; evaluation of proximal femoral, trochanteric, and proximal humeral physes is also important to monitor total growth.

Special Views

Occasionally special views of the spine are necessary to adequately demonstrate spinal anatomy.

OBLIQUE VIEWS

Oblique views of the spine are taken with the patient positioned on a wedge on the table; both right and left oblique views are taken. These films are used in the lumbar spine to evaluate the pars interarticularis in spondylolysis and spondylolisthesis. They are also used to evaluate the integrity of the fusion mass, as the oblique view places the fusion mass in profile.

SPOT VIEW

Spot coned down views are used to better demonstrate spinal anatomy. The most common one is a spot lateral standing view of the lumbosacral junction, which is used if this area is not adequately seen on the routine standing lateral radiograph.

FERGUSON VIEW

When there are abnormalities of the lumbosacral junction, a Ferguson view is used. This is a view taken with the x-ray tube tilted 30 degrees cephalad in a male and 35 degrees in a female. The x-ray beam goes through the lumbosacral intervertebral disc, and thus the anatomy of this junction is well shown (Fig. 5–14A). A similar view can be obtained in the supine anteroposterior film if the radiograph is taken with the hips flexed 90 degrees. This position eliminates the lordosis, and the lumbosacral anatomy is well seen (Fig. 5–14B and C). The Ferguson view should only be taken when the anatomy is poorly seen on other radiographs as the gonadal exposure for this single view is relatively high.

DEROTATED VIEW OF SPINE (PLAN D'ELECTION OF STAGNARA)[45]

In large curves (usually over 100 degrees), the posteroanterior radiograph does not show the true magnitude of the deformity because of accompanying spinal rotation. The rotation gives an appearance of kyphosis, and the deformity is called kyphoscoliosis when it is in actuality kyphosing scoliosis. The sagittal deformity is due to rotation and not to true kyphosis. If this rotation is eliminated, the scoliotic curve is much larger than seen on the posteranterior view. To achieve this an oblique radiograph of the curve is necessary. The ideal method would be to examine the spine with the aid of fluoroscopy, rotate the patient until the maximal curve is seen, and then take the radiograph. In practice, an oblique view is taken with the

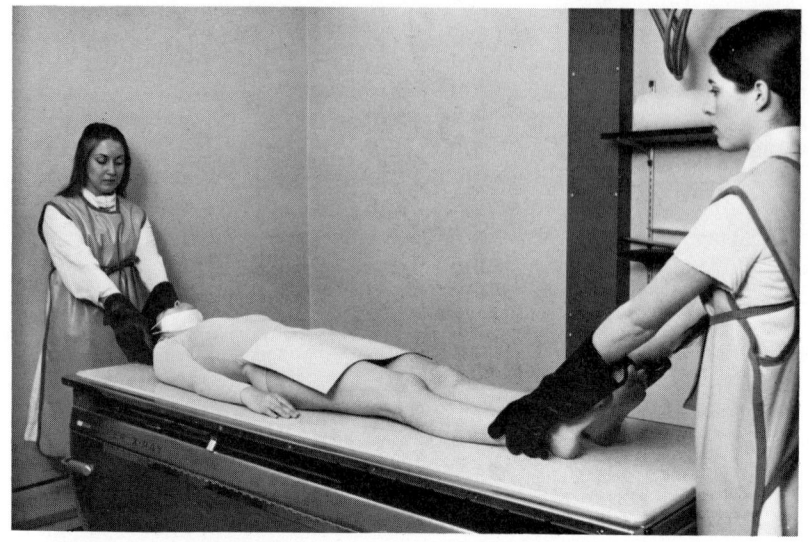

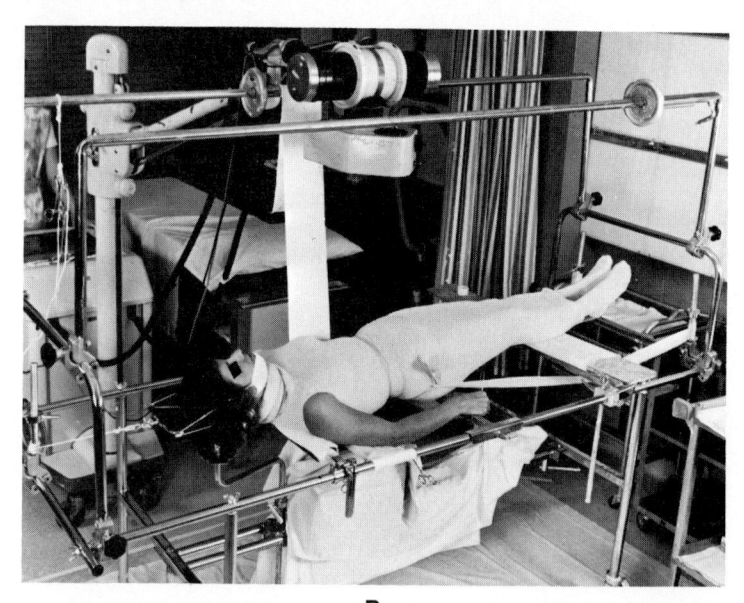

Figure 5–13. Traction film. This is used in patients with large curves (over 90 degrees) or in patients with neuromuscular scoliosis. *A*, Traction using a disposable head halter and leg traction. *B*, Traction film on the Risser-Cotrel frame using longitudinal traction and a thoracic localizer.

Illustration continued on opposite page

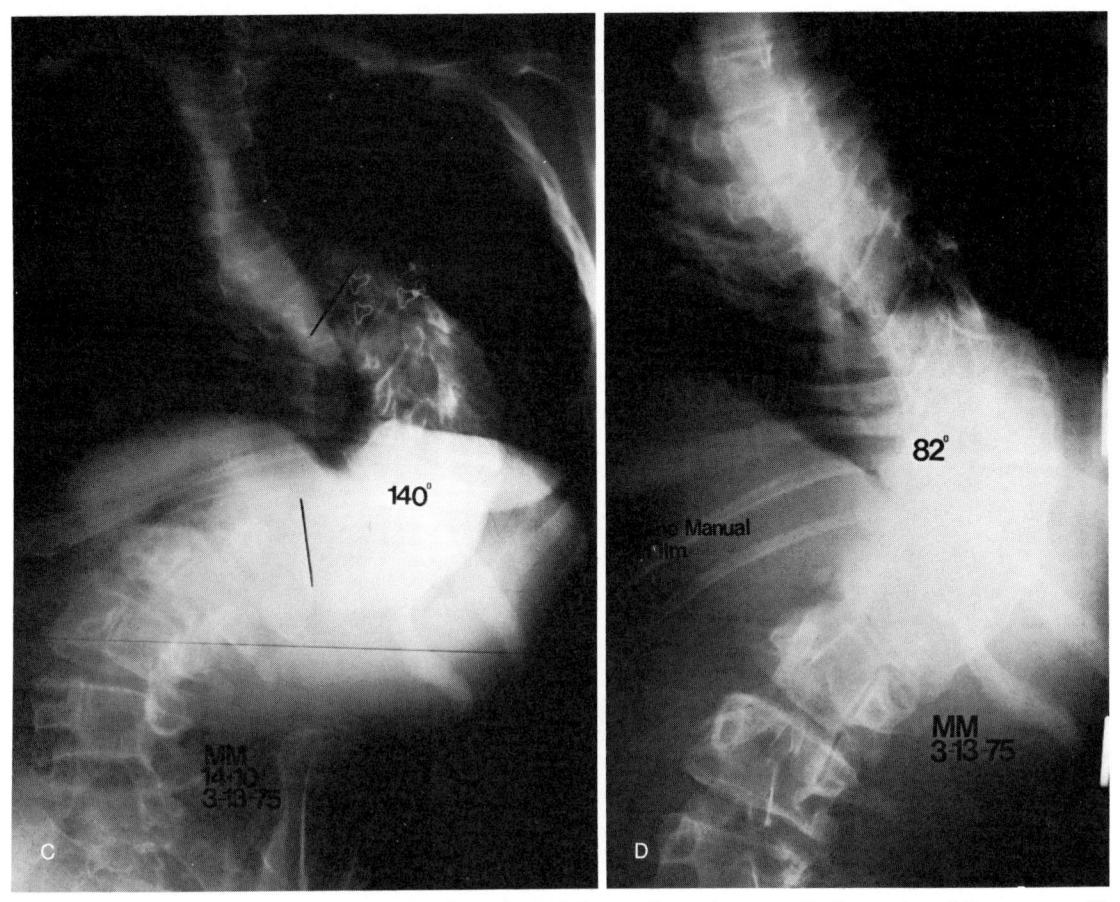

Figure 5-13 Continued. C, Posteroanterior view of a 140 degree thoracic curve. D, Correction of the curve to 82 degrees on a traction film.

cassette positioned parallel to the medial aspect of the rotational rib prominence. The x-ray beam is positioned at right angles to the cassette (Fig. 5-15). This technique gives a true coronal view of the apical vertebrae, revealing the true scoliosis. This view is also valuable in the evaluation of congenital anomalies and large curves. With the derotation of the spine, the vertebral anatomy is appreciated, and any anomalies or diastematomyelia are well seen.

CURVE EVALUATION

The radiographs taken are reviewed to evaluate the curve pattern, curve magnitude, curve flexibility, and the patient's maturity. The upright radiographs form the basis of evaluation and are examined first.

General Evaluation

The radiographs are evaluated to help determine the etiology of the spinal deformity. The presence of congenital anomalies is sought (e.g., hemivertebrae, wedge vertebrae, failure of segmentation, or block vertebrae). The length of the curve is noted; a short angular curve raises the possibility of neurofibromatosis, a long curve, neuromuscular deformity. The pedicles and the interpediculate distance are evaluated throughout the length of the spine and, where necessary, they are compared with normal ranges by age.[25] Widening of the interpediculate distance is seen in intraspinal lesions such as syringomyelia and spinal dysraphism. In the latter, a midline bony spur of diastematomyelia is often seen (Fig. 5-16).

In addition to the vertebrae, the remainder

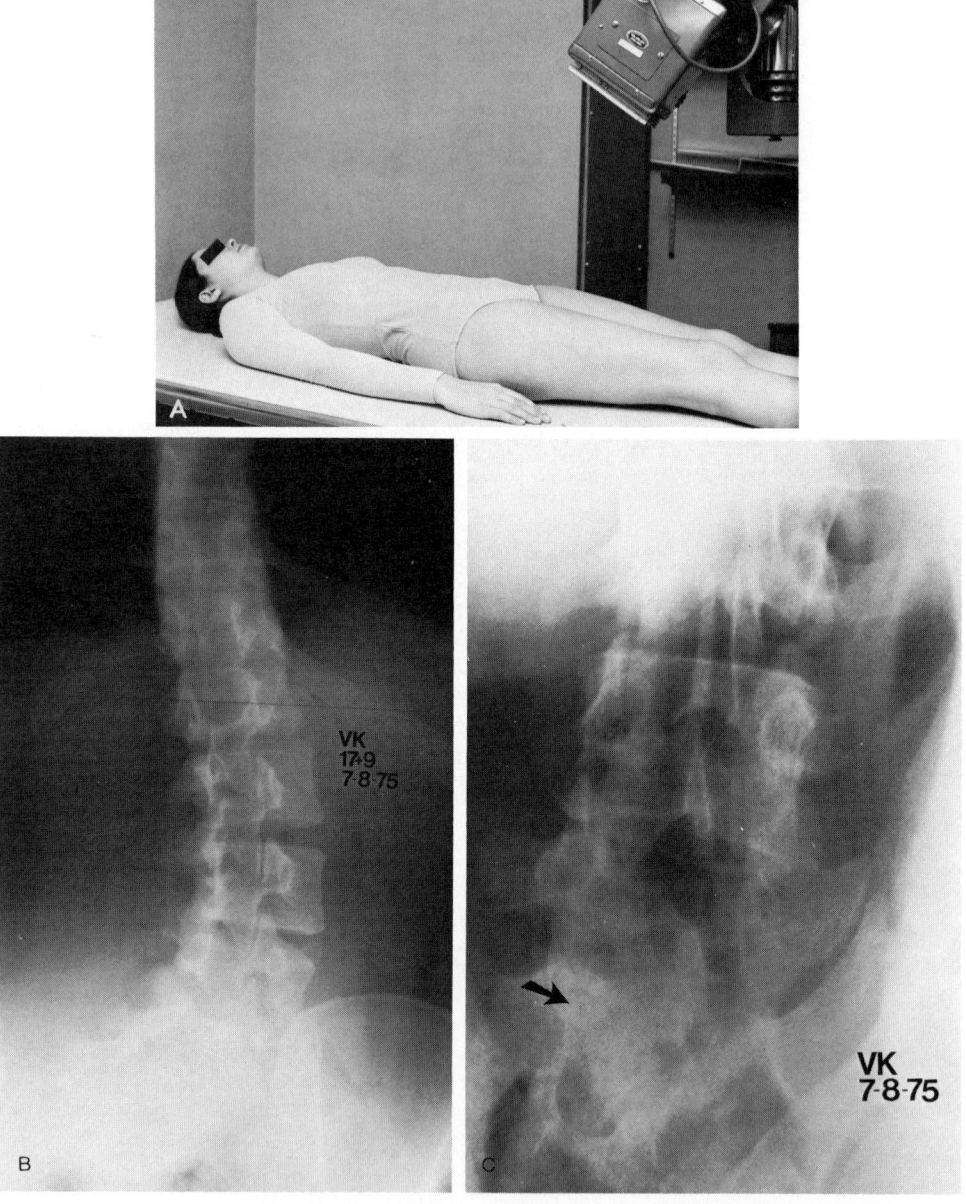

Figure 5–14. *A*, Position for Ferguson view. The patient is supine, and the tube is tilted cephalad so that the x-ray beam goes through the lumbosacral joint. *B*, Anteroposterior view shows a right lumbar curve, but the lumbosacral joint cannot be seen; a shift to the right is obvious. *C*, In the Ferguson view the anatomy of the lumbosacral area is seen. The sacrum is normal, and there is a hemivertebra at L6 with a tilt of the spine above.

PATIENT EVALUATION

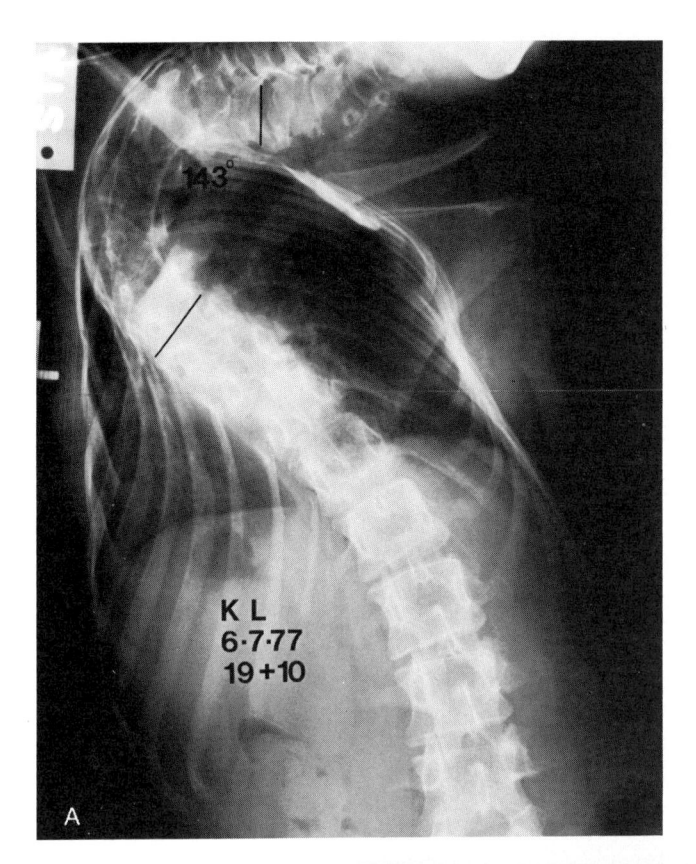

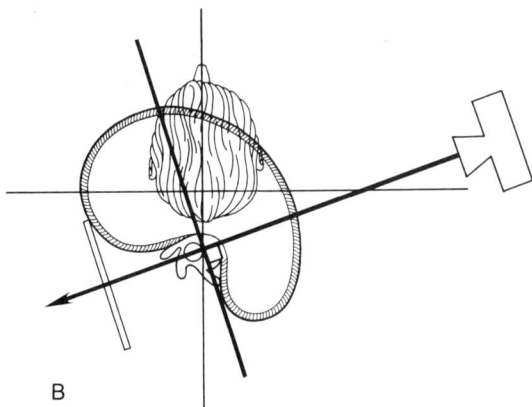

Figure 5–15. *A,* Derotated view of the spine. Standing posteroanterior view shows a severe 143 degree left thoracic curve. The anatomy of the curve is not visible. *B,* Diagram to demonstrate the derotation view. The cassette is positioned parallel to the medial aspect of the rib prominence and the x-ray beam is at right angles to the plate. *C,* This view eliminates the effect of rotation. The anatomy of the apical vertebrae is well seen with the fused bodies and a hemivertebra on the convexity.

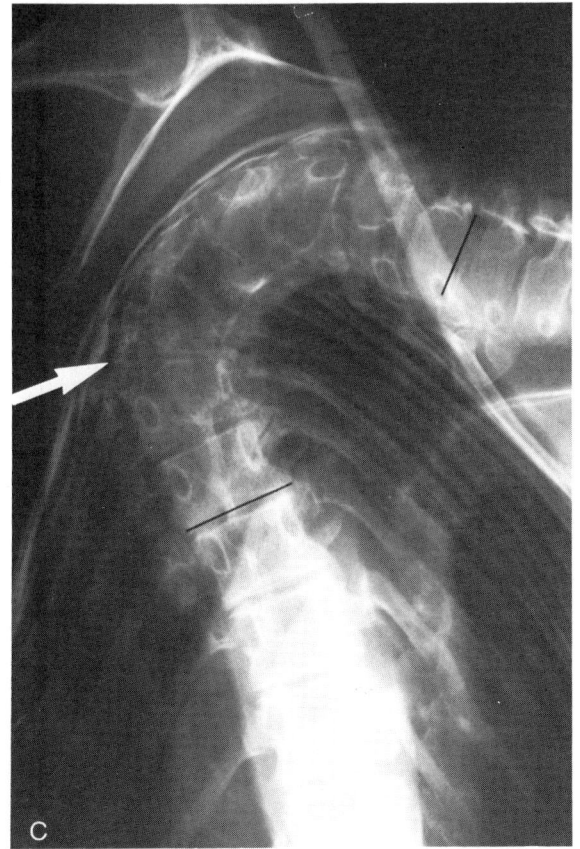

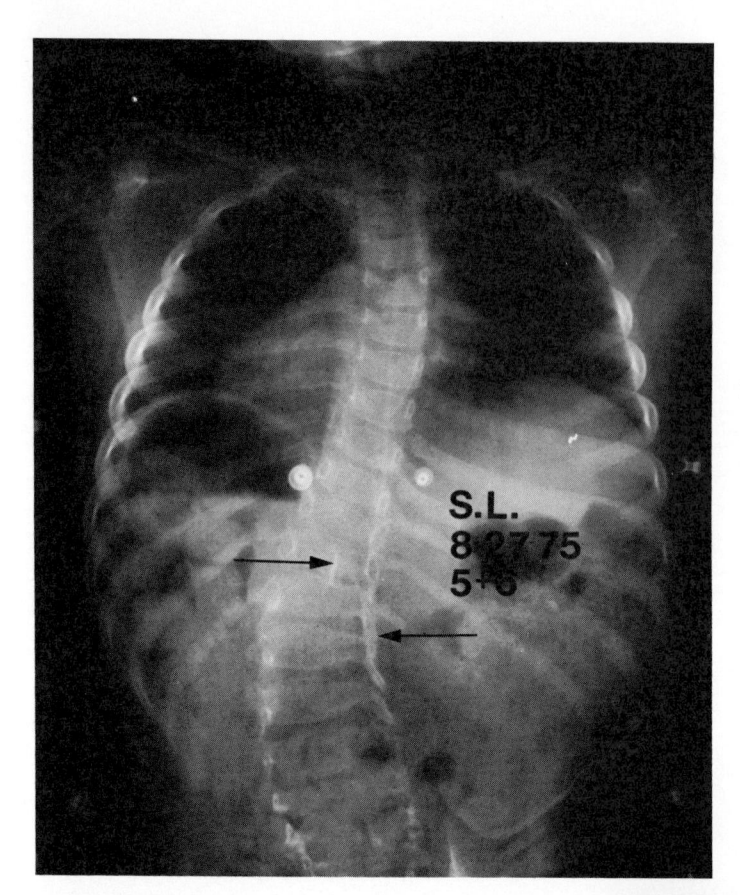

Figure 5–16. Standing x-ray of a 5 + 6 year old girl. Note the widening of the interpediculate distance from the lower thoracic area with the absence of laminae and spinous processes. A midline bony spur is well seen as is the fusion of the pedicles in the thoracolumbar area.

Figure 5–17. Rib droop due to intercostal paralysis. This is a radiographic indication of neuromuscular scoliosis.

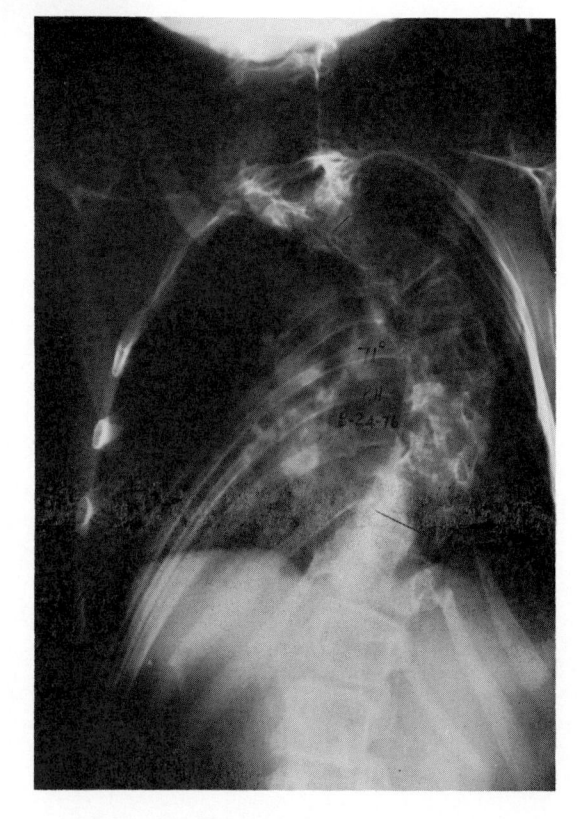

PATIENT EVALUATION

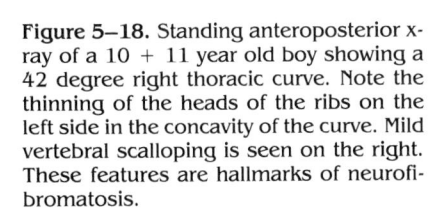

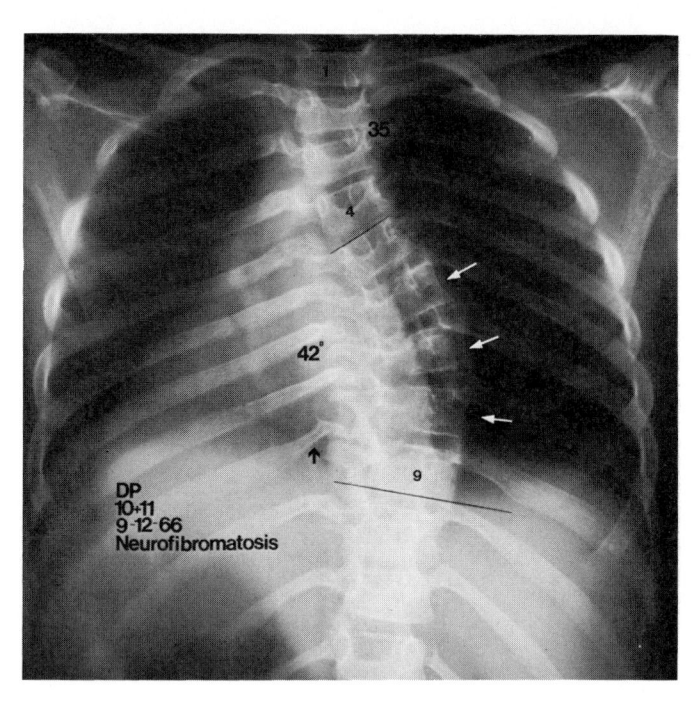

Figure 5–18. Standing anteroposterior x-ray of a 10 + 11 year old boy showing a 42 degree right thoracic curve. Note the thinning of the heads of the ribs on the left side in the concavity of the curve. Mild vertebral scalloping is seen on the right. These features are hallmarks of neurofibromatosis.

of the structures seen on the radiograph are examined. In paralytic spinal deformities, rib drooping due to intercostal paralysis is seen (Fig. 5–17). In neurofibromatosis there is vertebral body scalloping as well as pencilling or thinning of the ribs (Fig. 5–18). Rib synostosis frequently accompanies congenital anomalies of the spine. The humeral heads, scapulae, lung fields, heart, pelvis, and proximal femora are all examined.

Curve Pattern[38]

The curve pattern, as seen on the upright radiograph, is now evaluated. The curve site is classified according to the apical vertebra—cervical, thoracic, or lumbar. A junctional curve (cervicothoracic or thoracolumbar) must have the apex *at* the junction of the two areas. In a thoracolumbar curve the apex is either T12 or L1 or the disc between these two vertebrae.

In correct anatomic terms dorsal is *not* used interchangeably with thoracic. Dorsal is the opposite of ventral, and thus all the vertebrae are dorsal with reference to the body. Thoracic is the term used for the vertebrae of the thorax, the vertebrae with ribs articulating with them.

Curve Measurement

Once the curve pattern is noted, the extent and magnitude are determined. The site of the deformity, disc space or vertebral bodies, is noted (Fig. 5–19). The first step in curve measurement is the identification of the *end vertebrae* (Fig. 5–20A). The end vertebra is the last vertebra tilted into the concavity of the curve being measured. When the vertebrae are parallel, the one farthest from the apex

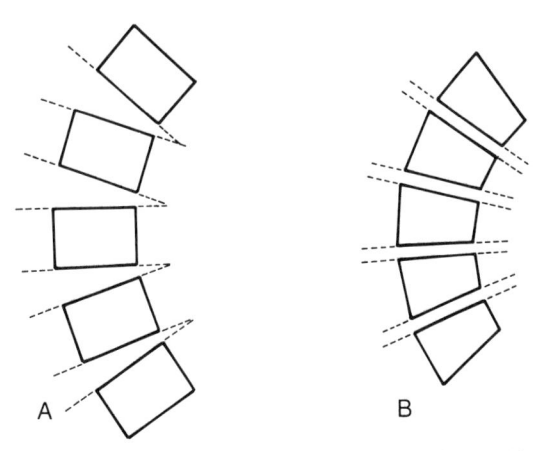

Figure 5–19. The spine deformity can be due to disc space wedging (A) or to vertebral wedging (B); the latter is usually accompanied by some disc space wedging.

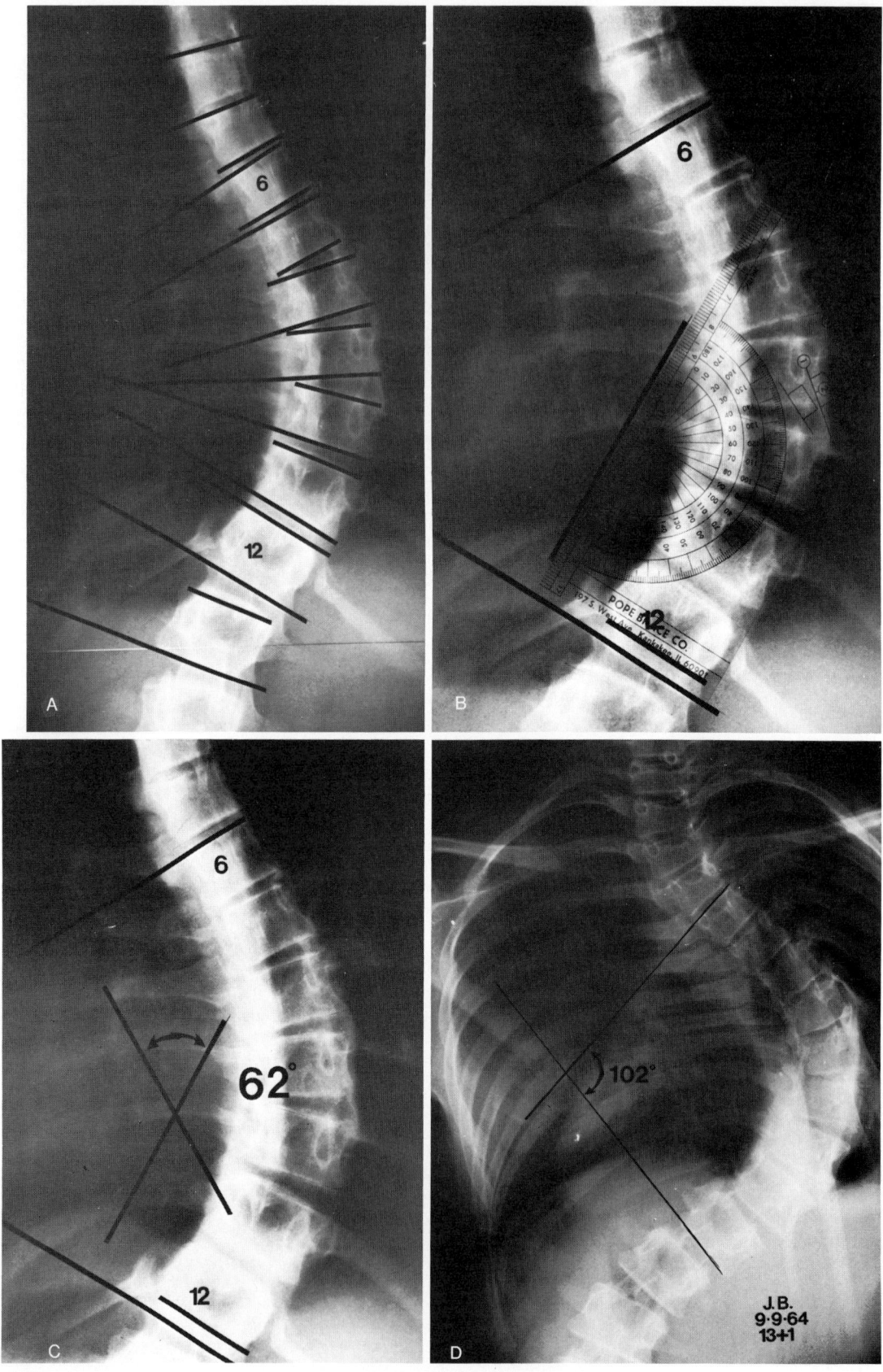

Figure 5–20. *See legend on opposite page*

72

is taken as the end vertebra. In a curve, the disc spaces are narrower on the curve concavity and wider on the convexity. In the transitional area between two curves the disc space next to the end vertebra is usually a parallel disc space. The end vertebrae are shared by adjacent curves; the lower end vertebra of one curve is the upper end vertebra of the next caudal curve. The curves, in a double thoracic and lumbar curve pattern, are thus T4-T12 right thoracic and T12-L4 left lumbar.

After the upper and lower end vertebra of each curve are identified, the curves are measured using the Cobb-Lippman technique.[10] A line is drawn at the upper end of the cranial end vertebra along the endplate or by marking the upper or lower margin of the pedicles. A line is then drawn at right angles to the vertebral line. A line is then drawn at the lower end of the caudal vertebra of the curve, using the end plate or pedicles. The pedicles are used when they are better visualized than the endplates. A right angle to this line is then drawn, (Fig. 5–20B). The angle to be measured is the angle formed by the two lines at the end vertebrae. Using the simple geometrical method with the right angle lines, the angle formed by these lines is measured, giving the magnitude of the curve (Fig. 5–20C). Only when large curves are measured is it possible to directly measure the angle formed by the end vertebral lines (Fig. 5–20D). This measurement technique has been shown to be highly accurate. Studies with the same examiner repeating measurements or with different examiners measuring the same films shows an error of no more than 3 degrees.[5, 24, 30, 36, 47] In addition, measurements of an anteroposterior versus a posteroanterior film have been compared and fall in the same error range.[13]

Vertebral Rotation[1, 40]

The shadows of the pedicles demonstrate the degree of vertebral rotation present. The amount of rotation of the apical vertebra of the curve is graded using the system described by Nash and Moe.[40] The rotation is divided into five grades, zero to IV (Fig. 5–21A). Zero rotation occurs when the pedicle shadows are symmetrical and equidistant from the sides of the vertebral body. In Grade I rotation, the pedicle shadow or the convexity has moved away from the side of the vertebral body. In Grade III rotation, the convex pedicle shadow is situated in the middle of the vertebrae, Grade II rotation is intermediate between Grades I and III. In Grade IV rotation the convex pedicle shadow is past the center of the vertebral body and closer to the concavity of the curve. The end vertebra of a curve is usually not rotated, but occasionally rotation in a curve continues beyond the end vertebra. This occurs more commonly on the caudal end on a curve. Alternate methods of measuring curve rotation have been described by Pedriolle (Fig. 5–21B),[41] Coetsier and coworkers,[11] and Bunnel.[8]

After the curves have been measured, the vertebral levels of the end vertebrae are marked on the radiograph. These must be counted carefully, as often there are 11 or 13 ribs. The correct vertebral level is more accurate if it counted from the cranial end to the caudal end. The magnitude of the curve and the end vertebrae are written on the radiograph with a soft-tip lead pencil, which is easily erasable from the radiograph using alcohol sponges. In addition, the patient's name, age, and date of the examination are written on the radiograph, usually in an area where they are easily seen—the upper ab-

---

Figure 5–20. Curve measurement. A, The first step is the identification of the end vertebrae; the last vertebra on each end that is tilted into the concavity of the curve cave is measured. The next vertebra tilts away from the curve concavity. The disc spaces are narrower on the concavity of the curve and parallel next to the end vertebra. T6 and T12 are the end vertebrae. B, A line is drawn at the lower end plate of T12 and a perpendicular line is drawn to this line. An alternate line at the lower end of the pedicles is shown. C, The procedure is repeated by drawing a line perpendicular to the upper end plate of T6, and the angles between the two perpendiculars are measured with a protractor. D, In larger curves, the perpendiculars need not be drawn, and the angle formed by the end vertebral lines is measured directly.

A ZERO

B GRADE I

C GRADE II

D GRADE III

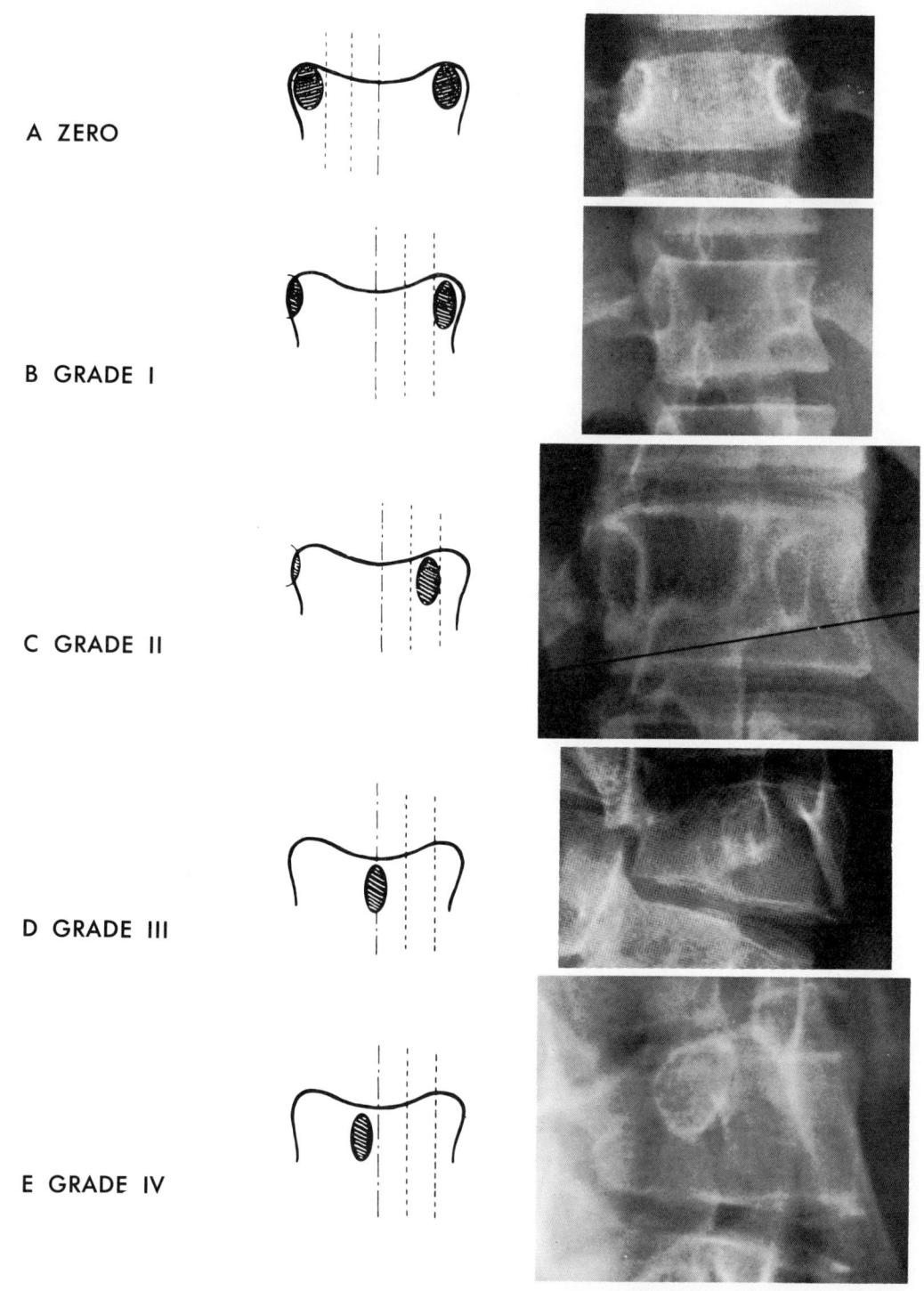

E GRADE IV

Figure 5–21. Evaluation of vertebral rotation. The rotation of the apical vertebra is evaluated using the system described by Nash and Moe. *A*, Zero rotation. The pedicle shadows are equidistant from the sides of the vertebral bodies. *B*, Grade I rotation. The pedicle shadow on the convexity has moved from the edge of the vertebral body. C, Grade II rotation. Rotation intermediate between Grade I and Grade III (*D*) rotation. The pedicle shadow is close to the center of the vertebral body. *E*, Grade IV rotation. The pedicle shadow is past the center of the vertebral body. (Reprinted with permission from Nash, C., and Moe, J.: A study of vertebral rotation. J. Bone Joint Surg., *51A*:223, 1969.)

Illustration continued on opposite page

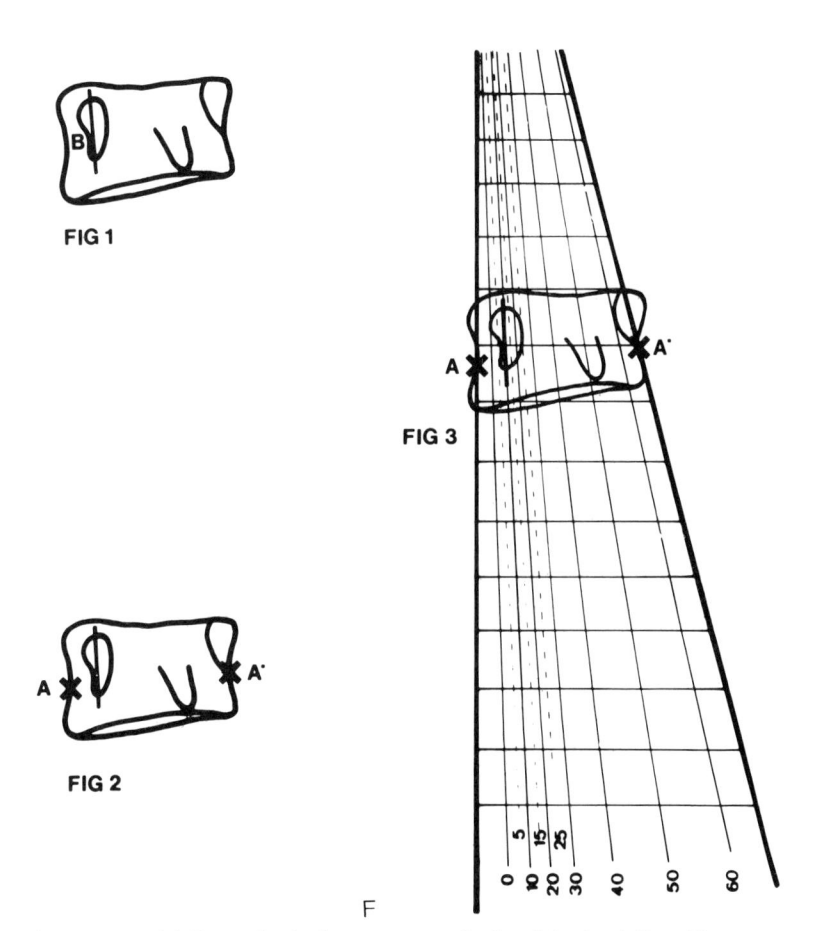

Figure 5–21 *Continued. F,* Pedriolle method of measurement of vertebral rotation. The measurement is made from the pedicle situated at the convexity of the apical vertebra under consideration. *Fig. 1,* Mark the greatest diameter of the pedicle (B). *Fig. 2,* Mark a reference at the waist of each lateral border of the vertebra (A and A'). *Fig. 3,* Superimpose the torsiometer on the vertebra so that the edges of the rule are at the sides of the vertebral body. The amount of rotation of the pedicle line is read from the rotation scale, 10 degrees in this example. (Redrawn from Pedriolle, R.: La Scoliose. Maloine, S. A. editeur, Paris, 1979.)

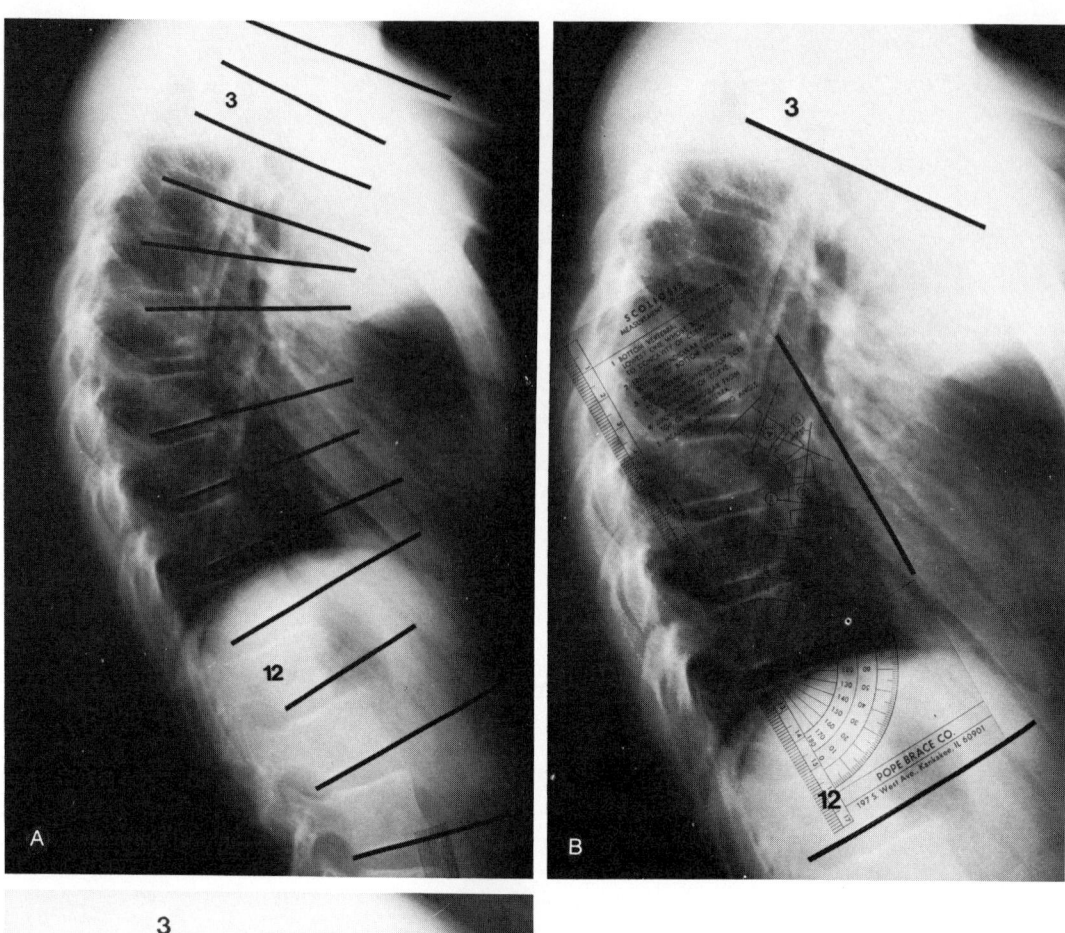

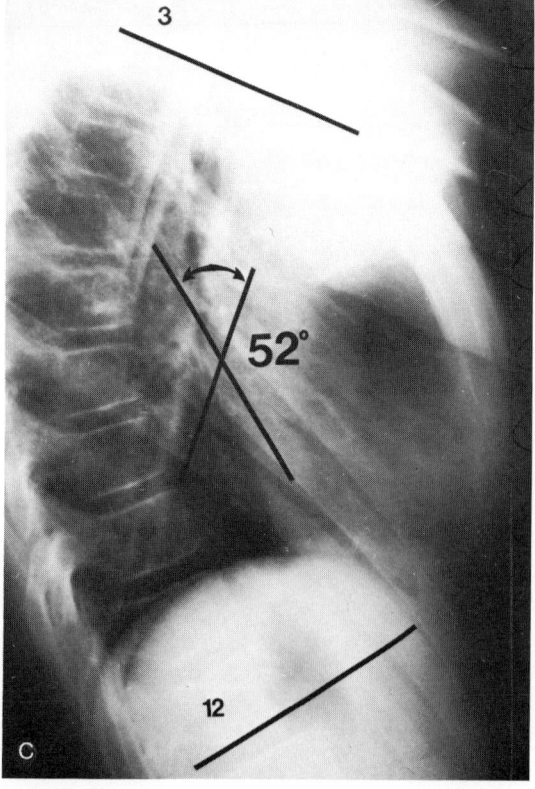

Figure 5–22. Kyphosis measurement. *A*, The end vertebrae are identified. These vertebrae are the last vertebrae that are tilted into the concavity of the kyphosis; the next vertebrae tilt away from the concavity. The end vertebrae are T3 and T12. *B*, A line is drawn perpendicular to the lower end plate of T12. *C*, A similar line is drawn perpendicular to the upper end plate of T3. The angle formed by these lines is measured.

domen or the pelvic area where the radiograph is lighter.

The lateral radiograph is measured in the same way, the end vertebrae are best identified as those vertebrae maximally tilted into the concavity of the curve (Fig. 5–22). All kyphotic angles are measured as positive (+) curves and all lordotic curves as negative (−), zero degrees being a straight spine. This system gives a standard nomenclature for curve evaluation.

In congenital anomalies, the description of the radiograph and anatomy are important, especially with reference to vertebral numbering in the case of a hemivertebra. All vertebrae, including any hemivertebrae, are numbered in a craniocaudal direction (Fig. 5–23). Thus in the case of a midthoracic hemivertebra, the anomaly is described as "a hemivertebra on the left at T9" *not* as "a hemivertebra on the left between T8 and T9." In difficult complex anomalies, evaluation of the ribs is important, since fewer ribs are present on the side opposite a hemivertebra, and vertebral body segmentation defects are often associated with congenital rib synostosis.

When all the curves have been identified and measured on the upright radiographs, the flexibility films are measured. The end vertebrae, identified on the upright view, are constant for the remainder of the radiographic evaluation. In addition, *these end vertebrae are constant for the remainder of the patient's treatment course.* The occasional exception is for curves treated orthotically, when the brace shortens the curves the shortened curve is measured subsequently. The other exception is in small curves that are followed for progression. Often the end vertebrae on these curves vary from one examination to the next.

The end vertebrae are identified on the flexibility views, and the curve is measured by the same method as before. In some cases the ends of the curve are more flexible than the apical segment, but the *whole* curve identified on the upright radiograph is measured. In these cases a note is made that the apical segment is less flexible, and this apical segment can be measured separately. In very flexible curves overcorrection is possible, which can be documented as a negative amount, for example, a 20 degree curve overcorrecting to −5 degrees. Only the side bending view towards the convexity of the curve is measured (i.e., the right side bending of a right thoracic curve). If any radiograph shows the left side bending of this curve, this bending is *not* measured. Similar measures are used for all flexibility evaluations—hyperextension for kyphosis and hyperflexion for lordosis and the traction film.

MATURITY

Bone Age

Bone age is evaluated on a radiograph of the left wrist and hand on all patients under the age of 18. The radiograph is compared to standards in the Greulich and Pyle Atlas.[23]

Iliac Epiphyses

The ossification of the iliac epiphysis is evaluated as originally described by Risser.[44]

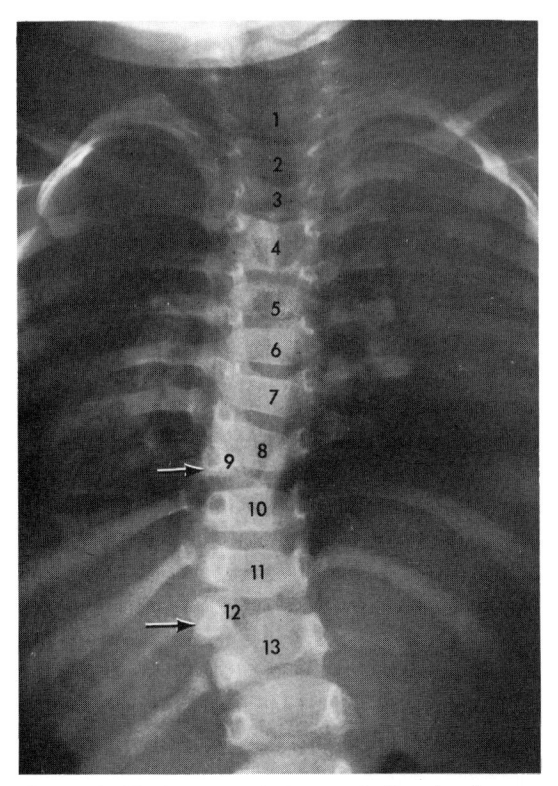

Figure 5–23. Anteroposterior projection to demonstrate numbering of hemivertebrae. There are two hemivertebrae on the left, and the vertebrae are numbered from cranial to caudal, each hemivertebra being numbered.

Ossification normally starts at the anterior superior iliac spine and progresses posteriorly to the posterior superior iliac spine. Once complete excursion of the ossification has occurred, fusion to the iliac crest occurs. Risser divided the excursion into four quarters—1 is 25 per cent excursion, 2 is 50 per cent, 3 is 75 per cent, 4 is complete excursion, and 5 is fusion to the ilium (Fig. 5–24). Zaoussis and James[51] found the range of time for completion of ossification was large, from 7 months to 3.5 years; 2 years was the average. The chronological age at appearance also varied, averaging 14.25 years in girls (range 11 to 18 years) and 15.4 years in boys (range 12.8 to 17.5 years). A Risser sign of 4 correlates with the cessation of spinal growth, and Anderson and coworkers have shown that a Risser sign of 5 correlates with cessation of height increase.[3]

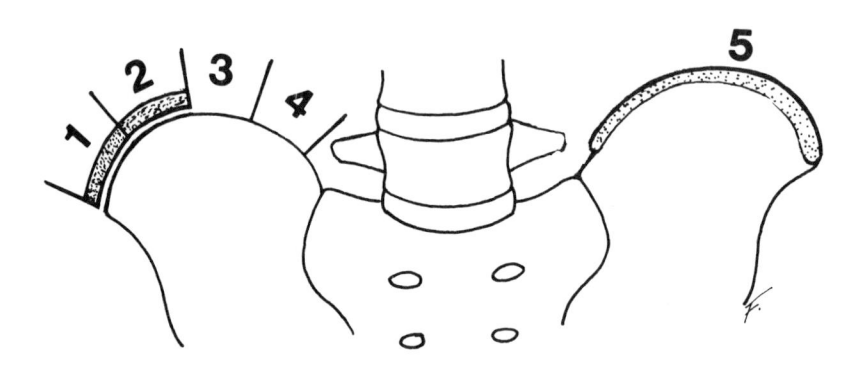

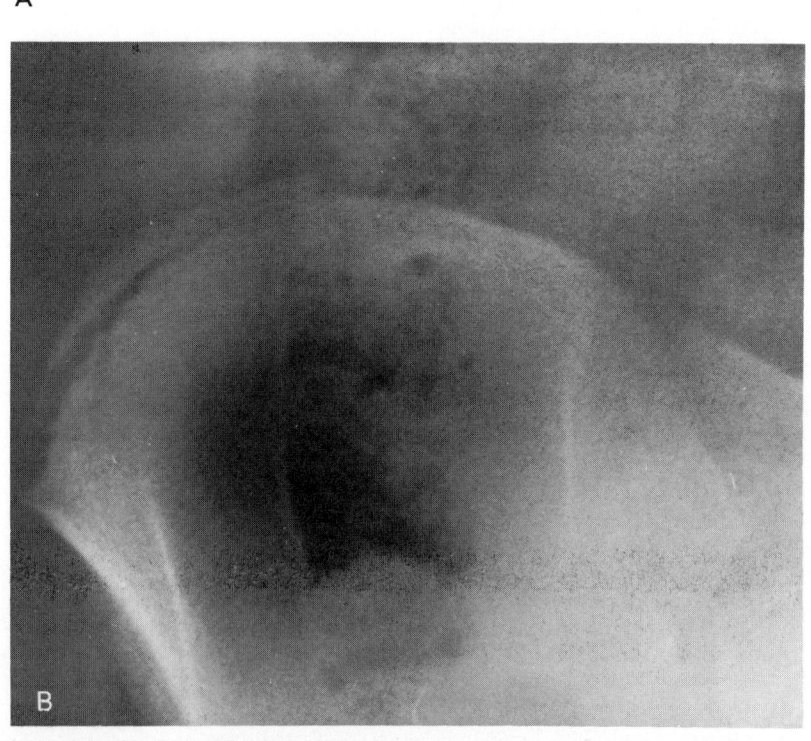

Figure 5–24. Iliac epiphysis. A, Ossification of the epiphysis usually starts at the anterior superior iliac spine and progresses posteriorly. The iliac crest is divided into four quarters, and the excursion or stage of maturity is designated as the amount of progression. In the example shown, the excursion is 50 per cent complete, and the Risser sign is thus 2. On the right, the excursion is complete and the epiphysis has fused with the iliac crest—a Risser 5. B, A Risser 2 excursion.

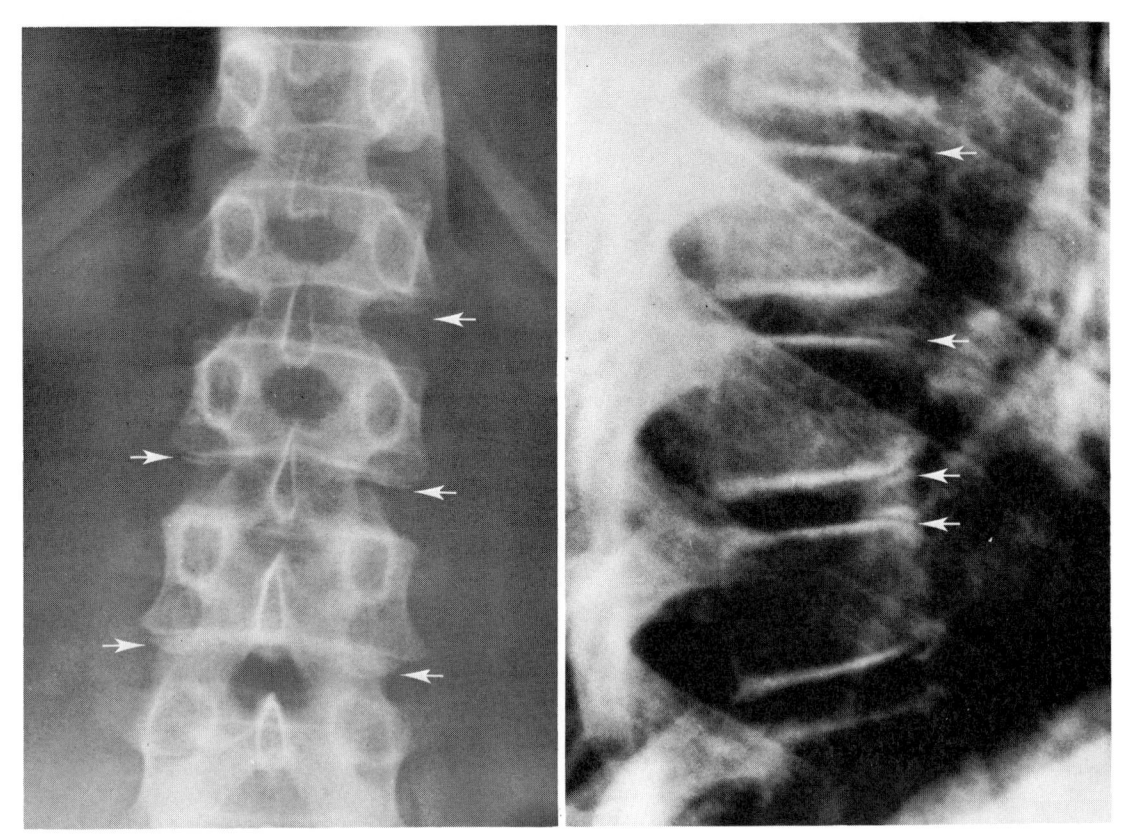

Figure 5–25. Anteroposterior and lateral x-ray films showing ring apophysis ossification adjacent to the vertebral end plates (*arrows*). The ossification is more easily seen on the lateral view.

Vertebral Ring Apophysis

The vertebral ring apophyses lie at the upper and lower margins of the vertebral body, overlying the cartilage growth plate. These initially appear as a separate secondary ossification center, and form a complete ring that fuses to the vertebral body (Fig. 5–25). They are seen most clearly on the lateral radiograph, but can be seen on the posteroanterior or anteroposterior projection. Fusion of the apophysis with the vertebral endplate indicates cessation of all vertebral body growth potential.

SPECIAL RADIOGRAPHIC STUDIES

In the evaluation and treatment of spinal deformities, special radiographic studies are occasionally necessary. These include laminogram, myelogram, CT scan (computerized tomography), discogram, intravenous pyelogram, "Rib hump" view, angiogram, and upper gastrointestinal evaluation.

Laminogram

A laminogram (tomogram) is used in cases in which the plain radiographs do not show good anatomic detail. It is thus used to delineate the anatomy in congenital spine anomalies, in some cases of anterior fusion to visualize the incorporation of bone graft, and in some cases to visualize anatomy poorly seen on plain radiographs (Fig. 5–26). The laminogram is obtained by having the x-ray source and x-ray plate moving during the exposure; only a specific area is in focus, and the remainder of the body is out of focus. By varying the focal point, a series of radiographic views or "cuts" .5 or 1.0 cm. apart are obtained of the desired area. In some cases the sagittal reconstruction in comput-

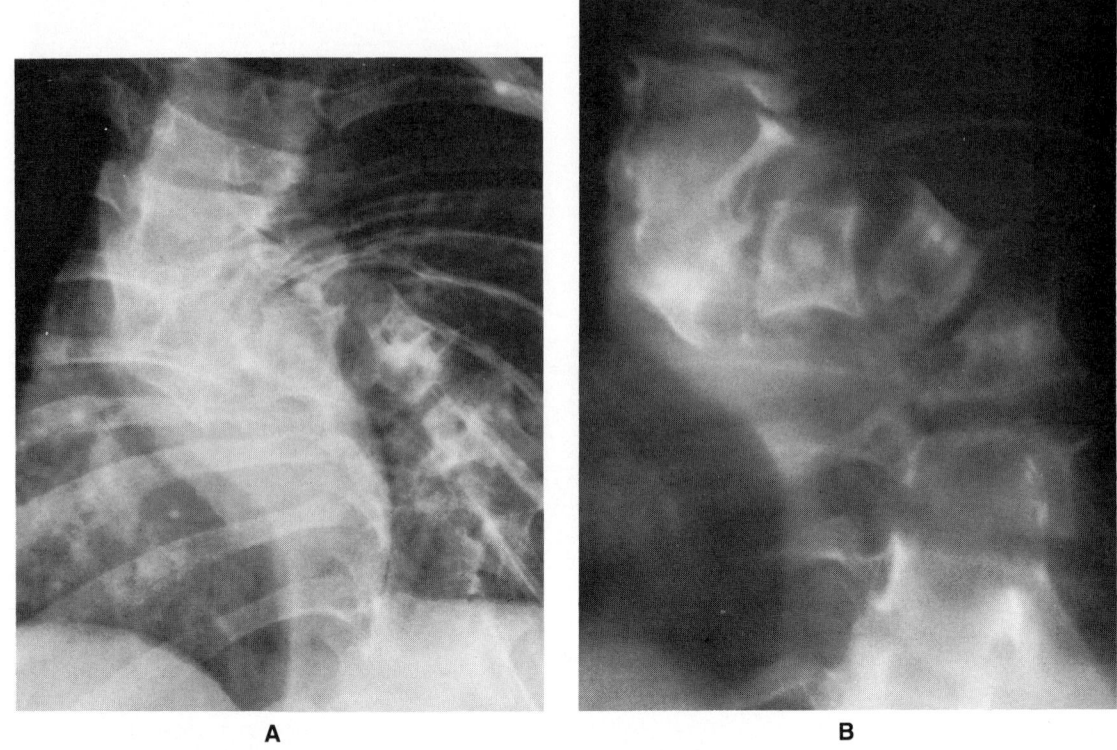

Figure 5–26. *A*, Anteroposterior x-ray of a case of a neurofibromatosis spine deformity. The vertebral anatomy is poorly visualized. *B*, Anteroposterior laminogram demonstrates the severe vertebral dysplasia caused by the neurofibromatosis.

erized tomography has replaced the laminogram (see subsequent section).

Myelogram (Spinogram)

A myelogram is not obtained in all cases of spine deformity, but rather in special cases. If widening of the interpediculate distance is seen, with or without erosion of pedicles, a myelogram is obtained to make the diagnosis (spinal dysraphism, diastematomyelia, syringomyelia, spinal cord tumor) (Fig. 5–27).

In cases of compression of the spinal cord, a myelogram will demonstrate the level of compression and will also exclude intradural pathology. Where a spinal cord tumor is suspected, (e.g., abnormal forward bending test or neurologic signs) a myelogram is mandatory.

A myelogram is also performed for cases in which a wedge excision of the spine for excision of a hemivertebra or correction of a severe deformity is planned. In these cases knowledge of the anatomy of the spinal canal is necessary. In congenital spine deformities, if there are any skin stigmata of a spinal dysraphism (hair patch, skin pigmentation, skin dimple), or any lower limb neurologic signs or foot deformity, or where distraction of the spine is planned, a myelogram is indicated.

Pantopaque or water soluble dyes can be used. When oil-based dyes (Hypaque or Pantopaque) are used to adequately visualize the canal to diagnose intraspinal pathology or spinal cord compression, large volumes of

---

Figure 5–27. Use of myelography. *A*, Metrizamide myelogram in a case of diastematomyelia showing the midline spur and split cord in this area. *B*, Metrizamide myelogram in a case of spinal dysraphism showing the low lying conus (dotted line) and the thick filum terminale (arrows). *C*, CT cut with metrizamide myelogram at the level of a fibrous septum splitting the spinal cord.

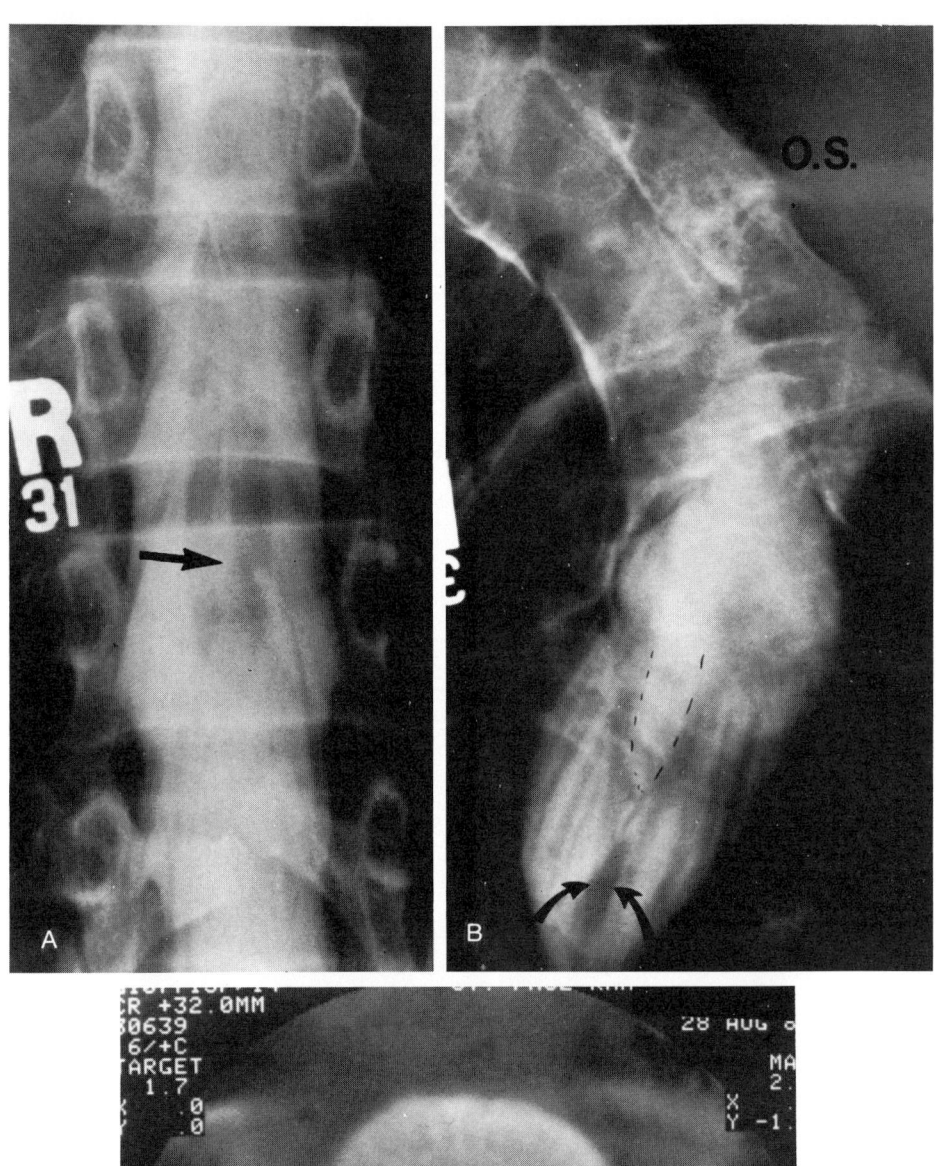

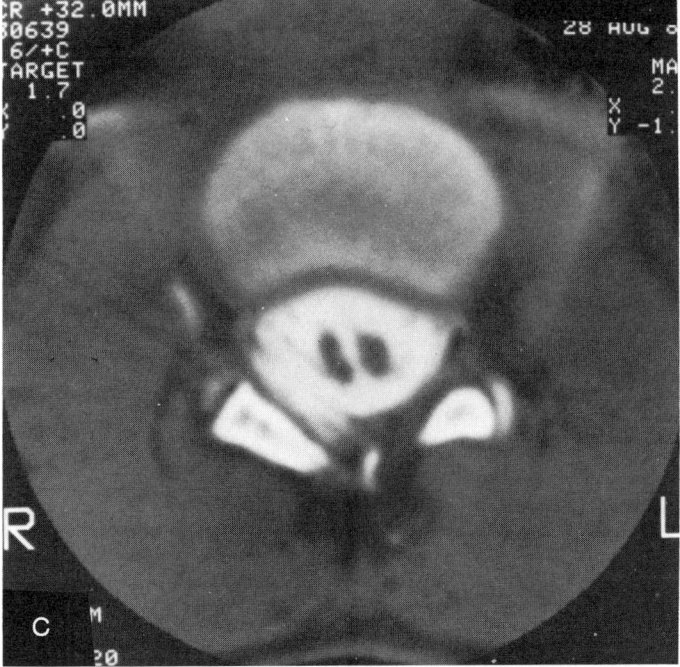

Figure 5–27. See legend on opposite page

dye, up to 90 cc., are used. This technique, developed by Gold and Leach,[20] adequately fills the subarachnoid space so that adequate visualization of pathology is obtained. In addition, it may be necessary to remove the needle after the dye is introduced so that the patient can be turned supine. In this position the dye pools in the area of a kyphotic deformity, allowing adequate visualization of the dural sac in the area of the kyphosis. Using this technique any obstruction to the dye column or intraspinal pathology in the area of the kyphosis is visualized. This technique also allows visualization of the distal sac and is useful in cases of spinal dysraphism.[42]

Water-soluble dyes are also used, but are not as useful as oil-based dyes in the upper thoracic or cervical area. These dyes are very useful in the thoracolumbar or lumbar areas and are commonly used in the evaluation of painful adult scoliosis with radiculopathy. In all myelograms performed in the presence of scoliosis, rotated or oblique views are necessary to demonstrate the anatomy and allow visualization of the unrotated subarachnoid space.[14, 37]

In very heavy or obese patients or in those in whom difficulty in obtaining an adequate radiograph of the myelogram is experienced, laminograms performed with the dye in place will help visualize the dye column. Computerized tomography performed with the dye in place is very useful in cases of spinal cord compression or intraspinal pathology to visualize the area of pathology and help plan the treatment approach (see Fig. 5–27C).

Air myelography is performed in some

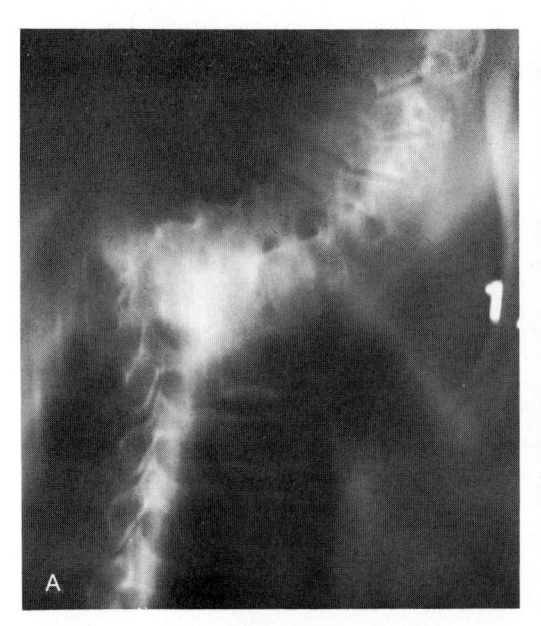

Figure 5–28. Use of CT scan and myelography in a case of spinal cord compression in a 13 + 6 year old boy with healed tuberculosis and paraparesis. A, The lateral laminogram shows the high thoracic kyphosis but the spinal canal anatomy is not well seen. B, A metrizamide myelogram was performed with computerized tomography. This CT cut at the apex of the kyphosis shows the large spinal canal, but the dural sac and spinal cord are tight against the vertebral body and the cord compression is well seen. C, A sagittal reconstruction of the CT shows the apical anatomy with the kyphosis and the spinal cord tight against the body at the apex of the kyphosis.

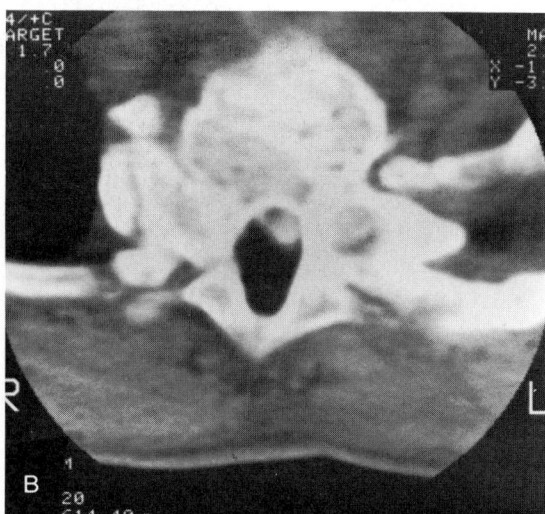

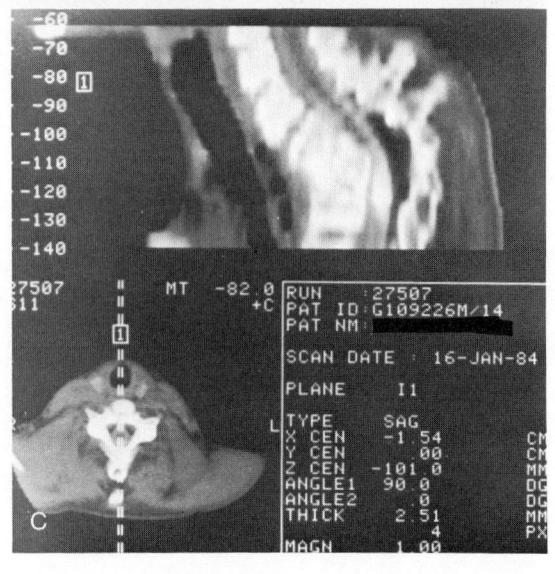

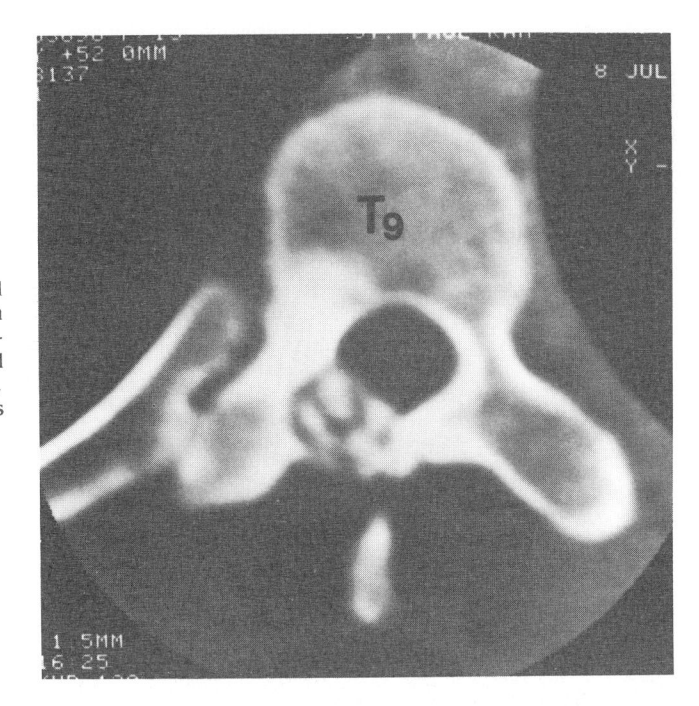

Figure 5–29. CT scan in a case of osteoid osteoma. The sclerotic pedicle was well seen on the plain radiographs. The CT scan localizes the tumor to the lamina so that a limited approach is possible to remove the nidus, and removal of the pedicle and facets is thus unnecessary.

centers; it is a very safe procedure that provides excellent visualization of the dural sac. We have little experience with this technique. However, it is being replaced by computerized tomography or by magnetic resonance imaging.

CT Scan (Computerized Tomography)[17, 24]

Computerized tomography is a useful technique in difficult cases. In cases of spinal cord compression or scoliosis with radiculopathy, the CT scan will demonstrate the area of compression of the neural tissue. In most cases this visualization is improved if the CT scan is performed after the myelogram with the myelographic dye still present. This addition of contrast shows the compression of the dural sac and of the spinal cord whereas the view without dye shows only encroachment into the spinal canal (Fig. 5–28). The CT scan is also useful in cases of bone tumors, either to accurately localize a benign lesion such as an osteoid osteoma so that the surgical approach can be planned (Fig. 5–29) or to visualize the extent of bony destruction with metastatic disease.

CT's ability to reconstruct the sagittal view of the spine is invaluable. It is used in the assessment of neural tissue cord compression, for example, root compression in adult scoliosis or spinal cord compression due to deformity. The reconstruction gives better detail of the anatomy than does lateral tomography, with a lower dose of irradiation. When performed after a metrizamide myelogram, the anatomic detail is improved (see Fig. 5–28C).

Magnetic Resonance Imaging (MRI)

This new technique has the ability to demonstrate spine and cord anatomy and pathology with great detail. Spinal cord tumors, syringomyelia, and bone lesions are seen in detail, with their extents well documented.

Discogram

Discography has proved to be useful in the assessment of painful adult lumbar or thoracolumbar scoliosis. It helps identify the source of pain, particularly in cases with unusual pain patterns, such as (1) pain above or below the curve, (2) lumbosacral pain, (3) pain in discs below a previous fusion, and (4), pain in discs above a previous lumbosacral fusion. In these discograms, the radiographic appearance is far less important than the symptoms reproduced on injection of the dye. In adults, discography will demonstrate a high percentage of degenerative discs, with or without dye leakage. If, on injection of the dye, pain occurs with the same character, site, and radiation as the patient's symptoms, then that disc is a source of the patient's problem.

Discograms are performed in painful adult scoliosis to help in the decision making process. In unusual pain problems, it is used to localize the source of the pain. In decision making it is used in the lumbosacral area to determine the extent of the fusion (see Chapter 17).

Intravenous Pyelogram (Urogram)

Because of the high incidence of renal tract anomalies associated with congenital spine deformities, an intravenous pyelogram is mandatory for all patients with congenital spine anomalies.[33, 46] The intravenous pyelogram is performed in the routine manner, with light anesthesia (Ketamine) being used in small children and infants.

An intravenous pyelogram is also used in cases of bladder paralysis (myelodysplasia, paraplegia) to evaluate the renal tract. The presence of any obstruction is seen as well as the anatomy of the kidneys, renal calyces, and ureters (Fig. 5–30).

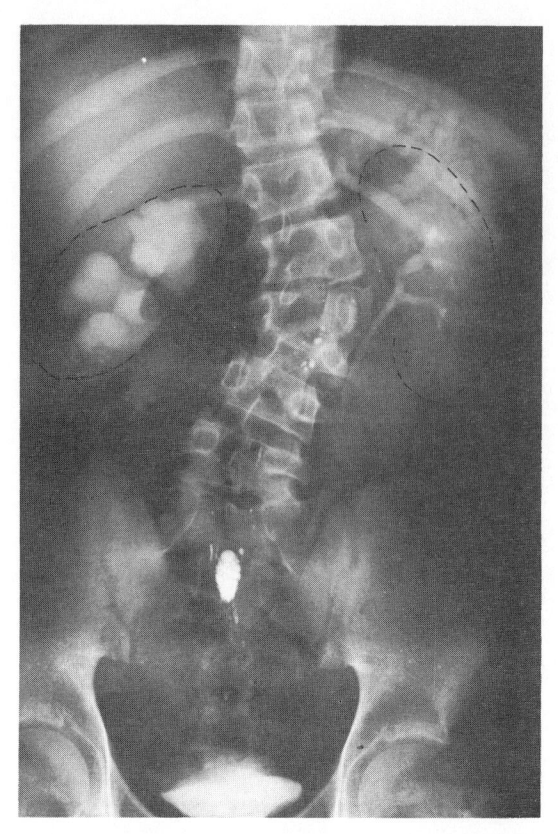

Figure 5–30. Sixteen year old boy diagnosed as having scoliosis on a routine school screening examination. The hemivertebra at L3 is seen. A routine intravenous pyelogram was performed and demonstrates the marked hydronephrosis on the right due to uterovesical obstruction. This congenital obstruction was treated surgically. The reduction of renal parenchyma on the right is also seen. (Reprinted with permission from Lonstein, J. E. et al.: School screening for the early detection of spine deformities. Minn. Med., 59:51, 1976.)

Tangential ("Rib Hump") View of the Rib Deformity

When surgery is performed on the rib prominence to reduce it, a tangential view

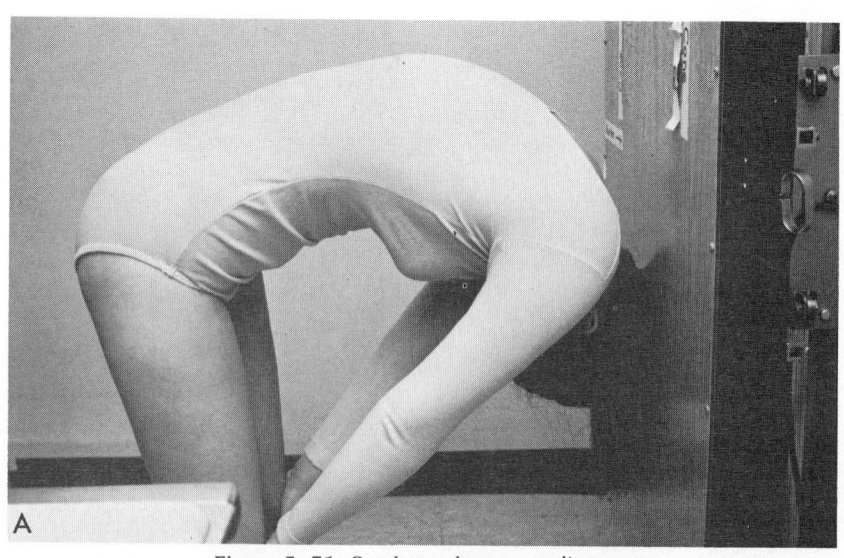

Figure 5–31. See legend on opposite page

Illustration continued on opposite page

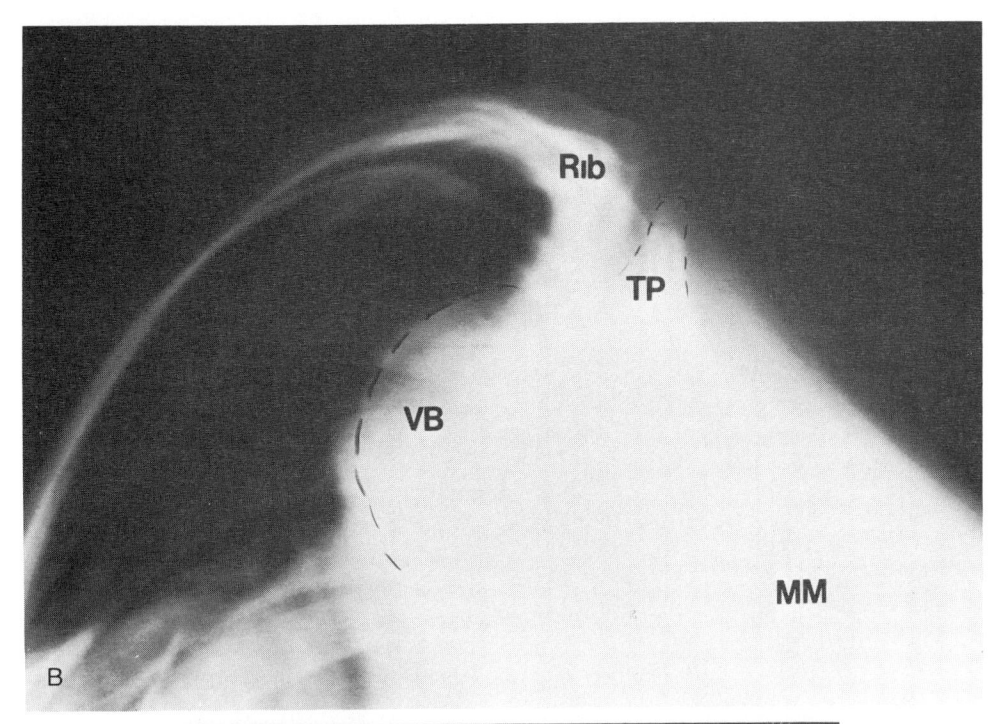

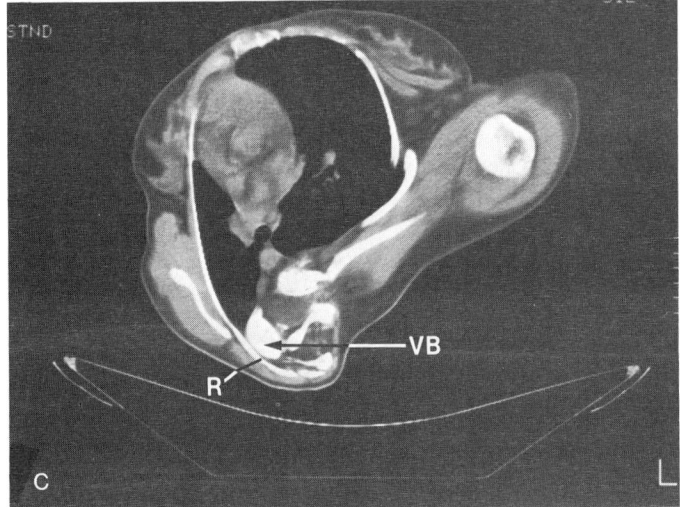

Figure 5–31. *A*, Tangential view of rib deformity. The patient bends forward and leans against the x-ray cassette. The x-ray beam is directed tangentially across the back. *B*, Tangential view of a severe rib prominence. Note the rotation of the vertebral body (*VB*) and the transverse process (*TP*) directed posteriorly. The marked upward slope of the head of the rib is well seen. *C*, Single CT cut at the apex of a rib prominence shows the anatomy, with the marked rotation of the vertebral body (*VB*) and the rib (*R*) adjacent to the body.

will demonstrate the prominence radiographically, showing the relationship of the vertebral body to the ribs. This view is taken with the patient bending forward, leaning on the cassette, and the x-ray beam directed tangentially across the back (Fig. 5–31*A* and *B*). A similar relationship of the ribs and vertebrae can be seen on a single CT cut taken at the apex of the spine deformity (Fig. 5–31*C*).

Angiogram[29]

A spinal cord angiogram has been used in some cases of spinal deformity. In the past

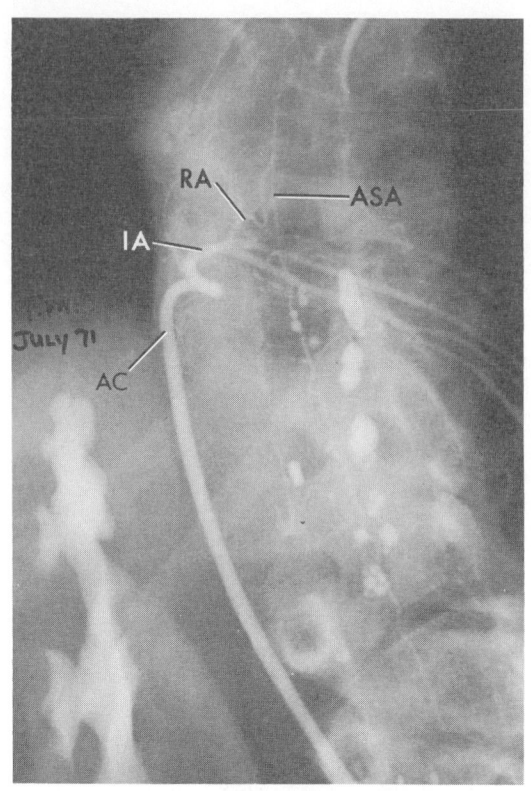

Figure 5–32. Anterior spinal artery angiogram. Retrograde arterial catheter (*AC*) is positioned in an intercostal artery (*IA*), which is well visualized. The radicular artery (*RA*) is a branch of the intercostal artery and supplies the anterior spinal artery (*ASA*).

intercostals bilaterally in the area under evaluation (Fig. 5–32). The dangers are damage to the intercostal artery or the femoral artery because of repeated manipulation of the intra-arterial catheter.

Upper Gastrointestinal Evaluation

The use of an upper GI evaluation is necessary in patients with suspected vascular obstruction of the duodenum (see Chapter 22). A Gastrografin (not barium) swallow is used to evaluate the outflow obstruction of the second part of the duodenum. Gastrografin is used because if vomiting and aspiration occur there is no irritation of the bronchial tree, whereas barium is very irritating to the lungs. The radiographs confirm the obstruction and also help differentiate between a complete and a partial obstruction (Fig. 5–33).

its use has been recommended for the evaluation of the site of the main blood supply of the spinal cord, the Artery of Adamkiewicz.[15] Some people have recommended its use in intraspinal space–occupying lesions or with cord compression. Because of the dangers of the procedure and the minimal additional knowledge gained in routine cases, we feel the procedure has few indications. It is useful in cases of an intraspinal vascular anomaly or a very vascular intraspinal or bone tumor. In these cases, a knowledge of the blood supply of the lesion for planning of the surgical approach or for embolization of feeding vessels is essential. There is wide variation in the blood supply of the cord, with no single feeding artery as has been shown by Dommisse.[15, 16] In addition, he demonstrated the numerous anastomoses at each level.

A transfemoral approach is used with retrograde cannulation of the aorta and cannulation of each intercostal artery. Dye is injected at each level and appropriate radiographs taken, with evaluation of the

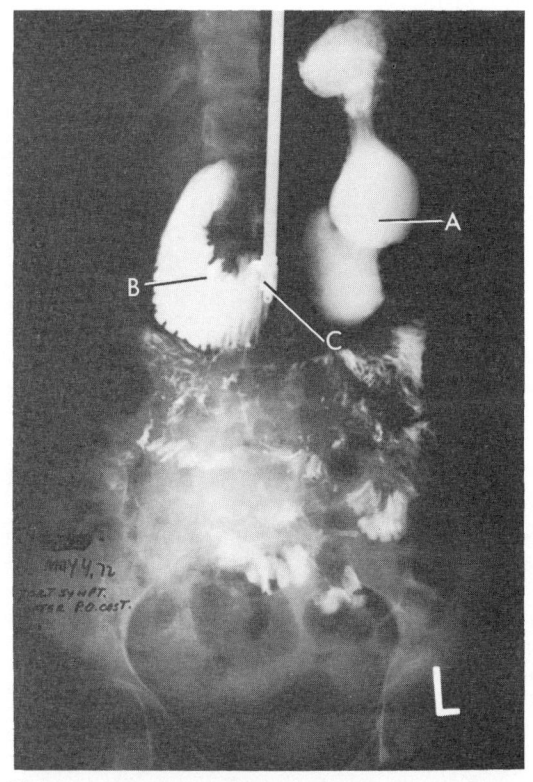

Figure 5–33. Gastrografin swallow in a 16-year old girl with vascular obstruction of the duodenum. One week postoperatively, after being placed in a postoperative cast and ambulated, she had nausea and vomiting. A Gastrografin swallow shows the slight distention of the stomach (*A*) and the marked distention of the duodenum (*B*). The obstruction is partial and at the third part of the duodenum (*C*). The cast was removed and the patient kept supine. A nasogastric tube was used to decompress the stomach, and resolution of the obstruction followed.

LABORATORY TESTS

The laboratory currently plays a very minor role in the diagnosis of the etiology of spinal deformities. In unusual cases in which a mucopolysaccharidosis or homocystinuria is suspected appropriate urine tests are helpful.

Laboratory tests play a larger role in the surgical treatment of patients with spinal deformities. Preoperative routine evaluation of hemoglobin and hematocrit and on urinalysis are essential in all cases. For adults, in addition, a BUN, creatinine, electrolytes, and electrocardiogram are ordered as necessary. In myelodysplasia and in cases of paralytic bladders, a knowledge of renal function and urine cultures are required preoperatively. If an infection is suspected a white cell count, differential count, and sedimentation rate are necessary. If the infection is postoperative, serial tests are necessary, as the results may be elevated owing to the surgical trauma alone.

PULMONARY FUNCTION EVALUATION

Pulmonary function evaluation and testing are important parts of patient assessment and are discussed fully in Chapter 22.

DOCUMENTATION

The accurate recording of all findings in the care of a patient with scoliosis is of utmost importance. Such documentation permits evaluation of the various treatment modalities available.

All pertinent findings on initial evaluation must be accurately recorded. All measurable physical findings should be noted. Documentation of findings such as "a little decompensation," "a moderately large rib prominence," or "right shoulder slightly elevated" is worthless without numerical amounts. It is impossible to compare the effect of treatment unless values are given to all measurable entities and the results recorded.

Dr. Paul Harrington developed a data storage and retrieval system utilizing electronic data procesing (computer). The system stores the data about the patient's history, physical examination, radiologic evaluation, surgical treatment, and response to surgery. This system has been expanded in the Twin Cities to include patients treated nonoperatively. Information about all patients treated by the authors has been placed on coding forms and stored for evaluation and retrieval utilizing electronic data processing. With the addition of the current status of the surgical, brace, and nontreated patients, a long-term evaluation of these groups will be possible.

The radiograph forms the basis for the treatment of all spinal deformities. All films should be marked with the patient's name, date of examination, and position of evaluation (see Fig. 5–8). In addition, the curves should be measured and the results recorded on the radiograph. These figures should also be recorded on the treatment chart, eliminating ambiguities such as "slight improvement," "a little loss of correction," or "a few degrees change." In addition, we place the pertinent radiographs of each patient in a special summary folder (see Fig. 5–8). This facilitates storage and retrieval of the important radiographs and allows easy comparison of current radiographs with the original presenting deformity so that progression or the effect of therapy, bracing, or surgery may be evaluated. We prefer not to destroy radiographs or transfer them to microfilm, but rather to keep and store all radiographs.

References

1. Aaro, S., and Dahlborn, M.: Vertebral rotation—estimation of vertebral rotation and spinal and rib cage deformity in scoliosis by computerized tomography. Spine, 6:460–467, 1981.
2. Andersen, P. E., Jr., Andersen, P. E., and van der Kooy, P.: Dose reduction in radiography of the spine in scoliosis. Acta. Radiol. [Diagn.], 23:251–253, 1982.
3. Anderson, M., Hwan, S., and Green, W. T.: Growth of the normal trunk in boys and girls during the second decade of life. J. Bone Joint Surg., 47A:1554, 1965.
4. Bachmann, M.: Die Varanderugen des Innern Ograne Bei Hochgradiger Skoliosen and Kyphoskoliosen. Stuttgart, 1899.
5. Beckman, C. E., and Hall, V.: Variability of scoliosis measurement from spinal roentgenograms. Phys. Ther., 59:764–765, 1979.
6. Binstadt, D. H., Lonstein, J. E., and Winter, R. B.: Radiographic evaluation of the scoliotic patient. Minn. Med., 61:474–478, 1978.
7. Board, R.: Radiography of the scoliotic spine. Radiol. Technol., 38:219, 1967.
8. Bunnell, W. P.: Vertebral rotation—a simple method of measurement in routine radiographs. Ortho. Trans. 9:114, 1985.
9. Calliet, R.: Scoliosis: Diagnosis and Management. Philadelphia, F. A. Davis Co., 1979.
10. Cobb, J. R.: Outline for the Study of Scoliosis in Instructional Course Lectures. The American

Academy of Orthopaedic Surgeons, Vol. 5, Ann Arbor, MI., J. W. Edwards Co., 1948.
11. Coetsier, M., Vercauteren, M., and Moerman, P.: A new radiographic method for measuring vertebral rotation in scoliosis. Acta. Orthop. Belg., 43:598–605, 1977.
12. DeSmet, A., Fritz, S. L., and Asher, M. A.: A method for minimizing the radiation exposure from scoliosis radiographs. J. Bone Joint Surg., 63A:156, 1981.
13. DeSmet, A. A., Goin, J. E., Asher, M. A., and Scheuch, H. G.: A clinical study of the differences between the scoliotic angles measured on PA vs. AP radiographs. J. Bone Joint Surg., 64A:489–493, 1982.
14. Devkota, J., Gammal, T. E., and Lucke, J. F.: Measurement of the normal cervical cord by metrizamide myelography. South. Med. J. 75:1363–1365, 1982.
15. Dommisse, G. F.: The blood supply of the spinal cord. J. Bone Joint Surg., 56B:225, 1974.
16. Dommisse, G. F.: The Arteries and Veins of the Human Spinal Cord from Birth. Edinburgh, Churchill Livingstone, 1975.
17. Donavan-Post, M. J.: Radiographic Evaluation of the Spine—Current Advances with Emphasis on Computer Tomography. New York, Masson Publishers, 1980.
18. Drummond, D., Ranallo, F., Lonstein, J. E., et al.: Radiation hazards in scoliosis management. Spine, 8:741–748, 1983.
19. Farren, J.: Routine radiographic assessment of the scoliotic spine. Radiography, 47:92–96, 1981.
20. Gold, L., Leach, D., Kieffer, S. A., et al.: Large volume myelography. Radiology, 97:531, 1970.
21. Gray, J. E., Hoffman, A. D., and Peterson, H. A.: Reduction of radiation exposure during radiography for scoliosis. J. Bone Joint Surg., 65A:5–12, 1983.
22. Gregg, E. C.: Radiation risks with diagnostic x-rays. Radiology, 123:447–453, 1977.
23. Greulich, W. W., and Pyle, S. I.: Radiographic Atlas of Skeletal Development of the Hand and Wrist, 2nd ed. Stanford, CA., Stanford University Press, 1959.
24. Gross, C., Gross, M., and Kuschner, S.: Error analysis of scoliosis curve measurement. Bull. Hosp. Jt. Dis. Orthop. Inst., 43:171–177, 1983.
25. Hinck, V. C., Clark, W. M., and Hopkins, C. E.: Normal interpediculate distances (minimum and maximum) in children and adults. Am. J. Roentgenol. Radium Ther. Nucl. Med. 97:141–153, 1966.
26. Hippocrates: On the Articulations. In Adams, F. (trans.): The Genuine Works of Hippocrates, Vol. 2. London, Sudenham Society, 1849.
27. Hopkins, R., Grundy, M., and Sherr-Mehl, M.: X-ray filters in scoliosis x-rays. Orthop. Trans., 8:148, 1984.
28. Houston, C. S.: Radiologists and thoughtful use of radiation. Can. Assoc. Radiol. J., 28:2, 1977.
29. Keim, H. A., and Hilal, S. K.: Spinal angiography in scoliosis patients. J. Bone Joint Surg., 53A:904, 1971.
30. Kittleson, A. C., and Lim, L. W.: Measurement of scoliosis. Am. J. Roentgenol., 108:775, 1970.
31. Kleinman, R. E., Csongradi, J. J., Rinsky, L. A., and Bleck, E. E.: A radiographic assessment of spinal flexibility in scoliosis. Clin. Orthop., 162:47–53, 1982.
32. Lonstein, J. E., Winter, R. B., Moe, J. H., et al.: School screening for the early detection of spine deformities. Minn. Med., 59:51, 1976.
33. MacEwen, G., Winter, R., and Hardy, J.: Evaluation of kidney anomalies in congenital scoliosis. J. Bone Joint Surg., 54A:1451, 1972.
34. Marshall, W. A., and Tanner, J. M.: Variations in Pattern of Pubertal Changes in Girls. Arch. Dis. Child., 44:291, 1969.
35. Marshall, W. A., and Tanner, J. M.: Variations in Pattern of Pubertal Changes in Boys. Arch. Dis Child., 45:13, 1970.
36. McAlister, W., and Shackelford, G.: Measurement of spinal curvatures. Radiol. Clin. North Am., 13:113, 1975.
37. McNeill, T. W., Huncke, B., Kornblatt, I., et al.: A new advance in water soluble myelography. Spine, 1:72, 1976.
38. Moe, J., and Kettleson, D.: Idiopathic scoliosis, analysis of curve patterns and the preliminary results of Milwaukee brace treatment in one hundred and sixty-nine patients. J. Bone Joint Surg., 52A:1509, 1970.
39. Nash, C. L., Gregg, E. C., Brown, R. H., and Pillia, M. S.: Risk of exposure to x-rays in patients undergoing long term treatment for scoliosis. J. Bone Joint Surg., 61A:371–380, 1979.
40. Nash, C., and Moe, J.: A study of vertebral rotation. J. Bone Joint Surg., 51A:223, 1969.
41. Pedriolle, R.: La Scoliose. Maloine S. A. Editeur, Paris, 1979.
42. Peterson, H., et al.: Conventional metrizamide myelography and computerized tomographic metrizamide myelography in scoliosis. Radiology, 142:111–114, 1982.
43. Raia, T. J., and Kilfoyle, R. M.: Minimizing radiation exposure in scoliosis screening. Appl. Radiol., 11:45–55, 1982.
44. Risser, J. C.: The iliac apophysis: an invaluable sign in the management of scoliosis. Clin. Orthop., 11:111, 1958.
45. Stagnara, P.: Examen du scoliotique. In Deviations Laterales du Rachis: Scolioses. Encyclopedie Mediocochirurgicale (Paris), Appareil Locomoteur, 7, 1974.
46. Tanner, J. M.: Growth and endocrinology of the adolescent. In Gardner, L. (ed.): Endocrine and Genetic Diseases of Childhood. Philadelphia, W. B. Saunders Co., p. 14, 1975.
47. Vitko, R., Cass, A., and Winter, R.: Anomalies of the genitourinary tract associated with congenital scoliosis and congenital kyphosis. J. Urol., 108:655, 1972.
48. Wilson, M. S., Stockwell, J., and Leedy, M. G.: Measurement of scoliosis by orthopaedic surgeons and radiologists. Aviat. Space Environ. Med., 54:69–71, 1983.
49. Winter, R. B., and Moe, J. H.: A plea for the routine school examination of children for spinal deformity. Minn. Med., 57:419, 1974.
50. Young, L. W., Oestreigh, A. E., and Goldstein, L. A.: Roentgenology in scoliosis: contribution to evaluation and management. Am. J. Roentgenol., 108:778, 1970.
51. Zaoussis, A. L., and James, J. P.: The iliac apophysis and the evaluation of curves in scoliosis. J. Bone Joint Surg., 40A:442–453, 1958.

6
NATURAL HISTORY OF SPINAL DEFORMITY

Robert B. Winter, M.D.

INTRODUCTION

One cannot study the treatment of spinal deformity without first knowing its natural history. If patients with spinal deformities never developed dyspnea, never died early, never developed pain due to the curve, never developed spinal cord or nerve compression, and never developed negative self-image problems, there would be no point in discussing treatment. This however is not the case. The astute physician or surgeon must therefore learn those situations in which the prognosis is benign versus those situations in which the prognosis is poor.

How do we know what the future of a given situation will be? We can learn *only* by studying those who were not treated in the past. Throughout this book we shall endeavor to provide for each etiology the natural history of that etiology. This chapter will deal only with some general topics common to all spinal deformities.

STUDIES OF THE PREVALENCE OF SCOLIOSIS

The prevalence of any condition can be established only by the application of mass screening techniques to large segments of the population. Prevalence refers to the number of individuals in a population having a condition at any one time. Incidence refers to the number of new cases occurring in a given time period. Figures based only on those patients seeking medical attention are quite unreliable.

Two types of prevalance studies have been performed—those based on chest radiographs taken for tuberculosis screening and those based on school screening. Shands and Eiseberg[20] reviewed chest minifilms of 50,000 people and noted scoliosis of 10 degrees or more in 1.9 per cent of those over age 14. Scoliosis of 20 degrees or more was observed in 0.5 per cent. Chest minifilms have the disadvantage of not showing the lumbar spine, but are highly accurate for thoracic scoliosis.

In another minifilm review, Duhaime, Archambault, and Poitras[10] noted scoliosis in 1.1 per cent of 14,886 people. The mean age was 14. Of the 164 patients detected, 108 were personally interviewed. Of these, 107 had idiopathic scoliosis, and the other had a congenital scoliosis. Eight patients had curves over 40 degrees, and 16 had curves of 20 to 39 degrees. The remaining 84 had curves between 5 and 19 degrees. Tulit[24] noted 337 cases of scoliosis (0.47 per cent) in 22,089 minifilms of persons over age 14.

Studies of the prevalence of scoliosis based on mass screening of school children began in North America in Delaware in 1962.[7] Hensinger and coworkers[12] reviewed the first 10 years' experience in Delaware. In this program 316,000 students (Grades 1 to 12) were examined. Of these, 1,109 were referred by the initial examiner to a physician for final evaluation of a possible spinal deformity. Of these 1,109, 599 were deemed to have true spinal deformity, 475 scoliosis, 47 kyphosis, 15 hyperlordosis, 18 poor posture, 17 back pain, and 27 torticollis.

Wynne-Davies[27] in a survey of 10,000 school children in Edinburg, noted scoliosis in 1.3/1000 under age 8 and 1.8/1000 over age

8. In children under age 8, the incidence was equal in males and females, but in those over age 8, females outnumbered males by 2.3 to 1.0.

Drummond, Rogala, and Gurr[9] examined 14,000 students in Montreal, Canada. The initial screeners (school nurses) felt that 1252 merited more detailed evaluation. Of the 1252, 821 (5.5 per cent of the 14,900 screened) were found to have a definite scoliosis. Of the 821 students, 610 had a structural scoliosis of 5 degrees or more, and 603 of the 610 were idiopathic scoliosis. Five had Scheuermann's kyphosis. Fifty-seven had a rotational prominence but no scoliosis on an x-ray, 16 had a nonstructural scoliosis due to leg length discrepancy, and four had spine deformity due to spondylolisthesis. Thus the prevalence of spine deformity was 4.6 per cent and of scoliosis 4.1 per cent. Curves of 5 to 10 degrees were found in 305 children, and in this group males equaled females. Curves of 11 to 20 degrees were seen in 244 children, and in this group there were 1.6 females to 1.0 male. Fifty-four patients had a curve of more than 20 degrees, and in this group there were 6.4 females to 1.0 male.

The largest study of school screening has been done in Minnesota and was reported in 1982 by Lonstein and associates.[16] Over a seven year period (1973 to 1980) 1,473,697 examinations were done of children aged 12, 13, and 14. Many of these children were examined more than once, since examinations were usually done consecutively in grades 6, 7, and 8. Very consistently, 3.4 per cent of the children were referred for more detailed evaluation, and 1.1 per cent had scoliosis confirmed. Subsequent to the reported study, an additional 1,000,000 examinations have been done in Minnesota with identical findings. This article contains a detailed bibliography of other school screening studies both from North America as well as other countries.

Is the prevalence of scoliosis the same worldwide? Are there differences based on country, nationality, or racial grouping? Inoue, Shinoto, and Ohki[13] screened 2000 school children in Chiba, Japan, and noted 1.37 per cent to have a structural scoliosis confirmed by x-ray. Takemitsu[23] screened 6949 school children in Hokkaido, Japan, and noted an incidence of 1.92 per cent with curves of 10 degrees or more.

In South Africa, Dommisse[8] noted 1.66 per cent of 50,000 white children in Pretoria to have scoliosis, 90 per cent of which were idiopathic. Segil, in Johannesburg,[19] reviewed both Caucasian and African Bantu (black) students. Curves of 10 degrees or more were noted in 2.5 per cent of the Caucasian students examined (929) and in only 0.03 per cent of the black students examined (1016).

Span, Robin, and Makin[22] reviewed 10,000 school children aged 10 to 16 in Jerusalem, and 300 (3 per cent) were found to have a definite scoliosis, 150 of these with curves of 10 degrees or more. The prevalence was twice as high in Jewish children as in Arabic children.

Smyrnis and coworkers[21] reported a study of school screening in Athens, Greece. Of 3494 children aged 11 and 12 that were screened, 10 per cent were positive for scoliosis on x-ray. A higher percentage of scoliosis was noted in fair-haired, blue-eyed children as compared to dark-complectioned children.

Willner and Uden[26] analyzed the prevalence of scoliosis in a very tightly controlled group of school children in Malmo, Sweden. Seventeen thousand children were screened yearly from age 7 to age 16 (1971 to 1980). For curves of 10 degrees or more, 3.2 per cent of the females and 0.5 per cent of the males had scoliosis. Only 1.1 per cent of the 17,000 had a curve of 20 degrees or more.

In summary, the prevalence of scoliosis is rather constant worldwide with the exceptions noted above. Figures vary considerably from one study to another, but most of these variances appear to be due to the criteria used in diagnosis. Considerable controversy exists as to what constitutes a spinal deformity versus what is a variation of normalcy. Kane[15] pointed out that if 5 degrees of scoliosis is considered significant, the prevalence is much higher than if 10 degrees is used as a definition of scoliosis, but can a 5 degree curve be considered pathology or only a variance of normal?

STUDIES OF UNTREATED CURVES DURING GROWTH

Instead of a detailed analysis of each different diagnosis in this chapter, the reader is referred to the various diagnostic chapters for this information. Rather than there being

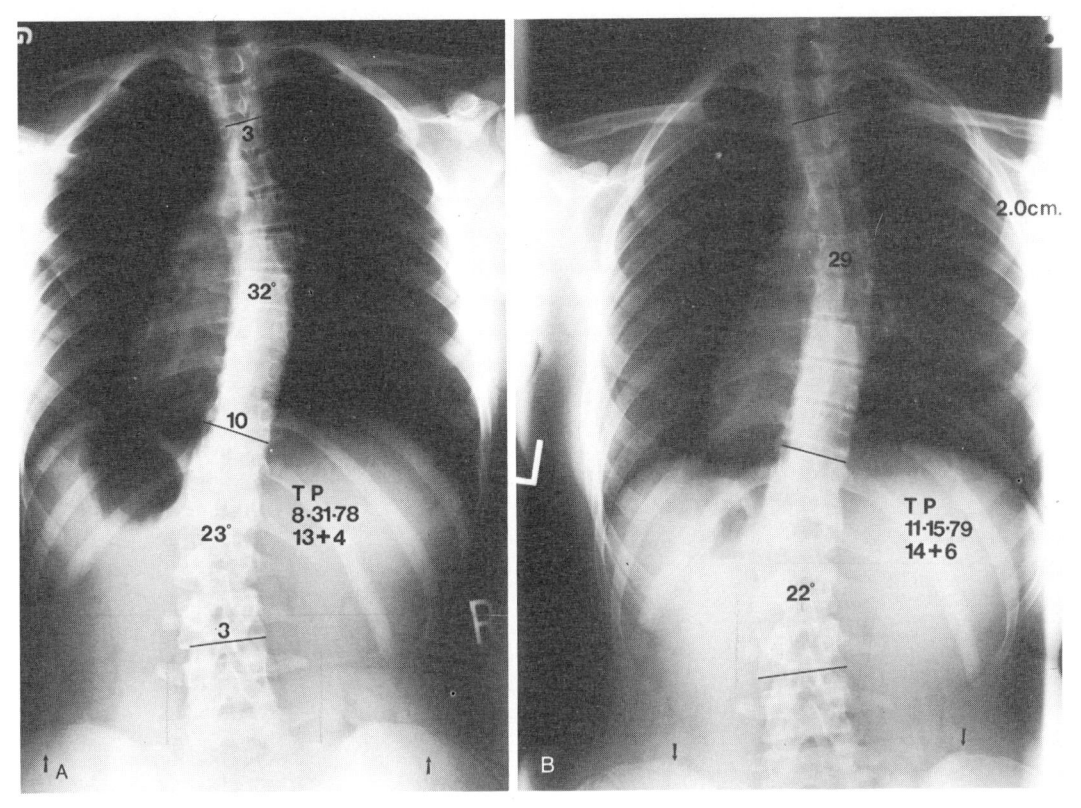

Figure 6–1. A, T. P., a 13 year old girl with a 32 degree right thoracic idiopathic scoliosis. Her menses had not yet begun. The Risser sign was 2+. Will this curve progress? A brace was recommended but it was refused by the family. No treatment of any kind was given. B, The same patient 14 months later. Her menses had begun, she is now Risser 3+ and the curve is 29 degrees. In retrospect, her curve had progressed to 32 degrees at some previous time, but was non-progressive when first seen by us. Her curve was 30 degrees on followup at age 17.

a single "natural history," there are a great variety of natural histories, depending upon a large number of different factors. These may include the specific etiology, the age at onset, the genetic "load" of the primary disease, the specific configuration of the deformed vertebrae, and the area of the spine in which the deformity occurs (Figs. 6–1 and 6–2).

THE EFFECTS OF SPINE DEFORMITY ON THE PATIENT

As stated earlier, there would be no cause for concern if patients with spinal deformity had no subsequent problems, but unfortunately this is not the case. Any center dealing with spinal deformities sees a large number of both children and especially adults presenting with very real problems. Among these problems are diminished pulmonary function, pain, neurologic compromise, and loss of self-image.

In 1968, two very important studies appeared. Nilsonne and Lundren[18] traced 113 patients who presented originally in the years 1913 to 1918. The study was done in 1963, providing follow-up of up to 50 years. No treatment had been given to these patients. Paralytic and congenital curves were excluded. Of the 113 patients, 88 were female and 25 male. The average age at first visit was 15.9 years. Only 11 of the 113 patients could not be traced. Of the rest, 56 were alive and 46 dead. The mean age at death was 47 years, and mortality was noted to be especially high after age 45. There were 31 actual deaths compared to 9.6 expected deaths for the Swedish population at that time. Cardiac or pulmonary disease ac-

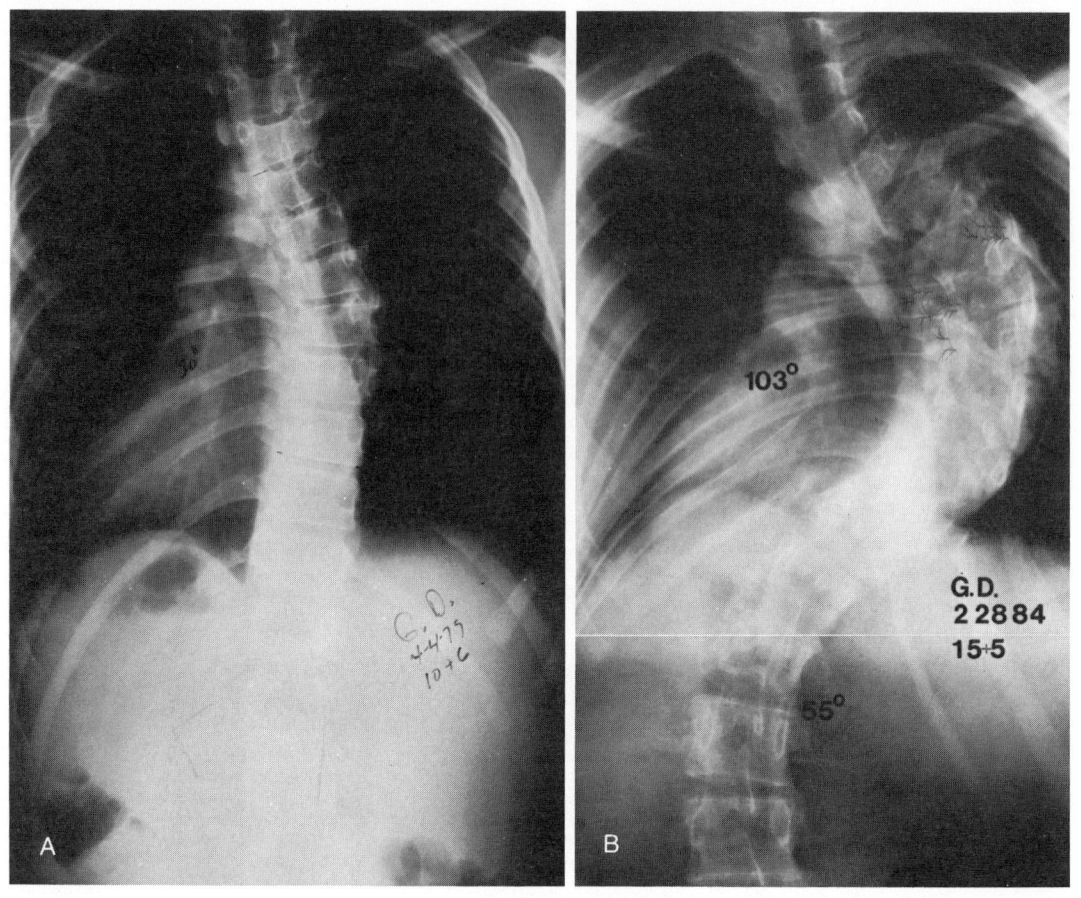

Figure 6–2. A, This boy, age 10, was seen elsewhere at a scoliosis clinic. He had a 30 degree T5 to T11 right thoracic idiopathic scoliosis. A Milwaukee brace was recommended, but refused by the parents. He was treated by the parents with stretching, massage, vitamins, and prayer. B, When seen by the author at age 15, his curve had increased to 103 degrees. Despite the obvious increase of his deformity, his parents had never consulted another doctor. The patient himself insisted on the evaluation at age 15 because he hated the way he looked.

counted for 60 per cent of the deaths, and 16 of the deaths were specifically caused by right heart failure.

In addition to mortality, social and sociomedical aspects were analyzed. It was noted that patients with scoliosis had a decreased work capacity, particularly in severe cases. Of the women studied, 76 per cent were unmarried. All the living patients were studied as to their work function and any subjective back trouble. Back symptoms were reported by 90 per cent of the patients, mostly in the form of a feeling of tiredness or pains in the thoracic or lumbar spine on exertion. Many of the patients had used some type of corset most of their lives. Thirty per cent had received a disability pension for their back trouble, while a further 17 per cent felt they were unable to work and had lived with parents or relatives most of their lives. Altogether 47 per cent of the living patients were disabled.

In a second study reported in the same journal, Nachemson[17] analyzed 130 scoliotic patients first seen in the years 1927 to 1936. No treatment had been given to these patients. The diagnoses included poliomyelitis, congenital scoliosis, idiopathic scoliosis, and miscellaneous causes. Of the group, 75 per cent were female and 25 per cent male. The average age at first visit was 14 years. Of the 130 patients, 117 were traced in 1966. Of these, 20 were dead, 16 having died of cardiopulmonary diseases that were probably related to the spine. Of the living, the average curve was 105 degrees and the vital capacity 50 per cent. Like that in the study of Nilsonne and Lundgren, the mortality rate in this study was twice normal for the Swedish population at that time. The 97 living patients were also surveyed as to disability and back pain. Twenty-four of the living patients were on disability compensation because of their back problems. The average age at which disability was claimed was 36. Another 15 patients reported serious heart and lung troubles. No patient was doing hard manual labor, 21 were in moderately active work, and 48 were in light occupations. Back pain was a relatively constant complaint in 39 of the 97 living patients, and a brace or corset was used by 24 patients. It was the conclusion by Nachemson that "this pain is probably due to the severe degree of osteoarthritic changes that will always occur in these patients."

The third major study on the late effects of nontreated scoliosis was that of Collis and Ponseti[5] from Iowa City. Of an original group of 358 patients with idiopathic scoliosis, 106 were examined personally and 109 more answered a questionnaire at an average follow-up of 24 years into adult life. This is only 60 per cent of the original group, a much lower retrieval rate than the 90 per cent in the two Swedish studies. The average age at follow-up was 42.

Of the 215 patients, 3 had undergone spine fusion as adults and 17 had died. In regard to back symptoms, 22 per cent had no back symptoms, 16 per cent had rare back pain, 31 per cent had occasional back pain, 16 per cent had frequent back pain, and 15 per cent had daily back pain. This result was not felt to be different than an age- and sex-matched control group.

Vital capacity was measured in 106 patients and was greater than 2 liters in all but 10 patients. Pulmonary symptoms were noted to correlate directly with diminished vital capacity. Sixty-six per cent of the patients with curves greater than 60 degrees had significantly decreased vital capacities.

In comparison with the Swedish studies, these curves were, on the average, much less severe, the follow-up was shorter, and the percentage of retrieval was much lower.

This study is the only one reported to date in which the original roentgenograms are available as well as the recent ones. Thoracic curves of 60 to 80 degrees at the end of growth progressed the most. This study was extended in 1981 by Weinstein, Zaval, and Ponseti[25] and is discussed in more detail in the chapters on Idiopathic Scoliosis and Adult Scoliosis (Fig. 6–3).

Fowles and associates[11] traced 221 patients in Canada, 117 of whom had not been treated. They were able to locate 55 patients who were alive and 10 who were dead. The average follow-up was 23 years, the average curve 60 degrees. Of those living, 40 per cent had intermittent pain, and 24 per cent had constant pain. The pain was correlated with the size of the curve and was more common after age 30. Of the group, 22 per cent were unemployed, 15 per cent had never worked, and none was doing heavy work. Nine per cent received pensions specifically for scoliosis. Sixty-seven per cent were psychologically embarrassed by their curves. There were fewer marriages in this scoliotic group as compared to nonscoliotics, and the curvature had a profound effect on self-image. Of the 10 dead, 4 had idiopathic, 3 congenital, and 3 paralytic scoliosis. Four of the deaths were from cardiopulmonary causes.

Berkreim and Hassan[2] reviewed 70 patients who were followed an average of 9 years after the end of growth. The majority of curves increased, the average being 3 degrees per year until age 20 and then 1 degree per year thereafter. Thoracic curves of 60 to 80 degrees progressed the most.

SUMMARY

What can be said about the natural history of scoliosis? The preceding studies are in some ways complementary and in some ways conflicting. The general trend is obvious; when there is a large (90 degrees or more) thoracic scoliosis, there will inevitably be a significant reduction in vital capacity, a twice normal likelihood of early death from cor pulmonale,[3] an increased amount of back discomfort, and a markedly reduced self-image leading to psychological (but not psychiatric) disturbance.[1, 4]

There is *no* evidence that curves of 45 degrees or less at the end of growth are at any particular risk for subsequent increase, pain, respiratory deficit, or decreased self-image. These figures are based, however, on averages of large groups and do not mean that there is not the occasional patient who will develop significant symptoms with a

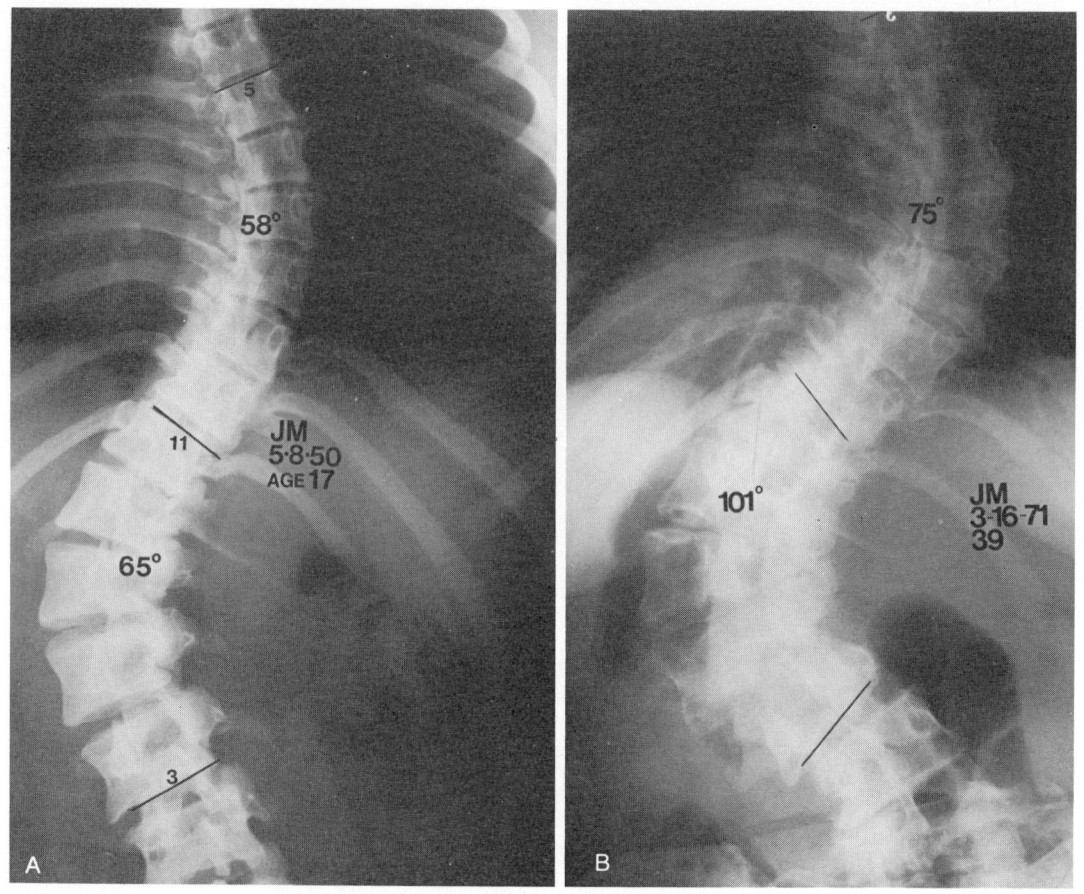

Figure 6–3. This 17 year old girl was seen in Iowa City in 1950, with a double major idiopathic scoliosis of 58 degrees and 65 degrees. She was Risser 4+ and growth was complete. No treatment was recommended. B, When first seen by the author in 1971 at age 39, this patent's curves had increased to 75 degrees and 101 degrees. She presented because of severe low back pain and left leg sciatica. Her back pain had begun at age 28 and had steadily increased to the point of markedly interfering with her daily activities.

curve of less than 50 degrees. Also, some curves of 50 degrees at maturity are quite stable and never progress while others do progress. Each patient must be taken as an individual and not treated as a statistic.

Another way to look at the natural history of the spine deformity problem is to look at the experience of large centers dealing with scoliosis patients. If adults with scoliosis had no problems, they would not seek medical attention. The reality of life is that all scoliosis centers are seeing large numbers of adults presenting with myriad problems.[6]

The most common problem is pain, followed by progressive deformity, decreased pulmonary function, loss of self-image, and neurologic deficits. All of these will be discussed in greater detail in the chapter on Adult Scoliosis.

References

1. Bengtsson, G., Fallstrom, K., Jansson, B., and Nachemson, A.: A psychological and psychiatric investigation of the adjustment of female scoliosis patients. Acta Psychiatr. Scand., 50:50–59, 1974.
2. Berkreim, I., and Hassan, I.: Progression in untreated idiopathic scoliosis after the end of growth. Acta Orthop. Scand., 53:897–900, 1982.
3. Bergofsky, E. H., Turino, G. M., and Fishman, A. P.: Cardiorespiratory failure in kyphoscoliosis. Medicine, 38:263–317, 1959.
4. Bjure, J., and Nachemson, A.: Non-treated scoliosis. Clin. Orthop., 93:44, 1973.
5. Collis D. K., and Ponseti, I. V.: Long-term followup of patients with idiopathic scoliosis not treated surgically. J. Bone Joint Surg., 51A:425–445, 1969.
6. Coonrad, R. W., and Feierstein, M. S.: Progression of scoliosis in the adult. J. Bone Joint Surg., 58A:156, 1976.

7. Cronis, A., and Russell, A. Y.: Orthopaedic screening of children in Delaware public schools. Del. Med. J., 37:89–92, 1965.
8. Dommisse, G.: A survey of spinal deformity in the child. J. Bone Joint Surg., 61B:259, 1979.
9. Drummond, D., Rogala, E., and Gurr, J.: Spinal deformity: natural history and the role of school screening. Orthop. Clin. North Am., 10:751–760, 1979.
10. Duhaime, M., Archambault, J., and Poitras, B.: School screening for scoliosis. Presented to the Quebec Scoliosis Society, Montreal, June 1976.
11. Fowles, J. V., Drummond, D. S., Ecoyer, S., et al.: The prognosis of untreated scoliosis in the adult. J. Bone Joint Surg., 58A:156, 1976.
12. Hensinger, R. N., Cowell, H. R., MacEwen, G. D., et al.: Orthopaedic screening of school-age children: review of a 10-year experience. Orthop. Rev., 4:23–28, 1975.
13. Inoue, S., Shinoto, A., and Ohki, I.: The Moire topography for early detection of scoliosis and evaluation after surgery. Presented to the Combined Meeting of the Scoliosis Research Society and Japanese Scoliosis Society, Kyoto, Japan, 1977.
14. Kane, W. J., and Moe, J. H.: A scoliosis prevalence survey in Minnesota. Clin. Orthop., 69:216–218, 1970.
15. Kane, W. J.: Editorial: A new challenge in scoliosis care. J. Bone Joint Surg., 64A:479–480, 1982.
16. Lonstein, J. E., Bjorkland, S., Wanninger, M. H., and Nelson, R. P.: Voluntary school screening for scoliosis in Minnesota. J. Bone Joint Surg., 64A:481–488, 1982.
17. Nachemson, A.: A Long-term followup study of non-treated scoliosis. Acta Orthop. Scand., 39:466–476, 1968.
18. Nilsonne, U., and Lundgren, K. D.: Long-term prognosis in idiopathic scoliosis. Acta Orthop. Scand., 39:456, 1968.
19. Segil, C. M.: The incidence of idiopathic scoliosis in the Bantu and white population groups in Johannesburg. J. Bone Joint Surg., 56B:393, 1974.
20. Shands, A. R., and Eisberg, H. B.: The incidence of scoliosis in the State of Delaware. A study of 50,000 minifilms of the chest made during a survey for tuberculosis. J. Bone Joint Surg., 37A:1243, 1955.
21. Smyrnis, P. N.: School screening for scoliosis in Athens. J. Bone Joint Surg., 61B:215, 1979.
22. Span, Y., Robin, G., and Makin, M.: Incidence of scoliosis in school children in Jerusalem. J. Bone Joint Surg., 58B:379, 1976.
23. Takemitsu, T.: Incidence of scoliosis in Japan by mass screening examination of school children. Presented at their Combined Meeting of the Scoliosis Research Society Kyoto, Japan, 1977.
24. Tulit, A.: Screening of vertebral scoliosis by mass x-ray pictures. Tuberk, Tudobet 22:44–45, 1969.
25. Weinstein, S. L., Zaval, D. C., and Ponseti, I. V.: Idiopathic scoliosis long-term followup and prognosis in untreated patients. J. Bone Joint Surg., 63A:702–712, 1981.
26. Willner, S., and Uden, A.: A prospective prevalence study of scoliosis in southern Sweden. Acta Orthop. Scand., 53:233–237, 1982.
27. Wynne-Davies, R.: The aetiology of infantile idiopathic scoliosis. J. Bone Joint Surg., 56B:565, 1974.

7
ORTHOTICS

James W. Ogilvie, M.D.

INTRODUCTION

Conceptually, a cost effective, complication free, noninvasive orthotic method for treating spine deformity is clearly desirable.[5, 7, 16, 17, 22, 39, 66, 70] Materials development and fabrication technology have allowed an expanded role for orthotic devices in the treatment of the misshapen spine.[48] Enthusiasm for the nonoperative treatment of scoliosis, however, should not obscure the questions that must be asked of any therapeutic approach: What is the natural history of the disease in question?[43] Can a favorable result be expected without any intervention? Will the proposed treatment prevent or alter an unfavorable outcome?[18] If results are favorable, are the orthotic system's physical and psychologic drawbacks acceptable?

GOALS

An orthosis should accomplish the following objectives: (1) It should initially improve the deformity.[57, 64] Large curves have a greater tendency to worsen with a given load than do small curves.[15] The resultant increased stability obtained by curve improvement increases the likelihood of long-term control of the deformity by the orthosis. (2) An orthosis should be capable of preventing curve progression for long periods of time, frequently until the patient reaches skeletal maturity or until a fusion heals. Orthoses should allow social and physical development, which may critically affect compliance to a bracing regimen.[69] In general, orthoses contain but do not correct spine deformities. Curve severity five years after treatment has ended is seldom substantially improved from the degree of deformity at the beginning of brace treatment.[19, 20, 27, 28, 30, 41, 42] In younger patients with flexible curvatures, there is more likelihood of achieving long-term improvement. However, if a scoliosis curvature is unacceptable at the beginning of brace treatment, it will often be so at the conclusion.[25] Subjecting a patient to years of brace treatment during the teenage period only then to have her undergo surgery may sometimes be avoided by understanding the indications and limitations of orthotic treatment.

HISTORY

Although traction had been a popular concept since Hippocrates' time for correcting spine deformities, orthotic treatment was not used until 1582, when Ambrose Paré advocated metal braces made by an armorer for the treatment of scoliosis.[49]

Louis Albert Sayre is credited in 1874 as the first to cast a spinal deformity.[58] His suspensory-plaster cast was followed in 1893 by the localizer cast of Bradford and Brackett, and the hinged or turnbuckle cast by Hibbs and Risser in 1920 and 1927.[11, 28] Blount and Schmidt first used the Milwaukee brace (cervical-thoracic-lumbar-sacral orthosis or CTLSO) in 1946 for postoperative poliomyelitis curves and subsequently advocated a CTLSO treatment protocol for idiopathic scoliosis.[10] The Milwaukee brace has become the standard of comparison for subsequent orthotic devices. The terms Milwaukee brace and CTLSO are used synonymously. Thermoplastics and brace technology have developed, leading to several different orthoses that are frequently designated by the city of origin, Boston, Wilmington, Miami, Pasa-

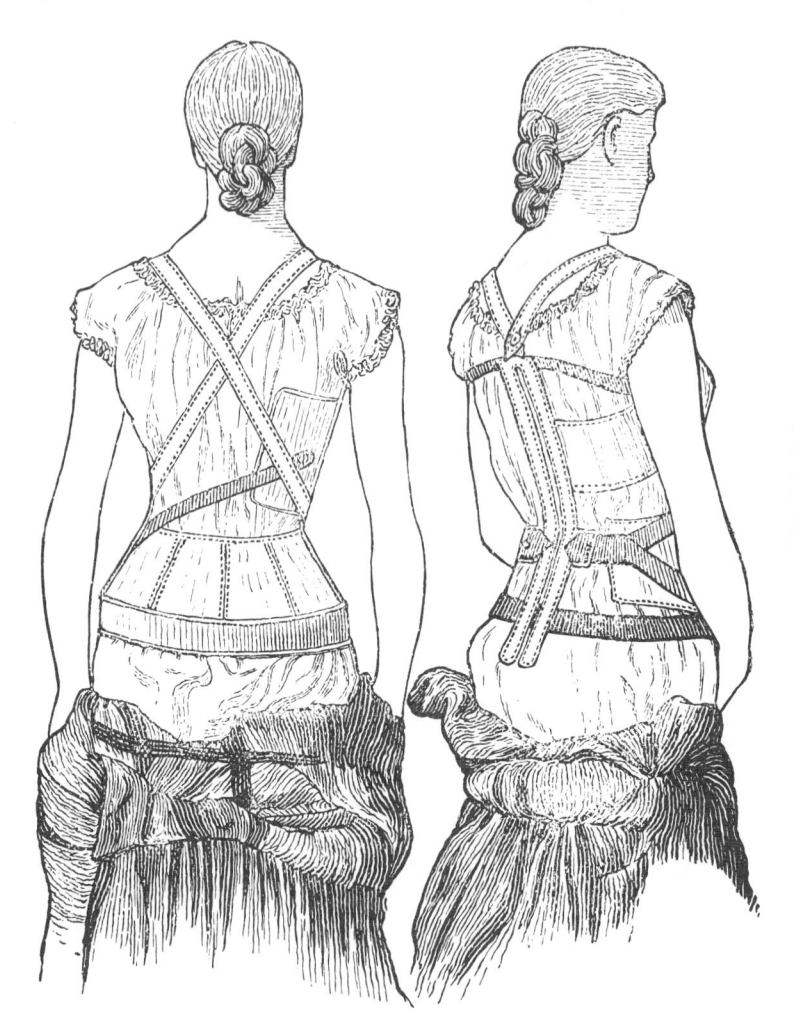

Figure 7–1. This scoliosis brace does not reduce lumbar lordosis but does apply force over the rib hump. Note the maturity of the patient. The brace was used by Bigg in 1882.

dena. Many present day thoracolumbar sacral orthoses (TLSO) have striking similarities to those of 100 years ago (Fig. 7–1).[9]

The success of orthotic treatment depends not only on the anatomy of a spinal deformity and the geometry of the orthosis, but also on the biology and maturation of the patient. Bampfield recognized in 1824 that skeletal growth and scoliosis progression were closely linked.[6] Growth potential determinations made according to biologic factors such as breast development, menarche, and pubic hair growth, as in the method of Tanner, and radiographs of selected physes are critical for decision making.[14, 24, 53, 61] Unsuccessful brace treatment of skeletally mature patients or of those with rigid congenital curves reflects on our misunderstanding of spine deformity, not on the inadequacy of orthotics. As the etiology, pathogenesis, and natural history of scoliosis are better understood, it will be possible to employ orthotic care with increasing selectivity and effectiveness.

BIOMECHANICS

Spinal contour can be influenced by four methods: (1) longitudinal traction, (2) transverse force application, (3) muscle contraction (compression), and (4) asymmetrical growth.

A spinal deformity can be improved by applying longitudinal traction. Because longitudinal traction is most efficient for large curves and large curves are not usually braced, traction provides only supplemental support to those forces generated by transverse force application. Andriacchi and coworkers demonstrated that the neck ring of a CTLSO acted as a fulcrum for the head to distract the vertebral column in the recumbent patient.³ That force was lost by the removal of the occiput piece. This mechanism is negated by gravity and the use of skeletal traction, such as provided by the halo device, is necessary for the application of sustained longitudinal traction in the upright patient.

Transverse forces applied at the apex of the scoliotic or kyphotic deformity are more efficient than traction when correcting a spinal deformity less than approximately 50 degrees. Three-point fixation is necessary for transverse force application. With the use of a CTLSO, the pelvic mold provides distal fixation and the cephalad component of the three- or four-point fixation is provided by the neck ring (Fig. 7–2). Initially, the Milwaukee brace was fitted with a mandibular rest, but dental deformities were caused in many patients.³⁶ Replacement of the mandibular rest with a throat mold eliminated the malocclusion that resulted from sustained pressure on the jaw. Trochanteric extensions on the pelvic portion may be added if the control of trunk decompensation is necessary. Reduction of lumbar lordosis is accomplished with gluteal extensions that tilt the pelvis and may thereby reduce lumbar scoliosis by coupled motion.⁶³ Transverse forces at the apex of lumbar curves are provided by the lumbar pad (Fig. 7–3). This pad tends to reduce the scoliosis and derotate the flexed lumbar spine.²,³⁵,⁶⁷ If the apical vertebra of the curve is above T12, a thoracic pad is placed over the posterolateral aspect of those ribs that articulate with the apex of the thoracic scoliosis (Fig. 7–4). This force, transmitted through the ribs to the thoracic spine, creates a vector, which can be separated into x and z components. The component acting medially (x axis) can decrease coronal plane

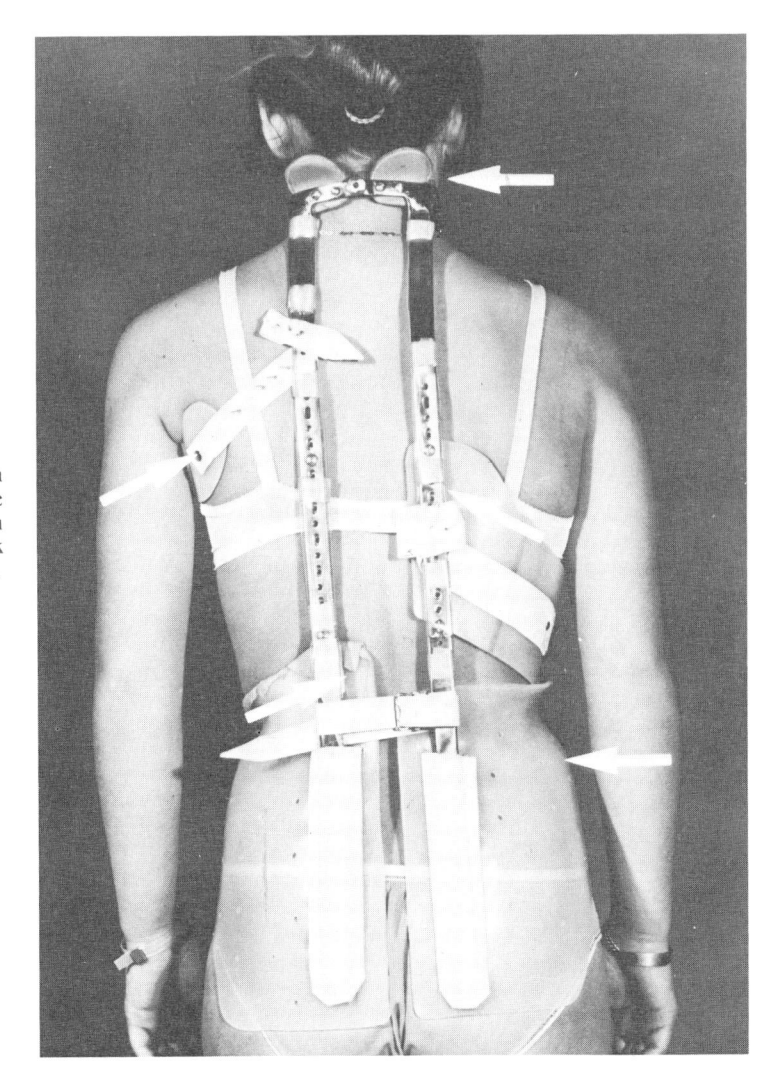

Figure 7–2. Posterior view of a CTLSO demonstrates the transverse forces that can be generated (from cephalad to caudad) with the neck ring, axillary sling, thoracic pad, lumbar pad, and the pelvic mold.

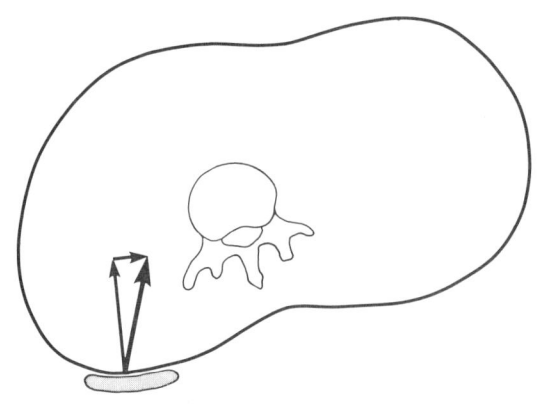

Figure 7–3. A cross-section through the L2 level of a left lumbar curve illustrates the anterior and medial forces that the lumbar pad generates.

deformities. It does not reduce rib hump deformity independently from correcting scoliosis in idiopathic curves.[62] This medially directed force can also deform the rib cage without controlling scoliosis in patients with spinal muscular atrophy or osteogenesis imperfecta.[52, 72] The vector directed anteriorly (z axis) is frequently undesirable, since thoracic idiopathic scoliosis is usually accomplished by a loss of physiologic thoracic kyphosis. Thus, an anteriorly directed vector tends to further accentuate hypokyphosis, and an anterior elastic gusset placed across the apex of the hypokyphosis may be needed to counter the anterior vector of the thoracic pad force. Modification of the standard TLSO by placing the thoracic pad area more laterally, allowing more lumbar lordosis, and contouring the

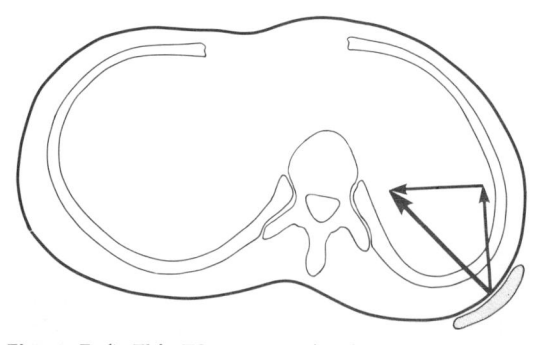

Figure 7–4. This T8 cross-section illustrates the thoracic pad of a CTLSO and separates the anteromedial force into its component vectors. Moved close to the midline, the anterior force is increased, but the tendency to decrease thoracic kyphosis may be undesirable. If the pad is lateral, there is no anterior force over the rib hump, and the straight lateral vector may further rotate the spine in a clockwise direction.

posterior uprights may also control the hypokyphotic spine.[26, 70] Anterior displacement of the neck ring may encourage a midthoracic flexion to reduce the tendency toward hypokyphosis if a CTLSO is used. Thoracic lordosis accompanying a scoliosis deformity usually militates against orthosis usage.

Mulcahy and others demonstrated in children with idiopathic adolescent scoliosis that the neck ring complex of a CTLSO can have a distractive function through the occiput pads and throat mold.[46] Removal of the thoracic pad in the TLSO increased pressure readings on the components of the neck ring. They concluded, however, that forces exerted through the chest pad made the major contribution to the passive correction of scoliosis deformity. Andriacchi and others used computer models of various scoliotic spines to demonstrate that midthoracic curves responded best to the corrective forces generated by a CTLSO and that lumbar curves responded only one-fourth as well as the thoracic curves,[3] an observation that has been confirmed clinically.[31, 44] Our preliminary observation has been that lumbar curves respond as well if not better than thoracic curves to the use of a TLSO. High thoracic curves responded poorly to a CTLSO, and in some instances they were made worse by forces applied to adjacent midthoracic curves. Andriacchi and associates also noted that the neck ring of the CTLSO had the chief function of centering the head, neck, and upper torso over the pelvis and did not exert any significant traction. Loosening of the pelvic portion of the CTLSO decreased the forces on the thoracic pad.

Scoliosis curvatures with an apex at T8 or above often require the CTLSO rather than a lower profile TLSO.[33, 37, 38, 50] Improvement and long-term control of right midthoracic idiopathic curves with the apical vertebra up to T6 treated with a TLSO has been reported.[25, 29, 33] An axillary extension is constructed on the concavity of the thoracic curve and a thoracic pad is used over the convexity. While not applicable to high thoracic or cervical-thoracic curves, it has been effective and has avoided the objections present with the neck ring of a CTLSO.

Adjunct points of fixation can be added to a CTLSO such as an axillary sling, lateral head restraint, or trapezius pad if it is necessary to control cervical-thoracic or high thoracic scoliosis. McMaster has reported on sitivity, these forces are best spread over a large area thereby reducing the force per unit area or pressure. A total contact molded body jacket, rather than the standard CTLSO with the smaller thoracic pad, is used in patients with decreased sensation or paralytic deformities.[21, 23, 40]

A CTLSO is usually required to treat thoracic kyphosis deformity.[55] The short upper lever arm between the posterior contact area and the sternal bar of a TLSO is inadequate to control Scheuermann's kyphosis (Fig. 7–6). Forward chin thrust, frequently associated with excessive cervical lordosis, is often present in the Scheuermann's patient, and this can only be controlled with the neck ring of a CTLSO. Pads are placed on the two posterior uprights at the apex of the kyphus, usually T6 to T8. No lateral pads are needed unless there is an accompanying scoliosis.

By relieving the asymmetrical loading of cartilaginous endplates in scoliotic and kyphotic deformities, an orthosis can minimize asymmetrical growth, which takes place in accordance with the Hueter-Volkman principle.[65] It is this biologic correction that provides the long-term benefit to the deformity.

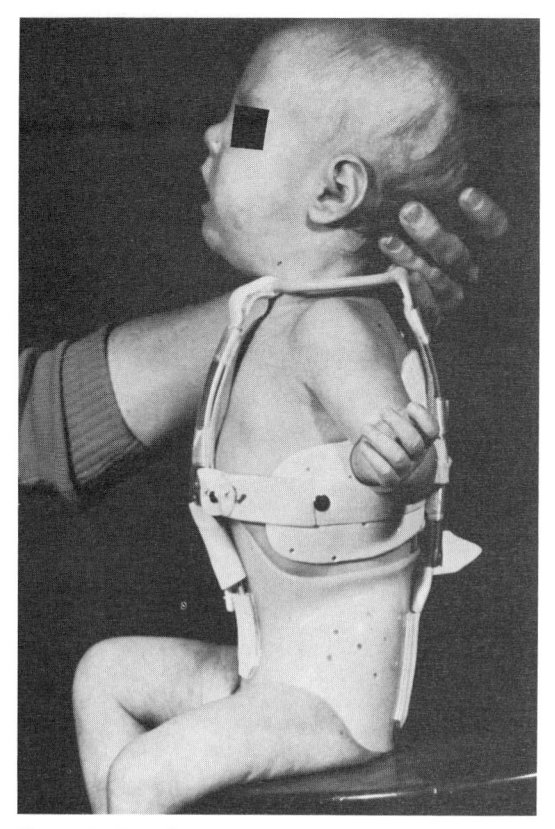

Figure 7–5. This seven month old infant has been fitted with a CTLSO for an infantile idiopathic scoliosis.

the use of a modified Milwaukee brace in the treatment of progressive infantile idiopathic scoliosis.[39] CTLSO application can be made in children at an early age and is usually limited only by the energy of the physician and orthotist (Fig. 7–5). In prescribing an orthosis, accurate pad placement is essential in order to maximize the transverse corrective forces that the brace generates and still not create hypokyphosis or accentuate trunk shift or high thoracic curves.[71]

The righting reflex is the major active stimulus to curve correction in the neurologically intact patient.[56] Neuromuscular impairment dictates that braces used in these patients not rely on principles of active correction. The neck ring of a CTLSO does not provide passive support, since sustained direct pressure on the anterior cervical soft tissue is not tolerated. Although pad irritation may induce some active correction, passive support rather than active muscle correction is the principle used in most orthotic applications.[13] In the patient with decreased cutaneous sen-

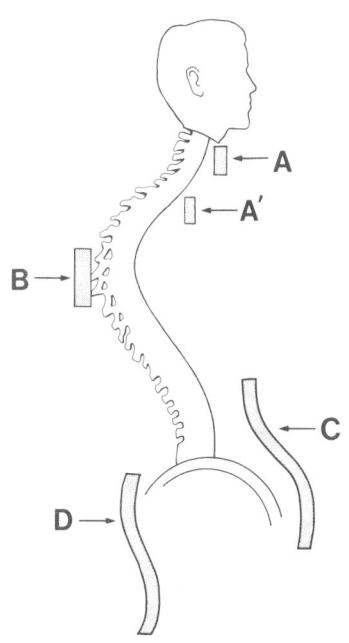

Figure 7–6. The lever arm A'B generated by the sternal bar of a TLSO (A') and the posterior pressure point (B) is not adequate to control most Scheuermann's kyphosis deformities. The neck ring of a CTLSO provides a longer lever arm (AB) and controls the forward head thrust often present with Scheuermann's deformity.

It also explains why bracing does not improve a deformity in the skeletally mature patient. If an orthosis is unable to overcome the asymmetrical forces acting on the growing skeleton with a progressive curvature, failure of brace treatment results.

Congenital scoliosis resulting, for example, from an unsegmented unilateral bar can produce severe deformity. Orthotic treatment cannot impart growth to a congenital growth deficiency. It is not indicated in the treatment of progressive congenital curves. There are often compensatory curves that accompany congenital spine deformity and these, however, may be amenable to brace control (see Chapter 12).

ELECTROSPINAL TREATMENT

Lateral bending is one of the physiologic planes of motion in the cervical, thoracic, and lumbar spine. This motion can be accomplished with muscles attached to the shoulder girdle, such as the latissimus dorsi, unilateral contraction of the abdominal wall musculature, intercostal muscles, or the numerous muscles of the paraspinous group. Intrinsic muscle contraction of the torso is both empirically and theoretically effective in changing the contour of scoliosis.[5, 41] Rab used a mathematical three-dimensional centroid line of the medial and lateral erector spinae, latissimus dorsi, and the multifidus and the semispinalis rotators to determine the theoretical forces that would be expected on the scoliotic spine by selective electrical stimulation (Fig. 7–7).[51] While noting that no group effectively derotated the scoliotic deformity, he determined that the lateral erector spinae muscles generated the most favorable forces for correction of the right thoracic curve of idiopathic scoliosis. Schultz and others further confirmed the theoretical basis of selective muscle stimulation for scoliosis correction by using computerized mathematical models of three different idiopathic scoliosis patterns: right thoracic, left lumbar, and left lumbar-right thoracic.[59] It was determined that the intercostal muscles were most effective for the right thoracic curve correction and that the lateral erector spinae group was most effective for correction of lumbar curves. Several other important observations were also made. They stressed that care should be taken to stimulate only those muscles spanning the curve, and thus avoid unwanted worsening of adjacent curves. Stimulation of the curve should be done in the recumbent position so that modest contraction of appropriate trunk muscles can affect a substantial change in spinal contour.

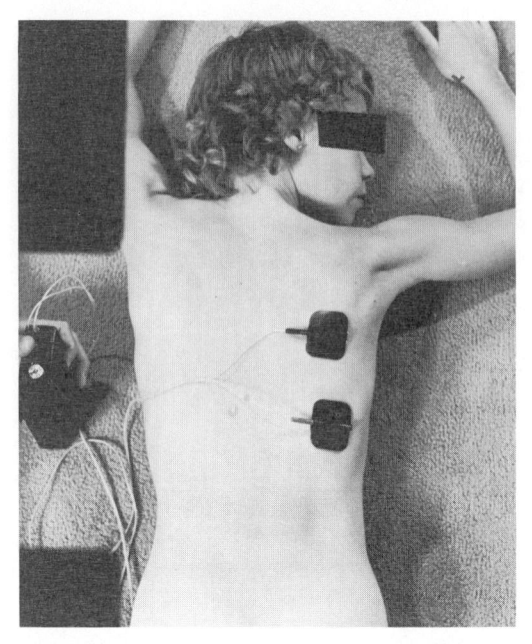

Figure 7–7. Surface electrode muscle stimulation for this right thoracic idiopathic scoliosis is applied in a position to utilize the intercostal and latissimus dorsi muscles in treating the curvature.

Numerous clinical trials dating from the mid-1970's have confirmed the premise that electrode stimulation of trunk muscles has the ability to control certain idiopathic scolioses.

Axelgaard and Brown reported the ability of transcutaneous muscle stimulation to arrest progression of idiopathic scoliosis in 95 per cent of patients who comply with their protocol.[5] To qualify for treatment, the patients must have the diagnosis of idiopathic scoliosis, have at least two years of skeletal growth remaining, and have documented progression of a curvature between 20 and 29 degrees or any curve between 30 and 45 degrees.

Subsequent reports from other centers have been much less optimistic about the ability of surface electrode muscle stimulation to control idiopathic scoliosis.[2a, 30a, 60a] Their failure rates ranged from 35 to 65 per cent.

Bradford and coworkers have reported that patients whose curvatures are unresponsive to treatment with an electrospinal orthosis do not respond to the subsequent use of a Milwaukee brace.[12]

Although considerable variation exists in the reported results of surface electrode stimulation of patients with idiopathic scoliosis, there emerges a pattern of rough equivalency in the effectiveness of surface electrode stimulation and orthotic treatment of idiopathic adolescent scoliosis. Additional evaluation of electrospinal stimulation is required before it can be considered the standard of care.

ORTHOTIC PRESCRIPTION

After determining the diagnosis and prognosis of a given spine deformity, a rigid orthosis may be the treatment of choice. The prescribing physician should then specify the particular aspects of the orthosis needed to treat that given deformity. In addition to providing radiographs for the orthotist, the physician should specify the exact type, a TLSO or a CTLSO, with its choices of thoracic pad, lumbar pad, axillary sling, trapezius flang, shoulder ring, kyphosis pads, anterior gussets, or trochanteric extensions, and the location, medial-lateral orientation of pads and placement over the apex of the deformity. Free communication must exist between the orthotist and the physician. In general, orthotic prescriptions should follow the patterns listed below. Curves best suited for the CTLSO are:

1. Cervicothoracic. Molded shoulder pad ring and head restraint.
2. High thoracic. Trapezius pad (Fig. 7–8).
3. Double thoracic. Trapezius pad for the high thoracic curve and contralateral thoracic pad for the midthoracic component.
4. Thoracic kyphosis. Paraspinous pads at the kyphus apex.

Curve patterns suitable for TLSO or modified TLSO treatment are:

1. Thoracolumbar. Low thoracic and lumbar oval pads and ipsilateral trochanteric extension.
2. Double curves, thoracic and lumbar (Fig. 7–9).
3. Lumbar. Lumbar pad ipsilateral trochanteric extension, and contralateral thoracic extension (Fig. 7–10).

Depending on the location of the curve and the supplemental features desired, we choose from one of five basic orthotic designs (Fig. 7–11). The choice between a CTLSO and the "low profile" TLSO is sometimes difficult. After effectiveness, the advantages and disadvantages of each orthotic type must be weighed. The TLSO with its low profile is more socially acceptable, but adjustments for longitudinal growth, changing curve pattern and weight gain cannot be made. Cervicothoracic and upper thoracic curves are poorly controlled with the underarm TLSO.

Patient acceptance is poorer with the CTLSO because of the visible neck ring. Adjustments are possible, however, and the CTLSO's capability for additional points of force application may allow control of upper spinal deformities, trunk tilt, elevated shoulder, and neck thrust. Because of its open design, the CTLSO is better tolerated in warm weather. Trunk decompensation was not improved with the CTLSO in a study by Radicel and Renshaw.[54] The braces used in this study, however, did not utilize trochanteric extensions, which can influence trunk compensation.

Fabrication of the orthosis follows one of two patterns. If a TLSO in one of its modifications is to be fitted, off-the-shelf blanks are available in different sizes, which can accomodate the trunk dimensions of 90 per cent of brace patients.[71] Measurements are taken of the torso, and the nearest fitting prefabricated blank is chosen. Small variations may be compensated for by a foam lining, but the control of lumbar lordosis is fixed. The prefabricated brace is then trimmed to meet the specifications of the spinal curvature, and inserts are added as needed. The pelvic girdle of a CTLSO may also be fitted in this manner, followed by the addition of anterior and posterior uprights and the neck ring.

For those patients who require a more custom fitting of the torso component, a mold of the trunk is taken. This may be done in the standing position, or if the patient is unable to stand, the mold may be obtained on the Risser casting table. If pelvic or cervical traction is needed or if correction of the deformity with the localizer is desired, it can be accomplished at the same time. From this mold a positive cast of the torso is made, and the brace is then fabricated on that model.

While the prefabricated orthosis has considerable advantages in construction time needed, it lacks the adaptability required for many spine deformities. The interest, skill, and innovativeness of the orthotist play a pivotal role, and it should not be assumed that one skilled in fitting lower limb orthotics,

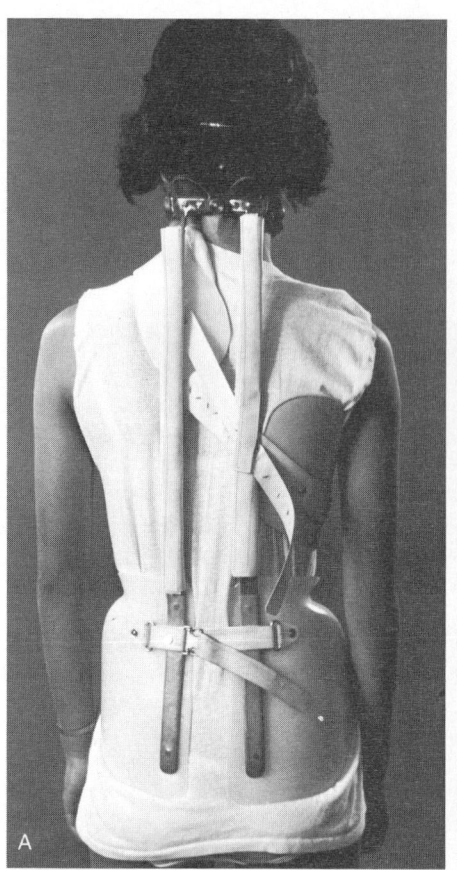

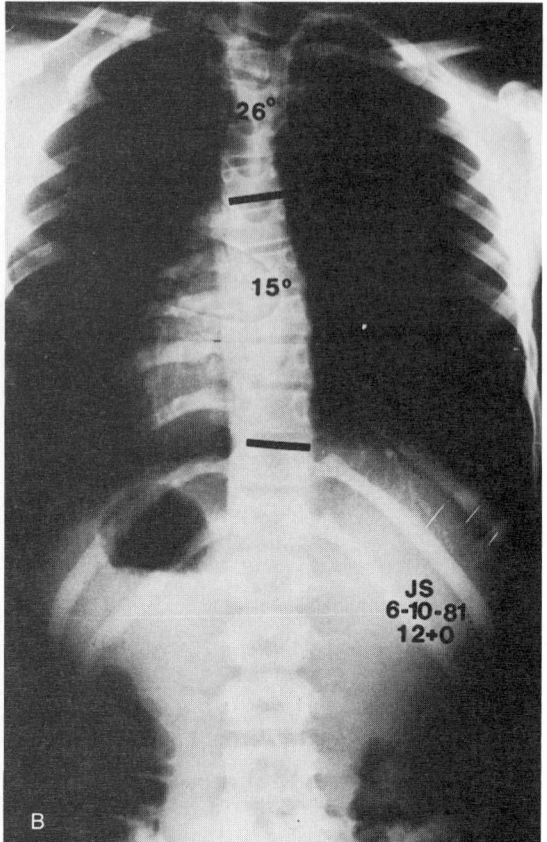

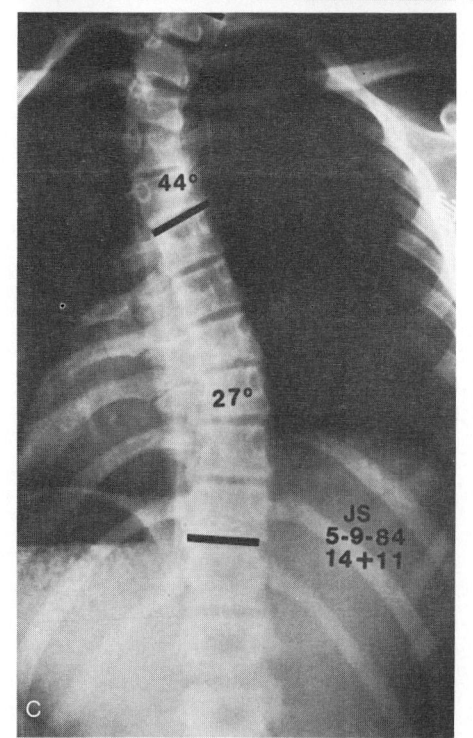

Figure 7–8. This 12+0 year old female received a CTLSO (A) with right thoracic pad and left trapezius pad for her idiopathic scoliosis (B). Note the left shoulder elevation on both the clinical photograph and her initial radiograph. At age 14+11 (C) her left upper thoracic curve had progressed from 26 degrees to 44 degrees while her left scapular elevation had improved slightly.

ORTHOTICS

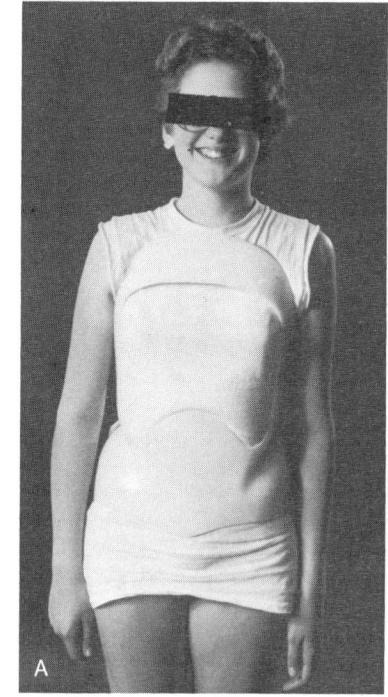

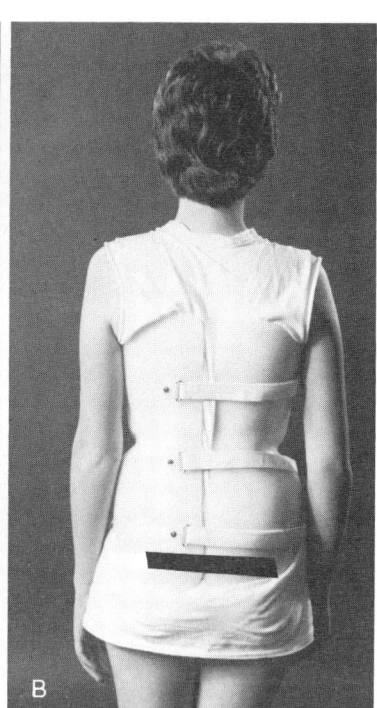

Figure 7–9. *A* and *B,* This standard TLSO is used for a right thoracic-left lumbar adolescent idiopathic scoliosis.

for instance, has an equal expertise in spinal orthoses.

After the orthosis is fitted, it is the physician's responsibility to evaluate the final product. Relieving specific pressure points and adjustments in brace length and pad placement are occasionally necessary and should be ordered without delay. The patient and family must understand and be in agreement with regard to the specific times and

Figure 7–10. *A* and *B,* A 13+2 year old female with left lumbar idiopathic scoliosis with apex at L2 is fitted with this modified TLSO. The left lumbar pad is countered with a right thoracic extension to prevent trunk tilt to the right.

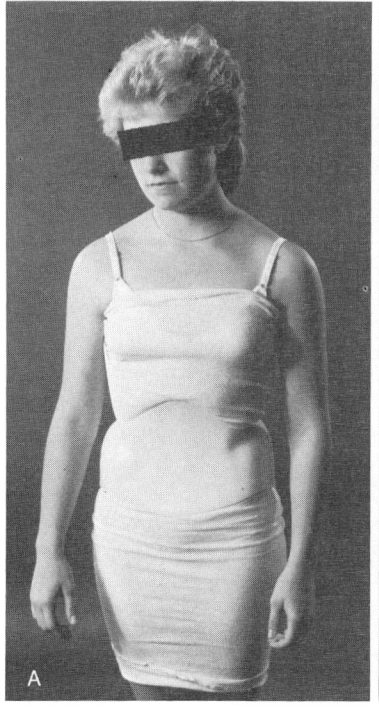

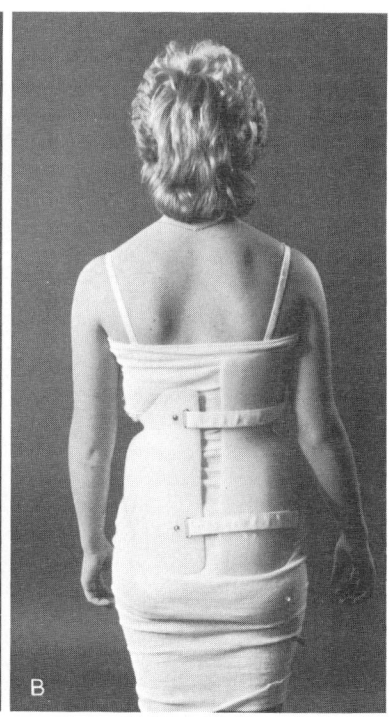

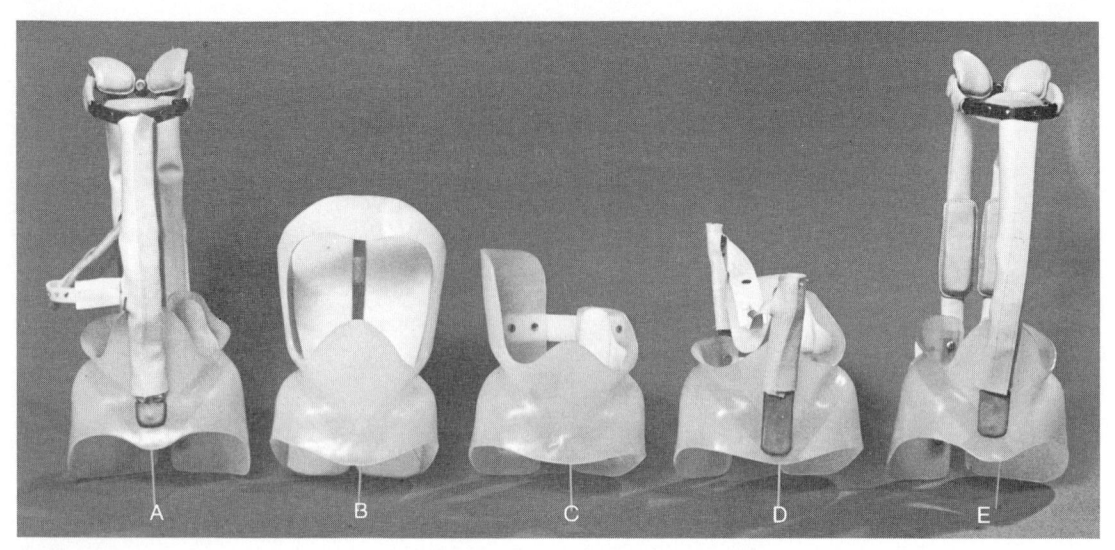

Figure 7–11. Five basic patterns of spinal orthoses can be modified as required. A, CTLSO (Milwaukee brace) with left lumbar pad and right thoracic pad used for s-shaped scoliosis. B, TLSO used in thoracic and thoracolumbar curves. C, Modified TLSO with left lumbar pad for lumbar curves. D, The extension on this modified TLSO provides a more open design and counteracts the left lumbar pad's tendency to right trunk tilt. E, CTLSO for thoracic kyphosis.

duration of brace wear. It seldom requires more than five to seven days for a patient to adjust to a brace. A snug fitting T-shirt is worn under the brace, and skin conditioning is initiated with alcohol rubs and corn starch or powder as needed. If the orthosis is too loose, skin irritation may result from shifting of the brace, and if too tight, pressure points may arise.

COMPLICATIONS

Orthotic treatment is not without potential complications and problems. Although usually mild and transient from a physical standpoint, both somatic and psychological changes can occur when orthotic treatment is elected.[34, 68] Compression of abdominal viscera is an invariable companion of a properly fitting TLSO. Increased intragastric pressure may result in reflux esophagitis.[32] A decrease in glomerular filtration rate and effective renal blood flow has also been noted.[1, 8] Although reversible with removal of the brace, this tendency toward sodium retention could be measured in certain patients even after four to twelve months of brace treatment. A slight decrease in total lung volume has been noted in patients wearing the CTLSO; however, there has been no significant effect on the vital capacity.[60] The circumferential fitting TLSO has more restriction of thoracic expansion than does the CTLSO, and prolonged wearing can produce a "tubular thorax" deformity.

Brace treatment in the adolescent can produce psychological disturbances that are measurable into adult life.[4] Self-image in adolescents is difficult to evaluate, but it is an important factor in compliance with brace wearing,[69] and it also affects whether the patient is satisfied with the cosmetic result following years of brace treatment. Orthosis patients in general have a less favorable outlook towards their body image than do surgery patients.[47]

SUMMARY

Brace treatment of curvatures known to be unresponsive to an orthosis should not be considered as conservative care. The decision of when to brace and whom to brace can be very complex. It depends on the biologic age of the patient, the location, severity and progression of the curve, the amount of cosmetic deformity, the preferences and psychological stability of patient and family, and skill and availability of the orthotist, but most of all on the specific diagnosis of the spine deformity. It is for this reason that the specific indications and contraindications for orthotic care of a spine deformity are included in the chapters dealing with each particular diagnosis.

References

1. Aaro, S., and Berg, U.: The immediate effect of Boston brace on renal function in patients with idiopathic scoliosis. Clin. Orthop., *170*:243–247, 1982.
2. Aaro, S., Burstrom, R., and Dahlborn, M.: The derotating effect of the Boston brace: a comparison between computer tomography and a conventional method. Spine, *6*:477–482, 1981.
2a. Akbaria, B. A., Keppler, L., Price, E. A., and Gotz, T.: Lateral electrical surface stimulation (LESS) for the treatment of adolescent idiopathic scoliosis. Proceedings of the Scoliosis Research Society, Coronado, CA, Sept. 17–20, 1985.
3. Andriacchi, T. P., Schultz, A. B., Belytschko, T. B., and DeWald, R. L.: Milwaukee brace correction of idiopathic scoliosis: a biomechanical analysis and a retrospective study. J. Bone Joint Surg., *58A*:806–815, 1976.
4. Apter, A., Morein, G., Munita, H., et al.: The psychological sequelae of the Milwaukee brace in adolescent girls. Clin. Orthop., *131*:156–159, 1978.
5. Axelgaard, J., and Brown, J. C.: Lateral electrode surface stimulation for the treatment of progressive idiopathic scoliosis. Spine, *8*:242, 1983.
6. Bampfield, R. W.: An Essay on Curvatures and Diseases of the Spine, Including All the Forms of Spinal Distortion. London, Longman, Hurst, Rees, Orme, Brown, and Greene, 1824.
7. Bancel, P., Kallin, A., Hall, J., and Dubousset, J.: The Boston brace: results of a clinical and radiologic study of 401 patients. Orthop. Trans., *8*:33, 1984.
8. Berg, U., and Aaro, S.: Longterm effect of Boston brace treatment on renal function in patients with idiopathic scoliosis. Clin. Orthop., *180*:169–172, 1983.
9. Bigg, R. H.: Spinal Curvature. London, Churchill, 1882.
10. Blount, W. P., Schmidt, A. C., Keever, E. D., and Leonard, E. T.: Milwaukee brace in the operative treatment of scoliosis. J. Bone Joint Surg., *40A*:511–525, 1958.
11. Bradford, E. H., and Brackett, E. G.: Treatment of lateral curvature by means of pressure correction. Boston Med. Surg. J., *CXXVIII*:463, 1893.
12. Bradford, D. S., Tanguy, A., and Vanselow, J.: Surface electrical stimulation in the treatment of idiopathic scoliosis: preliminary results in 30 patients. Spine, *8*:757, 1983.
13. Bunch, W. H.: The Milwaukee brace in paralytic scoliosis. Clin. Orthop., *110*:63–68, 1975.
14. Bunch, W. H., and Dvonch, V. M.: Pitfalls in the assessment of skeletal immaturity: an anthropologic case study. J. Pediatr. Orthop., *3(2)*:220–222, 1983.
15. Bunch, W. H., Patwardhan, A. G., Vanderby, R., and Knight, G. W.: Stability of scoliotic spines—part I: Single and double primary curves. Orthop. Trans., *8(1)*:145, 1983.
16. Bunnell, W. P.: Treatment of idiopathic scoliosis. Orthop. Clin. North Am., *10(4)*:813–827, 1979.
17. Carr, W. A., Moe, J. H., Winter, R. B., and Lonstein, J. E.: Treatment of idiopathic scoliosis in the Milwaukee brace. J. Bone Joint Surg., *62(4)*:599–612, 1980.
18. Dickson, J. H., Dericks, G. H., and Rossi, C. D.: Results in operated idiopathic scoliosis patients previously treated in the Milwaukee brace. Tex. Med., *77(8)*:45–47, 1981.
19. Edmonson, A. S., and Morris, J. T.: Follow-up study of Milwaukee brace treatment in patients with idiopathic scoliosis. Clin. Orthop., *126*:58–61, 1977.
20. Edmonson, A. S., and Smith, G. R.: Longterm follow-up study of Milwaukee brace treatment in patients with idiopathic scoliosis. Proceedings of the Scoliosis Research Society, Denver, Sept. 22–29, 1982.
21. Evans, G. A., Drennan, J. C., and Russman, B. S.: Functional classification and orthopaedic management of spinal muscular atrophy. J. Bone Joint Surg., *63B*:516–522, 1981.
22. Farady, J. A.: Current principles in the nonoperative management of structural adolescent idiopathic scoliosis. Phys. Ther., *63(4)*:512–523, 1983.
23. Fisk, J. R., and Bunch, W. H.: Scoliosis in neuromuscular disease. Orthop. Clin. North Am., *10(4)*:863–875, 1979.
24. Greulich, W. W., and Pyle, S. I.: Radiographic Atlas of Skeletal Development of the Hand and Wrist. London, Oxford University Press, 1950.
25. Hall, J. E., Emans, J. B., Kaelin, A., and Bancel, P.: Boston brace system treatment of idiopathic scoliosis. Follow-up in 400 patients finished treatment. Orthop. Trans., *8(1)*:148, 1983.
26. Hall, J. E., Mills, M. B., Lipton, H., and Gebhardt, M.: Treatment of hypokyphotic scoliosis: nonoperative and operative. Orthop. Trans., *8(1)*:154, 1983.
27. Hassan, J., and Bjerkreim, I.: Progression in idiopathic scoliosis after conservative treatment. Acta Orthop. Scand., *54*:88, 1983.
28. Hibbs, R. A., Risser, J. C., and Ferguson, A. B.: Scoliosis treated by the fusion method. An end-result study of 360 cases. J. Bone Joint Surg., *13*:91–104, 1931.
29. Jonassen-Rajala, E., Josefsson, E., Lundberg, B., and Nilsson, H.: Boston thoracic brace in the treatment of idiopathic scoliosis. Clin. Orthop., *183*:37, 1984.
30. Kahanovitz, N., Levine, D. B., and Lardone, J.: The part-time Milwaukee brace treatment of juvenile idiopathic scoliosis. Longterm follow-up. Clin. Orthop., *167*:145–151, 1982.
30a. Kahanovitz, N., and Weiser, S.: LESS compliance in adolescent female scoliosis patients. Proceedings of the Scoliosis Research Society. Coronado, CA, Sept. 17–20, 1985.
31. Keiser, R. P., and Shufflebarger, H. L.: The Milwaukee brace in idiopathic scoliosis: evaluation of 123 completed cases. Clin. Orthop., *118*:19–24, 1976.
32. Kling, T. F. Jr., Drennan, J.C., and Gryboski, J. D.: Esophagitis complicating scoliosis management with the Boston thoracolumbosacral orthosis. Clin. Orthop., *159*:208–210, 1981.
33. Laurnen, E. L., Tupper, J. W., and Mullen, M. P.: The Boston brace in thoracic scoliosis. A preliminary report. Spine, *8(4)*:388–395, 1983.
34. Lindh, M.: Energy expenditure during walking in patients with scoliosis. The effect of the Milwaukee brace. Spine, *3(4)*:313–318, 1978.

35. Lindh, M.: The effect of sagittal curve changes on brace correction of idiopathic scoliosis. Spine, 5(1):26–36, 1980.
36. Logan, W. R.: The effect of Milwaukee brace on the developing dentition. In Transactions of the British Society for the Study of Orthodontics. London, pp. 1–8, 1962.
37. Mariani, G., and DeGiorgi, G.: The treatment of lumbar scoliosis with a three piece brace. Ital. J. Orthop. Traumatol., 6(2):207–212, 1980.
38. McCollough, N. C., Schultz, M., Javech, N., and Latta, L.: Miami TLSO in the management of scoliosis: preliminary results in 100 cases. J. Pediatr. Orthop., 1(2):141–152, 1981.
39. McMaster, M. J., and MacNicol, M. F.: The management of progressive infantile idiopathic scoliosis. J. Bone Joint Surg., 61:36–42, 1979.
40. McMaster, W. C., and Clayton, K.: Spinal bracing in the institutionalized person with scoliosis. Spine, 5(5):459–462, 1980.
41. Mellencamp, D. D., Blount, W. P., and Anderson, A. J.: Milwaukee brace treatment of idiopathic scoliosis: late results. Clin. Orthop., 126:47–57, 1977.
42. Michel, C. R., Caton, J., Allegre, G., and Allegre, M.: The place of a 4 piece spinal support in the conservative treatment of scoliosis. A review of 700 cases over ten years. Orthop. Trans., 7:131, 1983.
43. Miller, J. A. A., Nachemson, A. L., and Schultz, A. B.: Effectiveness of braces in mild idiopathic scoliosis. Spine, 9:632, 1984.
44. Moe, J. H., and Kettleson, D. N.: Idiopathic scoliosis. J. Bone Joint Surg., 52A:1509, 1970.
45. Monticelli, G., Ascain, E., Salsano, V., and Salsano, A.: Experimental scoliosis induced by prolonged minimal electrical stimulation of the paravertebral muscles. Ital. J. Orthop. Traumatol., 1:39, 1975.
46. Mulcahy, T., Galante, J., DeWald, R., et al.: A follow-up study of forces acting on the Milwaukee brace on patients undergoing treatment for idiopathic scoliosis. Clin. Orthop., 93:53–68, 1973.
47. Nachemson, A. L., Cochran, T. P., Fallstrom, K., and Irstam, L.: Somatic, social and psychologic effects of treatment for idiopathic scoliosis. Orthop. Trans., 7:508, 1983.
48. Nash, C. L.: Current concepts review: scoliosis bracing. J. Bone Joint Surg., 62A:848, 1980.
49. Paré, A.: Opera Ambrosii Parei. Paris, Apud Jacobum. Du-Puys, 1582.
50. Park, J., Houtkins, S., Grossman, J., and Levine, D. B.: A modified brace (prenyl) for scoliosis. Clin. Orthop., 126:67–73, 1977.
51. Rab, G. T.: Muscle forces in the posterior thoracic spine. Clin. Orthop., 139:28, 1979.
52. Riddick, M. F., Winter, R. B., and Lutter, L. D.: Spinal deformities in patients with spinal muscle atrophy: a review of 36 patients. Spine, 7(5):476–483, 1982.
53. Risser, J. C.: The iliac apophysis: an invaluable sign in the management of scoliosis. Presented at the Annual Meeting of the American Academy of Orthopaedic Surgery, Chicago, 1947.
54. Rudicel, S., and Renshaw, T. S.: The effect of the Milwaukee brace on spinal decompensation in idiopathic scoliosis. Spine, 8(4):385–387, 1983.
55. Sachs, B. L., Bradford, D. S., Winter, R. B., et al.: Scheuermann's kyphosis: longterm results of Milwaukee brace treatment in 132 patients. Orthop. Trans., 9(1):108, 1984.
56. Sahlstrand, T., Ortengren, R., and Nachemson, A.: Postural equilibrium in adolescent idiopathic scoliosis. Acta Orthop. Scand., 49(4):354–365, 1978.
57. Salanova, C.: Les resultats lointains du corset de Milwaukee—les indications. Acta Orthop. Belg., 43:603, 1977.
58. Sayre, L. A.: Spinal Disease and Spinal Curvature: Their Treatment by Suspension and the Use of Plaster of Paris Bandage. London, Smith, Elder and Co., 1877.
59. Schultz, A., Haderspeck, K., and Takashima, S.: Correction of scoliosis by muscle stimulation: biomechanical analyses. Spine, 6:468–476, 1981.
60. Sevastikoglou, J. A., Linderholm, H., and Lindgren, U.: Effect of the Milwaukee brace on vital and ventilatory capacity of scoliotic patients. Acta. Orthop. Scand., 47(5):540–545, 1976.
60a. Sullivan, J. A., Renshaw, T. S., Eman, J. B., Johnston, C. E., Sussman, M., and Davidson R.: Further evaluation of the Scolitron treatment of idiopathic scoliosis. Proceedings of the Scoliosis Research Society, Coronado, CA, Sept. 17–20, 1985.
61. Tanner, J. M.: Some main features of normal growth in children. In Zorab, P. A. (ed.): Scoliosis and Growth. London, Churchill-Livingstone, 1971.
62. Thulbourne, T., and Gillespie, R.: The rib hump in idiopathic scoliosis. Measurement, analysis, and response to treatment. J. Bone Joint Surg., 58(1):64–71, 1976.
63. Uden, A., and Willner, S.: The effect of lumbar flexion and Boston thoracic brace on the curves in idiopathic scoliosis. Spine, 8:846, 1983.
64. Uden, A., Willner, S., Pettersson, H.: Initial correction with the Boston thoracic brace. Acta. Orthop. Scand., 53:907–911, 1982.
65. vonVolkman, R.: Chirurgische Erfahrungen uber Knochenuer-beigungen und Knochenwachsthum. Arch. Pathol. Anat. Physiol., 24:512–540, 1862.
66. Watts, H. G.: Bracing spinal deformities. Orthop. Clin. North Am., 10(4):769–785, 1979.
67. Watts, H. G., Hall, J. E., and Stanish, W.: The Boston brace system for the treatment of low thoracic and lumbar scoliosis by the use of a girdle without superstructure. Clin. Orthop., 126:87–92, 1977.
68. White, A. A., and Panjabi, M. M.: The clinical biomechanics of scoliosis. Clin. Orthop., 118:100–112, 1976.
69. Wickers, F., Bunch, W., and Barnett, P.: Psychological factors in failure to wear the Milwaukee brace for treatment of idiopathic scoliosis. Clin. Orthop., 126:62–66, 1977.
70. Willner, S.: Effect of the Boston thoracic brace on the frontal and sagittal curves of the spine. Acta. Orthop Scand., 55:457, 1984.
71. Winter, R. B., and Carlson, J. M.: Modern orthotics for spinal deformities. Clin. Orthop., 126:74–86, 1977.
72. Yong-Hing, K., and MacEwen, G. D.: Scoliosis associated with osteogenesis imperfecta. J. Bone Joint Surg., 64B:36–42, 1982.

8

TRACTION IN SPINE DEFORMITIES

James W. Ogilvie, M.D.

INTRODUCTION

Longitudinal traction of scoliosis deformities by suspension was advocated by Glisson in 1660, and in 1788, Venel suggested prolonged bedrest in traction for scoliosis treatment.[9, 14] In 1874, Professor Thomas Sayre, an American, applied spinal traction with a chin halter and axillary slings before fitting his scoliosis patient with a suspensory-plaster cast.[21] Technical advances over the years have given surgeons the ability, through skeletal traction, to exert sustained tensile forces when attempting to straighten the spine. Skeletal traction is a powerful treatment method whose indications and complications must be understood if it is to be properly employed.

When traction is considered for spinal correction, it must fulfill the following criteria.

1. It must be necessary and efficient when compared with exercise, brace, localizer cast, postural reduction, or intraoperative correction.
2. The tensile forces should act on the curve without unsafe tractive loads adversely affecting intervening structures, such as the cervical spine or spinal cord.
3. Possible complications of traction must favor the patient when considering the risk:benefit ratio.

Only when these criteria have been knowledgeably addressed and answered should one proceed with traction therapy.

MECHANICS

Longitudinal traction is an efficient means of mechanically correcting spinal curvatures greater than 53 degrees.[29] For curves less than this, transverse forces acting at the apex of the curve are a more efficient means of correction.

Postural reduction of kyphotic deformities uses the principle of transverse forces at the apex of the curve and should be considered in the treatment of fractures and other spine disorders that result in anterior angulation of the spine.[8, 28] Guerin advocated a form of hinged brace for applying a bending moment to correct scoliosis.[11] Turnbuckle casts and Risser's localizer cast both effectively apply transverse forces to a spine deformity and may be preferable to traction as the choice of nonoperative correction.[22]

The practical limitation of traction, in those deformities where it may be useful, is application of distractive vectors to the curvature without damage to the adjacent spine. It is technically possible with the utilization of skeletal traction (e.g., halofemoral, halopelvic, and halogravity) to apply forces in excess of the limits of safety. For instance, when applying traction to a thoracic curve of T5-T12 with the patient in the upright position, it is first necessary to overcome the force of gravity tending to worsen the curve. This necessitates lifting that portion of the body cephalad to T5. If this superincumbent force

109

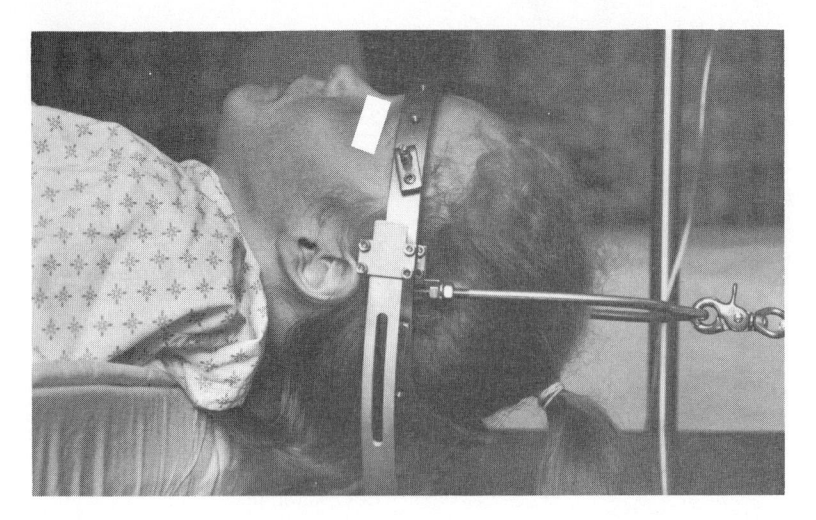

Figure 8–1. A split mattress and the use of a skid applied to the halo to reduce friction and allow side-to-side turning are shown.

exceeds the maximum traction force that can safely be applied to the cervical spine, then no distraction force reaches the thoracic curve. In general, cervical and upper thoracic deformities are the only locations that are amenable to halo traction. It is unreasonable to suppose that a halo traction force limited to a maximum of 15 kilograms would be able to effect any distraction of a low thoracic or lumbar curve when applied to the upright adult patient.

If the patient is horizontal, the compressive force of gravity is removed and traction must overcome the static friction generated between the bed and the patient before any force can act on the spine. The use of a split mattress or other means of reducing the halo-bed friction is helpful in achieving this (Fig. 8–1). Skeletal traction for spine deformities must have the resultant force vectors equal to zero if the patient is to be stationary. Since halo traction can reasonably apply up to 15 kilograms in the cephalad direction, this force must be counterbalanced by friction, restraint of the patient, or by skeletal traction applied to the pelvis or femur. When the patient is changed from halogravity traction to in-bed halo traction, the traction may need to be reduced, since the effects of gravity are no longer acting opposite to the traction force.

Takahashi studied the viscoelastic relaxation characteristics of human and animal spines under tensile stress.[25] He noted an improvement that was the expression of the force-deformation curve and soft tissue relaxation rate of the scoliotic spine. When traction was able to improve the nature of a spine deformity, he noted that most of the improvement appeared within the first week of treatment. Ex vivo studies on the relaxation characteristics of spinal soft tissue (creep) reveal that most of the changes occur in less than five minutes.[13]

CLINICAL EXPERIENCE

The halo device was introduced in 1959 by Perry and Nickel and is our choice for cranial traction.[18] Halo fixation can be used for postoperative immobilization through a variety of devices such as the halo cast or halo vest (Fig. 8–2). With a vest, the halo apparatus controls bending and rotational stresses on the spine. If properly fitted through a cast which is well molded to the iliac crest, it can counteract the compressive forces of gravity on uninstrumented cervical and upper thoracic spine surgeries or on fractures that are unstable. If previous spinal instrumentation has uncertain integrity because of poor bone stock or other technical factors, the halo cast apparatus provides the supplemental stability needed until biologic stability is achieved through healing.

We have, as reported by Swank and others, utilized halogravity wheelchair traction (Fig. 8–3) in evaluating changes of pulmonary function in patients with paralytic scoliosis.[24] Following 10 to 14 days of halo traction, there was a substantial improvement in vital capacity, increased PaO_2 from 55 to 64 mmHg, and decreased $PaCO_2$ from 52 to 43 mmHg in those patients with curves secondary to poliomyelitis. In those who did not experience respiratory improvement, surgery was not performed. Halo traction was thus a screening test for reversible cor pulmonale

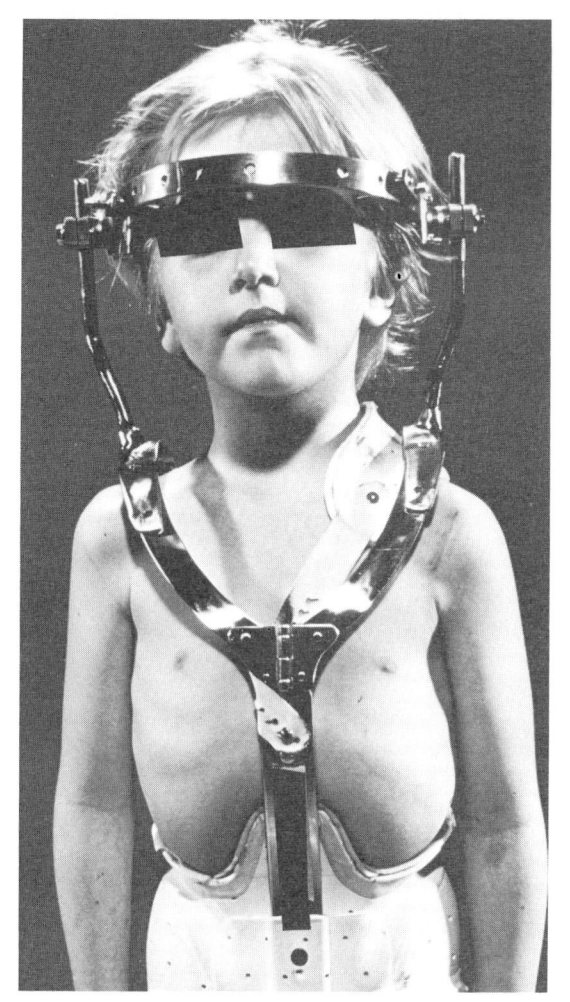

Figure 8–2. This halo cast reduces the axial compression of the spine and prevents bending or rotation. The patient has an uninstrumented cervicothoracic fusion for post-laminectomy kyphosis.

current halogravity traction following the initial surgery. This assumes two preconditions. First, if the patient has been rendered unstable by the initial procedure, it may be necessary to use traction to support the patient thus allowing improved pulmonary function and the psychological benefits of wheelchair mobility. Secondly, traction may improve the deformity between stages of surgery. In 43 patients undergoing two-stage surgery at the Twin Cities Scoliosis Center for failed scoliosis fusion, halofemoral traction after the initial stage resulted in an improvement of both thoracic and lumbar and thoracolumbar curves. The initial stage consisted of multiple osteotomies through the posterior fusion mass or resection of a pseudarthrosis.[3] This procedure provided the flexibility needed to allow improvement by traction. As noted in the section on complications, skeletal spinal traction is a critical maneuver and must be closely monitored to prevent neurologic dysfunction. Toledo and

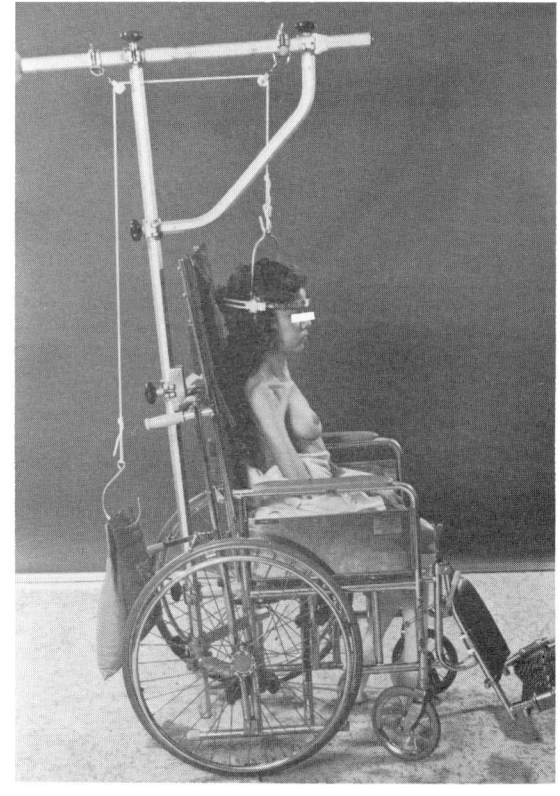

Figure 8–3. A modified halogravity traction has been advocated by Stagnara (Lyon). Progressive distraction is possible as demonstrated with the patient's body providing the necessary counterweight. This technique can be advantageous, since it allows the patient to be upright during the daytime.

rather than primarily for curve correction. When successful, the improved respiratory status allowed patients to tolerate spinal surgery.

Preoperative skeletal traction or traction by the method of Cotrel has not been shown to benefit patients with idiopathic scoliosis by decreasing intraoperative complications or increasing the amount of curve correction possible at surgery.[1, 5, 7, 10, 16, 17] In adult patients with spontaneously ankylosed or previously fused facets, preoperative traction does not result in any increased correction when compared with that obtained in side bending radiographs (Fig. 8–4).[23] When embarking on a multiple stage spine reconstruction, it may be advantageous to apply inter-

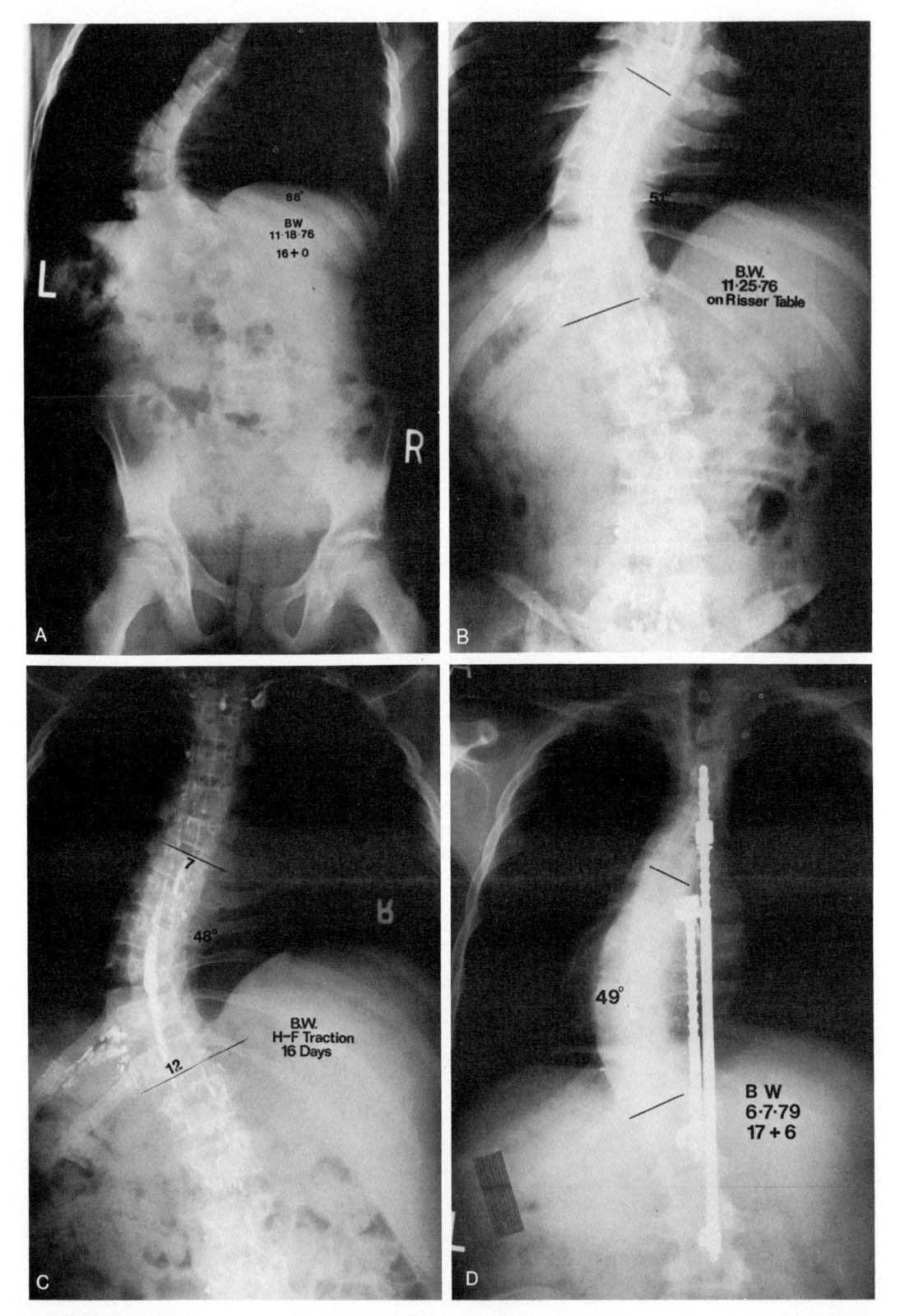

Figure 8–4. An 88° scoliosis in a 16 year old female (A) can be corrected to 51° on the Risser table with a localizer strap (B). After 16 days of halofemoral traction, correction was at 48° (C). Harrington distraction rods achieved correction to 49° (D). No benefit was achieved by the use of traction.

others have reported the use of halo traction on the circolectric bed as a means of applying intercurrent traction to staged spine surgery.[26]

If a curvature is not flexible and has not been made unstable by the initial stage of a multiple stage spine reconstruction, traction can only represent the risk factor of the risk-benefit ratio, without the accompanying possibility of benefit.

Halopelvic traction has also been used in the treatment and reduction of severe spondylolisthesis.[2] This is a specially adapted form of traction that not only applies tensile loads to the spine, but also produces a torsional moment on the pelvis, rotating it from the vertical toward the horizontal with a Hoffman pelvic fixator. Details of this treatment are contained in the chapter on spondylolisthesis (Chapter 19).

APPLICATION

Application of the halo device, although requiring attention to detail, is relatively simple. It can be applied under local anesthesia. Ideally, the halo is placed 1 to 2 centimeters above the eyebrow and the helix of the ear. It should be horizontal in anterior and lateral planes, but this may be altered if flexion or extension is desired. Six standard sizes of halos are available, which will accommodate the cranial circumference of most patients while leaving 1 to 2 centimeters of clearance. Four screws should be placed just below the crown of the head, which is the greatest diameter of the skull. Individual cranial variations often seen in hydrocephalus and other cranial dysplasias and dysostoses may make a compromise of halo placement necessary. With the patient supine, the head is supported by an assistant or a narrow metal extension, which is cupped to cradle the head. After antiseptic preparation of the scalp and instillation of local anesthetic down to the periosteum, four studded screws are advanced through the halo ring into the outer cortex of the cranium (Fig. 8–5). The anterior screws are placed in the hairline. If they are placed too far forward, unsightly scars are left on the forehead. Placement too far posterior involves the temporalis muscle, interfering with mastication, and may also lead to placement in the thinner temporalis bone rather than the more substantial frontalis. The posterior screws are behind the ear in approximately 180 degree opposition to the corresponding anterior screws. Opposite screws are sequentially tightened to 6 inch-pounds torque with either a torque wrench or thumb-index finger force. To relieve torque on the skin, which may result in an area of necrosis, each screw is backed off 1/4 turn after final tightening. Lock nuts are applied to each screw as a final step.

The halo is then attached either to the traction device or to a halo cast or vest. With good pin tract care the halo device can usually be maintained for 6 months or longer. In general, halo traction is initiated with 5 to 7 kilograms in the adult and less in a child. Progressive weight increases of 1/2 to 1 kilogram are added daily until the maximum limits are achieved; our upper limit is 10 to 15 kilograms in the adult and less in children.

At 7 to 10 days after initial application, the screws should be retightened. Daily pin tract cleansing and antibiotic cream application are imperative. If an individual pin becomes infected, the exudate must be cultured and appropriate antimicrobials initiated. Location of the pin to another site may be done or the halo discontinued entirely if pin tract infections indicate. Continued tightening of the halo pins risks penetration of the inner table of the cranium and subsequent brain abscess. Intracranial abscess, however, has been reported even without skull penetration of the halo screw.[12]

COMPLICATIONS

Small amounts of traction can be applied to the spine by devices requiring skin contact such as cervical halter or pelvic corset traction. Persistent cervical halter traction in excess of 2 to 3 kilograms or pelvic traction, if more than 15 kilograms, is rarely tolerated for extended periods. Superficial skin irritation and transient hypesthesia of cutaneous nerves may result but usually resolve when traction is discontinued. These devices are easy to apply and remove, thus allowing access for personal hygiene and permitting frequent ambulation. In general, the problems, the complications, and the resultant benefits to the spine are all minimal.

Halohoop traction, introduced by DeWald and Ray in 1970, is an extremely powerful method of distraction force application to the spine.[4] The problems and complications of this technique include bowel perforation

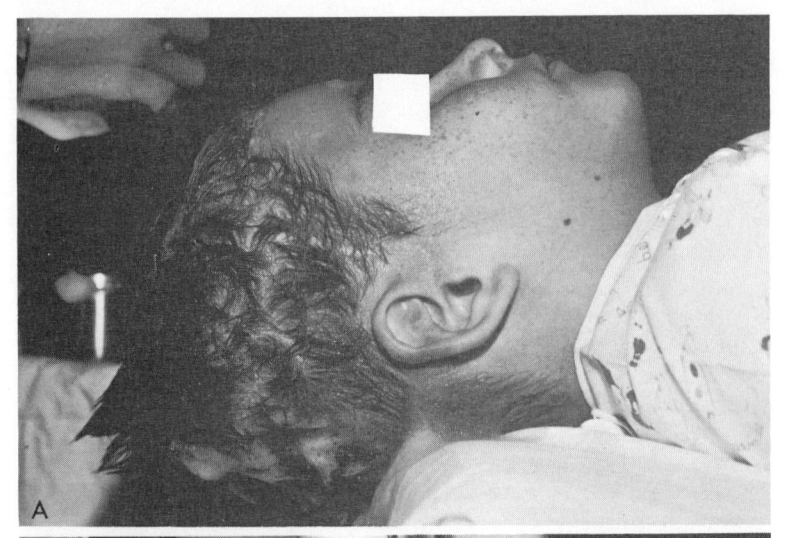

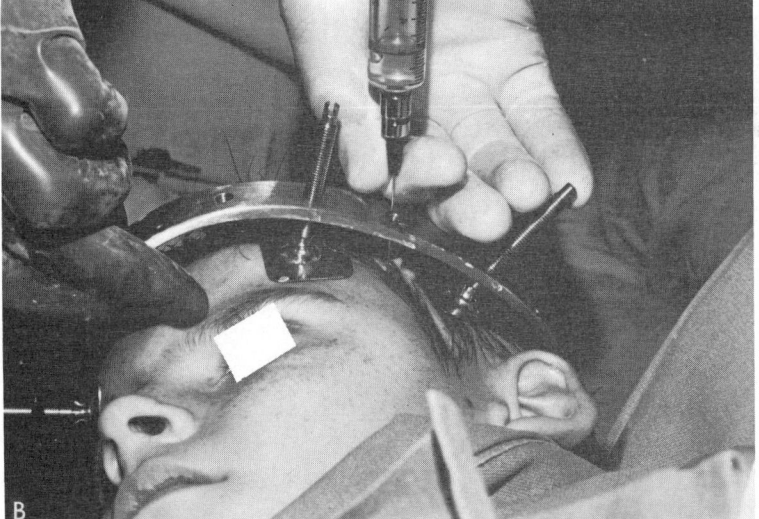

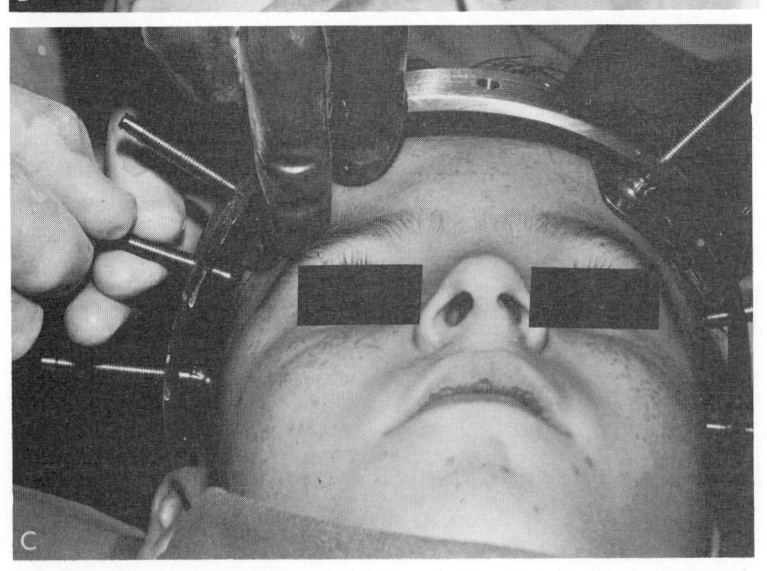

Figure 8–5. *A,* For the application of the halo the hair need not be shaved but should be shampooed with a surgical soap scrub and left wet. Local anesthesia is generally sufficient, provided the individual is cooperative and well sedated. The assistant positions the halo below the maximum diameter of the skull, approximately 1 centimeter above the eyebrows and the ear lobes. The skin is infiltrated with Xylocaine, 1 per cent, with epinephrine (*B*). The four pins are then inserted, two posterolaterally and two anterolaterally (*C*).

Illustration continued on opposite page

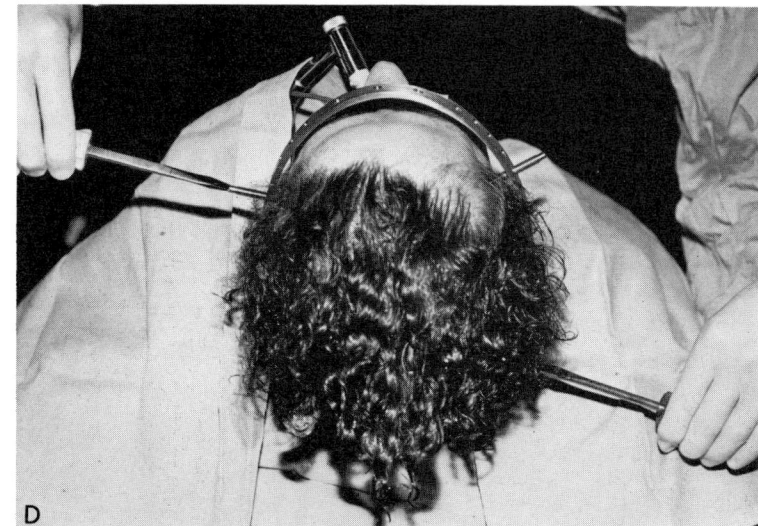

Figure 8–5 *Continued.* The assistant tightens one front pin and the diagonally opposite posterior pin simultaneously with the fingers to maximum finger tension (*D*). When maximum tension has been achieved, the pins are locked into position with special lock nuts (*E*). The final tension of 4 to 6 kilogram centimeters is achieved with a torque screwdriver. If a torque screwdriver is not available, however, a short-handled screwdriver may be used, taking care to apply force with two or three fingertips only.

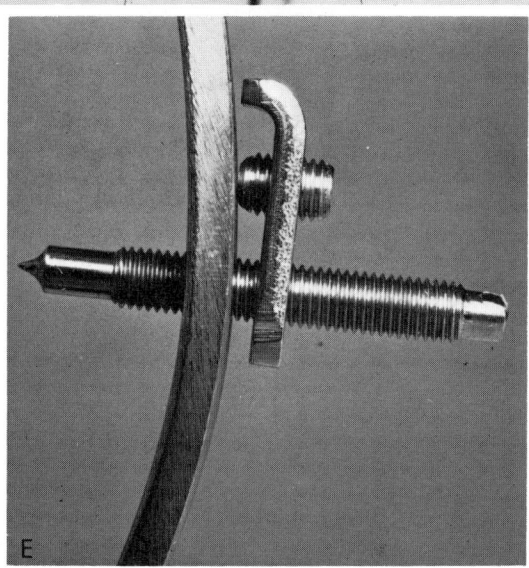

when inserting the pelvic fixator and pin tract infection. When this rigid traction device is left on for extended periods of time, especially in patients older than 15 years of age, chronic neck pain, spontaneous cervical fusion, degenerative joint changes in the cervical spine, and osteonecrosis of the dens can occur.[6, 19, 20, 27] We have not used the halohoop device at the Twin Cities Scoliosis Center since 1977.

Halofemoral traction can also exert strong tensile forces on the spine. With skeletal traction exerted from the caudad portion of the spinal column via pins in the distal femora, pelvic obliquity as well as scoliosis can be influenced. In adults, the possibility of complications is substantial. Deep vein thrombosis, stiffness of the hips, and psychological depression can all occur and thus the indications for halofemoral traction are limited (Fig. 8–6).[15]

Twice daily or more frequent neurologic examinations are mandatory for those undergoing skeletal traction of the spine. A knowledgeable nursing staff, fully alert to the potential dangers of skeletal traction on the spine and capable of responding independently if need be, is a prerequisite to its use. Inability to void or a heavy sensation in the thighs may herald impending neurologic deficit.[32] Each patient should be tested for long tract signs, hyperreflexia or Babinski reflex, and cranial nerve dysfunction. Dysfunction of cranial nerves six, nine, ten, and twelve may result in lateral gaze paralysis,

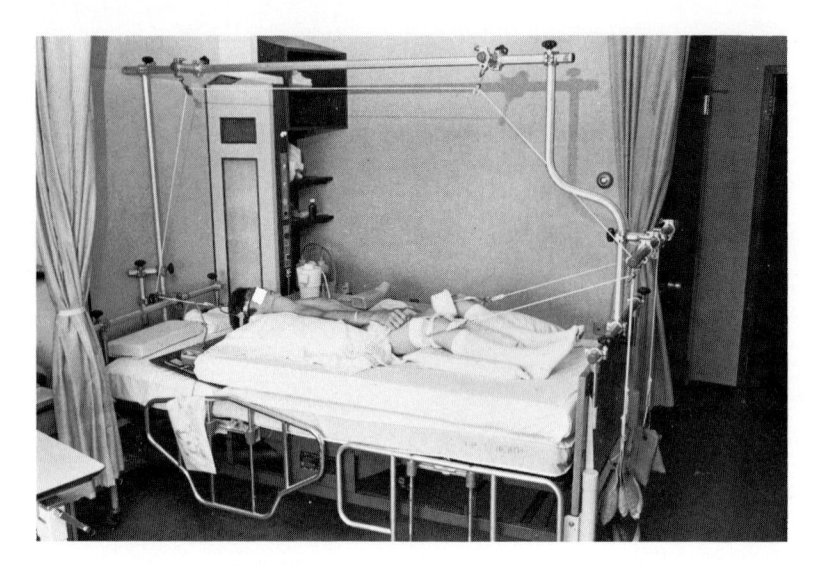

Figure 8–6. Halofemoral traction and the use of a split mattress are illustrated.

deglutition malfunction, speech difficulty, and asymmetric tongue protrusion.[30, 31] The combination can be irreversible and fatal but will usually resolve spontaneously if the traction is immediately reduced by 3 to 5 kilograms. Neck pain and hypesthesia in the upper limbs may also result from traction on the brachial plexus. Traction in excess of 15 kilograms results in an unacceptably high rate of complications and is not indicated. We seldom exceed 10 kilograms traction in the supine patient.

Permanent paralysis has resulted from spinal traction and use of this technique must be accompanied by a full knowledge of the potential risks and benefits. Congenital kyphosis is particularly sensitive to traction, and Winter has reported paraplegia in four patients, two of which cases were irreversible, treated by this method.[33] Wilkins and MacEwen have also noted the susceptibility of myelomeningocele and radiation spine deformities to halo traction-induced paresis.[31]

SUMMARY

As the technology of spinal deformity correction evolves, the role of skeletal traction on the spine has also changed.

Halo traction is not indicated in the following clinical circumstances:

1. Poor cranial bone stock such as in osteogenesis imperfecta or in children less than three to four years of age.
2. Rigid spine deformities. When traction is applied to a rigid curve, the spine proximal or distal to the curve may stretch and bow string the cord across the rigid segments.
3. Cervical and craniocervical junction instability. Tractive forces transmitted through incompetent spinal segments, such as Klippel-Feil deformity or Down's syndrome, can result in deformity and neurologic dysfunction.

Our use of skeletal spine traction is now generally limited to the following conditions:

1. Preoperative evaluation of flexible paralytic curves with pulmonary insufficiency.
2. Intercurrent halo traction in multiple stage spine reconstructive surgery. Halogravity traction can allow wheelchair mobility by stabilizing the spine between staged surgeries. This implies a degree of flexibility that would respond to traction in an upper thoracic or cervicothoracic curvature location.
3. Halo cast or vest application also is used for added external immobilization in cervical and upper thoracic deformities where surgery does not impart sufficient stability for the spine to be left unprotected until healing occurs.
4. Preoperative curve correction in severe flexible cervical and upper thoracic spine deformities such as neurofibromatosis and postlaminectomy kyphosis.
5. Selected cases of severe spondylolisthesis.

References

1. Bjerkreim, I., Carlsen, B., and Korsell, E.: Preoperative Cotrel traction in idiopathic scoliosis. Acta. Orthop. Scand., 53(6):901–905, 1982.
2. Bradford, D. S.: Treatment of severe spondylo-

listhesis. A combined approach for reduction and stabilization. Spine, 4:423, 1979.
3. Cummine, J. L., Lonstein, J. E., Moe, J. H., et al.: Reconstructive surgery in the adult for failed scoliosis fusion. J. Bone Joint Surg., 61A:1151, 1979.
4. DeWald, R. L., and Ray, R. D.: Skeletal traction for the treatment of severe scoliosis. The University of Illinois halo-hoop apparatus. J. Bone Joint Surg., 52A(2):233, 1970.
5. Dickson, R. A., and Leatherman, K. D.: Cotrel traction, exercises, casting in the treatment of idiopathic scoliosis. A pilot study and perspective randomized controlled clinical trial. Acta. Orthop. Scand., 49(1):46–48, 1978.
6. Dove, J., Hsu, L. C., and Yau, A. C.: The cervical spine after halo-pelvic traction. An analysis of the complications of 83 patients. J. Bone Joint Surg., 62B(2):158–161, 1980.
7. Edgar, M. A., Chapman, R. H., and Glasgow, M. M.: Preoperative correction in adolescent idiopathic scoliosis. J. Bone Joint Surg., 64(5):530–535, 1982.
8. Frankel, H. L., Hancock, D. O., Hyslop, G., et al.: The value of postural reduction in the initial management of closed injuries of the spine with paraplegia and tetraplegia. Paraplegia, 7:179, 1969.
9. Glisson, F.: De rachitide, sive morbo puerili qui volgo "The Rickets" dicitur, tractatus. 2.ed. 10. London, L. Sadler, 1660.
10. Goldberg, C., Dowling, F., Blake, N. S., and Regan, B. F.: A retrospective study of Cotrel dynamic spinal traction in the conservative management of scoliosis. Ir. Med. J., 74(12):363–365, 1981.
11. Guerin, J.: Memoire sur l'extension sigmoide et la flexion dans le traitement des déviations laterales de l'epine. Ed. 3. Paris, 1842.
12. Humbyrd, D. E., Latimer, F. R., Lonstein, J. E., and Samberg, L. C.: Brain abscess as a complication of halo traction. Spine, 6(4):364–368, 1981.
13. Kazarian, L. E.: Creep characteristics of the human spinal column. Orthop. Clin. North Am., 6:3, 1975.
14. Klemm, M.: Dr. med. Venel in Orbe, der Begrunder der modernen Orthopadie. Zentralbl. Chir. Mech. Orthop., vi:432, 1912.
15. Leslie, I. J., Dorgan, J. C., Bentley, G., and Galloway, R. W.: A prospective study of deep vein thrombosis of the leg in children on halo-femoral traction. J. Bone Joint Surg., 63B(2):168–170, 1981.
16. Letts, R. M., Palakar, G., and Bobecko, W. P.: Preoperative skeletal traction in scoliosis. J. Bone Joint Surg., 57(5):616–619, 1975.
17. Nachemson, A., and Nordwall, A.: Effectiveness of preoperative Cotrel traction for correction of idiopathic scoliosis. J. Bone Joint Surg., 59(4):504–508, 1977.
18. Perry, J., and Nickel, V. L.: Total cervical-spine fusion for neck paralysis. J. Bone Joint Surg., 41A:37, 1959.
19. Ransford, A. O., and Manning, C. W.: Complications of halo-pelvic distraction for scoliosis. J. Bone Joint Surg., 57(2):131–137, 1975.
20. Rozario, R. A., and Stein, B. M.: Complications of halo-pelvic traction. Case Report. J. Neurosurg., 45(6):716–718, 1976.
21. Sayre, L. A.: Spinal Disease and Spinal Curvature: Their Treatment by Suspension and the Plaster of Paris Bandage. London, Smith, Elder & Co., 1877.
22. Smith, A. D., Butte, F. L., and Ferguson, A. B.: Treatment of scoliosis by the wedging jacket and spine fusion. J. Bone Joint Surg., 20:825, 1938.
23. Swank, S., Lonstein, J. E., Moe, J. H., et al: Surgical treatment of adult scoliosis. J. Bone Joint Surg., 63A:268, 1981.
24. Swank, S. M., Winter, R. B., and Moe, J. H.: Scoliosis and cor pulmonale. Spine, 7:343, 1982.
25. Takahashi, K.: Biomechanical study of the deformed spine treated by Chiba University-type halo-pelvic distraction apparatus. Nippon Seikeigeka Gakkai Zasshi, 55(4):411–423, 1981.
26. Toledo, L. C., Toledo, C. H., and MacEwen, G. D.: Halo traction with the circolectric bed in the treatment of severe spinal deformities: a preliminary report. J. Pediatr. Orthop., 2(5):554–559, 1982.
27. Tredwell, S. J., and O'Brien, J. P.: Avascular necrosis of the proximal end of the dens. A complication of halo-pelvic distraction. J. Bone Joint Surg., 57(3):332–336, 1975.
28. Watson-Jones, R.: The results of postural reduction of fractures of the spine. J. Bone Joint Surg., 20:567, 1938.
29. White, A. A., and Panjabi, M. M.: Clinical Biomechanics of the Spine. Philadelphia, J. B. Lippincott Co., p. 105, 1978.
30. Wilkins, C., and MacEwen, G. D.: Halo-traction affecting cranial nerves. J. Bone Joint Surg., 56A:1540, 1974.
31. Wilkins, C., and MacEwen, G. D.: Cranial nerve injury from halo traction. Clin. Orthop., 126:106–110, 1977.
32. Winter, R. B.: In Chou, S. N., and Seljeskog, E. L. (eds.): Spinal Deformities and Neurological Dysfunction. New York, Raven Press, pg. 209, 1978.
33. Winter, R. B., Moe, J. H., and Lonstein, J. E.: The surgical treatment of congenital kyphosis: a review of 94 patients age five or older. Proceedings of the Scoliosis Research Society, Orlando, FL, Sept., 1984.

9
CAST TECHNIQUES

John E. Lonstein, M.D.

INTRODUCTION

Early medical writings contain many descriptions of crude and ingenious devices for distraction and straightening of spinal curvatures. There is no evidence that such devices were helpful until the introduction of plaster of Paris body casts during the latter part of the nineteenth century.[7, 8, 9, 10] Bradford and Brackett described correction on a distraction frame and holding of correction with a body cast. The correction was rarely maintained. Not until the technique of spinal fusion was introduced by Hibbs in 1911 was there any method with prolonged maintenance of correction.

Great strides have been made in the technique of cast correction. Hibbs invented the turnbuckle cast, which was perfected by Risser in 1927.[7] Risser combined the technique of distraction and lateral pressure with his "localizer cast" in 1952. This cast was used with early postoperative ambulation and is a widely used and effective method of maintaining correction obtained at fusion.[8] Dr. Yves Cotrel of Berck-Plage, France, developed the E.D.F. (elongation, derotation, flexion) cast, which in principle is similar to Risser's localizer cast.[2, 3]

The casts used at the Twin Cities Scoliosis Center embody some of the principles of the Risser and Cotrel casts. The use of this form of postoperative immobilization has been largely replaced by the postoperative TLSO (see Chapter 7).

Risser "Localizer" Cast (Fig. 9–1)

This cast extends from the mandible and occiput to the buttocks, sometimes being cut down to a low neck or shoulder straps. It is applied supine on a Risser frame, a well-molded pelvic portion being applied first. Traction is now applied via a disposable head halter and the pelvic section, and the remain-

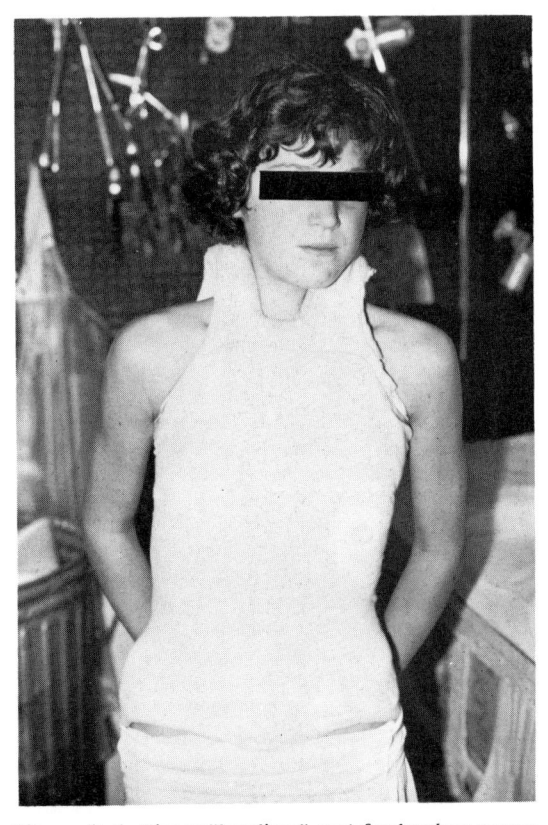

Figure 9–1. Risser "localizer" cast for lumbar curves with shoulder straps. The cast is applied in two sections with careful molding around the pelvis and upper thorax. A localizer device presses against the convexity of the curve. The cast is extended to the mandible and occiput for thoracic curves. (Published with permission of Dr. J. Risser.)

der of the cast is applied with careful molding around the mandible, occiput and upper thorax. A localizer device is attached that presses against the convexity of the curve, thus correcting the curve. The cast is trimmed and finished, allowing hip flexion to 100 degrees and adequate arm function. The fit over the anterior thorax is loose to allow chest expansion.

Cotrel E.D.F. Cast (Fig. 9–2)

The Cotrel E.D.F. cast is applied on a special frame, which is basically a Risser frame with an overhead attachment with numerous correcting pulleys. The patient is placed supine in traction using a Cotrel head halter and muslin straps passing around the waist, in much the same manner as the Cotrel pelvic straps (see page 122). The cast is applied in one piece, without adding a mandibular/occipital piece. Derotation straps are used, which pass under the patient and are attached to the frame next to and above the patient, creating a lateral and derotating force against the convexity of the curve. Additional straps correct shoulder elevation and help maintain torso balance. Correction is obtained by adjusting the traction and the tension in these straps with the aid of the ratchets and pulleys. The cast is trimmed, giving shoulder straps, an anterior chest window, and a posterior window on the concavity of the curve. In addition, an inflatable bladder is added over the convexity of the curve to correct the rotational prominence.

Dr. Stagnara, formerly of Lyon, France, used similar principles in his distraction cast and postoperative cast (Figs. 9–3 and 9–4).[6]

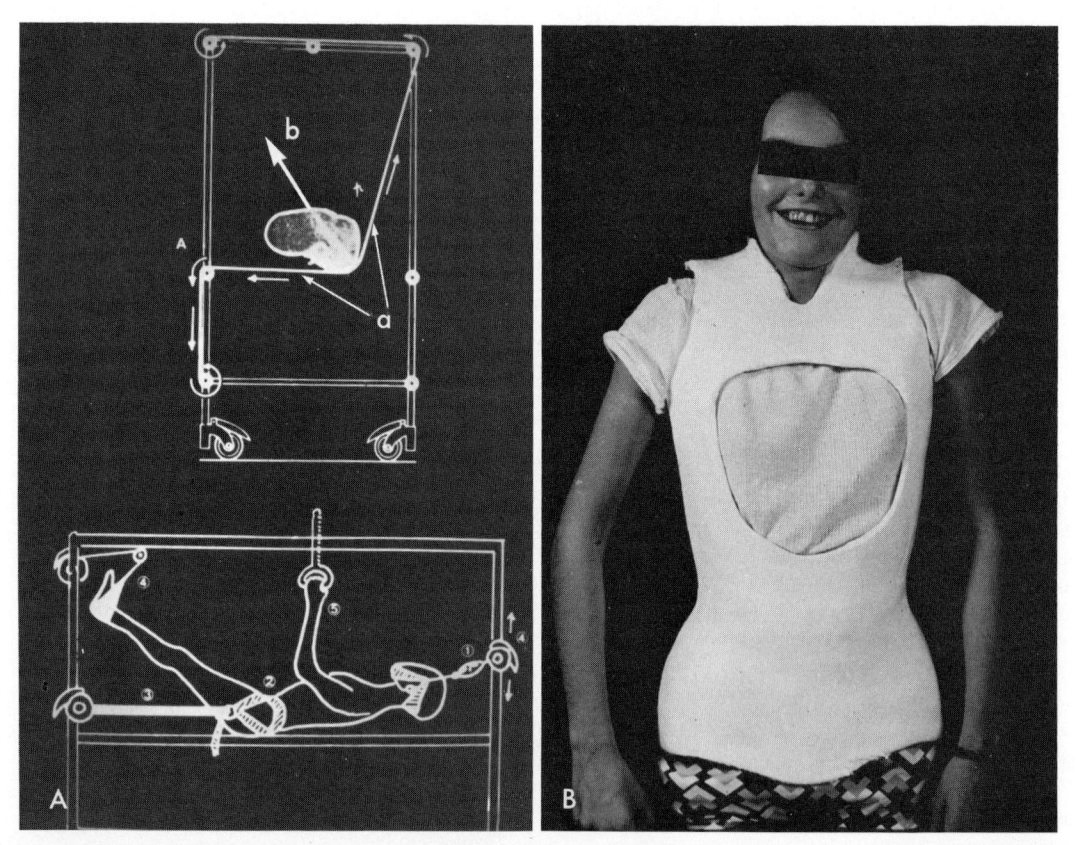

Figure 9–2. A, Cotrel E.D.F. (elongation, derotation, flexion) principle. The patient is positioned on a special frame and placed in longitudinal traction using a head halter and pelvic straps. The hips are flexed. After the cast has been applied a derotation strap (a) is added, which passes under the patient and then overhead on the side of the convexity of the curve. Tension in this strap gives a derotating corrective vector (b) on the rib prominence. B, The cast is applied in one piece on the Cotrel frame. There is a large chest window anteriorly. (Published with permission of Dr. Y. Cotrel.)

CAST TECHNIQUES

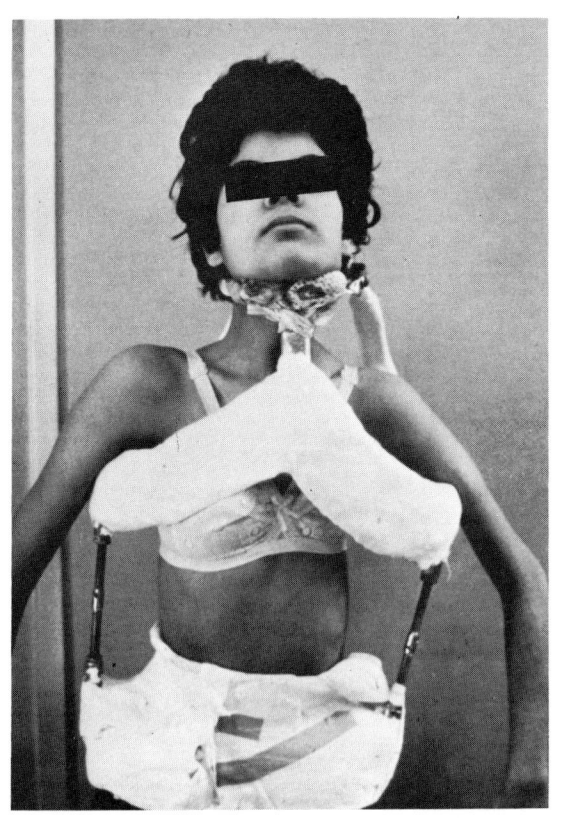

Figure 9–3. Distraction cast as used by Dr. Stagnara. Gradual distraction is applied over a number of months. When maximal correction is obtained, the two parts of the cast are attached and the turnbuckles removed. (Published with permission of Dr. P. Stagnara.)

Risser-Cotrel Cast

The cast used at the Twin Cities Scoliosis Center is a combination of the two casts and techniques just described. It is basically a Risser cast applied in one piece with a mandibular/occipital section, using the distraction technique of Cotrel plus his derotation strap and a posterior thoracic window (Fig. 9–5).

TECHNIQUES OF APPLICATION[5]

The Risser-Cotrel cast is rarely used today. The postoperative TLSO has replaced it; or the underarm cast is used. The full Risser-Cotrel cast is still used in children or in cases in which great control of the cervicothoracic area is desired. Since it encompasses all the principles of a cast, its application will be described first, and the modifications for applying other casts will follow.

Postoperative Risser-Cotrel Cast

The casting frame used is a modified Risser table (Fig. 9–6A). An overhead frame is added, with pulleys for the derotation strap. The removable shoulder bar has been replaced by a flat bar, which allows application of a total contact cast. The sacral bar has been modified by the addition of a rectangular sacral seat, which allows for better application of the cast around the pelvis. There is a windlass at the head end and two at the foot end of the table for longitudinal traction.

The patient lies on a cart and is placed in two layers of tubular stockinet. The stockinet must be long enough to extend from mid-thighs to over the head. The outer layer is rolled up to around the lower abdomen. The patient is placed on the Risser table and positioned so that the removable cross bar lies at the level of the axilla (Fig. 9–6B). The cross bar is padded with a strip of felt. The

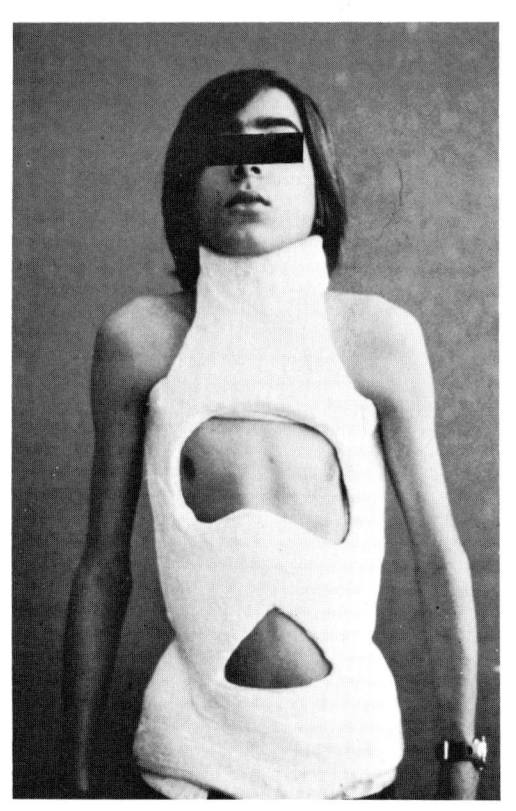

Figure 9–4. Postoperative cast as used by Dr. Stagnara. Note the head position, with the cast causing head extension. The cast has a small chest window and also a small abdominal window. (Published with the permission of Dr. P. Stagnara.)

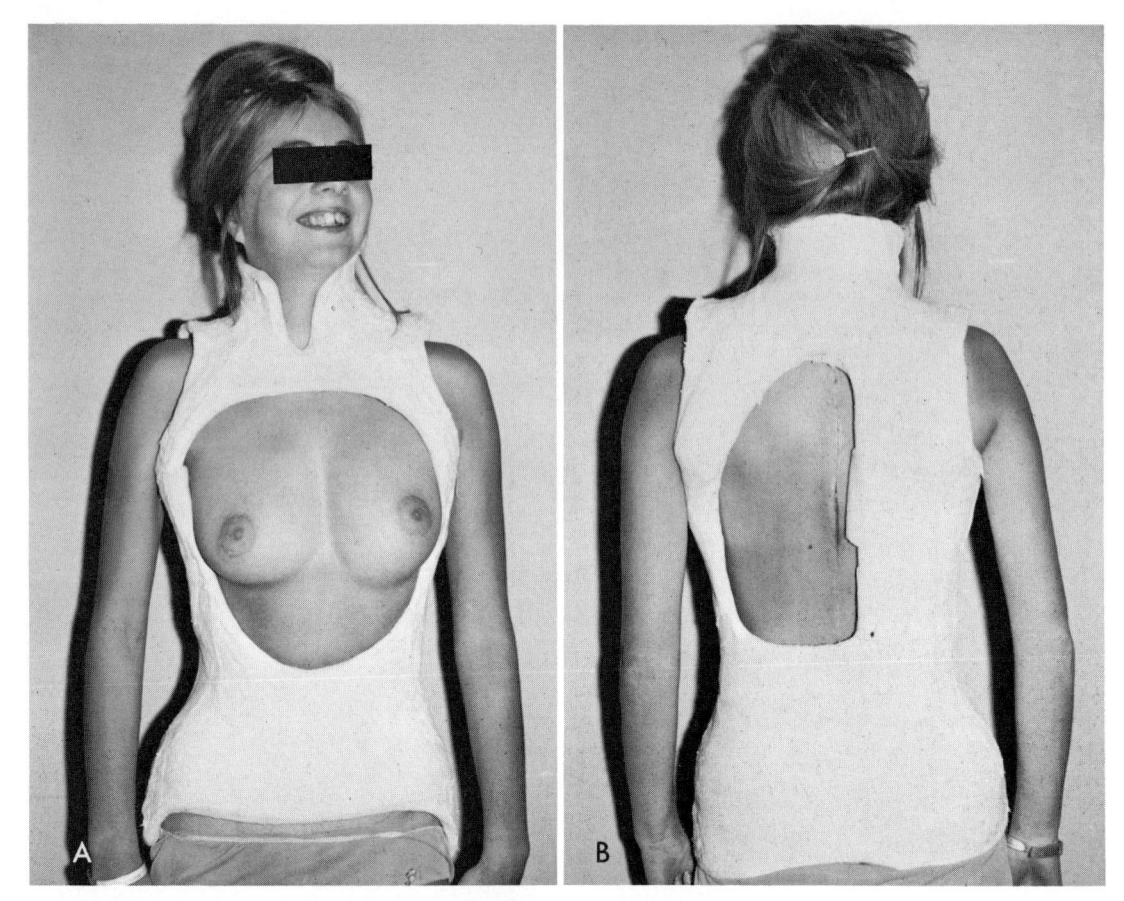

Figure 9–5. Risser-Cotrel cast. The cast is a combination of the principles of Risser and Cotrel. The cast extends from the mandible and occiput to the groin and buttocks. *A*, There is a large *thoracic* window anteriorly to allow full chest expansion. The cast is trimmed to allow full hip flexion and arm movement. *B*, Posteriorly the cast fits *under* the occiput and extends low over the buttocks to control pelvic tilt. A large window is removed over the concavity of the curve to allow expansion in this area with restriction over the rotational rib prominence.

sacral seat should comfortably support the pelvis, with the sacral bar lying below the buttocks. The legs are supported on a wooden leg support, which is not raised, maintaining the normal lumbar lordosis. A longitudinal canvas strap is *not* used in the postoperative cast.

Traction is applied with a disposable head halter, which is attached to the windlass at the head end of the frame. Muslin straps are passed around the waist over one layer of stockinet, positioned just above the iliac crest, and tied on the opposite side at the level of the greater trochanter. Both straps are passed under the leg support to the foot of the table. They are attached to separate windlasses, and longitudinal traction is applied. The outer layer of stockinet is rolled over the muslin straps. These straps thus lie *between* the two layers of stockinet, allowing easy removal after the cast is applied. Maximal tolerated distraction is applied. The patient is awake and not sedated. Ketamine anesthesia is used in smaller children or in patients unable to cooperate. A four or six inch canvas strap is attached to the frame so that it will pass under the patient and be applied to the convexity of the curve. Two straps are used for double curves.

The only padding used is ¼ inch foam rubber,* which is placed as a single sheet around the waist and hips and taped in place. No other padding is used. In very bony patients felt padding is added, being used as donuts *around* bony prominences. The stockinet must be free of wrinkles. The position

---

*"Profex" brand, Airfoam Splint & Cast Padding—¼", ½".

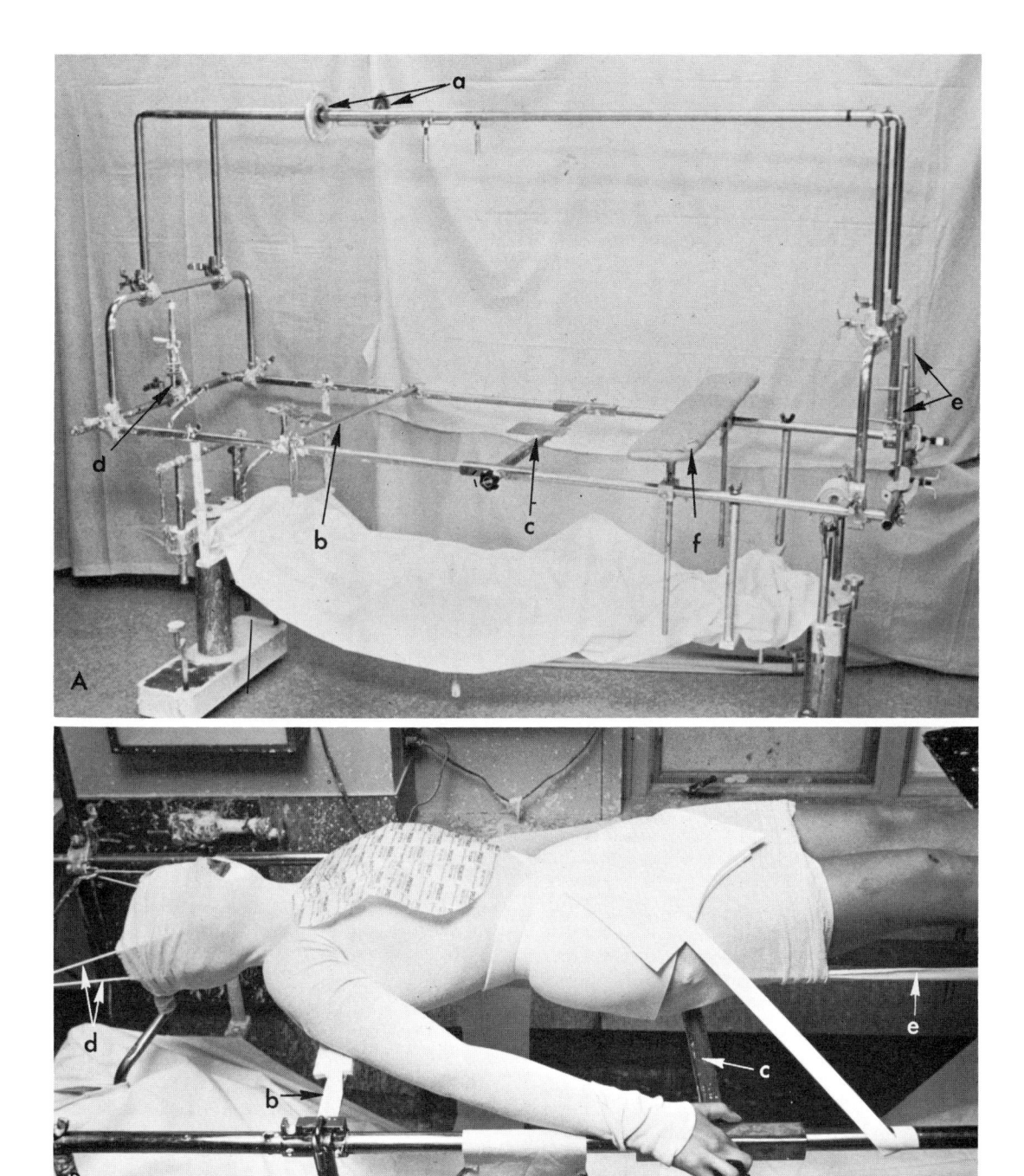

Figure 9–6. Technique of cast application. *A*, Casting frame. The frame is a modified Risser table with an overhead frame with pulleys (a) for the derotation strap. The patient lies on the shoulder bar (b) and sacral seat (c). Traction is applied via the windlass at the head of the table (d) and the two at the foot of the table (e). The feet are supported on the foot board (f), *no* hip flexion being used. *B*, The patient is placed in two layers of stockinet and positioned on the cast table. The shoulder bar (b) lies at the level of the axilla and the sacral bar and seat (c) lie just below the buttocks at the level of the greater trochanters. Longitudinal traction is applied via a disposable head halter (d), and muslin straps (e) are attached to windlasses. Note that the muslin straps pass around the pelvis between the two layers of stockinet and are tied at the level of the greater trochanter. The only padding used is ¼ inch foam around the pelvis.

Illustration continued on following page

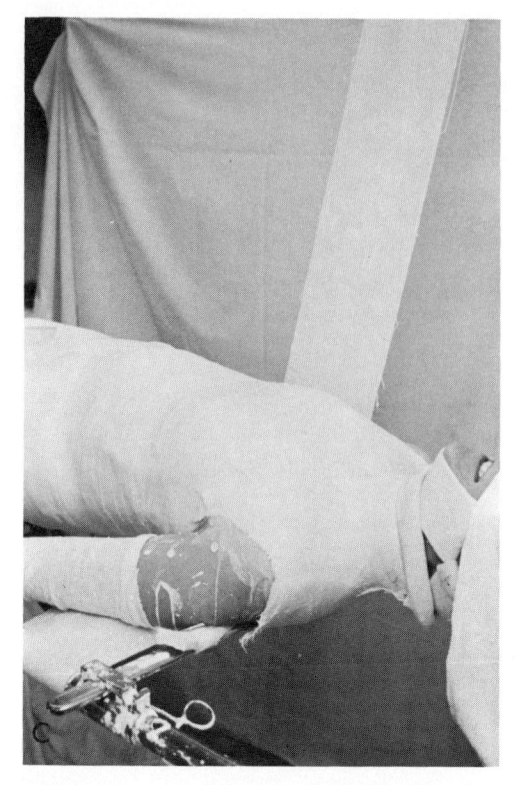

Figure 9–6 *Continued. C,* Derotation strap. The Cotrel derotation strap passes from the side bar on the concavity of the curve, under the patient and to the pulley on the overhead bar on the side of the convexity of the curve. The strap is applied after the whole cast is applied and the plaster is setting.

Illustration continued on opposite page

of the patient is checked. The pelvis must be level, with the torso and head in balance above it. The suprasternal notch lies over the pelvis. The head level is checked by elevating or lowering the head support, the head positioned so that the ears are over the middle of the shoulder.

Extra strong, resin-reinforced plaster is used, as it allows application of a thinner cast. Two six inch rolls are applied, rolling from the pelvis upward, covering the torso evenly and going over shoulders. Five by thirty-six inch splints (12.5 × 91 cm.) (five to six layers thick) are applied posteriorly, starting over the buttocks and extending up, each splint overlapping the one previously applied. Splints are placed over the shoulders, running from the pelvis, over the shoulder, and then down the back. While the splints are incorporated using one or two plaster rolls, the neck is added. A four inch plaster roll is placed around the neck and mandible and reinforced using four by fifteen inch splints placed obliquely. The upper end of these splints is *below* the mandible and occiput, at the final level of the neck piece. These splints are incorporated with a four inch plaster roll. The application of plaster is rapid so that all the plaster still is wet, allowing molding and incorporation of the layers.

The Cotrel strap is placed under the patient *outside* the plaster and attached to the windlass on the overhead frame on the convexity, and a derotation force is applied to the convexity of the curve (Fig. 9–6C). The plaster is carefully rubbed to incorporate layers. The cast is molded to the contours of the body, care being taken especially posteriorly with molding under the occiput (Fig. 9–6D). Care is taken to mold over soft tissues, with no pressure applied over bony prominences. In cases with a sharp "razor back" rib prominence, the Cotrel strap is not used, as localized pressure against the rib prominence can cause skin necrosis. Hand molding is used, ensuring that pressure on the apex of the kyphos is avoided, the molding being on the medial wall of the rib hump.

Once the plaster has set, the cast is trimmed. The neck is trimmed about half an inch below the mandible with an anterior notch for the trachea, the latter extending to the suprasternal notch. The pelvic section is trimmed above the pubis and laterally over the thighs to give enough room for 100 degrees of hip flexion. Note that the lower end of the cast is trimmed to resemble a Milwaukee brace pelvic section. The plaster is trimmed in the area of the shoulders, allowing full arm motion. A large thoracic window is removed, extending to the epigastrium but leaving plaster covering the lower abdomen. Enough plaster is removed laterally to allow full chest expansion. Plaster should not compress the breasts.

The patient is removed from the Risser frame. The removable cross bar at the shoulder, once removed, allows the patient to be easily lifted onto a cart. The back of the cast is trimmed below the occiput and low over the buttocks. In patients with a very bony sacrum, extra felt padding is added at the sides of the sacrum to remove any pressure over the midline of the sacrum. A window is removed posteriorly on the side of the concavity of the thoracic curve, allowing the "thoracic valley" to be expanded with the use of breathing exercises. Sharp areas are

CAST TECHNIQUES

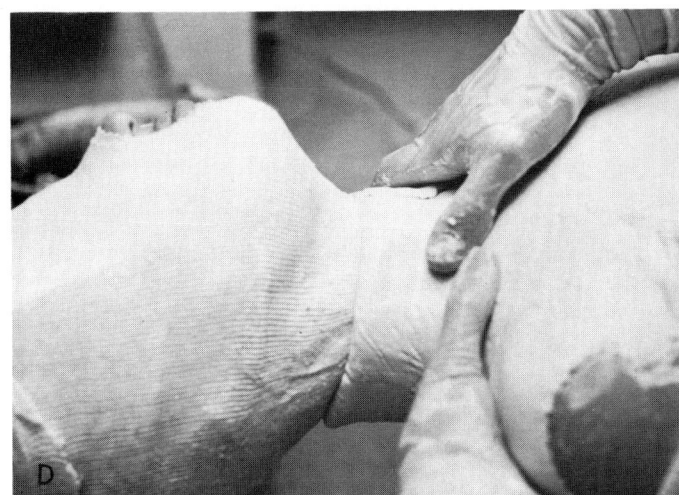

Figure 9–6 *Continued.* *D,* The neck is molded carefully to the contours of the patient. The plaster fits snugly around the neck and extends to below mandible and occiput with a fit the same as that of a well-fitting Milwaukee brace neck ring. *E,* The edges of the cast are finished by careful skiving. The cast is undercut to eliminate all sharp edges.

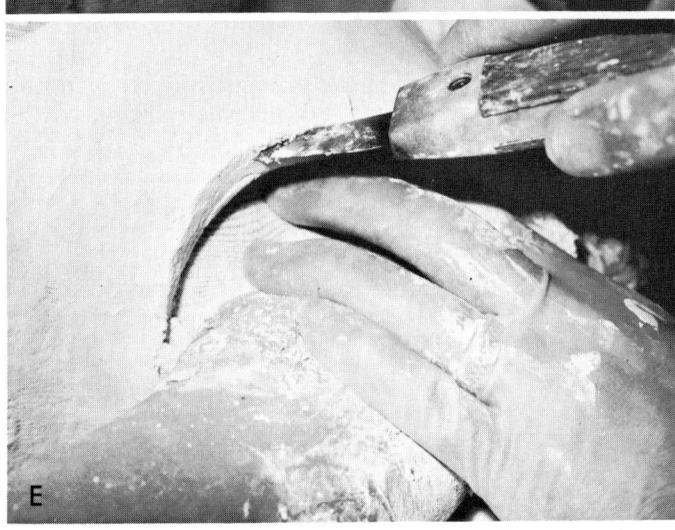

removed by skiving the edges (Fig. 9–6E). The two layers of stockinet are pulled taut and fixed in place to the cast, using half-length three inch wide splints. No sharp edges or rough areas should remain.

The cast is usually applied five to seven days postoperatively. Absorbable intracuticular skin sutures are used so there is no need to delay cast application to remove skin sutures. After the cast is applied the patient is x-rayed supine and then is ambulated the same day. Constant attention to cast fit is necessary. Any area of pain is inspected for redness. The cast must be relieved in this area or, when necessary, padding added. The padding is applied around but never *over* bony prominences. If pain occurs under the cast, the area is windowed to inspect the skin. With this careful attention to cast application and fit, pressure sores are unusual.

With early ambulation, not more than five degrees should be lost between the supine and standing x-rays, the supine film being usually equal to or a few degrees better than the correction obtained on the day of surgery. If more than five degrees are lost the cause is usually a poor cast, and a new cast should be applied. The average cast time is six to nine months, the cast being changed once. If the fusion extends above T4, a new Risser-Cotrel cast is usually applied. An underarm cast is used for the second cast if the fusion ends at T5 or below. With this technique, surgical correction is maintained, and five degrees loss between the day of surgery and one year postoperatively is average.[4]

Hyperextension Cast

The patient is placed in two layers of stockinet, positioned on the Risser frame as described above, and placed in traction (Fig. 9–7). A hyperextension strap is placed around the patient and attached to the two pulleys on the overhead frame. This strap consists of a long piece of four inch tubular stockinet with a strip of one quarter inch felt placed *in* the stockinet. This strap is positioned over the apex of the kyphosis and is tightened until it lifts the patient off the shoulder bar. The two straps are tied together to allow adequate fit around the thorax. This causes restriction of breathing, and the patient must be reassured during cast application. The shoulder bar is removed, the patient being supported on the strap and sacral seat (Fig. 9–7). The position of the head is checked, as is the balance of the patient. Foam padding is placed around the pelvis.

The cast is applied as described previously, with care being taken to place reinforcing four inch splints vertically along the lateral aspect of the thorax. Once the plaster is set, it is trimmed. The chest window is made large to allow full chest expansion. There is no posterior window, but the cast is windowed over the apex of the kyphosis, and the hyperextension strap is cut, the window being replaced. This prevents a ridge of pressure over the kyphosis and makes pressure sores over the kyphosis rare.

In cases with high thoracic kyphosis, the hyperextension strap is difficult to use. The patient is positioned with the apex of the kyphosis on the cross bar, and the latter is *not* removed. The bar then acts as the hyperextension force.

Underarm Cast (Fig. 9–8)

With the more common use of additional internal fixation, stabilization of the neck with a Risser-Cotrel cast has not been routinely necessary. When a postoperative cast is needed, the underarm cast is usually used. Occasionally, the neck is still included with instrumentation to T1 or T2 when no sublaminar wires are used.

The technique of application is similar to the postoperative cast with the following exceptions:

1. The cast extends only to the sternum anteriorly and upper back posteriorly.

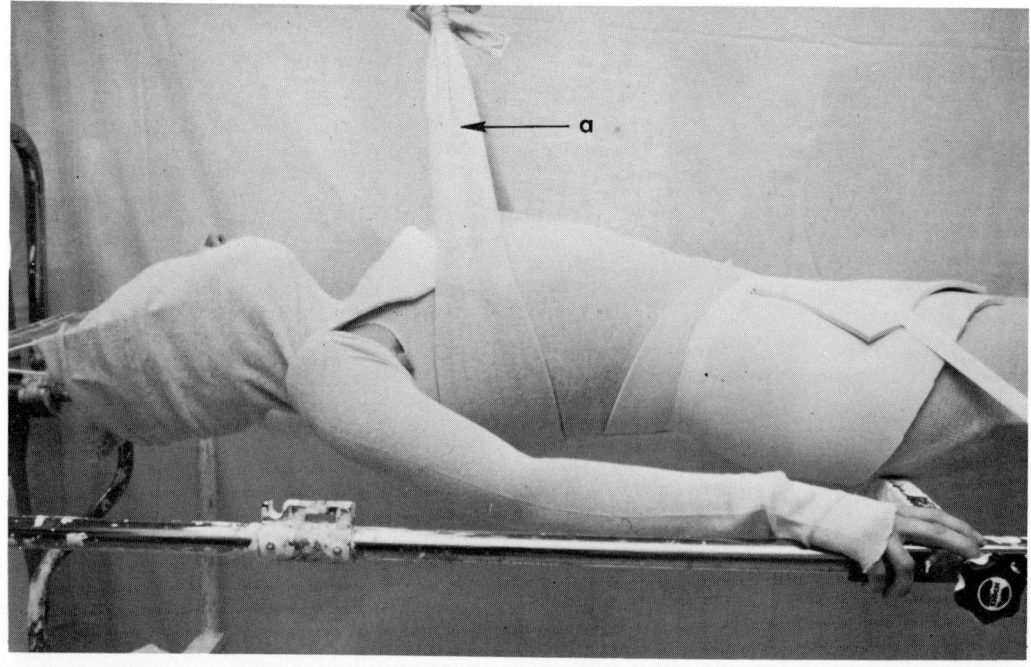

Figure 9–7. Position for hyperextension casting. The position is similar to that shown in Figure 9–6B for the Risser-Cotrel cast. The shoulder bar is removed after the patient is suspended by a hyperextension strap (a). This strap consists of a long piece of four inch tubular stockinet with a strip of ¼ inch thick felt in the stockinet. The strap is attached to the pulleys on the overhead frame and is positioned at the apex of the kyphosis.

CAST TECHNIQUES 127

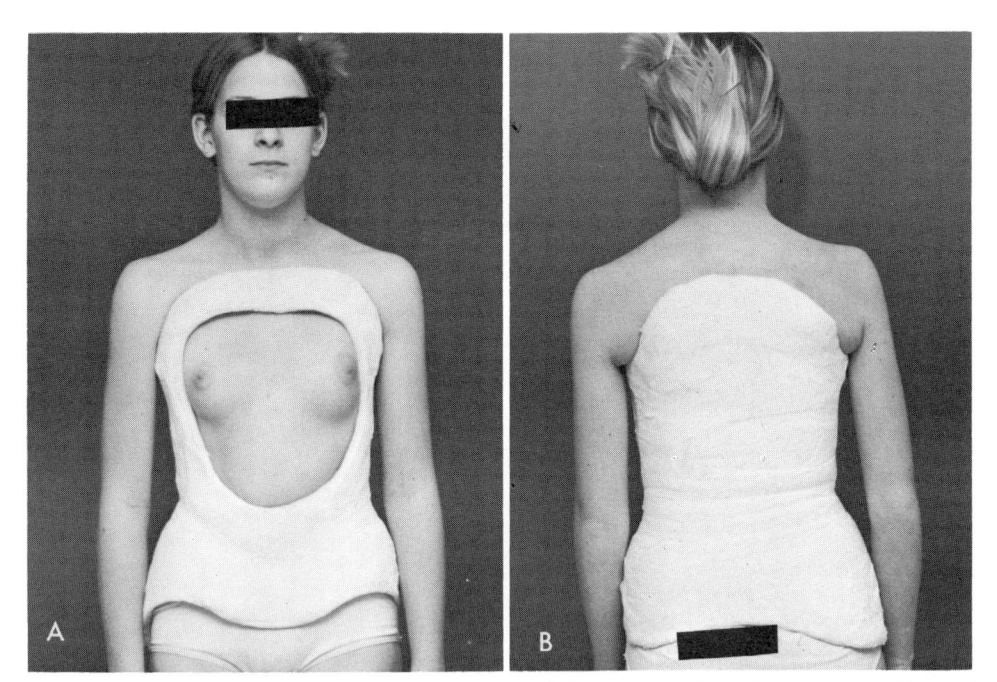

Figure 9–8. Underarm cast. *A,* Front view. *B,* Back view. This cast extends to the sternum with no shoulder straps. There is a large anterior thoracic window and *no* posterior window.

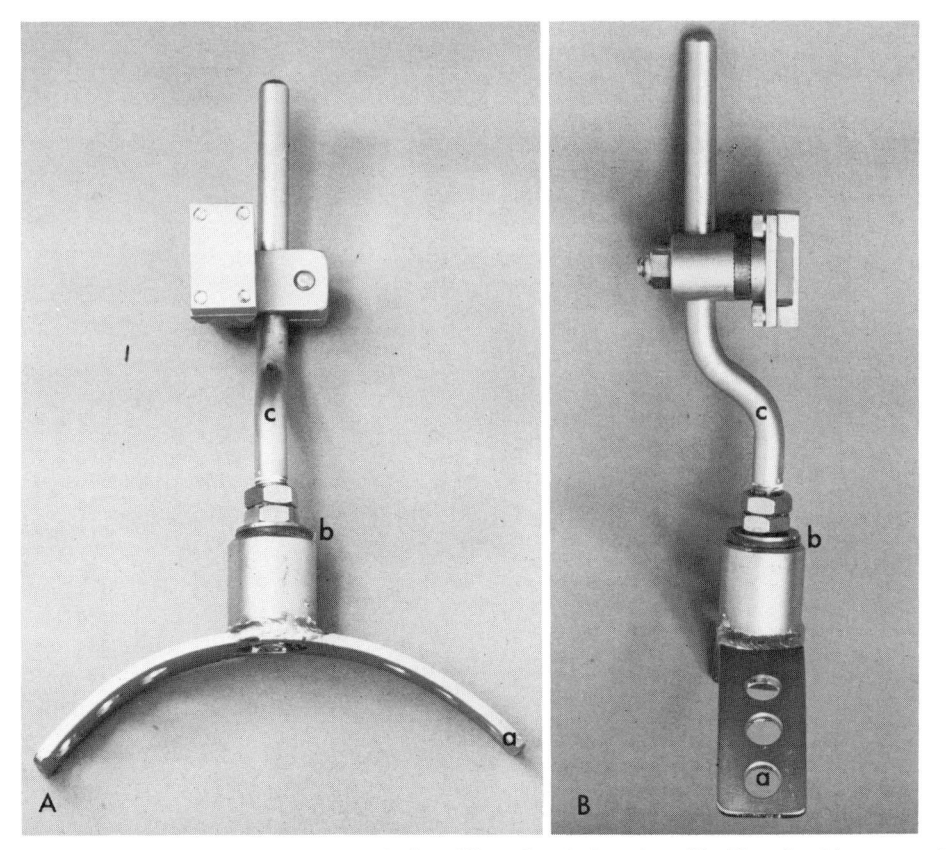

Figure 9–9. "Lo-Profile" halo supports. Lateral view (*A*) and anterior view (*B*). The shoulder support (a) is malleable and is contoured to the shoulder straps of the cast. A silicone bushing (b) allows some motion of the upright (c). This upright is either straight or bent; the latter, which is illustrated, is necessary for children. The halo attachment allows control of halo height, tilt, and anteroposterior position.

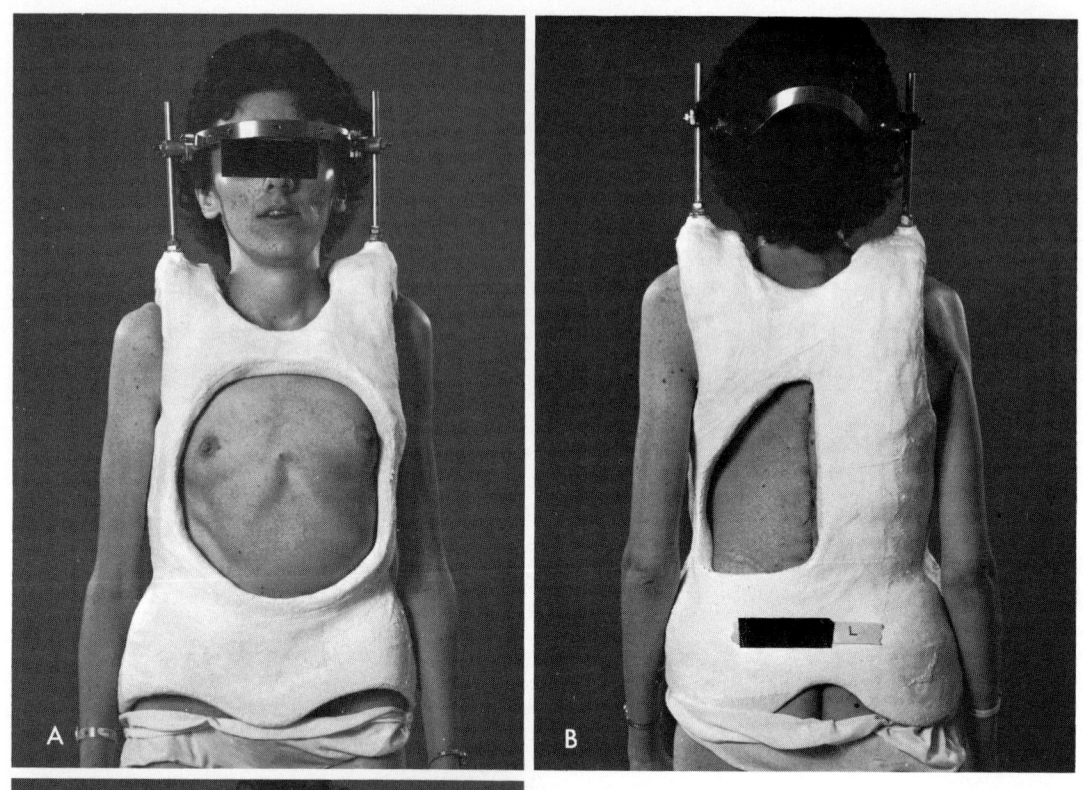

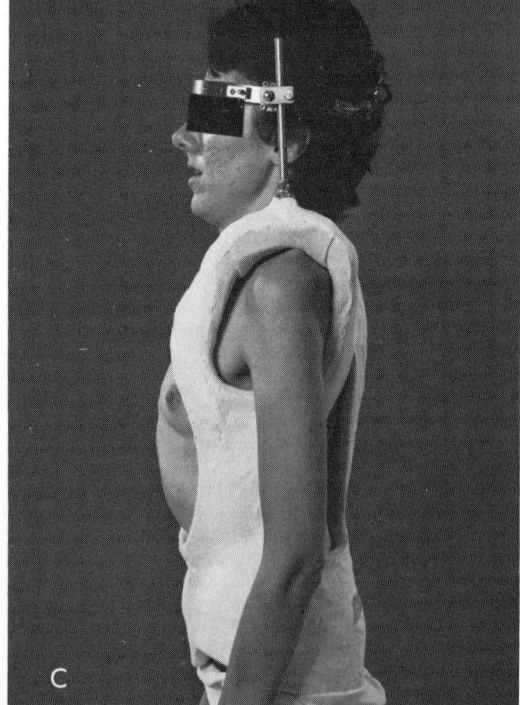

Figure 9–10. Halo cast. The cast portion consists of a Risser-Cotrel cast with shoulder straps and large anterior and posterior windows. The halo is attached to the cast with "Lo-Profile" halo supports.

CAST TECHNIQUES

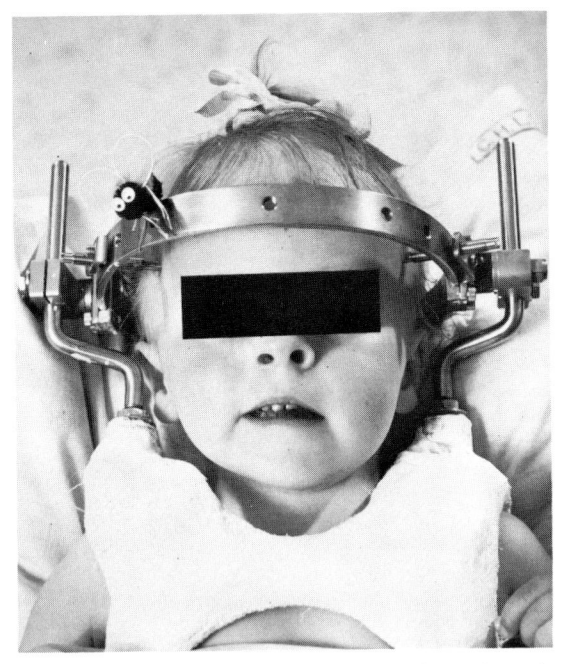

Figure 9-11. A child in a halo cast needs contoured "Lo-Profile" supports to attach the halo to the cast.

2. The patient is positioned low on the shoulder bar, which lies at the upper shoulders.
3. The arms are placed in a relaxed manner on the side bars and *not* pulled down.
4. Plaster is applied under the arms with reinforcement anteriorly over the sternum and posteriorly as high as possible.
5. The cast is well molded around the pelvis and iliac crests. The cast is trimmed at the suprasternal notch and then under the arms. A large thoracic window is removed leaving three to four inches (7 to 10 cm.) above the window. This portion is cut wider than necessary, the final trim being performed with the patient sitting. No posterior window is removed.

Halo Cast (Figs. 9–9 to 9–13)

The halo cast is used for immobilization of cervical fractures and fusions, and fusion of cervicothoracic curves. This cast also aids in

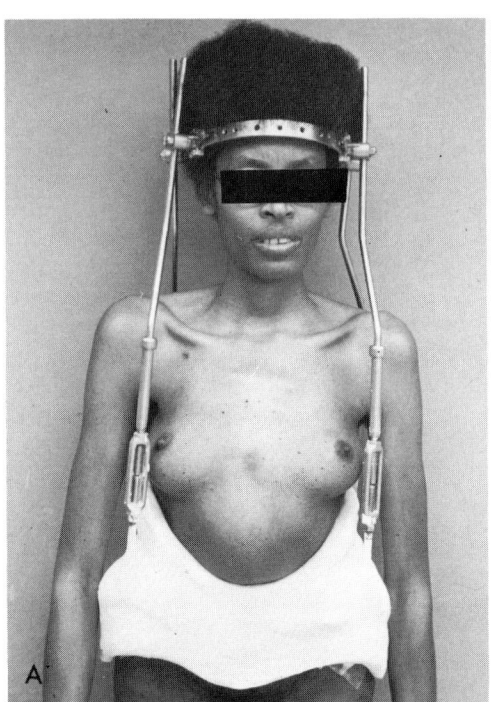

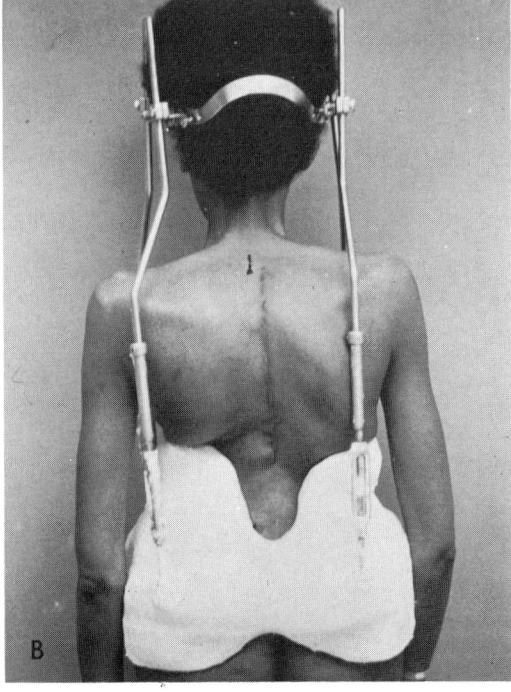

Figure 9-12. Halo pelvic cast. Alternative method of halo cast fixation when no thoracic pressure is desired or as a form of ambulatory distraction. A well-molded pelvic section is attached to the halo via four contoured uprights, with turnbuckles for distraction.

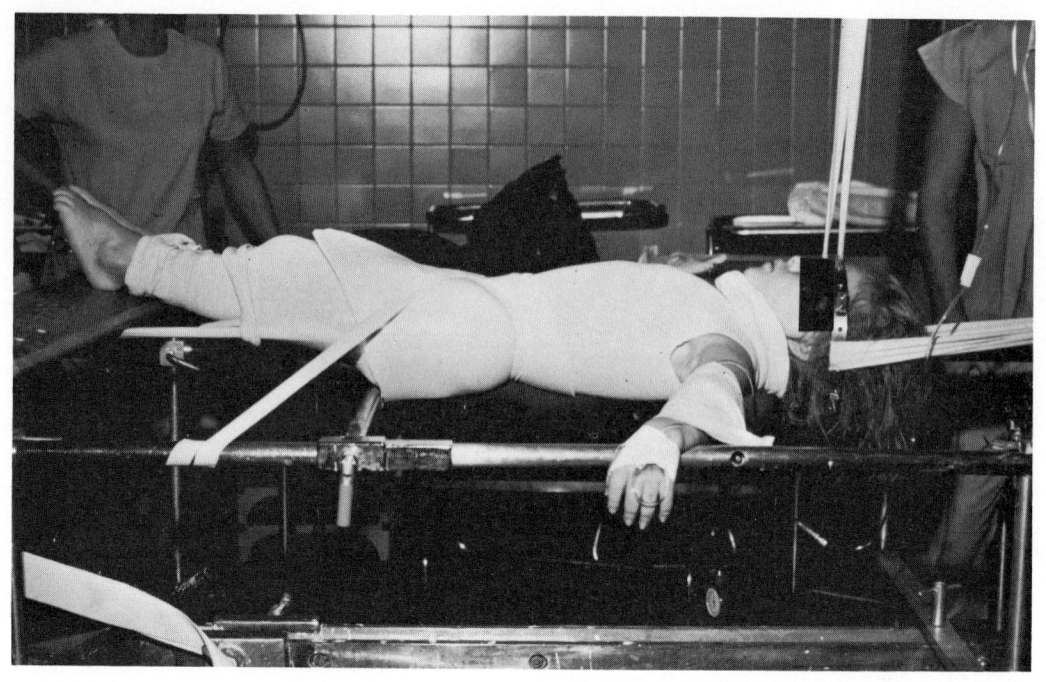

Figure 9–13. Position for halo cast application. The patient is positioned on the Risser frame as for the application of a Risser-Cotrel cast. The halo is supported from the overhead frame, and traction is applied to the halo via muslin straps or rope.

the postoperative immobilization of severe curves. The postoperative "old style" halo support consisted of two anterior uprights that extend to a frame to which the halo is attached. The new "lo-profile" supports extend from the shoulder of the cast to the halo with silicone bushings at the junction of the uprights and shoulder supports (Fig. 9–10).[1] Both these supports allow a little motion, thus preventing the pin-skull interface from being the main site of motion. Both the halo supports allow for adjustments in head position.

The fit of the cast is as the postoperative cast, the differences being as follows:

1. The halo, having previously been applied, is suspended from the overhead frame and traction is applied to the halo. Countertraction is supplied by the muslin straps as described previously (Fig. 9–13).
2. Felt padding is added over the shoulders and held in place with one or two turns of webril around the thorax.
3. The cast is applied extending over the shoulders, no neck being added.
4. The halo shoulder supports are contoured with bending irons to fit the shoulder sections of the cast. In children the uprights have a bend in them to allow the supports to be placed on the shoulders.
5. The connecting piece to the halo is applied, the uprights inserted and fitted to the shoulders. The head and uprights are positioned and the connecting pieces locked to the halo. The uprights are left loose while the shoulder portions are attached to the cast. Once this connection has completely set, the uprights are locked to the connecting pieces.
6. The cast is trimmed with anterior and posterior thoracic windows. A great deal of care is necessary to trim and skive the cast sufficiently over the shoulders (Fig. 9–10).
7. Final adjustments in halo and head position are performed the following day once the patient stands and ambulates. This position is critical for position of fusion, plus the fact that in the halo cast the head position is fixed and thus must be as functional as possible.

Cast With Leg Extension (Fig. 9–14)

Any of the above casts may be extended down one or both legs to the knee or foot to aid in stabilizing the pelvis with certain lumbosacral fusions. The most common use is in cases of lumbosacral fusions for spondylolisthesis in which cast reduction of the spondylolisthesis is performed. In these cases the leg extension can be unilateral or bilateral. Leg extension casts are also used to control pelvic obliquity, for lumbosacral fractures, after excision of lumbosacral hemivertebrae, or in any case where control of the pelvis is important postoperatively.

The application of a unilateral leg extension cast for the cast reduction of spondylolisthesis will be described. This consists of an underarm cast with a leg extension (Fig. 9–14B).

Positioning is the same as for an underarm cast with the following differences:

1. The sacrum is supported on a special sacral seat and not on the sacral bar. This allows the plaster to extend from the pelvis to the thigh.
2. The stockinet is long and is cut and taped around the thigh.
3. The leg support is placed to give hip hyperextension, supporting the calves behind the axis of the body.
4. Webril is applied on the thigh, extending to cover the foam rubber over the pelvis.

Cast application and trimming are the same as for an underarm cast, with the following differences:

1. Plaster rolls are applied from the thigh proximally to the pelvis.
2. Long splints (5 × 36 inches) are applied laterally, anteriorly, and posteriorly from the body portion to the thigh.
3. Additional long splints are applied in a spinal oblique manner from the thigh to the pelvis anteriorly and posteriorly to reinforce the hip joint area.
4. The cast is trimmed as described for an underarm cast.
5. The thigh portion is trimmed 3 to 4 cm. (1 to 1½ inches) above the patella.
6. Adequate trimming in the perineum anteriorly and posteriorly is essential.

Turnbuckle Cast (Fig. 9–15)

One of the most common methods of obtaining correction prior to the use of Harrington instrumentation was with cast correction and fusion in the corrected position. A method of obtaining cast correction was the turnbuckle cast. This is a cast that is wedged

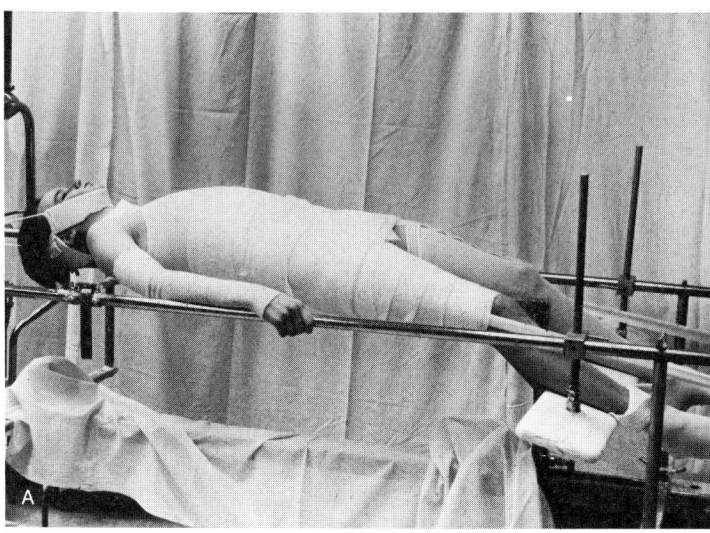

Figure 9–14. A, Position to apply an underarm cast with a right leg extension for reduction of spondylolisthesis. Note the absence of a sacral bar, the sacral seat being used, the lower part just being visible between the knees. The hips are hyperextended with the calves supported on the leg supports. B, Completed and trimmed cast. Note the large thoracic window and the adequate trimming in the perineal area.

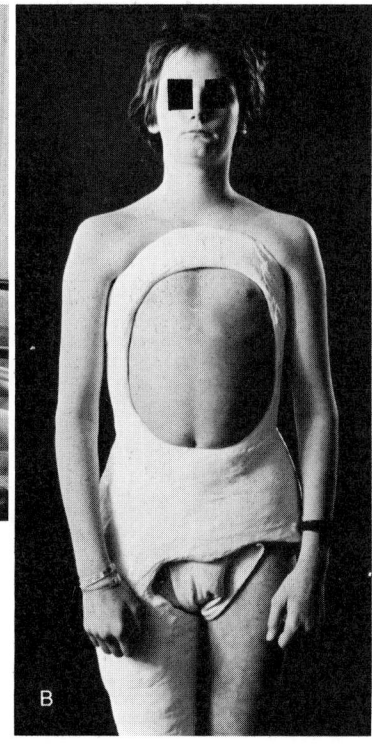

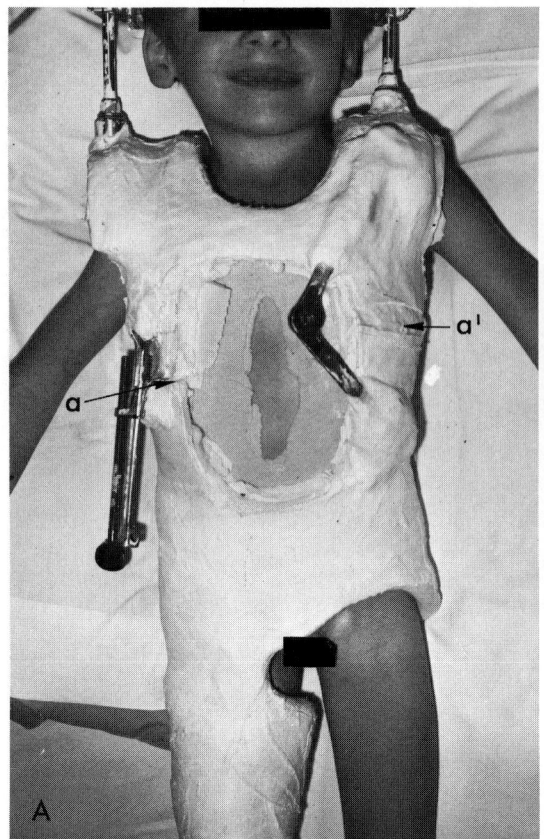

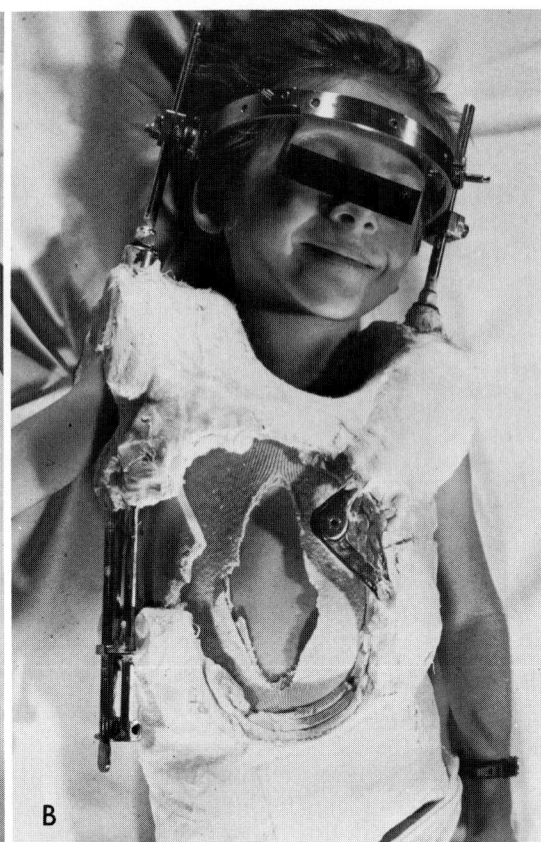

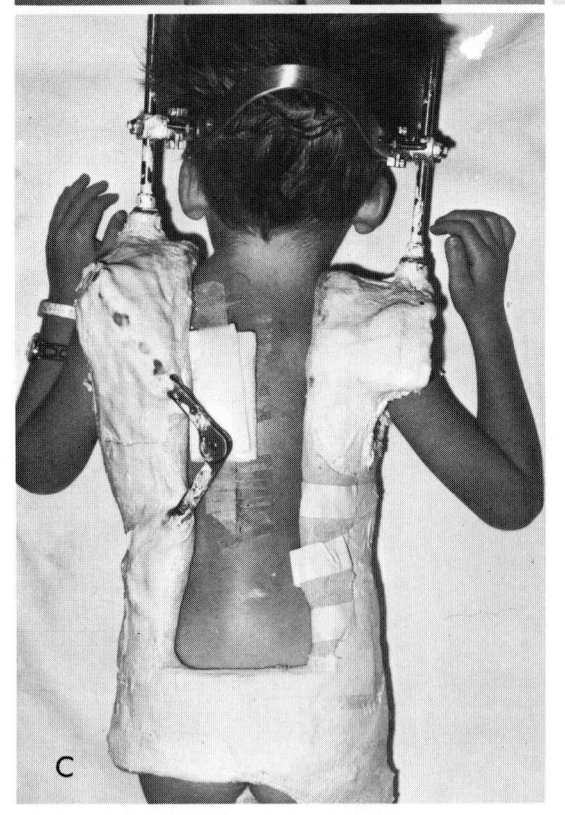

Figure 9–15. Halo turnbuckle cast with leg extension. This cast is used to correct a curve with control of the head via the halo and the pelvis via the leg extension. *A*, The cast with the turnbuckle on the side of the concavity of the curve and anterior and posterior hinges over the spine. Note the plaster removed on the two sides a and a^1. *B*, The turnbuckle has been gradually lengthened with opening on the concavity of the curve. The wedge of plaster removed on the convexity of the curve has been closed, and the angle of the hinge is decreased. *C*, Posterior view after the area of the hinge has been sealed with plaster. The turnbuckle is removed and the cast filled in and reinforced, maintaining the correction.

with the aid of turnbuckles incorporated in the cast. Guerin introduced the concept in 1842, and Risser modified it by moving the hinge from the side to over the spine.[7]

A cast is applied—either a Risser cast or halo cast with a leg extension to stabilize the pelvis where necessary. The cast is wedged opposite the apex with the hinges both in front and in back over the spine. Initial correction is obtained using a cast spreader. A turnbuckle is attached on the side of the concavity, and by gradual distraction on this side the curve is corrected. Once maximal correction has been obtained, the cast is held in this position by plastering the two sides in and removing the turnbuckle.

While correction is being obtained, great care must be exercised to protect the skin. The skin should be watched for pressure and care taken not to pinch the skin during the period of correction.

It must be remembered that there are numerous methods of postoperative immobilization as described above. Each case must be carefully evaluated and the most appropriate method of immobilization used.

References

1. Anderson, S., and Bradford, D. S.: Lo-Profile halo. Clin. Orthop., 103:72, 1974.
2. Cotrel, Y., and Morel, G.: Le technique de l' E.D.F. dans la correction des scolioses. Rev. Chir. Orthop., 50:59, 1964.
3. Cotrel, Y.: Le corset de platre E.D.F. dans le traitement de la scoliose idiopathique. Med. Hyg., 28:1032, 1970.
4. Leider, L. L. Jr., Moe, J. H., and Winter, R. B.: Early ambulation after the surgical treatment of idiopathic scoliosis. J. Bone Joint Surg., 55A: 1003, 1973.
5. Moe, J. H.: Methods of correction and surgical techniques in scoliosis. Orthop. Clin. North Am., 3:17, 1972.
6. Ollier, M.:Techniques des platres et corsets des scolioses. Paris, Masson et Cie., 1971.
7. Risser, J. C., Lauder, C. H., Norquist, D. M., and Craig, W. A.:Three types of body casts. Am. Acad. Orthop. Surg. Instructional Course Lect., 10:131, 1953.
8. Risser, J. C.: The application of body casts for the correction of scoliosis. Am. Acad. Orthop. Surg. Instr. Course Lect., 12:255, 1955.
9. Sayre, L. A.: Spinal Disease and Spinal Curvature. London, Smith-Elder & Co., 1877.
10. Wullstein, L., and Schulthess, W.: Die Skoliose in inner Behandlung und Entschung Nach Klinischen und Experimentellen Studien. Z. Orthop. Clin., 10:178, 1902.

10

TECHNIQUES OF SURGERY

David S. Bradford, M.D.

INTRODUCTION

At the time of this writing it is indeed unfortunate but nevertheless axiomatic that the long-term success of any spinal reconstructive procedure is only achieved by assuring a solid spinal arthrodesis with resultant loss of spinal mobility. In our experience at the Twin Cities Scoliosis Center a solid arthrodesis is best achieved by meticulous exposure of the bony elements, bony decortication, copious autogenous bone grafting, and adequate postoperative immobilization, depending upon the use and the type of spinal implant. If posterior arthrodesis is attempted, we favor facet joint excision. More recent accumulated experience with L-rod instrumentation over the past five to ten years has shown that fusion may be achieved by meticulous cleaning of the spine and grafting without either excision of the facet or decortication.[3, 4] These latter modifications, however, have not withstood the test of time, and in the adult particularly, we feel they may be associated with a higher incidence of pseudarthrosis. Decortication does, on the other hand, provide more bone bulk for surgical arthrodesis and does insure a denuded surface, free of any fibrous tissue that could jeopardize eventual arthrodesis. Therefore, at the Twin Cities Scoliosis Center, we have favored facet excision, decortication, and autogenous bone grafting on all spinal cases requiring arthrodesis. If autogenous bone grafting appears deficient, we favor supplementing the graft with allograft bone, either femoral head, rib, tibia, or pelvis from our bone bank (see Chapter 22).

POSITIONING THE PATIENT
(Fig. 10–1)

For adequate exposure of the spine with minimal blood loss the position of the patient at the time of surgery is most important. After intubation the patient is placed on a prone four-poster or Relton-Hall frame, which allows the abdomen to hang free. Intra-abdominal pressure is minimized and venous bleeding appreciably decreased. The arms should be carefully supported, the elbows well padded, and the shoulders should rest in no more that 90 degrees of abduction. The upper pads of the four-poster frame should rest on the chest and not in the axillae. The back is then scrubbed with a surgical soap solution for five to ten minutes and then painted with a dilute iodine solution. The wound is draped in a customary fashion; adhesive plastic drapes are useful in keeping the operative field and the cotton drapes dry. If the patient has some loss of lumbar lordosis or a spinal lumbar osteotomy is contemplated, it is desirable to position the patient with the lumbar spine and hip joint in an extended position.

INCISION

A straight or slightly curved incision is made through the dermis only. The intradermal and subcutaneous area is infiltrated with an epinephrine solution (1:500,000). The incision is deepened to the fascia, and the skin margins are retracted with self-retaining Adson or Weitlaner type retractors. The interspinous ligament overlying the spinous proc-

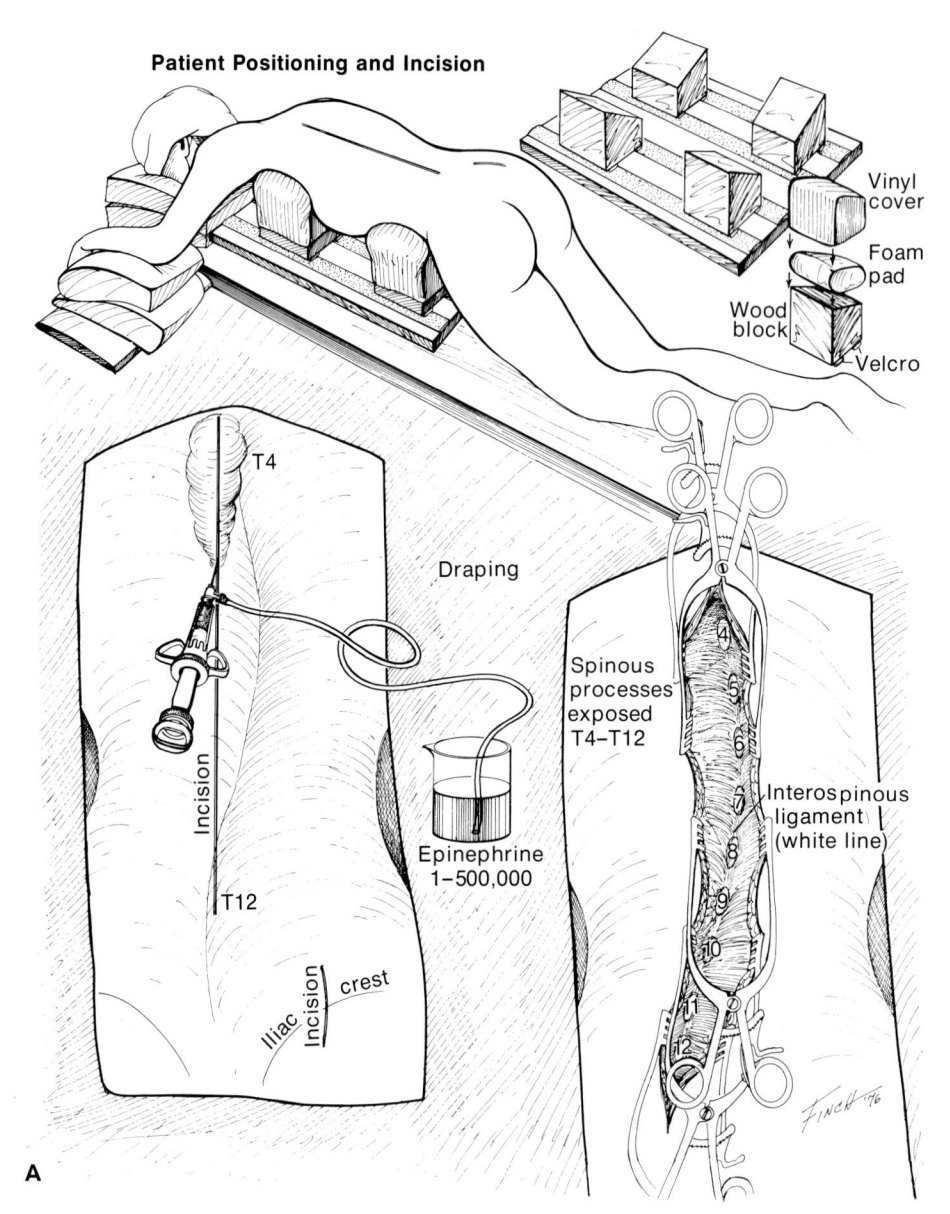

Figure 10–1. *A*, Patient is positioned on a well-padded four-poster frame, allowing the abdomen to remain completely free. Following the skin preparation, a midline skin incision is made over the area of the spine to be fused. The incision is made just into the dermis, and the dermal and subcutaneous tissues are infiltrated with epinephrine 1–500,000 solution. The skin incision is then deepened down to the linea alba, dissection being facilitated by use of Weitlaner self-retaining retractors. *B* and *C*, These figures demonstrate a useful technique to facilitate maintaining lumbar lordosis or closing a posterior osteotomy at the time of surgery after the wedge has been taken.

Illustration continued on opposite page

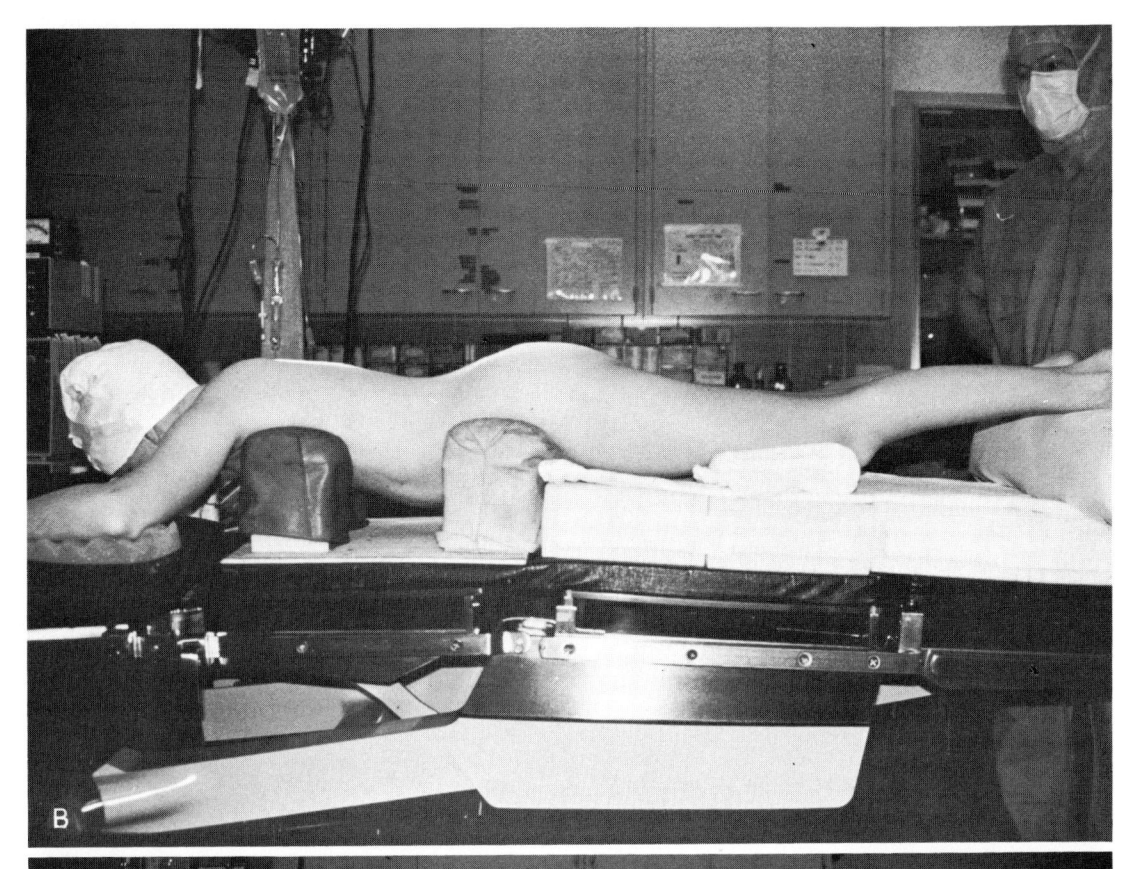

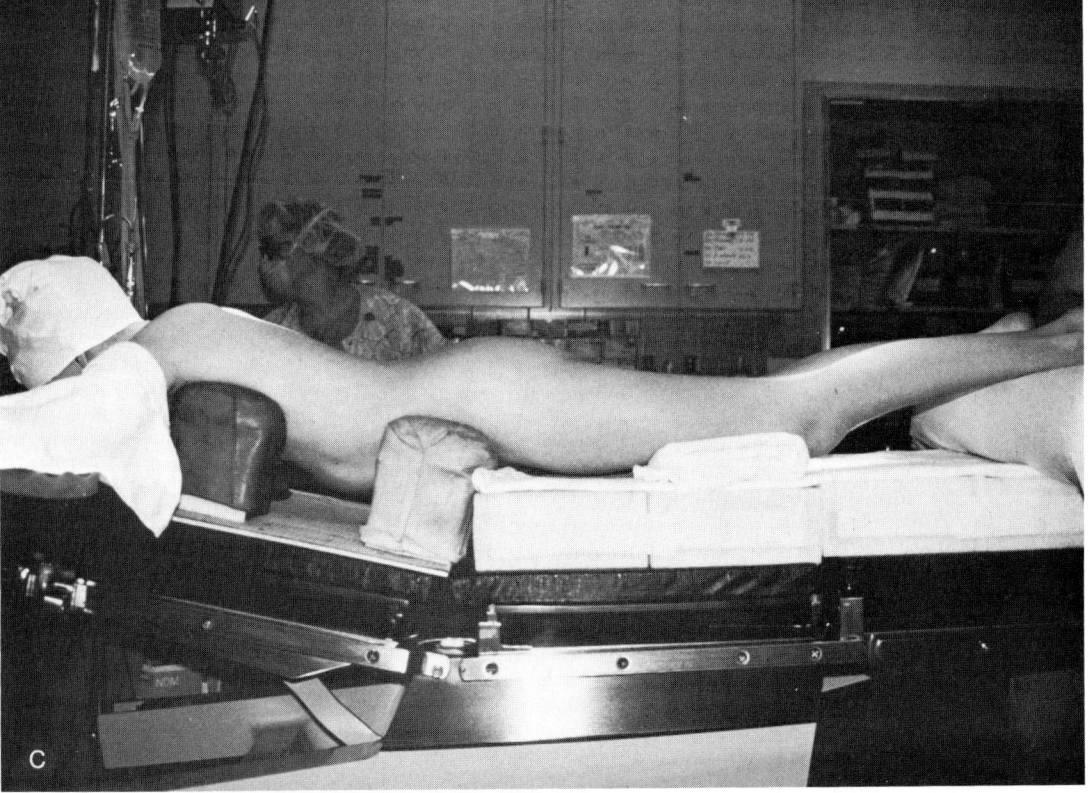

Figure 10–1 *Continued.*

esses is identified and dissection proceeds in this avascular plane; the cartilaginous cap overlying the spinous processes is incised. A Bovie's knife or a scalpel may be used. Each half of the cartilaginous cap is pushed aside with a Cobb elevator, exposing the spinous process and initiating the subperiosteal stripping.

After exposure of three or four spinous processes, the retractors are carefully introduced between the divided caps and spread slowly; excessive force and muscle tearing should be avoided. Continued dissection and retraction open up the soft tissues like a book. In the thoracic spine, it is most useful to begin distally and to work proximally, since the oblique attachments of the short rotator muscles and ligaments are most easily detached from the lamina in this direction (Fig. 10–2).

Liberal use of a scalpel to release tendinous and ligamentous attachments along the inferior margins of the lamina aids in the dissection. It is preferable to separate subperiosteally only to the facet joints on the first dissection with the Cobb elevator and then to continue the dissection laterally to the end of the transverse process on the second sweep with the Cobb elevator. Stripping too far laterally on the initial dissection often tears muscle as well as the branch of the segmental vessel just lateral to the facet joint.

The success of clean subperiosteal stripping of the spinous processes and laminae lies in gentle periosteal elevation, sharp division of resistant muscle insertions, and careful mechanical traction with the self-retaining retractors. Gauze packing should be used liberally to maintain hemostasis. We prefer not to remove the capsular covering of the facet joints until the exposure has been completed out to the ends of the transverse processes. A metallic marker may be placed in the spinous process of the lowest vertebra exposed and an x-ray then taken to confirm the correct level of exposure.

In the lumbar spine, a transverse process fusion is performed routinely on the concave

Exposure of T4–T12

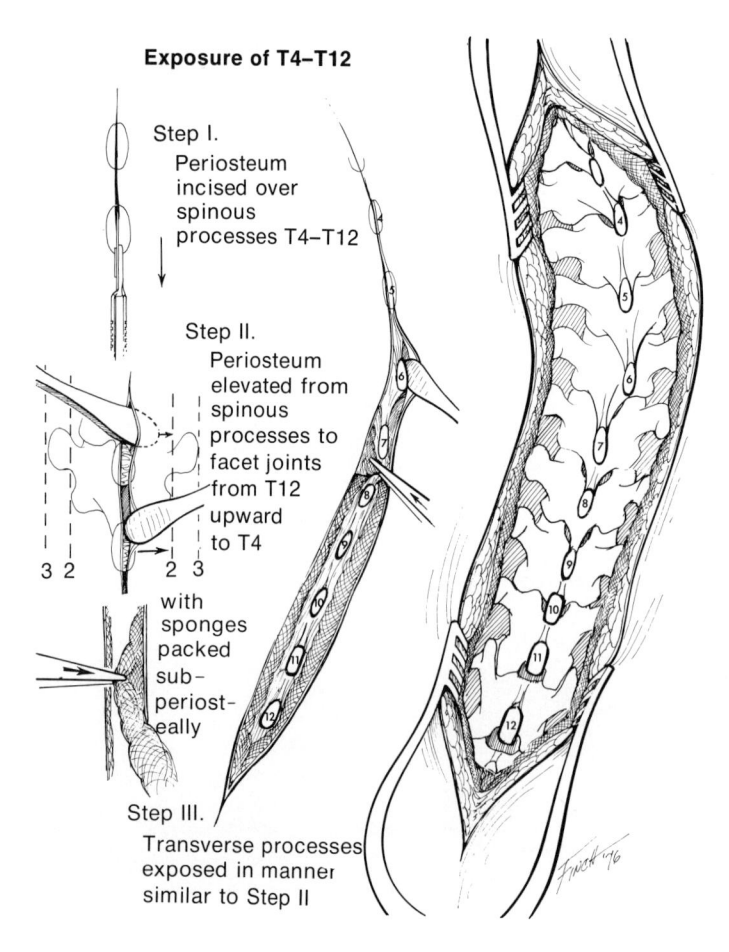

Step I. Periosteum incised over spinous processes T4–T12

Step II. Periosteum elevated from spinous processes to facet joints from T12 upward to T4 with sponges packed sub-periosteally

Step III. Transverse processes exposed in manner similar to Step II

Figure 10–2. After the spinous processes have been identified, the centers of the spinous processes are then incised with a sharp scalpel through the cartilage cap and down into the bony tip. A careful sharp subperiosteal dissection is then carried out, beginning at T12 and working proximally to the upper vertebra to be exposed. Hemostasis is facilitated by subperiosteal sponge packing. In general, it is preferable to expose the transverse processes only after all facet joints have been exposed throughout the area to be fused. Exposure too far laterally on the initial sweep often tears muscle, resulting in excessive blood loss. In the lumbar spine, the facet joint capsule is left intact. A sharp incision is made into the superior facet and the pars interarticularis, allowing the soft tissue with periosteum to then be dissected laterally out to the transverse process (see text).

side of the curvature, and therefore exposure should proceed laterally to the tips of the transverse processes. Again, it is easier to leave the joint capsule intact initially while this soft tissue is dissected and the periosteum is stripped from the spinous processes and lamina just lateral to the facet joint. The pars interarticularis is delineated, and a sharp incision is made from the pars interarticularis along the superior facet. The soft tissue with periosteum is then swept laterally over the superior process down to the lateral aspect of the transverse process.

At this stage of the procedure, the spinous processes are removed, saving the end ones to facilitate secure fixation with either the L-rod or the Harrington rod. In the thoracic spine the inferior articular facets are removed with a Capener gouge, removing a semicircular precise cut down to the superior articular process. The cartilage of the superior articular process is sharply curetted out and then a double-action Lexel rongeur is used to remove the remaining interspinous ligament, soft tissue debris, fat, and outer fibers of the ligamentum flavum. If L-rod instrumentation is planned, the double-action Lexel rongeur is used to remove the remaining fibers of the ligamentum flavum in the midline until the epidural fat is encountered. By removing the soft tissues from the lamina and the spinous processes and the transverse processes in this fashion, a very complete exposure is possible, and the stage is then adequately prepared for facet fusion, decortication, and Harrington instrumentation (or L-rod instrumentation and fusion with decortication lateral to the implant).

BONE GRAFTING

Before decortication is carried out, a bone graft is taken from the outer table of the ilium. The iliac crest is exposed through the same incision if exposure has already been extended into the lumbar spine or through a separate incision if the original exposure stopped at the T12-L1 level. A vertical incision over the iliac crest is preferable since this usually gives the best cosmetic scar. Subperiosteal dissection should expose at least 50 per cent of the ilium. Care is taken to avoid damaging the superior gluteal artery as it emerges from the sciatic notch. It may be helpful to identify the sciatic notch, as the bone immediately cephalad to the notch provides an optimal quantity of cancellous cortical grafts. Cortical and cancellous strips of bone are taken in a routine fashion and placed in a kidney basin and covered with a blood-soaked sponge. Bleeding may be controlled with bone wax as well as thrombin-soaked Gelfoam packs.

The success of an arthrodesis depends for the most part on the adequacy of bone grafting and the care with which the posterior elements have been meticulously cleaned of all soft tissue. A large amount of cancellous autogenous bone and cortical bone harvested just before use and maintained in as biologic a state as possible is desirable to the success of an arthrodesis. Bone grafts that are taken too early during the operative procedure, left exposed to operating room lights or laminar flow ventilation, or placed in sterile water or saline solutions will lose surface cell viability. They will thus offer little more than a bank bone allograft.

FACET JOINT FUSION

Facet joint fusion is carried out by a variety of techniques all of which are aimed at completely removing the cartilaginous material from the articular facet and placing cancellous bone within the remaining space. The Moe technique[88, 91] consists of elevating two hinge fragments of bone from adjacent transverse processes and moving them laterally to fill the intertransverse area. The joint surfaces are cleared of articular cartilage and a block of cortical cancellous bone is then placed in the defect (Fig. 10–3). The Moe technique has a disadvantage of being more time consuming than the simpler methods that will be described. Hall uses a similar technique, excising the joint surface totally and laying in a strip of cancellous iliac bone at each facet joint level (Fig. 10–4). Goldstein[53] removes the joint by decortication and fills the area with cancellous bone. Risser, using the Hibbs' technique,[61] curettes the dorsal margin of the cartilage from the joint, then interweaves flaps of bone into each other over the articulation. In his technique, decortication is complete but iliac bone is seldom added except sometimes in the lumbar spine. We prefer to remove the inferior articular process sharply with a gouge, curette out the superior articular cartilage, and then lay cancellous bone grafts into the roughened area.

In the lumbar spine the facet joints are

140   TECHNIQUES OF SURGERY

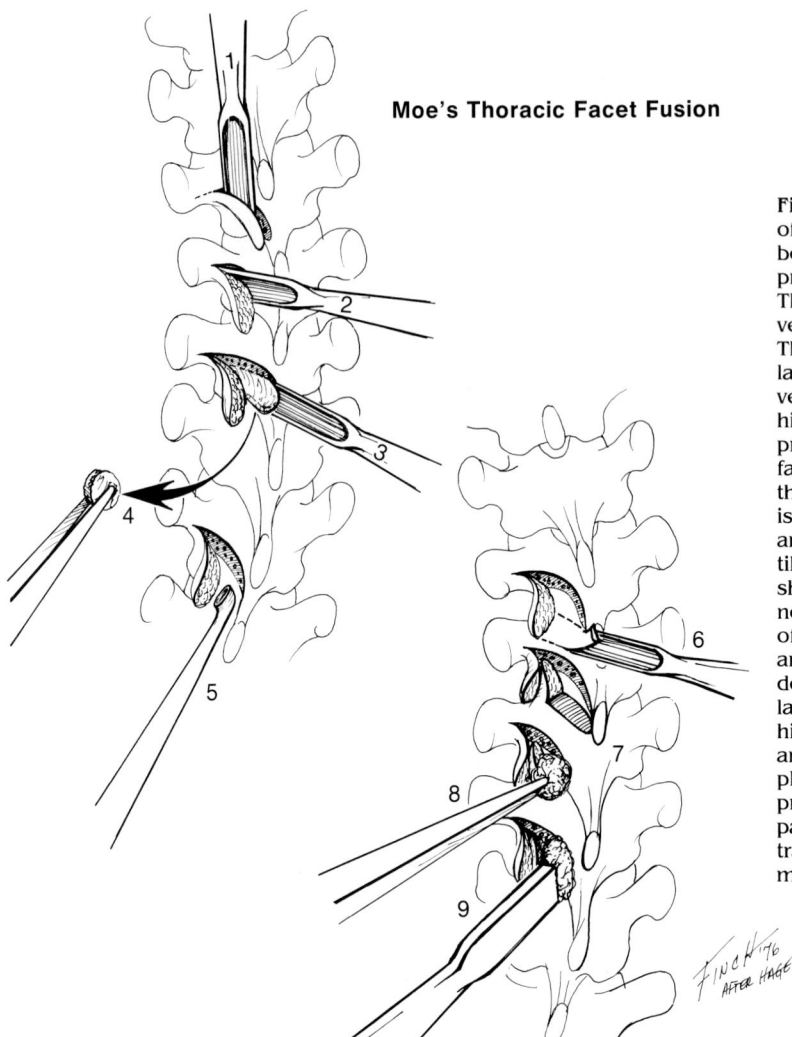

Moe's Thoracic Facet Fusion

Figure 10–3. The Moe technique of facet joint fusion. A cut is first begun over the cephalad articular process at the base of the lamina. This is carried along the transverse process almost to its tip. This fragment is bent and levered laterally to lie between the transverse processes. It should remain hinged to the superior transverse process. The superior joint surface should not be included in this fragment. The joint surface is removed with a separate cut and discarded. The articular cartilage, which is now visible, is sharply curetted out. The cut is next made into the mid-portion of the caudal transverse process and curved inward and outward, decorticating the superior articular facet so that it creates another hinge fragment. A cancellous and/or cortical bone graft is now placed in the defect, which was previously the joint, and impacted in place, moving the two transverse process fragments more laterally.

Figure 10–4. An excellent facet joint fusion may be achieved by the method described by Hall. In the first step, the inferior facet joint is sharply cut with a semicircular gouge in the manner outlined. The bone fragment with underlying articular cartilage is removed in one piece. The superior facet cartilage is then easily visualized and is removed with a sharp curette. A trough is created by removing the outer cortex of the superior facet. Cancellous bone is then taken from the outer table of the ilium and snugly impacted into the decorticated area previously created.

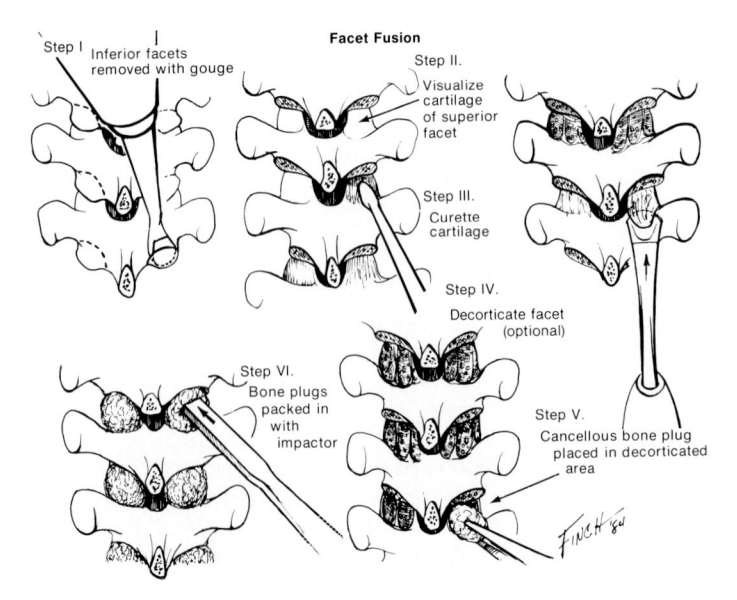

oriented in a sagittal direction. Facet fusion is best performed by cutting away the joint surface with a small thin osteotome, then sharply cutting the trough deeper with a thin Lampert rongeur and curetting out the floor of the joint with a small angled or straight curette. A block of cancellous bone from the ilium may then be firmly driven into the defect (Fig. 10–5).

As a final step, decortication is carried out over the entire exposed spine. Cancellous strips and then cortical strips of bone are placed from the tips of the transverse processes to the lamina.

CLOSURE

The deep tissues are approximated with a running absorbable suture, and a drain is placed in the subcutaneous tissue and put to Hemovac suction. The subcutaneous tissues are approximated with 2-0 suture and the skin with a running subcuticular 3-0 suture of self-absorbable material, such as Vicryl. A bulky dressing is applied. During the procedure, irrigation with an antibiotic is carried out every 30 minutes. Furthermore, all of our patients are placed on preoperative, intraoperative, and 48-hour postoperative intravenous antibiotic therapy.

POSTERIOR SPINAL OSTEOTOMY

Osteotomies through the posterior aspect of the spine may involve merely excising hypertrophic osteophytes that lie within the facet space, removing the facet joints completely, or cutting through the whole posterior elements down to the neural foramen in those cases in which the spine has been previously arthrodesed.

Osteotomies through facets alone may be carried out without difficulty provided the surgeon is cognizant of the anatomical landmarks and the variations associated with a malrotated spine (Fig. 10–6). Following exposure of the posterior elements as previously described, a sharp gouge may be placed at the junction of the transverse process and the inferior facet and oriented so that the concavity of the gouge covers a major portion of the inferior articular facet. A cut is then made perpendicular to the bony surface totally excising this osteophyte and a portion of the facet down to the superior articular facet. The remaining osteophyte may be removed with a gouge or a curette. A Blount spreader may then be placed between the two transverse processes or between the spinous processes and spread gently in order to determine if the facet joint has been completely released. If after excising the facet on the convex as well as the concave side, little mobility is possible, a laminotomy should be done between the two spinous processes. Angled Kerrison rongeurs are then used to cut away the superior articular facet, opening up the neural foramen; the emerging nerve root is then identified. A Blount spreader is again used to determine the mobility after this release has been completed. Residual tightness and lack of mobility at this point most probably denote spontaneous anterior interbody fusion. In cases of combined ankylosis, two-stage procedures (anterior and posterior) are recommended, and resection of both concave as well as

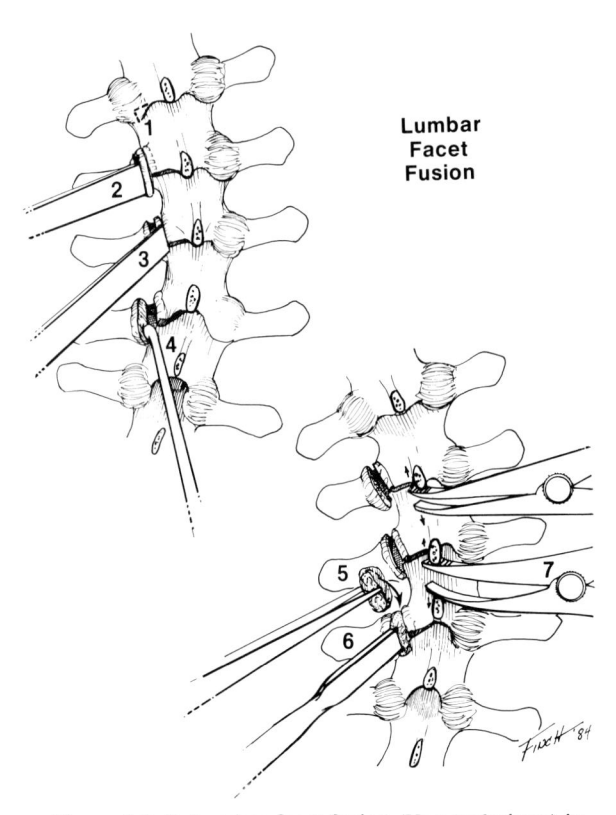

Figure 10–5. Lumbar facet fusion (Moe technique) is performed by cutting away the joint surfaces with a small thick osteotome. The floor of the joint is then curetted away. A block of the cancellous bone from the ilium is then firmly driven into the defect previously created. A Blount spreader applied between the spinous processes is helpful in visualizing the adequacy of facet joint removal.

Posterior Osteotomy for Ankylosed Facets.

Step I. Superior facets removed bilaterally with gouge

Step II. Ankylosed material gouged from inferior facets bilaterally

Step III. Blount spreader affords exposure of inferior facet

Step IV. Inferior facets rongeured

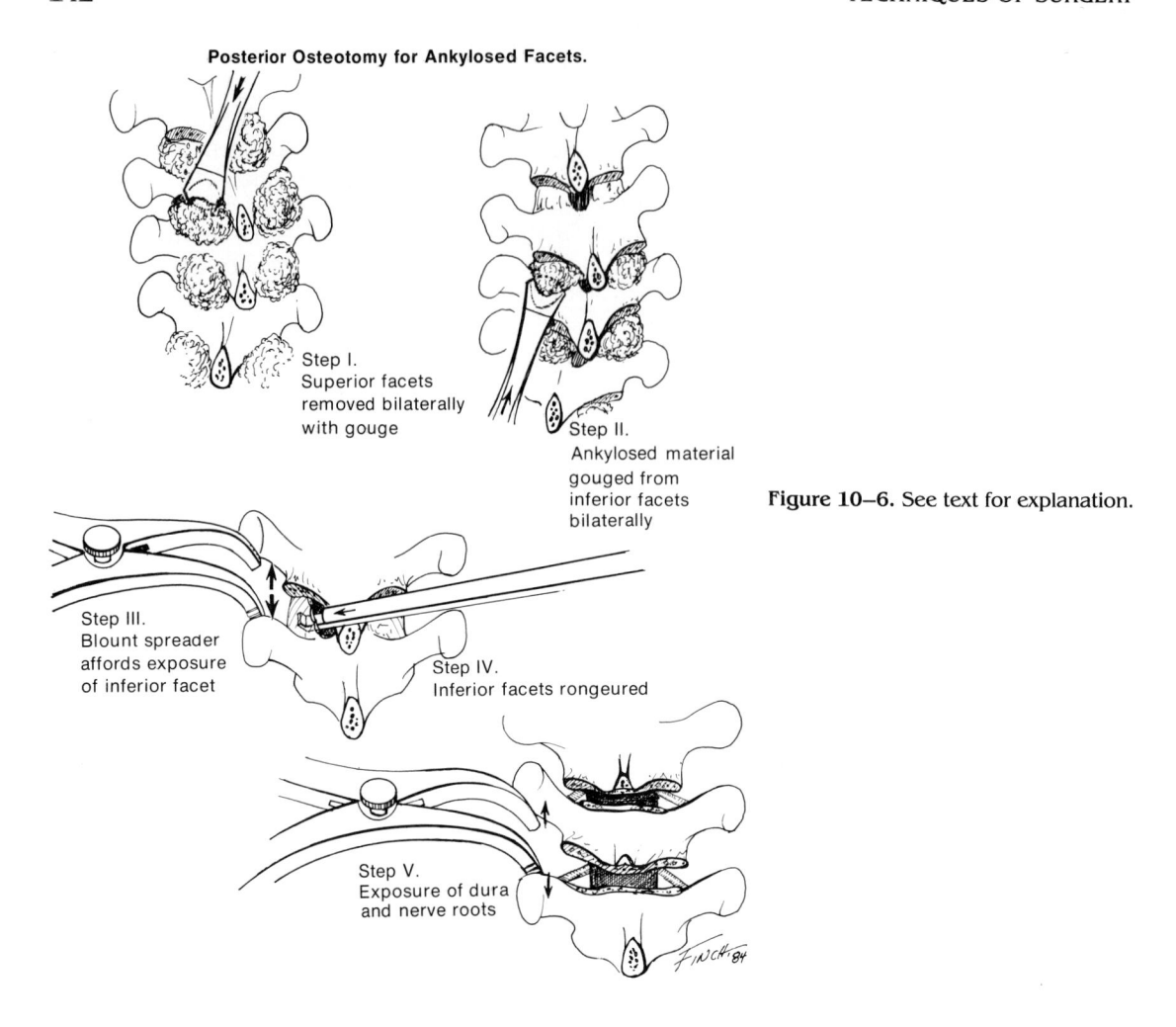

Step V. Exposure of dura and nerve roots

Figure 10–6. See text for explanation.

convex ribs must often be combined with a posterior approach to achieve correction (see Special Techniques).

POSTERIOR OSTEOTOMY OF A PREVIOUSLY FUSED SPINE
(Fig. 10–7)

Posterior osteotomy through an established posterior fusion mass, either in the presence or the absence of a pseudarthrosis, may be safely carried out provided careful attention to anatomic landmarks is observed. The transverse processes provide reliable anatomic landmarks to the facet area and the interpedicular location. A trough is cut at this site in the fusion mass with osteotomes, gouges, or rongeurs of appropriate sizes. An air-driven, high speed burr is particularly useful in performing an osteotomy. The outer cortical shell and the cancellous bone are removed down to the inner cortex, a small opening may be made with the air drill, and then appropriate rongeurs and gouges are used to complete the osteotomy. The dissection proceeds laterally toward the intervertebral foramen, making certain the dissection stays midway between the two pedicles and the transverse processes. A Blount spreader, again, is helpful in determining mobility after the osteotomy is complete. Hemostasis may be facilitated with Gelfoam soaked in a thrombin solution.

If subsequent fixation is anticipated, the outer cortex of the fusion mass will provide excellent fixation for a spinal implant, either the Harrington hooks or segmental instrumentation devices. In the latter circumstance wires may be passed underneath the outer cortex if the fusion mass is thick. If the fusion mass is thin, then it is preferable to pass the wires underneath the inner cortex of the fusion within the epidural space.

Figure 10–7. See text for explanation.

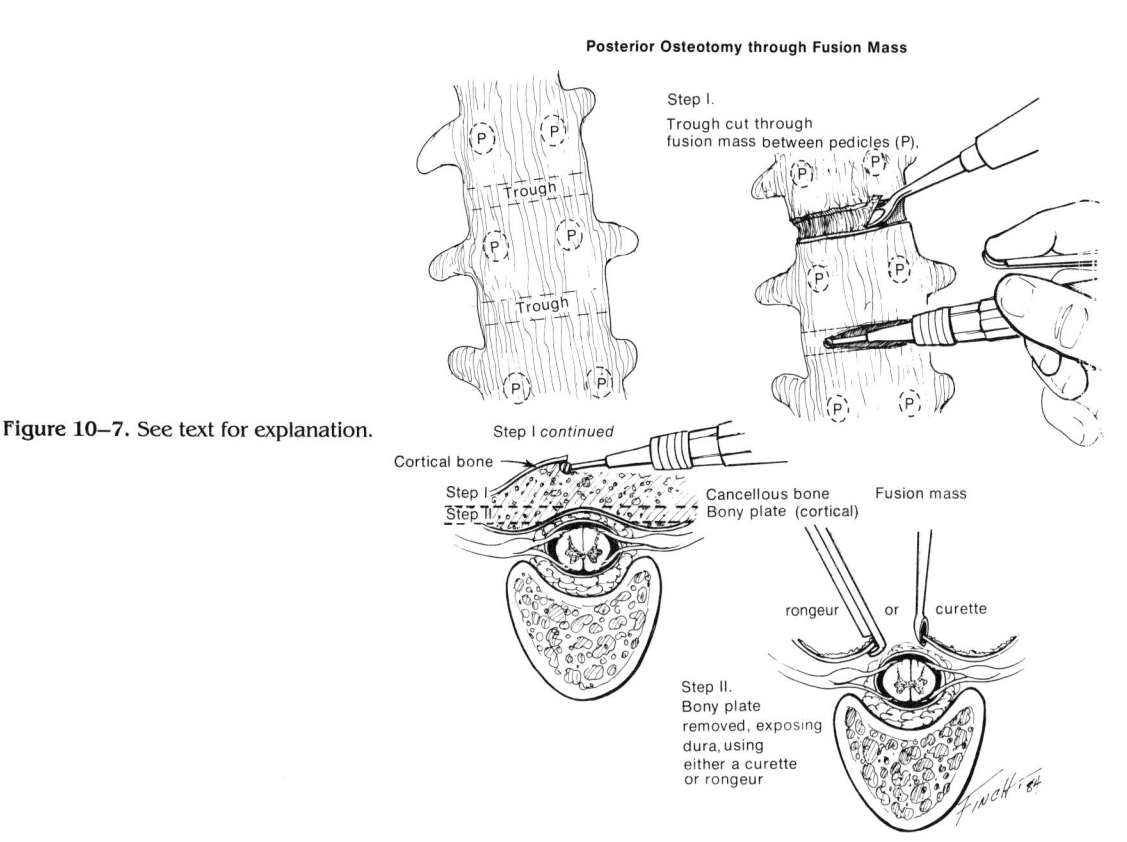

POSTERIOR SPINAL INSTRUMENTATION

Harrington Instrumentation[57, 58, 59, 88, 124]

The use of Harrington instrumentation in the treatment of scoliosis and allied spinal deformities has become a standard by which other forms of therapy are compared. Although limitations of the assembly are well appreciated, the usefulness of this device with or without segmental attachments is still apparent.

PLACEMENT OF THE HOOK
(Fig. 10–8)

After the initial exposure, the site for the upper hook is first prepared by squaring off the inferior facet joint with a small ¼-inch osteotome or a Capener gouge. The cut is made obliquely so that the medial margin is more cranially directed than the lateral margin. A No. 1251 hook is inserted into the facet interspace in the manner outlined subsequently. The hook should be tilted forward at least 45 degrees to avoid penetrating the inferior facet. When the hook has engaged the pedicle, it may be impacted with a mallet. The hook is then removed and a dull, flanged hook, No. 1262, or a dull, unflanged hook, No. 1253, is inserted and firmly impacted into the pedicle. A flanged hook, if properly placed, will not damage the lamina and will have a better grip into the bone. It is often preferable to have the medial one third of the hook lying medial to the facet joint. This serves to avoid a tendency for lateral hook displacement and subsequent dislodgement.

The lower hook, No. 1254, is inserted underneath the lamina of the selected vertebra (Fig. 10–9). The exposure is facilitated by removing a portion of the inferior facet, rongeuring or curetting the ligamentum flavum from its attachment to the lamina, and squaring off the superior facet with a Kerrison rongeur. A Blount spreader or a lamina spreader may facilitate hook insertion.

THE HARRINGTON OUTRIGGER

The use of the Harrington outrigger is elective. It may prove beneficial in more severe curvatures (>75 degrees) by facilitating correction, improving the exposure, and

Hook Insertion T4–T5

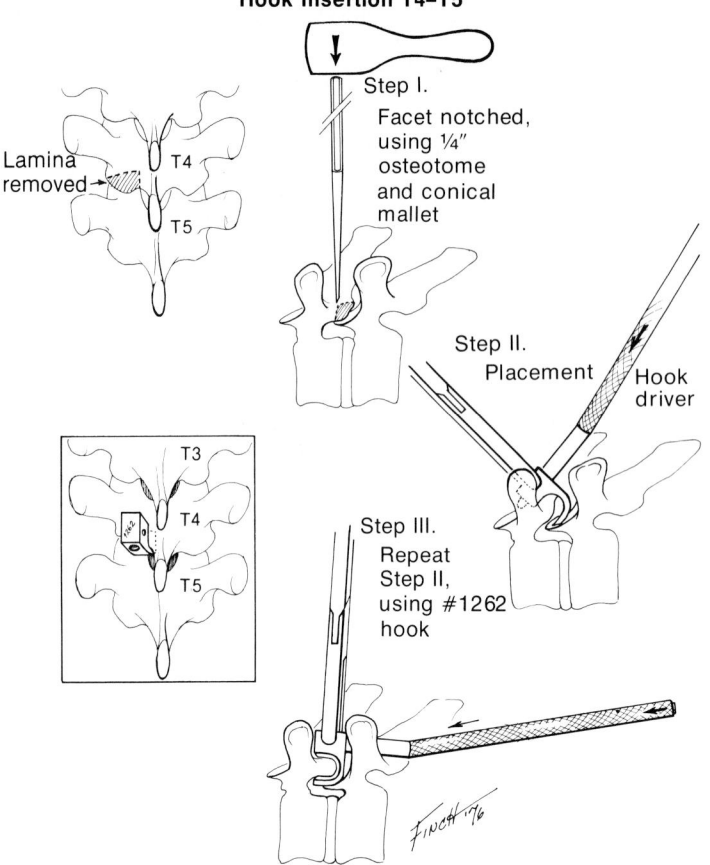

Step I. Facet notched, using ¼" osteotome and conical mallet

Step II. Placement — Hook driver

Step III. Repeat Step II, using #1262 hook

Lamina removed — T4, T5

Figure 10–8. Preparation for the insertion of the upper hook of the Harrington assembly. A small (¼ inch, 0.6 cm) osteotome is used to cut the inferior portion of the superior facet at a slightly oblique angle, as demonstrated. The facet joint is then easily identified and its most medial margin delineated. A #1251 hook is inserted into the facet interspace as demonstrated in Step II. The hooks should be tilted forward at least 45 degrees to assure proper placement and to prevent the tendency for the hook to improperly engage into the superior facet. Once the hook has engaged the pedicle, it may be impacted with a light mallet. This sharp hook is then removed and a flanged hook, #1262, is inserted and impacted into the pedicle, as demonstrated in Step III.

Hook Insertion T11–T12

Areas of lamina removed — T11, T12

Step I. Spread spinous processes of T11–T12, using Blount spreader

Step II. Portion of inferior facet excised; Portion of lamina removed with Kerrison rongeur

Step III. #1254 hook inserted under lamina, using hook clamp

Figure 10–9. Insertion of the lower hook assembly (#1254). It is best to curette out the ligamentum flavum from its attachment to the lamina. It is helpful to remove the most inferior portion of the inferior facet in order to better outline the limits of the ligamentum. A sharp curette or a knife may then be used to completely remove the ligamentum flavum and thus expose the dura. It is helpful to use a Blount spreader to obtain a wider exposure of this area. In Step II, portions of the lamina are removed with a Kerrison rongeur, giving a flat margin that extends to the pars interarticularis. It is easiest to prepare the facet joint at this level and pack it with cancellous bone prior to insertion of the Harrington outrigger or the Harrington rod. Insertion of the Harrington outrigger between the two hooks is demonstrated. Facet fusion is carried out as outlined in Figures 10–4 and 10–5.

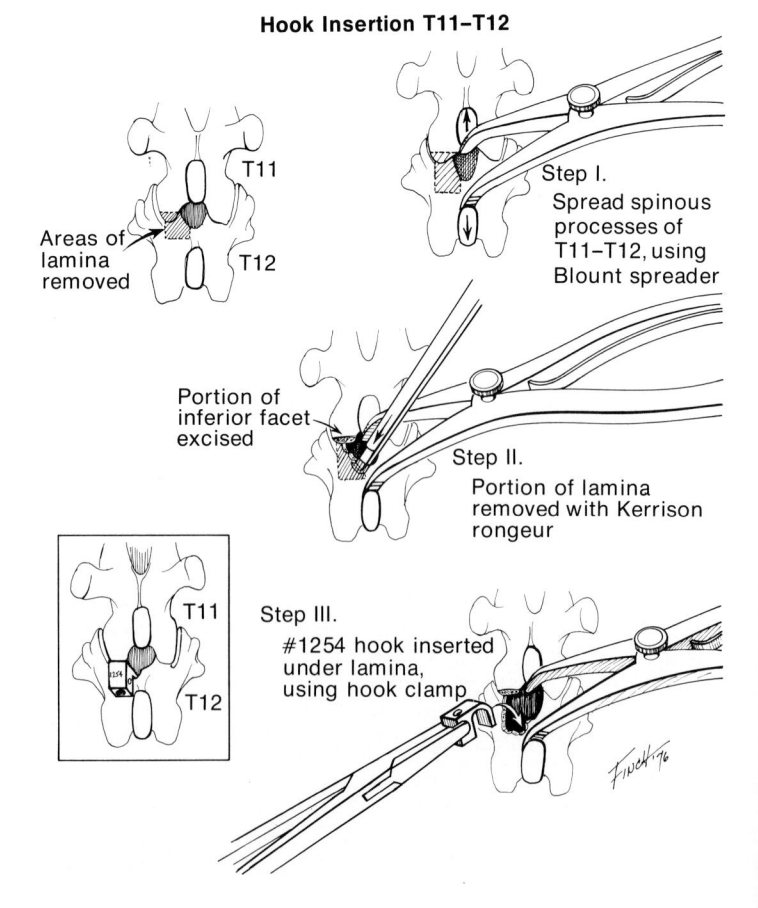

allowing the procedure to be performed while the spine is in the corrected position. It may also prove helpful in choosing optimal rod length prior to insertion.

HARRINGTON ROD INSERTION

After decortication and facet fusion on the concave side, the distraction strut bar is placed between the two hooks and distraction is carried out (Fig. 10–10). Only experience can indicate to the operating surgeon the point at which the safe maximum distraction has been obtained. Distraction should not be carried out to the point of bone disruption or to the point of rod bending. Decortication is then carried out on the convex side. An 18-gauge wire or a C-ring is threaded around the upper ratchet of the rod just below the hook to prevent the rod from telescoping within the hook. A Stagnara wake-up test[114] is then performed, and if spontaneous voluntary foot and leg movements are observed, anesthesia is deepened and closure then proceeds in a routine fashion. To maximize the usefulness of the test the distraction may be carried out while the patient is awake. It may also be useful to repeat the test several times during the procedure, particularly in those cases in which there is deformity or in which more radical combined techniques are being used.

HARRINGTON COMPRESSION ASSEMBLY

The compression rod assembly should be used along with the distraction bar in those cases in which there is a kyphosis associated with scoliosis, such as in Scheuermann's disease, in the lumbar spine to maintain lordosis, or alone in those cases of pure kyphosis. It may also be used in pure idiopathic scoliosis with a distraction assembly to increase fixation. The insertion of the compression assembly is more difficult (Figs. 10–11 and 10–12). The assembly consists of two sizes of hooks, No. 1256 and No. 1259, which adapt to two sizes of fully threaded rods, a larger rod, 1/8-inch, and a smaller rod, 5/11-inch. The smaller rod is easier to insert, as it is much more flexible and adapts readily to

Bony Decortication

Step I.
Spinous processes of T4–T12 cut

Step II.
Bony decortication on concave side, using Capener gouge

Step III.
Distraction rod inserted on concave side, using Harrington spreader

Step IV.
Bony decortication on convex side, using gouge

A

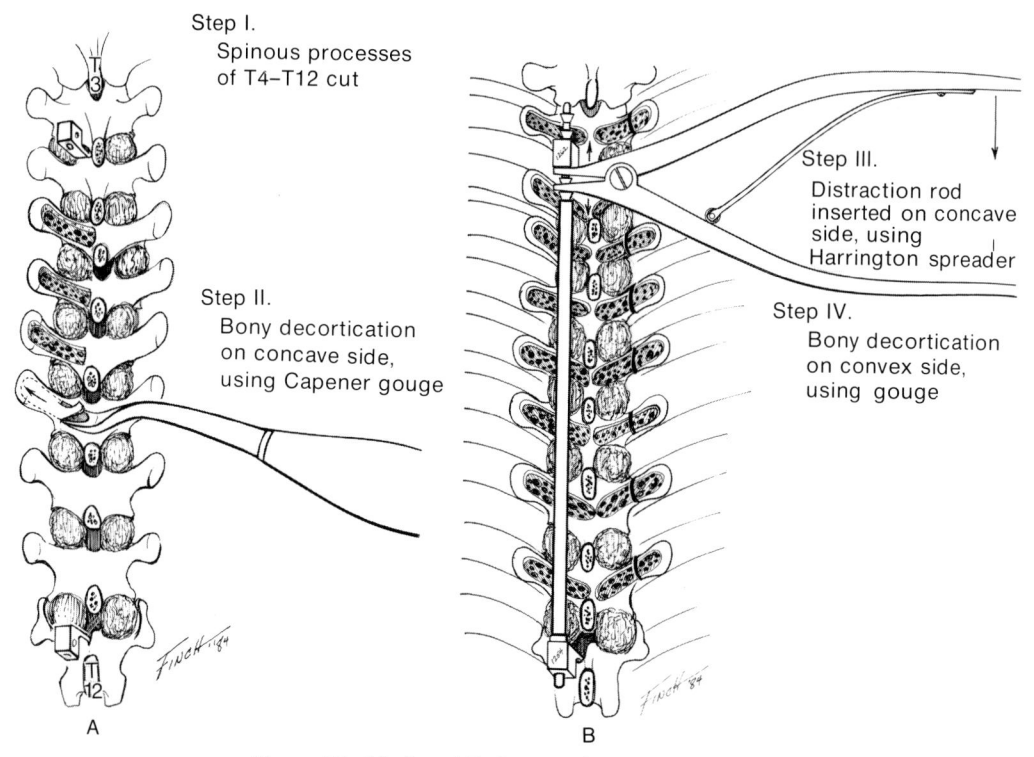

B

Figure 10–10. A and B, See text for explanation.

Insertion of Compression Assembly—Part 1

Step I.
#1259 hook inserted temporarily around transverse process of T5, T6, T7 on convex side, creating a bed for later permanent insertion.

Movement of hook to create insertion site

Step II.
Portion of lamina (on convex side) of T10, T11, T12 is removed, using osteotome, gouge, and rongeur to facilitate insertion of #1259 hooks

Blount spreader

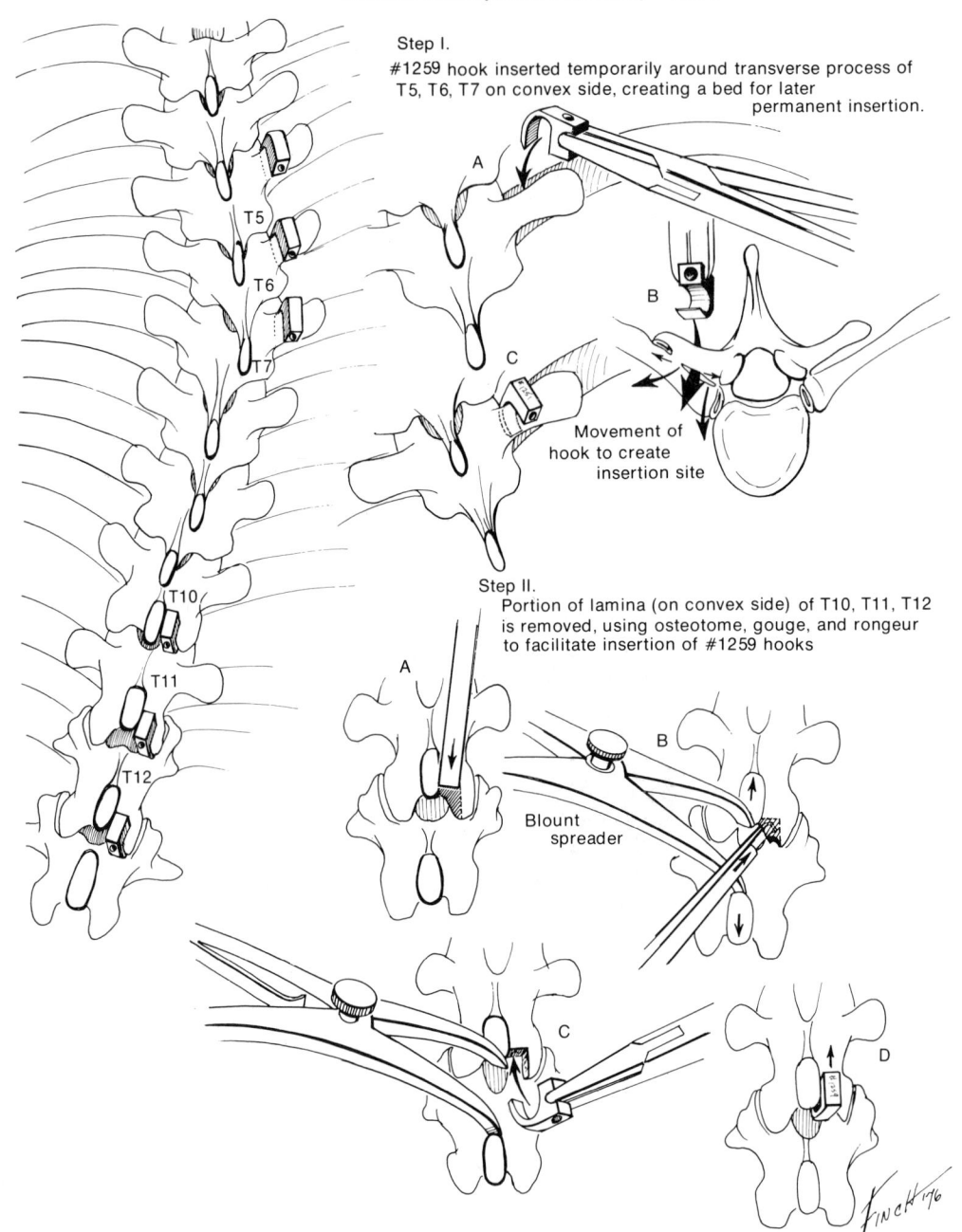

Figure 10—11. Procedure for insertion of the contracting assembly. The contracting assembly comes in two sizes, ⅛ inch and 5/11 inch. The smaller rod with the #1259 hook is generally more useful, since it is flexible and adapts readily to kyphosis. Insertion of this assembly is facilitated by careful and thorough preparation of the spine. The #1259 hooks should be placed individually under the selected transverse processes at the junction of the transverse process and the lamina. The sharp edge of the hook cuts the costotransverse ligament. Care should be taken to ensure that the hook does not cut into the transverse process and the seating is carried out easily in a horizontal fashion. If the hook must be tilted to slide under the transverse process, insertion will be extremely difficult once the rod is attached to the hook. Below T11 there are no suitable transverse processes, so the hooks must be placed under the lamina at this area. Appropriate amounts of bone are cut from the inferior lamina and inferior facet with an osteotome and Kerrison rongeur. A Blount spreader is then placed between the two spinous processes, and the #1259 hook is carefully inserted into place. Again, one should strive for placement of this hook in a horizontal fashion to facilitate its insertion once the rod is attached to the hook.

TECHNIQUES OF SURGERY

Insertion of Compression Assembly—Part 2

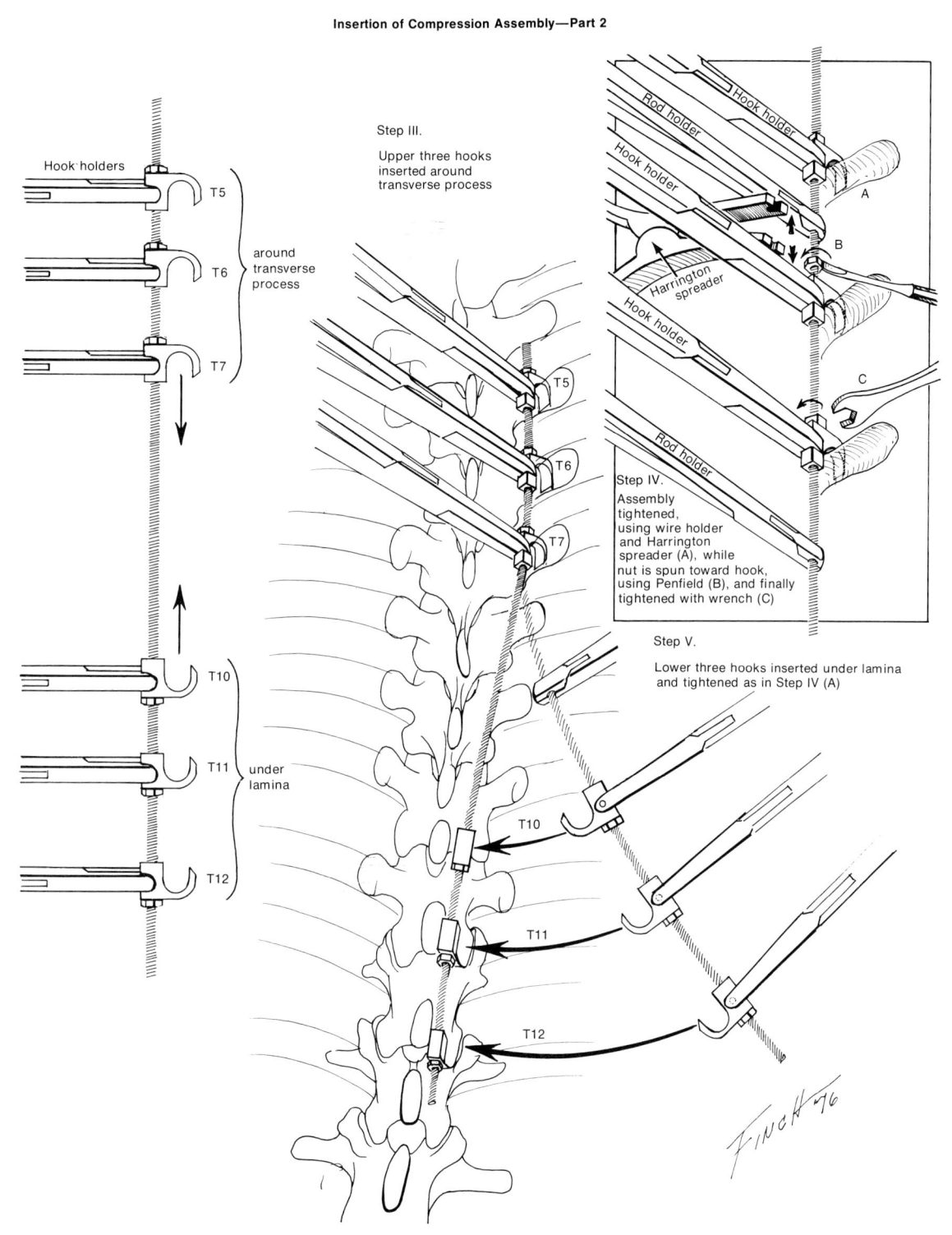

Step III. Upper three hooks inserted around transverse process

Step IV. Assembly tightened, using wire holder and Harrington spreader (A), while nut is spun toward hook, using Penfield (B), and finally tightened with wrench (C)

Step V. Lower three hooks inserted under lamina and tightened as in Step IV (A)

Figure 10–12. Insertion of the contraction assembly (continued from Fig. 10–11). After the transverse processes and laminae have been prepared as outlined, a threaded rod with the appropriate size hooks attached to it is then inserted. It is generally easier to insert the cranially directed hooks first, followed by insertion of the more caudally directed hooks in a single step. After the hooks are securely in place, they may be tightened with either a wrench or a spreader placed between a rod holder and a hook holder. The Moe elevator is used to tighten the nut between the hook holder and the rod holder after the distraction has taken place. After maximal contraction, the central threads adjacent to the nuts on the rod must be damaged with a clamp close to the nut to prevent them from unwinding and becoming loose.

a kyphosis, but it will undergo a fatigue failure in tension much more readily than the larger rod.

To facilitate insertion, the hook is first placed temporarily under the selected transverse process at the junction of the transverse process and the lamina. The sharp edge of the hook cuts into the costotransverse ligament. It is imperative that the hook not penetrate the transverse process, otherwise insecure fixation results and hook pull-out is inevitable. From T11 caudally the hook is preferably placed underneath the lamina as close to the facet joint as possible (see Fig. 10–11), the facets having been previously prepared and cleaned of soft tissue.

After the transverse processes and the lamina have been prepared to accept the contraction assembly, a threaded rod of appropriate size with hooks attached along with the nuts is inserted. It is often easier to begin insertion of the assembly at the upper level of the spine to be instrumented, then work distally. It is essential that the hook sites be well prepared so the hooks can be inserted perpendicular to the spine, since once the hooks are attached to the rod it is not feasible or possible to tilt the hook for insertion. If the larger rod is being used, which we generally recommend under all possible circumstances, a slight kyphotic bend to the rod facilitates insertion. The compression assembly is tightened by using appropriate rod holders and the Harrington spreader, then spinning the nuts using a Penfield elevator. The hooks may also be tightened by turning the nuts with a hexagonal wrench. If one is using the compression assembly in conjunction with a distraction rod, the contraction rod ought to be put on first to facilitate correction of the scoliosis as well as the kyphosis.

In patients with true kyphosis without significant scoliosis, two compression assemblies are used. In these cases it may be desirable to have the head elevated or slightly extended during the operation by the use of skeletal traction with a halo attachment, since this position facilitates exposure to the C7 to T3 area as well as hook insertion.

HARRINGTON INSTRUMENTATION TO THE LOWER LUMBAR SPINE AND SACRUM

Distraction implants to the lower lumbar spine and sacrum should be avoided at all costs. It is our combined and recurring experience at the Twin Cities Scoliosis Center that distraction instrumentation across the lumbar spine, and particularly into the sacrum, invariably produces a loss of lumbar lordosis, sacral malrotation, and a high likelihood of pseudarthrosis, implant failure, or hook dislodgement.[11, 92] In idiopathic scoliosis, fusions distal to L4 are rarely necessary. If the lumbar curve must be fused and instrumented and the Harrington implant is preferred, a compression assembly should be placed on the convex side of the lumbar curve to produce and maintain lordosis prior to placement of the distraction implant. In cases in which instrumentation distal to L4 is necessary (e.g. paralytic obliquity, degenerative osteoarthritis), L-rod, transpedicular, or Cotrel-Dubousset instrumentation with maintenance of lumbar lordosis is preferable. Lumbar lordosis may be facilitated by bending a square-ended Harrington rod and forcefully driving the lumbar spine into lordosis by three-point fixation. This, however, assumes that the lateral curvature of the lumbar spine is quite flexible or that it is partially corrected by the convex contracting assembly so that the posterior elements of the lumbar spine on the concave side lie underneath the Harrington distraction implant and are in effective contact. This is usually difficult to achieve and alternative fixation implants would appear more desirable.

Wake-up Test

We have found that the best technique for monitoring neurologic function following corrective spinal surgery is the wake-up test first described by Drs. Vanzelle, Stagnara, and Jouvinroux.[114] This provides an effective means of neurologic evaluation of the patient immediately after implant insertion or other manipulative spinal procedures. The wake-up test may be performed repetitively throughout the surgery by carefully controlling the anesthesia. Voluntary foot and leg movement will not occur until voluntary hand movement is elicited. If hand movement returns in the absence of foot and ankle motion, one presumes that the possibility of neurologic damage is present and removes the distraction implant. At the Twin Cities Scoliosis Center we have several patients who have been unable to move their feet after distraction implant insertion, but motor function has returned with rod removal at the time of surgery. Patients rarely, if ever, have adverse reactions to this procedure provided the anesthesia is well controlled and proceeds without consequence.

Spinal cord monitoring (by evoked potentials) is likewise a useful adjunct for neurologic assessment. It has the advantage of being continuous but the disadvantage of being expensive. It requires a team of experienced personnel, and at the present time it monitors posterior column function only (see Chapter 22, Anesthesia subchapter).

Segmental Spinal Instrumentation

Segmental spinal instrumentation is a form of instrumentation that allows interlocking fixation of vertebral components over multiple levels. The concept is not a new one. Fritz Lange described wiring a rod to the spine in 1902.[70]

In 1963, Resina[97] described a technique for fixation of a rod to the spine with wires passed through the base of the spinous process at each vertebral level. In 1972, he and Ferreira-Alves reported on 100 cases using this technique. A. Hernandez-Ros,[60] in 1965, reported a similar technique using a tibial strut graft that was wired into the bases of the spinous processes as well as the transverse processes. Excellent correction and fixation of the deformity were possible. Morscher,[93] in 1972, described the use of sublaminar wires attached to a Harrington distraction rod. Beginning in 1973, Eduardo Luque and his colleagues began using sublaminar wiring attached to a Harrington rod to strengthen fixation.[76-78, 80, 81]

Subsequently, Luque developed a more flexible rod, shaped in an L configuration and attached to the spine at each level by sublaminar wiring. An operation, using this instrument, was first performed by him in August of 1976. By trial and error it became apparent that this type of segmental fixation of the spine was secure enough that the use of a postoperative cast or orthotic immobilization was not necessary.[28] To Dr. Ben Allen and his associates great credit should be given for further development, modification, and standardization of the L-rod instrumentation technique.[3-8] In the following description we will focus primarily on the L-rod system, recognizing again that segmental spinal instrumentation includes any implant attached over multiple vertebrae, for example, the Harrington compression system,[57] transverse coupling with the Harrington rod,[9, 10] the Harrington rod augmented with sublaminar wiring, or the techniques described by Resina,[97] Zielke,[129] and Drummond.[39]

L-ROD INSTRUMENTATION

The L-rod instrumentation system consists of stainless steel wires, 18 (.040 mm.) or 16 (.048 mm.) gauge, and rods of stainless steel measuring 4.8 mm. (3/16 in.) or 6.4 mm. (¼ in.) diameter. This technique has proved to be one of the most difficult and demanding of spinal reconstructive procedures. It is a procedure that should not be undertaken lightly. The surgeon should have had extensive spinal reconstructive experience, and it is preferable that the surgeon has had hands-on experience while working with others well versed in this technique.

DETERMINATION OF THE LEVEL OF INSTRUMENTATION

As a general rule, the instrumented level should go from end vertebra to end vertebra determined by neutral rotation or, preferably, the vertebra transected by the vertical C7 mid-sacral line as described by King and workers.[69] It is generally preferable to add an additional vertebra proximally, as fixation and correction appear to be improved. It may be useful to determine preoperative correctability by either a side-bending film or a stretch film plus a surcingle single strap while the patient is on the plaster table (Fig. 10–13). Allen uses this x-ray to determine how closely the tips of the spinous processes can be made to approximate a straight line when the deformed segment is maximally corrected.[4] When the spinous processes do not align straight on the bending or the combined stretch-bend x-ray, a line is drawn from the tip of the spinous process of the uppermost vertebra in the deformed segment to the tip of the lowermost vertebra. A perpendicular distance from this line to the tip of the spinous process of the apical vertebra is measured. This value consists of "lateral deviation" and is used to determine preoperatively how much to pre-bend the rod at the time of surgery (Fig. 10–13). This is less critical when one is using the 3/16 inch (4.8 mm.) diameter stainless steel rod, since this

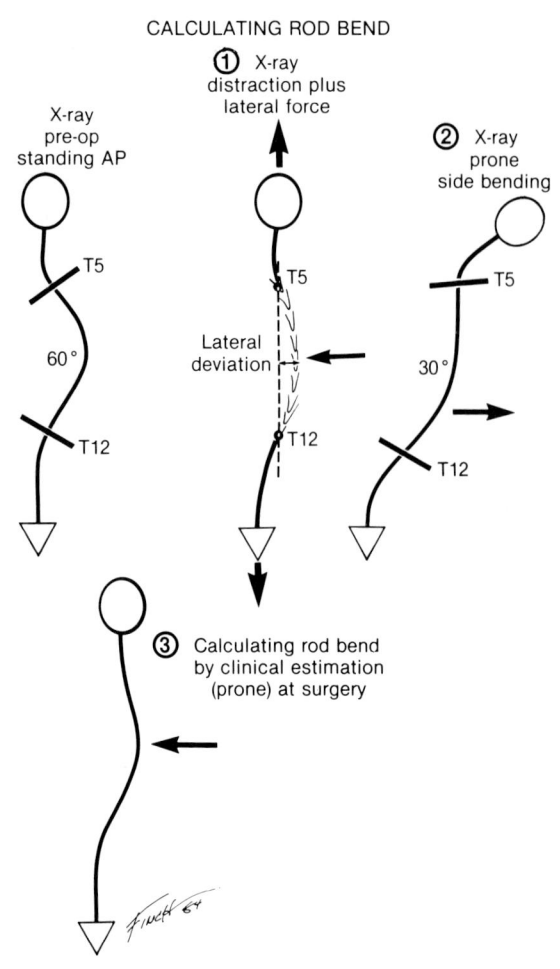

Figure 10–13. If using the L-rod segmental instrumentation system, three techniques are useful in determining the amount of bend to place into the rod prior to insertion. One may use the lateral deviation line as determined by x-ray taken under distraction, or calculate the rod bend directly from a side bending x-ray, or make a clinical estimation of the amount of curvature of the spine at the time of surgery after a lateral force is placed over the apex of the curvature (see text).

rod has considerable flexibility. However, if one is using the ¼ inch (6.4 mm.) diameter rod, a more precise prebend determination should be made. With either rod, the lateral deviation should be slightly less than the x-ray determination. Attempts to place a sagittal curvature in the rod to correct thoracic lordosis are certainly feasible, but the amount of correction that is possible to achieve and hence the amount of pre-bend to place into the rod are at best estimates. With the smaller 3/16 inch rod, the production of normal thoracic kyphosis in a previously lordotic spine is unlikely. Rod bending usually occurs before any substantial correction is achieved. On the other hand, using a ¼ inch stainless steel rod will result in some improvement of the sagittal curve, but restoration of normal kyphosis, especially in a skeletally mature individual with minimal spinal flexibility is most likely to be achieved with a combined surgical approach (see Special Techniques).

EXPOSURE

For optimal exposure a partial excision of the inferior facet as previously described is most worthwhile. The ligamentum flavum is then excised with a rongeur placed between the spinous processes parallel to the lamina. By progressively cutting away the fibers of the ligamentum flavum along with the attached bone the epidural fat is exposed. The fat may then be separated from the underlying remaining ligamentum flavum with a Penfield dissector. The remainder of the ligamentum flavum may be excised with a rongeur; care should be taken to avoid damaging the dura and the epidural vessels.

Stainless steel wire measuring either 18 (.040 mm.) or 16 (.048 mm.) gauge is shaped in an S-fashion as shown in Figure 10–14. The diameter of the first bend should be slightly larger than the lamina, and the tip of the wire should be bent slightly greater than the smooth contour of the primary bend. The second portion of the S contour should be a mirror image of the first bend in order for the wire to be easily passed underneath the lamina. Since this is the most crucial portion of the operation and the one that is most likely to produce neurologic damage if inadvertent contusion of the cord occurs, it is extremely important if not crucial to develop a failsafe system to minimize this eventuality. For wire passage, the tip is first placed into the neural canal at the inferior lamina edge toward the midline. The tip is then directed parallel; the surgeon holds the long end of the double looped wire in the left hand and advances the tip with the right hand, which is supported on the spine. Passage should be easy, the wire may be advanced in this position parallel to the inner cortex of the lamina. The wire is rotated slowly with continued advancement after the tip has advanced at least half the width of the lamina. When the tip of the wire presents above the lamina, a needle holder or a secure wire holder that will not spring off is attached to the tip of the loop. By pulling the wire

TECHNIQUES OF SURGERY

Luque wire passage

A. Shape wire

B. Insert wire under lamina

C. Grasp emerging wire end

D. Gently bend each wire ...medial one

E. ...lateral one

F.

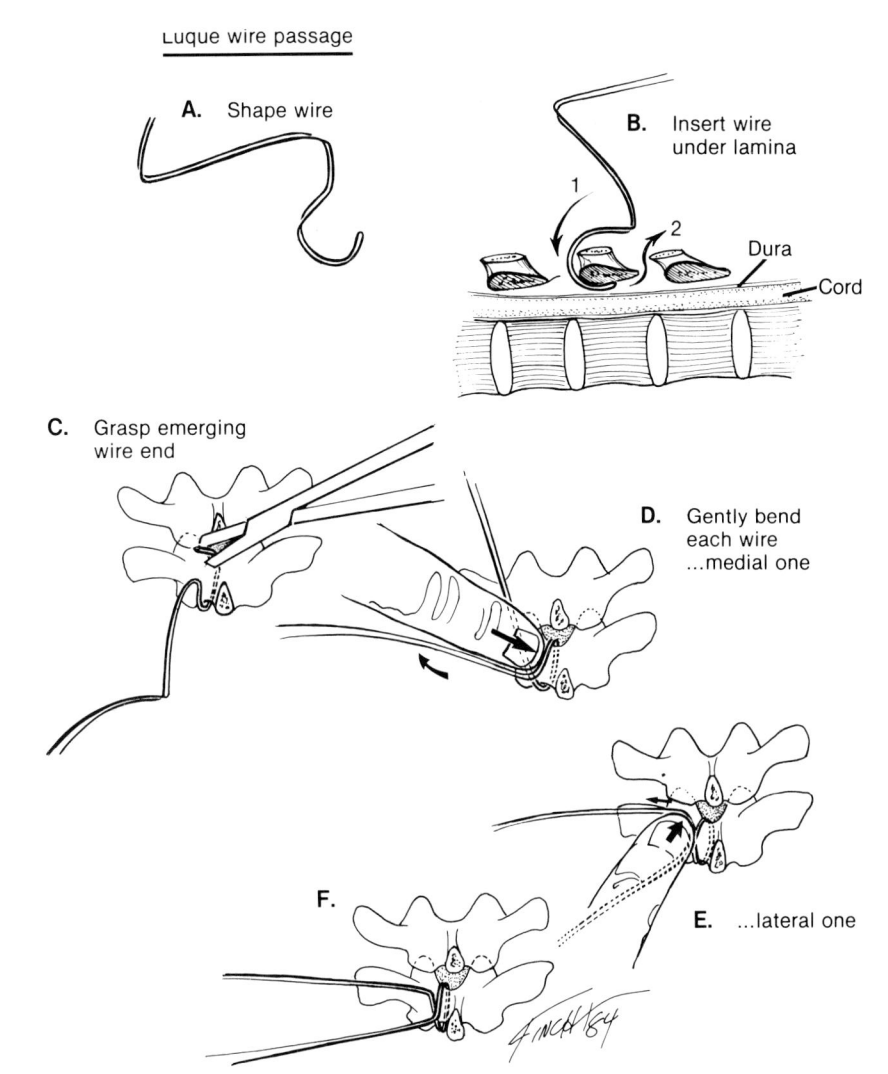

Figure 10–14. A useful technique for passing the sublaminar wire. Carefully bend the wire into an S shape. Advance the tip of the wire underneath the lamina; rotate and advance it carefully. Grasp the emerging tip (C) with a clamp. Then, pull the tip in a very gentle and controlled fashion. Bend each end carefully over the top of the lamina to prevent the wire from telescoping within the canal (see text).

with the clamp carefully and gently feeding the long end of the wire with the opposite hand, the wire is advanced until half the length protrudes above the lamina and half below. Again, it is helpful to support the hand on the patient while these maneuvers are taking place. Exerting too great a force to pull the wire through may result in the clamp being dislodged from the tip of the wire and the wire springing back into the canal against the dura and cord. After the wire has been satisfactorily advanced, it is then crimped over the top of the lamina, the superior portion being crimped toward the midline and the inferior half laterally. A second wire is placed in a similar fashion on the convex side resulting in double-stranded wires being placed on each half of the lamina. At the extreme cephalad and caudal laminae the wire is bent over the laminae so that the superior portion is crimped lateral to the inferior exiting wire (Fig. 10–15). As Allen has pointed out,[4] this arrangement provides a more secure fixation at the points of rod overlap proximally and distally. Some authors have preferred cutting the tip of the double wire at each level, passing one length on the right side and the other length on the left side. I have generally preferred using two double wires of 18 gauge (.040 mm.)

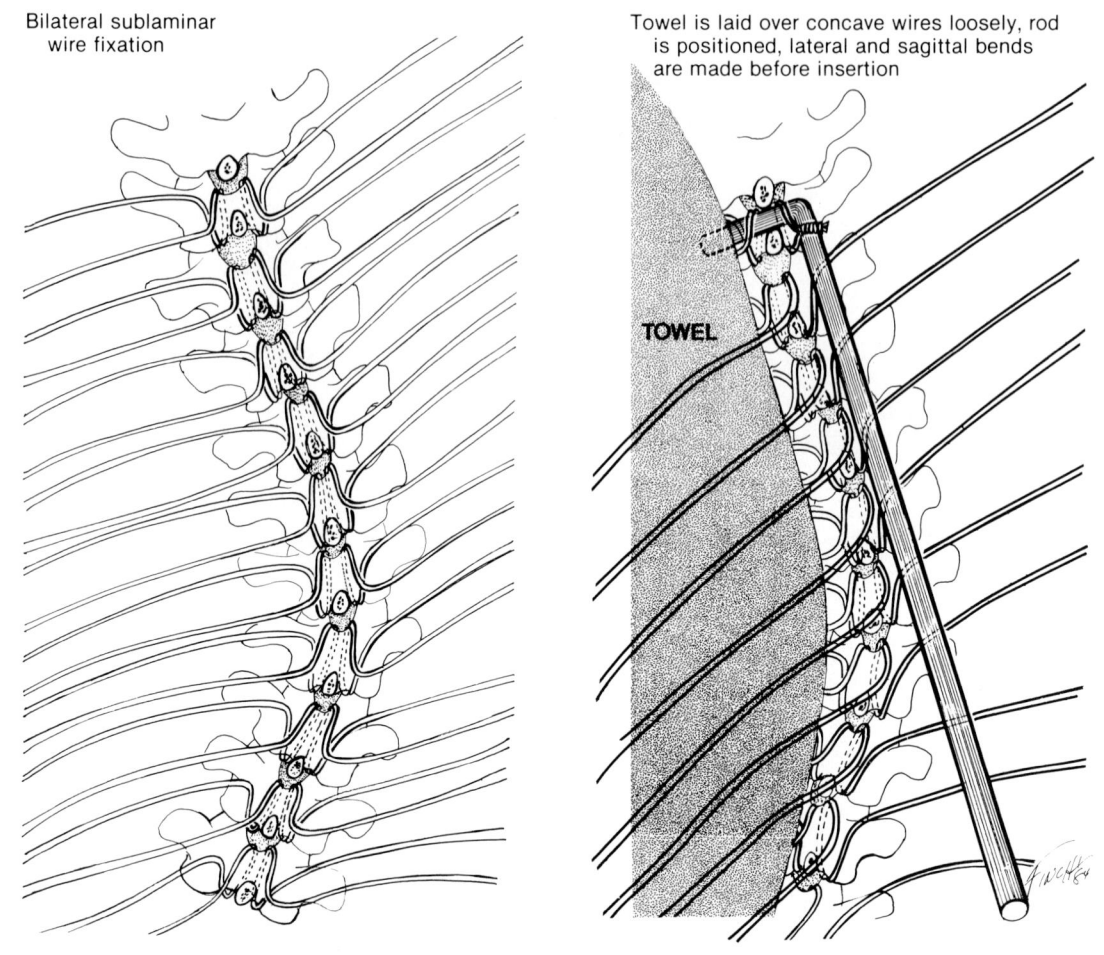

Figure 10–15. Continued from Figure 10–14. After all wires are passed and bent over the top of the lamina as noted, it is helpful to place a towel over the concave wires while the convex rod is positioned; and the wires on the convex side are tied over the top of the rod.

width for the right and for the left side of the lamina, whereas my associates have generally preferred using double wires of 16 gauge (.048 mm.) size.

Techniques of Correction

Correction with the L-rod system may be carried out in two fashions (Fig. 10–16). (1) The first rod may be applied to the convex side of the curvature or, (2) the first rod may be applied to the concave side of the curvature; hence, the terms convex technique and concave technique.[4, 5] In general, the convex technique is more useful to maintain or correct thoracic kyphosis, whereas the concave technique is more helpful when attempting to correct thoracic lordosis with scoliosis or to correct more extreme degrees of lumbar lordosis. This ability to build in secondary curvatures is particularly important when the fusion extends below the second or third lumbar vertebra. It is much easier with this technique to promote lumbar lordosis than it is to produce normal thoracic sagittal kyphosis in the presence of a thoracic lordosis. As Allen has pointed out,[4] providing secondary contours in the L-rod system introduces considerable torsion or stress into the implant. It is crucial, therefore, that firm fixation at the rod ends be achieved to prevent rod rotation with loss of fixation.

CONVEX TECHNIQUE

With the convex technique, the initial rod is placed on the convex side of the scoliotic

TECHNIQUES OF SURGERY

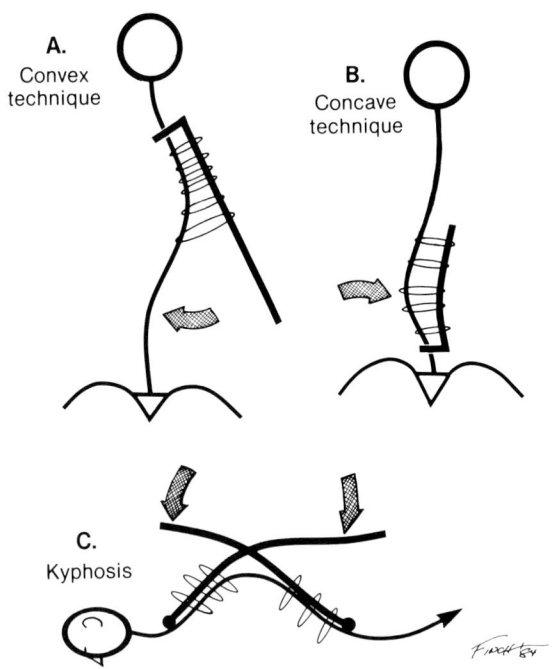

Figure 10–16. Diagrammatic demonstration of the convex (A) and concave (B) techniques for L-rod instrumentation of the spine. C, The useful technique of placing L-rods to correct kyphosis. (See text for details.)

curvature. For thoracic scoliosis in which lordosis is not a major component, the initial L-rod is attached to the first lamina above the superior end vertebra of the measured curve, the short arm of the L lying above the spinous process in a small groove across the lamina. Sequential wires secure the rod to the first four or five laminae. At this point the second rod is positioned on the concave side of the curvature with the L lying inferior to the lamina to be instrumented, underneath the spinous process, or in a groove or hole cut into the spinous process. This rod is tied down over the distal four to five laminae working distally to proximally. By gently levering the rods in a parallel fashion, positioning the long limb over the short L-limb, correction of the curvature is achieved and the remaining wires are tied to the rod. After the wires are fastened by progressive twisting, they are trimmed to approximately ½ inch (1 cm.) in length and then bent over the top of the rod towards the midline, away from the site of the arthrodesis. The end wires are cut slightly longer and bent toward the midline over the top of the short L-limb. A double wire is then passed underneath both rods, and the rods are secured together by twisting this wire.

CONCAVE TECHNIQUE

In the lumbar spine, as previously mentioned, the concave technique is usually preferable. Also in the thoracic spine in the presence of significant lordosis, this sequence of L-rod placement works best. The distal segment of the rod is attached to the lamina by passing the short limb through a notch made in the spinous process of the most caudad vertebra to be instrumented. The inferior double end wire on the concave side of the curvature is tied down over the rod to secure fixation at the distal site. If extreme degrees of lordosis have been pre-bent into the rod, it may be necessary to temporarily secure the short end on the convex side as well. The convex rod is attached proximally after the short end is placed loosely underneath the long limb of the concave rod. The convex rod is rotated superiorly to lie out of the field, while the remaining concave wires are tied to the rod and sequentially tightened. Maximum correction is best achieved by pushing over the apex of the curvature while sequential tightening occurs. Following this initial tightening, the lamina and spinous processes, particularly over the apex of the curve, may not lie juxtaposed to the concave rod. The second rod is then tied securely from cephalad to caudad, bringing both rods into contact with the laminae and spinous processes. This is facilitated using a rod approximator. Following convex rodding, the concave wires are now loose and must be tightened again. It is noted that the short limb of the L lies underneath the long limb for both the concave and the convex technique. The wires are then trimmed again to approximately 1 cm. in length and bent toward the midline, and the end wires are bent toward the opposite rod and secured together with a single double-stranded wire passed circumferentially around each rod.

PELVIC FIXATION

Pelvic fixation of the L-rod system may be provided by the short arm bent at a right angle to the long arm and passed in a bicortical fashion through the posterior iliac spine. However, this fixation is usually deficient especially in the osteoporotic patient, and the technique of pelvic fixation described first by Allen and Ferguson (referred to as the Galveston technique) is preferred.[5,6] Although the exposure is a bit more cumbersome, this technique appears to provide the best available fixation for L-rod instrumentation to the sacrum. It is helpful to expose both iliac crests and identify the sciatic notch. For fixation to the pelvis a ¼ inch (6.4 mm.) rod is preferable. The sacral-iliac articulation is exposed at the level of the posterior-superior iliac spine; this is best accomplished by elevating the erector spinal musculature off the midline and posterior iliac crest. A pelvic pin is driven into the ilium at the level of the posterior-superior iliac spine and passes within the diapole of the ilium, just cephalad to the sciatic notch for depth of approximately 6 to 9 cm. (Fig. 10–17). The pelvic pin used measures 3/16 inch (4.8 mm.). If a ¼ inch (6.4 mm.) rod is to be used, this pin is removed and the initial one third of the hole is drilled with a ¼ inch (6.4 mm.) drill bit. A pin is laid in place to serve as a guide for rod contouring. This may prove a most cumbersome procedure, especially if ¼ inch (6.4 mm.) stainless steel stock is being used. Contours must be made in three planes. We prefer to make the initial bend at a right angle, leaving the short arm approximately 12 cm. in length. A second bend is made approximately 2 to 3 cm. distal to the first bend at a 50 to 75 degree angle, depending on the angle of the ilium to the midsagittal plane. Lordosis is then bent into the long limb of the rod, tilting the short limb to the desired orientation. The short limb is measured again to be certain that iliac penetration is no greater than the initial guide insertion, and this should be no greater than 9 to 10 cm. in the adult patient.

Special Considerations

KYPHOSIS

L-rod instrumentation may prove particularly useful in the correction of kyphosis. It is necessary in these cases, however, to use ¼ inch (6.4 mm.) stainless steel rods, since the smaller rod is unable to produce and maintain correction. Cases of posterior correction with the L-rod system must usually be proceeded by an anterior discectomy and interbody fusion. At the second stage posterior procedure a halo may prove useful in maintaining head and upper thoracic spine position as well as maximum intraoperative correction. Gauging the amount of rod pre-bend may prove difficult. In general, the rod is pre-bent to that amount calculated on the hyperextension x-ray. Following exposure, Allen prefers to place the short limbs of the L-rod at the caudal extreme of the instrumentation.[4] We have preferred to place the short limbs at opposite ends of the curvature, similar to the placement for correction of scoliosis. In order that the short limb be placed under the long limb of the opposite rod, the second rod should be placed into position before the first rod is completely tied down. In kyphosis we would prefer to use double wires at each segmented level.

LORDOSIS

As mentioned earlier, kyphosis may be built into the implant as a secondary curvature. For correction of mild degrees of thoracic lordosis, less than −20 degrees, and particularly in patients who are skeletally immature, some apparent correction of the thoracic lordosis on the lateral x-ray may be possible with the L-rod system. Again in these cases it is best to place the initial rod on the concavity, pulling the spine up to the pre-bent rod (concave technique). For a more substantial correction of thoracic lordosis (greater than −30 degrees) particularly in the skeletally mature patient with decreased pulmonary function, a combined approach may be preferable (see Special Techniques).

PELVIC OBLIQUITY

Pelvic fixation according to the Galveston technique is particularly useful in correcting pelvic obliquity.[6, 7] In patients with paralytic scoliosis, correction is possible by using a first stage anterior release by discectomy with interbody fusion followed by a second stage posterior Luque rod instrumentation with pelvic fixation ("Galveston" technique). At the first stage, anterior approach discectomy and fusion to the sacrum is desirable. At the second stage, complete release of the attached musculature to the contracted high riding iliac crest facilitates correction. For total correction of the obliquity the long limb of the rod should be aligned perpendicular to the sacrum. This may not be possible, and lateral as well as sagittal bends must be placed into the rod to allow the rod to be in firm contact with the base of the spinous process and lamina. Correction may be facilitated by applying a distraction implant of Harrington outrigger to the concave side of

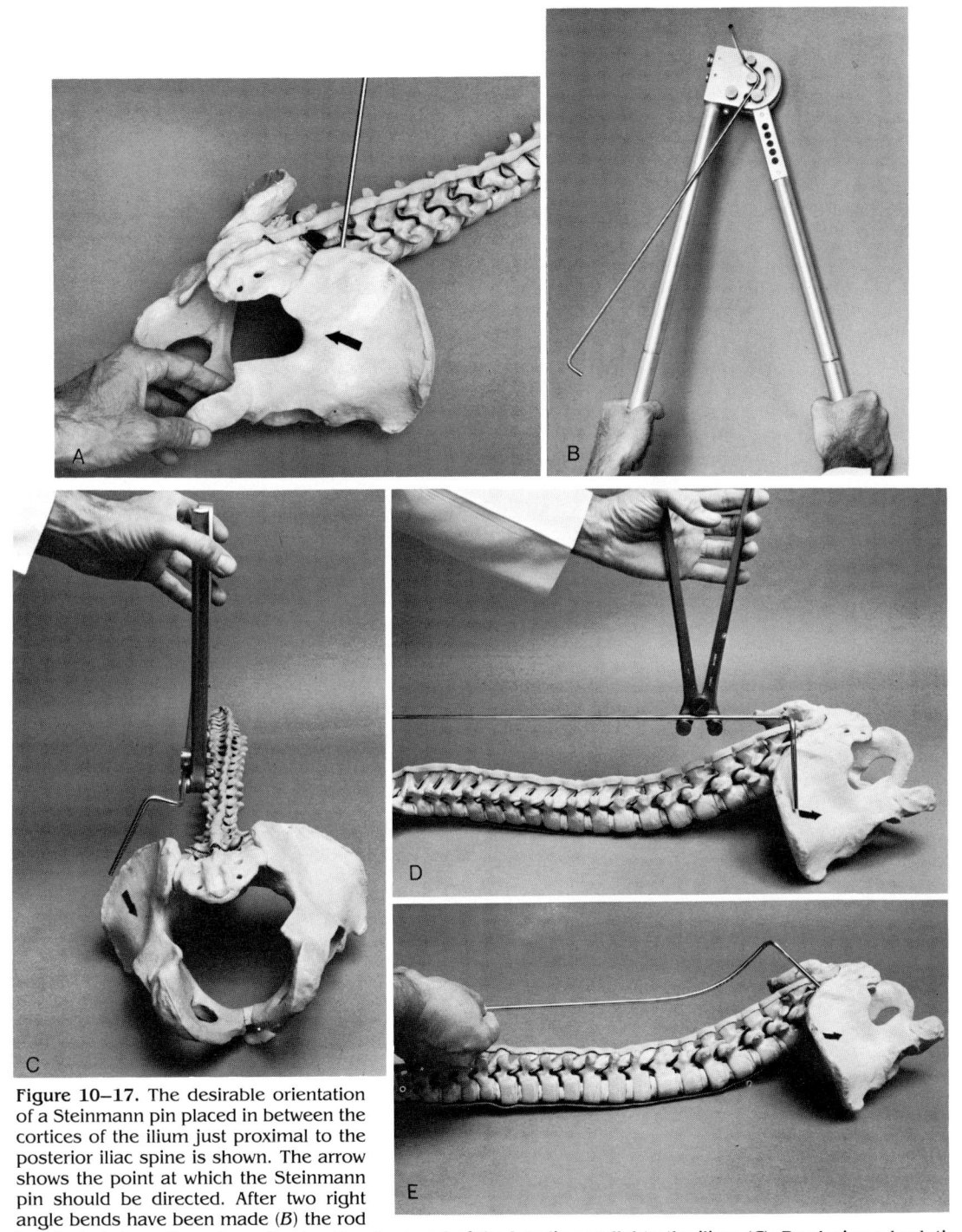

TECHNIQUES OF SURGERY

Figure 10–17. The desirable orientation of a Steinmann pin placed in between the cortices of the ilium just proximal to the posterior iliac spine is shown. The arrow shows the point at which the Steinmann pin should be directed. After two right angle bends have been made (*B*) the rod is oriented along the spine, allowing the short end of the L to lie parallel to the ilium (*C*). By placing a lordotic bend into the rod (*D*) the short end of the arrow then becomes oriented in the correct plane and the sagittal correction and proper lordosis have been produced (*E*).

the curve (using a sacral hook) as a temporary correcting force while the Luque rod is positioned into the convex ilium and maneuvered to the spine.

MYELOMENINGOCOELE

The attachment of the L-rod system to the spine in a patient with myelomeningocoele may prove somewhat more difficult. Since the laminae are usually absent, the wires must be placed around the base of the pedicles. The wire may have to be first twisted around the base of the pedicle with the knot facing laterally prior to attachment to the rod.[8] Pelvic fixation may prove difficult because of the deficient and osteopenic nature of the pelvis in these patients. Dunn[42] has described a useful technique for pre-bending rods in the myelomeningocoele patient, providing essentially a 180 degree loop that attaches over the sacral alar providing pelvic purchase and support (Fig. 10–18).

GENERAL COMMENT ON L-ROD INSTRUMENTATION

Although L-rod instrumentation is still in its developmental stage, as of this writing it has proved to be a major and important adjuvant in the management of spinal deformity patients. The greatest benefit of L-rod instrumentation is the ability of this implant to furnish secure fixation, allowing patients to go without postoperative cast or orthoses.[120] In some patients, such as those with idiopathic scoliosis, this may prove only a small and at times insignificant convenience. In patients with paralytic deformity associated with insensitive skin, this implant system is clearly advantageous. When fusion to the sacrum is necessary, this technique provides the most secure pelvic fixation currently available and at the same time allows maintenance and even production of normal lumbar lordosis, a major advantage not offered by a pure distraction implant system.

Disadvantages of the L-rod instrumentation system include a greater possibility of neurologic damage, a more demanding surgical technique, greater blood loss, a prolongation of the operative time, and potential problems if implant removal is necessary.[74] Complications from broken wires have been reported, and extraction of the wire, either in a controlled fashion by cutting the wires and then using needle-nose pliers to wind the wire around the tip or using a more rapid

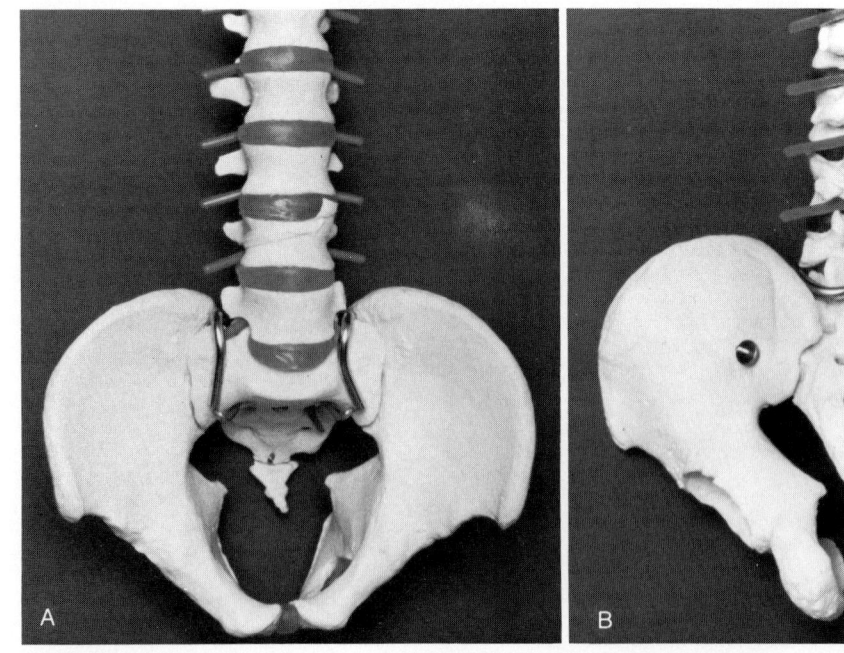

Figure 10–18. The Dunn technique for contouring a Luque rod for alar purchase. The anterior loop of the L-rod as shown in A is somewhat longer than is necessary but is useful for visualization. This technique is particularly helpful in instrumenting to the sacrum in patients with myelomeningocoele, in whom pedicular fixation may be more difficult.

extraction force may result in wire migration into the dura and spinal cord.[94] The author has seen two such substantial dural leaks from wire extraction. If rod removal is necessary in the lumbar spine below the conus, the author would favor controlled extraction with the needle-nose plier technique. In areas involving the thoracic cord and conus, the author would prefer to remove the implant but tie the ends of the wire over the lamina leaving them in place. If wire removal is nonetheless necessary, a small laminectomy (a longitudinal slit in the lamina) can be made over the affected segment if possible, and wires removed under direct vision. In light of these possible complications and disadvantages, one should proceed with caution in using this system for the patient with adolescent thoracic idiopathic scoliosis. Clear advantages over the Harrington system for the treatment of adolescent thoracic idiopathic scoliosis have yet to be established.

Harrington Rod Instrumentation With Sublaminar Wires

The degree of fixation and versatility of Harrington distraction rod implants may be increased greatly by the addition of sublaminar wiring. Greater stability may be achieved with this adjunct, and in patients in whom the risk of pseudarthrosis is greater (e.g., adult scoliosis, thoracolumbar or lumbar curves, or reoperation for previously failed surgery), this adjunct may ultimately prove beneficial. Again, by bending secondary curves in the implant and using a square-ended lower hook, some correction in sagittal malalignment may be possible. It should be recognized, however, that torsional stresses, particularly at the end hook purchase sites, may prove substantial and result in hook pull-out. The author has found that this tendency may be lessened by wiring the inferior two spinous processes together, creating a

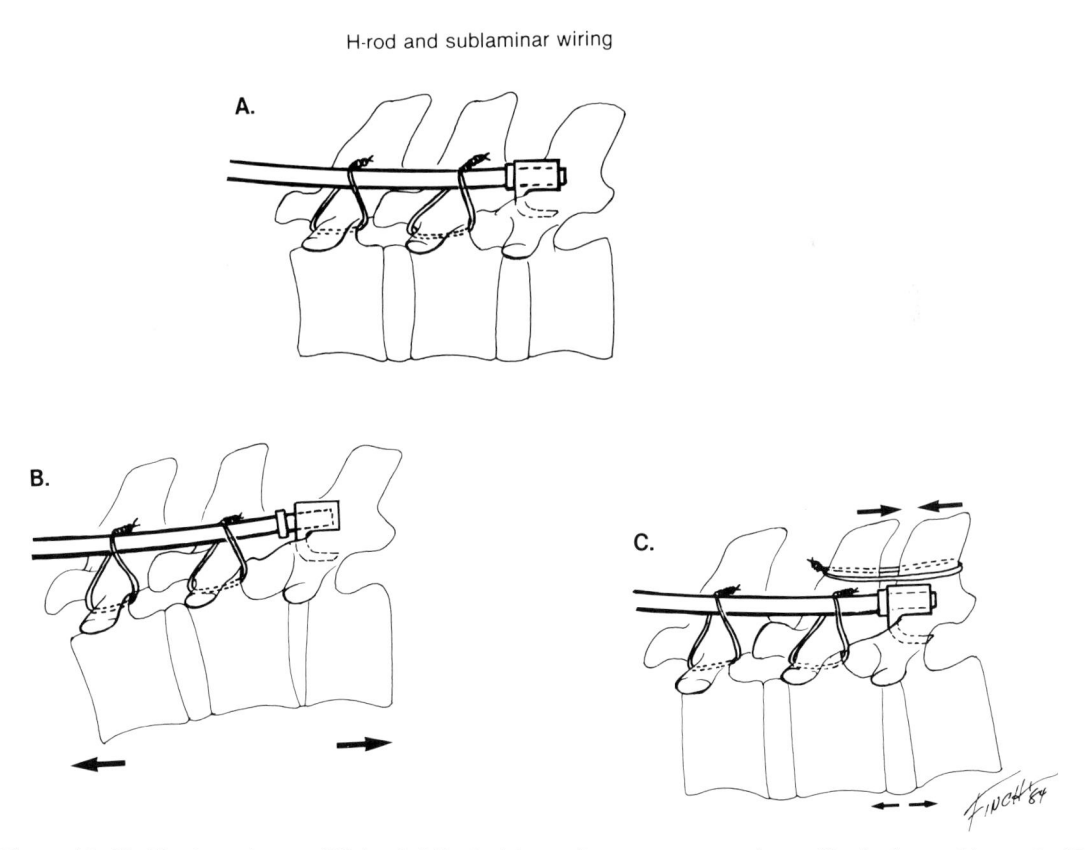

Figure 10–19. The importance of "tying in" the last two spinous processes when a Harrington rod is used with sublaminar wiring is shown. *B,* If this is not done, loosening of fixation by flexion will occur. *C,* If the spinous processes are locked together, loss of fixation distally should not occur and, more importantly, maintenance of lordosis at the lower fixation point is possible. This is particularly beneficial in the lumbar spine.

compression force across the last two vertebrae and locking the inferior hook in place (Fig. 10–19). This adjunct will also maintain some lordotic tilt to the inferior lumbar vertebra and may avoid the tendency of the distraction implant to flatten the lumbar spine (Fig. 10–20). The implant in this system rarely lies in firm contact with the spinous processes or the lamina throughout the curved segment, especially in the more severe single curve pattern where correction to less than 40 to 50 degrees is not possible. This lack of firm contact has theoretical disadvantages but has not proven of practical consequence in our experience. An attempt to make the rod fit into firm contact with the lamina is ill advised, particularly in the most cephalad lamina, as excessive wire tightening may force the upper hook through the facet into the spinal canal. As stated, this system provides more secure fixation than a Harrington device alone, results in less metal residing in the spinal canal than classical L-rod instrumentation, and frees one side of the spine for bone grafting, unimpeded by the metallic implant, and may allow some correction of sagittal plane deformity. Following this procedure, patients may be treated in an underarm brace that may be removed for bathing. Whether these advantages outweigh the disadvantages of the system so described in the treatment of idiopathic scoliosis is not known at this time. Further experience will be necessary to delineate the usefulness of this adjunct.

The use of Harrington rods with sublaminar wiring for the management of spinal fractures, however, does appear to have definite advantages over Harrington distraction fixation alone. Distraction implants serve to maintain vertebral height, and associated with sublaminar wiring, provide superb fixation for the neurologically injured patient. We have found this implant system most useful in patients with complete loss of neurologic function who have sustained fractures requiring open reduction of internal fixation (see Spinal Trauma section).

Cotrel-Dubousset Instrumentation
(Fig. 10–21)[34]

New forms of instrumentation are continuously being developed. Most recent at the time of this writing is that originated by Drs. Yves Cotrel and Jean Dubousset of Paris, France. Developed in 1981, the C-D system appears a useful and helpful addition to the surgical armamentarium. The C-D rod is ¼ inch solid, knurled; it is threaded into open-ended hooks as well as closed hooks, similar to Harrington hooks. The open-ended hooks facilitate placement of the rod into the hook at multiple sites along the curvature. The rod is pre-bent to conform to the partially corrected curve and is then locked into position in the hooks with rod sleeves that fit into the open-ended hooks. The rod is distracted slightly and then rotated approximately 90 degrees, achieving a three dimensional correction of the curvature. The rod is locked into the hooks by set screws that prevent it from rerotating. A second rod is placed on the convex side as a compression implant and the two rods are then coupled with two small transverse traction rods and hooks. This creates a fixed rectangular structure that provides tremendous stability to the implant. The major advantage of this system is the ability to mobilize the patient after surgery without a postoperative cast or brace. Fixation appears secure enough, and the patient may return to a more normal lifestyle sooner

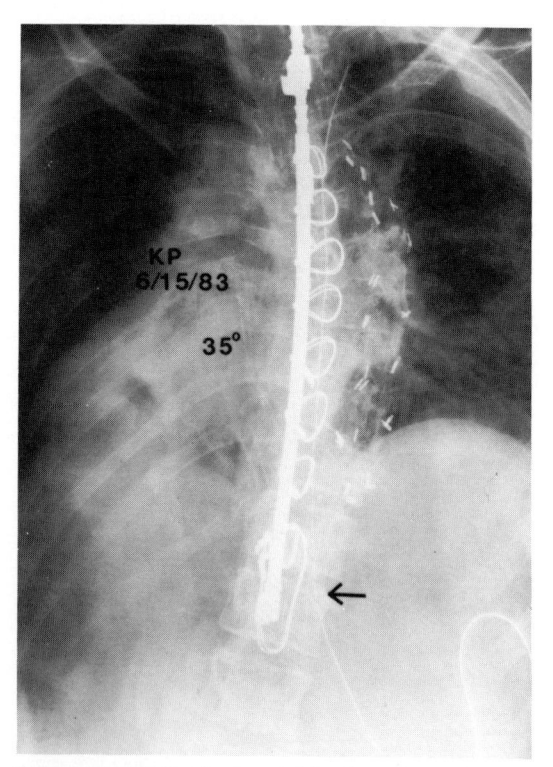

Figure 10–20. Harrington rod fixation with sublaminar wiring. The last two spinous processes have been locked together, preventing loss of fixation distally.

than would be allowed by other implant systems, without the need for an external orthosis. Partial correction of the spine deformity is achieved not only in the AP plane but also in the lateral plane, as well as to some degree in the axial plane with derotation of the vertebra to a more normal orientation. Further experience and longer follow-ups are necessary before a definitive statement can be made concerning the future role of this implant sytem. The early results, however, look most encouraging and provide the surgeon with another means of correcting and stabilizing spinal deformity.

PROCEDURE

Surgeons contemplating the use of this device are encouraged as a first step to obtain hands on experience. The instrumentation is more complex than Harrington implants, the options are greater, and the tools, upon initial use, are more cumbersome. The instrumentation consists of two types of rods; a ¼ inch diameter with a knurled surface in varying lengths, and a transverse loader rod which is ⅛ inch in diameter and serves to interlock the two rods. There are three types of hooks: a pedicle hook which has a bifid foot and two lamina hooks, one for the thoracic area which has a smaller foot and one for the lumbar area which has a larger foot. The three types of hooks come either open or closed. The rod is held into the open hooks by means of a hook blocker. The closed hooks as well as the blockers are furnished with set screws to prevent the rod from rotating once the position has been set. The instrumentation is unique as well and consists of a variety of inserters, pushers, holders, spreaders, rod tighteners, and drivers.

The fusion area is determined in the customary fashion, using neutral rotation and the end vertebra according to Cobb measurements. On the lateral x-ray, thoracic lordosis should be taken into consideration and it may be necessary to instrument from one to two segments more cephalad, depending on the end lordotic vertebra. Preoperative bending films or traction films are necessary. The hook sites are chosen on the end vertebra that would correspond to the stable zone of Harrington, considering neutral rotation as well as the end vertebra from the Cobb measurement. The apical vertebra and the intermediate vertebrae levels are also determined. The apical vertebra is the vertebral body with the most rotation on the standing x-ray, and it has a vertical convex side. The intermediate vertebrae are those two vertebra, one or two vertebral bodies on each side of the apical vertebra that show the least mobility on side bending or traction x-rays. It is extremely helpful to mark out on the preoperative x-rays the hook placement according to the principles as outlined. Four hooks would be placed on the concave side. The cephalad end vertebra would receive a closed pedicle hook, the cephalad intermediate vertebra would receive an open pedicle hook, the caudal intermediate vertebra would receive a sublaminar thoracic open hook, and the caudal vertebra would receive a closed sublaminar lumbar or thoracic hook. On the convex side, the cephalad vertebra would receive a closed lamina hook on the transverse process and a closed pedicle hook at the facet joint. The apical vertebra would receive an open pedicle hook into the facet joint and the caudal vertebra of the convexity would receive a closed lumbar hook or a closed pedicle hook if the end vertebra remained in the thoracic spine.

TECHNIQUE

After the patient is anesthetized, he or she is placed on the operating table; a head halter and leg traction may be used, depending upon the wishes of the operating surgeon. If traction is used, it is usually 25 to 30 lbs. or up to one third of body weight. The incision is made in a routine fashion and exposure is carried out as previously described. The pedicle hook sites are prepared with a sharp osteotome, and a pedicle finder is inserted into the facet joint until it is seated on the pedicle. It is important that the seating be solid, otherwise fixation will be jeopardized. The pedicle hook is then seated using the appropriate holder and inserter, making certain that the bifid portion of the hook engages the pedicle. The lamina hooks are placed in a routine fashion using a thoracic lamina hook with a smaller foot for the thoracic spine. The hook sites are prepared for the lamina hook with either a transverse process elevator or a lamina elevator. The concave hooks are placed in first. A malleable rod is used as a template, and a C-D rod is bent accordingly. Decortication is carried out on the concave side prior to placing the rod. The rod is positioned into the hooks, hook blockers are pushed into the open pedicle and lamina hooks on the concave side of the intermediate vertebra, but the set screws are not tightened. The blockers are locked into place with a C-ring. Using the rod holders, the spine is then derotated approximately 90 degrees, correcting the scoliosis and producing kyphosis. If traction has been used, it is decreased by about 50 per cent prior to derotation. After the rod has been rotated, the hooks are more snugly seated with the spreader and the set screws are tightened to prevent the rod from re-rotating. The two C-rings are removed from the intermediate hook sites and the convex hooks are positioned, locking in the blocker over the apical pedicle open hook. Compression is carried out, and the set screws are tightened. Distraction should again be carried out on the concave side to be sure that all hooks are snug in their fixation sites and then compression should be checked again on the convex side. Once all screws are tightened, two transverse loaders are applied near the end of the rods, and a Stagnara wake-up test is carried out. Following a satisfactory wake-up test, the anesthesia is deepened and the set screws are overtightened until they shear off, locking the system into place and preventing loss of fixation. Copious bone grafts from the iliac crest should be added around the implants, and decortication should have been carried out prior to fixation. Postoperatively, the patient is log-rolled in bed usually for two days, and mobilization and ambulation are begun when the drains have been removed. No postoperative immobilization is generally necessary.

The technique as described would apply primarily to a thoracic curve pattern. Double curve patterns, either double thoracic or tho-

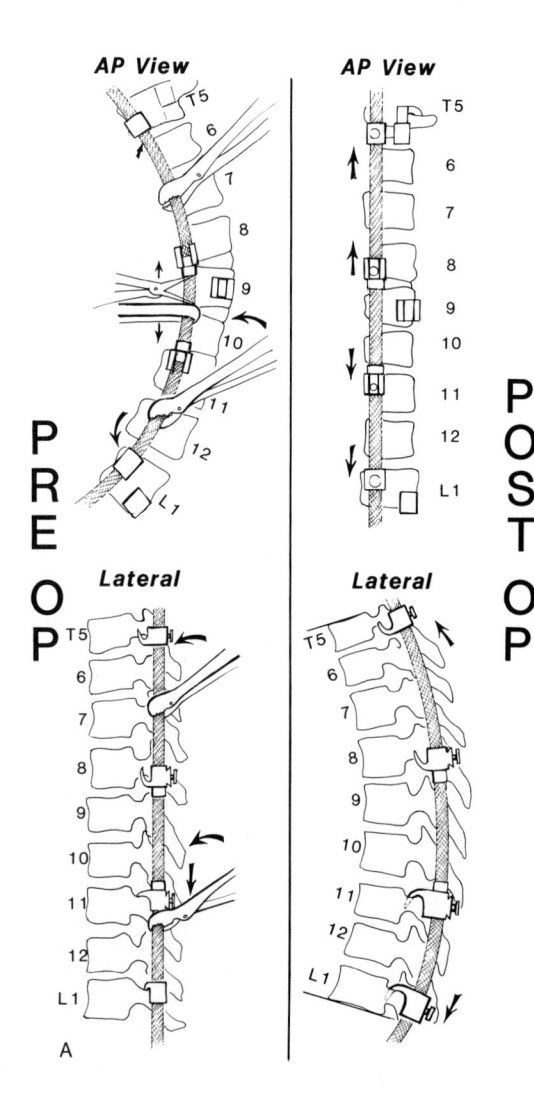

Figure 10–21. A, Note the appearance of the spine in the AP and lateral planes. By laying the rod in the AP plane to conform to the scoliotic curve and then rotating the rod counterclockwise while the rod is locked into the hooks, as shown, correction of the lateral plane deformity is possible. In patients with hypokyphosis the rotation of the rod will serve to produce a more normal kyphosis, restoring sagittal plane alignment (see text). B, L-rod shows the correction and stability of correction possible with the C-D implant for not only single thoracic curves, but also double thoracic and lumbar curves. B and C, Preoperatively the patient had a rigid high thoracic curve with an asymmetrical neckline. Both curves were instrumented using the C-D implant. D and E, Substantial correction was possible. Because of the nature of the rod, the same rod may be used for distraction as well as compression simultaneously. Sagittal plane alignment has likewise been maintained, and the rib asymmetry was significantly improved.

Illustration continued on opposite page

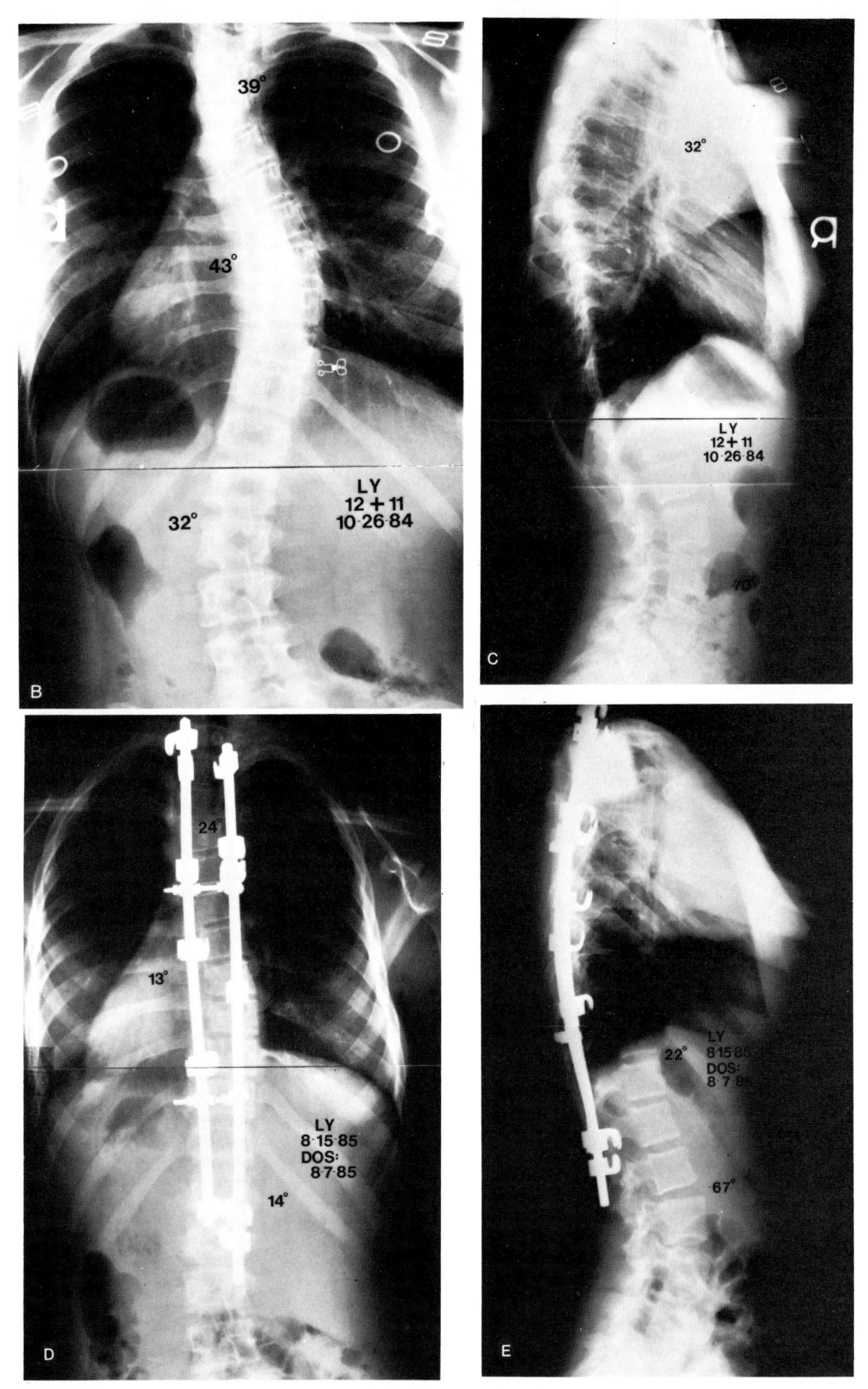

Figure 10-21 Continued.

racic and lumbar are more complex and would require more hooks at more fixation points. It is important to realize that a meticulously carried out fusion is the most important part of any procedure, and even the best implant will fail if this point is not taken into consideration.

ANTERIOR APPROACH TO THE SPINE

Although occasional attempts were made to approach the spinal column through the anterior route over 200 years ago,[52, 100] it is only recently that anterior approaches to the spine have become more widely appreciated and indeed, used rather commonly. In 1922, MacLennan[81] first described an anterior approach by costotransversectomy in a patient with congenital scoliosis. His work was subsequently followed by reports from Royle,[102] Compere,[32] VonLackum and Smith,[117] and Wiles[122] and Roaf.[99] Hodgson popularized the transthoracic approach to the spine for the management of spinal tuberculosis when he first published his work in 1956.[62] With the advent of Dwyer's instrumentation, newer implants[106, 129] have proven immensely helpful to surgeons in managing deformities of the thoracic and lumbar spine.

Transthoracic Approach[15, 19, 24, 25, 33, 56, 67, 98]

The transthoracic approach to the spine may be made from the right or the left side, depending primarily upon the discretion of the operating surgeon and the anatomy of the deformity. In the absence of scoliosis or a rotatory spinal deformity the great vessels will lie anterior to the spine and therefore, in either a right or a left sided approach, they will not interfere with the exposure. In the presence of a scoliosis greater than 30 degrees, the great vessels will lie on the concavity of the curvature and therefore exposure through the concavity may prove difficult if not impossible.

The level of the approach is determined by the procedure to be performed. The rib selected for removal should be that one lying above the most cephalad vertebral body to be exposed. If a lower rib is chosen, it will be difficult to reach the upper portion of the deformity since the downward inclination of the ribs usually interferes with visualization. For example, if one removes the fifth rib, access from T5 to T11 can be accomplished without problems. Similarly, removal of the sixth rib gives access from T6 to T12. There are exceptions to this rule. If patients have horizontally oriented ribs, removal of the sixth rib gives access from T5 to T11. In patients with severe sloping ribs, removal of the fifth rib may give access only from T6 to T11. If after rib removal it is apparent that a higher exposure is necessary, one may divide the rib above at the angle without removing it, facilitating the more cephalad exposure.

It is possible to go as cephalad as the third rib through this approach by careful mobilization and displacement of the scapula upward and forward. Approach to the first thoracic vertebra through the third to fifth rib is possible. It is also possible to reach T1 to T4 through a sternal spreading incision of the suprasternal notch to the xiphoid.[29] The thymus may be retracted, the innominate vein is divided, and the trachea and esophagus are displaced to the left. This approach may be a formidable one, and maneuverability is limited. The risk of complications would appear to be high. For these reasons, we have not used this approach and have preferred to approach the highest thoracic vertebra through a thoracotomy incision.

After preparation of the skin, the incision is made from the posterior angle of the rib to the tip of the costal cartilage (Fig. 10–22). The incision is carried down to the rib, and the rib is exposed subperiosteally and then detached anteriorly from the costochondral junction and as far posteriorly as possible (at least to the costotransverse articulation). The chest is entered by incising the pleura along the rib bed. The edges of the wound are covered with moist sponges, and rib retractors are positioned.

The parietal pleura is now incised along the vertebral bodies throughout the length of the spine to be exposed (Fig. 10–23). The discs will appear as prominences and the vertebral bodies as depressions. The pleura may be easily dissected off the anterior longitudinal ligament. The segmental vessels will be visualized as they cross over the vertebral bodies. The vessels should be secured and ligated over the midportion of the vertebra at its anterior lateral edge. If the vessels are ligated too far laterally next to the intervertebral foramen, the collaterals from foramen to foramen may be disrupted and damage to the segmental feeder vessels to the spinal cord may result.[37] We have not seen this occur.

TECHNIQUES OF SURGERY

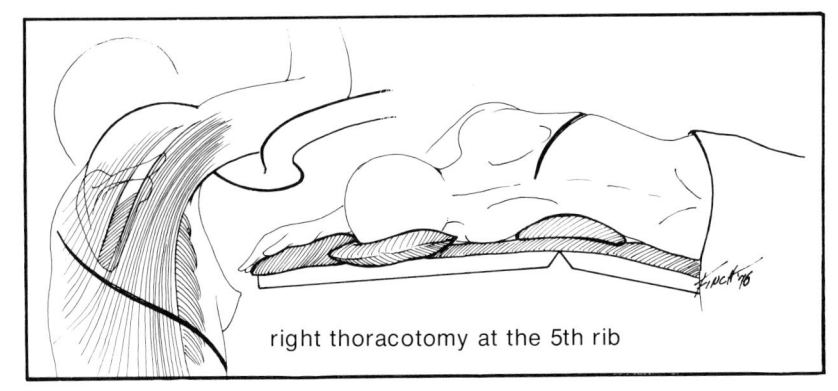

right thoracotomy at the 5th rib

Figure 10–22. The correct positioning for a patient undergoing a thoracotomy for exposure of the anterior spine at T5.

The dissection proceeds along either of two routes: (1) the areolar extraperiosteal plane, or (2) the subperiosteal plane. Generally, the extraperiosteal plane is more common, but for inlay strut grafting the subperiosteal plane is preferable. If the extraperiosteal route is chosen, the areolar tissue with the divided vessels is stripped off the vertebral

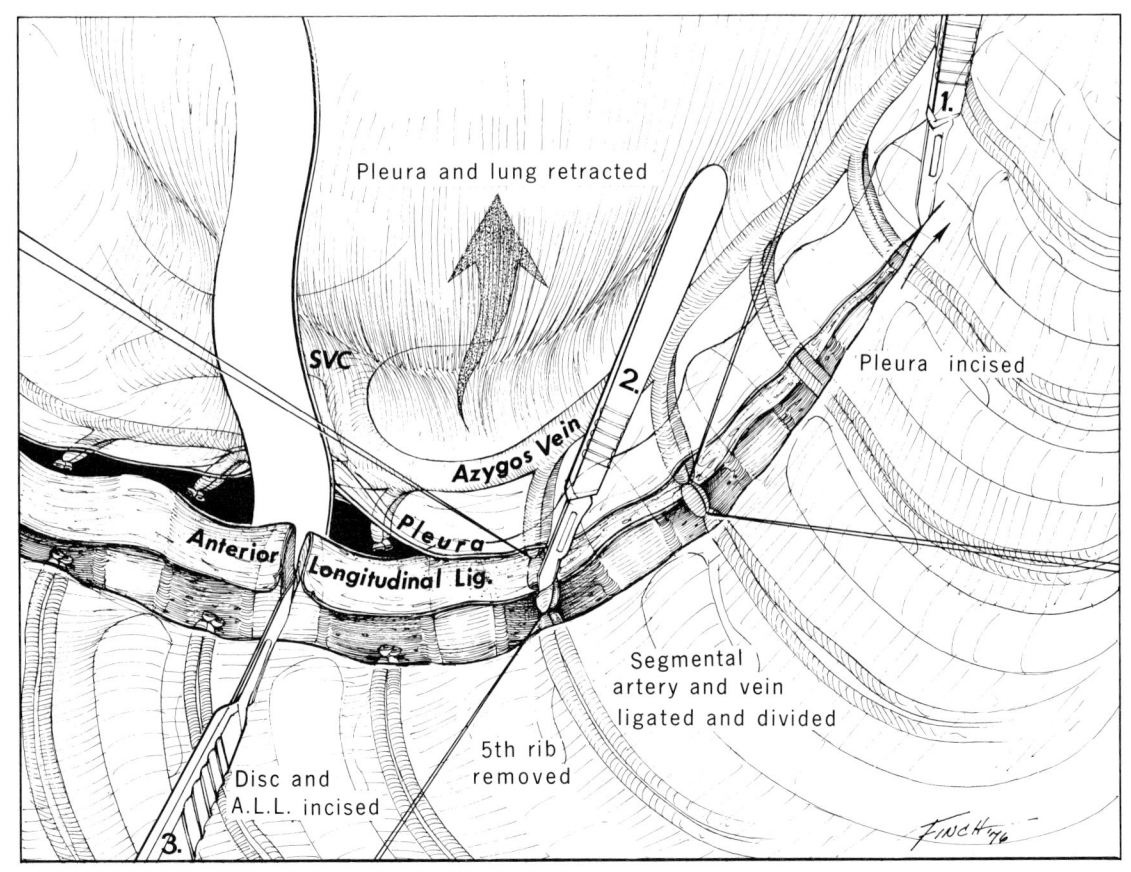

Figure 10–23. The exposure to the spine following removal of the fifth rib. First the parietal pleura is incised along the length of the spine to be exposed. The segmental vessels are identified overlying each vertebral body and are ligated and divided anterolaterally at least 1 centimeter away from the intervertebral foramen. By staying outside the periosteum, the areolar tissue with the divided vessels is pushed off the vertebral bodies and the anterior longitudinal ligament around to the opposite side and into the angle between the vertebral body and the transverse process. A malleable retractor provides excellent exposure. The disc and anterior longitudinal ligament may be incised and completely removed as necessary.

body and away from the anterior longitudinal ligament to the opposite side of the body. This exposure will be done blindly; the soft tissue will be carefully separated manually from the spine. The sponge may be packed into the area and a malleable retractor inserted to the opposite side of the vertebral bodies. This provides excellent exposure and separates the great vessels from the operating field. No attempt is made to preserve the splanchnic nerve chain. Division causes no problems. However, if the thoracic duct is inadvertently divided, it should be ligated.

Thoracoabdominal Approach

Exposure to the thoracic and lumbar spines conjointly may be accomplished through a single incision by dividing the diaphragm from its costal attachments. For this approach, removal of the ninth or tenth rib is generally preferred. The incision is extended along the costocartilage junction across the upper abdomen to the lateral edge of the rectus abdominus sheath, toward the symphysis pubis, depending upon the length of the lumbar spine to be exposed. Through this incision it is possible to expose all the way to the sacrum (Fig. 10–24).

After the tenth rib is removed from its costal attachments, the retroperitoneal entry into the abdominal cavity is carried out. This is facilitated by blunt dissection with the fingertips between the cut edges of the cartilage, peeling off the peritoneum from the underside of the diaphragm. As this dissection proceeds laterally and posteriorly, the diaphragm will become free of its peritoneal attachment and the viscera will fall forward, away from the vertebral column. The diaphragm may then be detached, leaving about

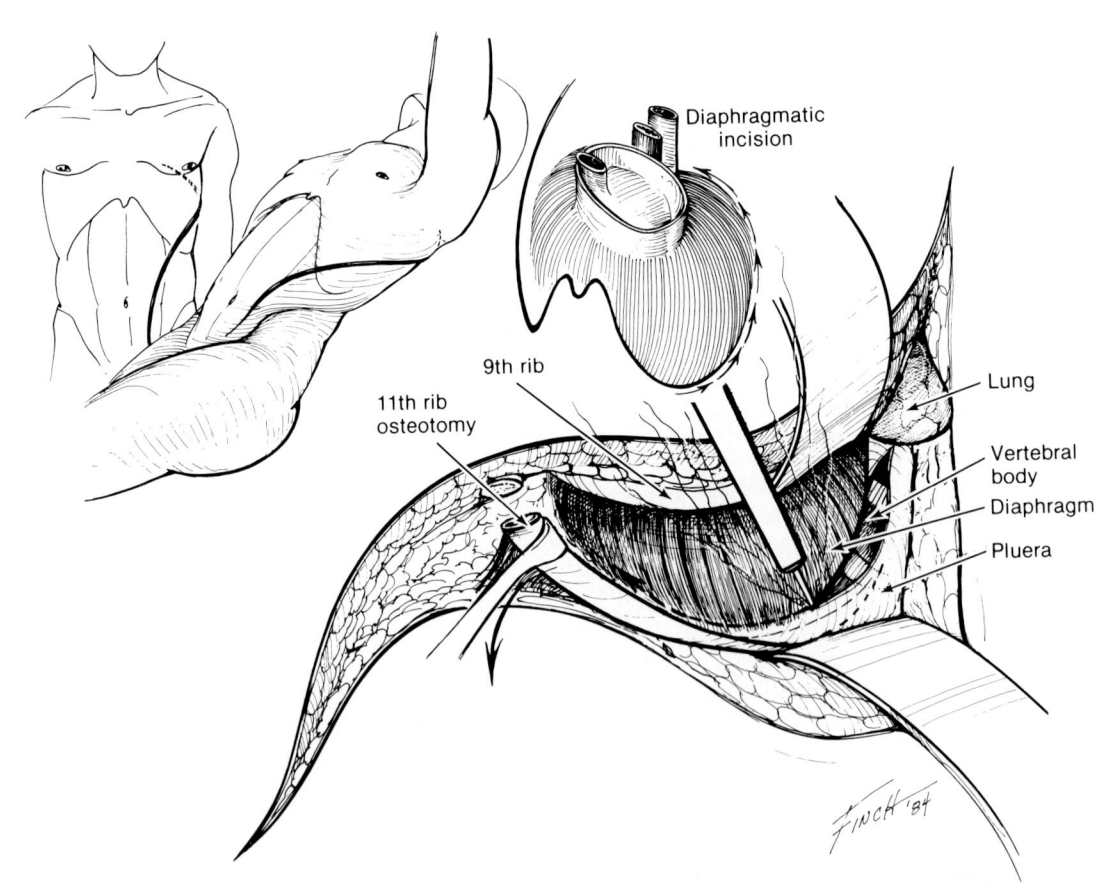

Figure 10–24. Exposure is facilitated by detaching the diaphragm along its costal margin; one literally falls into the peritoneum, providing easy access to the retroperitoneum and a relatively bloodless field. Reattachment of the diaphragm following surgery poses no problem.

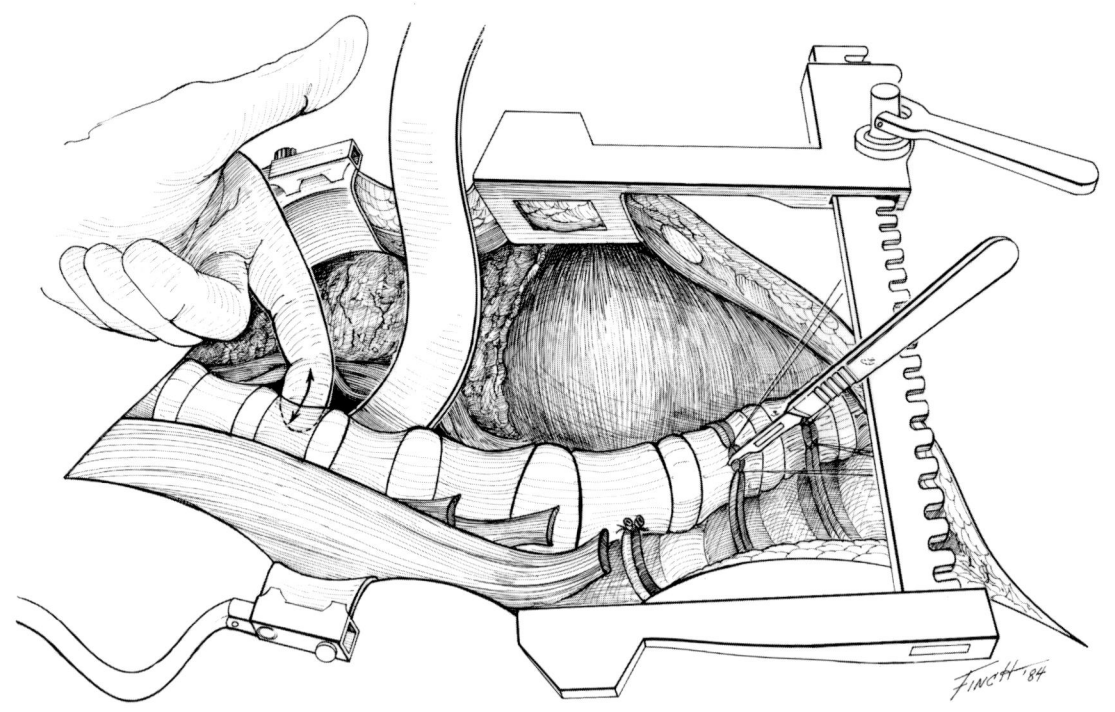

Figure 10–25. Exposure (see Fig. 10–24) now proceeds proximally and distally along the spine from the areas to be visualized. The segmental vessels are identified and ligated in the manner previously described. In the lumbar spine the exposure is more difficult, since the psoas muscle overlies the anterior lateral aspect of the vertebral body. With careful dissection, however, more than adequate visualization is possible. The vessels may be freed and displaced anterior medially or laterally for exposure to the L5-S1 disc.

1 cm. of tissue along its costal insertion. Over the last several years we have preferred to enter the retroperitoneum by dividing the diaphragm from the thoracic side along its costal attachment using the Bovie knife. This may be done without leaving any diaphragmatic tissue, and the exposure is relatively bloodless. Reattachment has not proven to be a problem, and postoperative atelectasis appears to be lessened. Once the retroperitoneum is entered, the vertebral bodies are identified and the psoas muscle is carefully dissected laterally off the intervertebral disc spaces. Segmental vessels overlying each vertebral body are exposed, ligated, and divided. As one proceeds more distally, the iliac vessel will overly the intervertebral disc at L4-L5. By careful dissection and ligation and division of the recurrent lumbar vein, these vessels may be freed and displaced anteriorly and medially, allowing exposure to the intervertebral disc at L5-S1 (Fig. 10–25). One may also go anterior to the iliac vessels, dividing the middle sacral vessels thereby furnishing excellent exposure to L5-S1.

Retroperitoneal Approach

The retroperitoneal approach to the lumbar spine may be satisfactorily accomplished through a T11 rib approach, first described by Fey.[46] The exposure may be maintained in an extrapleural retroperitoneal fashion. Exposure to the lower lumbar spine may be accomplished through a twelfth rib incision described by Digby,[36] which is similar to the exposure described by Fey through the eleventh rib. It is not necessary to excise the twelfth rib if one is approaching the lower lumbar spine, and in those cases a routine sympathectomy type approach is sufficient.

Transperitoneal Approach

The anterior transperitoneal approach to the lumbar spine described by Freebody, Bendall, and Taylor[49] has been most useful in our experience. The incision may be made transversely (Pfannensteil) or midline. Adequate bowel preparation along with Foley catheter insertion and complete relaxation of the patient by the anesthesiologist facilitates the exposure. A transverse incision furnishes a superior cosmetic result with more than adequate exposure at the L4 to S1 area, and that is the one we prefer. Following the transverse incision, the rectus muscles may be divided transversely as well, and after the peritoneum is entered and the bowel is packed out of the field, the retroperitoneum from the level of the aorta and vena cava bifurcation distally is injected with epinephrine solution (concentration 1:500,000). The retroperitoneum is then incised along the midline, above the bifurcation of the great vessels caudally, along the right common iliac artery. Cautery should be limited. The middle sacral artery and vein are ligated. The presacral plexus should be displaced bluntly to the left side to avoid damaging the nerve supply to the bowel, bladder, and genitalia.[47, 68]

Costotransversectomy Approach

The costotransversectomy approach to the spine may prove particularly useful for limited biopsy of tumors, drainage of abscesses, or for more extensive debridement and anterior decompression.[26] For a limited exposure for biopsy, a paravertebral incision can be made over the side of the spinous process and over the laminal plate of the affected vertebra. By exposing the transverse process and performing a transverse osteotomy at the base of the transverse process a biopsy of the vertebral body directly through the pedicle can be done, or after exposure of the junction of the pedicle with the vertebral body, a trephine may be used to penetrate the junction at a 45 degree angle toward the centrum of the vertebral body. This approach was first described by Michelle and Krueger[86] and is most useful for an extrapleural vertebral body biopsy. For more extensive exposure, which is necessary for decompression, the Hyndman-Schneider exposure[66] is most useful.

ANTERIOR FUSION

An anterior arthrodesis may either be accomplished by an interbody technique, an inlay strut fusion technique, or an anterior strut fusion technique.[17, 21, 24, 63, 127] Each of these procedures has a place and a use, depending upon the magnitude of the deformity and the preference of the surgeon. In general, the interbody technique is most useful for moderate degrees of kyphosis (less

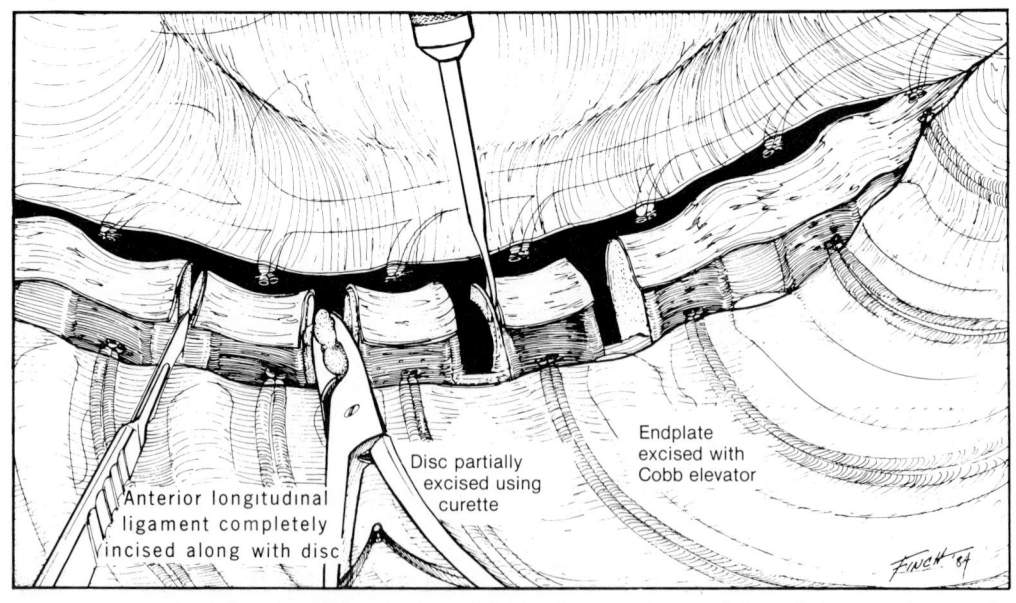

Figure 10–26. Anterior interbody fusion is accomplished by complete excision of the anterior longitudinal ligament along with removal of the disc. The disc is removed to the posterior annulus, and the intervening cartilage is removed to the bony endplates. If correction of the kyphosis is necessary, one should remove the posterior annulus along with the endplates up to the posterior longitudinal ligament. Generally, however, this will not be essential, since removal of the disc material up to the posterior annulus will make it possible to hinge open the kyphosis and significantly correct the angular deformity.

TECHNIQUES OF SURGERY 167

than 80 degrees) in which a substantial correction is possible and a second stage posterior arthrodesis is contemplated.

Interbody Technique

Following exposure of the spine, as previously outlined, it is often desirable to expose the anulus from the edge of one intervertebral foramen around anteriorly to the opposite foramina. Disc removal is done in two stages (Fig. 10–26). The outer fibers of the anulus are first dissected out sharply with a scalpel and the remaining anulus with a portion of the nucleus is removed with double action rongeurs. The cartilage endplates are then elevated off the vertebral body with a sharp periosteal elevator; then this cartilage plate, along with attached remaining anulus, is removed with a rongeur. Angle curettes and thin osteotomes are useful in removing the remaining portion of the posterior anulus along with the cartilage endplates from the posterior longitudinal ligament. It is desirable to remove all anular material back to the posterior ligament for correction of kyphosis, whereas in scoliosis correction the opposite outer fibers of the anulus may be left intact, functioning as a hinge, since a closing wedge osteotomy will not require the convex anulus removal. Hemostasis is facilitated with the use of Gelfoam soaked in thrombin solution or topical collagen. The rib that has been removed for the thoracotomy is cut into small pieces, which are then wedged into the anterior portion of the inner space to achieve partial correction of the kyphosis (Fig. 10–27). The remaining portions of the rib are cut into small match sticks. A trough is then cut approximately 1 cm. in width along the lateral aspect of the vertebral bodies and deepened at least one-half way through the vertebral body at each level. The cancellous bone

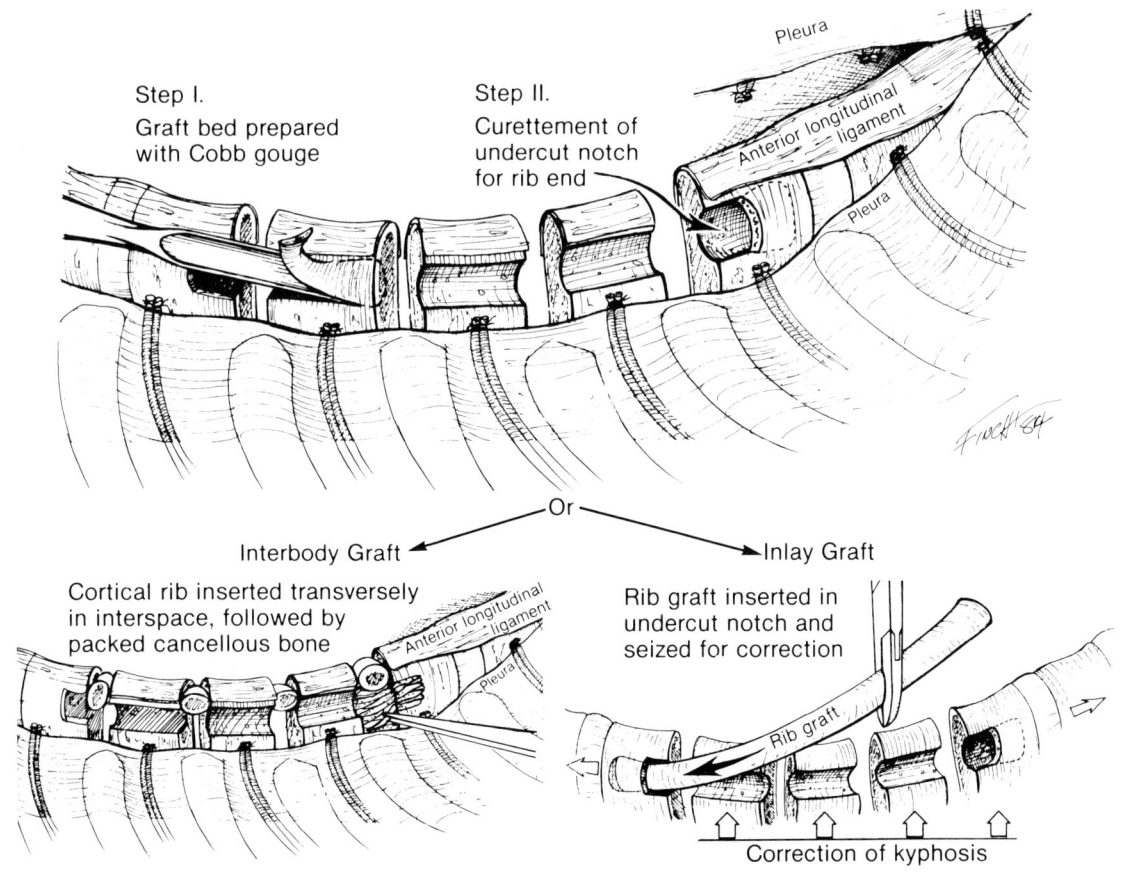

Figure 10–27. Technique of vertebral body preparation for either an interbody graft or an inlay graft. After the trough has been cut, the disc space is wedged open anteriorly with the rib bone for the interbody graft. The bone chips are packed loosely in the trough. If an inlay graft is used, the rib may be inserted as shown.

Strut Graft Technique—Part 1

Step I.
Intercostal arteries and veins ligated and divided

Step II.
Incise reflected pleura and intercostal vessels

Aorta

Azygos v.

Step III.
Elevate anterior longitudinal ligament and periosteum

Step IV.
Excise discs

A

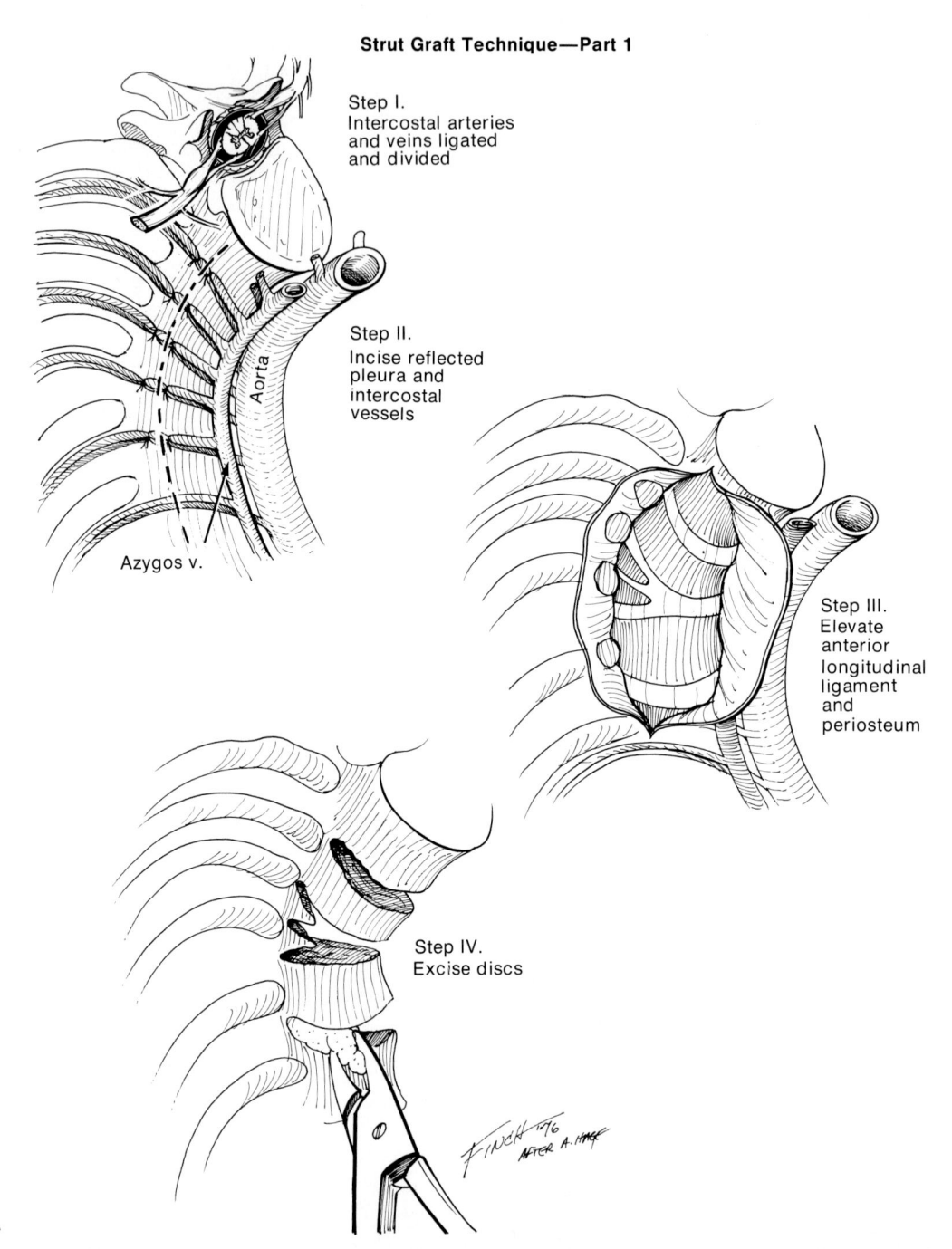

Figure 10–28. Anterior strut fusion. A, The length of the strut graft depends upon the severity of the kyphotic deformity. In general, the strut should extend from the end vertebra above to the end vertebra below the structural part of the kyphosis and lie in the weight-bearing line of the spine if possible. The most common error is placement of grafts between the apical two or three vertebrae only. Progression of the deformity is then possible as a result of an anterior fusion that is too short. After the vessels are ligated as previously described, the periosteum with the anterior longitudinal ligament is elevated as a single flap of tissue.

Illustration continued on opposite page

TECHNIQUES OF SURGERY

Strut Graft Technique—Part 2

Step V. Curettement of notches for strut graft insertion

Step VI. Strut inserted superiorly as kyphosis correction is made

Step VII. Strut graft 1 is inserted

Step VIII. Two additional strut grafts are inserted in a similar manner, with increase in kyphosis correction

Step IX. Interspaces packed with cancellous "matchstick" bone

Step X. Rib strut graft wedged in slots

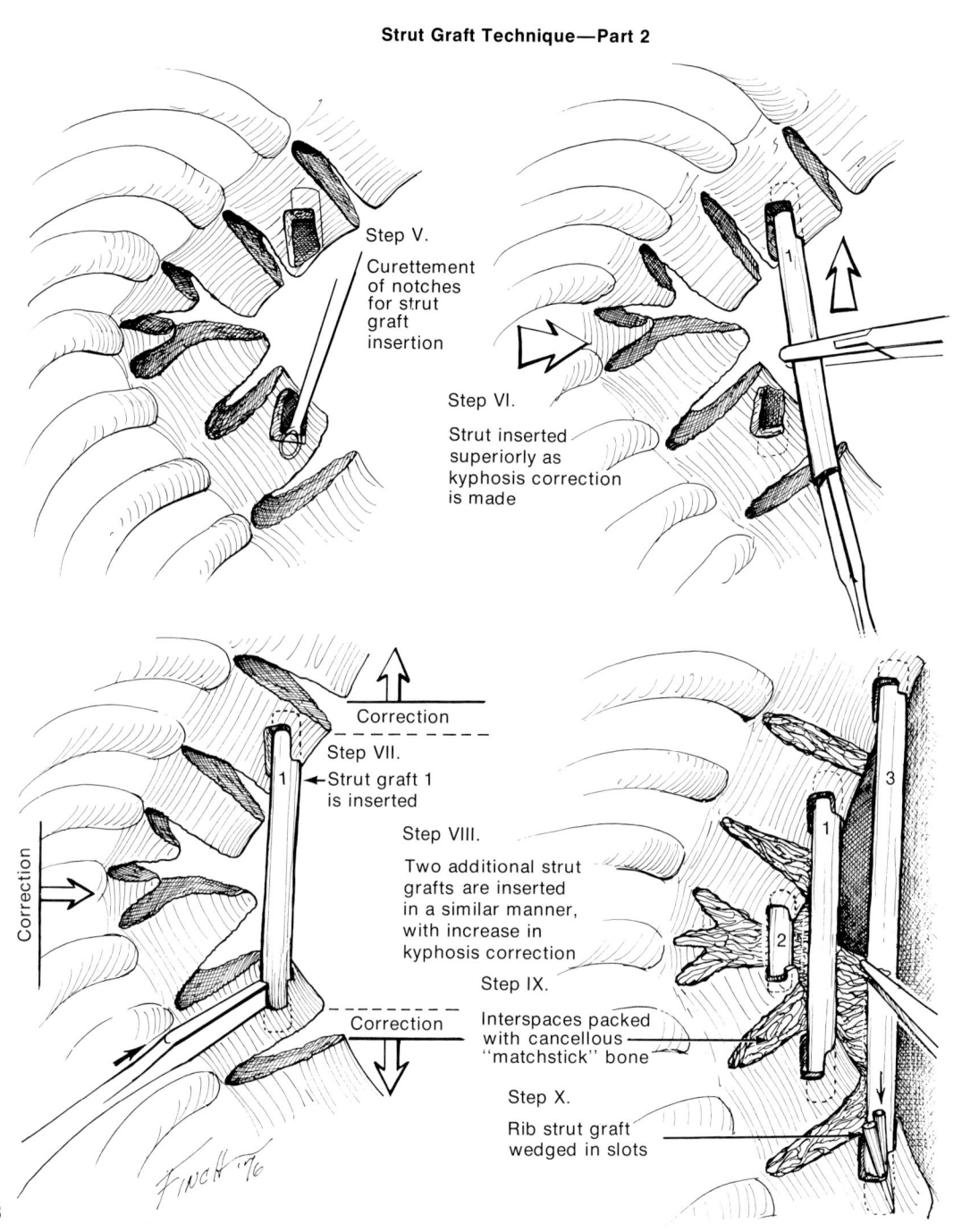

Figure 10–28 *Continued. B,* The intervertebral discs are removed as previously described, and a tunnel is carved into the anterior body of the end vertebra below and above the apex of the curvature. Rib or fibula or even iliac strut is then cut to the appropriate length and wedged into place, applying a force over the apex of the curve as well as longitudinal traction on the head. Additional strut graft can then be inserted as outlined, and cancellous and remaining rib bone may then be inserted in each intervertebral disc space and on top of the periosteum between the strut graft and anterior cortex of the vertebral bodies. No attempt is made to reattach the periosteum.

that is removed is cut into small pieces and mixed with the match stick pieces of rib bone. Hemostasis is, again, secured with thrombin-soaked Gelfoam. This bone is packed into the inner space and into the trough. This assures a more rapid arthrodesis with early incorporation of bone grafts. If additional bone is necessary, cancellous and cortical bone can be taken from the iliac crest. The parietal pleura is now sutured over the vertebral bodies, separating the dissection from the pleural cavity.

It should be stressed that all cartilage from the vertebral bodies should be removed during the dissection, especially in children. If an anterior strut fusion is carried out in the presence of residual cartilage in a growing child, progressive deformity will occur since in effect a type II congenital kyphosis has been produced.

Inlay Strut Fusion (see Fig. 10–27)

When a major portion of a vertebral body has been removed, an inlay strut fusion graft is desirable to support the adjoining vertebral bodies and to prevent collapse into kyphus, and at the same time to achieve satisfactory spinal stability. Exposure proceeds as described previously. Again a trough is cut out, but the trough at this time is packed with one, two, or even three rib strut grafts that act as supporting bone. It is important to undercut each trough back to the edge of the subchondral bone. The surgical assistant may facilitate graft placement by forcefully pushing on the apex of the kyphus while the anesthesiologist pulls gently on the head, correcting the deformity as the surgeon keys the graft into place. The remaining portion of rib bone may be cut into small pieces and wedged around the edges of the strut graft, further locking the graft into position. A fibular graft may be used in place of the rib for support and again, iliac bone graft may be necessary to provide additional cancellous bone. If total vertebrectomy has been done, additional support may be furnished by fashioning a femoral head allograft using the calcar portion as a spacer. A trough then may be cut into the allograft along with the adjoining vertebral bodies into which can be positioned a fibular, a rib, or a vascularized rib graft (see Anterior Vascularized Rib Grafting).

Anterior Strut Fusion (Fig. 10–28)

In the presence of an angular structural kyphosis, where a radical resection and total correction is not deemed indicated, it may be necessary to place the supporting strut grafts anterior to the vertebral bodies in order to achieve maximum stability.[23, 30, 35, 54, 107, 109, 110, 112] The length of the arthrodesis and the strut graft depends on the severity of the kyphotic deformity. In general, the graft should extend from end vertebra to end vertebra of the structural part of the kyphosis and lay in the weight-bearing axis of the body if possible. The most common technical mistake is placement of the graft between the apical two or three vertebra; progression of the deformity proximally or distally to the fusion with graft failure and pseudarthrosis is the possible result. If there is associated scoliosis, it is desirable that the graft lie on the concave side of the curvature. If the scoliosis is greater than 40 degrees, it is much easier to approach the spine on the convex side away from the great vessels, although it should be recognized that the graft will, by necessity, lie somewhat out of the weight-bearing axis of the spine.

After the vertebral bodies are visualized, a subperiosteal rather than an extraperiosteal exposure for this procedure is preferable, since bone grafts must be placed between the vertebral bodies and the anterior strut graft. The intervertebral discs are removed as previously described. A tunnel, approximately 1 to 2 cm. in length, is then cut into the anterior body of the end vertebra above, as well as the end vertebra below the apex of the kyphus. A rib or a fibular strut is then cut to the appropriate length. The fibula may provide greater strength than rib, and therefore, it may be preferable particularly in severe kyphosis. The strut graft is then keyed into the vertebral bodies after the anesthesiologist has pulled on the head and the assistant has placed pressure over the apex of the kyphus. A temporary or permanent distractor[51, 96, 106] may be positioned, providing partial correction of the deformity and facilitating strut graft placement. After the graft is in place, the temporary implant may be removed. The anterior surfaces of the vertebral bodies that face the bone graft may be further curetted of all soft tissue debris that remains after the subperiosteal dissection. The intervening space between the vertebral bodies and the strut graft is then packed with cancellous or rib bone. The elevated periosteum lying deep to the strut graft acts as a protective wall, preventing the chips of additional bone from falling free into the thorax and acting as a source of osteogenesis.

Usually, two or more strut grafts are inserted, depending on the severity and the length of the kyphosis. No attempt is made to reattach the periosteum. Gelfoam may be placed over the lateral aspects of the graft at the completion of the procedure to prevent small bone chips from dislodging. Provided the strut is well keyed into place, no problem results from the graft lying against lung tissue.

A more rapid revascularization may be possible by using the Stagnara technique of raising an osteoperiosteal flap with a sharp osteotome prior to the removal of the intervertebral disc.[108, 109] With strut grafts that are positioned only 2 to 3 cm. anterior to the vertebral bodies, this may be helpful. With strut grafts positioned more anterior to the apical vertebral bodies, the cancellous periosteal flap will not reach the strut graft.

ANTERIOR OSTEOTOMY (Fig. 10–29)

An osteotomy from an anterior approach may be carried out with minimal difficulty provided circumferential exposure to the opposite foramen is carried out prior to beginning the osteotomy. In a type II congenital kyphosis, for example, a bony bar may be present at the most anterior portion of the vertebral body. Here disc material is absent anteriorly but is present laterally and posteriorly. It is relatively easy to remove the bony bar anterior to the disc, completely excising the disc space using appropriate shaped gouges, rongeurs, and curettes. An anterior fusion, as previously described, is then performed. Occasionally, the bony ridge may be complete all the way back to the posterior longitudinal ligament. In these cases it may be easier to do the osteotomy using a high speed drill. As one approaches the posterior cortical shell the transection between cancellous and cortical bone is easily visualized. A Blount spreader or laminectomy type spreader placed between the two vertebral bodies at that point will complete the osteotomy, fracturing the posterior cortex and allowing the vertebral bodies to open anteriorly like clam shells. Angle curettes and angle rongeurs are particularly useful for completing the osteotomy.

ANTERIOR CORD DECOMPRESSION
(Fig. 10–30)

Decompression of the spinal cord anteriorly is not an unduly difficult procedure provided that the exposure is adequate and the surgeon experienced with the anterior approach.[17, 75] Decompression may be carried out posteriorly as previously outlined by the Hyndman-Schneider procedure[66] via the pedicle,[86] or the Capener approach[26] as modified and nicely described by Bohlman.[13] This approach may be particularly useful in patients with traumatic paraplegia, but in the presence of a kyphus that requires longer strut grafts with greater exposure, an anterior transthoracic or the anterior thoracoabdominal approach would be preferable.[19] It is appreciated that in those cases with severe vertebral body rotation and angulation, cord impingement may be secondary to pressure from the pedicle and the head of the rib on the concave side of the curve. This situation may occur in patients with neurofibromatosis. In such cases, decompression may still proceed anteriorly followed by fusion, and then completion of the decompression during the second stage posterior approach by the Hyndman-Schneider method.[66]

Following a thoracotomy or a thoracoabdominal incision, the apical vertebra or the site of the compression is identified and the intervertebral disc on each side of the vertebral body or the vertebral bodies in question is completely removed back to the posterior longitudinal ligament. It is much easier to do a vertebrectomy after the discs are removed than before the discs are removed. The vertebral body between the excised disc is then rongeured away with double action large tooth rongeurs, removing the major part of the vertebral body and leaving only a thin cortical cancellous rim of the opposite lateral cortex. A high speed air drill is particularly useful in completing the exposure. With the use of the drill it is possible to safely remove all of the cancellous bone back to the posterior cortex of the vertebral body from pedicle to pedicle, leaving this thin rim comparable to an egg shell. After the cancellous bone has been removed bleeding is rarely a problem. Beginning on the far lateral side, the posterior cortical shell of bone is pryed away using

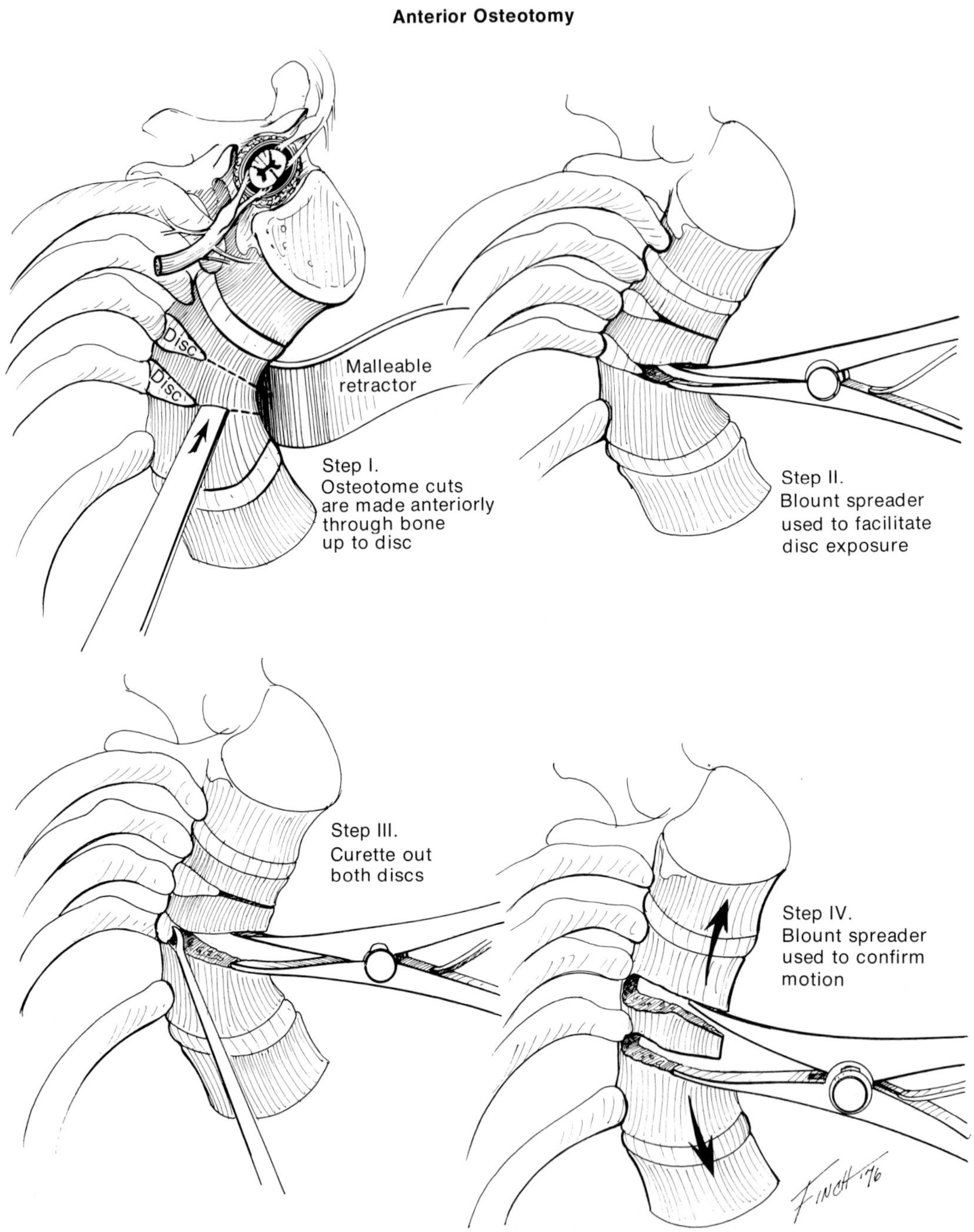
Anterior Osteotomy
Disc
Disc
Malleable retractor
Step I.
Osteotome cuts are made anteriorly through bone up to disc
Step II.
Blount spreader used to facilitate disc exposure
Step III.
Curette out both discs
Step IV.
Blount spreader used to confirm motion
FINCH '76

Figure 10–29. The technique for anterior osteotomy. In Type II congenital kyphosis, as noted, a bony bar may be present in the most anterior portion of the vertebral body. The bony bar is removed, using a sharp osteotome, beginning anteriorly and working posteriorly until the remaining disc material is entered. A Blount spreader may facilitate exposure, making it possible to completely remove the disc material back to the posterior longitudinal ligament. If the bony bridge is complete to the posterior longitudinal ligament, osteotomy must be complete through the posterior cortex. By use of the Blount spreader, the posterior cortex remaining may be fractured, allowing the vertebral bodies to open anteriorly, like a clamshell.

TECHNIQUES OF SURGERY

Anterior Cord Decompression

Step I. Trough cut through bodies and discs laterally at apex of kyphosis, using gouge and curette

Apex of kyphosis

Step I

Steps II and III. Curette posterior sheet of bone and remove discs

Step II

Cord

Step III

allows for anterior cord displacement

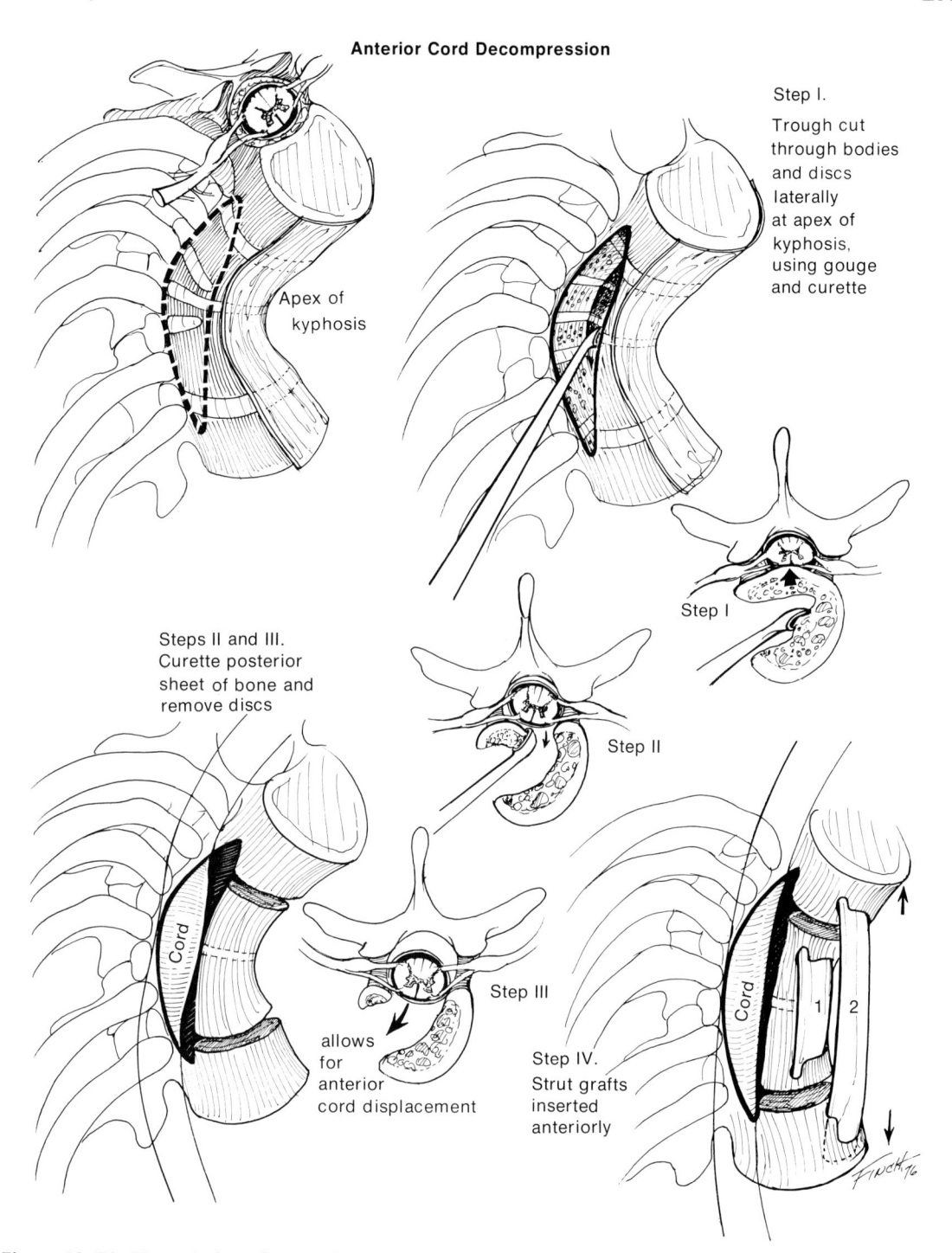

Step IV. Strut grafts inserted anteriorly

Cord

Figure 10–30. The technique for anterior cord decompression. The exposure should be on the concave side of the curvature for mild degrees of scoliosis, less than 20 to 25 degrees. For more severe degrees of scoliosis the spine should be approached on the convexity. The trough is cut into the vertebral bodies, using either a gouge or a highspeed burr. Cancellous bone is removed down to the posterior cortical shell, which is fractured first from the far side of the field, using a reverse angle curette. The thin cortical shell is then removed on the proximal side, using angled curettes, starting first away from the apex of the kyphosis and then working toward the center. It will become apparent that the dura begins to move anteriorly into the space thus created. This may make exposure difficult, and it may be prevented by beginning the decompression as noted from the far side of the field and away from the apex of the deformity, working finally toward the apex. The procedure is completed by anterior strut graft fusion.

a sharp reverse angle curette. By proceeding in this fashion and maintaining the cortical shell on the proximal anterior and lateral side, the more difficult portion of bone removal proceeds first before the spinal cord falls into the bony cavity thus created. Regular angle curettes will then facilitate removal of the proximal posterior-lateral shell of bone, working toward the apex. The posterior longitudinal ligament is removed routinely during this procedure if there is any question that it prevents adequate decompression. Removal of portions of the vertebra above and below the apex may be necessary if the angulation is acute. Epidural bleeding is sometimes troublesome, but it may be controlled with thrombin-soaked Gelfoam or topical collagen solution. When doing this decompression, the author prefers to use hypotensive anesthesia, maintaining a mean arterial pressure of 65 mm. of mercury. Even in the presence of an incomplete neurologic deficit, effective blood flow to the cord has not been clinically compromised and no patients have lost neurologic function with this technique to date. Blood loss has been minimized.

After the decompression has been completed, strut grafts are then placed across the spine at the site of decompression and anteriorly if a greater distance of fusion is indicated. Large fat grafts taken from the retroperitoneal area are placed loosely over the dura to prevent excessive scarring postoperatively. The fusion is completed as previously described, and the chest cavity is closed and drained in a customary fashion.

VERTEBRAL BODY RESECTION

Vertebral body resection was first described by MacLennan in 1922.[81] Since this time several authors have described resection with varying results.[14, 27, 64, 71, 72, 84, 99, 104, 105, 115, 117, 122, 123] In our experience at the Twin Cities Scoliosis Center a two-stage hemivertebra excision and fusion has given the best results. The first stage is carried out through a transthoracic or retroperitoneal approach, removing first the intervertebral disc on each side of the hemivertebra, and then removing the vertebra completely as described for anterior cord decompression. The pedicle is removed as completely as possible through the anterior approach, back to its junction with the posterior neural arch. It is important that complete anterior excision is carried out, otherwise, a compromised result is preordained. The posterior procedure may be carried out at the same sitting after repreparing and draping and repositioning the patient, or as a separate procedure one to two weeks later. At the second stage the portion of the remaining arch is completely removed and posterior instrumentation if feasible is done to complete the correction. In very young children in whom this is not possible, lateral bending correction and postoperative casting are necessary. It is important to state again that anterior arthrodesis is essential and the cartilage must be completely removed from the adjoining endplates in order that fusion may occur. Cancellous bone may be packed loosely into the interspace during the anterior procedure, and the cord may be protected with a fat graft. It is also possible to cut a slot into the vertebra above and below the resected segment and lay in loosely a rib graft, which is shorter than the slot. Following the posterior procedure and correction of the deformity, the vertebral bodies may angulate to a corrected position as the rib strut remains in place.

ANTERIOR INSTRUMENTATION

Anterior metallic implants have proven useful in the correction or stabilization of spinal deformity. Compression implants, as described first by Dwyer[43] and more recently by Zielke[48, 55, 129] have proven particularly valuable in the management of scoliosis. Newer types of distraction implants, as described by Slot,[106] Zielke,[129] and Dunn[40] to mention a few, demonstrate that anterior instrumentation of the spine has a definite role not only in the correction and stabilization of scoliosis but also in the management of kyphosis.

With the advent of Zielke instrumentation, we have all but given up use of the Dwyer implant. The disadvantages of the Dwyer implant include inability to modulate the correction at each segmental level, a high incidence of post-instrumentation kyphosis, and a greater degree of difficulty in achieving spinal derotation.[45] The Zielke implant with a flexible rod system, a derotating bar, and threaded nuts at each screw site has overcome many of the disadvantages of the Dwyer system. In the use of all anterior implants care must be taken to ensure that the vascular structures do not lie on the

TECHNIQUES OF SURGERY

implant, otherwise vessel rupture may subsequently develop.[38, 44]

The selection of vertebral levels to be instrumented for the anterior compression system of Zielke is based on the configuration of the intervertebral disc spaces and the degree of vertebral body translation on the standing AP x-ray. We have found as a general rule that all vertebral bodies adjacent to the intervertebral interspaces that are wedged open into the convexity of the curve should be instrumented.[90] It may be possible to shorten the instrumented levels and include only those discs and attached vertebra that remain wedged on side bend x-rays. If a vertebral body has a rotatory translation, that is a lateral spondylolisthesis of greater than 0.5 cm. from the subadjacent vertebra, we feel likewise it should be instrumented. Finally, as a rule of thumb, one may anticipate that approximately 15 degrees of correction is possible at each instrumented level and this may prove an aid in calculating the desired correction (Fig. 10–31).

Disc removal proceeds according to the technique as previously described. A sharp periosteal elevator is used to facilitate cartilage removal from the endplates, and the cartilage along with the remaining nucleus and anulus is removed back to the posterior longitudinal ligament. The opposite outer fibers of the anulus, that is the concave side, may be left intact. This may act as a hinge and prevent overcorrection of the spine. Calipers may be used to assess the transverse diameter of the vertebral body, and an awl is used to make a hole in the side of the vertebral body at its midlateral portion. The Zielke screw of the appropriate length with an attached staple is inserted across the midportion of the vertebral body (Fig. 10–32). The flange of the staple used on the end vertebrae should not penetrate into the normal intervertebral disc space above but only into the vertebral body. The screw is inserted through the hole in the staple and rotated firmly until it has just engaged the opposite cortex, which is felt with the index finger. If stability is questioned, that is the screw appears to cut through the cancellous bone, then the screw is removed, the hole is irrigated with antibiotic solution, liquid methylmethacrylate is injected into the hole and allowed to partially set up, and the screw is reinserted. This provides increased implant-bone contact and lessens the likelihood of screw cut out.[41] As the instrumented spine is approached at each level more distally, the more distal screw sites should be placed more posteriorly in the vertebral body. This lessens

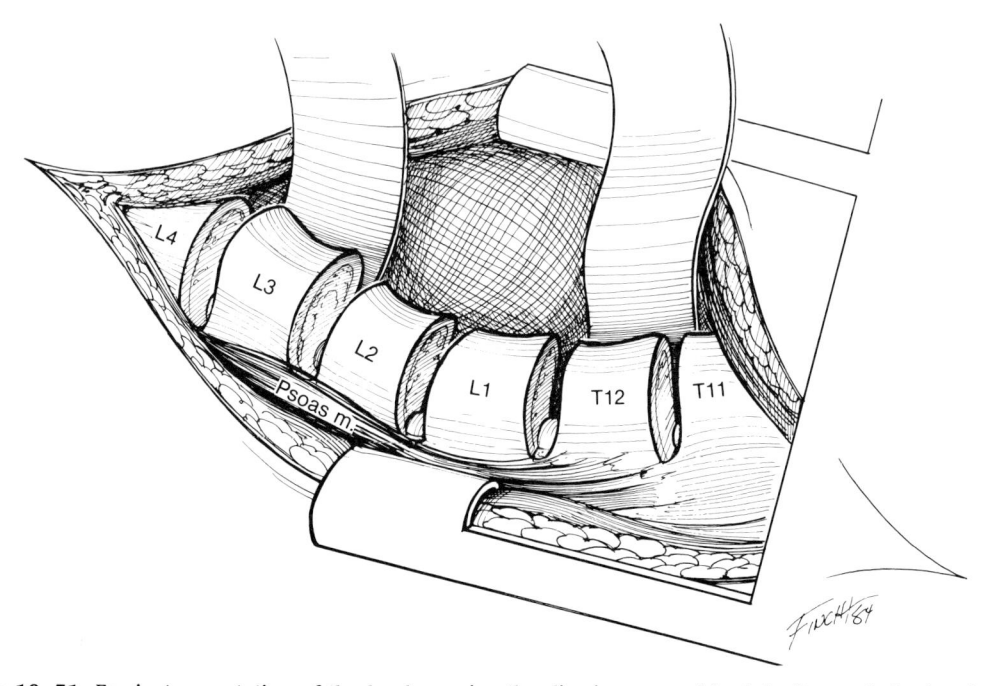

Figure 10–31. For instrumentation of the lumbar spine the disc is removed back to the posterior longitudinal ligament, completely removing cartilaginous endplates. The annulus on the concavity may be left intact.

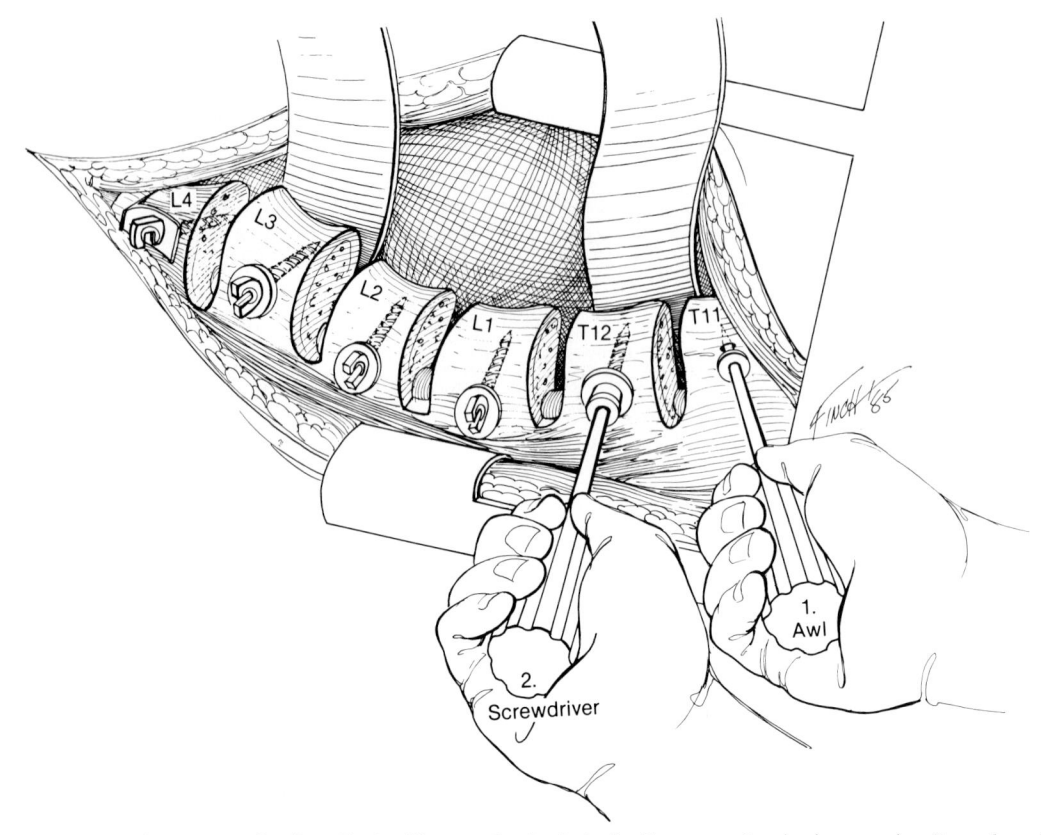

Figure 10–32. Zielke screw fixation. First, with an awl cut a hole for the screw, beginning proximally and working distally. It is important to assure bicortical fixation at each level and to assure that the screws are properly directed to prevent canal penetration. Finally, the end screws lie in the mid-lateral portion of the vertebral bodies, whereas the apical screw lies more to the posterior-lateral edge. This arrangement will facilitate derotation and the production of lumbar lordosis (see text).

the tendency for postinstrumentation kyphosis and facilitates greater derotation and correction of deformity. The screws should be directed in a slight posterior to anterior direction across the midportion of the vertebral body likewise to enhance the derotation effect. Each screw should penetrate the opposite cortex for maximum fixation. The most proximal and distal screws should be inserted approximately 1 cm. more anteriorly than the apical screws, forming a general C-shaped curve when viewed laterally. As the spine is derotated the rod will assume a straight position and as described, facilitate greater derotation in the process. At the more distal screw insertion, a flange may again be used. If hyperlordosis is present, the screws may be directed more in an anterior-posterior plane.

Following insertion of the screws, a flexible stainless steel threaded rod of appropriate length is inserted into the notches of each screwhead. The most proximal and distal screws should be side-opening, whereas the middle screws between the extremes should be top-opening. The most proximal and distal screws should have double nuts, one facing the other, whereas the intervening screws need only have one locking nut facing the apex of the deformity. After the rod is engaged, the derotator is applied, using the handle device for leverage (Fig. 10–33). The spine is derotated toward a more anatomic position. This produces a lordosis. At this stage, the rib is then cut into 1 to 2 cm. pieces and wedged anteriorly between each vertebral body at its most anterior lip. This prevents instrumentation kyphosis, and facilitates the production of a lumbar lordosis. The vertebral endplates may then be roughened up at this point with a sharp curette or a thin osteotome. The remaining portions of rib bone are then cut into very small pieces and packed loosely into the intervertebral

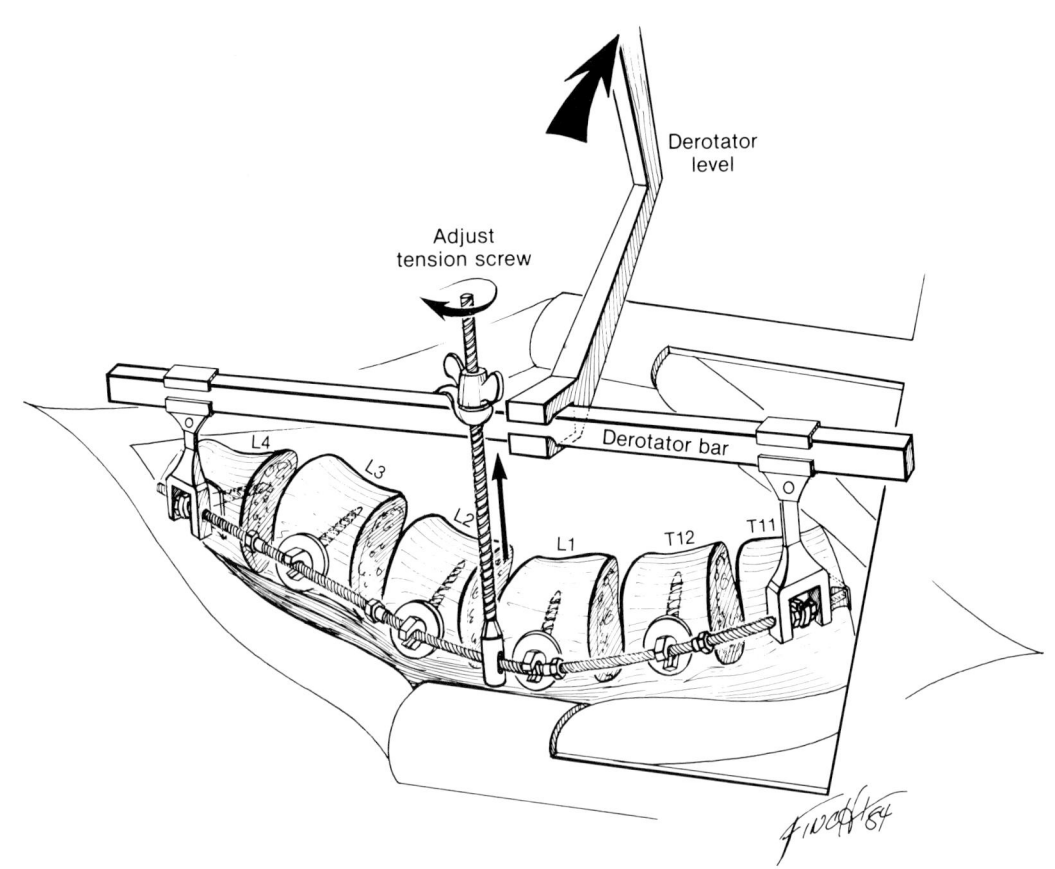

Figure 10-33. The application of the derotating bar and outrigger. Tension is directed to the compression rod system by exerting a force on the derotator lever; derotation of the apical vertebra occurs, with the disc spaces opening anteriorly. Bone grafts may then be placed between the vertebral bodies anteriorly, maintaining the lordosis.

disc spaces to insure complete bone to bone contact. With the spine held in the derotated position, the locking nuts are sequentially tightened, approximating the vertebral bodies and correcting the curve (Fig. 10–34). Total correction is possible with this technique, provided close attention to detail is followed. The weak link of the chain, so to speak, is that interspace of the most cephalad instrumented level. To prevent screw pullout at this point, Zielke has advocated only a blocked fusion across the disc space without total disc excision.

To prevent the lock nuts from unwinding, the threads of the compression rod may be destroyed with a mallet and impactor. The vertebral tissues are reapproximated over the instrumentation, and reattachment of the diaphragm and wound closure is performed in a routine fashion.

With Zielke instrumentation it is possible to reach L4 without difficulty, L5 with some difficulty, and sacrum never. It is important to stress that with this implant as well as other anterior implants, the ultimate success is only as good as the arthrodesis. All implants will eventually fail if complete removal of soft tissue and adequate arthrodesis is not carried out. To facilitate anterior fusion, it has proven useful to peel back the anterior periosteum and the anterior longitudinal ligament from the margin of the vertebral endplate approximately 1.5 cm. to ensure no soft tissue interposition between rims of the vertebral bodies.

SPECIAL TECHNIQUES

Posterior Instrumentation Without Fusion

Internal fixation without fusion was first described by Harrington in 1962.[57] This technique failed because partial fusion resulted from subperiosteal exposure of the spine and

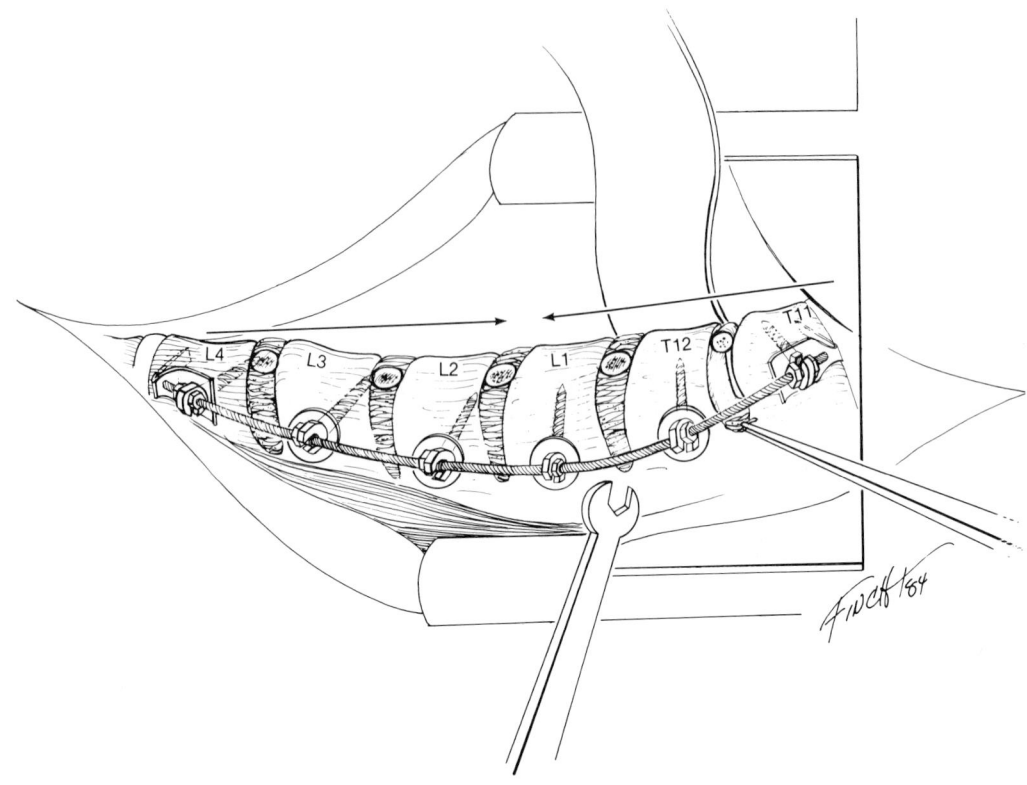

Figure 10–34. A single set of nuts is secured on each side of the screwhead, working from the apex to each end of the instrumented spine, aggressively correcting the scoliosis. More bone chips may be placed into the interspace as the vertebral bodies are pulled together. A double set of nuts is placed on each side of the screwheads of the end vertebra to prevent slippage.

the lack of postoperative external support, which led to hook dislocation and rod breakage. In a subsequent report by Marchetti and Valdini in 1977,[83] instrumentation without fusion was again recommended. Subsequent reports by other authors have suggested that this technique may be useful in the young patient, under ten years of age, with more severe deformities not amenable to brace treatment, and in whom early arthrodesis will result in significant trunk shortening.[89]

For this technique to be most successful it appears desirable to perform dissection only down to the lamina and spinous processes on the concave side of the curvature at the precise levels to be instrumented. Subperiosteal exposure to the remainder of the spine on the concave as well as the convex side of the curvature is best avoided. Pediatric size hooks may be necessary in the very small child. The hooks are applied in a routine fashion, and distraction is carried out with a wake-up test being performed. Postoperatively the patient is maintained in an orthosis. At four to six month intervals or if the curvature has lost more than 10 degrees of correction, the rod should be lengthened over a small incision at the site of the upper hook if a distraction implant is used, or over either the upper or the lower hook if a Harrington compression rod has been used as a distracting implant. At the time of initial surgery if the bone and lamina appear to be deficient, a localized fusion may be performed around the placed hooks and instrumentation carried out two to three months later. Methacrylate may be used to facilitate better hook fixation.[118] If the bone is less precarious, a localized fusion may be carried out along with rod placement at the initial procedure. At the time the patient reaches the pre-adolescent growth spurt, surgical arthrodesis is carried out.

In the experience reported at our Center the average gain over the instrumented area in nine patients who ultimately underwent surgical arthrodesis is 3.8 cm.[89] Complications, however, were frequent, with hook dislocation and rod breakage being the most common. This technique appears to be particularly useful in the management of neuromuscular curves not controlled by an orthosis or in congenital scoliosis secondary to hemivertebra where combined anterior and posterior hemiepiphysiodesis is planned.[18]

Luque and Cardoso[79] have also used this technique with segmental posterior instrumentation. It has remained our concern that segmental instrumentation in a young child will often be associated with spontaneous fusion because of the subperiosteal stripping that is necessary with this technique. Furthermore, fusion at a later time is certainly more difficult.

Anterior Vascularized Rib Grafting

Anterior strut grafting with either rib grafts or fibular grafts may provide excellent support. It is known however that the rib or fibula placed anterior to the spine may take up to two years for replacement and that it is weakest at approximately six months postoperatively. In fact, we have found 50 per cent fracture during the process of bone consolidation and healing[23] in grafts placed greater than 4 cm. from the apical vertebral body. More rapid consolidation may be facilitated by the osteoperiosteal flap described by Stagnara.[110] A vascularized graft would solve this problem. This could be accomplished by a fibular strut graft with microvascular anastamosis towards the juxtaposed intercostal artery and vein. A much simpler procedure is a rib transfer on its neurovascular pedicle, avoiding microvascular anastomosis. This procedure was first described in a brief report by Rose and associates in 1975[101] and subsequently in more detail by Bradford in 1980.[16] At the time of this writing the author has performed this procedure on 43 patients with at least a one year followup. Graft fracturing during the healing phase has not occurred. Shaffer[103] has recently reported on the favorable flow gradient between rib to vertebral body no doubt accounting for the high success of this procedure.

The technique may be performed by removing the rib that may easily be maneuvered to span the kyphosis (Fig. 10–35). For a kyphosis with an apex from T2 to T5, one should remove the rib two or three segments below the apex, rotating the distal rib segment to the superior vertebral body to be fused. If the kyphosis is at an apex of T6 below, one can remove a rib two or three segments more proximal to the apex and rotate the distal segment to the distal vertebral body to be fused. After making a skin incision overlying the rib to be used for grafting, a cautery knife is then used to detach the intercostal muscle at its junction to the superior surface of the rib. The rib is then detached distally at its costochondral junction. The intercostal muscle is next divided on the inferior aspect of the rib, distally to proximally, leaving approximately 3 to 4 mm. of intercostal muscle attached to the rib. This assures that the intercostal vessels will not be damaged by the cautery. Once this dissection has proceeded to the angle of the rib, the chest retractors may be placed into the wound, allowing better exposure to the thorax and, hence, better identification of the intercostal vasculature. Just proximal to the angle of the rib, a subperiosteal dissection is done. The rib is divided, keeping the neurovascular pedicle intact. The pedicle may then be stripped carefully from the remaining proximal rib section and dissected back to the neural foramen. The remaining avascular segment of proximal rib is then detached and used for a second strut graft. One may continue dissection of the vessel, mobilizing the segment overlying the vertebral body by detaching the foramenal branch. It is usually not necessary to do this, however, as ample pedicle is available. The vasculature of the rib is confirmed by observing periosteal bleeding along its surface or by observing bleeding from the distally divided intercostal vessel. This vessel should be carefully ligated or troublesome oozing will continue after the completion of the procedure.

The rib may now be placed out of the way into the superior portion of the chest cavity while the vertebral bodies to be fused are identified, exposed, and prepared for strut grafting as previously described. The segmental vessels overlying the vertebra need not be divided, and the intervertebral discs need not be excised if an in situ fusion is planned and if the patient is skeletally mature. On the other hand, if the patient still has skeletal growth remaining and one wishes to mobilize each intervertebral disc space to obtain some correction of the kyphus, the segmental vessels overlying the vertebral bodies are ligated and the spine is prepared for an interbody fusion as previously noted. It is essential, however, that the segmental vessels supplying the intercostal vessels of the rib that have been mobilized

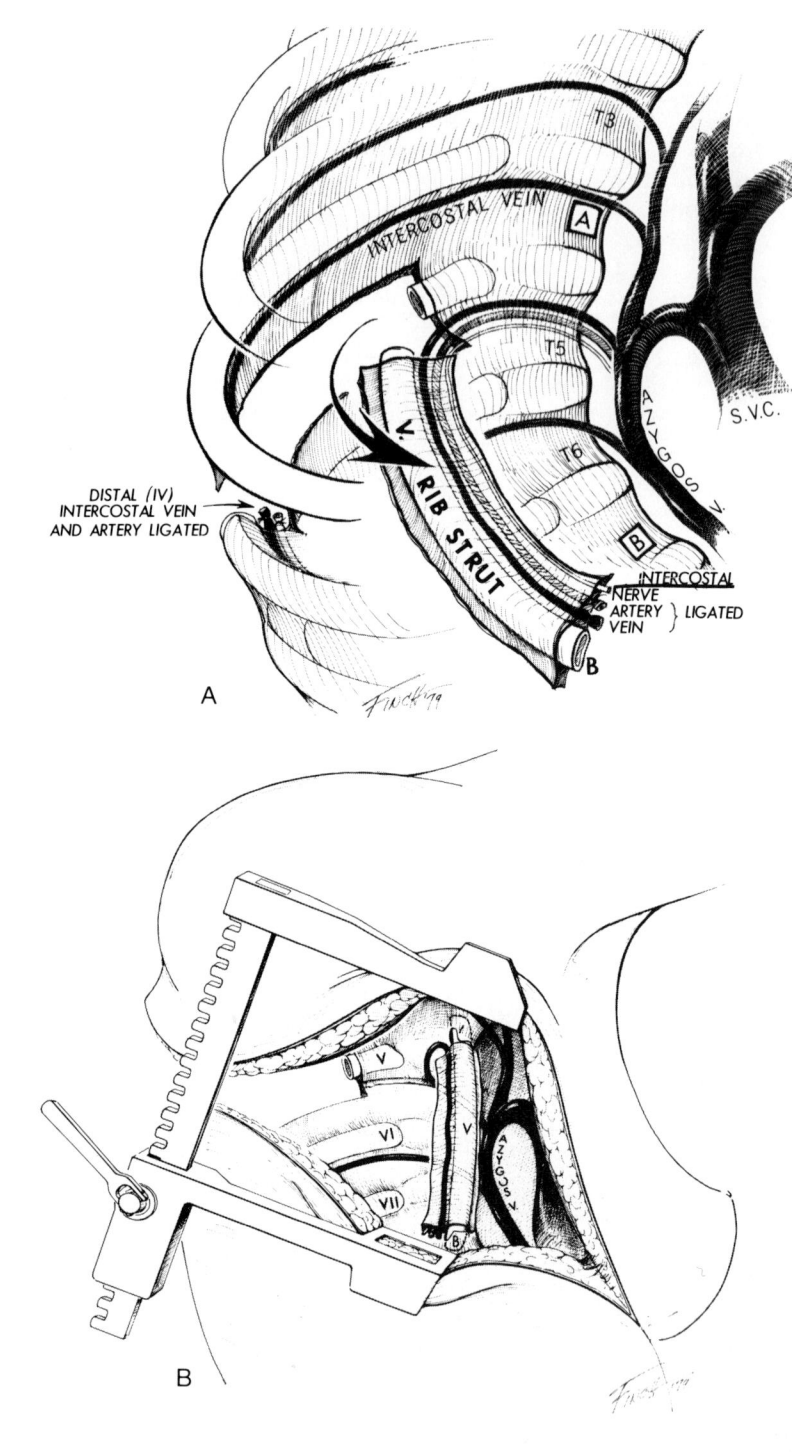

Figure 10–35. The technique of taking a rib from its neurovascular pedicle and using it as a vascularized graft is demonstrated. It is important that the distal artery and vein be ligated. Otherwise excessive bleeding will occur in the chest after wound closure.

for the vascularized strut not be violated or jeopardized. Prior to insertion of the strut graft, the soft tissue is peeled back approximately 1 cm. from each end of the rib. The distal intercostal vessel is divided again just proximal to the vascular cleft to double check for bleeding. Once the intact circulation is visualized, the distal vessel is again ligated and the strut graft is inserted in a routine fashion.

Postoperative management depends on the indications of the techniques of surgery. If surgery has been performed to correct a kyphus and interbody fusions have been done at each level, posterior arthrodesis with or without Harrington or segmental instrumentation may be carried out as a second stage. If, on the other hand, surgery has been carried out to stabilize a kyphus without attempt at correction, vascularized pedicle strut graft without interbody fusion should be sufficient (Fig. 10-36).[85] It should be stressed again that this latter alternative would be ill-advised in a child—progressive deformity may result since, in effect, a Type II "congenital" deformity has been produced. Immobilization for approximately 6 to 8 weeks in a body jacket made of polyproplene is all that is required for graft consolidation to the vertebral bodies.[20]

Management of Thoracic Lordosis[22]

The management of severe thoracic lordosis associated with scoliosis in the skeletally mature patient may pose a special problem. Treatment of scoliosis by Harrington rod instrumentation may partially correct the deformity and prevent its progression but will not lead to a normal kyphosis (Fig. 10-37). If the lordosis is of a congenital nature, the problem is not well managed by posterior surgery alone.[126] If an anterior fusion is extended above and below the deformity, improvement will occur with growth.[18] However, the production of normal kyphosis is not possible. Segmental sublaminar wiring with instrumentation according to the technique described by Luque or a modification using sublaminar wiring with a sagittally convex bent Harrington or L-rod can improve the lordosis in idiopathic cases and even lead to a minimal kyphus in young patients with minimal deformity. However, the results of this correction are inconsistent and a restoration to a normal kyphosis in a mature individual with more severe degrees of lordosis (-30 degrees) is unlikely. CD instrumentation is also helpful but rotation of the rod to correct the lordosis for fixed scoliosis curvatures >60 degrees in the adult is usually not feasible. Since partial correction of lordosis in patients with a decrease in vital capacity has been shown to often increase lung volumes,[126] attempts to

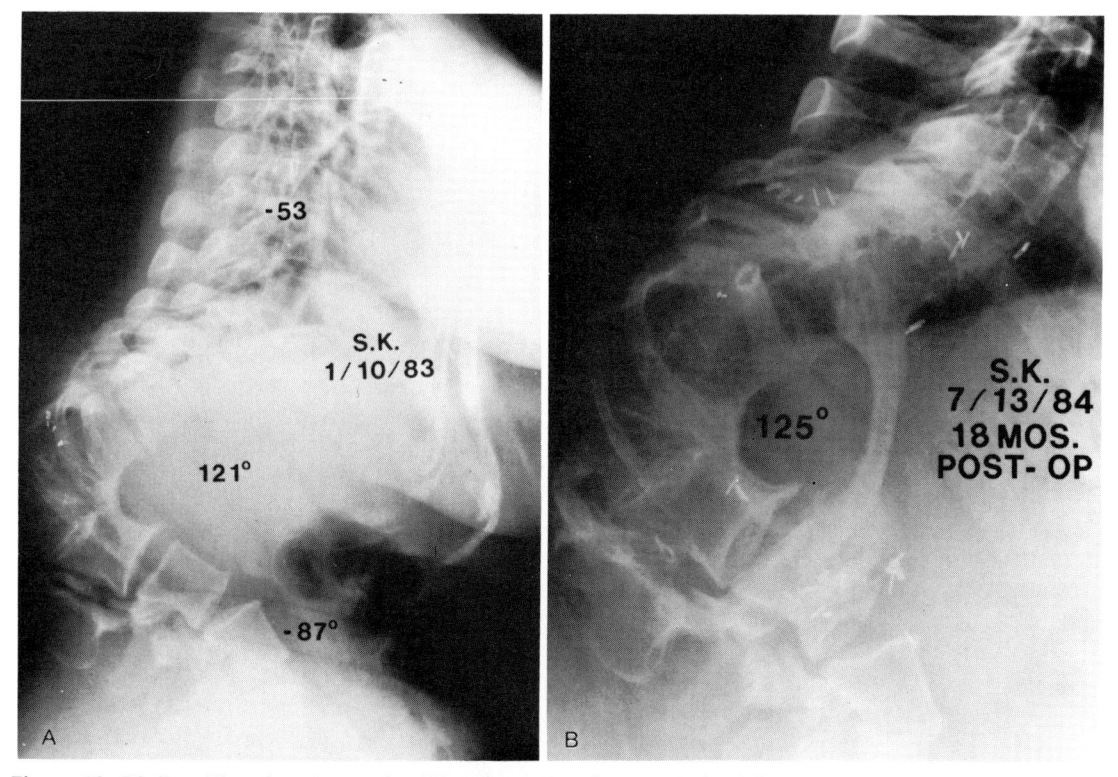

Figure 10-36. Pre- (A) and postoperative (B) radiographs of a vascularized rib graft used in treating a congenital kyphosis in a patient with achondroplasia. Fusion in situ was carried out without attempts at correction.

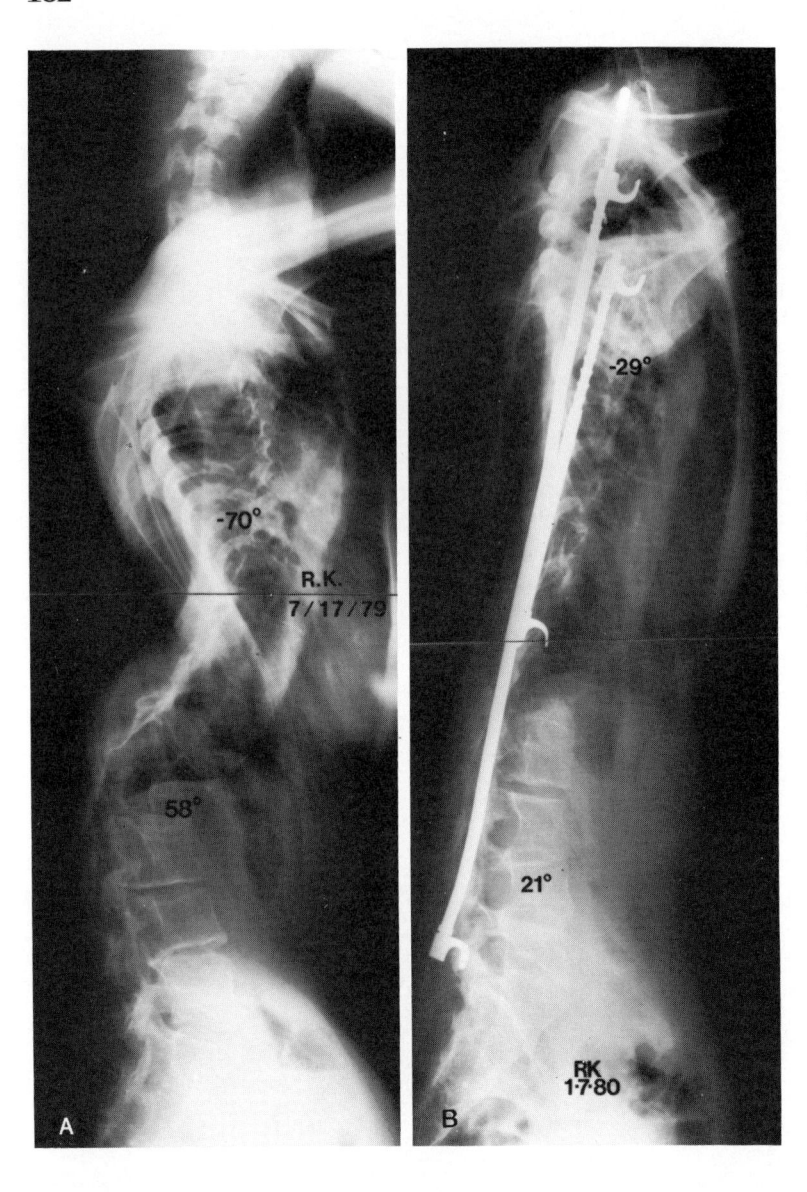

Figure 10–37. Pre- (A) and postoperative (B) lateral x-rays of a patient with severe thoracic lordosis and scoliosis. Note that with distraction, improvement of thoracic lordosis was possible but restoration to normal thoracic kyphosis was not.

correct the lordotic component of this deformity in patients with more severe degrees of pulmonary insufficiency may occasionally be indicated.

The surgical technique[22] is based on two principles (1) complete removal of the intervertebral discs through an anterior approach and performance of bilateral rib osteotomies at multiple levels over contiguous segments posteriorly, and (2) creation of a kyphosis by pulling the spine and the attached posterior rib cage to the pre-bent convex oriented distraction or L-rods (Fig. 10–38). Each vertebra is pulled to the rods by bilateral segmental sublaminar wires. The surgical correction is staged. The first stage includes a transthoracic approach to the convex side of the scoliotic curvature. The intervertebral disc is completely removed back to the posterior longitudinal ligament, which should be removed if it is tight and thickened. Anterior-based wedges are cut in the vertebral bodies at each disc level in order to facilitate correction of the lordosis during the posterior procedure. A trough is cut in the lateral aspect of each vertebral body, and the bone that was taken while creating the trough is minced into small pieces along with the rib that was removed. These bone chips are laid back into the trough to facilitate fusion. The disc spaces are not packed with bone, since this would jeopardize correction during the posterior procedure. The ribs on the convex side of the chest that were exposed are cut

TECHNIQUES OF SURGERY

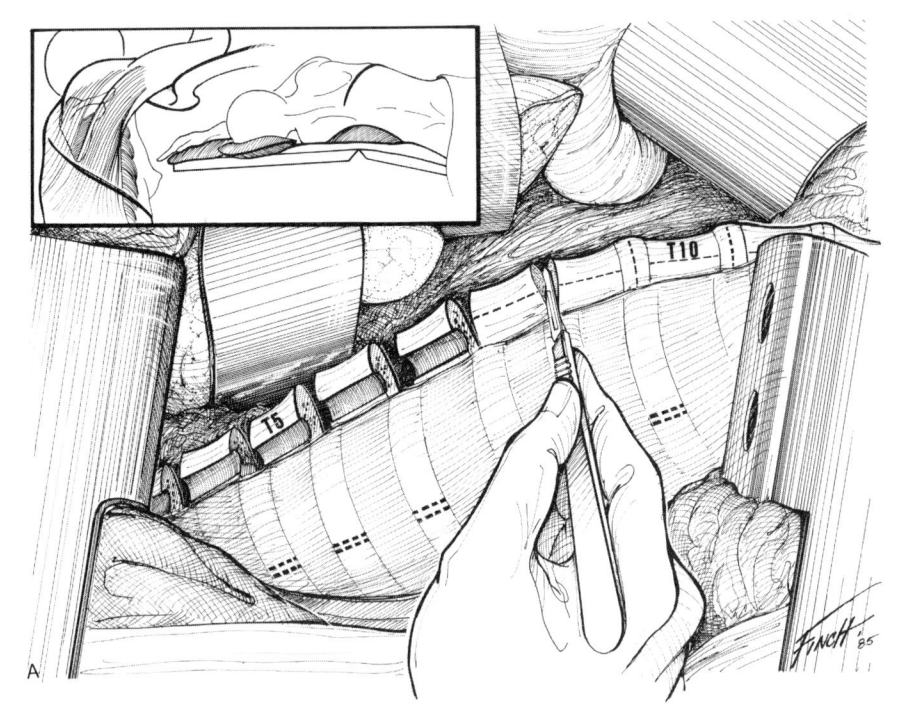

**Ribs 4–11 Transected Bilaterally
H or L Rods From T3–T12 Bilaterally**

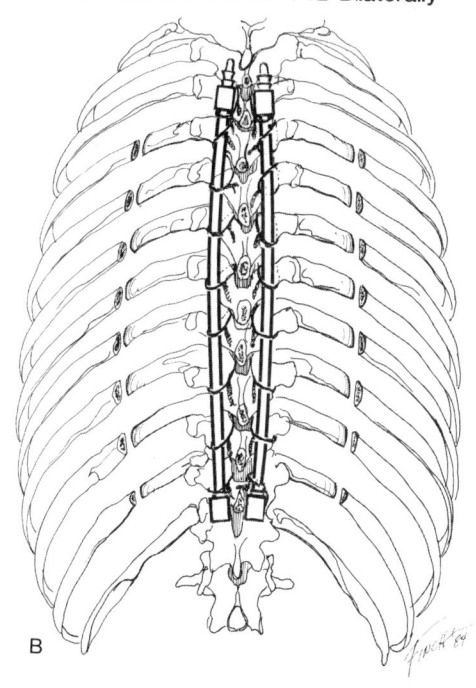

Figure 10–38. *A,* For correction of thoracic lordosis a first stage anterior discectomy with interbody fusion is carried out, cutting the ribs on the side of the thoracotomy incision. *B,* One week later a posterior procedure is carried out. When the rib osteotomies are carried out on the side away from the thoracotomy, sublaminar wires are passed, and the spine segment with detached ribs is pulled posterior to the bent convex oriented Harrington or L-rods. Complete correction of thoracic lordosis with restoration of normal kyphosis is possible with this procedure.

approximately 10 to 15 cm. lateral to the insertion into the vertebral body, removing about a 0.5 to 0.75 cm. section.

A second stage is carried out 7 to 14 days later and consists of rib osteotomies on the concave side of the curvature, approximately 10 to 15 cm. lateral to the rib vertebral body junction. Sublaminar wires are then passed, and two square-ended Harrington distraction rods, bent in the sagittal plane to fit a normal kyphosis, are placed between the hooks and distracted only enough to obtain fixation. An alternative is to use ¼ inch L-rods, pre-bent into a normal kyphotic contour. The segmental wires are then looped around the rods and are tied down, pulling the spine and the affected posterior chest wall to the rod. Posterior fusion is then completed by careful decortication and addition of cancellous and cortical iliac bone grafts. A brace is applied postoperatively, and the patient is ambulated on the fourth to seventh postoperative day.

This is a formidable surgical procedure, but may prove particularly useful in those patients with structural rigid lordosis greater than −30 degrees who are skeletally mature and present with pulmonary dysfunction (Fig. 10-39).

Thoracoplasty (Rib Resection)

Patients who present with a scoliotic deformity complain not so much of the deformity of the spine per se, the abnormal body symmetry, or the shoulder elevation, but of the rib deformity, referred to as the rib hump.[65] In fact, this is often the problem for which the patients seek help. Correction of the deformity by instrumentation techniques associated with spinal fusion may improve the clinical appearance of the rib elevation or rib hump to some degree,[50] but more often than not the patient is left with an improved x-ray appearance of better spinal balance in the AP plane, but significant rib prominence

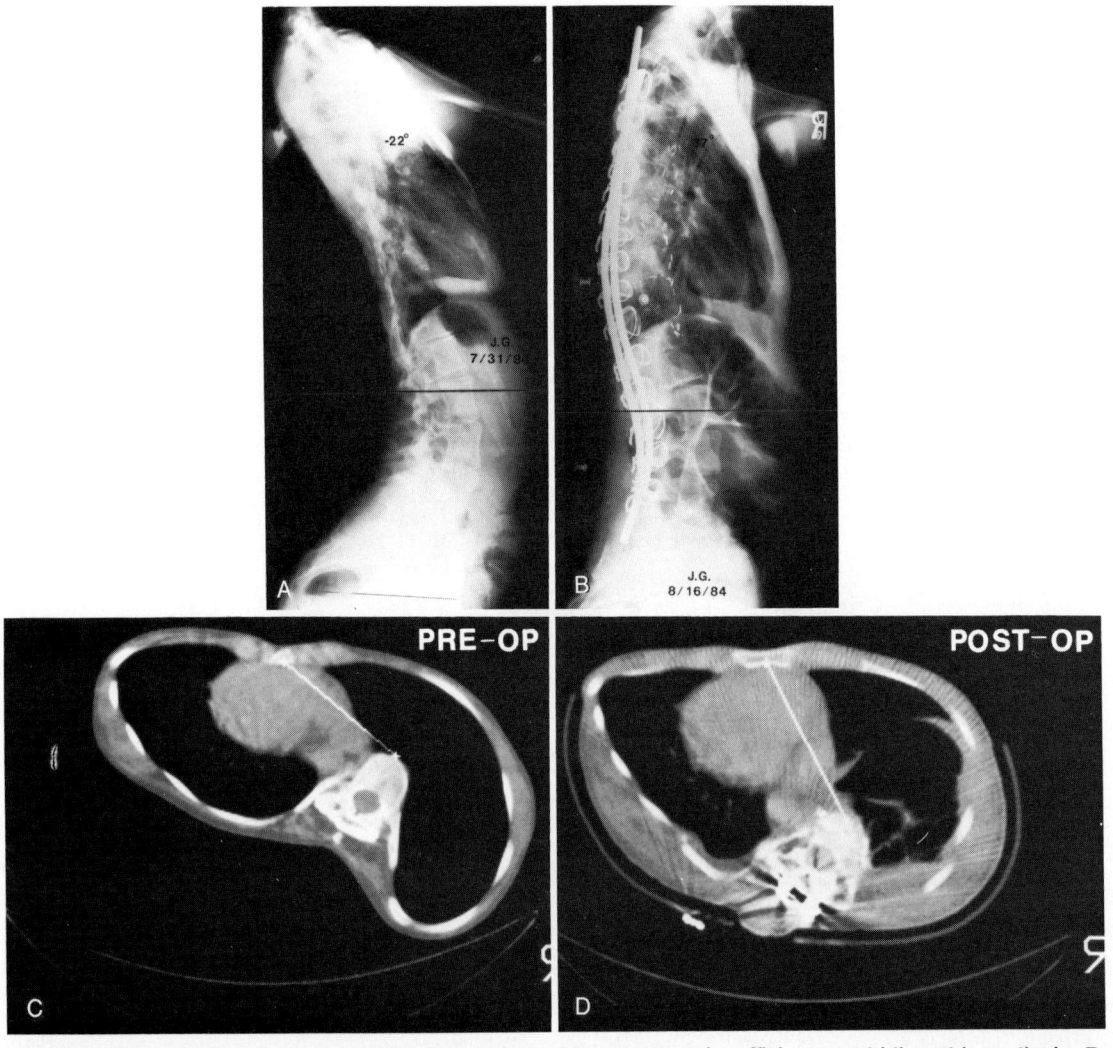

Figure 10-39. A, Marked thoracic lordosis in a patient with pulmonary insufficiency and idiopathic scoliosis. B, Following combined anterior surgery and rib osteotomies, restoration to a normal thoracic kyphosis was possible for a total of 59 degrees of correction. The patient's pre- (C) and postoperative (D) CT scans show marked increase in the AP diameter of her thoracic cage.

that is cosmetically undesirable, if not unacceptable.[1, 2, 113] Furthermore, early posterior fusions may be associated with increasing rib prominence until skeletal growth is complete.[73]

Resection of the rib hump deformity was first carried out by Volkman in 1899.[116] Other authors have likewise published their experiences with this procedure.[12, 31, 82, 95] Steel,[111] more recently, has presented a definitive work. The procedure is best performed through the same midline incision used to expose the spine. The rib resection may precede the spinal fusion with instrumentation or it may follow. It is the author's prejudice that the correction of the curvature may be enhanced by doing the rib resection first, but that is impossible to determine statistically. In any event, after the midline incision is made, the trapezius muscle is detached from the midline fascia and dissection proceeds dorsal to the paraspinal musculature to the rib prominence. With careful dissection a wide exposure is achieved, allowing visualization of the ribs to the posterior axillary line. The periosteum overlying the prominent ribs to be excised is incised in a longitudinal fashion. The subperiosteal exposure is then carried out, first detaching the ribs distally at the posterior axillary line, and then continuing the exposure proximally, retracting the paraspinal musculature immediately. A sharp elevator may facilitate detachment of the rib from the transverse process, and by carefully rotating the rib it can be extracted from its insertion into the vertebral body disc junction. It is preferable to remove the rib intact, since residual rib attached to a transverse process may prove prominent and limit the result. The number of ribs removed depends upon the appearance of the deformity. In general, the mistake is to remove too few ribs or to leave residual rib prominences either proximally or distally. In the author's experience, removal of six to eight ribs is usual for the thoracoplasty. Following rib removal, the wound is irrigated to check for any air leaks. If they are present, a chest tube is inserted and brought out through the skin laterally. In the absence of a pleural leak, a large hemovac drain is placed into the wound and brought out through the skin laterally. The trapezius muscle is reattached to the midline. The spine is prepared for arthrodesis and the transverse processes over the apex of the curvature are completely removed. Failure to do this leads to a continued prominence over the apex of the curvature and again compromises a result. The ribs may be cut into small match sticks and then used as bone grafting material.[121] Additional iliac bone is not necessary.

Postoperatively, the patients may have some transient decrease in pulmonary function; this averaged 12 per cent in Steel's series, but three months after operation pulmonary function approached the preoperative level and at the end of one year the pulmonary function level had equaled or was improved from the preoperative measurement in 90 per cent of Steel's patients. There was no evidence in any of his patients that rib resection caused a decrease in pulmonary function. Radiographically it is interesting to notice how frequently and quickly rib regeneration occurs after surgery. Following rib resection if the scapula appears to be prominent, a reduction scapuloplasty may be carried out.

References

1. Aaro, S., and Dahlborn, M.: The effect of Harrington instrumentation on the longitudinal axis rotation of the apical vertebra and on the spinal and rib-cage deformity in idiopathic scoliosis studied by computer tomography. Spine, 7:456–462, 1982.
2. Aaro, S., and Ohlen, G.: The effect of Harrington instrumentation on the sagittal configuration and mobility of the spine in scoliosis. Spine, 8 (6):570–575, 1983.
3. Allen, B. A. Jr.: Segmental spinal instrumentation. Instructional Course Lectures, Vol. 32. Am. Acad. Orthop. Surgeons, St. Louis, C. V. Mosby Co., p. 202, 1983.
4. Allen, B. L. Jr.:Segmental instrumentation of the spine—indications, results and complications. In Dickson, R., and Bradford, D. (eds.): Management of Spinal Deformities. London, Butterworths, pp. 162–192, 1984.
5. Allen, B. L. Jr., and Ferguson, R. L.: Basic considerations in pelvic fixation cases. In Luque, E. R. (ed.): Segmental Spinal Instrumentation. Thorofare, N. J., Slack, pp. 185–220, 1984.
6. Allen, B. L. Jr., and Ferguson, R. L.: The Galveston technique for L-rod instrumentation of the scoliotic spine. Spine, 7:119–127, 1982.
7. Allen, B. L. Jr., and Ferguson, R. L.: L-rod instrumentation (LRI) for scoliosis in cerebral palsy. J. Pediatr. Orthop., 2:87–96, 1982.
8. Allen, B. L. Jr., and Ferguson, R. L.: The operative treatment of myelomeningocele spinal deformity. Orthop. Clin. North Am., 10:845–862, 1979.
9. Armstrong, G. W. D.: Application of SSI to the lumbosacral spine. In Luque, E. R. (ed.): Segmental Spinal Instrumentation. Thorofare, N. J., Slack, pp. 235–254, 1984.

10. Armstrong, G. W. D., and Connock, S. H. G.: A transverse loading system applied to a modified Harrington instrumentation. Clin. Orthop., *108*:70, 1975.
11. Balderston, R., Winter, R., Moe, J., et al.: Fusion to the sacrum for non-paralytic scoliosis in the adult. Orthop. Trans. *8*:170, 1984.
12. Barnes, J.: Rib resection in infantile idiopathic scoliosis. J. Bone Joint Surg., *61B*:31–35, 1979.
13. Bohlman, H. H., and Eismont, F. J.: Surgical techniques on anterior decompression and fusion for spinal cord injuries. Clin. Orthop. Rel. Res., *154*:57, 1981.
14. Boling, D., Taxdal, D., and Robinson, R. A.: Six case histories demonstrating the feasibility of partial or total replacement of vertebral bodies by bone grafts. Am. Surg., *26*:236, 1960.
15. Bradford, D. S.: Anterior spinal surgery in the management of scoliosis—indications, techniques, results. Orthop. Clin. North Am., *10*:801–812, 1979.
16. Bradford, D. S.: Anterior vascular pedicle bone grafting for the treatment of kyphosis. Spine, *5 (4)*:318–323, 1980.
17. Bradford, D. S.: *In* Kane, W. J. (ed.): Kyphosis: Current Orthopaedic Management. New York, Churchill Livingstone, 1981.
18. Bradford, D. S.: Partial epiphyseal arrest in supplemental fixation for progressive correction of congenital spine deformity. J. Bone Joint Surg., *64A*:610, 1982.
19. Bradford, D. S.: The role of the anterior approach in the management of spinal deformities. *In* Dickson, R., and Bradford, D. (eds.): Management of Spinal Deformities. London, Butterworths, pp. 275–302, 1984.
20. Bradford, D. S.: Vascularized rib grafts for stabilization of kyphosis. Presented at the AOA Annual International Symposium on Limb Reconstruction/Micro or Macro Surgery. Boca Raton, Florida, Nov. 7–11, 1984.
21. Bradford, D. S., Ahmed, K. B., Moe, J. H., et al.: The surgical management of patients with Scheuermann's disease. A review of twenty-four cases managed by combined anterior and posterior spine fusion. J. Bone Joint Surg., *62A*:705–712, 1980.
22. Bradford, D. S., Blatt, J. M., and Rasp, F. L.: Surgical management of severe thoracic lordosis: a new technique to restore normal kyphosis. Spine *8(4)*:420–428, 1983.
23. Bradford, D. S., Ganjavian, S., Antonious, D., et al.: Anterior strut grafting for the treatment of kyphosis. J. Bone Joint Surg., *64A*:680–690, 1982.
24. Bradford, D. S., Winter R. B., Lonstein, J. E., and Moe, J. H.: Techniques of anterior spine surgery for the management of kyphosis. Clin. Orthop., *128*:129–139, 1977.
25. Burrington, J. D., Brown, C., Wayne, E. R., and Odom, J.: Anterior approach to the thoracolumbar spine: technical considerations. Arch. Surg., *111*:456, 1976.
26. Capener, N.: The evolution of lateral rachotomy. J. Bone Joint Surg., *36B*:173, 1954.
27. Carcassone, M., Gregoire, A., and Hornung, H.: L'ablation de L'hemivertebre libre: traitement preventif de la scoliose congenitale. Chirurgie, *103*:110–115, 1977.
28. Cardoso, A. M., Tojonar, F. A., and Luque, E. R.: Osteotomias de columna nuevos conceptos. Ann. Orthop. Traumatol., *12*:105–113, 1976.
29. Cauchoix, J., and Binet, J. P.: Anterior approaches to the spine. Ann. R. Coll. Surg. Engl., *21*:237–243, 1956.
30. Cervenansky, J., Skroving, B., and Moor, D.: Use of fibular bone grafts in reconstructive surgery. Chir. Narzadow Ruchu Ortop. Pol., *27*:297, 1962.
31. Chopin, D., Briard, J. L., and Seringe, R.: Surgery for thoracic deformity in scoliosis. *In* Zorab, P. A., and Siegler, D. (eds.): Scoliosis 1979. London, Academic Press, pp. 161–168, 1980.
32. Compere, E. L.: Excision of hemivertebrae for correction of congenital scoliosis. J. Bone Joint Surg., *14*:555–562, 1932.
33. Cook, W. A.: Transthoracic vertebral surgery. Ann. Thorac. Surg., *12*:54–68, 1971.
34. Cotrel, Y., and Dubousset, J.: New segmental posterior instrumentation of the spine. Orthop. Trans., *9*:118, 1985.
35. Deloste, J. Y.: L'osteoplastie vertebrale anterieure par la convexite pour le traitement des cyphoscolioses severes (a propos de 26 observations du Centre des Massues). Thèse Médécine, Lyon, 1980.
36. Digby, K. H.: Twelfth rib incision as approach to kidney. Surg. Gynecol. Obstet., *73*:84–85, 1941.
37. Dommisse, G. G.: The blood supply of the spinal cord. J. Bone Joint Surg., *56B*:225–235, 1974.
38. Dove, J., Lin, Y. T., Shen, Y. S., and Ditmanson, M. L.: Aortic aneurysm complicating spinal fixation with Dwyer's apparatus. Report of a case. Spine, *6*:524–526, 1981.
39. Drummond, D., Narechania, R., Wenger, D., et al.: Wisconsin segmental spinal instrumentation. Orthop. Trans., *6*:22–23, 1982.
40. Dunn, H. K.: Spinal Instrumentation, Part I: Principles of posterior and anterior instrumentation. *In* McCollister Evarts, C. (ed.): Instructional Course Lectures, Am. Acad. Orthop. Surg., Vol. XXXII, St. Louis, C. V. Mosby, pp. 192–209, 1983.
41. Dunn, H. K., and Bolstad, K. E.: Fixation of Dwyer screws for the treatment of scoliosis. J. Bone Joint Surg., *59A*:54–56, 1977.
42. Dunn, H. K.: Kyphosis in myelodysplasia; operative treatment based on pathophysiology. Orthop. Trans., *7*:19, 1983.
43. Dwyer, A. F., Newton, N. C., and Sherwood, A. A.: An anterior approach to scoliosis—a preliminary report. Clin. Orthop., *62*:192–202, 1969.
44. Dwyer, A. P.: A fatal complication of paravertebral infection and traumatic aneurysm following Dwyer instrumentation. J. Bone Joint Surg., *61B*:239, 1979.
45. Dwyer, A. P., O'Brien, J. P., Seal, P. P., et al.: The late complications after the Dwyer anterior spinal instrumentation for scoliosis. J. Bone Joint Surg., *59B*:117, 1977.
46. Fey, B.: L'abord du rein par voie thoraco-abdominale. Arch. Urologicale Clin. Necker, *5*:169–178, 1925.
47. Flynn, J. C., and Hoque, M. A.: Anterior fusion of the lumbar spine. J. Bone Joint Surg., *61A*:1143–1150, 1979.
48. Fountain, S. S., Hsu, L. C. S., Yau, A. C. M. C.,

and Hodgson, A. R.: Progressive kyphosis following solid anterior spine fusion in children with tuberculosis of the spine. J. Bone Joint Surg., 57A:1104–1107, 1975.
49. Freebody, D., Bendall, R., and Taylor, R. D.: Anterior transperitoneal lumbar fusion. J. Bone Joint Surg., 53B:617–627, 1971.
50. Gaines, R. W., McKinley, L. M., and Leatherman, K. D.: Effect of the Harrington compression system on the correction of the rib hump in spinal instrumentation for idiopathic scoliosis. Spine, 6(5):489–493, 1981.
51. Gardner, A. D. H.: Four year's experience with an anterior spinal distraction device for the correction of kyphotic deformities and its use as a permanent implant. Orthop. Trans., 7:30, 1983.
52. Geraud: Observation sur un corp de feu a l'epine. Medicale Acad. R. Chir., 2:414, 1750.
53. Goldstein, L. A.: Surgical management of scoliosis. J. Bone Joint Surg., 48A167–196, 1966.
54. Gonon, G. P., DeMauroy, J. C., Frankel, P., et al.: Greffes anterieures en etai dans le traitment des cyphoses et cyphoscolioses. Revue Chir. Orthop., 67:731–742, 1981.
55. Griss, P., Harms, J., and Zielke, K.: Ventral derotation spondylodesis (VDS). In Dickson, R., and Bradford, D. (eds.): Management of Spinal Deformities. London, Butterworths, pp. 193–236, 1984.
56. Hall, J. E.: The anterior approach to spinal deformities. Orthop. Clin. North Am., 3:81–98, 1972.
57. Harrington, P. R.: Correction and internal fixation by spine instrumentation. J. Bone Joint Surg., 44A:591, 1962.
58. Harrington, P. R.: Surgical instrumentation for management of scoliosis. J. Bone Joint Surg., 42A:1448, 1960.
59. Harrington, P. R.: Technical details in relation to the successful use of instrumentation in scoliosis. Orthop. Clin. North Am., 3:49, 1972.
60. Hernandez-Ros, A., and Codorniu, Y.: Nuevas tactica y tecnica operatorias en el tratamiento de las escoliosis. Scritti Medici in Onore Di P. Del Torto, 1965.
61. Hibbs, R. A.: An operation for progressive spinal deformities. N. Y. Med. J. 93:1013–1019, 1911.
62. Hodgson, A. R., Stock, F. E.: Anterior spine fusion. Br. J. Surg., 44:266, 1956.
63. Hodgson, A. R., Stock, F. E., Fang, H. S. Y., and Ong, G. B.: Anterior spine fusion. Br. J. Surg., 48:172–178, 1960.
64. Hoffa, A.: Operative behandlung einer schweren skoliose (resection des rippenbuckels). Zeitschur. Orthop. Chir., 4:402–408, 1896.
65. Houghton, G. R.: Cosmetic surgery for scoliosis. In Dickson, R., and Bradford, D. (eds.): Management of Spinal Deformities. London, Butterworths, pp. 237–251, 1984.
66. Hyndman, O. R.: Transplantation of the spinal cord: the problem of kyphoscoliosis with cord signs. Surg. Gynecol. Obstet., 84:460–464, 1947.
67. Jackson, J. W.: Surgical approaches to the anterior aspects of the spinal column. Ann. R. Coll. Surg., 48:83–98, 1971.
68. Johnson, R. M., and McGuire, E. J.: Urogenital complications of anterior approaches to the lumbar spine. Clin. Orthop., 154:114–118, 1981.
69. King, H. A., Moe, J. H., Bradford, D. S., and Winter, R. B.: The selection of the fusion levels in thoracic idiopathic scoliosis. J. Bone Joint Surg., 65A:1302–1314, 1983.
70. Lange, F.: Operative Behandlung der Spondylitis. MMW, 56:1817, 1909.
71. Langenskiold, A.: Correction of congenital scoliosis by excision of one half of a cleft vertebra. Acta Orthop., 38:291–300, 1967.
72. Leatherman, K. D.: Resection of vertebral bodies. J. Bone Joint Surg., 51A:206–208, 1969.
73. Leatherman, K. D.: Results of questionnaire of fusion-in-situ for congenital scoliosis. Orthop. Trans., 6:12–13, 1982.
74. Leatherman, K. D., Johnson, J. R., Holt, R. T., and Broadstone, P.: A clinical assessment of 357 cases of segmental spinal instrumentation. In Luque, E. R. (ed.): Segmental Spinal Instrumentation. Thorofare, N. J., Slack, pp. 165–184, 1984.
75. Lonstein, J. E., Winter, R. B., Moe, J. H., et al.: Neurologic deficits secondary to spinal deformity: a review of the literature and report of 43 cases. Spine, 5:331–355, 1980.
76. Luque, E. R.: Segmental spinal instrumentation: a method of rigid internal fixation of the spine to induce arthrodesis. Orthop. Trans., 4:391, 1980.
77. Luque, E. R. (ed.): Segmental Spinal Instrumentation. Slack, Thorofare, N. J., 1984.
78. Luque, E. R.: Segmental spinal instrumentation for correction of scoliosis. Clin. Orthop., 163:192–198, 1982.
79. Luque, E. R., and Cardoso, A.: Paralytic scoliosis in growing children. Clin. Orthop., 163:202, 1982.
80. Luque, E. R., and Cardoso, A.: Segmental correction of scoliosis with rigid internal fixation. Orthop. Trans., 1:136–137, 1977.
81. MacLennan, A.: Scoliosis. Br. Med. J., 2:864–866, 1922.
82. Manning, C. W., Prime, F. J., and Zorab, P. A.: Partial costectomy as a cosmetic operation in scoliosis. J. Bone Joint Surg., 55B:521–527, 1973.
83. Marchetti, P. G., and Valdini, A: End fusions in the treatment of severe progression or severe scoliosis in childhood or early adolescence. Orthop. Trans., 2:271, 1978.
84. Mayer, L.: Treatment of congenital scoliosis due to hemivertebrae. J. Bone Joint Surg., 17:671–678, 1935.
85. McBride, G. G., and Bradford, D. S.: Vertebral body replacement with a femoral neck allograft and vascularized rib strut graft—a technique for treating post-traumatic kyphosis with neurologic deficit. Spine, 8:406–415, 1983.
86. Michelle, A. A., and Krueger, F. J.: Surgical approach to the vertebral body. J. Bone Joint Surg., 31A:873–878, 1949.
87. Moe, J. H.: A critical analysis of methods of fusion for scoliosis. J. Bone Joint Surg., 40A:529, 1958.
88. Moe, J. H.: Methods of correction and surgical technique in scoliosis. Orthop. Clin. North Am., 2:17, 1972.

89. Moe, J. H., Kharrat, K., Winter, R. B., and Cummine, J. L.: Harrington instrumentation without fusion plus external orthotic support for the treatment of difficult curvature problems in young children. Clin. Orthop. Rel. Res., 185:35, 1984.
90. Moe, J. H., Purcell, G. A., and Bradford, D. S.: Zielke instrumentation (VDS) for the correction of spinal curvature. Clin. Orthop., 180:133, 1983.
91. Moe, J. H., Winter, R. B., Bradford, D. S., and Lonstein, J. E.: Scoliosis and Other Spinal Deformities. Philadelphia, W. B. Saunders, 1978.
92. Morscher, E.: Experiences with the transthoracic hemilateral epiphyseodesis in the treatment of scoliosis. In Chapchal, G. (ed.): Operative Treatment of Scoliosis. Stuttgart, Thieme Stratton, 1973.
93. Morscher, E.: International Congress Series 291. Orthopaedic Surgery and Traumatology (Amsterdam, Holland, 1972, pp. 1102–1105.) Amsterdam: Excerpta Medica, 1972.
94. Nicastro, J. F., Traina, J., Lancaster, M., and Hartjen, C.: Sublaminar segmental wire fixation: anatomic pathways during their removal. Orthop. Trans. 8:172, 1984.
95. Piggott, H.: Posterior rib resection in scoliosis. J. Bone Joint Surg., 53B:663–671, 1971.
96. Pinto, W. C., Avanzi, O., and Winter, R. B.: An anterior distractor for the intraoperative correction of angular kyphosis. Spine, 3:309, 1978.
97. Resina, J., and Ferriera-Alves, A. F.: A technique of correction and internal fixation for scoliosis. J. Bone Joint Surg., 59B:159–165, 1977.
98. Riseborough, E. J.: The anterior approach to the spine for the correction of deformities of the axial skeleton. Clin. Orthop., 93:207–214, 1973.
99. Roaf, R.: Wedge resection for scoliosis. J. Bone Joint Surg., 37B:97–101, 1955.
100. Rodolfi: Palla de fucile penetrata nel cello e incuneata al lato destro della solonna vertebrale. Extrazione del proiettile. Gazzetta Medicala Italia (Lombardia), 4:404, 1859.
101. Rose, G. K., Owen, R., and Sanderson, J. M.: Transposition of rib with blood supply for the stabilization of spinal kyphosis. J. Bone Joint Surg., 57B:112, 1975.
102. Royle, N. D.: The operative removal of an accessory vertebra. Med. J. Aust. 1:467, 1928.
103. Shaffer, J. W.: Rib transposition vascularized bone grafts—hemodynamic assessment of donor rib graft and recipient vertebral body. Orthop. Trans., 8:153, 1984.
104. Simmons, E. H.: Observations on the technique and indications for wedge resection of the spine. J. Bone Joint Surg., 50A:847–848, 1968.
105. Slabaugh, P. B., Winter, R. B., Lonstein, J. E., and Moe, J. H.: Lumbosacral hemivertebrae: a review of 24 patients, with excision in eight. Spine, 5(3):234–244, 1980.
106. Slot, G. H.: A new distraction system for the correction of kyphosis using the anterior approach. Orthop. Trans., 6:29, 1982.
107. Stagnara, P., DeMauroy, J. C., Gonon, G. P., and Campo-Paysaa, A.: Scolioses cyphosantes de l'adulte et greffes anterieures. Intl. Orthop., 2:149–165, 1978.
108. Stagnara, P., Gonon, G. P., and Fauchet, P.: Surgical treatment of idiopathic rigid lumbar scoliosis in the adult. In Dickson, R., and Bradford, D. (eds.): Management of Spinal Deformities. London, Butterworths, pp. 303–321, 1984.
109. Stagnara, P., Gounot, J., Campo-Paysaa, A., et al.: Arthrodesis transthoraciques dans le traitement des cyphoses et des cyphoscolioses. Intl. Orthop., 1:199–214, 1977.
110. Stagnara, P., Gounnot, J., Fauchet, R., and Jouvinroux, P.: Les greffes anterieures par voie thoracique dans le traitement des deformations et dislocations vertebrales epiphyphose et cyphoscoliose. Revue Chir. Orthop., 60:39–56, 1974.
111. Steel, H. H.: Rib resection and spine fusion in correction of convex deformity in scoliosis. J. Bone Joint Surg., 65A:920–925, 1983.
112. Streitz, W., Brown, J. C., and Bonnett, C. A.: Anterior fibular strut grafting in the treatment of kyphosis. Clin. Orthop., 128:140, 1977.
113. Thulbourne, T., and Gillespie, R.: The rib hump in idiopathic scoliosis. Measurement analysis and response to treatment. J. Bone Joint Surg., 58B:64–71, 1976.
114. Vanzelle, C., Stagnara, P., and Jouvinroux, P.: Functional monitoring of spinal cord activity during spinal surgery. Clin. Orthop. Rel. Res., 93:173, 1973.
115. Van Loon, L., and Hoogmartens, M.: Technique of combined anterior and posterior wedge resection for fixed lumbar scoliosis. Acta Orthop. Belg., 42:75–83, 1976.
116. Volkman, R.: Resektion von Rippenstucker bei Skoliose. Berl. Klin. Wochenschr., 26:1097–1098, 1889.
117. VonLackum, H. L., and Smith, A.: Removal of vertebral bodies in the treatment of scoliosis. Surg. Gynecol. Obstet., 57:250–256, 1933.
118. Waugh, T. R.: The biomechanical basis for the utilization of methylmethacrylate in the treatment of scoliosis. J. Bone Joint Surg., 53A:194, 1971.
119. Wenger, D., and Carollo, J.: Biomechanics of segmental spinal instrumentation. In Luque, E. R. (ed.): Segmental Spinal Instrumentation. Slack, Thorofare, N. J., pp. 31–48, 1984.
120. Wenger, D. R., Carollo, J. J., Wilkerson, J. A., et al.: Laboratory testing of segmental spinal instrumentation versus traditional Harrington instrumentation for scoliosis treatment. Spine, 7:265–269, 1982.
121. Whitman, A.: Rib grafting for scoliosis. Am J. Surg., 6:801–803, 1929.
122. Wiles, P.: Resection of dorsal vertebrae in congenital scoliosis. J. Bone Joint Surg., 33A:151–154, 1951.
123. Winter, R. B.: Congenital kyphoscoliosis with paralysis following hemivertebra excision. Clin. Orthop., 119:116–125, 1976.
124. Winter, R. B.: Posterior spinal fusion in scoliosis: indications, techniques, and results. Orthop. Clin. North Am., 10:787, 1979.
125. Winter, R., Lovel, W. W., and Moe, J.: Excessive thoracic lordosis and loss of pulmonary function in patients with idiopathic scoliosis. J. Bone Joint Surg., 57A:972–977, 1975.
126. Winter, R. B., Moe, J. H., and Bradford, D. S.:

Congenital thoracic lordosis. J. Bone Joint Surg., *60A*:806–810, 1978.
127. Yau, A. C., Hsu, L. C. S., O'Brien, J. P., and Hodgson, A. R.: Tuberculous kyphosis: correction with spinal osteotomy, halopelvic distraction and anterior and posterior fusion. J. Bone Joint Surg., *56A*:1419–1434, 1974.
128. Zielke, K., and Pellin, B: Neue Instrumente und Implantate zur Erganzung des Harrington Systems. Z. Orthop. Chir., *114*:534–537, 1976.
129. Zielke, K., Stundat, R., and Beaujean, F.: Ventrale derotationsspondylodese. Vorlaufiger Ergebnissbericht uber 26 operierte Falle. Arch. Orthop. Unfallchir., *85*:257–277, 1976.

11

IDIOPATHIC SCOLIOSIS

John H. Moe, M.D. • J. Abbott Byrd, III, M.D.

Idiopathic scoliosis is the most common of all forms of lateral deviation of the spine. It occurs during the growing years and is customarily divided into three categories: infantile, juvenile, and adolescent. These are classified according to the age at which the deformity is first noted, which does not necessarily coincide with the time the spinal curvature first appears.

The term scoliosis was first used by Galen (A.D. 131–201),[37] although spinal deformity had been previously described by Hippocrates. The differentiation into idiopathic, paralytic, congenital, and other forms came only after the discovery of x-rays by Roentgen in 1895. Many more years elapsed before a more definitive classification was recorded in the orthopaedic literature. Even in 1924 when Hibbs[44] reported on 59 cases of scoliosis operated on by his method, the case reports in the series included several obviously idiopathic curvatures that he grouped with the rest, all of which he said were paralytic in origin.

ETIOLOGIC INVESTIGATION AND GENETIC ASPECTS

The etiology of idiopathic scoliosis has long been sought, but despite years of research no single causative factor has been identified.

In 1979, Sahlstrand and coworkers[93] examined postural equilibrium in patients with adolescent idiopathic scoliosis, using tests of postural sway and the electronystagmographic evaluation of labyrinthine function. They found increased postural sway and nystagmus in the scoliosis group; this was interpreted as showing a difference in postural equilibrium between normal children and those with scoliosis. The authors were unable to conclude whether the vestibular dysfunction was the cause or merely a result of the spinal deformity. Investigation by Herman and associates,[43] also in 1979, strongly suggested that vestibular function is functionally impaired in patients with idiopathic scoliosis. Samberg and workers[94] used electronystagmography to evaluate the vestibular function of 41 patients with adolescent idiopathic scoliosis and came to the same conclusion—abnormalities exist in vestibular end organ function. In 1984, Yamada and coworkers[121] examined the equilibrium function of 150 patients with idiopathic scoliosis using tests for righting reflex, drift reaction, and optokinetic nystagmus. Seventy-nine per cent of the patients showed marked equilibrium dysfunction in at least one of the tests compared with only 5 per cent of 20 control subjects.

Wyatt and coworkers[118] have investigated posterior column function in patients with idiopathic scoliosis by evaluating vibration sensation, which is felt to be the most sensitive indicator of posterior column function. Reporting their findings to the 1984 SRS meeting, they noted a significant asymmetry in the ability to detect vibration in scoliotic patients compared with normal controls. These findings occurred in both the upper and lower extremities, suggesting a central aberration in the posterior column pathway.

The intervertebral disc has been examined in idiopathic scoliosis. Both Pedrini[86] and Taylor[102] have documented a rise in nucleus pulposus collagen in adolescent idiopathic scoliosis. It was Taylor's opinion that the increased collagen level was related to the degree of curvature at each disc. His data support the view that this change is secondary rather than primary, reflecting effect rather than cause. Zaleske[124] has examined the hexosamine content of the intervertebral disc and found it to be decreased by approximately 25 per cent in the nucleus pulposus of idiopathic scoliosis discs. Conversely, the acid phosphatase level was elevated. Examination of discs from patients with scoliosis secondary to myelomeningocele revealed the same pattern, with even greater changes than those seen in the idiopathic discs. Because similar nucleus changes are seen in both myelomeningocele and idiopathic scoliosis, Zaleske concluded that the disc changes are secondary to and not the primary cause of idiopathic scoliosis. Oegema and associates[85] have studied the proteoglycan content of discs obtained from patients with idiopathic scoliosis, scoliosis secondary to cerebral palsy, and age matched controls. While differences between anular and nuclear proteoglycan structure were found for each disc there was no significant difference between discs from patients with idiopathic scoliosis and those with cerebral palsy related scoliosis. However, they both differed from control values, having significantly higher levels of aggregate and larger non-aggregating monomers, although there was no significant differences in proteoglycan monomer chemistry. These results suggest that the curve itself, regardless of etiology, may lead to similar alterations in proteoglycan composition.

The observation that patients with idiopathic scoliosis are taller[110] than healthy non-scoliotic controls has led many investigators to evaluate growth-promoting hormones as possible etiologic factors. There are conflicting reports. Skogland's[98] prospective study of 95 patients with idiopathic scoliosis and 60 controls found a higher sensitivity of the pituitary release mechanism of growth hormone and elevated concentrations of testosterol in 12 year old pubertal females. Misol and coworkers[70] found no difference in serum growth hormonal levels in their prospective study of 15 patients with idiopathic scoliosis using the insertion stimulator test. The study of Willner and associates[114] found an elevated serum level of somatomedin in the scoliotic female, which they felt supported the assumption that growth hormone secretion is higher in females with adolescent idiopathic scoliosis as compared with age and sex matched controls. On the other hand, Skogland and workers[99] did not find a significant difference in the somatomedin levels when comparing patients with idiopathic scoliosis and controls. While a question regarding the levels of growth-promoting hormones still remains, most authors agree that regardless of the levels the etiologic importance of these hormones remains to be proved.

Much has been written about skeletal muscle and its relationship to idiopathic scoliosis. Various areas examined include: the muscle spindle;[59, 123] morphology of individual muscle fibers;[92, 125] histochemistry;[100, 109] electromyographic activity of the paraspinal musculature;[2, 89] abnormalities of the sarcolemma at the myotendon junction;[52] calcium, copper, and zinc concentrations in paraspinal musculature;[122] and platelet abnormalities as they relate to skeletal muscle.[36] Although abnormalities have been found, there is no definite proof that idiopathic scoliosis is caused by a defect in skeletal muscle.

Abnormalities in the vertebral bodies themselves with asymmetrical growth at the paired neurocentral junction have also been proposed as a cause of scoliosis.[54] It has been postulated but not proved that asymmetrical growth might produce rotation, leading to scoliosis.

Previous research has suggested that a collagen abnormality may be the underlying cause of idiopathic scoliosis. Works by Bradford and coworkers[6] and Venn and coworkers[107] do not support this, and in fact state that the collagen metabolism of both spinal ligaments and skin in patients with idiopathic scoliosis is normal.

One of the more promising areas of etiologic research appears to be in the genetic aspects of idiopathic scoliosis. In 1968, Wynne-Davies[119] reported on 180 case records from the Edinburgh scoliosis clinic. She concluded that idiopathic scoliosis was familial. Her findings suggested either a dominant or multiple gene inheritance, but she noted that a large study was needed before a firm conclusion could be reached. A study by Riseborough and Wynne-Davies[90] in 1973 reviewed the families of 207 indexed patients in Boston and compared the results with those of the Edinburgh study to see whether differences existed. The Boston study revealed a much more precipitous drop in proportions of affected first, second, and third degree relatives (11.1 per cent, 2.4 per cent, and 1.4 per cent respectively) compared with the Edinburgh survey (7.0 per cent, 3.7 per cent, and 1.6 per cent respectively). Although a definite statement regarding inheritance could not be made, it was felt that this study supported a multifactorial mode of inheritance. Cowell and coworkers'[23] study of 590 parents and siblings of 110 scoliosis patients in an unselected group suggested a dominant mode of inheritance in idiopathic scoliosis, with a sporadic incidence of 20 per cent. DeGeorge and Fisher,[24] because of the results of their study of monozygotic and dizygotic twin pairs, feel that there is no single genetic basis for idiopathic scoliosis. They suggest that maternal factors predominate, as their study showed a statistically significant excess of children with scoliosis born to mothers age 30 to 39 years old.

In summary, although much research into possible etiologies has been performed, the cause of idiopathic scoliosis remains unknown.

NATURAL HISTORY

Studies that show the deleterious effects of the severe curve on the adult have been done.[20, 77, 82, 108] While these studies have provided a reason to prevent curve progression they have not answered two pertinent questions: (1) Which curves will progress? and (2) of these, which curves will progress into the deleterious range? These questions remain to be conclusively answered; recent studies, however, have provided more insight into the problem.

In attempting to distinguish the progressive from the non-progressive curve, Clarisse (1974)[17] reviewed 110 patients with 10 to 29 degree idiopathic curves presenting during growth. Patients were not treated unless the curves progressed past 30 degrees. Curve progression past 30 degrees occurred in 53 per cent of patients presenting between the ages of 3 and 11; curves in patients presenting between the age of 11 and the onset of menses progressed past 30 degrees only in 15 per cent. Evaluating the progression of individual curve patterns in the pre-menstrual patient, Clarisse found that thoracic curves progressed in 42 per cent of patients, lumbar curves in 12 per cent, and double major curves in 67 per cent.

Rogala, Drummond, and Gurr[91] reported their natural history findings in 1978 based on 603 adolescent patients who had idiopathic scoliosis detected by school screening with a follow-up of two years. Progression was defined as a 5 degree curve increase into the range of a 20 degree curvature or more. Increasing curves of less than 20 degrees did not meet the criterion for progression. Curves less than 10 degrees progressed in 1.9 per cent of males and 4 per cent of females; curves of 11 degrees or more progressed into the 20 degree range in 15.4 per cent of females and 3.8 per cent of males. They concluded that the curve at risk was one measuring 11 degrees or more in a growing female.

Bunnell[11] reviewed 123 patients who met the following criteria: (1) the presence of a curve showing less than 50 degrees at the time of diagnosis, (2) a radiograph taken at skeletal maturity, and (3) a minimum follow-up of one year prior to skeletal maturity. The average curvature in this group was 33 degrees, with a range of 10 to 49 degrees. Progression of at least 10 degrees prior to skeletal maturity was seen in 44 per cent of curves measuring 10 to 20 degrees, 28 per cent of curves measuring 20 to 30 degrees, 48 per cent of curves measuring 30 to 40 degrees, and 61 per cent of curves measuring between 40 and 50 degrees. The risk of at least 5 degrees of progression was correlated with the curve pattern; 77 per cent of thoracic, 67 per cent of thoracolumbar, 66 per cent of double-major, and 30 per cent of lumbar curves progressed. Patients diagnosed prior to age 10 had had a 76 per cent risk of progression of 10 degrees or more, while patients older than 15 years when diagnosed had a 14 per cent risk. The onset of menarche also correlated with curve progression. Patients diagnosed prior to menarche progressed in 53 per cent of cases, whereas only 11 per cent of patients diagnosed after menarche progressed. Patients whose iliac crests showed a Risser 0 had a 68 per cent risk of curve progression, while those with a Risser 3 or 4 had an 18 per cent risk. In summary, Bunnell found that curve severity, curve pattern, age at diagnosis, onset of menses, and the Risser sign were prognostic indicators. Factors such as a positive family history, thoracic kyphosis, lumbar lordosis, and trunk imbalance were not helpful in predicting outcomes.

Lonstein and Carlson[58] further delineated the risk factors for curve progression in their 1984 review of 727 patients with idiopathic scoliosis presenting initially with 5 to 29 degree curves. The patients were followed until the end of growth or until curve progression was detected. Progression was defined as a curve increase of 10 degrees or more for curves less than 19 degrees and a curve increase of 5 degrees or more for curves of 20 to 29 degrees. Using their criteria, progression was found in 23 per cent of patients. The incidence of curve progression was related to curve pattern and magnitude. Double curves progressed more than single curves. Curve progression was found to increase with increasing curve magnitude at initial detection. The average non-progressive curve initially measured 15 degrees, whereas the progressive curves averaged 19.7 degrees at initial detection. The incidence of progression also decreased with increasing age and Risser sign at initial diagnosis. Similarly, the onset of menses had occurred by the time of the initial visit in 68 per cent of patients with non-progressive curves as opposed to 32 per cent with progressive curves.

While each patient is a unique individual and cannot be treated indiscriminately according to group statistics, the above studies do aid in identifying the patient with a curve that is likely to progress. While no single factor determines curve progression, one is able to predict with some accuracy which curves will progress by combining different pieces of information. The most important of these are curve magnitude, the patient's Risser sign, and skeletal bone age at diagnosis; secondary are knowledge of curve pattern and the menarchal status. For example, an 11 year old, premenarchal, Risser 0 patient having a 20 degree thoracic curve is at high risk for progression and must be closely followed. If this same 20 degree curve is found in an 18 year old, post-menarchal, Risser 4 patient, the risk of progression is quite low. The chance of progression still exists, but the follow-up need not be so often. These two examples point out extremes but illustrate that by combining available pieces of information it is possible to make a reasonable estimate regarding the risk of curve progression. It is not possible, though, to predict the amount of curve progression regardless of what factors are used.

CURVE PATTERNS

Classification of curve patterns is necessary to allow comparisons and prognostication of various patients. In idiopathic scoliosis the curve pattern generally does not change from that noted at the onset of the deformity. Confusion has existed in the past regarding the terminology of different curves (see Glossary in Chapter 4). Terms such as primary and secondary are probably more confusing than Cobb's[18, 19] descriptive terms of major and minor curves. A major curve is more structural and deforming, whereas a minor curve is less structural and deforming and is often called the compensatory curve. Currently, using these terms and the location of the apical vertebrae, we have found the following classification to be most helpful in outlining treatment and prognosis.

> Single major high thoracic curve
> Single major thoracic curve
> Single major thoracolumbar curve
> Single major lumbar curve
> Major thoracic and minor lumbar curves
> Double major thoracic and lumbar curves
> Double major thoracic and thoracolumbar curves
> Double major thoracic curves
> Multiple curve patterns

Single Major High Thoracic Curve Pattern

The upper vertebra of this curve is generally T1 or T2, but rarely may be C7. This pattern has been erroneously termed cervicothoracic, however, the apex actually lies in the upper thoracic spine. The high thoracic curve may appear without a lower thoracic curve or with a small completely flexible curve below.

Single Major Thoracic Curve Pattern

This pattern is one of the most deforming of idiopathic spinal curvatures. The apex lies within the thoracic spine and the upper end vertebra is either T4, T5, or T6, and the lower end vertebra, T11, T12, L1, or L2. The most common end vertebrae are T5 and T12. The great majority of these curves are convex to the right. In the lateral projection the thoracic spine usually has decreased kyphosis or may actually be lordotic. It is this lordosis that may play a significant role in deceasing pulmonary function.[17]

This pattern is usually associated with a rotational prominence; the magnitude varies significantly from curve to curve and is not related to the degree of the curve or to the rotation seen on the frontal radiograph.[9] Using a forward bending test, a 40 degree curve may be associated with a 1 to 2 cm. rib elevation, whereas a 25 degree curve may have a 3 to 4 cm. rib elevation.

Single Major Thoracolumbar Curve Pattern

This is a single curve with its upper end vertebra at T8, T9, or T10 and the lower end vertebra at L3. The apical vertebra is T12 or L1. Both the upper thoracic and lower lumbar spine may show small compensatory curves, which are usually completely flexible. This pattern is often associated with decompensation of the spine from the midline. Although frequently seen as a small curve in school screening programs, the thoracolumbar curve pattern is not a common pattern in surgical experience.

Single Major Lumbar Curve Pattern

This pattern is frequently found as a small flexible curve in the early school screening program. The apex is usually at L2. The upper end vertebra is T11, T12, or L1, and the lower end vertebra, L4 or L5; the most common end vertebrae are L1 and L4. There is a fractional curve between the lower end vertebra and the sacrum. The pelvic brim is often not level in patients with this pattern and is most often lower on the convex side. Leveling the pelvis with standing blocks prior to radiography may diminish the apparent severity of this curve. These curves seldom measure more than 60 degrees during adolescence but may markedly distort the waistline.

Major Thoracic and Minor Lumbar Curve Pattern

This curve pattern, which is commonly seen, consists of an upper curve with the upper end vertebra at T4 or T5 and the lower end vertebra at T12 and a lower curve with the upper end vertebra at T12 and the lower end vertebra at L4 or L5. The upper curve is the larger and more structural of the two. As time passes the lumbar curve may increase and become more rigid, though it usually remains more flexible than the thoracic curve above.

Double Major Thoracic and Lumbar Curve Pattern

This pattern consists of a thoracic and a lumbar curve both of which appear at the same time, usually during the juvenile years. Both curves are of nearly the same degree and rigidity. Because of this, the spine is usually compensated with regard to the midline and the cosmetic appearance is good. The thoracic curve is generally convex to the right with the apical vertebra at T7 or T8 and the upper end vertebra at T4, T5, or T6 and the lower end vertebra at T10, T11, or T12. The lower curve is convex to the left, having its apical vertebra at L1 or L2 and extending to L4 or occasionally L5.

Double Major Thoracic and Thoracolumbar Curve Pattern

The thoracic curve extends from T4 to T9 or T10 with its apex at T6 or T7. The convexity is usually to the right with minimal associated rib prominence. The thoracolumbar curve has as its end vertebra T9 or T10 and L3, with an apex at the T12-L1 disc space.

Double Major Thoracic Curve Pattern

A left upper and right lower thoracic curve is typical of this pattern, which has been described by Moe.[72] The upper curve has its apex at T3 or T4 and extends from T1 or T2 to T5 or T6. The lower curve has its apex within the thoracic spine and extends from T5 or T6 to T11 or as low as L2.

The upper curve may cause marked deformity owing to elevation of the first rib, its associated neck muscles, and the shoulder; this deformity of the neckline is often overlooked in patients with long hair. The upper thoracic curve may also be missed on the routine 14 × 17 inch radiograph, which fails to include the upper curve. Therefore, a 36 inch film taken at 6 feet is recommended. Omission of the upper curve from the side bending film may also cause its structural nature to be overlooked.

Multiple Curve Patterns

Multiple curves other than those described above do occur, but they tend to be short and non-deforming. Travaglini[106] was the first to give a detailed analysis of these curves. Progression of the curves in this pattern is unusual but may occasionally occur, requiring treatment.

Lumbosacral curves

Idiopathic lumbar curves usually have L4 as their end vertebra. It has been discussed in the past whether or not the curve between this end vertebra and the sacrum is significant. This curve has sometimes been called the "oblique take off," and in the past was seen as the basis for the curves above. In fact, orthopaedic surgeons in the past have attempted to treat thoracic curves by performing an L3 to sacrum fusion, using an obliquely placed tibial strut graft between the ilium and the convexity of the lumbar curve, reasoning that correction of the lumbar curve by the strut graft would secondarily produce correction of the thoracic curve.

It has been shown that the lumbosacral curve is compensatory to those above it. A study of 800 idiopathic curves by Fisk, Moe, and Winter[35] has shown that this area is not the cause of either lumbar or thoracic curves. The key point regarding the lumbosacral curve is related to its flexibility as seen on side-bending radiographs. In the young adolescent, a lumbosacral curve will readily straighten with side bending thereby centralizing L4 and L5 on the sacrum. In adults, the lumbosacral curve may become partially fixed, preventing a full return of L5 to the horizontal position.

TYPES OF IDIOPATHIC SCOLIOSIS

Infantile Idiopathic Scoliosis

Infantile idiopathic scoliosis is classically described as a lateral curvature of the spine that is structural and has its onset in patients under 3 years of age. Rare in the United States, most cases of infantile scoliosis occur in Europe.

One of the first reports in the literature is by Harrenstein of Amsterdam in 1929;[39] in 1936[40] he enlarged upon this and reported on 46 cases. Harrenstein considered rickets to be the etiology. He noted an onset at age two, a preponderance in girls, and satisfactory outcome of patients with a single curve treated in plaster. The first description of infantile scoliosis as it is understood today was made by James in 1951.[48] He presented 33 cases of idiopathic scoliosis with an onset before age 3, noting that as opposed to adolescent idiopathic scoliosis, boys outnumbered girls, with the curves being primarily thoracic and convex to the left. Four curves of less than 20 degrees resolved, eleven remained stationary during the period of observation, and the remaining 18 progressed with 12 of them exceeding 50 degrees.

In 1955, Scott and Morgan[95] analyzed 28 cases of progressive and seven cases of resolving infantile scoliosis; their results confirmed the findings of James. Boys were affected more frequently than girls, and the majority of curves occurred in the thoracic spine and were convex to the left.

James, Lloyd-Roberts, and Pilchers' review[46] of 212 patients and Lloyd-Roberts and Pilchers' 1965 review[55] of 100 patients further substantiated the previous observations concerning infantile scoliosis. Perhaps the most significant point brought out in all four of these studies is the fact that two types of infantile scoliosis exist, resolving and progressive. Occurrence of the progressive type ranged from 8 to 64 per cent of patients studied.[46, 55] The investigators were not able to distinguish the two groups of infantile scoliosis using various factors, including age of onset, curve length, degree of rotation, rate of progression, and the presence of a compensatory curve. Conner's study[21] of 61 patients in 1969 found a higher incidence of developmental anomalies in patients with the progressive type. He suggested that this could possibly be used to identify the patient with progressive infantile scoliosis.

In 1972, Mehta[67] reviewed the charts and radiographs of 361 patients with infantile scoliosis seen at the Royal National Orthopaedic Hospital in London. By contacting the mothers, she located 138 patients who returned for follow-up study consisting of clinical and radiologic examinations. Mehta noted certain differences between the resolving and progressive types of curves concerning the relationship between the rib and vertebral body as seen on the PA radiographs. Despite the similarity of the early curves in both groups, she was able to distinguish the progressive from the resolving curve by measuring the rib-vertebral angle difference (RVAD) at the apical vertebra of the thoracic curve. The rib-vertebral angle (RVA) is constructed by the intersection of a line perpendicular to the apical vertebral endplate with a line drawn from the midneck to the midhead of the corresponding rib. The rib-vertebral angle difference is the difference between the RVA of the concave and convex ribs of the apical vertebra. In a straight spine the RVAD is zero. In a scoliotic spine the convex ribs form a more acute angle with the vertebral body than do the concave ribs, thereby producing a RVAD that is greater than zero.

In addition to the RVAD, Mehta described two phases that helped distinguish between progressive and resolving infantile curves. Phase I is the early stage of infantile scoliosis in which the convex rib head does not overlap the vertebral body on the PA radiograph. Phase II is the next stage of progressive deformity in which the rib head overlaps the vertebral body on the PA radiograph (Fig. 11–1).

Mehta used the Phase and RVAD systems to distinguish the progressive from the resolving infantile curve. Eighty per cent of resolving curves had an initial RVAD of less than 20 degrees; the remaining 20 per cent had a RVAD greater than 20 degrees. On follow-up examination three months later, the RVAD decreased even if the curve itself showed an increase. Eighty per cent of progressive curves had an initial RVAD of greater than 20 degrees; the remaining 20 per cent had an initial RVAD of less than 20 degrees. At the three month follow-up, the RVAD was either the same or had increased. In addition, the transition from Phase I to Phase II signalled a progressive curve. Follow-up observations by Mehta have shown that the use of the RVAD and Phase systems as curve predictors have a 20 per cent inaccuracy rate.[66] Further studies[16, 103] using the RVAD and Phases I and II to determine the prognosis of infantile scoliosis have confirmed the usefulness of these criteria.

Wynne-Davies'[120] 1975 review of 134 patients with infantile scoliosis added further insight into this condition. Ninety-seven of the patients developed a curve in the first six months of life. Three per cent of parents and three per cent of siblings had the same deformity. This was 30 times the expected rate for the normal population.[119] The male-to-female ratio was 3:2. Ninety-eight per cent of the curves were thoracic, and 76 per cent were convex to the left. Six curves were present at birth, 91 developed between one and six months, the remaining 37 appeared between seven months and three years.

Other defects were associated with infantile scoliosis, the most common of which was plagiocephaly. This occurred in all 97 patients who had the appearance of scoliosis in the first six months of life. The flattened side of the head corresponded to the convexity of the curve in all cases. Mental retardation was the next most common abnormality affecting 13 per cent of males with progressive scoliosis. No patient with resolving scoliosis was mentally retarded. Congenital dislocation of the hip affected 3.5 per cent of all patients, while congenital heart disease was present in 2.5 per cent.

TREATMENT

In examining a patient with infantile idiopathic scoliosis the rigidity of the curve should be assessed by holding the infant suspended under the arms. It has been noted that the small, rigid curve may progress very rapidly.[64] A thorough neurologic evaluation of the patient should be performed. The presence or absence of hypotonia should be noted. The radiographic evaluation should include both suspended and supine films in the PA and lateral projections. All vertebrae

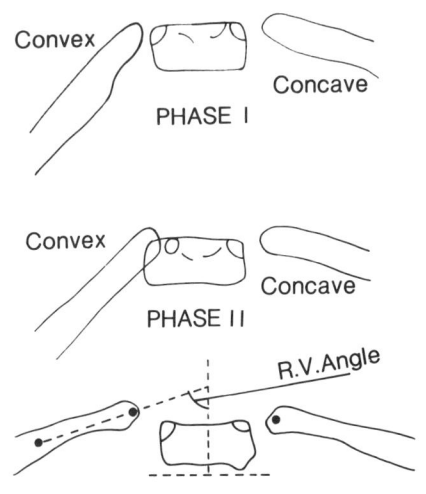

Figure 11–1. Phase I and Phase II, Method of measuring R-V angle (see text). (Redrawn from Mehta, M. H.: The rib-vertebra angle in the early diagnosis between resolving and progressive infantile scoliosis. J. Bone Joint Surg., 54B:230–243, 1972.)

must be seen and the presence of a possible congenital abnormality of the spine sought. The Cobb measurement of the curve as well as the RVAD and Phase of Mehta should be determined.

In addition to evaluating infantile scoliosis, the orthopaedist must also be aware of and look for associated anomalies. A heart murmur may signal the presence of congenital heart disease. The hips must be examined to assure that they are not dislocated. The presence of an inguinal hernia should be searched for, and some assessment as to the patient's mental status should be made.

Once the patient has been clinically and radiographically assessed, a treatment plan must be made. Resolving curves are noted radiographically by the presence of Phase I and a RVAD difference of less than 20 degrees. Patients who fall into this category and have curves that measure less than 25 degrees require no active treatment. Follow-up examination and radiographs should be performed every four to six months until the curve has resolved. Once the curve has resolved follow-up should continue at one to two year intervals until skeletal maturity, as occasional recurrences have been noted (Fig. 11–2).

The progressive-type of infantile idiopathic scoliosis is noted on the PA radiograph by the presence of Phase II and a RVAD greater than 20 degrees. Early detection and treatment are necessary to prevent these curves from progressing to significant levels. An attempt should be made to control the curve non-operatively until the patient has grown sufficiently to allow spinal arthrodesis without significant shortening of the spinal column.[63] A short straight spine is preferable to a still shorter crooked one, and if curve progression cannot be halted by non-operative methods, then either instrumentation without arthrodesis or immediate arthrodesis is indicated (Fig. 11–3).

In infants and toddlers the curve is best controlled by a well applied body cast, which is fitted while the child is under anesthesia. As the patient grows older, has more body definition, and becomes more cooperative, the Milwaukee brace is used. If the curve is controlled non-operatively, bracing may be continued throughout growth or until control is lost, often at the adolescent growth spurt.

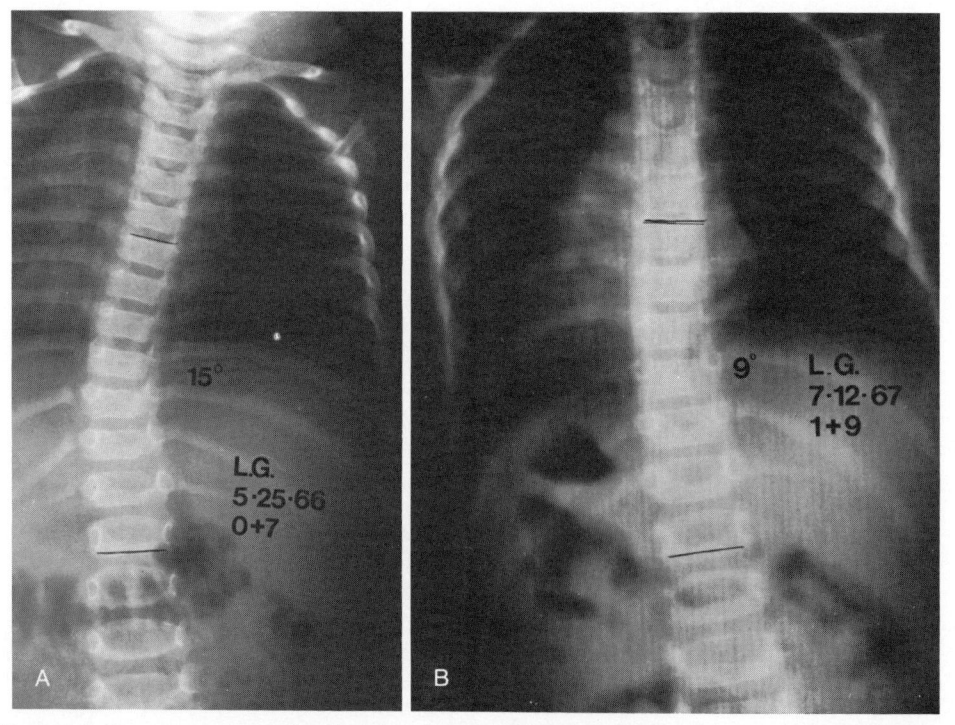

Figure 11–2. A, L.G., age seven months. Note the characteristic left thoracic curve, the RVAD of 5 degrees at the apical vertebra, and the Phase. B, L.G., age 1+9 years. Fourteen months later the curve had improved without treatment.

IDIOPATHIC SCOLIOSIS

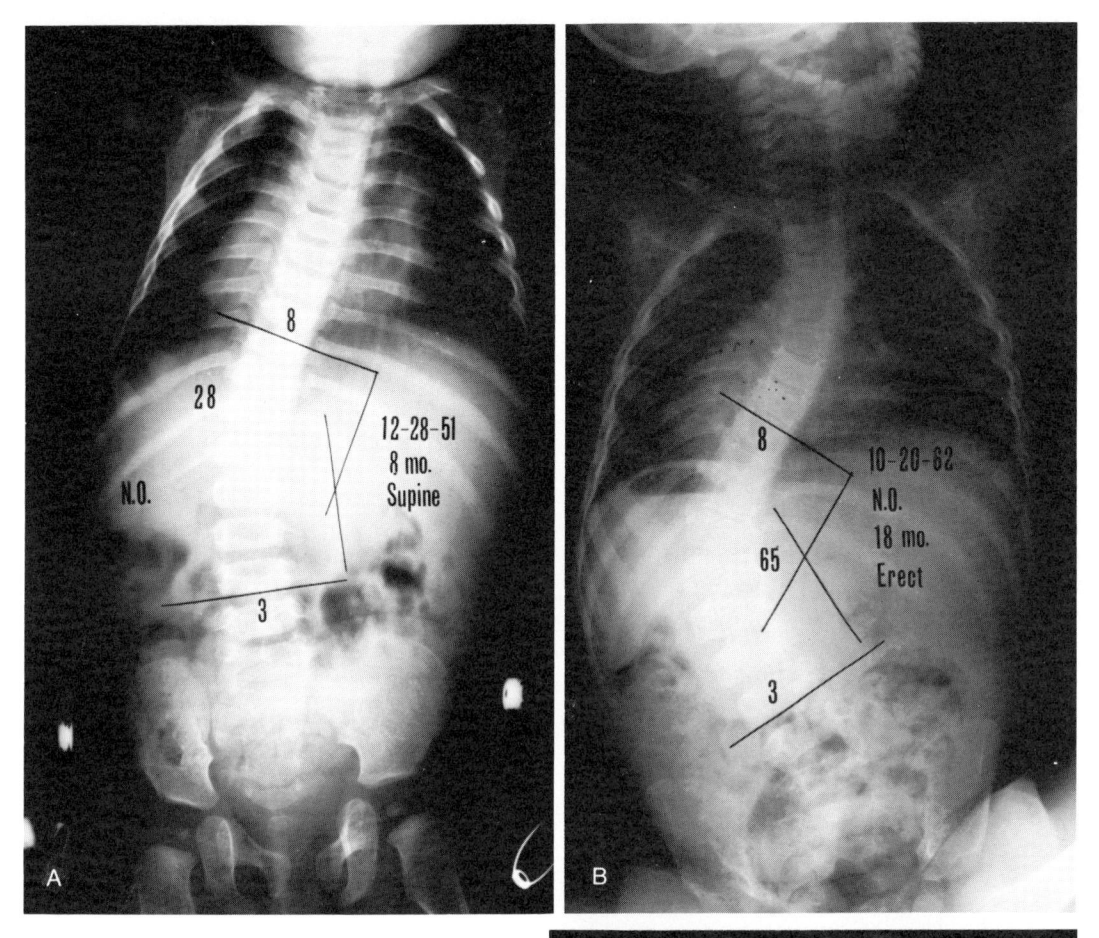

Figure 11–3. A, N.O., an eight month old female with an infantile idiopathic curve. Note the RVAD of 39 degrees at the apical vertebra. B, N.O., age 18 months. Note curve progression. C, N.O. age 4 + 11 years. Curve has progressed despite Milwaukee brace treatment. The patient was then placed in a Risser localizer cast with correction of the curve at 40 degrees. Patient wore the cast for six months and a second attempt was made to treat the curve with the Milwaukee brace. Progression of the curve continued in brace, requiring fusion at age 11 + 8 years at 60 degrees. Loss of correction followed to 73 degrees in 1972, with no further loss of correction.

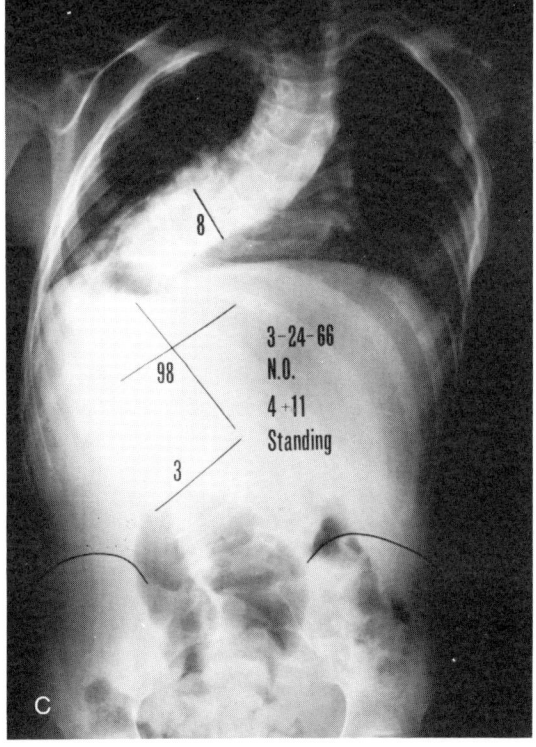

Mehta has recently observed that some curves falling into the progressive category may not require surgery because of satisfactory and lasting correction obtained from repeated casting.[65] Serial corrective casts are applied every two to three months in an attempt to straighten the curve and decrease the RVAD to zero. Once the curve is straightened and the RVAD is zero, casting is continued, allowing the spine to grow in a corrected position for three to six months. This is followed by a period of bracing to maintain the curve in its corrected state. If no evidence of relapse occurs, as indicated by an unchanging Cobb angle and RVAD, the brace is discontinued and the patient is observed to maturity. Mehta and Morel[68] have observed that if the curve is totally corrected prior to the pre-pubertal growth spurt, there will be no relapse during adolescence. If full correction has not been obtained, a small relapse may occur.

If curve control cannot be maintained with bracing, then there is no viable treatment option other than surgical stabilization of the curve. One must not continue to follow these patients with the hope that the scoliosis will improve with time. There are two surgical options (1) instrumentation without fusion (see Chapter 10), and (2) fusion of the curve. The surgeon must decide between these two options based on the flexibility of the curve. A flexible curve that partially corrects on a traction radiograph or a side-bending film is suitable for instrumentation without fusion. The rigid curve that shows little flexibility probably will not benefit from this approach and should be fused posteriorly. The selection of the fusion levels and instrumentation will be discussed later in the chapter.

Juvenile Idiopathic Scoliosis

Idiopathic scoliosis appearing between the ages of four and the beginning of adolescence is designated juvenile idiopathic scoliosis and is found in 12 to 16 per cent of all patients with idiopathic scoliosis. Ponseti and Friedman's review[88] of 335 scoliotic patients found 13 per cent occur in patients less than 10 years old. James'[47] evaluation of 134 patients with thoracic curves found 16 cases to occur in patients under 10 years of age. Twenty-six cases of juvenile scoliosis were found by Moe and Kettleson[74] in their review of 169 patients. Keiser and Shufflebarger[51] reported 20 patients with juvenile scoliosis out of 123 cases.

Various male-to-female ratios have been reported, but all authors agree that juvenile idiopathic scoliosis occurs in girls more frequently than in boys.[33, 47, 105] If different age groups are examined within the juvenile category, it becomes apparent that the sex ratio in patients age 4 to 6 is nearly equal. This is probably because this age group represents the infantile idiopathic classification, which began before age 3 and progressed to a substantial curve after age 4 or 5 years. The preponderance of female patients occurs in the 7 to 10 year old age group.

Various curve patterns occur in juvenile idiopathic scoliosis, and there is no consensus as to which one is most common. James[47] reported that combined thoracic and lumbar curves occur most frequently, whereas Figueiredo and James[33] found the single right thoracic curve to predominate. Tolo and Gillespie[105] found the right thoracic curve to predominate in the 4 to 6 year old age group; in older children the number of double curves equaled single thoracic curves. There is general agreement that the convexity of the thoracic curve is predominantly to the right. There is also agreement that the borderline between late infantile and early juvenile idiopathic scoliosis is hazy. Likewise, many and perhaps a majority of adolescent idiopathic patients have small curves during their juvenile years that are not recognized until adolescence.

TREATMENT

Observation is the preferred treatment for curves of less than 20 degrees. Following the initial evaluation, patients should be seen every four to six months for an examination and a standing PA radiograph. Follow-up should be continued until the patient has reached skeletal maturity and the risk of curve progression low. Special attention should be paid to the patient during the time of the adolescent growth spurt, since there is an increased chance of curve progression during this period (Fig. 11–4).

If definite curve progression past 20 to 25 degrees is documented radiographically, brace treatment should be initiated. The examiner must be sure that he or she is not misled by a change in posture during the radiographic examination. Unequal weight-bearing or torso rotation may give a false

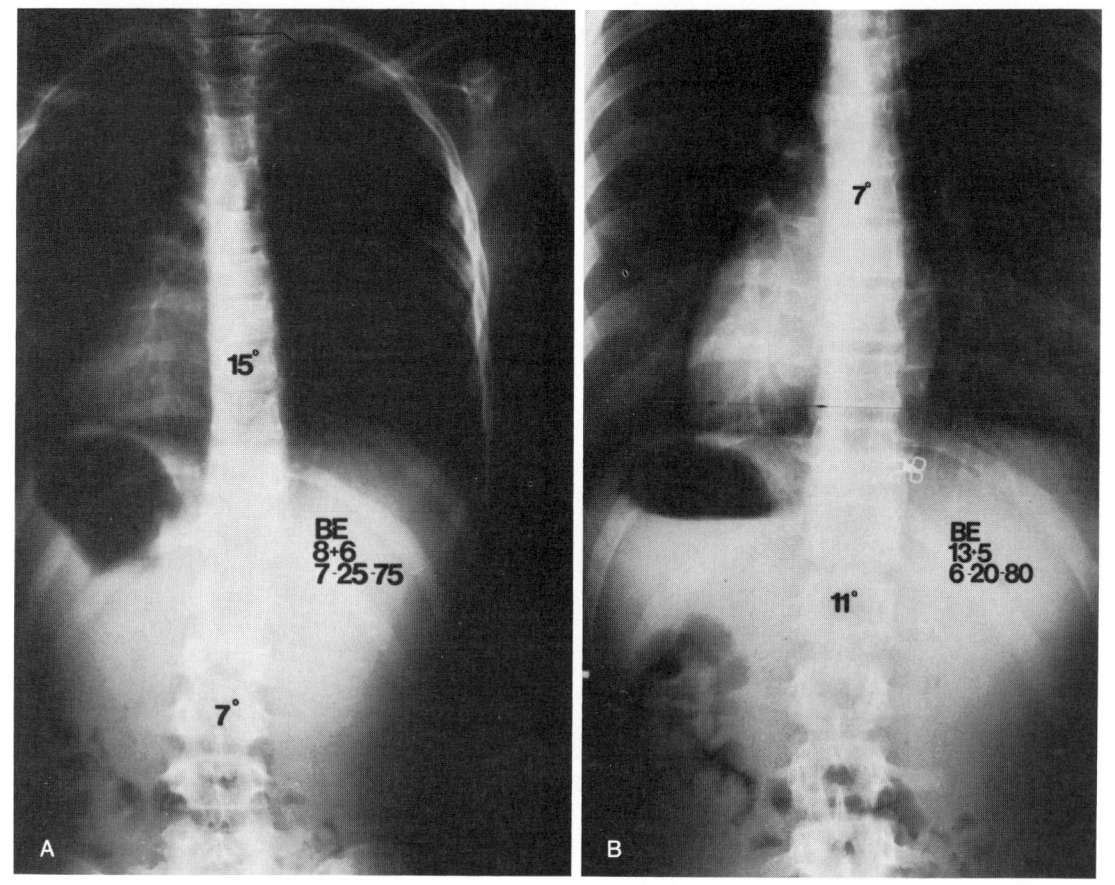

Figure 11–4. *A*, B.E., an 8+6 year old female, was referred for evaluation. Observation only was recommended. *B*, Patient is now 13+5 years old and a Risser 3. The thoracic curve has decreased and there is only a minimal increase in the lumbar curve.

impression of curve increase. We favor the Milwaukee brace for thoracic curves or double major curves and the TLSO for thoracolumbar curves or lumbar curves. Fulltime wear of the orthosis is begun initially. If the curve stabilizes or improves after fulltime bracing for a year or more, the patient may go to part-time bracing. Routine follow-up must be continued, and the wearing time is increased if curve progression occurs (Fig. 11–5). The success of non-operative treatment is variable. Forty-four per cent of Figueiredo's[33] series of 98 patients were managed by bracing or observation. Seven cases showed spontaneous resolution of the curve. In Tolo's[105] series of 59 patients, 73 per cent were managed non-operatively, while 16 patients required surgical treatment for progressive curves. Unfortunately, accurate predictors of curve progression have not been found to exist; therefore, all patients must be closely followed.

SURGICAL TREATMENT

If orthotic treatment with the Milwaukee brace or TLSO does not halt curve progression, surgical stabilization of the curve is indicated. It has been established that a solidly fused spine does not lengthen during growth; therefore, fusion should be avoided if possible during the earlier juvenile years. Moe, Sundberg, and Gustilo[76] reviewed 78 spine fusions after a period of several years in patients with an average age at fusion of 7.5 years. Only those showing no increase in the curvature were included in the study. They found that on the PA radiograph taken at a 6 foot distance, almost none showed an increase in length of the fusion mass and the few that did could be ascribed to an increase in the size of the thorax.

In 1984, Moe and coworkers[75] reported on the Twin Cities Scoliosis Center experience with distraction instrumentation without fu-

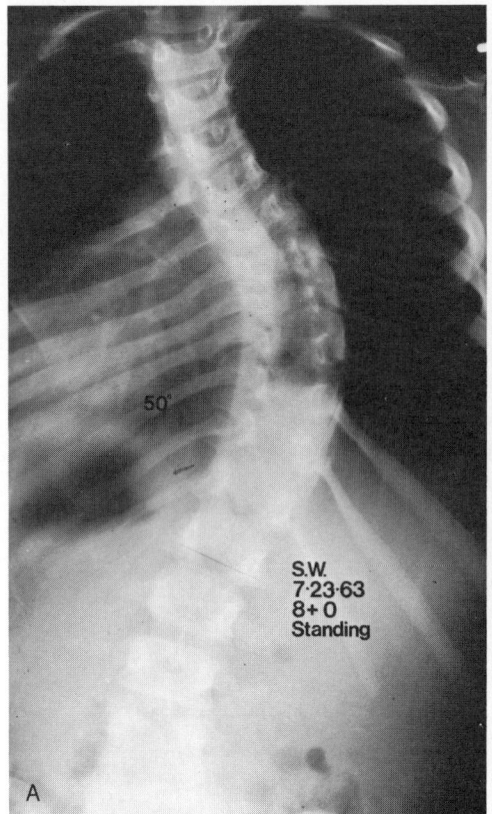

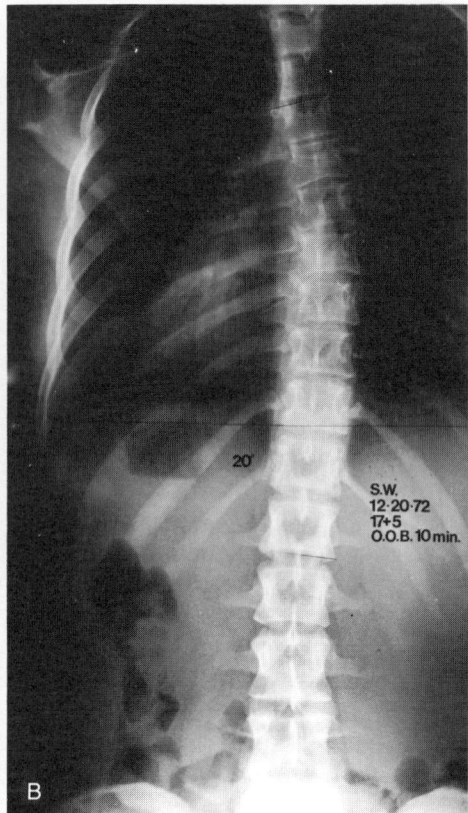

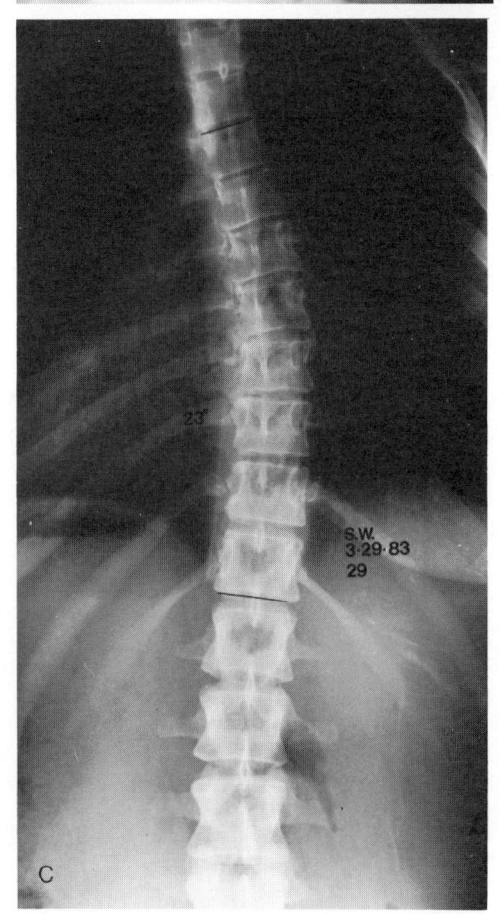

Figure 11–5. *A*, S.W., an 8+0 year old female with a juvenile idiopathic curve. Patient was placed in a Milwaukee brace. *B*, S.W., age 17+5 years. Weaning from the Milwaukee brace began at this time. *C*, S.W., age 29 years. Patient has now been out of the brace 11 years without significant increase in her curve.

sion in an attempt to prevent the shortening of the trunk that an early fusion produces. Internal fixation of the spine without fusion was first described by Harrington in 1962.[42] His technique failed for two reasons: (1) the spine was subperiosteally exposed for rod placement, which produced spontaneous fusion; and (2) no external support was used, resulting in hook slippage and rod breakage. In 1977, Marchetti and Faldini[61] described the "end fusion" technique, which consisted of posterior fusion of two vertebrae at each end of the curve followed six months later by the subperiosteal placement of a distraction rod between the two end fusions without further fusion. Although the Milwaukee brace was used postoperatively, problems still existed with spontaneous fusion due to the subperiosteal stripping. Moe and coworkers'[75] technique consisted of end fusion with placement of a distraction rod during the same surgery. Unlike the techniques previously described, in Moe's technique[75] only the end vertebrae were subperiosteally exposed for fusion and hook placement, leaving the remainder of the curve undisturbed by the distraction rod lying in the subcutaneous tissue.[75] The Milwaukee brace was used postoperatively. Using this technique, Moe and associates[75] reported on 20 patients, nine of whom had undergone definitive fusion at the time of the report. The average growth of the area instrumented in these nine patients was 3.8 cm., and no spontaneous fusions at the curve apices were noted prior to the definitive fusion. This technique allows the spine to grow in length while maintaining the curve at an acceptable level prior to a more optimal time for fusion (Fig. 11-6).

If a curve continues to progress beyond 60 degrees despite the use of an orthosis or distraction instrumentation without fusion, then spinal arthrodesis should be performed (Fig. 11-7). The fusion area in the juvenile curve should follow the rules set forth in the section *Selection of the Fusion Area* (see page 216). Currently recommended is the use of the Harrington distraction instrumentation and a facet fusion. On occasion, sublaminar wires are added to increase the stability of the implant. A solid fusion will usually prevent curve progression, although protection of the fusion mass by a brace may be necessary since the immature fusion mass in the young patient is plastic and may further rotate and deform with growth. Progression of the curve postoperatively in the brace probably indicates a pseudarthrosis or "adding on" of vertebrae to the curve. The spine should be re-explored and any pseudarthrosis repaired with or without extension of the fusion level as indicated.

In summary, curves less than 20 to 25 degrees may be observed, while those progressing beyond this point should be braced. An attempt is made to halt progression of the curve past 50 to 60 degrees using bracing with or without a subcutaneously placed distraction rod while awaiting a more optimum age for fusion. This allows the spine time to reach maturity and full growth. If, however, a curve continues to progress beyond 60 degrees despite bracing and subcutaneous rod placement, fusion of the major curve should be done.

Adolescent Idiopathic Scoliosis

Most cases of idiopathic scoliosis in the United States fall into the adolescent category because they are discovered during the pubertal growth spurt. A majority of these curves probably begin during the juvenile years and become apparent only after they increase during adolescence. Curves tend to increase during adolescence because of the rapid growth that is occuring and the destabilizing effect this has on the curved spine.[10] Not all adolescent curves progress, and it is this variability in behavior that poses problems to the physician caring for a patient with adolescent idiopathic scoliosis (Fig. 11-8).

GENERAL INFORMATION

Many studies have been done since Shands and Eisberg's 1955 review of 50,000 minifilms in an attempt to accurately determine the prevalence rate of adolescent idiopathic scoliosis.[97] Confusion has persisted; there has been a misuse of terms with regard to incidence rate versus prevalence rate. Most of the data has been generated through school screening surveys, which attempt to determine the number of a select group of people who have a lateral curvature of the spine at one point in time. This is a prevalence rate—not an incidence rate as it has been called by some. The magnitude of curvature that constitutes idiopathic scoliosis has also varied between examiners. This has produced prevalence rates that vary greatly. Another problem is that most of the studies lack

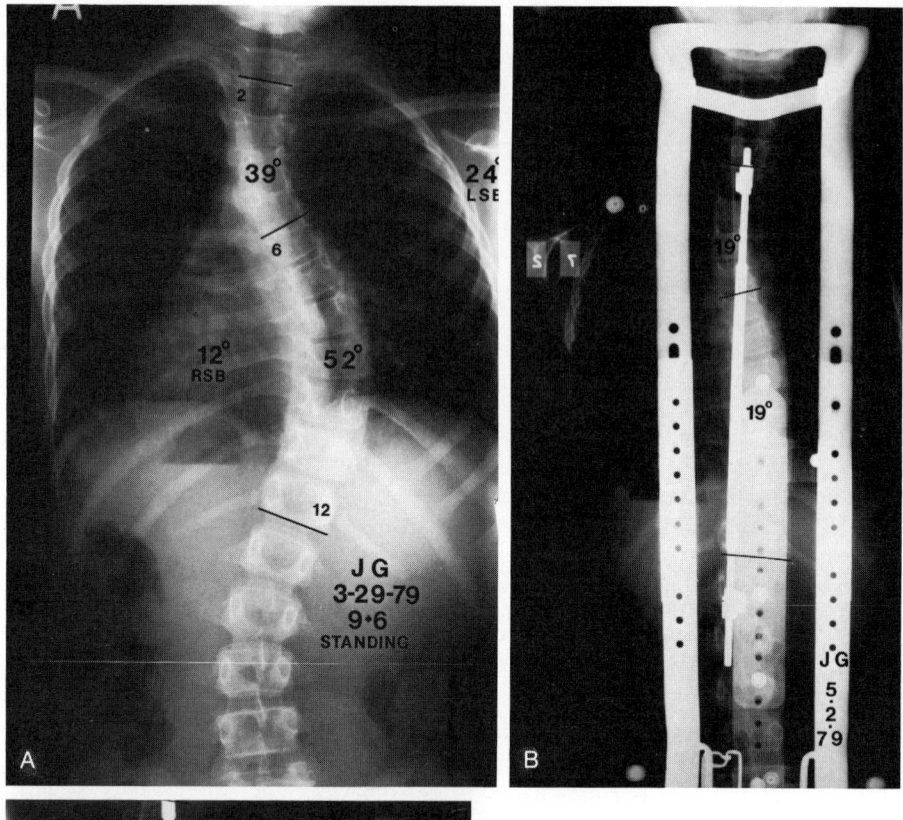

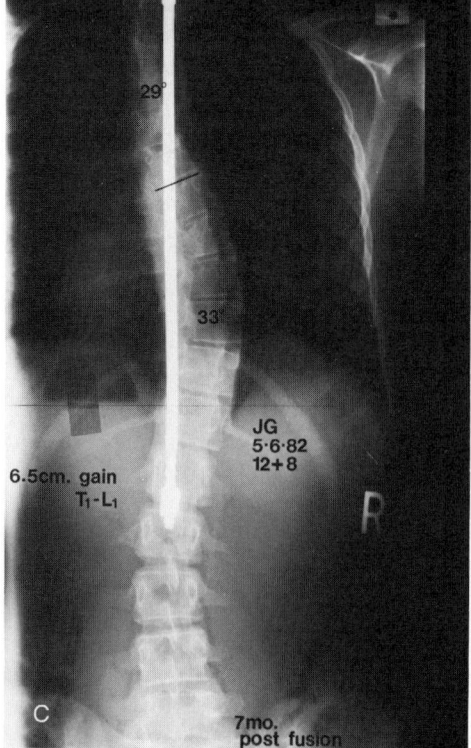

Figure 11–6. *A*, J.G., a 9+6 year old female with juvenile idiopathic scoliosis, was first seen with this curve. Because of the magnitude of the curve, instrumentation without fusion was recommended. *B*, This is the patient's film prior to discharge after placement of the Moe distraction rod without fusion of the curve. *C*, Patient underwent three lengthenings of the subcutaneous rod prior to her definitive fusion on October 26, 1981. Placement of the subcutaneous rod allowed a spinal growth of 6.5 centimeters prior to the definitive fusion.

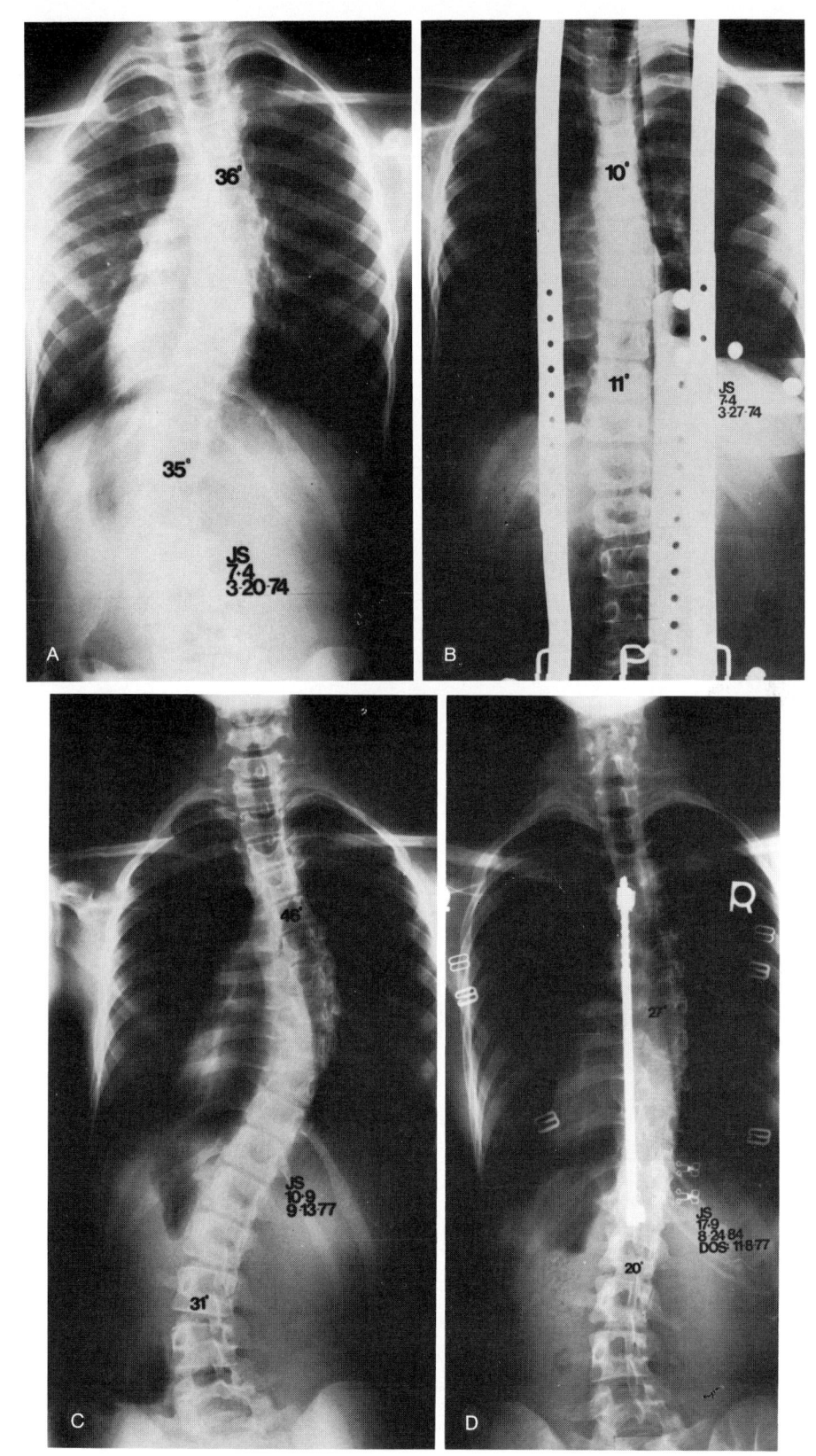

Figure 11–7. J.S. is a 7+4 year old female with juvenile idiopathic scoliosis who was placed in a Milwaukee brace when initially seen. *B,* The patient's curve corrected to 10 degrees and 11 degrees respectively in brace. *C,* Despite compliance, the patient's curves increased, necessitating fusion. *D,* The patient, nearly 7 years following surgery, has a solid fusion without curve progression.

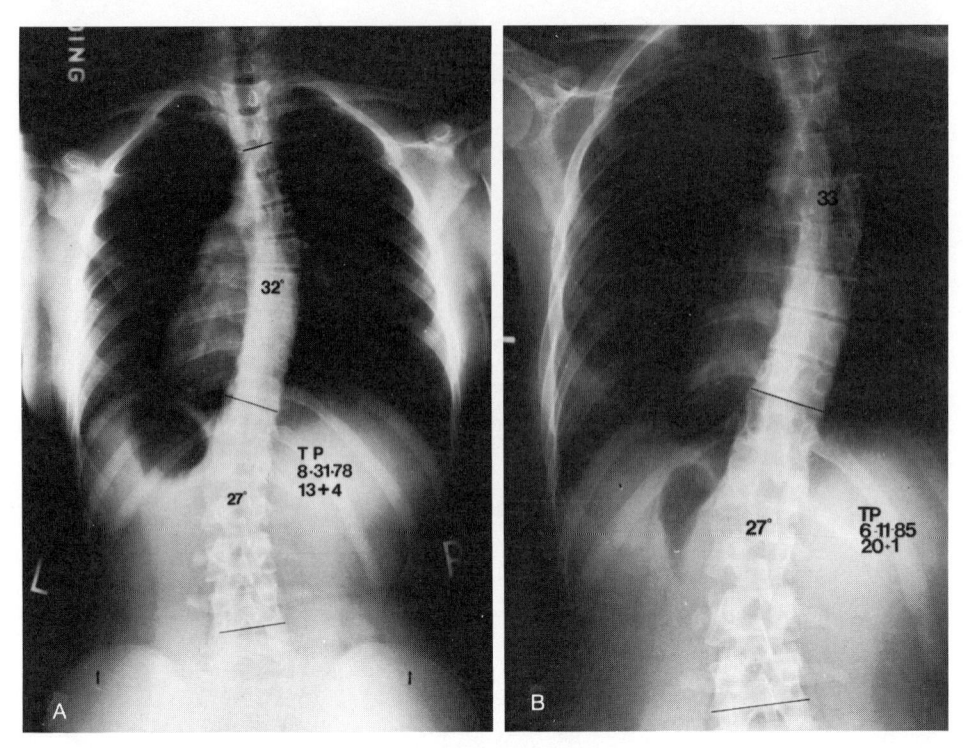

Figure 11–8. A, T.P., a 13+4 year old female, was first seen in the clinic with these curves. A Milwaukee brace was recommended; however, because of religious beliefs this was not placed. B, The patient is now 20+1, a Risser 5, and shows only a 1 degree increase in her right thoracic curve and no change in the lower curve.

sufficient data to allow extrapolation in an attempt to reach a consensus.

Most studies reflect a prevalence rate of approximately 2 to 4 per cent of the population for curves of at least 10 degrees.[27, 45, 47, 56, 84] Also of importance is the prevalence rate for curves with magnitudes greater than 20 degrees, because these patients are the ones who will possibly require treatment. Again, there is some discrepancy in the reported rates, with most falling into the 0.13 to 0.30 per cent range.[25, 50, 91] In other words, one to three patients per thousand screened will have adolescent idiopathic curves greater than 20 degrees.

In the past, adolescent idiopathic scoliosis has been considered a disorder primarily of females. Female:male sex ratios have been reported ranging from 5:1 to 10:1.[34, 50, 119] No allowance has been made for curve magnitude when calculating this ratio. Two more recent reviews[25, 91] have found that the ratio is quite dependent on curve magnitude. For curves in the 10 degree range the ratio approaches 1:1. As the degree of lateral curvature increases so does the female:male ratio.

Rogala, Drummond, and Gurr[91] report a 5.4:1 ratio for curves greater than 21 degrees.

The various curve patterns encountered in idiopathic scoliosis have been described earlier in the chapter. Most researchers agree that thoracic curves are usually convex to the right, whereas lumbar curves are usually convex to the left. Dickson[26] has stated that right thoracic curves occur eight times more frequently than left thoracic curves. A recent study by Coonrad, and associates[22] has shown that idiopathic-appearing left thoracic curves have an increased incidence of syringomyelia. This suggests that patients with left thoracic curves must be thoroughly evaluated and a myelogram obtained if there is any evidence of a neurologic abnormality. Thoracolumbar curves are usually convex to the left; double major thoracic curves usually consist of a convex left upper and a convex right lower thoracic curve. Double major thoracic and lumbar curves are usually composed of a right thoracic and a left lumbar curve.

The frequency of the different patterns varies considerably, according to which study one reviews.[12, 17, 58, 88, 91, 111] There is no clear consensus whether the thoracic or thoracolumbar pattern occurs most frequently. Four of the seven studies indicate that the lumbar curve pattern occurs least frequently. Lonstein's review[58] of 727 patients found the following frequency of curve patterns: 31 per cent thoracic, 11 per cent lumbar, 10 per cent thoracolumbar, and 48 per cent double major.

The growth pattern of patients with adolescent idiopathic scoliosis has been shown o differ significantly from age matched non-scoliotic controls. Willner[112, 113] and Nordwall[83] have found that scoliotic girls are on the average taller than a control population even if the height loss due to the deformity is considered. Their body weight does not differ from controls and thus they are relatively leaner. The ratio of sitting-to-standing height is the same between the two groups. Buric and Momcilovic's review[14] of 207 scoliotic girls found that the standing and sitting heights were 5 cm. and 2 cm. greater, respectively, than 21 age matched controls. Drummond and Rogala[28] have reported that when the measurement of height and weight is corrected for skeletal age, both boys and girls with scoliosis are taller and heavier than normal. These studies as well as the one by Low and associates[60] have shown that early in adolescence (age 10 to 14) the girls with scoliosis are skeletally more mature than their non-scoliotic counterparts. After this period of time the patients with scoliosis appear to have slightly retarded skeletal development when compared to normal subjects.

DETERMINATION OF MATURATION

An increase in the rate of curve progression is often associated with the increased growth velocity seen during adolescence.[29] Knowledge of this allows the orthopaedist to follow the patient closely during this period of increased risk. If all patients matured at the same chronological age and with the same rate, this task would be quite easy; unfortunately this is not the case. In 95 per cent of males, the onset of puberty varies between the ages of 9 1/2 and 13 1/2 years and ends between 13 and 17 years. In a small percentage, the onset may not begin until age 15 years with a similar delay in the end. The duration of puberty in males also differs between patients with some maturing in 2 years whereas others may take longer than 4 1/2 years. Similarly, in females the age at the onset of puberty may also differ considerably. While the average age of menarche in American girls is 12 1/2 to 13 1/2 years, the range of normal is quite wide, and 1 to 2 per cent of normal girls have not menstruated by 16 years of age.[81]

The various determinants of maturation such as skeletal bone age, the Risser sign, and the Tanner classification are discussed in other chapters.

SCHOOL SCREENING

Idiopathic scoliosis is a treatable condition that should be detected early in order to prevent the progression of small deformities and assure optimum treatment results. One means of doing this is through the School Screening Program, which is conducted for children 10 to 16 years of age who are most at risk for progressive adolescent idiopathic scoliosis. Though controversy exists, we feel that school screening is an effective method of doing this. School screening is becoming widespread in the United States, Canada, and other countries but is mandatory only in Japan at present. Our first screening in Minnesota was begun in 1947.

Lonstein and coworkers' 1982 review[57] of Minnesota's voluntary school screening for students in Grades 5 to 9, age 10 to 16, indicated that the number of patients requiring surgery for idiopathic scoliosis has decreased since 1970; similarly, the average curve requiring surgery decreased from 60 to 42 degrees. Of this group, 3.4 per cent were referred for evaluation, and scoliosis was present in 1.2 per cent of the one and one quarter million students screened. The program was cost-effective based on 1980 medical rates, averaging 6.6 cents per student. While many screening techniques are available, such as Moire topography used in Canada and Japan, the Adams[1] forward bending test of the bare back was chosen in Minnesota because it is accurate, inexpensive, and easily taught to screening personnel.

Problems Lonstein reported during the statewide, voluntary screening program were over and under referral, lack of compliance by parents, and inaccurate opinions by physicians unaware of scoliosis problems; the cost factor was minimal and not a problem. The solution to these problems is education of everyone from the screening staff to the students, parents, and primary care physicians through workshops, PTA presentations, audiovisual demonstrations for students, and scientific lectures and displays.

It is hoped that school screening will ultimately prove to be an effective tool for the early recognition of adolescent idiopathic scoliosis and that through the early treatment of the progressive curve the incidence of those patients requiring surgery will be decreased.

TREATMENT

The need for follow-up of patients with curves less than 10 degrees depends on their age and degree of maturity. Patients who are mature need not be seen again. If the patient is physically immature, a follow-up examination and radiograph are recommended in six months.

For curves felt to be greater than 10 degrees, standing PA and lateral radiographs are obtained on the first visit. The degree of thoracic kyphosis and lumbar lordosis and the presence or absence of spondylolisthesis are evaluated on the lateral view. After the first visit, patients should be seen at four to six month intervals for a clinical evaluation and standing PA radiograph to monitor the curve for progression. Follow-up is continued until the patient reaches skeletal maturity. Patients with curves of 10 to 20 degrees at the time of skeletal maturity are discharged from future follow-up. Patients with curves greater than 20 degrees who have not required treatment are seen at one and two years after skeletal maturity to evaluate possible progression. If none is detected, the patient is discharged.

A curve greater than 20 degrees in an immature adolescent places that patient at an increased risk for curve progression. A follow-up clinical examination and standing PA radiograph are recommended at four month intervals. Indication for non-operative treatment is a curve of 25 to 30 degrees that has progressed more than 5 degrees in a patient who has at least one year of growth remaining. An increase of 2 to 3 degrees between a series of films may be interpreted as measurement error. To avoid this, the current radiograph should always be compared to the initial film as well as the last film. Occasionally, a patient may be treated on the basis of an increasing rib prominence even though the Cobb measurement does not change. Treatment is also recommended for the immature patient seen for the first time with a 30 to 40 degree curve. Waiting for curve progression might place this patient in the surgical category without ever giving the orthopaedist a chance to control the curve non-operatively. Non-progressive curves of 20 to 40 degrees in skeletally mature patients do not require treatment.

NON-OPERATIVE TREATMENT OF ADOLESCENT IDIOPATHIC SCOLIOSIS

While exercises may be prescribed as an adjunct to the non-operative treatment of idiopathic scoliosis, they are not in and of themselves therapeutic. Exercises will not prevent curve progression and should not be expected to do so.

Ten years ago the Milwaukee brace was routinely used at our center to treat the progressive curve in an immature patient. Since that time other treatment modalities have been introduced, making the treatment decision somewhat more complicated. Among these new treatment options are the TLSO and transcutaneous electrical muscle stimulation. While all three modalities are used to treat idiopathic scoliosis, each method has its own guidelines for use.

Orthotic Treatment. Orthoses used to treat idiopathic scoliosis may be divided into two general categories. One is the CTLSO as represented by the Milwaukee brace, first introduced by Blount and Schmidt at the 1946 Academy of Orthopaedic Surgeons. The other is the TLSO, of which there are many varieties. We reserve the use of the TLSO for thoracolumbar and lumbar curves. Thoracic and double-major thoracic and lumbar curves should be treated with a Milwaukee brace because it is difficult to control a thoracic curve with an apex higher than T8 with a TLSO. Others, however, have reported the treatment of thoracic curves with a TLSO.[13, 49] It is also our impression that chest expansion is limited, and therefore pulmonary function may be altered when a TLSO is properly constructed to control a thoracic curve. Conversely, the Milwaukee brace allows chest expansion away from the pads and straps and thus interferes little with pulmonary function.

The primary goal of orthotic treatment is to prevent curve progression and secondarily to achieve some curve correction (Fig. 11–9). While initial curve correction may be significant in an orthosis, this correction may be lost after the brace is removed. Carr and

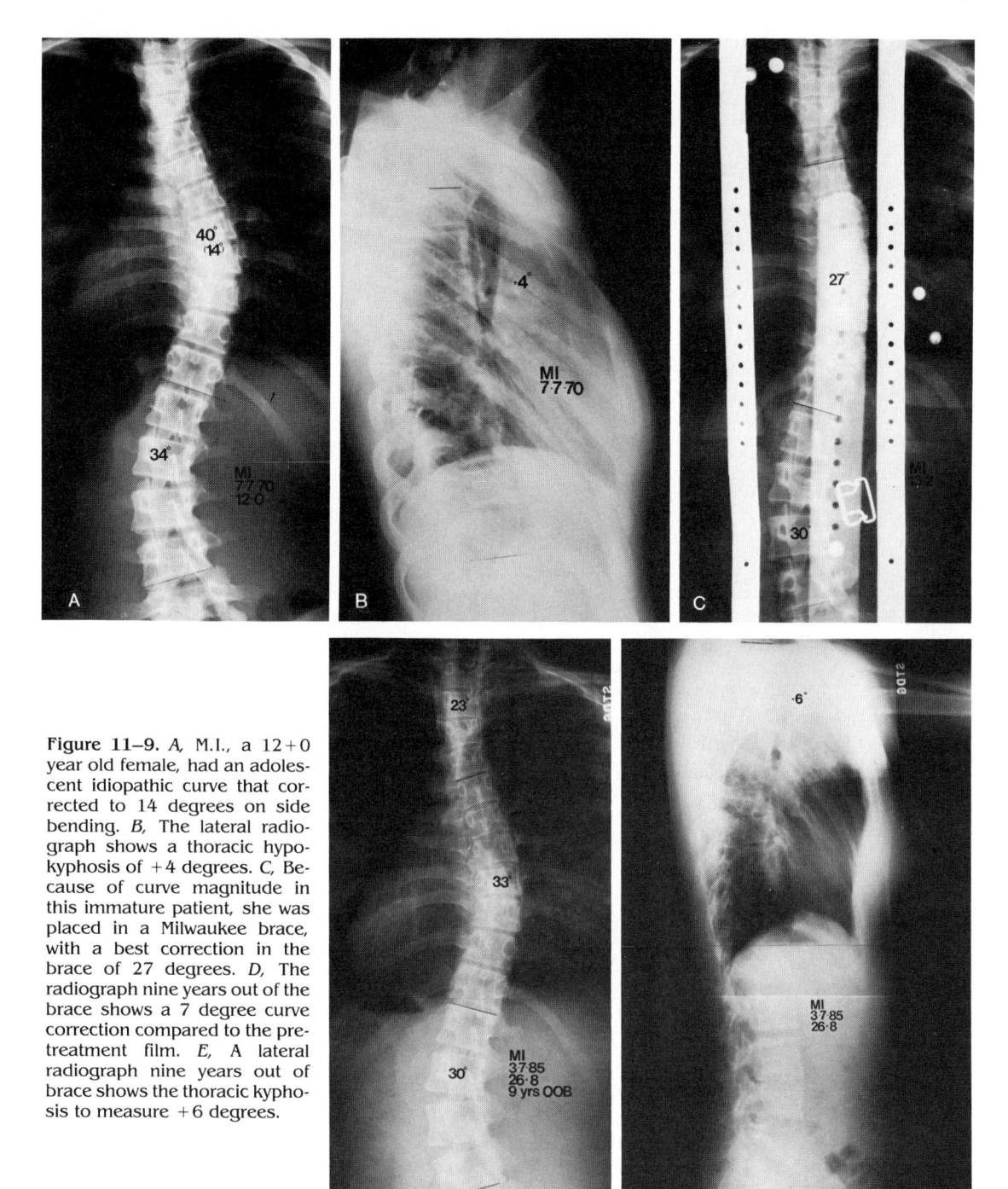

Figure 11–9. A, M.I., a 12+0 year old female, had an adolescent idiopathic curve that corrected to 14 degrees on side bending. B, The lateral radiograph shows a thoracic hypokyphosis of +4 degrees. C, Because of curve magnitude in this immature patient, she was placed in a Milwaukee brace, with a best correction in the brace of 27 degrees. D, The radiograph nine years out of the brace shows a 7 degree curve correction compared to the pretreatment film. E, A lateral radiograph nine years out of brace shows the thoracic kyphosis to measure +6 degrees.

coworkers[15] reviewed 133 patients treated for idiopathic scoliosis with a Milwaukee brace, 74 of whom had at least a five year follow-up. The average correction for a thoracic curve was 2 degrees (range −18 to 24 degrees) and 4 degrees for thoracolumbar and lumbar curves (range −11 to 17 degrees). Eighty-six patients with curves greater than 40 degrees were treated. Of these, 30 (35 per cent) eventually required surgical stabilization because of curve progression. It was found that brace treatment is most effective for curves less than 40 degrees. The best predictor of successful brace treatment was the initial correction achieved in the brace. If a curve was corrected by 50 per cent or more, there was a good chance that the orthotic treatment would be successful. Age, curve pattern, and the status of the iliac and ring apophyses did not correlate with a successful result.

Mellencamp and coworkers[69] reviewed 47 patients with a five year follow-up treated by Milwaukee bracing and came to similar conclusions. One third of the patients lost 5 degrees or less after bracing was stopped at skeletal age 18. The other two-thirds continued to progress until the curves stabilized when the patients reached their mid or late twenties. The average improvement at follow-up was 3 degrees compared to the pretreatment curvature, although there was a range from a gain of 40 degrees to a loss of 26 degrees.

In 1984 Winter and associates[116] reported on 95 growing patients with 30 to 39 degree idiopathic thoracic curves treated by Milwaukee bracing. All patients were managed by the same protocol, including exercises, a 23 hour per day wearing schedule, and weaning only after all growth had ceased and the Risser sign was at least 4. Follow-up averaged 2.5 years out of brace or until surgery. Of the 95 patients treated, only 14 (16 per cent) went on to surgery. For the 81 patients not requiring surgery, the average pretreatment curve was 33 degrees, the best in-brace curve was 21 degrees, the curve at brace discontinuance was 29 degrees, and the curve at follow-up was 31 degrees. For the 14 patients who went on to surgery, the average pretreatment curve was 33 degrees, the best corrected curve was 26 degrees, and the curve at the time surgery was decided upon was 40 degrees. In conclusion, this study showed an 84 per cent success rate for the treatment of high risk thoracic curves by the Milwaukee brace. Others have also reported good results with the Milwaukee brace though their follow-up is less than two years.[31, 51]

Within the past five years there has been a revival of the use of the TLSO or body jacket for non-operative treatment of scoliosis in this country (Fig. 11–10). The most popular of these is the Boston prefabricated module system. Review of the literature of the last century reveals many varieties of these external supportive jackets and braces; most of the recently described "new" body braces and jackets are copies of some of these, with the exception of those now manufactured with some form of plastic.

In 1984, Emans and coworkers[32] reported their results of 295 patients with idiopathic scoliosis treated by the Boston bracing system. Criteria for inclusion in this study were: (1) age 4 to 18 years at the initiation of bracing, (2) pre-brace curve of 20 to 59 degrees, and (3) follow-up greater than one year after cessation of bracing. Initial or best in-brace correction averaged 55 per cent. Average time in brace was 2.9 years. Mean final correction at follow-up was 10 per cent. Eleven per cent of patients required surgery before the end of bracing, and 1 per cent required surgery after the cessation of bracing. At follow-up 52 per cent of patients were within +/− 5 degrees of the initial pre-brace curve, 38 per cent showed correction of greater than 5 degrees, and 10 per cent had lost more than 5 degrees. Early in this study, braces with superstructures were used to treat thoracic curves. Later the superstructures were abandoned. Equal results were noted for similar thoracic curves treated by the Boston prefabricated module system both with and without the superstructures. Another published report[13] has also shown the TLSO to stabilize thoracolumbar and lumbar curves; however, the follow-up for this study was quite short. There have been no five year follow-up studies in this country to allow comparison of the TLSO with the Milwaukee brace. Even the studies noted above use different indications for bracing and different evaluation criteria, making comparison of the different treatment methods even more difficult.

No brace has proved to be of real value in controlling or improving the double thoracic curve pattern. The lower thoracic curve may respond to bracing, but there does not seem to be a brace capable of improving the high thoracic structural curve. This is due to the fact that this curve is usually short and that it is difficult to apply a corrective force to the apical rib because of interference from the scapula. If the high thoracic curve remains small and the neck deformity minimal, no treatment is required. Some curves do progress creating a high rib elevation and noticeable neck asymmetry and necessitating surgical treatment.

Extreme care must be used when bracing the hypokyphotic spine to prevent further flattening by posterior pad placement. To

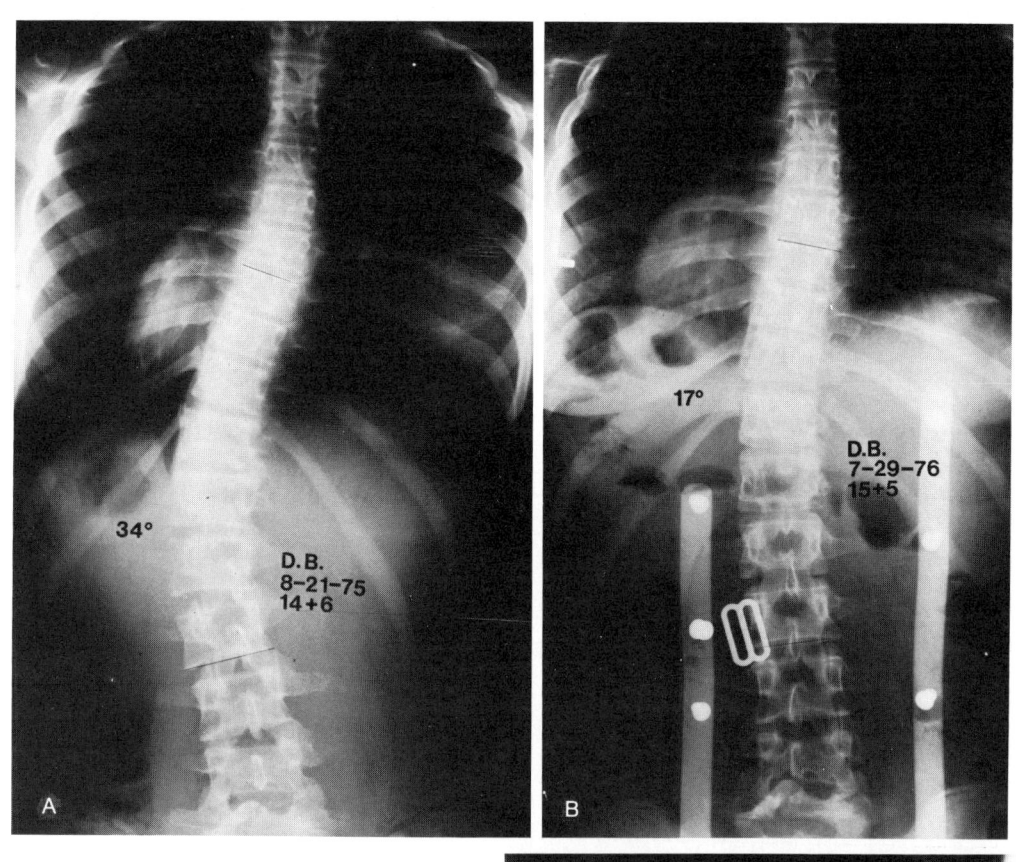

Figure 11–10. *A*, D.B. is a 14+6 year old female with a left thoracolumbar curve. Despite her advanced Risser sign, the patient was placed in a TLSO because of curve progression from 24 degrees when first seen on December 19, 1974. *B*, Best correction in brace was 17 degrees. *C*, The patient wore the brace until July 5, 1979, and on this follow-up radiograph three years later, no loss of correction is evident.

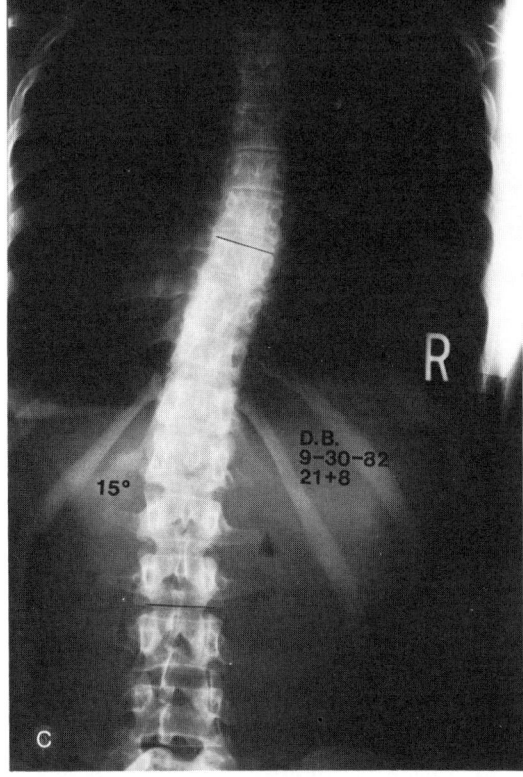

prevent this, the pads should be placed as far laterally as possible to prevent transmission of any anteriorly directed force to the already flattened spine.

The main function of orthotic treatment of juvenile and adolescent idiopathic scoliosis is to prevent progression of the curve. If the orthosis halts progression of curves of 25 to 35 degrees, bracing may be continued during adolescence; however, long-term brace wear may not be well tolerated emotionally by the adolescent, and the patient may prove to be totally uncooperative. In such an event, there is no alternative other than to watch carefully, to prescribe brace wear after school and at night, and to perform surgery if the curve increases beyond 40 to 50 degrees.

Weaning the patient from the brace depends upon the stability of correction achieved. From experience, it has been shown that the orthosis must be worn for at least a year on a full-time basis before considering weaning. Full-time wearing allows removal for one hour a day for bathing. Criteria for weaning include: (1) no increase in height over a four month period, and (2) a Risser sign of at least 4. Once these criteria are met, a PA standing radiograph is scheduled four hours after the brace is removed; this is then compared to a recent standing PA film in the brace. If there is no loss of correction or if there is only a three to five degree loss, the patient is allowed four hours out of the brace daily.

The patient is brought back for a four month follow-up evaluation, at which time the same test is repeated after eight hours out of the brace. Once stability of correction has been established for 12 hours out of brace following this pattern for weaning, night use only of the brace is allowed. This is continued for an additional three months at which time a film is taken after the patient has been out of the brace for 24 hours. If the curve is stable, bracing is discontinued. If loss of correction is noted at these weaning trials, continued full-time use of the brace is required until such time as trials out of the brace demonstrate stability of correction or until progression of the curvature demonstrates the need for surgical stabilization.

These same general principles of brace wear and weaning apply equally well to the Boston-type brace. Because of its constriction of torso activity, however, time out of this brace should begin at once after its application for inclusion of vigorous exercise, particularly swimming, in the patient's daily schedule.

All patients undergoing orthotic treatment for scoliosis should be encouraged by their physicians to participate in outdoor activities, excluding body contact sports. If they are active participants in skiing, skating, or tennis, they should continue to be involved in these activities. The patient may remove the orthosis for swimming, which is an excellent exercise for maintaining strong trunk muscles.

Electrical Surface Stimulation Treatment. Although the treatment of idiopathic scoliosis by electrical stimulation was described as early as 1857 by Seiler[96] of Paris, its use has only become more popular on this continent during the last 10 years. Some of the initial research began in the early 1970's when two methods of using electrical stimulation to correct idiopathic scoliosis were described. Bobechko and Herbert's[5] early work consisted of implanting paraspinal electrodes in growing pigs. Stimulation was accomplished through the use of an external transmitter. After the initial animal studies were conducted, the method was extended to use in humans.

McCollough and associates[62] described surface electrical stimulation using electrode pads placed on the skin over the paraspinal muscles on either side of the rib leading to the apical vertebrae. Since these initial reports on electrical stimulation have appeared, other studies have been done. Axelgaard, Nordwall, and Brown[4] used a cat model to determine that lateral placement of the surface electrodes produced more spinal deformity than did electrodes placed over the paraspinal muscles. They attributed this to the added biomechanical advantage of the long lever arms of the ribs and pelvis upon which the lateral muscles were acting. This concept was then extended to the treatment of idiopathic scoliosis. Through a clinical trial, it was found that lateral placement of the electrodes rather than over the paraspinal muscles improved the curve correction threefold. Further studies using thermography have shown that the most lateral fibers of the latissimus dorsi and the lateral abdominals contract when the electrodes are placed in the lateral position.[38]

Mechanism of Action. Many theories as to how electrical stimulation works have been advanced, including remodeling of bone due to muscle contraction, strengthening of possibly weak muscles on the convexity of the curve, and the effect electrical stimulation might have on the central nervous system. However, at the present time the mechanism of action is unknown.

Patient Selection. The criteria for treating idiopathic scoliosis with an electrical stimulator are the same as for treating a patient with an orthosis. The patient should also have a reliable family that is willing and able to accurately place the electrodes each evening. When patients requiring non-operative treatment are initially seen they are given a choice of using either the stimulator or an orthosis. An attempt is made to present both treatment options without bias. While an occasional patient chooses the orthosis, most select the stimulator because of the minimal alteration in life style it requires.

Although the stimulator was initially restricted to treating single major thoracic, thoracolumbar, and lumbar curves, double major curves are now being treated at the Twin Cities Scoliosis Center by the use of dual channel stimulators. Stimulators are rarely used to treat thoracic curves with an apex higher than T5 because the scapula interferes with placement of the electrode pads (Fig. 11–11).

Treatment Methods. When the decision has been made to treat with an electrical stimulator the patient is seen by the physical therapist who supervises the placement of the electrode pads under the physician's direction. For thoracic curves the pads are placed on either side of the rib leading to the apical vertebrae and adjusted from a medial to lateral position, depending upon which location yields the best clinical correction. The distance between the electrode pads varies with curve length, using the following guidelines.[3] For patients with a normal trunk length and curves of 5 to 7 segments 10 cm. is the distance used. For curves less than 5 segments 7 to 9 cm. is appropriate, and for curves greater than 7 segments 10 to 14 cm. is used. The electrode pads should not be placed closer together than 6 cm. as this distance limits the strength of the muscular contraction. The pads must also be placed so that the muscle contractions produced do not worsen any existing thoracic hypokyphosis.

Lumbar curves are treated by placing the pads on either side of the apical vertebrae again adjusting the medial-to-lateral position to produce the best clinical results and using the aforementioned guide to determine the distance between pads. If a double major curve is treated, two sets of pads are placed on each curve as described.

We use two stimulating systems, both of which consist of a stimulator containing its own battery power source connected by a set of wires taped to carbon electrode pads; a conducting gel is also used.

The initial intensity is set at a level that is comfortable for the patient. The stimulator is used only during bedtime for a minimum of six hours per night. Patients are encouraged to gradually increase the intensity of the stimulation as their tolerance increases. Most patients eventually tolerate an intensity of 35 to 40 mA with little difficulty. No specific exercise therapy is prescribed for these patients though they are encouraged to maintain their general physical fitness.

After the initial fitting of the stimulator, the patient is seen in one month for a clinical evaluation and radiographs. Two films are taken in the prone position, one with the stimulator turned off and the other with the stimulator on. Electrodes are checked for satisfactory positioning, and the percentage of correction obtained with the stimulator on is recorded. Bradford and coworkers[7] have noted that it is preferable to have an initial curve correction of at least 50 per cent on the radiograph with the stimulator on. While some of the 25 patients in their review had less than 50 per cent correction and did well, all of the failures showed less than 50 per cent initial correction when stimulated.

The patients are seen at three month intervals for clinical evaluation and a standing PA radiograph with the pads in place and the stimulator turned off. Pad placement is noted and adjustments made as necessary. Curve measurements are determined and compared with the initial films, with the goal of treatment being the prevention of curve increase. Follow-up is continued at three month intervals until skeletal maturity.

Use of the stimulator is stopped without a weaning process when the patient reaches skeletal maturity. Criteria for stopping the stimulator are (1) a Risser sign of 4, and (2) cessation in height growth over a three month period. After the stimulator is discontinued, the patient is seen twice a year in follow-up until there is a Risser sign of 5. Follow-up then continues yearly for five years, with the patient discharged from care if curve progression has not occurred.

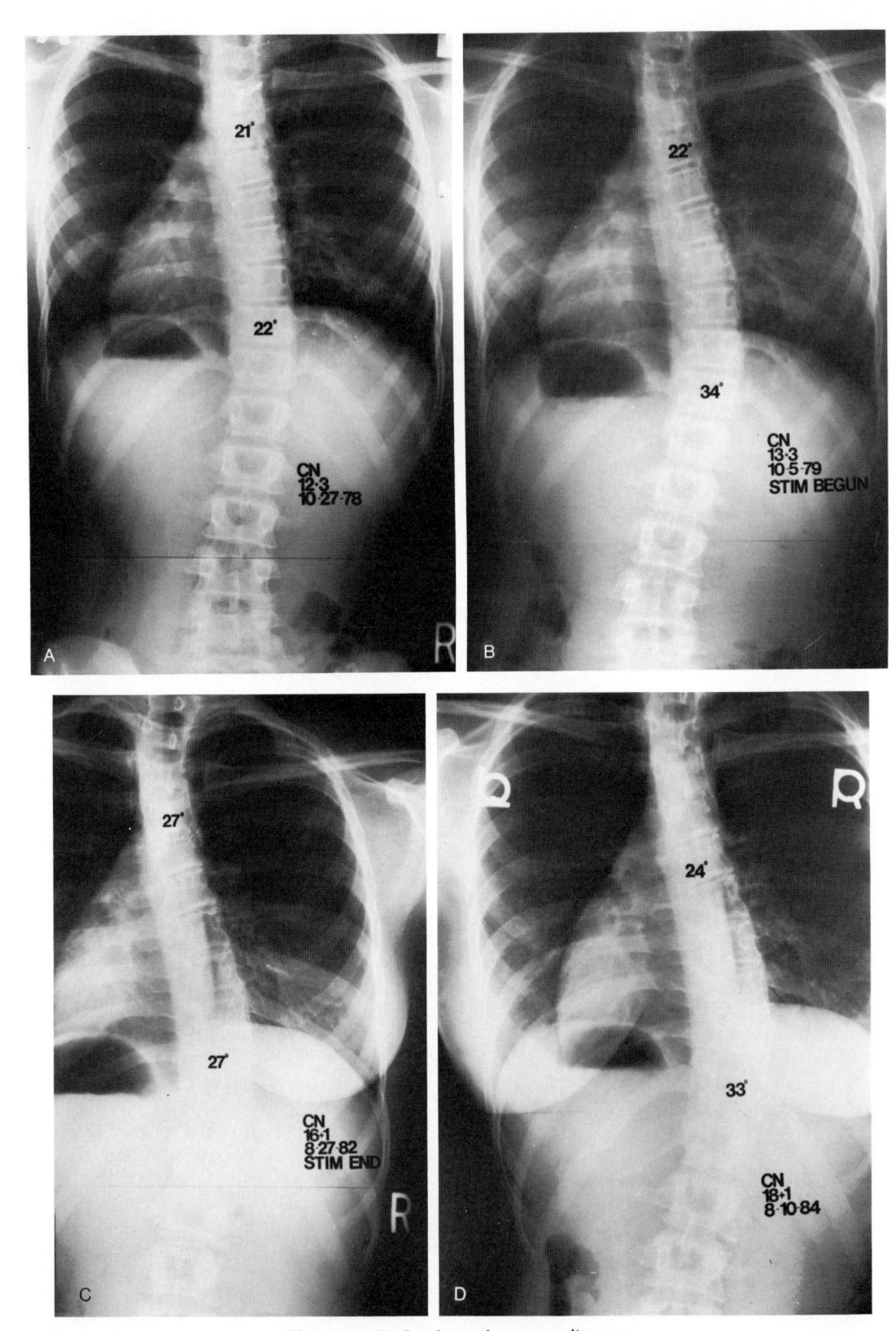

Figure 11–11 *See legend on opposite page.*

Results of Electrical Stimulation. It must be emphasized that electrical stimulation is still in its infancy at this time. There has not been sufficient follow-up to allow an adequate comparison between electrical stimulation and brace treatment. Some of the early results do appear promising. In 1980, McCollough and coworkers[62] reviewed 16 patients with idiopathic scoliosis treated by electrical stimulation during sleeping hours, ranging in age from 8 to 15 years at the patient's onset of stimulation. Curvatures ranged from 15 to 31 degrees and progression of 5 degrees or more was documented in 10 of the 16 patients. Criteria for patient selection included single primary lumbar or thoracolumbar curves of 30 degrees or less and at least two years of spinal growth remaining. Average stimulation time was 27 months. Average follow-up was 30 months, with the longest follow-up being 62 months. Of the 16 curves, 8 improved, 5 exhibited no change, and 3 became worse. Of the 3 curves that worsened, maximum progression was 9 degrees, with an average of 7.6 degrees. No significant difference was observed in the results obtained between thoracolumbar and lumbar curves.

In 1983, Brown and associates[9] reviewed 548 stimulator patients who are a part of the multicenter trial by 58 principal investigators in North America and Western Europe. One hundred of these patients met stringent criteria, including curves of 20 to 45 degrees, documentation of progression, Risser 0 to 1, and were premenarchal with skeletal ages less than 13 + 0 for females and 14 + 6 for males. The remaining 448 patients had less rapid progression and were more mature. Of 170 patients starting treatment at least two years before the review, 51 (30 per cent) were dropped before completing treatment. Ten were dropped because of non-compliance and 26 (15 per cent) showed curve progression of more than 5 degrees. Only 28 patients had completed treatment and were skeletally mature at the time of this review. The longest follow-up was 12 months after stimulation was completed. Of these 28 patients, four showed more than 5 degrees total progression after beginning stimulation. In 1983, Bradford and coworkers[7] reviewed their early electrical stimulation results. Of 25 patients treated between 1978 and 1981 one was improved, 14 were stable, two had mild acceptable progression, and eight had progression greater than 10 degrees that required an alternative form of treatment.

The evaluation of long-term results and the comparison of these results with the natural history of scoliosis as well as the known benefits of brace treatment will be necessary before the efficacy of surface electrical stimulation can be determined.

Complications. Complications of electrical stimulation treatment are minimal; the most common adverse effect is skin irritation from the electrode pads. The skin problems usually respond to local care or to a change in the type of electrode pad. In the review of 548 patients by Brown and coworkers[9], only three cases of skin irritation were not successfully handled by these means.

While not a strict complication of electrical stimulation, the question arises concerning the patient who has shown progression despite electrical stimulation treatment. If these patients still fulfill the criteria for brace treatment, they should be placed in an orthosis in an attempt to avoid surgery, although Bradford and coworkers[7] found in their review that curvatures not responding to electrical stimulation are less likely to respond to Milwaukee brace treatment than those placed directly into a brace.

SURGICAL TREATMENT

Despite the best non-operative treatment efforts some idiopathic curves progress. Other curves are so severe when initially seen that treatment by an orthosis or stimulator is useless. It is for these cases that surgical treatment is appropriate.

It is quite difficult to select patients suitable for surgical intervention based solely on the Cobb measurement of the deformity. Each patient and each curve is unique and must

---

Figure 11–11. *A,* C.N. is a 12 + 3 year old female with idiopathic scoliosis who had these curves when first seen. *B,* Stimulation was begun at this time because of the increase in the right thoracolumbar curve. *C,* Stimulation was stopped at this time when her Risser sign was 4 and her height was not increasing. *D,* Follow-up two years after the end of treatment shows no increase in the thoracolumbar curve compared to the pre-treatment film in 1979.

be treated as such. The 12 year old, skeletally immature female with an unbalanced 40 degree right thoracic curve unresponsive to brace treatment is quite different from the 17 year old, mature female with a stable, balanced 40 degree right thoracic, 40 degree left lumbar curve. Although both patients have curves with the same Cobb measurement, one has a high risk for curve progression and the other does not. One patient is decompensated with an objectionable cosmetic appearance while the other is balanced and appears almost normal. To treat both of these patients by strict Cobb measurement guidelines would possibly result in unnecessary surgery.

Principles must guide the orthopaedic surgeon in the selection of a patient for surgical stabilization. The goal of operative intervention is to partially correct and stabilize the uncontrollable curve. Knowledge of the risk factors for curve progression allows one to formulate guidelines to assist in patient selection. Curves with Cobb measurements of 40 to 45 degrees fall into a gray zone. Certainly, surgery is very rarely indicated for curves less than 40 degrees, as they are unlikely to progress. Curves that progress past 40 degrees in the skeletally immature patient warrant surgery, because it is probable that curve progression will occur as the patient continues to grow. Curves of 40 to 45 degrees in the mature teenager may be observed, depending on the deformity they produce; if curve progression is noted, then fusion is recommended. Curves greater than 50 degrees will often increase throughout adulthood and for this reason we would usually recommend surgery.

It is often possible to brace a 10 or 11 year old patient with a progressive curve thereby preventing further progression while awaiting the completion of spinal growth. However, if curve progression continues beyond 40 degrees despite non-operative treatment, one should not hesitate to either place a subcutaneous rod or fuse the patient's spine. Procrastination will not allow normal spinal growth but rather permit worsening of the curve.

There is an indication for surgical stabilization of a curve of less than 40 degrees. This is the patient who has progressive true thoracic lordosis and resultant decreasing anteroposterior diameter of the chest. Because of a concern for future respiratory and cardiac compromise as the result of decreased intrathoracic volume, it is felt best to stabilize and correct these curves. Patients who fall into this category usually have a thoracic kyphosis of +5 to +10 degrees when initially seen and on follow-up are noted to have progressed to a thoracic lordosis of 0 to −5 degrees.

Preoperative Distraction and Casting. In 1948, scoliosis correction was done by casting, and then surgery was carried out to stabilize the curve. The Hibbs-Risser turnbuckle cast, as modified by Cobb, was used initially, but in 1953 the Risser localizer cast was introduced and found to give more satisfactory curve correction with better tolerance. Serial casts were very occasionally applied preoperatively. Once maximum correction had been achieved, the patient was operated upon and the spine fused while still in the body cast. In 1960, the Harrington instrumentation was introduced, allowing intraoperative curve correction.[41] Although not abandoned immediately, it became apparent that pre-operative casting and traction produced no better results than did curve correction by Harrington instrumentation alone.

In 1976, Nachemson and Nordwall[78] evaluated the effects of Cotrel traction on curve correction in patients with idiopathic scoliosis undergoing posterior spinal fusion and Harrington rod instrumentation. They found that preoperative traction produced no better curve correction than did Harrington instrumentation alone.

Today preoperative casts are not used at our center. Preoperative halo gravity traction is occasionally used for the patient with a severe curve and associated pulmonary compromise. The traction partially corrects the patient's deformity, allowing the abdominal contents to fall out of the chest cavity, permitting the diaphragm to descend, and allowing a more vigorous preoperative pulmonary toilet.

Selection of the Fusion Area in Adolescent Idiopathic Scoliosis. Since Hibbs[44] published his first report in 1924 on the treatment of 59 cases of scoliosis by spinal fusion, no definite conclusions have been reached in the scoliosis literature concerning the best method for selecting fusion levels that will always lead to balanced and stable correction of the curvature. Hibbs considered all 59 cases to be the result of post-poliomyelitis scoliosis; however, when reviewed, several case reports were found to be definitely idiopathic scoliosis. Hibbs stated, "fusion should extend from the neutral vertebra above to the neutral vertebra below the apex." While Hibbs failed to specify his definition of "neutral vertebra," a similar concept has been the basis for most of the subsequent authors' opinions on this subject. The desired end-result is to fuse between stable vertebrae. If this is done correctly, no additional vertebrae will be added to the curve beyond the fusion; "adding on" signifies too short a fusion.

Since the earliest days of the Scoliosis Service founded at Gillette Children's Hospital by Moe in 1948, the development of a standard for selection of the proper fusion area in idiopathic scoliosis has been researched. It has become apparent that the selection of stable end vertebrae for fusion is a three step procedure: (1) the major curve(s) must be identified, (2) one must determine the neutrally rotated end vertebrae for each major curve as these are felt to be stable vertebrae, and (3) the relationship of a vertically drawn midsacral line to the major curve should be determined.

Major curves are identified by determining curve flexibility as described by Moe.[71, 72] Supine side bending radiographs are obtained of each curve. By calculating the percentage of correction for each curve, one arrives at the flexibility for that curve. Curves with low flexibility are stiff and structural and are therefore major curves. Curves with high flexibility are less structural or minor curves. When two curves have nearly the same flexibility both are equally structural implying a double curve pattern (Fig. 11–12). The lower end vertebra of a major curve usually coincides with the lower neutrally rotated vertebra, but on occasion may be one of several vertebrae in which rotation continues until the neutrally rotated vertebra is reached lying in the concavity of the curve below. In this situation, the extension of rotation may be reversed by the application of a strong distraction force on a horizontal frame such as a Risser frame. In this event, then neutrally rotated vertebra will be moved upward even to the point of coinciding with the lower end vertebra of the thoracic curve. The fusion area will then be shortened, usually by one vertebra.

Neutrally rotated vertebrae at the end of each major curve are then determined by noting the relationship of the pedicle shadows to the vertebral body margins on the PA radiograph, as described by Moe.[76] Both pedicle shadows will be equidistant from the vertebral margins at the neutrally rotated vertebrae (Fig. 11–13).

The third stage in this process involves drawing a line across the tops of the iliac crests and then erecting a perpendicular line from the midpoint of the sacrum.[53] The stable lower vertebra is identified as the vertebra that lies closest to the end vertebra of the curve and is most nearly bisected by this line (Fig. 11–14).

It is our impression at this time that only major curves require fusion from stable end vertebra to stable end vertebra. Once the major curve is identified it is necessary to determine the stable end vertebrae for that curve. When the neutrally rotated end vertebrae coincide with the end vertebrae as determined by the midsacral line, the decision for fusion level is simple; when they do not, only the good judgment and experience of the surgeon will result in the correct selection of the fusion area. Fusion to the stable end vertebra as determined by the midsacral line usually produces the best result.

Any correction achieved when fusing a major curve by the above guidelines is usually balanced by a similar correction in any associated, more flexible minor curves. This is what prevents decompensation when only the major curve is fused. However, if more correction of the major curve is obtained than can be compensated for by the minor curve then decompensation of the spine will result. It is for this reason that "total correction" of the major curve is often not desirable.

Selection of Instrumentation. There are so many ways to instrument the spine that selecting one often poses a problem. The surgeon must not become enamored with the instrumentation itself and forget that its role is primarily twofold: (1) partial correction of the deformity, and (2) immobilization of the spine until a solid arthrodesis occurs. It is imperative that a meticulous arthrodesis be performed regardless of what instrumentation is used.

There is some difference of opinion throughout the country as to the role Luque instrumentation plays in the treatment of juvenile and adolescent idiopathic scoliosis. Some feel that the secure fixation obtained with this technique warrants its routine use despite the increased risk of neurologic injury, others only employ the Luque system for special cases. The Harrington distraction rod in combination with the Harrington

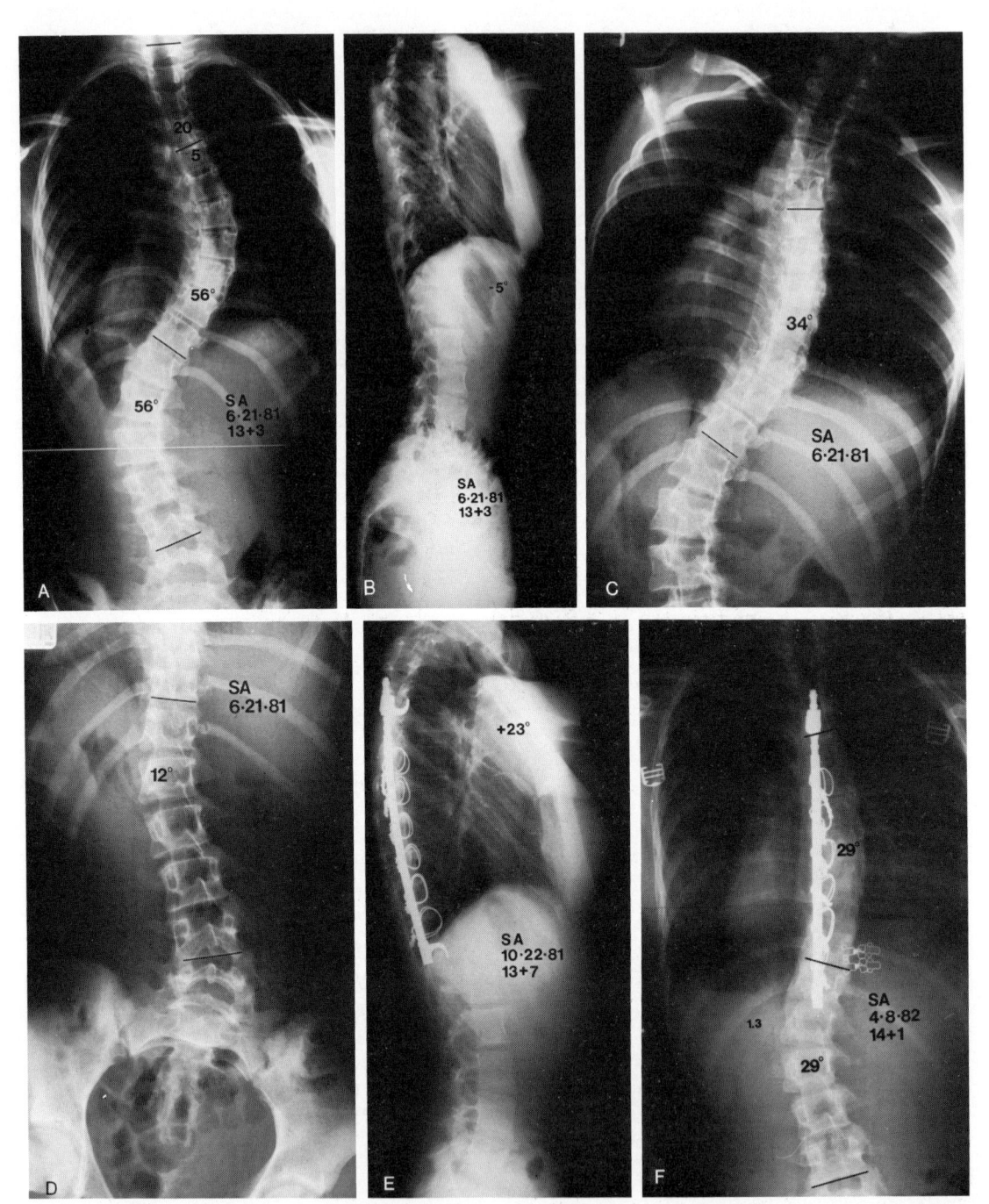

Figure 11–12. *A*, S.A. is a 13+ 3 year old female with a progressive curve. *B*, The lateral radiograph shows true thoracic lordosis. *C* and *D*, Right and left side bending radiographs were obtained as part of the preoperative evaluation. Note that the left lumbar curve is much more flexible than the right thoracic curve, indicating that this is a right thoracic curve pattern with a compensatory left lumbar curve, not a double major curve. *E*, The patient underwent posterior spinal fusion of the right thoracic curve, with Harrington-Luque instrumentation on June 22, 1981. This lateral radiograph shows the improvement in sagittal contour obtainable with this system. *F*, Standing PA radiograph ten months after surgery shows a balanced spine with a solid fusion. Note that the left lumbar curve has corrected to balance the correction obtained in the right thoracic curve.

IDIOPATHIC SCOLIOSIS

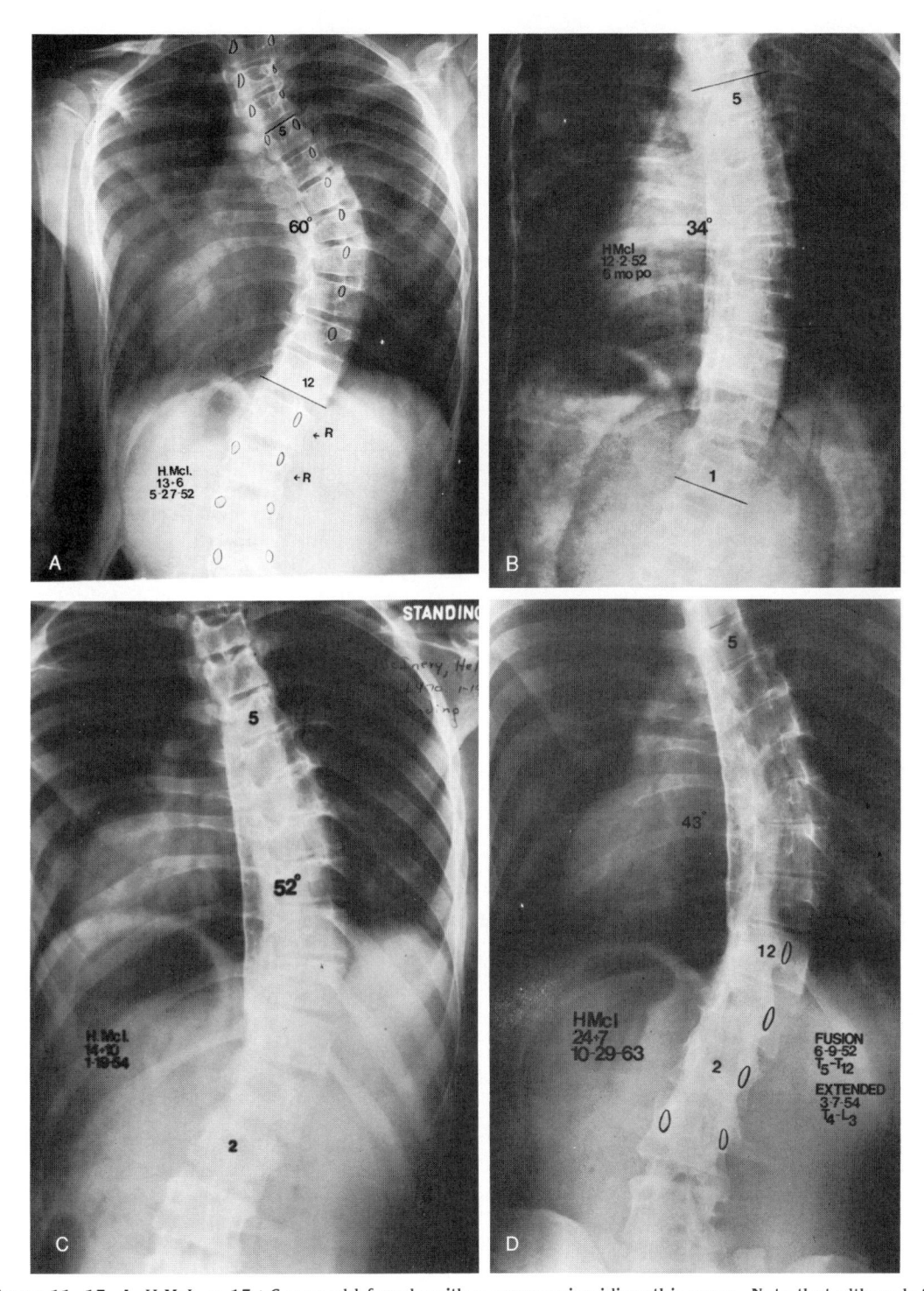

Figure 11–13. *A*, H.McI., a 13+6 year old female with a progressive idiopathic curve. Note that although the curve ends at T12, vertebral rotation continues until L3, which is the neutrally rotated vertebra, indicating that L3 should be the end point of fusion. *B*, The six month postoperative film in cast following a T5 to T12 fusion shows correction to 34 degrees. *C*, Follow-up radiographs 18 months postoperatively shows that despite a solid fusion from T5 to T12, the curve has increased to 52 degrees. This is due to the addition of L1 and L2 to the curve. Note that L3 is still neutrally rotated. *D*, Because of progression the patient underwent extension of her fusion to L3. This radiograph nine years postoperatively shows a solid fusion with a curve that has not increased.

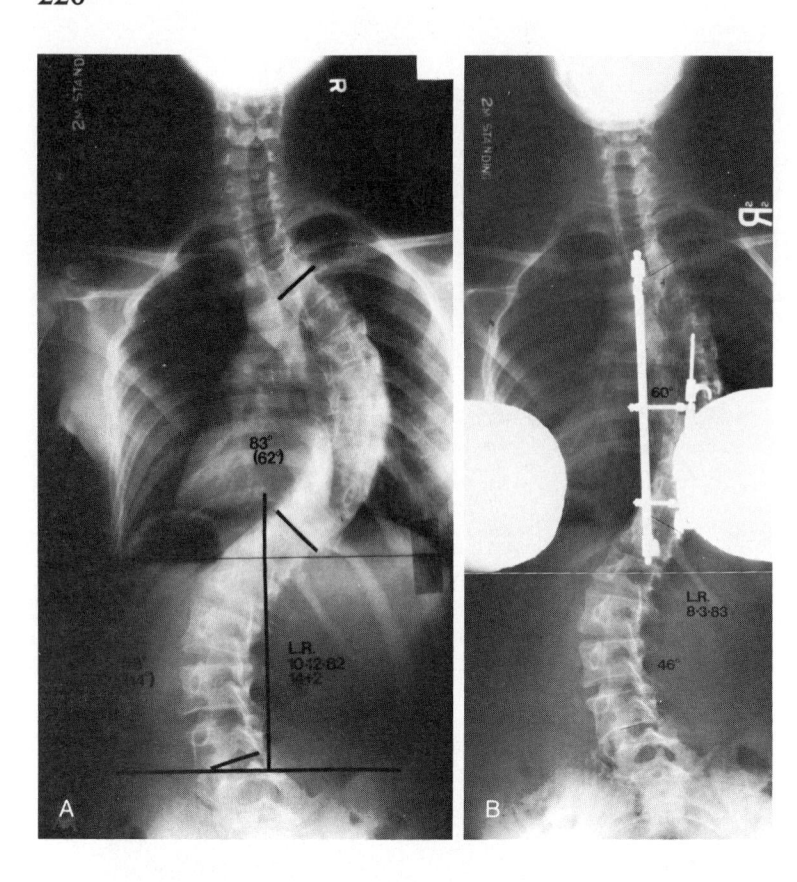

Figure 11–14. *A,* L.R. is a 14 + 2 year old female with a progressive idiopathic curve. Note that the vertical mid-sacral line falls on T12 and the neutrally rotated vertebra is T12. Correction on side bending radiographs is shown by the figures in parentheses. *B,* This radiograph shows the patient 10 months after surgery. Note that the lower level chosen for fusion is T12 as indicated by the mid-sacral line and vertebral rotation. Also note that the upper hook has been placed under the left lamina of L3 in an attempt to elevate the left shoulder, which was lower than the right preoperatively.

compression system produces correction and stabilization equal to that obtainable with the Luque system while allowing a solid fusion to develop with minimal risk of neurologic injury. More currently, the Cotrel-Dubousset system appears to offer some advantages over other systems.

Harrington instrumentation is suitable for most thoracic curves. The upper distraction hook should be placed in the facet joint on the side of the low shoulder to prevent increasing the shoulder asymmetry. Addition of a Harrington compression system provides segmental fixation and increases the rigidity of the spine prior to solidification of the fusion (Fig. 11–15). Regardless of whether Harrington or Luque instrumentation is used, the postoperative result is enhanced by three to six months in an orthosis.[8, 19, 101, 115] The Luque instrumentation or the Harrington-Luque combination provides better sagittal plane correction than Harrington instrumentation alone in the patient with severe hypokyphosis or even true lordosis of the thoracic spine. By using sublaminar wiring in conjunction with a contoured rod, one is able to create more thoracic kyphosis than with distraction instrumentation alone. For this reason, the use of sublaminar wires may be preferable to distraction instrumentation alone in this situation (Fig. 11–16). The Cotrel-Doubousset system appears to offer even better sagittal plane correction and possibly some improvement in rotation, and no postoperative casting or bracing is generally necessary.

Instrumentation of thoracolumbar and lumbar idiopathic curves is more complicated than instrumentation of thoracic curves for two reasons: (1) distraction of the lumbar spine may reduce the normal lumbar lordosis, which then subjects the patient to the problems of the flattened lumbar spine, and (2) extension of the fusion distally decreases the number of open segments between the end of the fusion mass and the pelvis, thereby possibly increasing the patient's chance of developing degenerative spine disease. Selection of instrumentation for thoracolumbar and lumbar curves must be made with the thought of decreasing or eliminating these problems.

Our recommended approach for flexible idiopathic thoracolumbar and lumbar curves is an anterior fusion with Zielke instrumentation (Fig. 11–17). This instrumentation usually limits the distal extent necessary for an adequate fusion by one or two vertebrae when compared with Harrington distraction or Luque instrumentation because of the superb correction obtainable and the excellent control over the vertebral bodies provided by the Zielke instrumentation. It is usually only necessary to fuse the structural vertebrae of the curve as determined on side-bending films. If properly used, preservation of normal lumbar lordosis is possible along with excellent curve correction. On occasion, Zielke instrumentation will not be possible, and in this case we recommend Luque instrumentation for the thoracolumbar or lumbar curve (Fig. 11–18).

The Harrington distraction rod may be used for the thoracolumbar or lumbar curve; however, it is important not to place the lower hook distal to L4 in an attempt to preserve motion segments. Lumbar lordosis should be contoured into the rod, which should be square-ended, in an attempt to prevent rotation of the contoured rod. Addition of a compression system will not only provide segmental fixation but also will help maintain lumbar lordosis (Fig. 11–19).

The selection of instrumentation for double major curves generally follows the guidelines previously noted. Double major thoracic curves may be treated with Harrington instrumentation or Luque instrumentation, although the Harrington system is generally preferred. A distraction rod is usually placed in an S-shaped configuration with the upper hook in the concavity of the upper curve. The upper hook should never be placed in the convexity of the upper curve, as this will worsen the neck and shoulder deformity. The Harrington compression system is usually not used for double major thoracic curves because each curve is short, making effective placement of the compression system difficult.

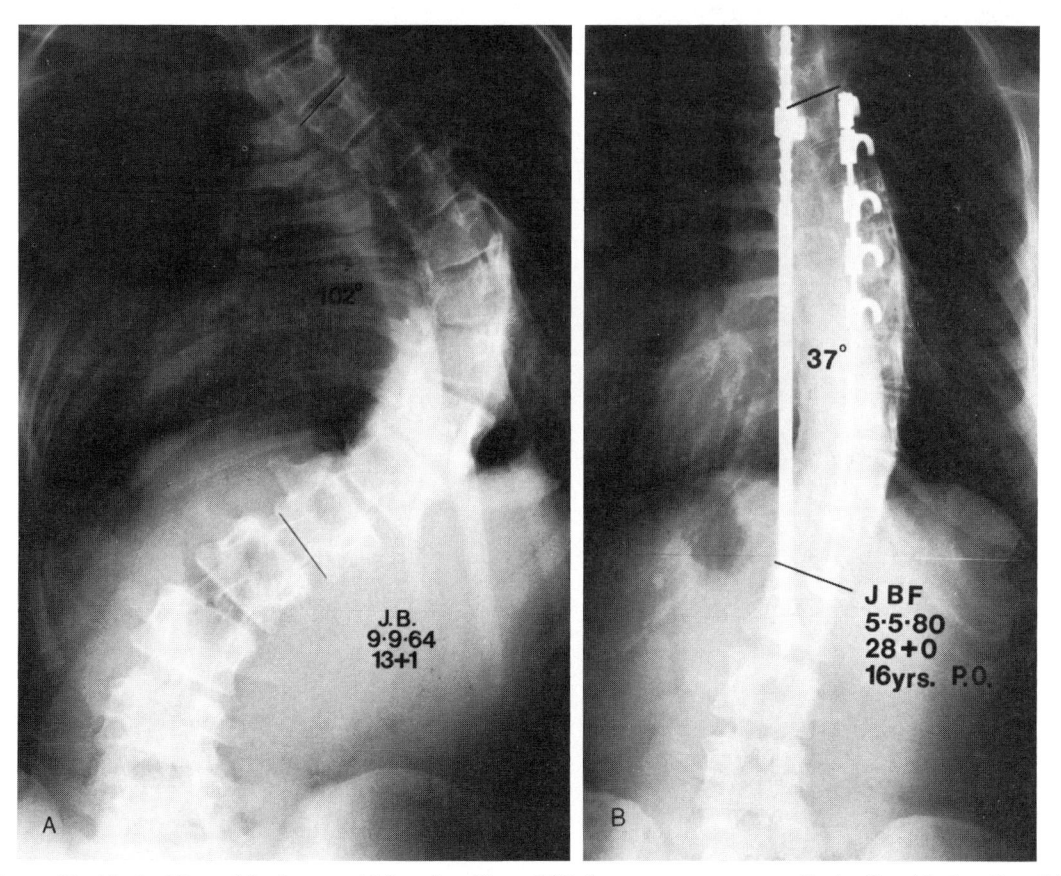

Figure 11–15. A, J.B., a 13+1 year old female with an 102 degree curve preoperatively. On side bending this curve corrected to 65 degrees. B, This radiograph shows the correction obtained with Harrington distraction and compression instrumentation. Only 2 degrees of correction have been lost since the fusion 16 years ago.

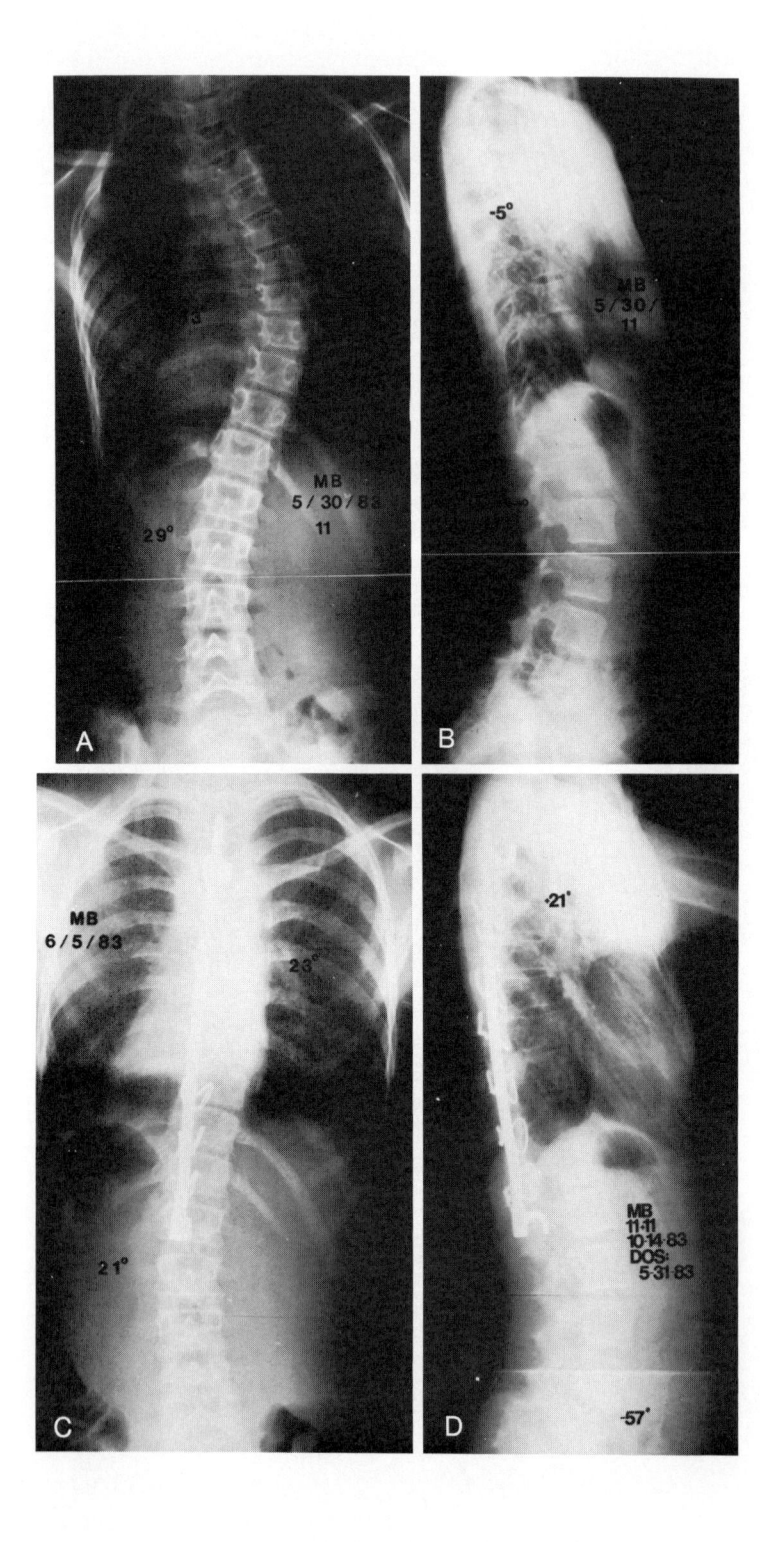

Figure 11–16. *A*, M.B. is an 11 year old female with a 53 degree right thoracic curve. *B*, The lateral film shows an associated 5 degree thoracic lordosis. Because of the thoracic lordosis it was decided to treat this curve with sublaminar wiring in an attempt to produce a more normal thoracic sagittal contour. *C*, Postoperative PA radiograph shows correction of the scoliosis to 23 degrees. *D*, A lateral radiograph shows a thoracic kyphosis of +21 degrees, which is a 26 degree improvement in the sagittal contour of the thoracic spine compared to the preoperative film.

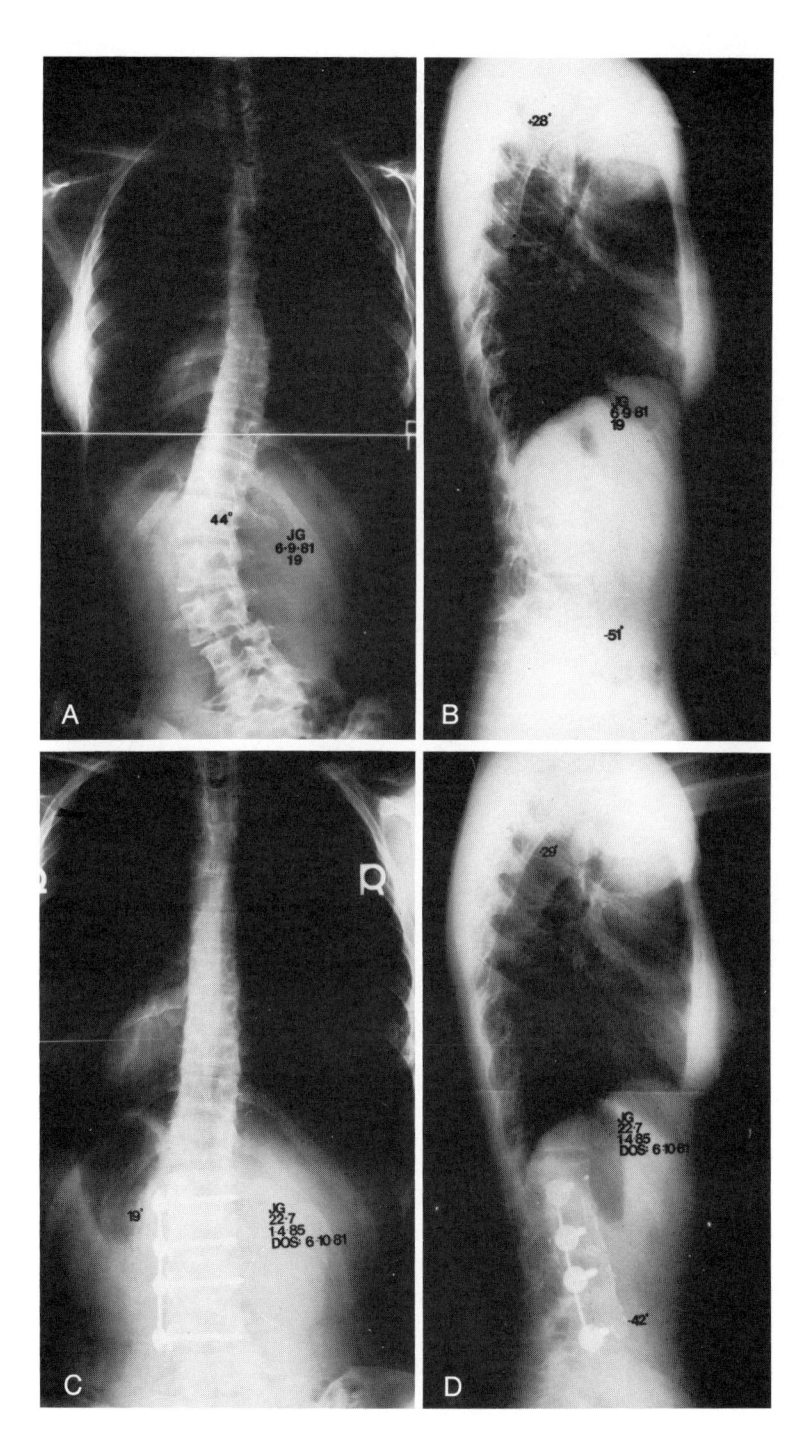

Figure 11–17. *A,* J.G. is a 19 year old female with a progressive 44 degree left lumbar curve. *B,* The lateral radiograph shows a −51 degree lumbar lordosis. *C,* It was elected to treat this patient with anterior spinal fusion and Zielke instrumentation. This film 3½ years after surgery shows a solid fusion and satisfactory curve correction. *D,* The lateral radiograph again shows a solid fusion and a −42 degree lumbar lordosis.

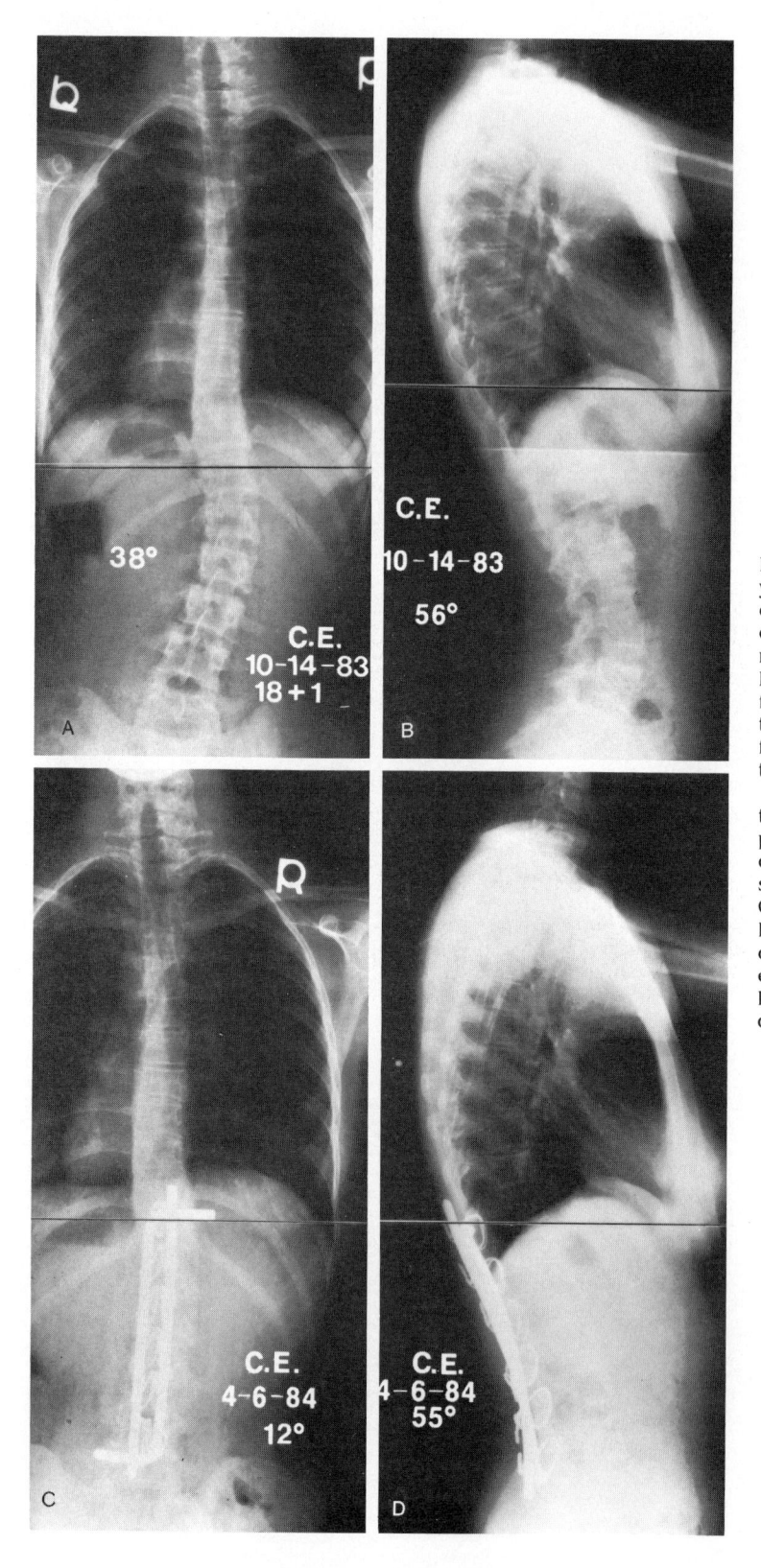

Figure 11–18. *A,* C.E. is an 18+1 year old female with a painful idiopathic right lumbar curve. Because of the pain it was recommended that she undergo fusion. Because of the incision necessary for Zielke instrumentation, the patient elected to have a posterior fusion. *B,* This radiograph shows the patient's sagittal contour with a −56 degree lumbar lordosis prior to the surgery. *C,* In an attempt to preserve the patient's lumbar lordosis she underwent posterior fusion with Luque instrumentation. Care was taken to contour the Luque rods to prevent loss of lordosis. *D,* Postoperatively, the lateral radiograph shows a lumbar lordosis of −55 degrees. Note the contouring of the Luque rods.

Figure 11–19. *A*, This radiograph shows the straightening of the lumbar spine that occurs when a straight Harrington distraction rod is used. *B*, In contrast, this radiograph demonstrates that it is possible to maintain lumbar lordosis through the use of a Harrington compression system as well as sublaminar wiring to a contoured distraction rod.

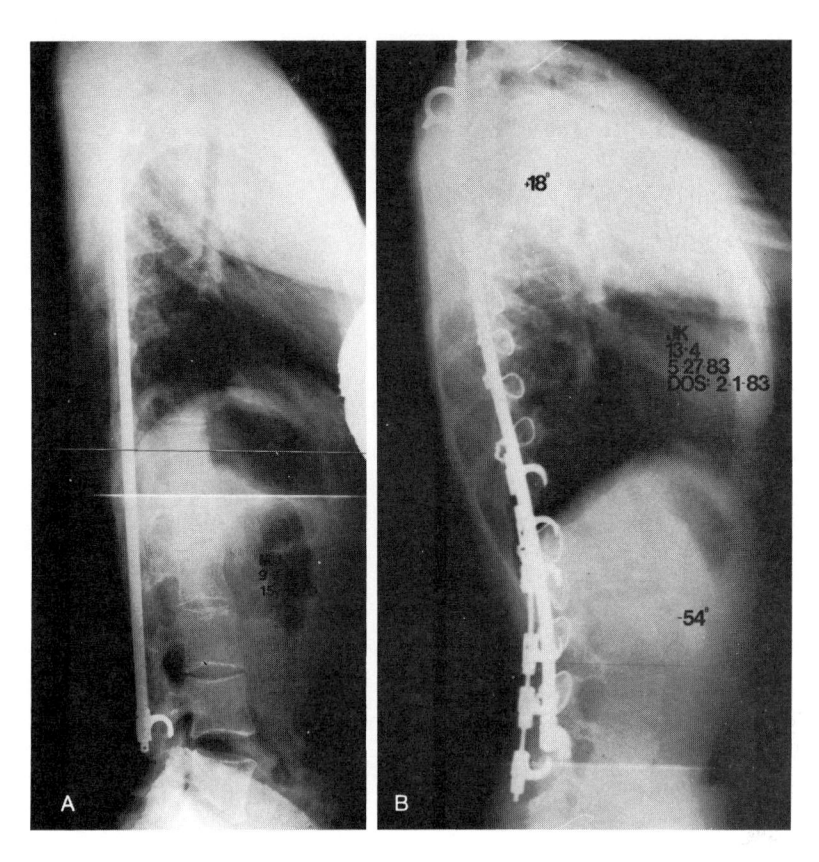

Double major thoracic-thoracolumbar and thoracic-lumbar curves may be instrumented with either Harrington instrumentation, the Luque system, or the Cotrel-Dubousset system (Fig. 11–20). The lower distraction hook should not be placed distal to L4, and lumbar lordosis should be contoured into a square-ended rod. Use of the square-ended rod will help prevent rotation of the contoured distraction rod. If used, Luque instrumentation should not extend distal to L4 either. The distal extent of the fusion necessary to treat these double major curves may be limited by combining Zielke instrumentation anteriorly with either Harrington or Luque instrumentation posteriorly. This technique involves two separate operations, with fusion and Zielke instrumentation of the thoracolumbar or lumbar curve during the first stage. Seven to 10 days later a second stage is performed posteriorly. Although both curves are instrumented, it is not necessary to place the posterior instrumentation distal to the lowest Zielke screw. This technique of combined instrumentation does require two operations; however, more motion segments distal to the fusion are preserved than if posterior instrumentation alone were used. This technique should be considered for double major curves requiring fusion to L5 if treated by posterior instrumentation and fusion alone.

Two-Stage Anterior and Posterior Fusions.[30] Although most idiopathic curvatures that require surgery prior to adulthood are satisfactorily treated by posterior fusion alone, there are instances in which a neglected curve may require a two-stage anterior and posterior fusion to achieve a satisfactory result. These patients generally have curves greater than 100 degrees that are very stiff and that would correct little with posterior instrumentation and fusion alone. Anterior discectomy and fusion followed seven to ten days later by posterior instrumentation and fusion usually results in partial curve correction, a balanced spine, and a solid arthrodesis.

Postoperative Treatment. Probably no changes in scoliosis treatment have meant more to the patient than the recent advances made in the area of postoperative management. While the goal of obtaining a solid arthrodesis has remained constant, the

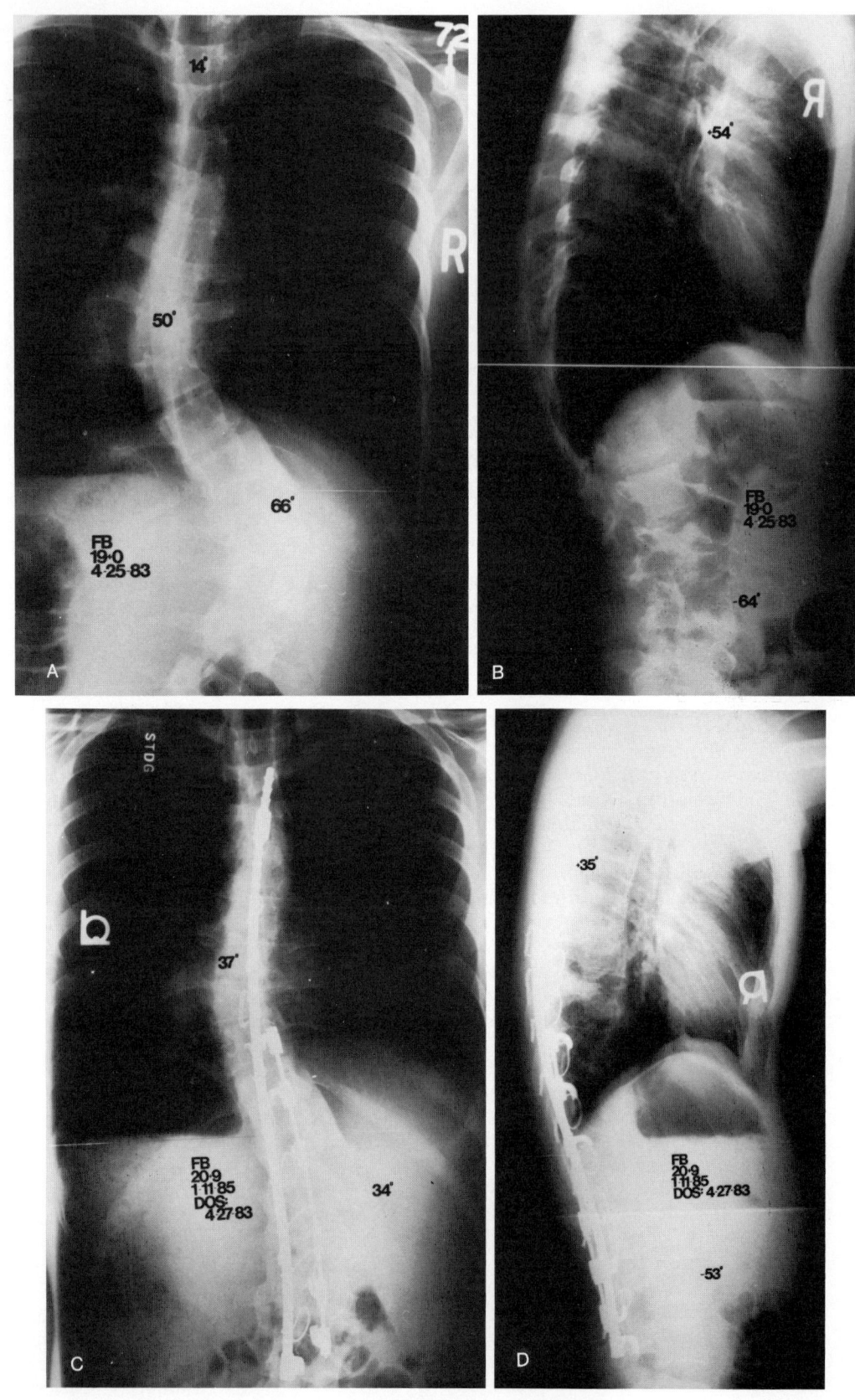

Figure 11–20 *See legend on opposite page.*

method of postoperative immobilization has changed from plaster casts to custom molded polypropylene body jackets. This change has come about as a result of more secure internal fixation of the spine, better surgical techniques, and improved fabrication of the TLSO. The TLSO has several advantages over the plaster cast. It is much lighter than the cast, weighing only 1 1/2 to 2 pounds, compared to the 8 to 10 pound body cast; the brace is more cosmetic and permits showering. Casts are still used for the non-compliant patient who cannot be trusted to wear the orthosis consistently as prescribed.

Following posterior spinal fusion, patients are kept supine for the first four to six postoperative days without immobilization. They are allowed to be logrolled and have a 35 degree back rest. Standing at the bedside with assistance begins on the third or fourth postoperative day, in preparation for taking a standing plaster mold of the body on the fifth or sixth postoperative day; the patient receives the orthosis the following day. Mobilization of the patient then begins, followed by discharge usually on the seventh to tenth day following a routine posterior spinal fusion. Prior to discharge, brace patients are instructed in showering, which is allowed one time per day. They remove the brace prior to stepping into the shower and then shower without bending. The brace is replaced after thorough drying. This regimen has improved the patient's attitude toward postoperative care and has not produced a noticeable increase in postoperative complications. If the Cotrel-Dubousset system has been used, no postoperative bracing is generally necessary, and the patients can be ambulated within two days of surgery.

Six weeks postoperatively the patient returns for a clinical evaluation and standing PA and lateral radiographs in the brace. The next visit is at four months at which time supine oblique radiographs of the fusion mass are taken out of brace in addition to the standing PA and lateral films. If the arthrodesis appears solid, bracing is discontinued; if not, the patient is seen at two month intervals until there appears to be a solid fusion. Most fusions in the adolescent patient become solid within six months of the time of surgery.[87] Restrictions after the fusion becomes solid vary from physician to physician. Generally it is our policy to allow all activities except perhaps football and gymnastics.

ASSOCIATED PROCEDURES

Thoracoplasty. It is becoming more and more obvious that cosmesis is one of the main factors that motivate patients to seek treatment. Many will not openly discuss this aspect of their scoliosis, but once the subject of cosmesis is raised most patients show interest in improving their body image. Perhaps the most disfiguring aspect of idiopathic scoliosis is the associated rotational prominence, especially in a single major right thoracic curve. The deformity is unsightly, interferes with the proper fit of clothing, and makes driving a car or sitting in hard-backed chairs difficult.

The exact etiology of the rib prominence is unknown, although Thulborne and Gillespie[104] postulate that it is due to an asymmetrical relationship between the pedicles, laminae, and transverse processes on the convex versus the concave side of the curve. They have shown that there is no linear relationship between the rib prominence and either the vertebral body rotation, Cobb measurement of the curve, or rib-vertebral angle difference.

As with all surgical procedures, patient selection is most important. Determining factors are not only the height of the deformity itself but the overall contour of the patient's back combined with the patient's desire for correction. Rib elevations of less than three centimeters rarely require correction, whereas prominences greater than six centimeters should be corrected if desired by the patient. Deformities of three to six centimeters fall into a gray zone, with some requiring correction and others not. The Techniques of Surgery chapter dis-

---

Figure 11–20. *A*, F.B. is a 19+0 year old male who was first seen with these curves. *B*, Lateral radiograph. On side bending both the left thoracic and the right lumbar curves had similar flexibility, and this was felt to represent a double curve pattern. *C*, This radiograph taken nearly two years following surgery shows satisfactory correction with a solid fusion. *D*, The Harrington compression instrumentation along with the contoured distraction rod and sublaminar wiring were chosen in an attempt to preserve this patient's lumbar lordosis.

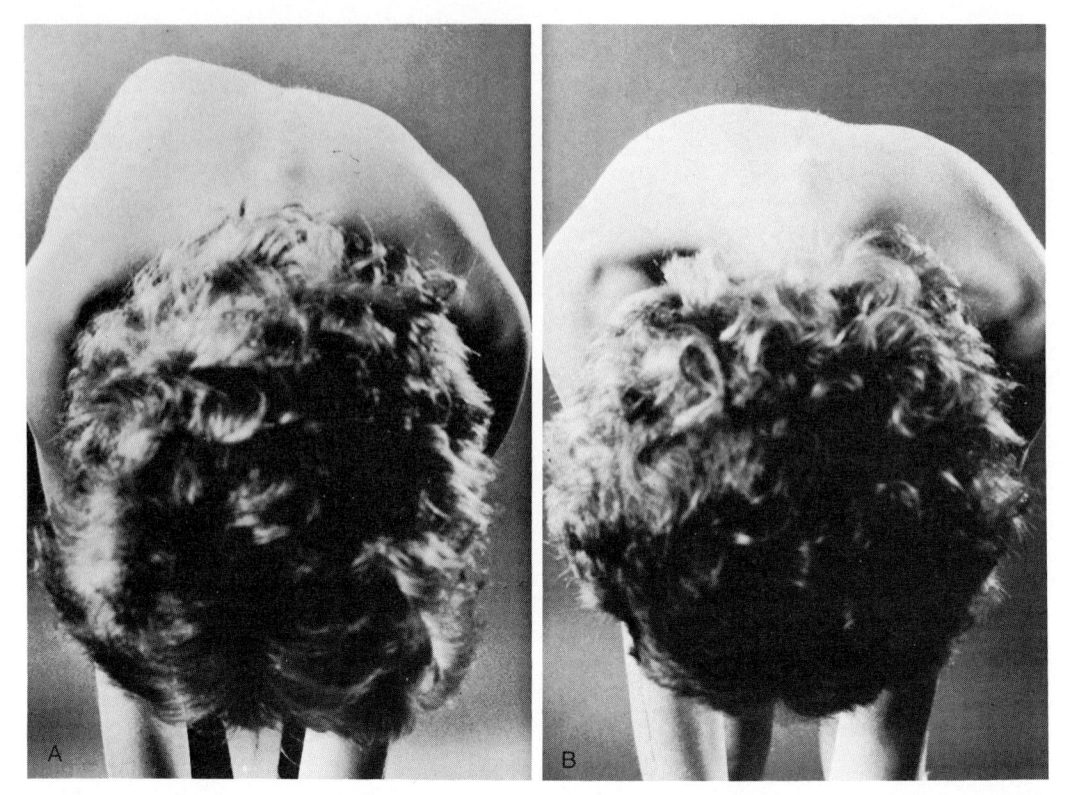

Figure 11–21. A, K.A. is an 18+0 year old white female; her status is three years post posterior spinal fusion for idiopathic scoliosis. Though the fusion was solid and there was no curve progression, the patient was bothered by the cosmetic aspect of her 4.5 centimeter right thoracic prominence. B, This photograph shows the cosmetic result following partial removal of right ribs T6 to T10.

cusses the thoracoplasty technique used at the Twin Cities Scoliosis Center (Fig. 11–21).

SUMMARY

Idiopathic scoliosis encompasses a wide age range of patients and may be subdivided into infantile (onset at less than 3 years of age), juvenile (onset between age 3 and adolescence), and adolescent (onset at the time of adolescence) groups. While it is easy to arbitrarily divide idiopathic scoliosis into these three types, clinically the dividing line is not always clear and there is often overlap.

The etiology of idiopathic scoliosis is unknown; however, research into the vestibular function and genetic patterns of patients with idiopathic scoliosis appears to hold the most promise for unraveling the mystery. The various curve patterns seen most frequently in patients with idiopathic scoliosis have been well described. Any deviation from these patterns should trigger a diligent serach for a possible underlying cause of the curve.

Infantile scoliosis may be divided into progressive and resolving types based on the RVAD and Phase of the curve as described by Mehta. The progressive curve is identified by a RVAD greater than 20 degrees and a shift from Phase I to Phase II. Progressive curves are best treated by serial casting under anesthesia in an attempt to correct the deformity. After correction is maintained for six months, casting may be discontinued, but the patient must be followed to skeletal maturity. Failure to control the curve by casting warrants operative intervention by either the placement of a subcutaneous rod or spinal fusion.

Juvenile idiopathic scoliosis occurs in patients from the age of 3 to the onset of adolescence. The ratio of affected males to females varies according to the age of the patient. There is no consensus as to which curve pattern is most common, although most agree that the thoracic curves are convex to the right. The threshold for treatment of patients with juvenile idiopathic scoliosis is lower than for those with adolescent idiopathic scoliosis because of the increased tendency for juvenile curves to progress. Curves that progress past 20 to 25 degrees should be braced using the Milwaukee brace for thoracic and double major curves and a TLSO for thoracolumbar and lumbar curves. If curve progression past 40 degrees cannot be prevented through bracing, then the curve must be treated surgically by either the placement of a subcutaneous rod if the curve is flexible or fusion if the curve is rigid.

Adolescent idiopathic scoliosis is the most common form of scoliosis in this country. The female to male ratio of affected patients varies according to the magnitude of the curve, but curves requiring treatment occur most commonly in females. Certain curve patterns exist, but there is no agreement as to which pattern is most common. Most thoracic curves are convex to the right.

To be adequately treated idiopathic adolescent scoliosis must first be detected. It appears that school screening programs set up throughout the country are doing this. Curve progression is closely linked to patient maturity.[110] Thus, to most effectively treat patients with idiopathic scoliosis it is important to accurately assess the patient's developmental status. This is probably best done through the use of the Tanner Classification and the Risser sign.

Adolescent idiopathic curves should be treated if progression past 25 degrees is documented or if a curve greater than 30 degrees is seen for the first time and one year of skeletal growth remains. Treatment may take several forms, including Milwaukee bracing, bracing with a TLSO, or the use of an electrical stimulator. Full-time treatment should be continued until all spine growth has ceased and the patient has a Risser sign of at least 4. Either a brace weaning process or stopping the use of the electrical stimulator should occur at this time.

Curve progression past 40 degrees in a growing adolescent despite non-operative treatment is an indication for spinal fusion. This is best accomplished through an articular fusion and instrumentation. The selection of instrumentation depends upon the specific case and the training of the surgeon. At the present time, the Harrington instrumentation is the standard by which all other implants are measured.

The most important fact the orthopaedist treating idiopathic scoliosis must remember is that each case is different. A successful outcome depends upon recognizing these subtleties and responding appropriately.

References

1. Adams, W.: Lectures on Pathology and Treatment of Lateral and Other Forms of Curvature of the Spine. London, Churchill Livingstone, 1865.
2. Alexander, M. A., and Season, E. H.: Idiopathic scoliosis; an electromyographic study. Arch. Phys. Med. Rehabil., 59:314–315, 1978.
3. Axelgaard, J., and Brown, J. C.: Lateral electrical stimulation for the treatment of progressive idiopathic scoliosis. Spine, 8:242–260, 1983.
4. Axelgaard, J., Nordwall, A., and Brown, J. C.: Correction of spinal curvatures by transcutaneous electrical muscle stimulation. Spine, 8:463–481, 1983.
5. Bobechko, W. P., Herbert, M. A., and Friedman, H. G.: Electrospinal instrumentation for scoliosis: current status. Orthop. Clin. North Am., 10:927–941, 1979.
6. Bradford, D. S., Oegema, T. R., and Brown, D. M.: Studies on skin fibroblasts of patients with idiopathic scoliosis. Clin. Orthop. Rel. Res., 126:111–118, 1977.
7. Bradford, D. S., Tanguy, A., and Vanselow, J.: Surface electrical stimulation in the treatment of idiopathic scoliosis: preliminary results in 30 patients. Spine, 8:757–764, 1983.
8. Broadstone, P., Johnson, J. R., Holt, R.T., and Leatherman, K. D.: Consider post-operative immobilization of double L-rod S.S.I. patients. Orthop. Trans., 8:171–172, 1984.
9. Brown, J. C., Axelgaard, J., and Howson, D. C.: Multicenter trial of a noninvasive stimulation method for idiopathic scoliosis. Orthop. Trans., 7:10, 1983.
10. Bunch, W. H.: Scoliosis can be explained with mechanical concepts and mathematical functions. In: Supplementary Program, 19th Annual Meeting of the Scoliosis Research Society, Orlando, Florida, pp. 39–48, 1984.
11. Bunnell, W. P.: The natural history of idiopathic scoliosis. In: Supplementary Program, 19th Annual Meeting of the Scoliosis Research Society, Orlando, Florida, pp. 49–52, 1984.
12. Bunnell, W. P.: A study of the natural history of idiopathic scoliosis. Presented at the 19th Annual Meeting of the Scoliosis Research Society, Orlando, Florida, 1984.
13. Bunnell, W. P., MacEwen, G. D., and Jayakumar, S.: The use of plastic jackets in the non-operative treatment of idiopathic scoliosis. J. Bone Joint Surg., 62A:31–38, 1980.
14. Buric, M., and Momcilovic, B.: Growth pattern and skeletal age in school girls with idiopathic scoliosis. Clin. Orthop. Rel. Res., 170:238–242, 1982.
15. Carr, W. A., Moe, J. H., Winter, R. B., and Lonstein, J. E.: Treatment of idiopathic scoliosis in the Milwaukee brace. J. Bone Joint Surg., 62A:599–612, 1980.
16. Ceballos, T., Ferrer-Torrelles, M., Castillo, F., and Fernandez-Paredes, E.: Prognosis in infantile idiopathic scoliosis. J. Bone Joint Surg., 62A:863–875, 1980.

17. Clarisse, P.: Prognostic evolutif des scolioses idiopathiques mineures de 10 degrees to 29 degrees en periode de croissance. Doctoral thesis, Univ. Claude Bernard, Lyon, 1974.
18. Cobb, J.: Instructional Course Lecture—Outline for Study of Scoliosis. Vol. V. Am. Acad. Orthop. Surg., J. W. Edwards, 1948.
19. Cobb, J.: Spine arthrodesis in treatment of scoliosis. Bull. Hosp. Joint Dis., 29:187–209, 1958.
20. Collis, D. K., and Ponseti, I. V.: Long-term follow-up of patients with idiopathic scoliosis not treated surgically. J. Bone Joint Surg., 51A:425–445, 1969.
21. Conner, A. N.: Developmental anomalies and prognosis in infantile idiopathic scoliosis. J. Bone Joint Surg., 51B:711–713, 1969.
22. Coonrad, R. W., Richardson, W. J., and Oakes, W. J.: Left thoracic curves can be different. Presented at 19th Annual Meeting of the Scoliosis Research Society, Orlando, Florida, 1984.
23. Cowell, H. R., Hall, J. N., and MacEwen, G. D.: Genetic aspects of idiopathic scoliosis. Clin. Orthop. Rel. Res., 86:121–131, 1972.
24. De George, F. V., and Fisher, R. L.: Idiopathic scoliosis: genetic and environmental aspects. J. Med. Genet., 4:251–257, 1967.
25. Dickson, R. A.: Scoliosis in the community. Br. Med. J., 286:615–618, 1983.
26. Dickson, R. A., and Archer, I. A.: Scoliosis in the community. In Dickson, R. A., and Bradford, D. S. (eds.): Management of Spinal Deformities. Boston, Butterworths, pp. 77–100, 1984.
27. Dickson, R. A., Stamper, P., Sharp, A. M., and Harker, P.: School screening for scoliosis: cohort study of clinical course. Br. Med. J., 281:265–267, 1980.
28. Drummond, D. S., and Rogala, E. J.: Growth and maturation of adolescents with idiopathic scoliosis. Spine, 5:507–511, 1980.
29. Duval-Beaupere, G.: Growth and its relationship to bone deformities. In Zorab, P. (ed.): Scoliosis and Growth. Edinburgh, Churchill Livingstone, 1971.
30. Dwyer, A. F., and Schager, M. F.: Anterior approach to scoliosis; results of treatment in 51 cases. J. Bone Joint Surg., 56B:218–224, 1974.
31. Edmonson, A. S., and Morris, J. T.: Follow-up study of Milwaukee brace treatment in patients with idiopathic scoliosis. Clin. Orthop. Rel. Res., 126:58–62, 1977.
32. Emans, J. B., Kaelin, A., Bancel, P., and Hall, J. E.: Boston brace treatment of idiopathic scoliosis. Submitted for publication.
33. Figueiredo, U. M., and James, J. I. P.: Juvenile idiopathic scoliosis. J. Bone Joint Surg., 63B:61–66, 1981.
34. Filho, N. A., and Thompson, M. W.: Genetic studies in scoliosis. J. Bone Joint Surg., 53A:199, 1971.
35. Fisk, J., Moe, J. H., and Winter, R. B.: Lumbosacral joint in idiopathic scoliosis. Presented at the Scoliosis Research Society, Goteberg, Sweden, 1974.
36. Floman, Y., Liebergall, M., Robin, G. C., and Eldor, A.: Abnormalities of aggregation, thromboxane A2 synthesis, and 14C serotonin release in platelets of patients with idiopathic scoliosis. Spine, 8:236–241, 1983.
37. Galen: De Moto Maerculorum.
38. Gradillas, E., Axelgaard, J.: Thermography for muscle contraction mapping. Rancho Los Amigos Rehabilitation Engineering Center, Annual Reports of Progress, Downey, CA. pp. 27–28, 1978.
39. Harrenstein, R. J.: Die skoliose bei Sauglingen und ihre Behandling. Z. Orthop. Chir. L., 11:1, 1929.
40. Harrenstein, R. J.: Sur la scoliose des nourressons et des jeunes enfants. Rev. Orthop., 23:289, 1936.
41. Harrington, P. R.: Surgical instrumentation for management of scoliosis. J. Bone Joint Surg., 42A:1448, 1960.
42. Harrington, P. R.: Treatment of Scoliosis: correction and internal fixation by spine instrumentation. J. Bone Joint Surg., 44A:591–610, 1962.
43. Herman, R., Maulucci, R., Stuyck, J., et al.: Vestibular functioning in idiopathic scoliosis. Orthop. Trans., 3:218, 1979.
44. Hibbs, R. A.: A report of 59 cases of scoliosis treated by fusion operation. J. Bone Joint Surg., 6:3–37, 1924.
45. Innoue, S.: Moire topography for the early detection and postoperative evaluation of scoliosis. Presented to the American Orthopaedic Research Society, 1978.
46. James, J. I. P., Lloyd-Roberts, G. C., and Pilcher, M. F.: Infantile structural scoliosis. J. Bone Joint Surg., 41B:719–735, 1959.
47. James, J. I. P.: Idiopathic scoliosis: the prognosis, diagnosis, and operative indications related to curve patterns and the age at onset. J. Bone Joint Surg., 36B:36–49, 1954.
48. James, J. I. P.: Two curve patterns in idiopathic structural scoliosis. J. Bone Joint Surg., 33B:399–406, 1951.
49. Jonasson-Rajala, E., Josefsson, E., Lundberg, B., and Nilsson, H.: Boston thoracic brace in the treatment of idiopathic scoliosis. Clin. Orthop. Rel. Res., 183:37–41, 1984.
50. Kane, W. J., and Moe, J. H.: A scoliosis-prevalence survey in Minnesota. Clin. Orthop. Rel. Res., 69:216–218, 1970.
51. Keiser, R. P., and Shufflebarger, H. L.: The Milwaukee brace in idiopathic scoliosis; evaluation of 123 completed cases. Clin. Orthop. Rel. Res., 19–24, 1976.
52. Khosla, S., Tredwell, S. J., Day, B., et al.: An ultrastructural study of multifidus muscle in progressive idiopathic scoliosis: changes resulting from a sarcolemmal defect at the myotendinous junction. J. Neurol. Sci., 46:13–31, 1980.
53. King, H. A., Moe, J. H., Bradford, D. S., and Winter, R. B.: The selection of fusion levels in thoracic idiopathic scoliosis. J. Bone Joint Surg., 65A:1302–1313, 1983.
54. Knutsson, F.: Vertebral genesis of idiopathic scoliosis in children. Acta Radiol. (Diagn.) 4:395–402, 1966.
55. Lloyd-Roberts, G. C., and Pilcher, M. F.: Structural idiopathic scoliosis in infancy; a study of the natural history of 100 patients. J. Bone Joint Surg., 47B:520–523, 1965.
56. Lonstein, J. E.: Screening for spinal deformities in Minnesota schools. Clin. Orthop. Rel. Res., 126:33–42, 1977.
57. Lonstein, J. E., Bjorklund, S., Wanninger, M. H., and Nelson, R. P.: Voluntary school screening for scoliosis in Minnesota. J. Bone Joint Surg., 64A:481–488, 1982.

58. Lonstein, J. E., and Carlson, J. M.: The prediction of curve progression in untreated idiopathic scoliosis during growth. J. Bone Joint Surg., 66A:1061–1071, 1984.
59. Low, W. D., Chew, E. C., Kung, L. S., et al.: Ultrastructures of nerve fibers and muscle spindles in adolescent idiopathic scoliosis. Clin. Orthop. Rel. Res., 174:217–221, 1983.
60. Low, W. D., Mok, C. K., Leong, J. C. Y., et al.: The development of southern Chinese girls with adolescent idiopathic scoliosis. Spine, 3:152–156, 1978.
61. Marchetti, P. G., and Faldini, A.: End fusions in the treatment of severe progressing or severe scoliosis in childhood or early adolescence. Orthop. Trans., 2:271, 1978.
62. McCollough, N. C., Friedman, H., and Bracale, R.: Surface electrical stimulation of the paraspinal muscles in the treatment of idiopathic scoliosis. Orthop. Trans., 4:29, 1980.
63. McMaster, M. J., and Macnicol, M. F.: The management of progressive infantile idiopathic scoliosis. J. Bone Joint Surg., 61B:36–42, 1979.
64. Mehta, M. H.: Infantile idiopathic scoliosis. In Bradford, D. S., and Dickson, R. (eds.): Management of Spinal Deformities. Boston, Butterworths, pp. 101–120, 1984.
65. Mehta, M. H.: Infantile idiopathic scoliosis. In Bradford, D. S., and Dickson, R. (eds.): Management of Spinal Deformities. Boston, Butterworths, p. 114, 1984.
66. Mehta, M. H.: Personal communication.
67. Mehta, M. H.: The rib-vertebra angle in the early diagnosis between resolving and progressive infantile scoliosis. J. Bone Joint Surg., 54B:230–243, 1972.
68. Mehta, M. H., and Morel, G.: The non-operative treatment of infantile idiopathic scoliosis. In Zorab, P. A., and Siezler, D. (eds.): Scoliosis. London, Academic Press, pp. 71–84, 1979.
69. Mellencamp, D. D., Blount, W. P., and Anderson, A. J.: Milwaukee brace treatment of idiopathic scoliosis. Clin. Orthop. Rel. Res., 126:47–57, 1977.
70. Misol, S., Ponseti, I. V., Samaan, N., and Bradbury, J. T.: Growth hormone blood levels in patients with idiopathic scoliosis. Clin. Orthop. Rel. Res., 81:122–125, 1971.
71. Moe, J. H.: Methods of correction and surgical techniques in scoliosis. Orthop. Clin. North Am., 3:17–48, 1972.
72. Moe, J. H.: Methods and technique of evaluating idiopathic scoliosis. Academy of Orthopaedic Surgeons Symposium on the Spine, St. Louis, C. V. Mosby, pp. 196–240, 1969.
73. Moe, J. H.: Modern concepts of treatment of spinal deformities in children and adults. Clin. Orthop. Rel. Res., 150:137–153, 1980.
74. Moe, J. H., and Kettleson, D. N.: Idiopathic scoliosis: analysis of curve patterns and the preliminary results of Milwaukee brace treatment in 169 patients. J. Bone Joint Surg., 52A:1509–1533, 1970.
75. Moe, J. H., Kharrat, K., Winter, R. B., and Cummine, J. L.: Harrington instrumentation without fusion plus external orthotic support for the treatment of difficult curvature problems in young children. Clin. Orthop. Rel. Res., 185:35–45, 1984.
76. Moe, J. H., Sundberg, B., and Gustilo, R.: A clinical study of spine fusion in the growing child. J. Bone Joint Surg., 46B:784–785, 1964.
77. Nachemson, A.: A long term follow-up study of nontreated scoliosis. Acta Orthop. Scand., 39:466–476, 1968.
78. Nachemson, A., and Nordwall, A.: The Cotrel dynamic spine traction—an ineffective method for preoperative correction of scoliosis. J. Bone Joint Surg., 58A:158, 1976.
79. Nasca, R. J.: Early experience with segmental spinal instrumentation. Orthop. Trans., 8:207, 1984.
80. Nash, C. L., and Moe, J. H.: A study of vertebral rotation. J. Bone Joint Surg., 51A:223–229, 1969.
81. Nelson, W. E.: Nelson Textbook of Pediatrics. Philadelphia, W. B. Saunders Co., 1979.
82. Nilsonne, U., and Lundgren, K. D.: Long-term prognosis in idiopathic scoliosis. Acta Orthop. Scand., 39:456–465, 1968.
83. Nordwall, A., and Willner, S.: A study of skeletal age and height in girls with idiopathic scoliosis. Clin. Orthop. Rel. Res., 110:6–10, 1975.
84. O'Brien, J. P., and Van Akkerveeken, P. F.: School screening for scoliosis: results of a pilot study. Practitioner, 219:739–742, 1977.
85. Oegema, T. R., Jr., Bradford, D. S., Cooper, K. M., and Hunter, R. E.: Comparison of the biochemistry of proteoglycans isolated from normal, idiopathic scoliotic and cerebral palsy spines. Spine, 8:378–384, 1983.
86. Pedrini, V. A.: Glycosaminoglycans of intervertebral disc in idiopathic scoliosis. J. Lab. Clin. Med., 82:938–950, 1973.
87. Ponseti, I. V., and Friedman, B.: Changes in the scoliotic spine after fusion. J. Bone Joint Surg., 32A:751–766, 1950.
88. Ponseti, I. V., and Friedman, B.: Prognosis in idiopathic scoliosis. J. Bone Joint Surg., 32A:381–395, 1950.
89. Reuber, M., Schultz, A., McNiell, T., and Spencer, D.: Trunk muscle myoelectric activities in idiopathic scoliosis. Spine, 8:447–456, 1983.
90. Riseborough, E. J., and Wynne-Davies, R.: A genetic survey of idiopathic scoliosis in Boston, Massachusetts. J. Bone Joint Surg., 55A:974–982, 1973.
91. Rogala, E. H., Drummond, D. S., and Gurr, J.: Scoliosis: incidence and natural history, a prospective epidemiological study. J. Bone Joint Surg., 60A:173–176, 1978.
92. Sahgal, V., Shah, A., Flanagan, N., et al.: Morphologic and morphometric studies of muscle in idiopathic scoliosis. Acta Orthop., 54:242–251, 1983.
93. Sahlstrand, T., and Petruson, B.: A study of labyrinthine function in patients with adolescent idiopathic scoliosis. Acta Orthop. Scand., 50:759–769, 1979.
94. Samberg, L. C., Benitez, J. T., Leisz, M. C., and Mulawka, S. M.: Study of vestibular function as a prognostic aid in adolescent idiopathic scoliosis. Presented at the 19th Annual Meeting of the Scoliosis Research Society, Orlando, Florida, 1984.
95. Scott, J. C., and Morgan, T. H.: The natural history and prognosis of infantile idiopathic scoliosis. J. Bone Joint Surg., 37B:400–413, 1955.
96. Seiler, X.: Dilatation artificielle du thorax, et traitement des deviations de la colonne verte-

brale, pour une nouvelle methode d'appliquer le courant d'induction galvanique. Bull. Acad. R. Med. Belg., *16*:69–74, 1856–1857.
97. Shands, A. R., and Eisberg, H. B.: The incidence of scoliosis in the state of Delaware; a study of 50,000 minifilms of the chest made during a survey for tuberculosis. J. Bone Joint Surg., *37A*:1243–1249, 1955.
98. Skogland, L. B., and Miller, J. A. A.: Growth related hormones in idiopathic scoliosis. Acta Orthop. Scand., *51*:779–789, 1980.
99. Skogland, L. B., Miller, J. A. A., Skottner, A., and Fryklund, L.: Serum somatomedin A and non-dialyzable urinary hydroxypoline in girls with idopathic scoliosis. Acta Orthop. Scand., *52*:307–313, 1981.
100. Spencer, G. S. G., and Zorab, P. A.: Spinal muscle in scoliosis. Part 1. Histology and histochemistry. J. Neurol. Sci., *30*:405–410, 1976.
101. Taddonio, R. F., Weller, K., and Appel, M.: A comparison of patients with idiopathic scoliosis managed with and without postoperative immobilization following segmental spinal instrumentation with Luque rods. Orthop. Trans., *8*:172, 1984.
102. Taylor, T. K. F., Phil, D., Ghosh, P., and Bushell, G. R.: The contribution of the intervertebral disk to the scoliotic deformity. Clin. Orthop. Rel. Res., *156*:79–90, 1981.
103. Thompson, S. K., and Bentley, G.: Prognosis in infantile idiopathic scoliosis. J. Bone Joint Surg., *62B*:151–154, 1980.
104. Thulbourne, T., and Gillespie, R.: The rib hump in idiopathic scoliosis: measurement, analysis, and response to treatment. J. Bone Joint Surg., *58B*:64–71, 1976.
105. Tolo, V. T., and Gillespie, R.: The characteristics of juvenile idiopathic scoliosis and results of its treatment. J. Bone Joint Surg., *60B*:181–188, 1978.
106. Travaglini, F.: Multiple primary idiopathic scoliosis. Ital. J. Orthop. Traumat., *1*:67–80, 1975.
107. Venn, G., Mehta, M. H., and Mason, R. M.: Characteristics of collagen from normal and scoliotic human spinal ligament. Biochim. Biophys. Acta *757*:259–267, 1983.
108. Weinstein, S. L., Zavala, D. C., and Ponseti, I. V.: Idiopathic scoliosis. J. Bone Joint Surg., *63A*:702–712, 1981.
109. Whalen, R. G., and Ecob, M. S.: Two-dimensional electrophoretic analysis of muscle contractile proteins in patients with idiopathic scoliosis. Clin. Chem., *28*:1036–1040, 1982.
110. Willner, S.: A study of growth in girls with adolescent idiopathic scoliosis. Clin. Orthop. Rel. Res., *101*:129, 1974.
111. Willner, S.: Prospective prevalence study of scoliosis in southern Sweden. Acta Orthop. Scand., *53*:233, 1982.
112. Willner, S.: A study of height, weight and menarche in girls with idiopathic structural scoliosis. Acta Orthop. Scand., *46*:71–38, 1975.
113. Willner, S.: The proportion of legs to trunk in girls with idiopathic structural scoliosis. Acta Orthop. Scand., *46*:84–89, 1975.
114. Willner, S., Nilsson, K. O., Kastrup, K., and Bergstrand, C. G.: Growth hormone and somatomedin A in girls with adolescent idiopathic scoliosis. Acta Pediatr. Scand., *65*:547–552, 1976.
115. Winter, R. B., Anderson, M. B.: Spinal arthrodesis for spinal deformity using posterior instrumentation and sublaminar wiring: a preliminary report of 100 consecutive cases. *In*: Supplementary Program, 19th Annual Meeting of the Scoliosis Research Society, Orlando, Florida, 1984.
116. Winter, R. B., Lonstein, J. E., and Noren, C. A.: Effectiveness of the Milwaukee brace in the nonoperative treatment of thoracic idiopathic scoliosis. Presented at the 19th Annual Meeting of the Scoliosis Research Society, Orlando, Florida, 1984.
117. Winter, R. B., Lovell, W. W., and Moe, J. H.: Excessive thoracic lordosis and loss of pulmonary function in patients with idiopathic scoliosis. J. Bone Joint Surg., *57A*:972–977, 1975.
118. Wyatt, M. P., and Barrack, R. L.: Posterior column function in idiopathic scoliosis. Presented at the 19th Annual Meeting of the Scoliosis Research Society, Orlando, Florida, 1984.
119. Wynne-Davies, R.: Familial (idiopathic) scoliosis: a family survey. J. Bone Joint Surg., *50B*:24–30, 1968.
120. Wynne-Davies, R.: Infantile idiopathic scoliosis: causative factors, particularly in the first six months of life. J. Bone Joint Surg., *57B*:138–141, 1975.
121. Yamada, K., Yamamoto, H., Nakagawa, Y., et al.: Etiology of idiopathic scoliosis. Clin. Orthop. Rel. Res., *184*:50–57, 1984.
122. Yarom, R., Robin, G. C., and Gorodetsky, R.: X-ray fluorescence analysis of muscles in scoliosis. Spine, *3*:142–145, 1978.
123. Yekutiel, M., Robin, G. C., and Yarom, R.: Proprioceptive function in children with adolescent idiopathic scoliosis. Spine, *6*:560–566, 1981.
124. Zaleske, D. J., Ehrlich, M. G., and Hall, J. E.: Association of glycosaminoglycan depletion and degradative enzyme activity in scoliosis. Clin. Orthop. Rel. Res., *148*:177–181, 1980.
125. Zetterberg, C., Aniansson, A., and Grimby, G.: Morphology of the paravertebral muscles in adolescent idiopathic scoliosis. Spine, *8*:457–462, 1983.

12

CONGENITAL SPINE DEFORMITY

R. B. Winter, M.D.

INTRODUCTION

Congenital spine deformities, long ignored because of the large number of tuberculous, paralytic, and idiopathic problems, has only recently been scientifically analyzed as to the natural history and results of various forms of treatment. Congenital deformities can be very benign or incredibly severe, can result in death from cor pulmonale, can cause paraplegia, and can be associated with a multitude of other problems.

CLASSIFICATION AND TERMINOLOGY

Congenital spine deformities are, by definition, those due to congenitally anomalous vertebral development; the anomalies are visible either on roentgenograms or on exposure at the time of surgery. A curvature appearing within the first few months of life is not necessarily congenital, as it may be an infantile idiopathic scoliosis.

Congenital deformities may be classified in several ways including: (1) area of spine involved, (cervical, cervicothoracic, thoracic, thoracolumbar, lumbar, lumbosacral), (2) pattern of deformity (scoliosis, kyphoscoliosis, lordoscoliosis, kyphosis), and (3) specific type of anomalous malformation.

The two basic types of malformation are (1) defects of segmentation and (2) defects of formation. It is rare, however, to see one of these in a pure form; most patients have a mixture of deformities, with one type predominating. Defects of segmentation may be lateral causing scoliosis (the unilateral unsegmented bar), posterolateral causing lordoscoliosis, purely posterior causing lordosis, or purely anterior causing kyphosis, (the anterior unsegmented bar). Some segmentation defects are circumferential in which case no deformity is created, but there is loss of segmental motion and loss of vertical growth (Fig. 12–1).[50]

Defects of formation are the failure of nature to provide all of the embryonic material for the normal development of a vertebra. An inadequate posterior element formation is seen in spina bifida, and these problems are discussed in the chapter on myelomeningocoele. The failure of one side of a vertebra to form results in a hemivertebra. It is important to realize that the hemivertebra is not an "extra" piece of bone thrust into the spine but rather is the normal half of that vertebra, the opposite side being absent or hypoplastic.

If the entire body of a vertebra is absent or hypoplastic and the posterior elements are normally developed, a kyphosis will result. One often sees the situation in which there are defects of formation both laterally and anteriorly, leaving only the posterolateral quadrant of the vertebra present. This produces a true kyphoscoliosis, and is often termed a "posterior quadrant vertebra" (Fig. 12–2).

Hemivertebrae can be seen in many forms and combinations, and it is important to recognize these varieties because of the differences in natural history. A hemivertebra can exist in a spine without causing any curvature owing to corresponding malformation of the adjacent vertebrae. This is called an incarcerated hemivertebra, and this situation is usually benign as far as curve progression is concerned.

A hemivertebra can be non-segmented from either one or both of its adjacent vertebrae. If separated by a disc from one adja-

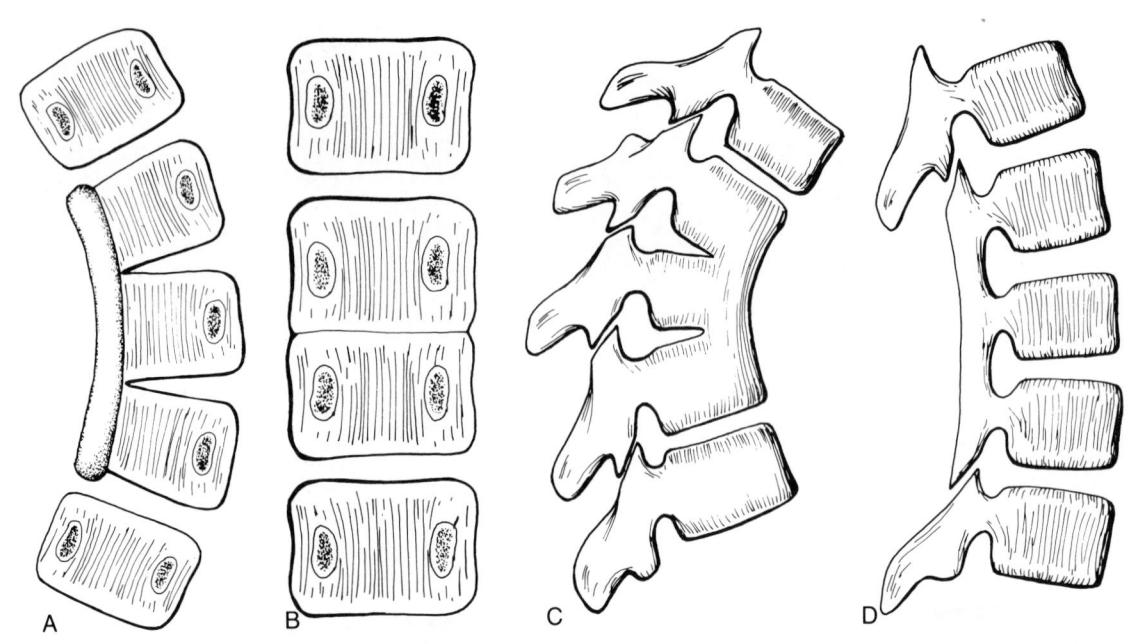

Figure 12–1. *A*, A unilateral defect of segmentation, frequently called a "unilateral unsegmented bar." This is a malformation that is highly likely to lead to a severely progressive scoliosis. *B*, A bilateral and symmetrical failure of segmentation. This is usually called a "bloc" vertebra and does not cause progressive deformity. *C*, An anterior defect of segmentation. This causes a progressive kyphosis. *D*, A bilateral posterior defect of segmentation with resulting lordosis. (Reprinted with permission from Winter, R. B.: Congenital Deformities of the Spine. New York, Thieme-Stratton, 1983.)

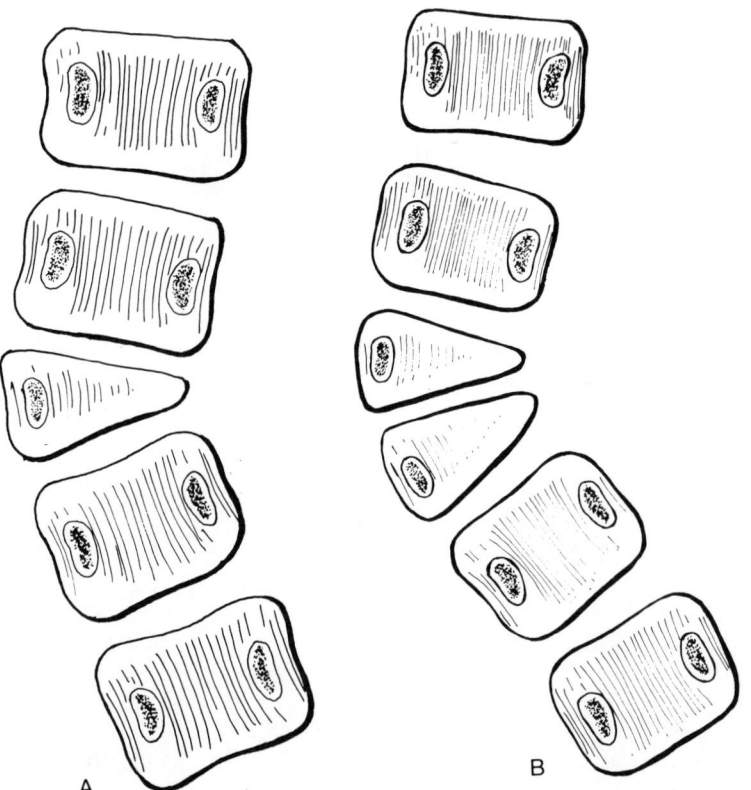

Figure 12–2. *A*, A unilateral defect of formation, commonly called a hemivertebra. In this case, a scoliosis is present and the hemivertebra is fully separated (segmented) from the adjacent vertebrae. *B*, A scoliosis with two convex hemivertebrae, which implies a very significant growth discrepancy between the convex and concave sides. Such situations are usually progressive. (Reprinted with permission from Winter, R. B.: Congenital Deformities of the Spine. New York, Thieme-Stratton, 1983.)

cent vertebra, it is called a semisegmented hemivertebra. If not separated from either adjacent vertebrae, it is called a non-segmented hemivertebra. If fully separated from both adjacent vertebrae, it is called a free hemivertebra or a fully segmented hemivertebra.

There can be more than one hemivertebra, and if both are on the same side of the spine, the prognosis is poor. These can be either adjacent to one another or separated. The two hemivertebra can also be on opposite sides of the spine, producing a more balanced situation, but they can also produce two progressive curvatures.

Finally, hemivertebrae can be combined with a segmentation defect such as a unilateral unsegmented bar. This is the most devastating of all scoliosis-producing situations (Fig. 12–3).[35]

GENETICS

Relatively little has been reported concerning the genetic nature of congenital spine deformities. Wynne-Davies[69] analyzed the families of 337 patients with congenital spine anomalies, 118 of which were myelomeningocoele. She found that an isolated hemivertebra or similar localized defect was a sporadic lesion that carried no risk to subsequent siblings or offspring. Patients with multiple anomalies, even if there were no spina bifida cystica, carried a 5 to 10 per cent risk to subsequent siblings. We have not noticed this relationship at our center except for two children (out of 1250 seen).

Most studies of identical twins have shown one twin to have a congenital defect and the other to be without a defect.[3, 4, 18, 42] There are two reports in which both twins had congenital anomalies.[1, 14]

One syndrome, spondylothoracic dysplasia (also known as costovertebral dysplasia, spondylocostal dysplasia, and Jarcho-Levin syndrome), has several reports in the literature of positive family histories.[5, 7, 25, 45] This syndrome has multiple levels of non-segmentation, multiple fused ribs, and often absent segments. Some, but not all, children die early of respiratory insufficiency. Both recessive and dominant patterns have been reported.

At our center, only about 1 per cent of our patients with congenital spine deformity

Figure 12–3. *A*, A scoliosis due to a hemivertebra, which is non-segmented from the adjacent superior vertebra. This is a "semi-segmented" hemivertebra. There is less chance of progression than with a fully segmented hemivertebra. *B*, A scoliosis due to a hemivertebra, which is non-segmented from both of its adjacent vertebra. This is called a "non-segmented" hemivertebra and does not by itself cause a progressive curve. (Reprinted with permission from Winter, R. B.: Congenital Deformities of the Spine. New York, Thieme-Stratton, 1983.)

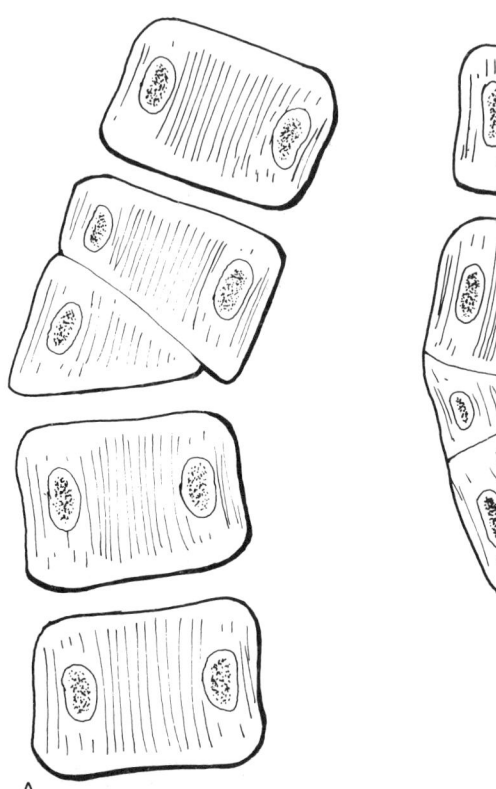

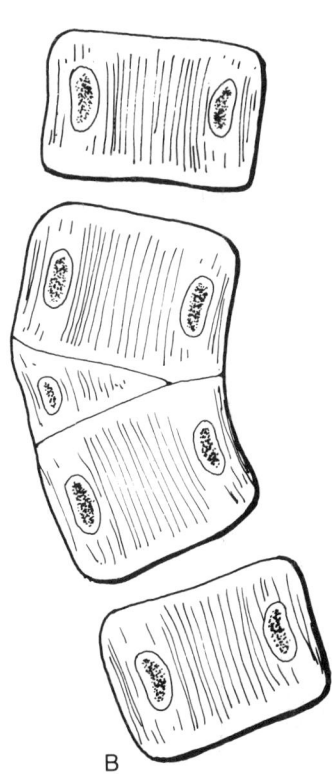

have a known relative with the problem.[58] In eight families siblings were involved. In two families a child and parents were involved. In three families first cousins were involved.

PATIENT EVALUATION

In addition to the general features of patient evaluation presented in Chapter 3, there are some special features that are particularly relevant to the patient with a congenital spine deformity. These special features have to do with associated congenital malformations of the neural axis (spinal dysraphism) and nonspinal congenital anomalies.

For the detection of the dysraphic spine, special attention must be paid to the skin of the back, looking for dimples, nevi, hair patches, lipomata, and scars of previous meningocoele or myelomeningocoele closures. These signs may sometimes be quite obvious, and at other times quite subtle.

One must also carefully examine the extremities, especially the lower extremities, for evidence of neurologic impairment. The more obvious signs are club foot, vertical talus, cavovarus foot, gross thigh or calf atrophy, and absent reflexes. The more subtle findings might be a slight degree of calf atrophy, a diminished reflex, or one foot smaller than the other (Fig. 12–4).

The routine roentgenograms should be carefully examined for evidence of widening of the pedicles, midline bony defects, and spina bifida. Myelograms (especially with water-soluble contrast media and simultaneous CT scanning) should be liberally ordered if there is any possibility of such a defect (Fig. 12–5).

There are a host of other anomalies to look for, including Klippel-Feil syndrome, preauricular ear tags, mandibular hypoplasia, ocular dermoids, cleft lip, cleft palate, congenital heart defect, anal atresia, absent uterus and/or vagina, and absent kidney or obstructive uropathy. The most common associated anomaly is in the urinary system. About 25 per cent of congenital spine patients have some type of genitourinary anomaly.[32] This high frequency of urinary tract problems indicates that all children with congenital spinal anomalies should have an intravenous pyelogram. There is no correlation between the area, size, or type of spinal lesion and the frequency of these urinary tract problems except that congenital kyphotics seem to have fewer problems than do scoliotics. The highest incidence is in those with Klippel-Feil syndrome (Fig. 12–6).

Congenital cardiac defects are also common, occurring in about 10 per cent of patients.[44] There is a strong correlation of Klippel-Feil anomaly, Sprengel's deformity, and

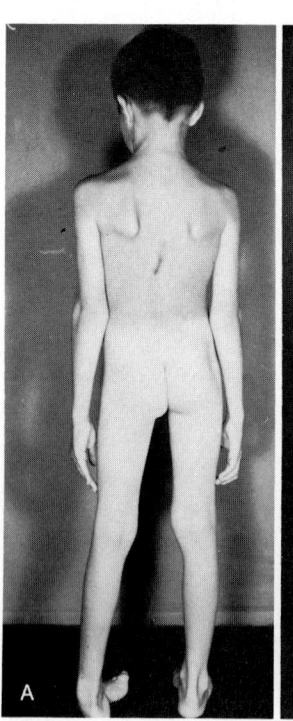

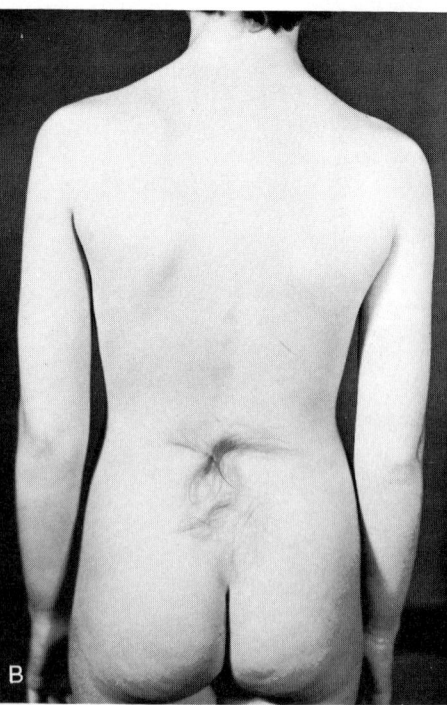

Figure 12–4. *A,* A boy who presented with a severe cavovarus left foot deformity. Examination of the back revealed a small lower thoracic hair patch. A myelogram shows a diastematomyelia. *B,* A girl with no curvature, but a lumbar hair patch and a history of bedwetting. She had a tethered cord due to a fibrous band. Release of the band solved the neurological problem.

Figure 12–5. A, This x-ray shows a congenitally anomalous lumbar spine. There is marked widening of the pedicles and a midline bony defect at L2-L3. B, An oil-soluble myelogram of the same patient showing the mid-line division of the dura, the two halves of the spinal cord, and the coming together of the two divisions distal to the bony spur (a low-lying conus). (Reprinted with permission from Winter, R. B.: Congenital Deformities of the Spine. New York, Thieme-Stratton, 1983.)

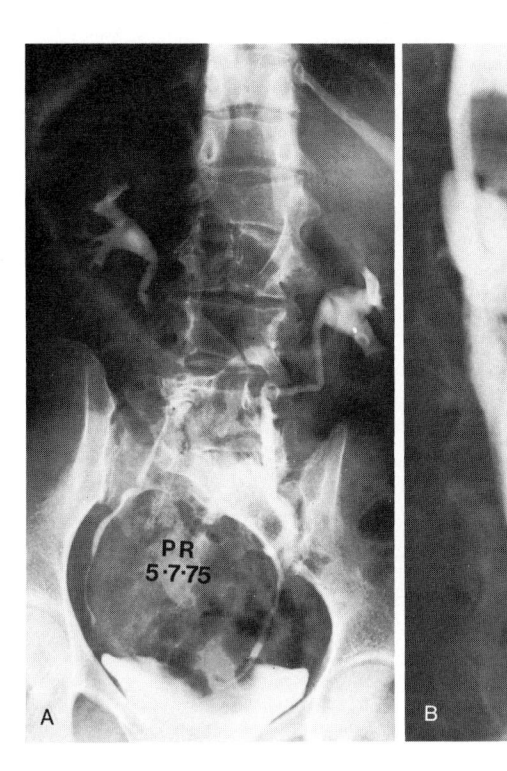

cervicothoracic congenital scoliosis. A diligent search for all possible anomalies is obviously indicated.

THE NATURAL HISTORY OF CONGENITAL SPINE DEFORMITY

It is best to subdivide this discussion first by the pattern of deformity (scoliosis, kyphosis), and second by the type of anomaly present (segmentation defect, formation defect, mixed defect). Other factors of significance will be mentioned in these separate areas.

Congenital Scoliosis

For congenital scoliosis, the most severely progressive deformities are those due to unilateral defects of segmentation. The severity of the deformity is related to the length of the area involved as well as the quality of convex growth. The more active and normal the convex growth, the more severe the problem. It is thus important to look not only at the concave unilateral bar, but also to closely examine the quality of bone and disc space development on the convexity. If the spaces are present and clearly defined and the pedicles crisply formed, the prognosis is bad. If the convex discs are only vaguely formed and the convex pedicles poorly delineated, the prognosis is not as bad.

Unilateral unsegmented bars are most common in the thoracic and thoracolumbar areas. Unilateral bars are rare in the cervical spine and slightly more common in the lumbar spine. In the lumbar spine they may produce pelvic obliquity, and in the cervical spine torticollis.

The earliest review of the natural history was that by Kuhns and Hormell in 1952.[26] They reviewed 85 children and found only 13 (15 per cent) to show no progression. Thirty-two showed severe progression, and these were most often thoracic curves with multiple unbalanced anomalies.

MacEwen, Conway, and Miller[31] reviewed 88 patients at the Dupont Institute. In the 10 patients with unilateral unsegmented bars, they noted an average progression of 5 degrees per year, the typical curve beginning at about 30 degrees and progressing to about 100 degrees.

Rathke and Sun[43] reviewed the natural history of 39 congenital patients. Only two showed no progression. Once again thoracic curves were the worst, and females were noted to have a worse prognosis than males.

At our center, 57 patients were reviewed as to the natural history.[64] Ten per cent progressed 5 degrees or less, 21 (37 per cent)

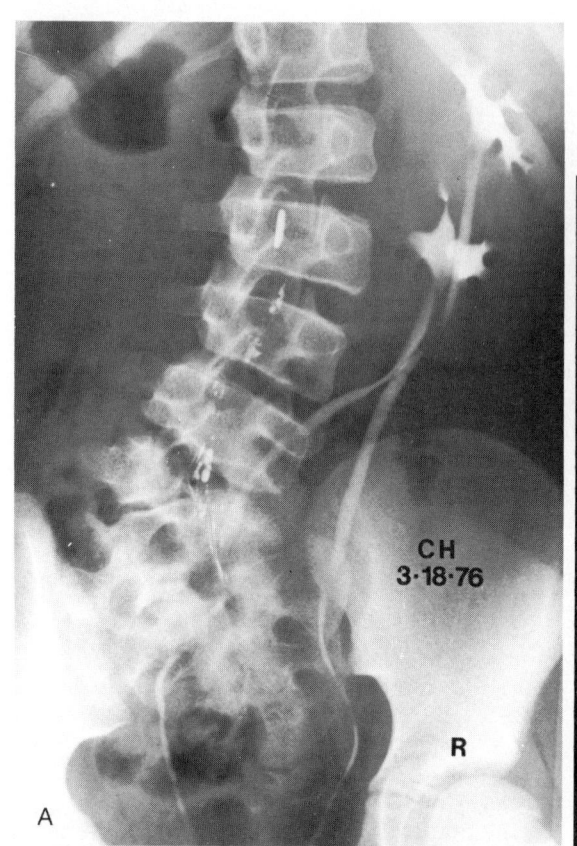

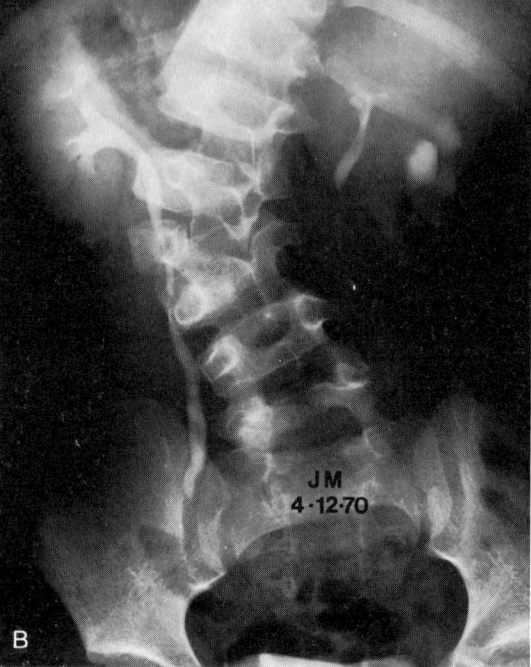

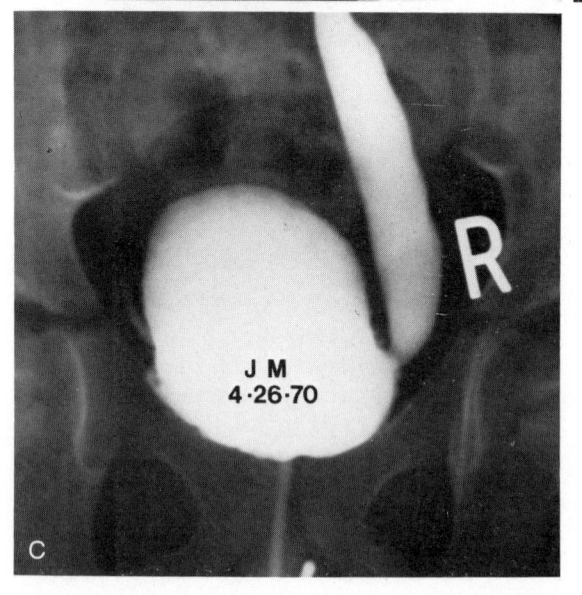

Figure 12–6. *A*, An intravenous pyelogram shows a crossed fused ectopia, both renal masses being on the same side, but with separate collection systems. There is no obstruction. (Reprinted with permission from Winter, R. B.: Congenital Deformities of the Spine. New York, Thieme-Stratton, 1983.) *B*, An intravenous pyelogram showing hydronephrosis of the left kidney. This patient had no renal or urinary symptoms and the urinalysis was normal. *C*, A retrograde study shows the dilated ureter and a stenosis at the ureterovesical junction. The patient's scoliosis surgery had to be delayed until this lesion was repaired.

progressed from 6 to 30 degrees, and 26 (45 per cent) progressed 31 degrees or more. As in the other studies, we also noted a high progression rate for thoracic curves, all 28 progressed and half of these progressed more than 30 degrees.

Other studies of the natural history have been reported by Tsou, Yau, and Hodgson,[55] Nasca, Stelling, and Steel,[40] and Touzet and coworkers.[54]

An excellent recent study of the natural history of congenital scoliosis is that of McMaster and Ohtsuka.[35] They reviewed 202 patients followed past age 10 without treatment. Only 11 per cent of the curves were non-progressive, 14 per cent progressed slightly, and 75 per cent progressed significantly. Thirty-six per cent of the patients had a curve of between 40 and 60 degrees, and 28 per cent had a curve of 61 degrees or more. The rate of deterioration depended upon the area of the spine and the type of anomaly. The worst anomaly was the unilateral unsegmented bar with a convex hemivertebra, followed by the unilateral unsegmented bar, double convex hemivertebra, a single free convex hemivertebra; the least progressive was the bloc vertebra (Figs. 12–7 to 12–9).

Congenital scoliosis due to formation defects is less easy to predict. Some hemivertebrae can cause extermely severe curves and others are quite benign. As indicated previously, if one carefully examines the roentgenogram for evidence of segmentation versus non-segmentation of the hemivertebra, one can predict with better accuracy the likelihood of curve increase.

As in all congenital spine problems, it is essential to obtain good quality films and to measure them accurately. In young children, supine films are preferable. If a patient is progressing at the rate of 6 degrees per year and the physician sees the patient three times a year, he is being expected to appreciate an increase of only 2 degrees per visit, an amount well within the error of measurement. It is thus important to compare the current roentgenogram not only with one taken at the last visit, but with the roentgenogram from a year ago and especially with the roentgenogram taken at the first visit (Figs. 12–10 to 12–13).

Congenital scoliosis due to mixed anomalies are especially difficult to predict, and treatment almost always depends upon serial observations rather than certainty based on a single visit. It seems best to form an overall opinion as to the quality of growth potential on one side as compared to the other.

Finally, it is as important to evaluate the secondary or compensatory curves as it is to monitor the primary curve. Quite often the secondary curve can become the more progressive and more deforming of the two curves (Fig. 12–14).

Congenital Kyphosis

Kyphotic deformities are less common than scoliotic deformities, but unfortunately their consequences may be more severe. Contrary to scolioses, segmentation defects are less progressive and less ominous than formation defects. The greatest danger of neglected congenital kyphosis is paraplegia. Unfortunately, congenital kyphosis is the most likely cause of paraplegia of all non-infectious spinal deformities. Worldwide, tuberculosis still ranks as the number one deformity-causing paraplegia.[30]

Paraplegia is most common with defects of formation, and especially with defects having an apex between T4 and T9 (the watershed area of spinal cord blood supply). Although paraplegia may occur earlier, it is most common during the adolescent growth spurt (Figs. 12–15 and 12–16).[9, 10, 30, 68]

Kyphosis due to defects of segmentation tends to be less progressive, produces less deformity, and does not cause paraplegia. It is most common in the lower thoracic spine or at the thoracolumbar junction. It necessitates a compensatory hyperlordosis of the lumbar spine and this may be far more symptomatic than the primary kyphosis (Fig. 12–17).[34]

NON-OPERATIVE TREATMENT OF CONGENITAL SPINE DEFORMITIES

Congenital Scoliosis

There is only one form of non-operative treatment of congenital scoliosis that has had any positive effect—bracing. The only brace with documented successful results is the Milwaukee brace. Underarm braces achieve curve control at the expense of thoracic constriction, a very undesirable effect in a patient whose respiratory capacity is already affected by the curve. Treatment by exercise, electrical

Text continued on page 250

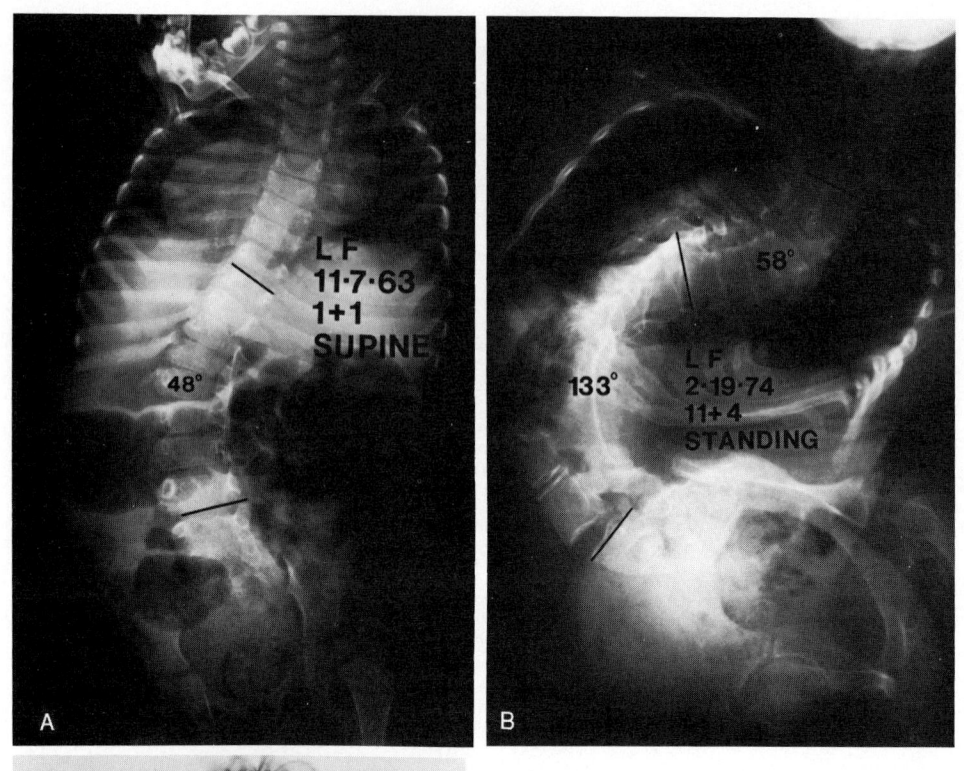

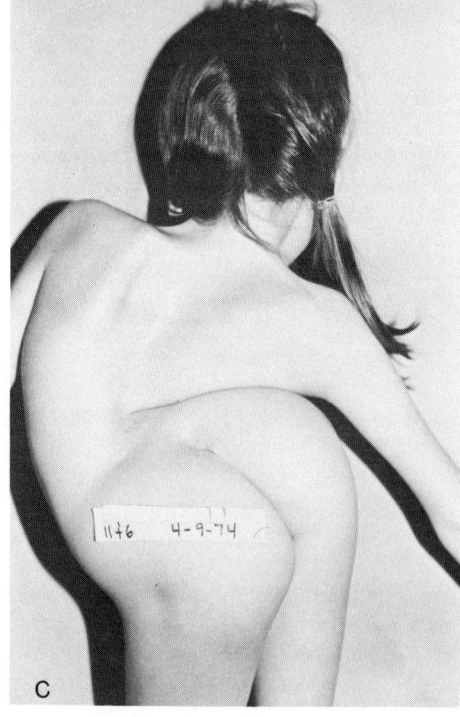

Figure 12–7. *A,* This one year old girl, who was seen elsewhere, had a 48 degree congenital scoliosis due to a unilateral unsegmented bar involving T11 through L3. There are bilateral defects of segmentation of T3 through T6 and L5 through S1. *B,* The same patient at age 11 when she presented to our center. The curve is now 133 degrees with a severe pelvic obliquity. Despite a completely "uncovered" right hip, it was not dislocated. *C,* A clinical photograph of the patient at age 11. (Reprinted with permission from Winter, R. B.: Congenital Deformities of the Spine. New York, Thieme-Stratton, 1983.)

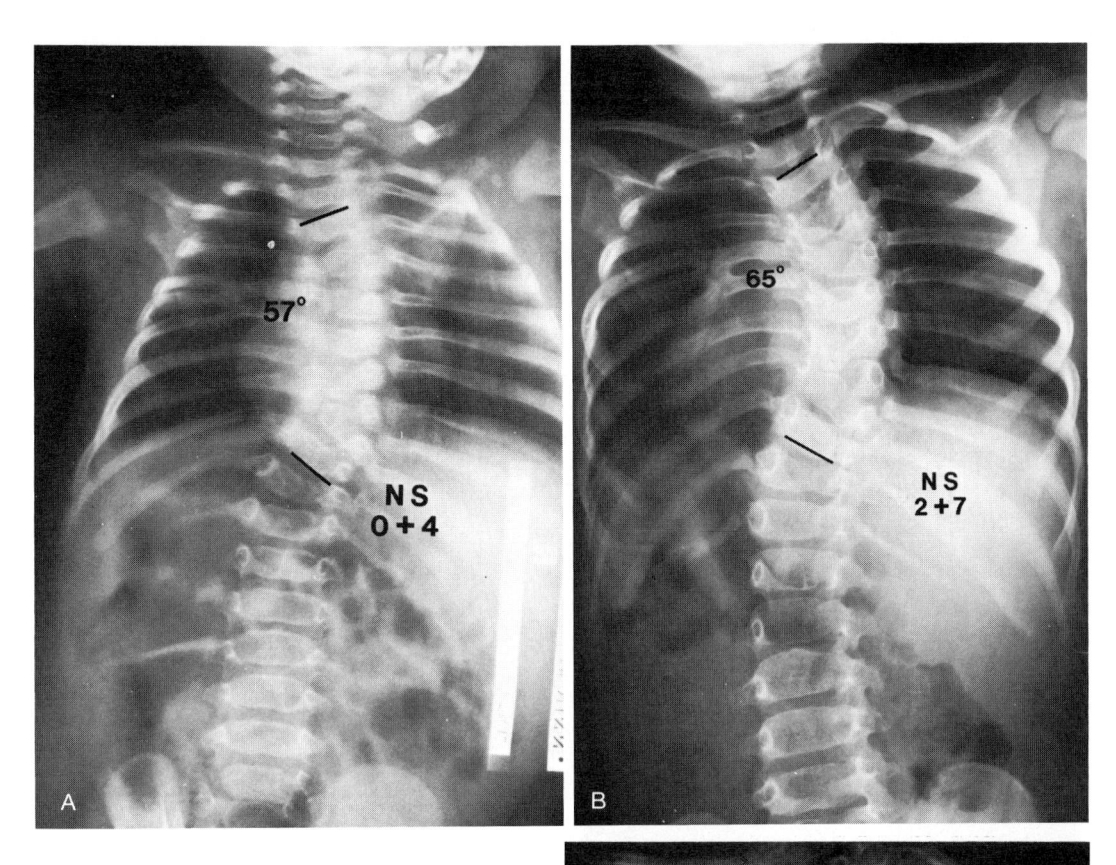

Figure 12–8. A, A four month old girl with a 57 degree right thoracic congenital scoliosis from T2 to T10. Note the straight lumbar spine. At first glance this appears to be a formation defect problem with two convex hemivertebrae, but note the concave synostosis of ribs 4, 5, and 6. One must also remember that at this age, much of the vertebrae are still cartilaginous. B, The same patient at age 2+7 years. The curve has increased to 65 degrees and now the bones are much better developed. The concave pedicles have coalesced into a unilateral bar from T3 to T9. The convex pedicles are clear and crisp. C, The same patient at age 14, with her curve now measuring 142 degrees. A secondary lumbar curve of 117 degrees has developed and with it a significant pelvic obliquity. She had been seen at an orthopaedic hospital once a year, but the x-rays had never been measured. No treatment had even been given. (Reprinted with permission from Winter, R. B.: Congenital Deformities of the Spine. New York, Thieme-Stratton, 1983.)

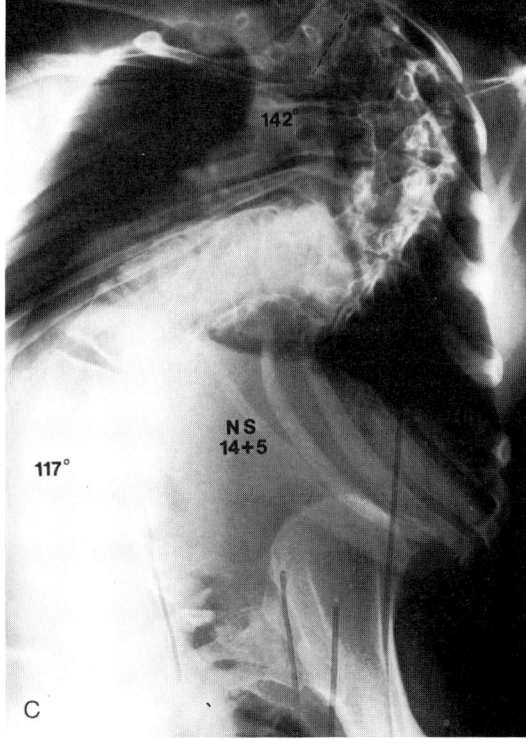

Figure 12–9. A, This 1+8 year old boy was seen with a 33 degree T1 to T6 right thoracic congenital scoliosis. There is a massive rib synostosis on the left and none on the right. Will this be progressive? B, The same patient at age 8+11 years. The curve is only 37 degrees and now it is possible to see that there is a bilateral failure of segmentation, not a unilateral one. No treatment was given. C, The same patient at age 27. The curve remains unchanged despite no treatment of any kind. Careful observation can sometimes be the best treatment of all. (Reprinted with permission from Winter, R. B.: Congenital Deformities of the Spine. New York, Thieme-Stratton, 1983.)

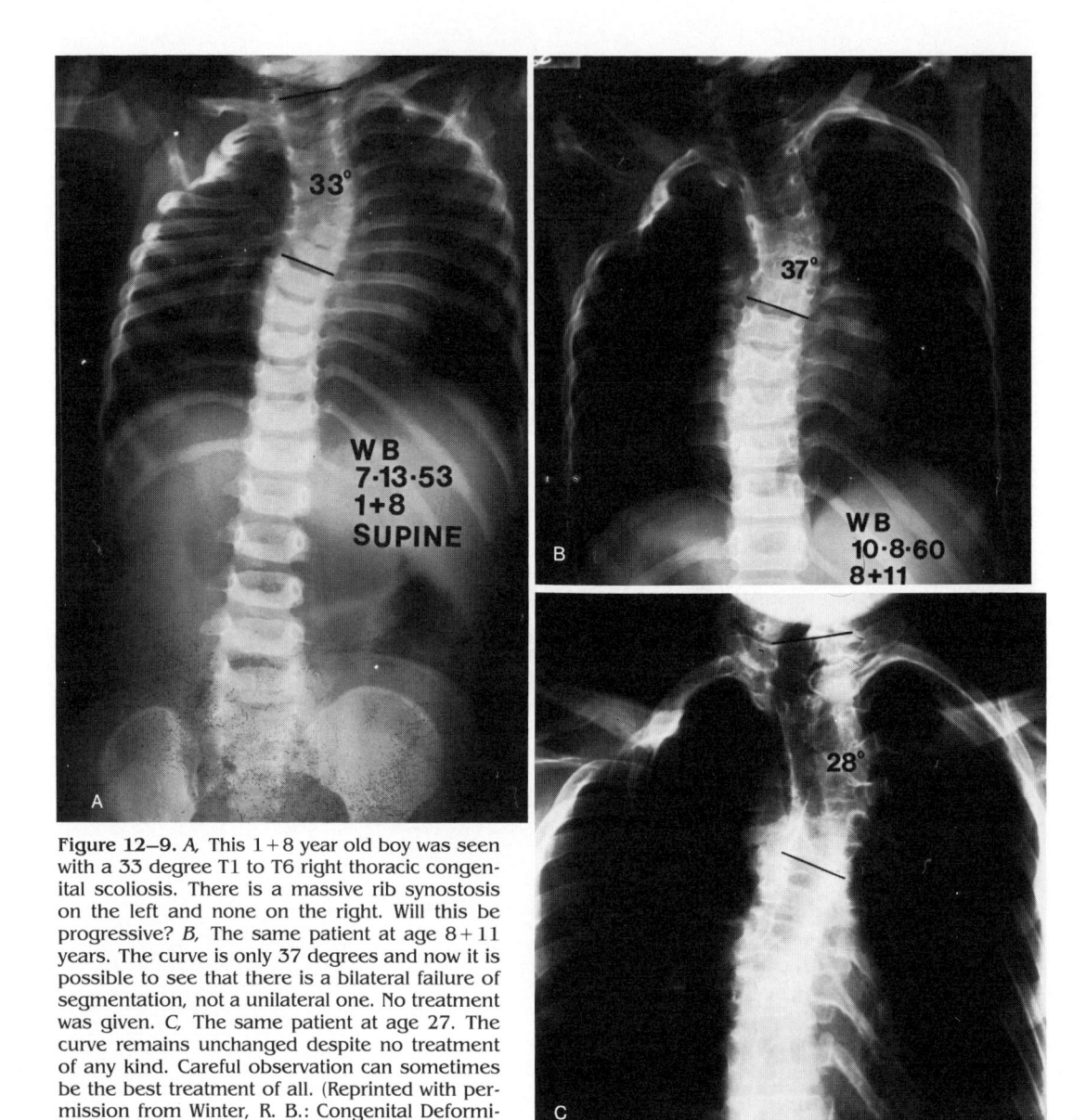

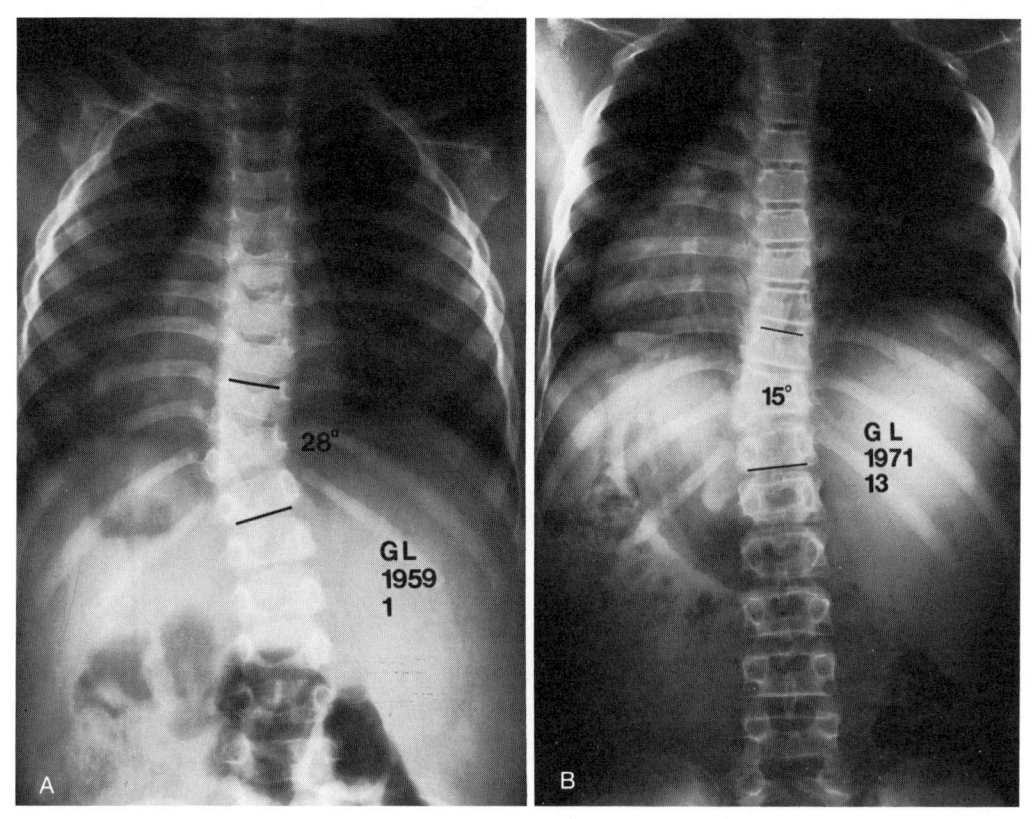

Figure 12–10. A, This patient was first seen in 1959 at the age of one year. There was a 28 degree scoliosis due to a hemivertebra on the left at T11. B, The same patient at age 13, twelve years later. There was no treatment. The curve measures 15 degrees and the hemivertebra is nearly non-segmented from the adjacent superior vertebra. (Reprinted with permission from Winter, R. B.: Congenital Deformities of the Spine. New York, Thieme-Stratton, 1983.)

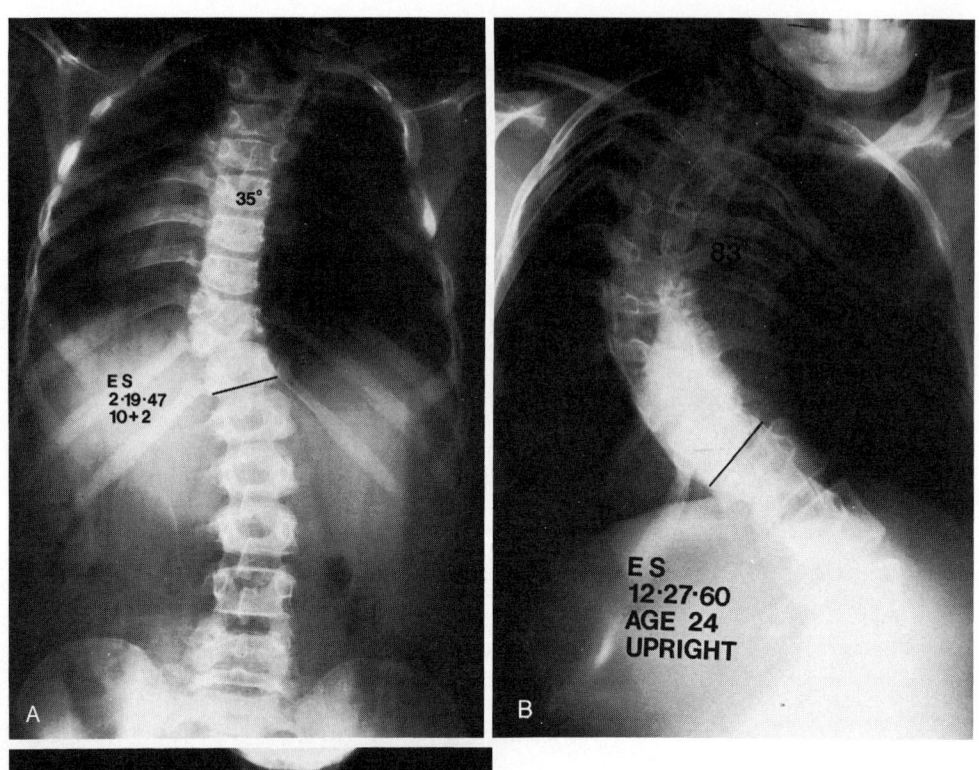

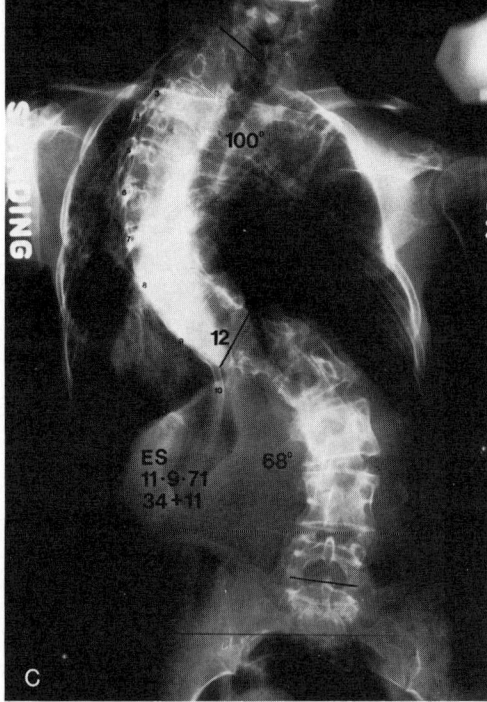

Figure 12–11. *A*, This ten year old girl presented to Gillette Children's Hospital with a 35 degree thoracic curve in 1947. No treatment was given, the family refusing the fusion recommended. *B*, She was next seen in 1960 at age 24 when she delivered a baby and went into cor pulmonale. Her curve now measured 83 degrees. Medical treatment was given and the heart failure resolved. *C*, When last seen in 1971 at the age of 35, she was in terminal cor pulmonale. Despite medical and surgical treatment, she expired in 1974 at the age of 38. (Reprinted with permission from Winter, R. B.: Congenital Deformities of the Spine. New York, Thieme-Stratton, 1983.)

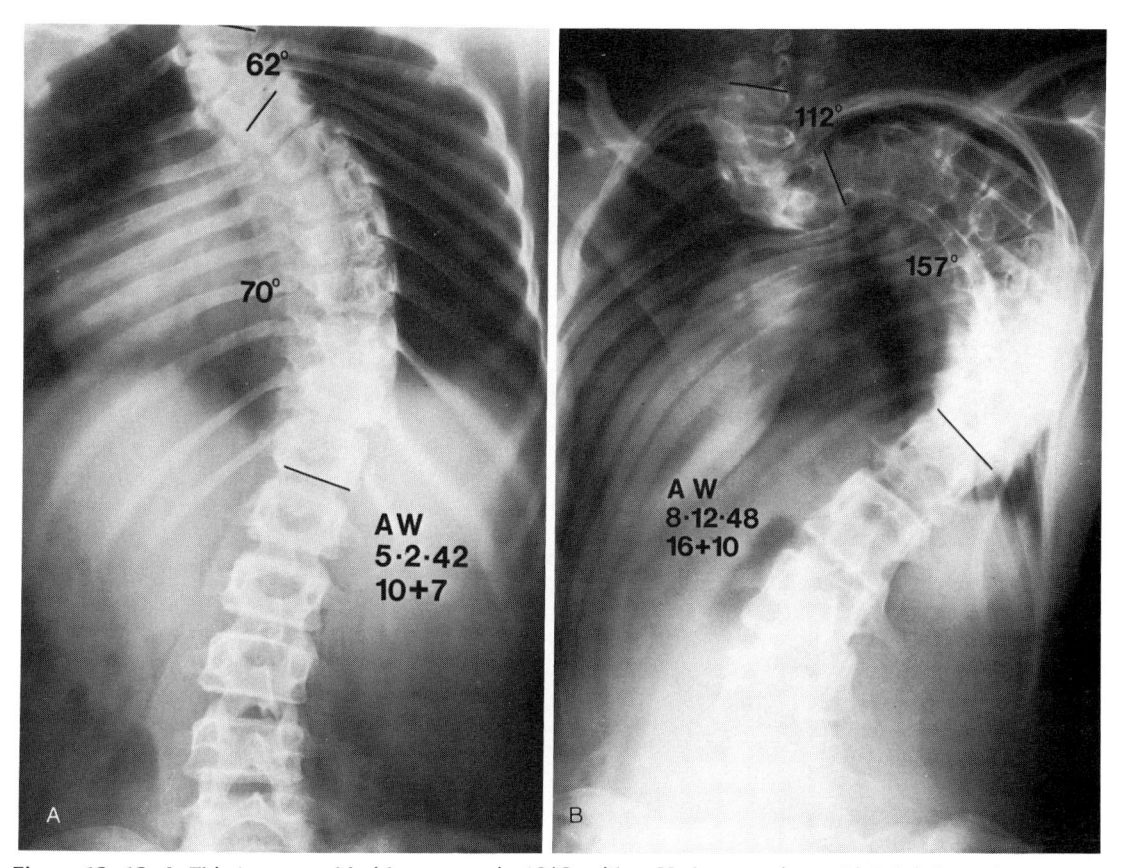

Figure 12–12. *A*, This ten year old girl was seen in 1942, with a 62 degree primary high left thoracic curve due to a single "free" hemivertebra at T3. There was already a 70 degree right thoracic compensatory curve. No treatment was given. *B*, The same patient at age 16. There was an increase of the primary congenital curve to 112 degrees, and the secondary curve was now 157 degrees. She was already dyspneic at this time. (Reprinted with permission from Winter, R. B.: Congenital Deformities of the Spine. New York, Thieme-Stratton, 1983.)

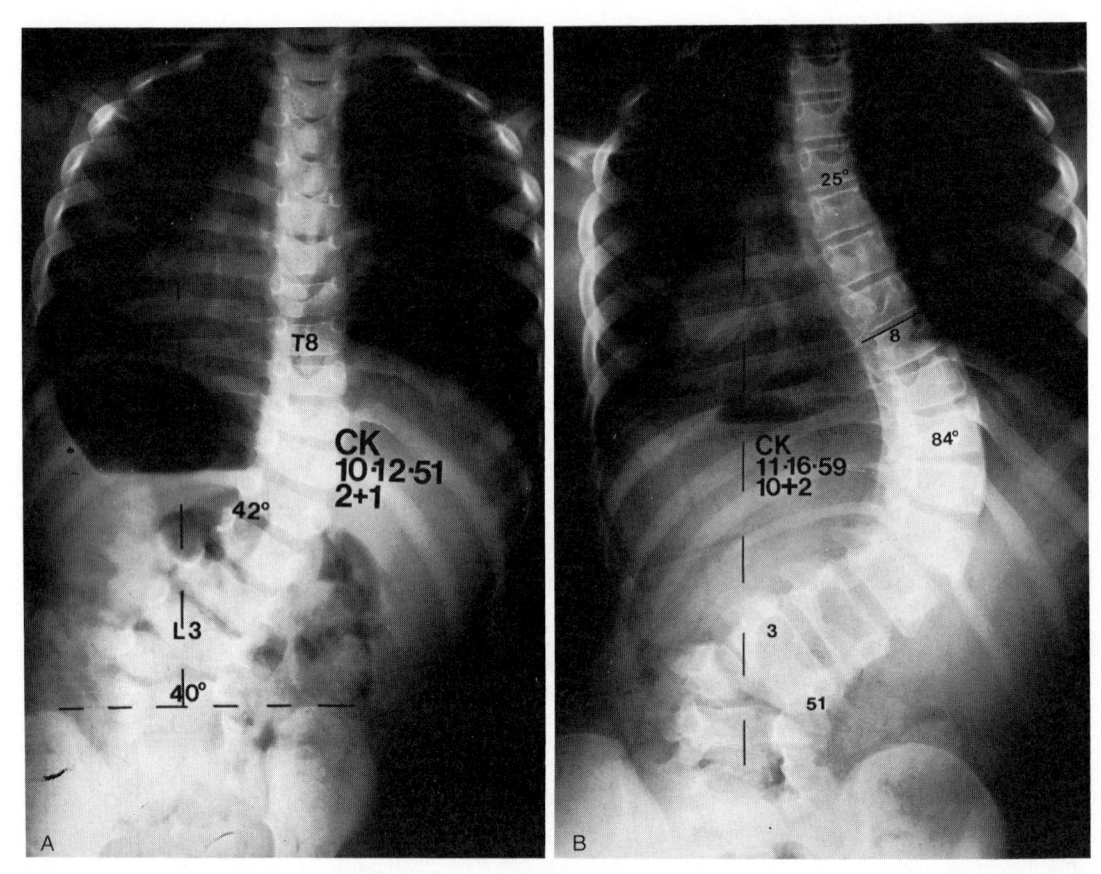

Figure 12–13. *A*, This two year old girl was seen elsewhere and was found to have a marked decompensation of the spine due to a hemivertebra on the left at L4. No treatment was given. *B*, When first seen by the authors in 1959 at the age of 10, the secondary T8 to L3 curve had doubled in magnitude and the primary L3 to L5 curve had also increased. At this point in time, it was necessary to correct and fuse both curves. (Reprinted with permission from Winter, R. B.: Congenital Deformities of the Spine. New York, Thieme-Stratton, 1983.)

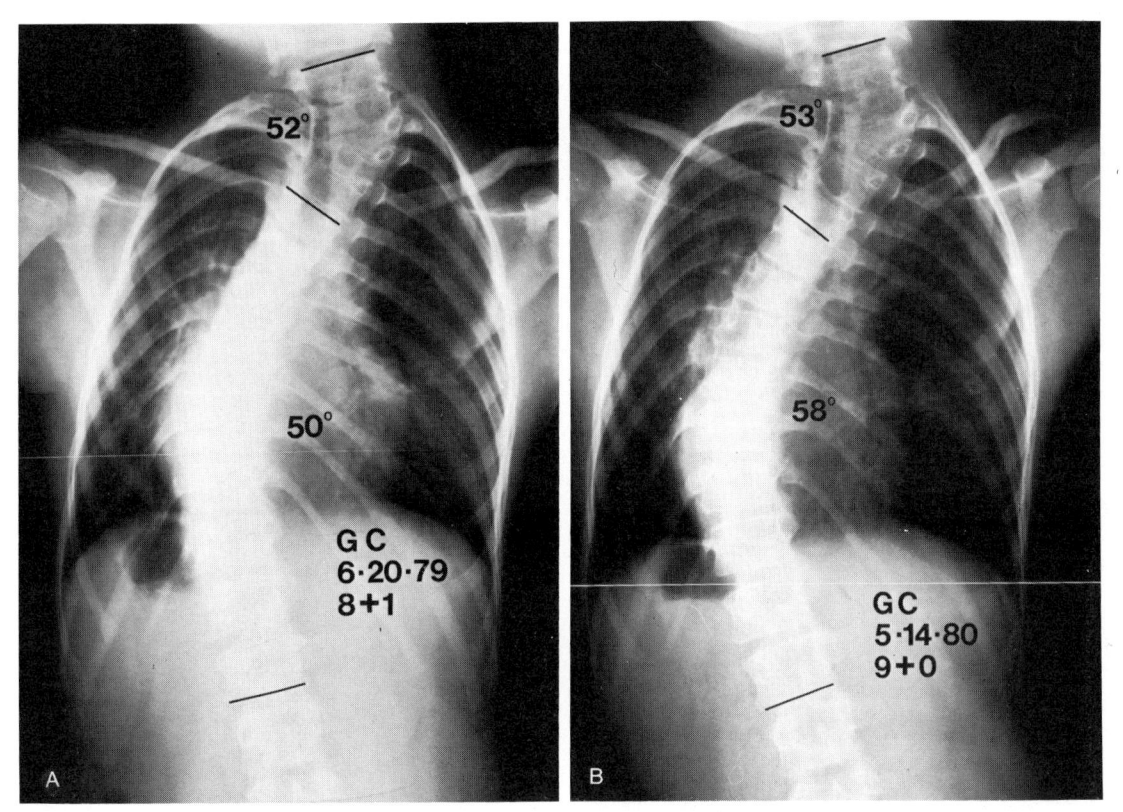

Figure 12–14. A, An eight year old girl with a 52 degree primary congenital cervicothoracic curve and a 50 degree T5 to L2 secondary curve. No treatment was given. B, The same patient a year later. The primary curve has increased only one degree, but the secondary curve has increased 8 degrees. (Reprinted with permission from Winter, R. B.: Congenital Deformities of the Spine. New York, Thieme-Stratton, 1983.)

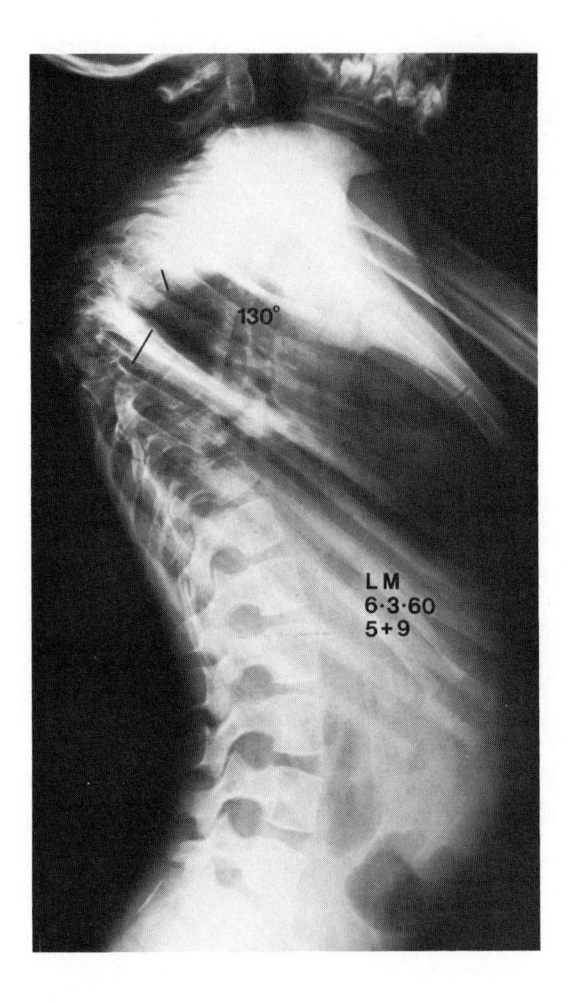

Figure 12–15. This five year old girl had a 130 degree congenital kyphosis due to defects of formation. She became paraplegic at the age of nine and died of respiratory insufficiency at age 10. (Reprinted with permission from Winter, R. B., et al.: Congenital kyphosis. J. Bone Joint Surg., 55A:223–256, 1973.)

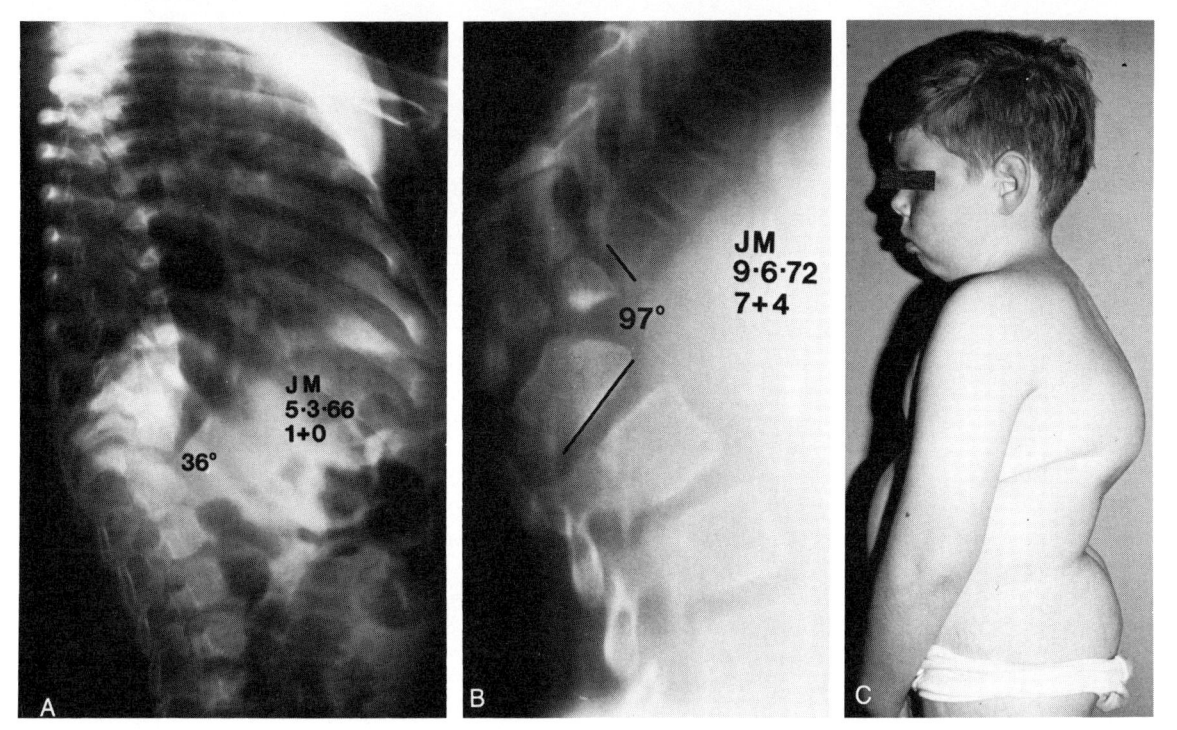

Figure 12–16. A, This one year old boy was seen elsewhere because of a "bump" on the back. There is a 36 degree congenital kyphosis due to a defect of formation. No treatment was given. B, When first seen by the author at age seven, this patient's kyphosis measured 97 degrees and he was showing the early signs of paraparesis. (For the subsequent treatment see Figure 12–31.) C, The clinical appearance of the patient at age seven. (Reprinted with permission from Winter, R. B.: Congenital Deformities of the Spine. New York, Thieme-Stratton, 1983.)

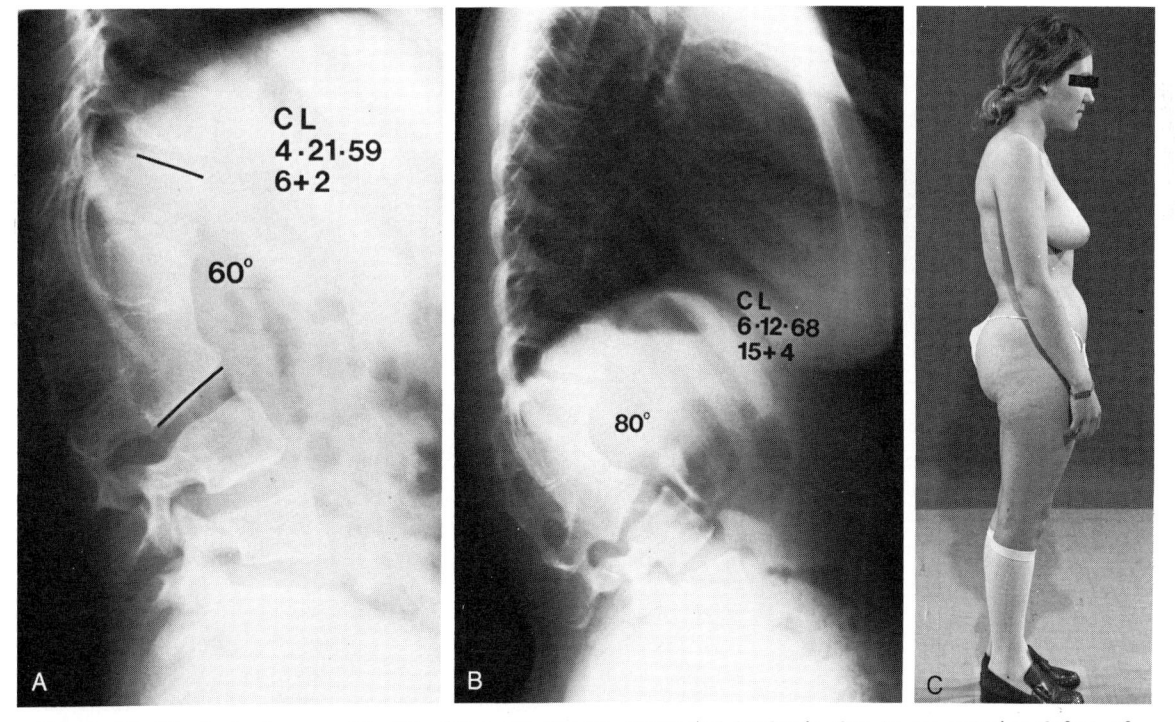

Figure 12–17. A, A six year old girl with a 60 degree congenital kyphosis due to an anterior defect of segmentation. No treatment was given. B, The same patient at age 15, showing an 80 degree kyphosis. She was beginning to have a significant amount of lumbar back pain. C, A clinical photograph at age 15 showing remarkably little external deformity. (Reprinted with permission from Winter, R. B.: Congenital Deformities of the Spine. New York, Thieme-Stratton, 1983.)

stimulation, massage, manipulation, and anything else have never been shown to be of any value whatsoever.

The treatment of congenital scoliosis by bracing (orthotics) is applicable only to a limited number of situations. It is incorrect to say that brace treatment is totally worthless. It is also incorrect to say that bracing is effective in "a large percentage" of patients. The only study of bracing in congenital scoliosis was published by Winter, Moe, MacEwen, and Peon-Vidales in 1976.[67] In this analysis of 63 patients seen at both the Twin Cities Scoliosis Center and the Dupont Institute, several examples of successful treatment are shown. The best results were seen with mixed anomalies and with the progressive secondary curve.

Bracing is seldom the only form of treatment, and even when successful, it usually only delays the fusion until adequate spinal growth has occurred (the onset of the adolescent growth spurt). A scoliosis that is completely rigid cannot be benefited by a brace, and thus a bending or traction film is useful in determining flexibility. The more flexible the curve, the more likely it is to be benefitted by a brace. Long curves (10 or more vertebrae) are more responsive to a brace than short curves. A curve with its apex at the thoracolumbar junction that is long and flexible (50 per cent or more correction on bending films) is an excellent candidate for bracing, particularly if the child has documented evidence of progression and several years of growth remaining before reaching the adolescent growth spurt (Fig. 12–18).

Congenital Kyphosis and Lordosis

Contrary to the situation with congenital scoliosis, there is no evidence of any kind of successful non-operative treatment of congenital kyphosis or lordosis.[63, 68] Braces, exercise, manipulation, vitamins, and massage will *not* alter the natural history of these deformities.

OPERATIVE TREATMENT OF CONGENITAL SPINE DEFORMITIES

Congenital Scoliosis

There is no one single form of operative treatment that is ideal for congenital scoliosis. The prudent surgeon must select the form of operative treatment that is best for the specific patient. This, of course, depends upon the age of the patient, the type of deformity,

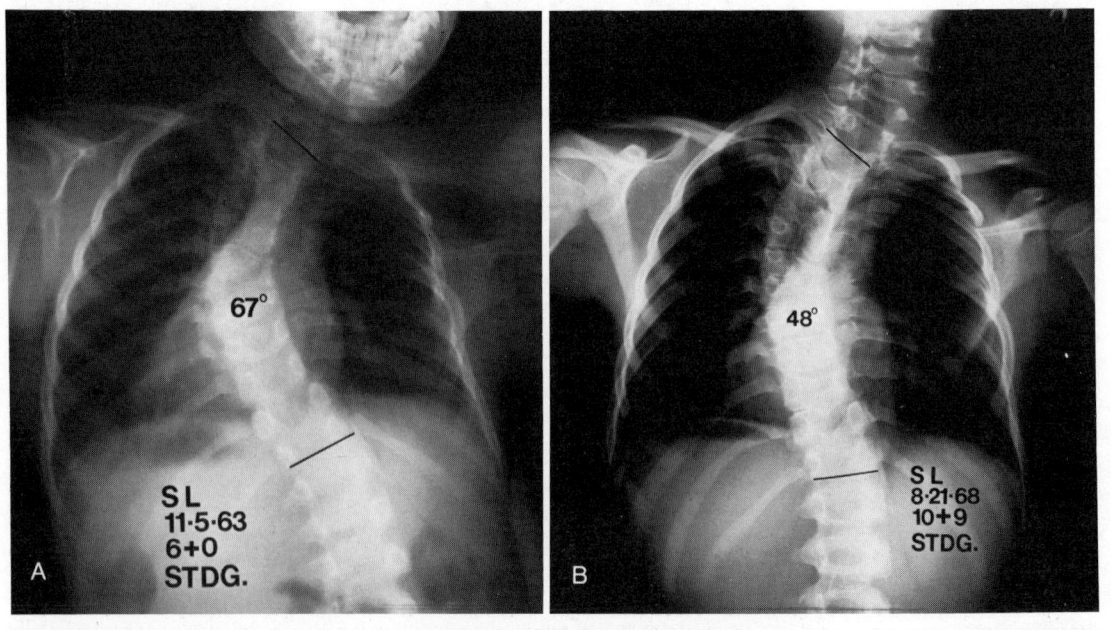

Figure 12–18. A, This six year old boy was seen in 1963; he presented with a progressive congenital thoracic scoliosis of 67 degrees. A Milwaukee brace was applied at this time. B, The same patient four years later, showing a curve of 48 degrees. Not only had the progression been halted, but some improvement had been obtained. He did well until age 12, at which time the curve increased and a fusion was done. (Reprinted with permission from Winter, R. B.: Congenital Deformities of the Spine. New York, Thieme-Stratton, 1983.)

the area of deformity, the natural history of the deformity, the pattern of curvature, and the presence or absence of other congenital anomalies.

The types of surgery available are: (1) posterior fusion in situ, (2) posterior fusion with external correction by cast or brace, (3) posterior fusion with correction by traction and maintenance by casting, (4) posterior fusion with correction by instrumentation, (5) posterior fusion with correction by traction and stabilization by instrumentation, (6) anterior and posterior convex fusion with epiphyseodesis, (7) hemivertebra excision with fusion, and (8) combinations of one or more of these procedures.

FUSION IN SITU

Fusion in situ is best for the curve that has either demonstrated progression, or is of such a nature that progression is inevitable, but at the same time, is so stiff and rigid that correction is not realistic. The classic example of such a curve is the unilateral unsegmented bar. A posterior fusion is done, incorporating all of the bar plus one mobile segment above and one below the bar. An abundant autogenous bone graft should be utilized. If not enough autogenous bone is available because of the child's young age, bank bone can be used (Fig. 12–19).

POSTERIOR FUSION WITH CAST CORRECTION

Posterior fusion with cast correction is best for situations in which the curve is flexible enough to improve with cast correction, but the bones are so small or formed in such a way as to make correction by instrumentation impractical. A good example is a curve due to one or two hemivertebrae, demonstrated to be progressive, but in a patient younger than age eight. Avoiding rods also reduces the risks of paraplegia (Fig. 12–20).

If it is noted on subsequent follow-up that a fused curve is bending, it should be treated by an anterior convex fusion combined with refusion posteriorly. This will promptly stop the bending process.

In the past, "protection" of the young fusion with many years of bracing was advocated. There was, however, no scientific evidence to support this program. Furthermore, a child's life is far happier if it is free of a brace. I personally feel it is better to do an anterior convex fusion that place a child in a Milwaukee brace for eight years.

Another complication of early fusion is curve lengthening. This can be easily solved by lengthening the fusion at a later time.

The results of posterior spine fusion without instrumentation are excellent as long as the surgeon realizes that a large amount of correction is not the main goal. The chief purpose of the operation is *stabilization*, that is, the prevention of further curve increase.[37] If a child of age 6 is seen with a 25 degree thoracic T5 to T11 scoliosis due to mixed anomalies, and if on follow-up over two years shows an increase of the curve to 32 degrees then it is best to fuse the curve promptly. The only thing to be gained by further procrastination is more curvature. Furthermore, because congenital curves tend to be rigid, there will be little chance of any significant correction unless heroic anterior and posterior wedge osteotomy surgery is performed.

A quality posterior fusion and localizer cast correction is a very low risk, high gain procedure, as shown by the recent study at our center. Of 163 patients having posterior fusion without rods, there were no paralyses, no infections, only one case of thoracic lordosis due to the fusion, and only a 14 per cent chance of bending of the fusion.[65] In other words, 86 per cent of the patients did *not* show bending of the fusion (average follow-up of 7 years following surgery).

It is often said that you should not do fusion in a young patient because it will stunt the child's spinal growth. It is true that a solid spine fusion will not elongate with growth, but is must be remembered that in congenital scoliosis *the area being fused is devoid of normal vertical growth potential*. It is mother nature that makes the spine short, not the surgeon!

POSTERIOR FUSION WITH CORRECTION BY TRACTION

Posterior fusion with correction by traction is reserved for more major curves, especially those in which there is a strong desire to avoid the sudden elongation or correction that is done by instrumentation. It is especially beneficial for patients with unsegmented bars in which osteotomy of the bar is part of the fusion procedure.[64] It has also proven of benefit in those children in whom a preliminary removal of a tethering structure

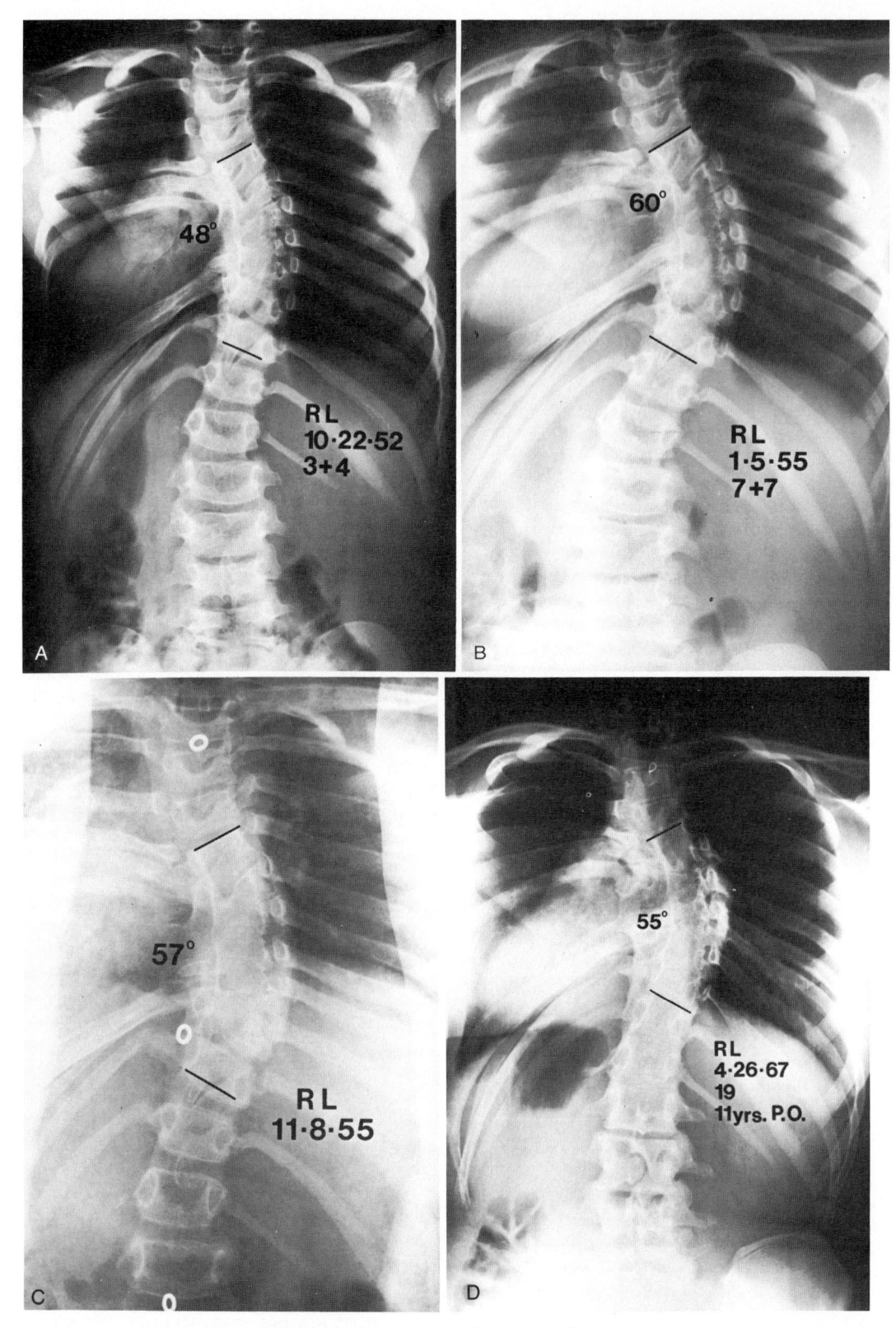

Figure 12–19. *See legend on opposite page.*

is necessary before curve correction can be done (Fig. 12-21).

POSTERIOR FUSION WITH CORRECTION BY INSTRUMENTATION

Posterior fusion with correction by instrumentation is appropriate for those curves in which it is safe to achieve correction at one time under anesthesia (no evidence of dysraphism). The curve must be small enough that anterior surgery (wedge osteotomy or multiple disc excision) is not necessary. The traditional form of instrumentation has been Harrington rods, but more recently the Luque rods have been introduced.[53] Congenital curves are difficult to instrument with Luque rods because of the frequent lack of normal interlaminar spaces. On the positive side, there is less distraction force with Luque rods than with Harrington rods and thus perhaps less risk of stretching the neural tissue. A preoperative myelogram is appropriate if rod use is planned. A localized spinal stenosis must be ruled out, and no tethering structures must exist.

Wake-up tests are mandatory when instrumenting congenital spines. Electronic cord monitoring can augment, but not replace the wake-up tests.[17] *Congenital scoliosis is the most common etiology in which Harrington rods create paraplegia* (Figs. 12-22 to 12-24).[29]

In our review of 127 patients with congenital scoliosis treated by posterior fusion and

Text continued on page 258

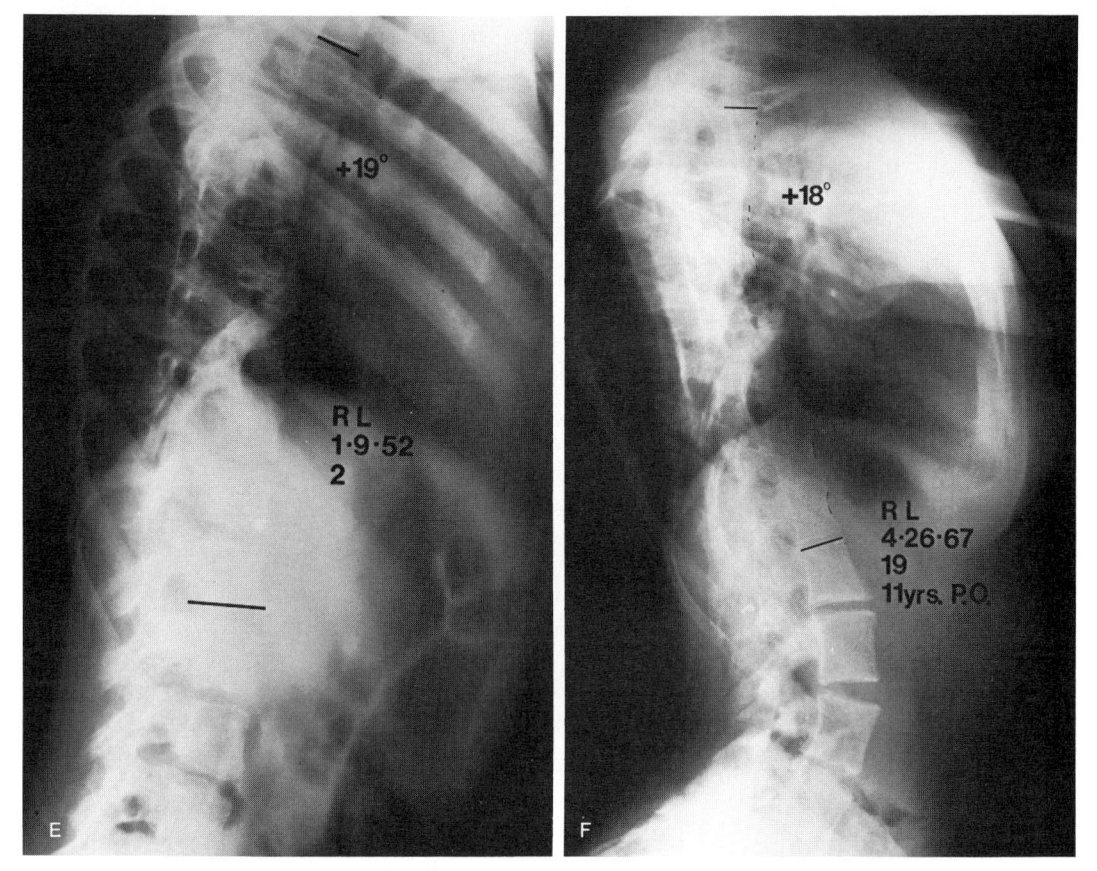

Figure 12-19. *Continued.*

Figure 12-19. *A*, This three year old girl was first seen in 1952 with a 48 degree thoracic curve due to a unilateral unsegmented bar. No treatment was given. *B*, By age seven, her curve had increased to 60 degrees. *C*, She was fused at Gillette Hospital in 1955. Because of the rigidity of the curve, she was essentially fused in situ. *D*, When last seen at age 19, 11 years after surgery, the curve was 55 degrees, not one degree of loss since the time of fusion. *E*, A lateral x-ray at age two, showing +19 degrees, a slight thoracic hypokyphosis. *F*, A lateral x-ray at age 19, 11 years after surgery, shows no change, the measurement being +18 degrees. Congenital scoliosis patients, unlike paralytic ones, do not show progressive lordosis after posterior fusion. (Reprinted with permission from Winter, R. B.: Congenital Deformities of the Spine. New York, Thieme-Stratton, 1983.)

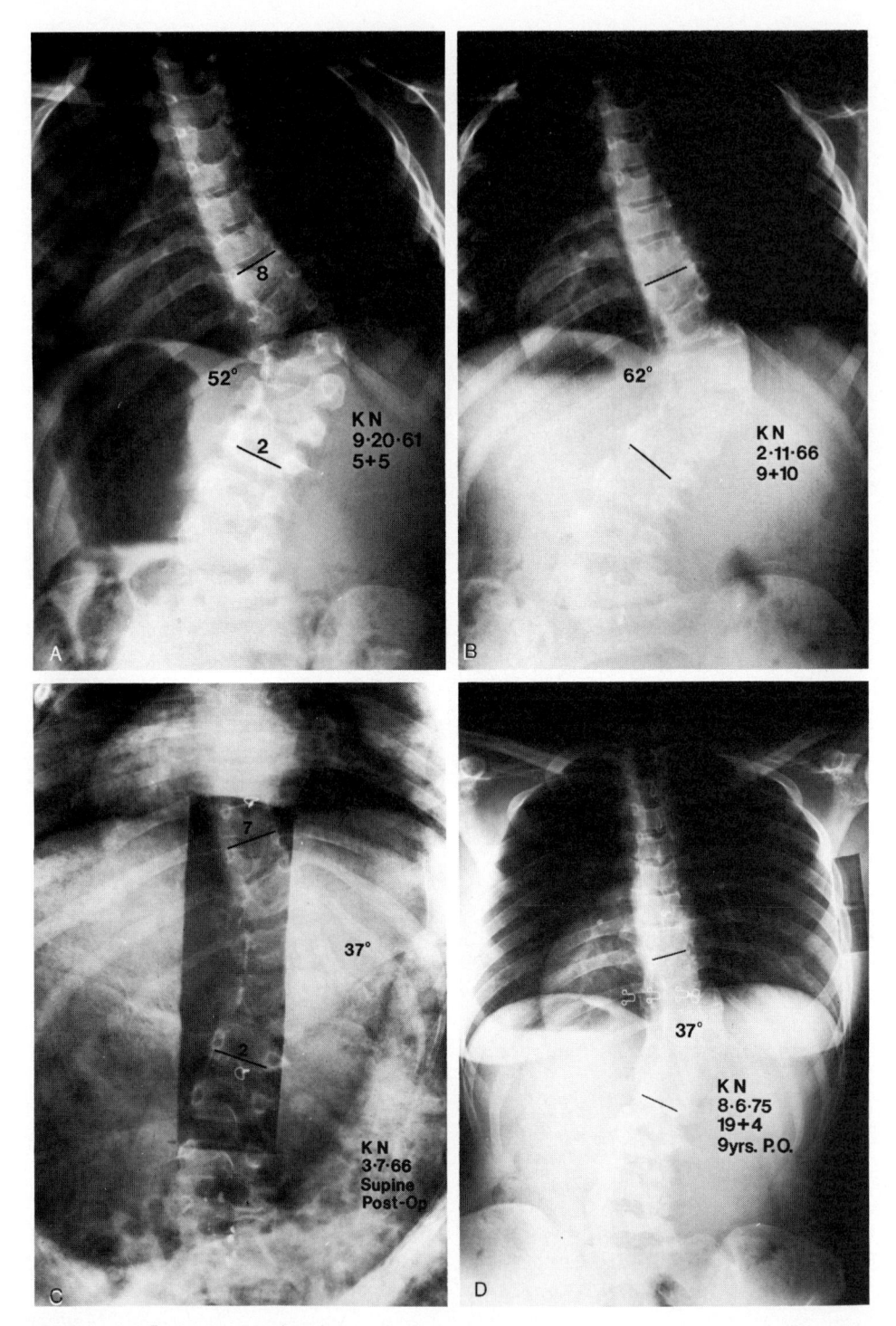

Figure 12–20. A, A five year old girl with a 52 degree scoliosis from T8 to L2. There is a semi-segmented hemivertebra at T11 and a fully segmented hemivertebra between T12 and L1. Treatment with a Milwaukee brace was attempted. B, After four years of bracing the curve was worse, now measuring 62 degrees. It is tempting to think hemivertebra resection is indicated, but it was not necessary in her case. C, She had a posterior arthrodesis from T6 to L2 in 1966 at Gillette Children's Hospital. An abundant autogenous iliac bone graft was added, and correction to 37 degrees was done with a Risser localizer cast. She remained recumbent for six months and in a cast for one year. There was no other treatment given. D, At her final follow-up at age 19 in 1975, nine years after surgery, the curve remained at 37 degrees, without any loss of correction. Such excellent results require massive bone grafting and prolonged casting until the fusion mass demonstrates vertical trabecular patterns. (Reprinted with permission from Winter, R. B.: Congenital Deformities of the Spine. New York Thieme-Stratton, 1983.)

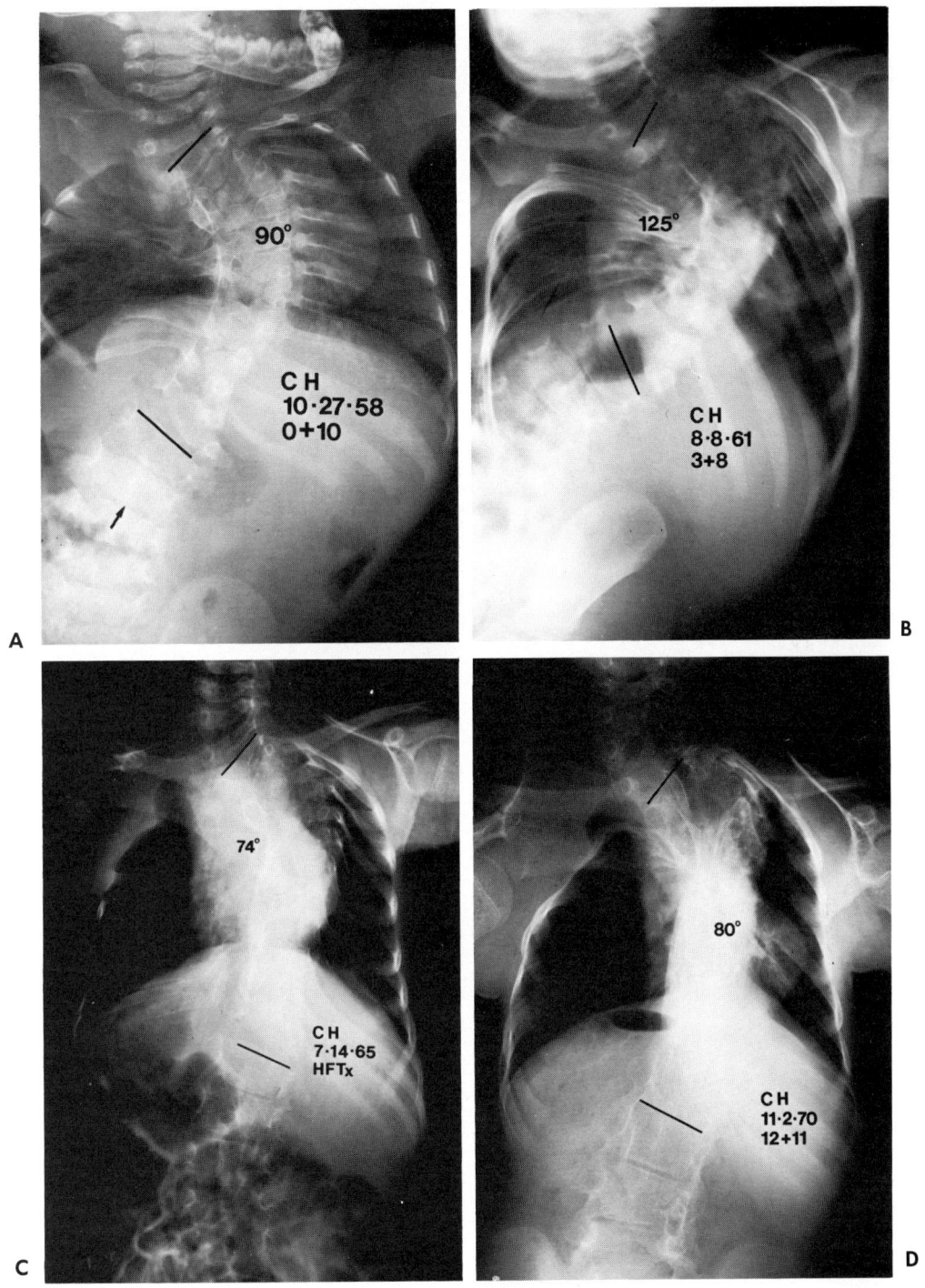

Figure 12–21. *A*, This ten month old girl was seen elsewhere and was found to have a 90 degree congenital scoliosis due to a severe defect of segmentation on the left, involving the whole thoracic spine. She also had a diastematomyelia at L2 to L3 (*arrow*). No treatment was given. *B*, The curve progressed to 125 degrees by the time the patient was 3+8 years old. An attempt was made elsewhere to treat this curve with a Harrington rod, a very foolish thing to do with a child so small and with a diastematomyelia. *C*, When first seen at our center in 1965, the curve was 138 degrees, the rod had dislocated, and a very serious situation existed. She was treated by concave rib resection, osteotomy of the unsegmented bar, excision of the diastematomyelia, posterior fusion, and correction by halofemoral traction to 74 degrees, as seen here. She was recumbent in a halo cast for six months, and then upright in a Risser cast for 12 months. *D*, When last seen in our clinics at age 13, her curve was 80 degrees. A pseudarthrosis had been detected in the upper lumbar spine and repaired before loss of correction happened. (Reprinted with permission from Winter, R. B.: Congenital Deformities of the Spine. New York, Thieme-Stratton, 1983.)

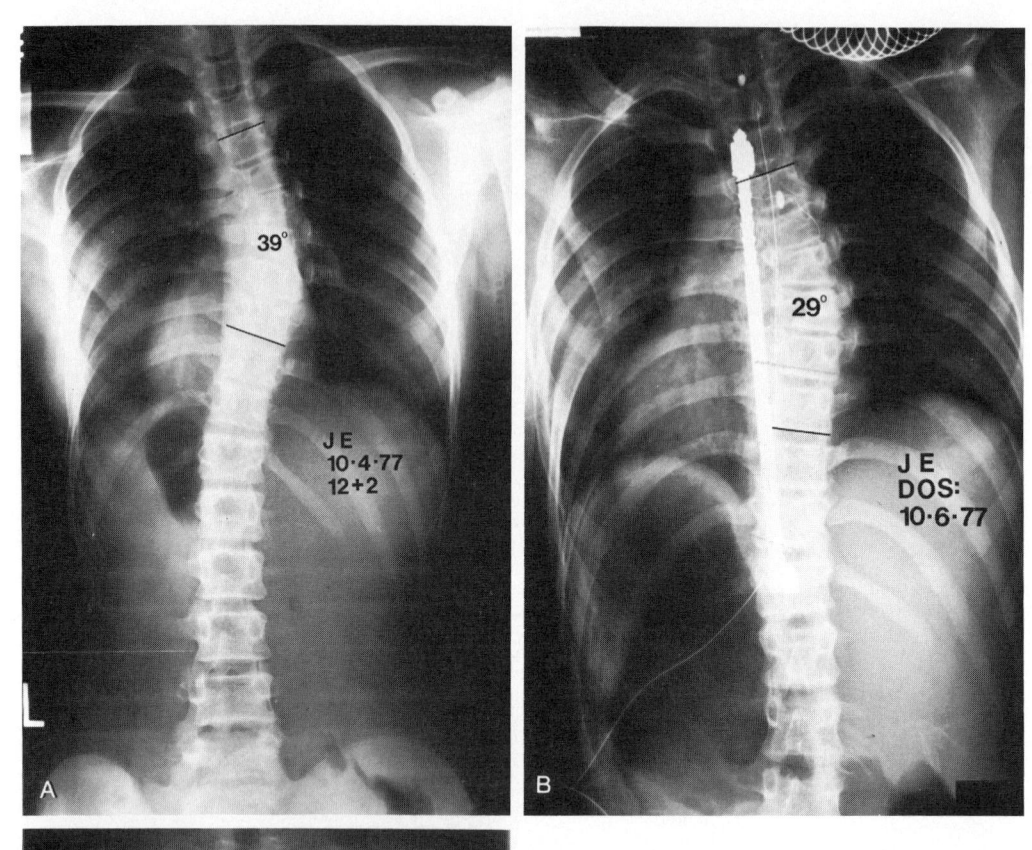

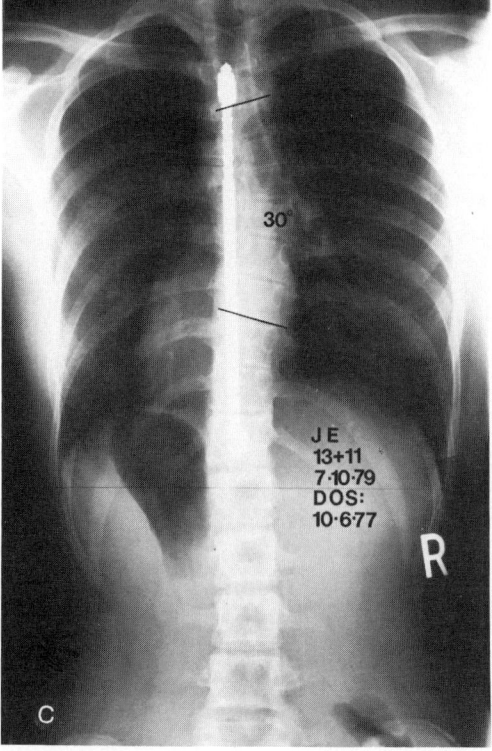

Figure 12–22. *A,* This 12 year old girl presented with a 39 degree thoracic curve due to a unilateral unsegmented bar of T5, T6, and T7. The curve was progressive, and brace treatment of such a curve is impossible. *B,* At surgery, a single Harrington distraction rod was used. She had had a myelogram before surgery, which did not show any abnormality. At the time of surgery, a wake-up test was done and was normal. *C,* At follow-up two years later, the curve was 30 degrees, showing no loss of correction. Postoperative treatment was in an ambulatory Risser cast for nine months. (Reprinted with permission from Winter, R. B.: Congenital Deformities of the Spine. New York, Thieme-Stratton, 1983.)

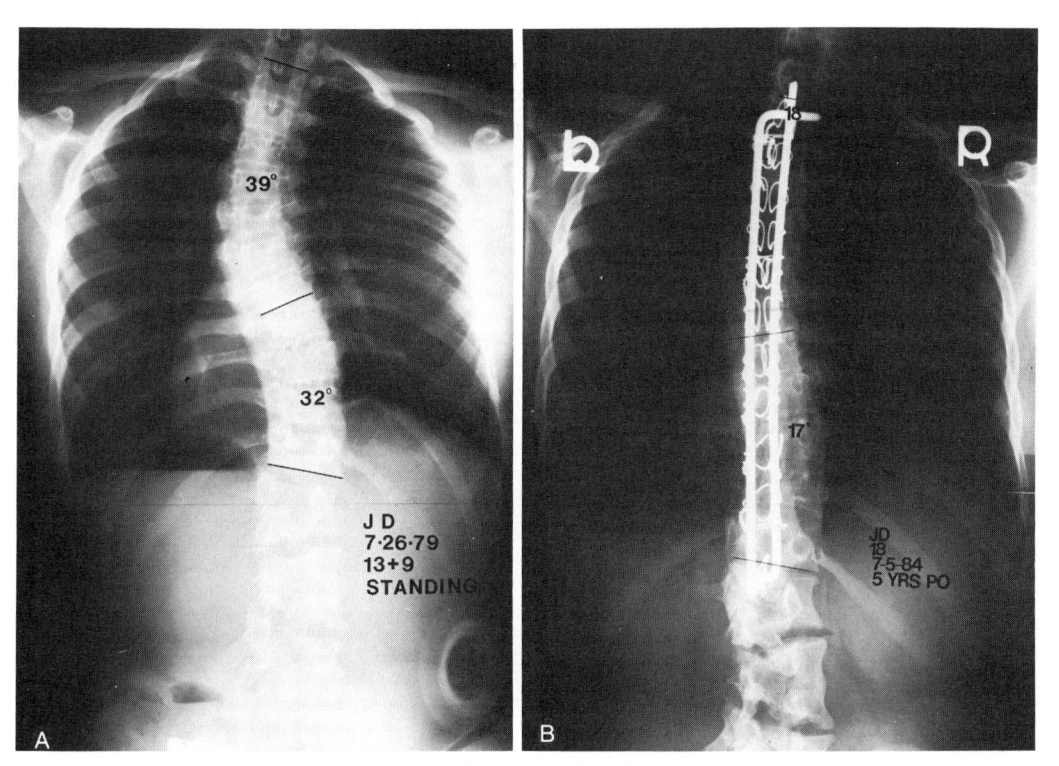

Figure 12–23. *A*, A 13 year old girl with congenital anomalies of the lumbar spine, exstrophy of the bladder, vaginal agenesis, and anal atresia. She had progressive thoracic scoliosis, and because of two ostomies on the abdominal wall, there was no chance for bracing. A Luque procedure was done in 1979. *B*, At five years post surgery, there has been no loss of correction, the curves measuring 18 degrees and 17 degrees.

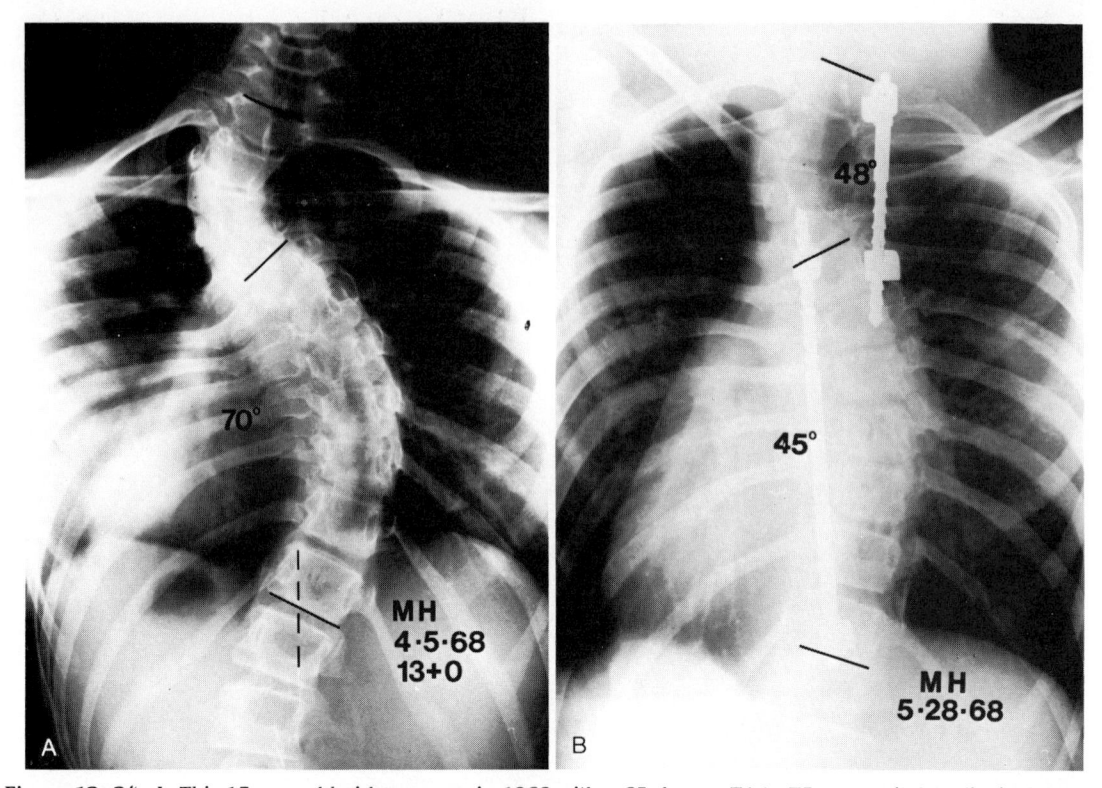

Figure 12–24. *A,* This 13 year old girl was seen in 1968 with a 65 degree T1 to T5 congenital scoliosis due to a hemivertebra at T3. This T5 to T12 curve was compensatory. No myelogram was done, and in 1968 we had neither the wake-up test nor electronic spinal cord monitoring. *B,* This film was taken immediately following surgery when the patient was discovered to be paraplegic. She was returned immediately to the operating room, where the rods were removed. The ligamentum flavum was found to be torn at T3, and there was an epidural hematoma. She never recovered. (Reprinted with permission from Winter, R. B.: Congenital Deformities of the Spine. New York, Thieme-Stratton, 1983.)

Harrington instrumentation, the average preoperative curve was 58 degrees, at surgery it was 37 degrees (21 degrees of correction), and at follow-up it was 43 degrees.[65] The average loss of correction was thus only 6 degrees (average follow-up of 5 years). This, however, was the same loss as seen in those cases (163) done without rods. It should be noted that the average curve at follow-up in those treated without rods was 44 degrees, just one degree of difference (the average preoperative curve was 53 degrees). Two patients developed paraplegia after rodding.

CORRECTION BY TRACTION FOLLOWED BY FIXATION BY INSTRUMENTATION AT FUSION

Correction by traction followed by fixation by instrumentation at the time of the fusion is a very reasonable approach in congenital scoliosis.[52] It is highly desirable to achieve correction in a slow and gradual manner so as to avoid sudden stretching of the neural tissue. The correction is achieved while the patient is awake and able to tell the surgeon or nurses of any numbness, tingling, or weakness. Once the correction has been achieved by traction it is stabilized by instrumentation. This avoids the need for prolonged traction, either in bed or in a halo cast (Fig. 12–25).

COMBINED ANTERIOR AND POSTERIOR CONVEX FUSION

Combined anterior and posterior convex fusion (and epiphyseodesis) is appropriate for those situations in which there is either a chance for concave growth after convex fusion, or such a severe potential for bending of the solid fusion that elimination of the convex growth forces is essential. The concept of arresting the excessive convex growth and allowing the lesser concave growth to take place is quite appealing. It was first reported by MacLennan in 1922[3] and subsequently pursued by Roaf,[46, 47, 48] Winter,[60] and

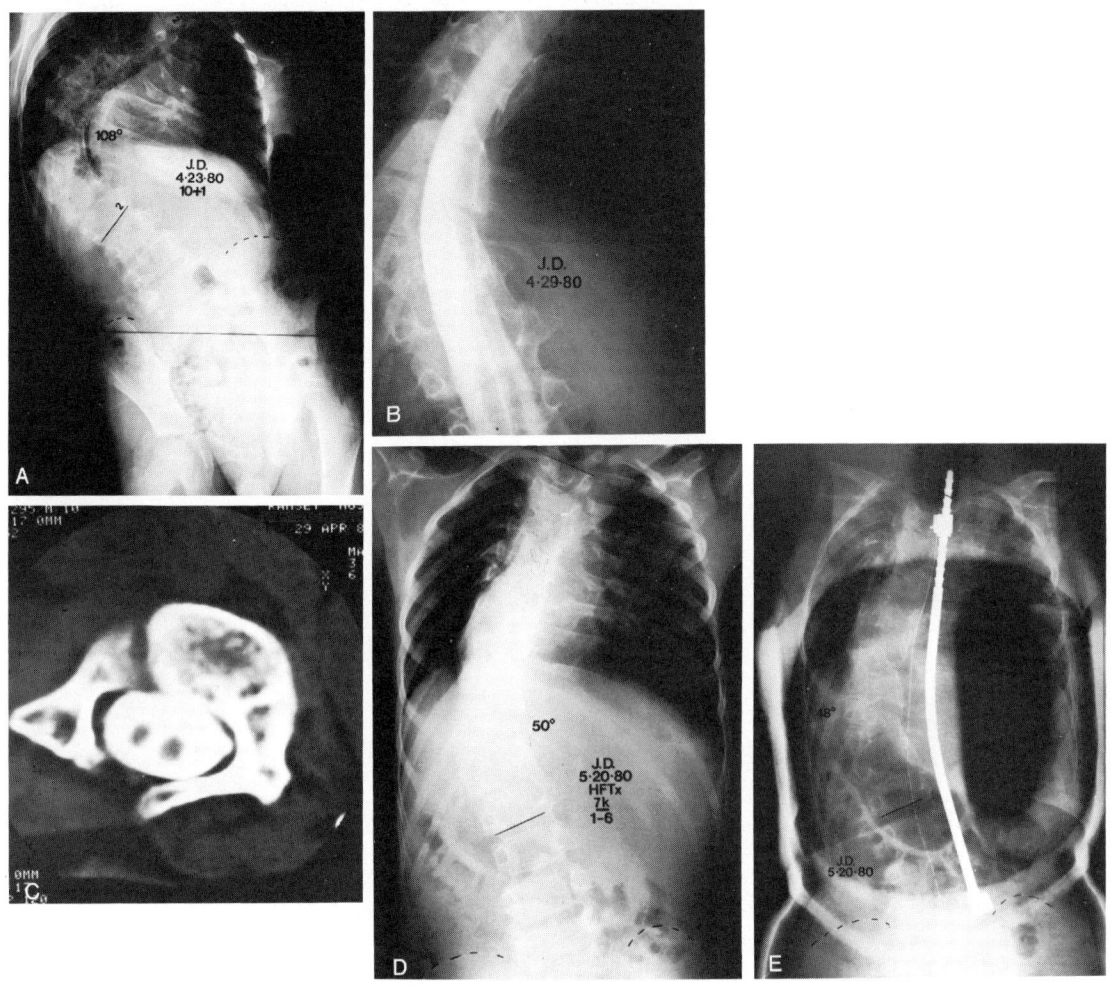

Figure 12–25. A, This ten year old boy presented with a 108 degree congenital scoliosis. He was neurologically normal but had a hair patch in the mid-lumbar spine. B, A metrizamide myelogram revealed a divided spinal cord with the conus at the L3 to L4 level. C, A CT scan of the myelogram demonstrates very well the divided spinal cord within a single dural sheath. D, After neurosurgical removal of a fibrous band between the halves of the spinal cord, the spine was slowly corrected by halofemoral traction. There were 7 kilograms of traction on the halo, 1 kilo on the left leg, and 6 kilos on the right leg. E, After correction by the traction, the curve was stabilized with a Harrington rod and a Risser cast. No attempt was made to gain additional correction. A wake-up test was done at the time of rod tightening. (Reprinted with permission from Winter, R. B.: Congenital Deformities of the Spine. New York, Thieme-Stratton, 1983.)

others.[2, 4, 39] To be successful, the surgery must be done when there are many years of growth remaining; it is contraindicated if there is an abnormal kyphosis (Fig. 12–26).

ANTERIOR AND POSTERIOR OSTEOTOMY WITH CORRECTION AND FUSION

Anterior and posterior osteotomy with correction and fusion has always been appealing, especially for a significant curve due to a hemivertebra. The first hemivertebra excision was reported by Royle in 1928,[49] but the procedure did not gain acceptance until the refinement of anterior spinal surgery in the 1960's and 1970's.[6, 8, 15, 16, 20, 27, 41, 51, 57] Even at the present time there is considerable controversy as to the indications for its use, since many hemivertebra problems can be solved by less complex methods.

As a general principle, wedge osteotomy surgery should be reserved for those rigid and angular scolioses in which adequate compensation cannot be achieved by any other method.[28] Hopefully, the prompt treatment of younger children will prevent the need for such major surgery in older children (Fig. 12–27).

A hemivertebra at the lumbosacral junction

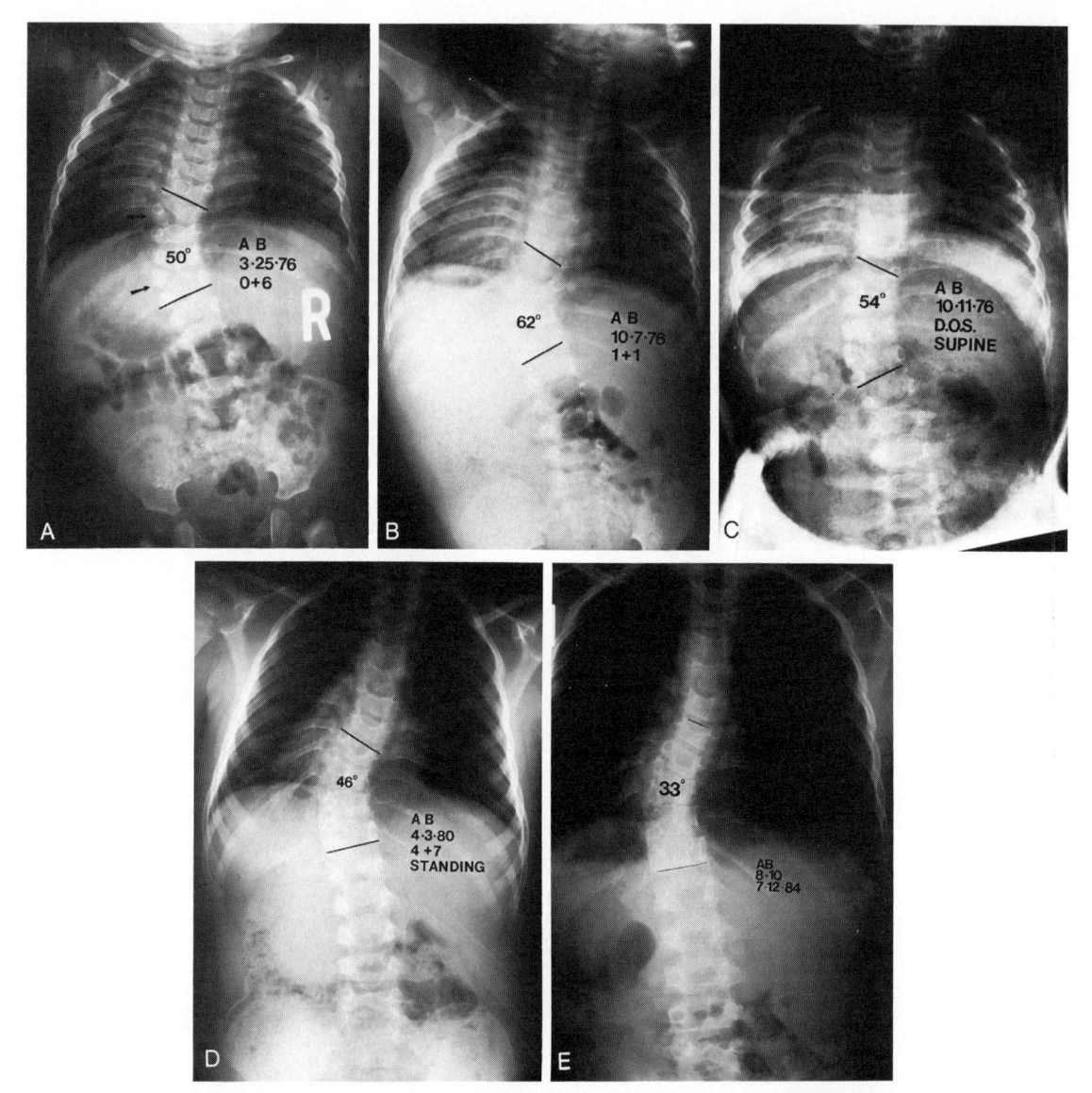

Figure 12–26. A, This six month old girl had a 50 degree curve due to two convex hemivertebrae. B, By age 13 months, the curve had increased to 62 degrees. Immediate treatment was indicated. Treatment consisted of anterior and posterior hemi-arthrodesis and epiphyseodesis from T7 to T12 (one vertebra above the upper hemivertebra to one vertebra below the lower one). C, At the time of surgery, a cast correction was done, improving her curve only to 54 degrees. She wore this cast for six months and has had no further treatment. D, At age 4+7 years, the curve was 46 degrees. (A, B, C, and D reprinted with permission from Winter, R. B.: Congenital Deformities of the Spine. New York, Thieme-Stratton, 1983.) E, At age 8+10 years, the curve had spontaneously improved to 33 degrees.

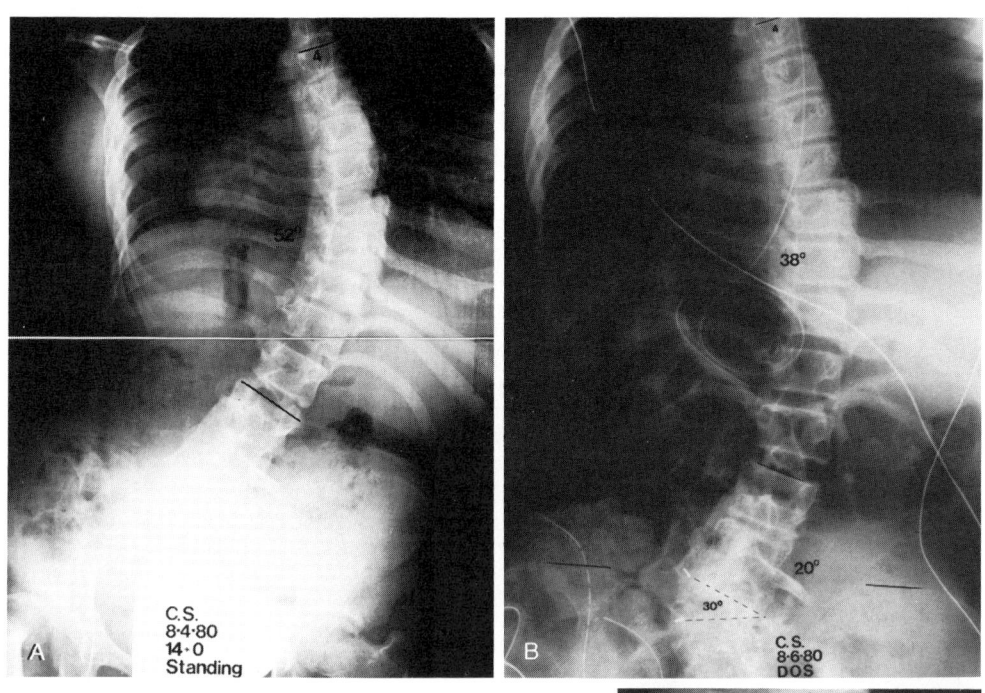

Figure 12–27. *A,* This 14 year old girl presented with a long, sweeping, 52 degree thoracolumbar scoliosis and a history of a fusion from L2 to the sacrum for a congenital lumbosacral curve due to hemivertebra at L5. A right side-bending film showed correction of the 52 degree thoracic curve to zero. *B,* An anterior wedge of bone was removed at the lumbosacral junction through a left retroperitoneal exposure. The area of the wedge is shown with the dotted lines. *C,* One week later, the same wedge was removed posteriorly and the gap was closed with a Harrington compression rod, the hooks being inserted into the previous fusion mass. (Reprinted with permission from Winter, R. B.: Congenital Deformities of the Spine. New York, Thieme-Stratton, 1983.)

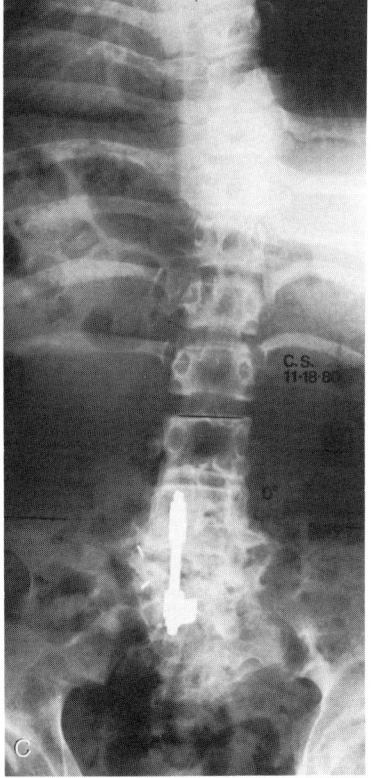

can create a major decompensation problem (see Natural History and Fig. 12–13). There is no way to achieve a compensated alignment other than with wedge excision. This is preferably done early (before age 5) so that the secondary curve above has not developed structural changes.

Often there are dystrophic changes (spina bifida occulata, lipoma, etc.) at the same level, making the bone stock insufficient for compression rodding. This can be overcome by a preliminary L4 to S1 hemifusion (convex), so that a year later, the wedge is removed through this solid area and good bone is available for hook placement.

Congenital Kyphosis[9, 34, 38, 56, 59, 66, 68]

Since the natural history of congenital kyphosis is usually bad and there is no known successful non-operative treatment, the treatment of choice is thus surgical. But what is the appropriate surgical treatment? The proper treatment depends upon the type of anomaly, the age of the patient, and the severity of the deformity.

DEFECTS OF SEGMENTATION

If detected early, the procedure of choice is posterior fusion, extending the fusion to one vertebra above, and one below the extent of the segmentation defect. This will not provide any correction, but will prevent any further curve increase.

If the problem has gone undetected and a significant deformity exists, then the procedure of choice is anterior osteotomy of the unsegmented areas followed by posterior fusion with instrumentation to achieve correction and stabilization. For severe deformities, halofemoral traction can be utilized between stages (Fig. 12–28).[34]

DEFECTS OF FORMATION

These are more common than defects of segmentation and can lead to much more severe deformities and even to paraplegia.[9, 10, 24] Thus their prompt treatment is of the utmost importance. The procedure of choice is posterior fusion at a young age, the best age being between one and three years. A simple posterior fusion is done with no instrumentation. The author prefers to use homologous bank bone because of the difficulty of obtaining an adequate amount of autogenous bone in these very young children. Postoperative support is best done with a cast, which is changed at frequent intervals to accommodate growth and soiling. An underarm cast can be used for thoracolumbar kyphoses, but a full Risser hyperextension cast is necessary for thoracic deformities. Casting must be for at least six months and should be followed by bracing for another six months. If a pseudarthrosis is seen on follow-up radiographs, it must be surgically repaired without delay. Routine exploration and augmentation of the graft at six months is also an accepted method of management.

This early posterior fusion, coupled with some anterior growth, usually results in a slow but steady decrease in the angle of the kyphosis. It is tempting to do an anterior fusion also to ensure a solid union, but this will eliminate the anterior growth plates, preventing progressive correction.

In a review of 17 congenital kyphosis patients fused before age 5, and followed for an average of nine years, Winter and Moe[62] noted this steady improvement in the 12 treated by posterior fusion only. The average preoperative kyphosis was 58 degrees; it was corrected in the cast to 38 degrees, and at follow-up it was 26 degrees (Fig. 12–29).

For children older than age 5, posterior fusion can be successful if the kyphosis is not too severe, the dividing line being about 50 to 55 degrees. For kyphoses greater than 55 degrees, both anterior and posterior surgery become necessary.[65] For adults, combined anterior and posterior surgery is necessary in virtually every patient needing surgical treatment.

The techniques of anterior surgery are outlined in Chapter 10, page 162 and need not be repeated here. There are two general principles that are important, (1) the release of the anterior tethering structures that prevent the correction of the kyphosis, and (2) the insertion of adequate bone grafts in order to achieve solid union.

The anterior tethering structures are the short and thick anterior longitudinal ligament, the anulus fibrosus, and the abnormal cartilagenous material that lies in the place of the absent bone. These must all be thoroughly removed back to the posterior anulus and all the way across from right to left. There is no need to remove any bone other than that necessary to remove these tethering

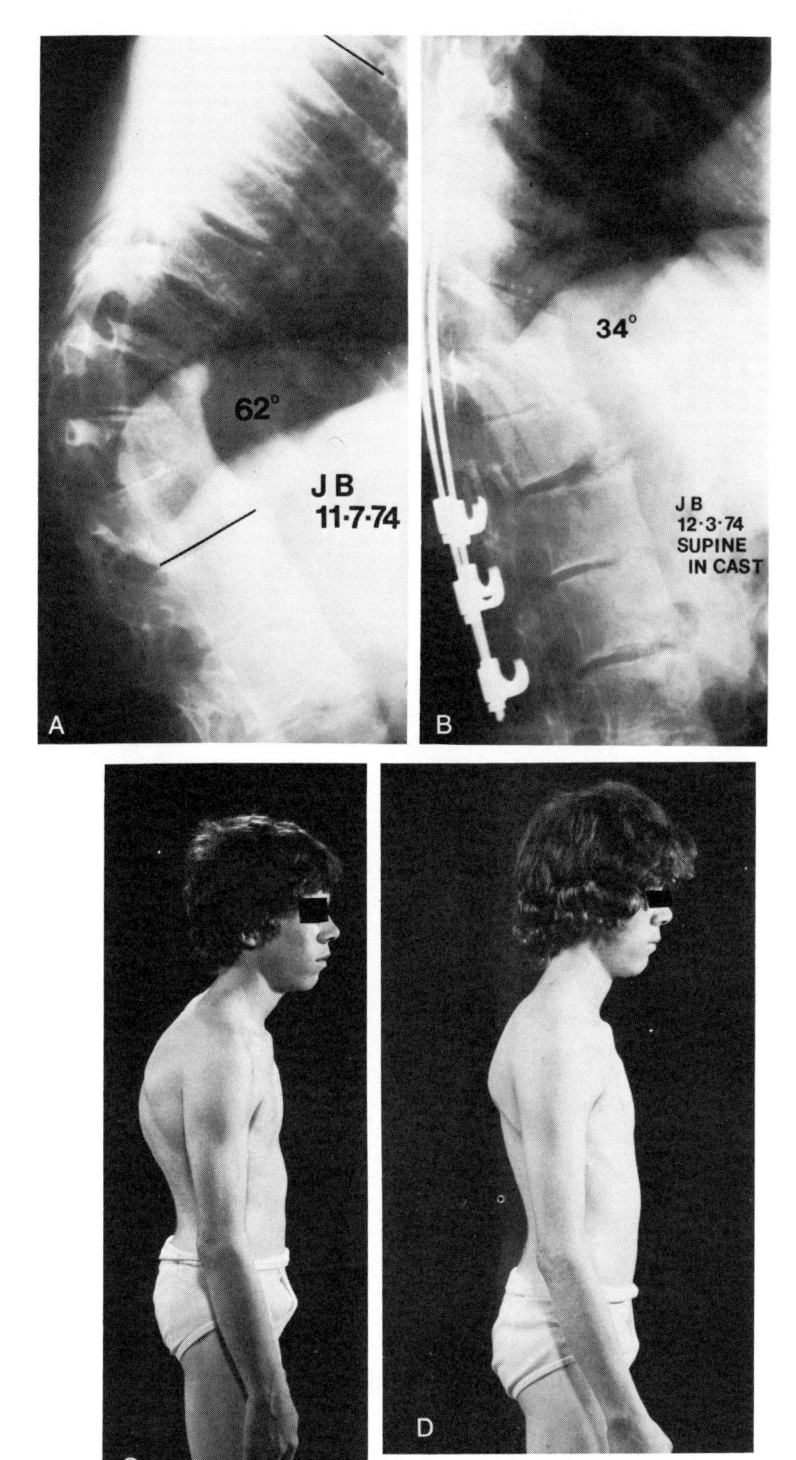

Figure 12–28. A, This 14 year old boy had a 62 degree kyphosis, which on physical examination looked exactly like Scheuermann's disease. Treatment consisted of anterior osteotomy of the bar, two weeks of halofemoral traction, and then posterior fusion with dual compression rods. B, This detailed x-ray taken in his postoperative cast best shows the levels of osteotomy, the anterior bone chips (from the resected rib), and the posterior instrumentation. C, A lateral preoperative photograph; the appearance is identical with Scheuermann's disease. D, A postoperative lateral photograph.

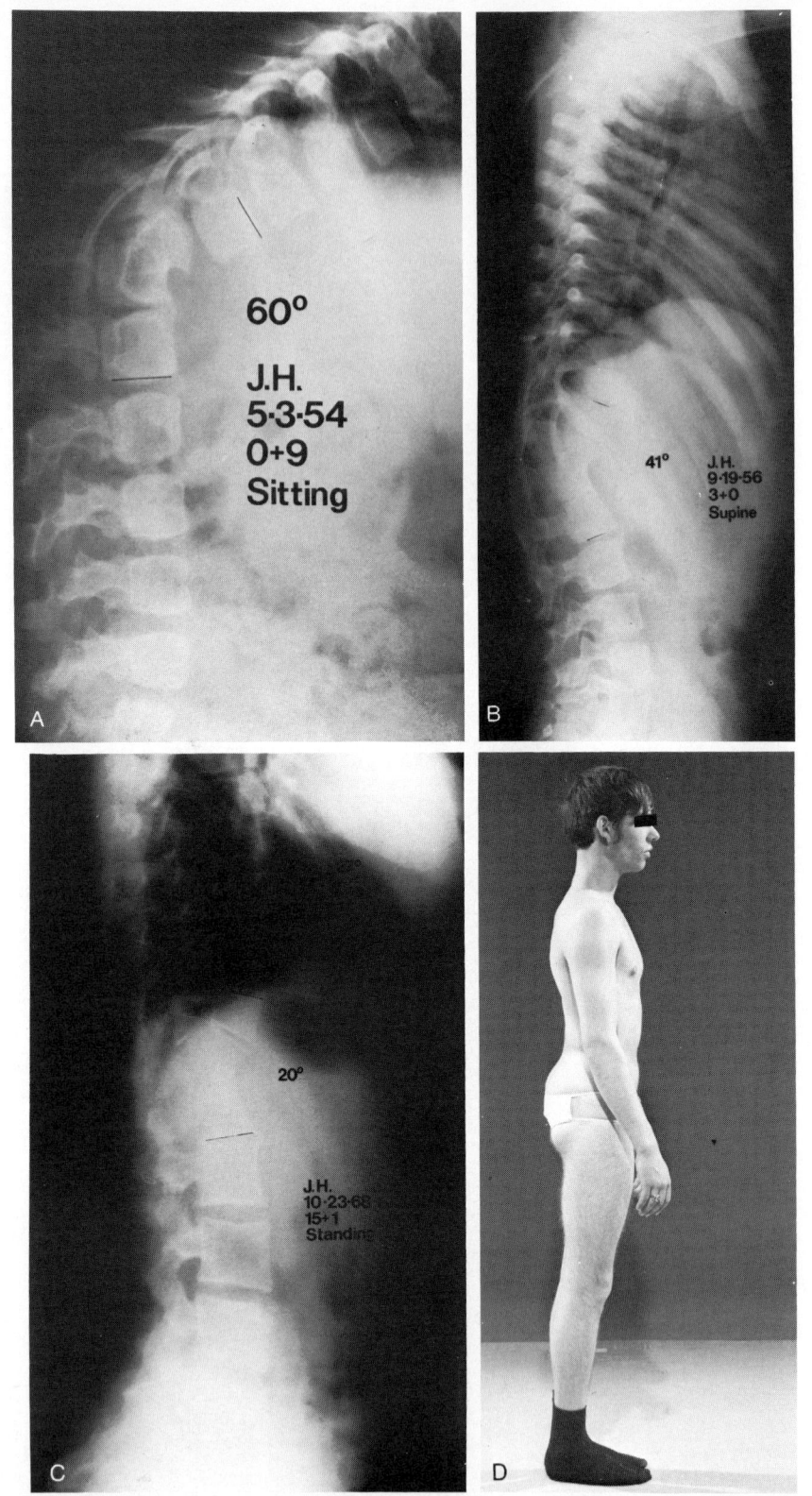

Figure 12–29. A, A three year old boy with a 60 degree congenital kyphosis who had posterior fusion and cast correction at age 16 months in 1955. B, At age three his kyphosis measured 41 degrees, the amount achieved by the cast correction. A pseudoarthrosis had been detected and repaired six months after the fusion. C, At follow-up in 1968 at age 15, the kyphosis measures only 20 degrees, a classic demonstration of the posterior growth arrest effect. D, A clinical photograph of the patient at age 15, showing a normal lateral contour, and a virtually normal torso-leg relationship. (See also Fig. 7–15E.) (Reprinted with permission from Winter, R. B.: Congenital Deformities of the Spine. New York, Thieme-Stratton, 1983.)

structures. There is no need to visualize the dura.

In some cases, correction is best done at the time of the anterior surgery, using metallic anterior distracting devices such as the Santa Casa or Slot distractors. The amount of correction is maintained by autogenous strut grafts, using rib or fibula. In other cases, a bone graft of many small chips is inserted, with correction taking place at the time of the posterior instrumentation.

The posterior instrumentation has traditionally been with Harrington compression devices, using dual compression rods for pure kyphosis or a single compression rod and a bent distraction rod for a kyphoscoliosis, the compression rod always being inserted first. More recently, there have been advocates for the use of Luque rods, but as yet there is no documentation of their superiority.

Correction by skeletal traction, that is, halofemoral or halopelvic, is attractive at first glance, but has been complicated by a *very high incidence of paraplegia*. In the series of 94 surgically treated congenital kyphosis patients by Winter, Moe, and Lonstein,[66] there were three paraplegias, one due to Harrington distraction rodding and the other two due to halofemoral traction (Fig. 12–30).

For the patient presenting with a congenital kyphosis and a developing paraparesis, a myelogram should be performed to rule out a tethered cord (a rare event), and to examine the area of the kyphosis to see precisely where the compression exists. This is followed by an anterior cord decompression and anterior fusion (see Chapter 10, page 171 for technique). A posterior fusion with or without instrumentation should also be done.

There are a few patients with fairly flexible kyphoses (as shown on a hyperextension film) with mild paraparesis in which it is not necessary to expose the dura in order to "decompress" the spinal cord. By reduction of the spinal angulation, pressure is removed from the cord, and the patient requires only anterior and posterior fusion (Fig. 12–31).[30]

SPINAL DYSRAPHISM[11, 12, 13, 21, 22, 23, 36]

Dysraphism is a broad term used to indicate a condition in which there is some evidence of nerve tissue anomaly in addition to bony anomalies of the spine. At its most severe, it is a myelomeningocoele, and at the other end of the spectrum, an asymptomatic lipoma or fibrous band in the spinal canal. In between there are such lesions as meningocoele, filum terminale, neurenteric cysts or bands, fibrous bands, diplomyelia, and diastemratomyelia.

The incidence of one or more of these lesions in congenital spine deformities is quite high, being between 10 and 20 per cent in most reported series.[22, 36, 61] In our experience, about one-half have been diastematomyelias and the other half a scattering of other lesions.

The key is to maintain a high index of suspicion. Anytime a congenital spine deformity is seen, the physician should ask himself (herself) if a dysraphic lesion is present. Is there a hair patch, a nevus, a dimple, a lipoma, or anything abnormal about the skin of the back? Is there any abnormality of the lower limbs? On review of the plain radiographs, is there a localized spina bifida, an area of increased interpediculate distance, or a midline bony defect?

If any of these are present, a myelogram should be performed. A water-soluble contrast medium (e.g., Metrizamide) should always be used, since the oil-soluble media are too thick and prevent an adequate view of the contents of the canal.[21] One must always examine the area of the conus and cauda equina in addition to more obvious areas above.[23] When a specific lesion is identified, then CT scanning of that area can give additional information (see Figs. 12–24 and 12–32). More than one diastematomyelia can exist in the same patient, so it is important to survey the entire spinal canal. Rotation of the spine caused by the curvature may confuse the radiologic evaluation, and the patient should be turned so that the spine is seen in its true anteroposterior projection.

Should these lesions be surgically removed? Considerable controversy exists in this area. At the present time, it is felt that while not all such lesions need be removed some should be. If the lesion is causing a neurologic defect, either static or progressive, it should be removed. If there is to be a correction of a spinal deformity by any kind of method (e.g., Harrington distraction rods, Luque rods, or traction), the lesion should be removed. If there is no neurologic defect and no stretching of the spine is contemplated, then the defect need not be removed, but careful neurologic monitoring must be done throughout growth. Even the end of

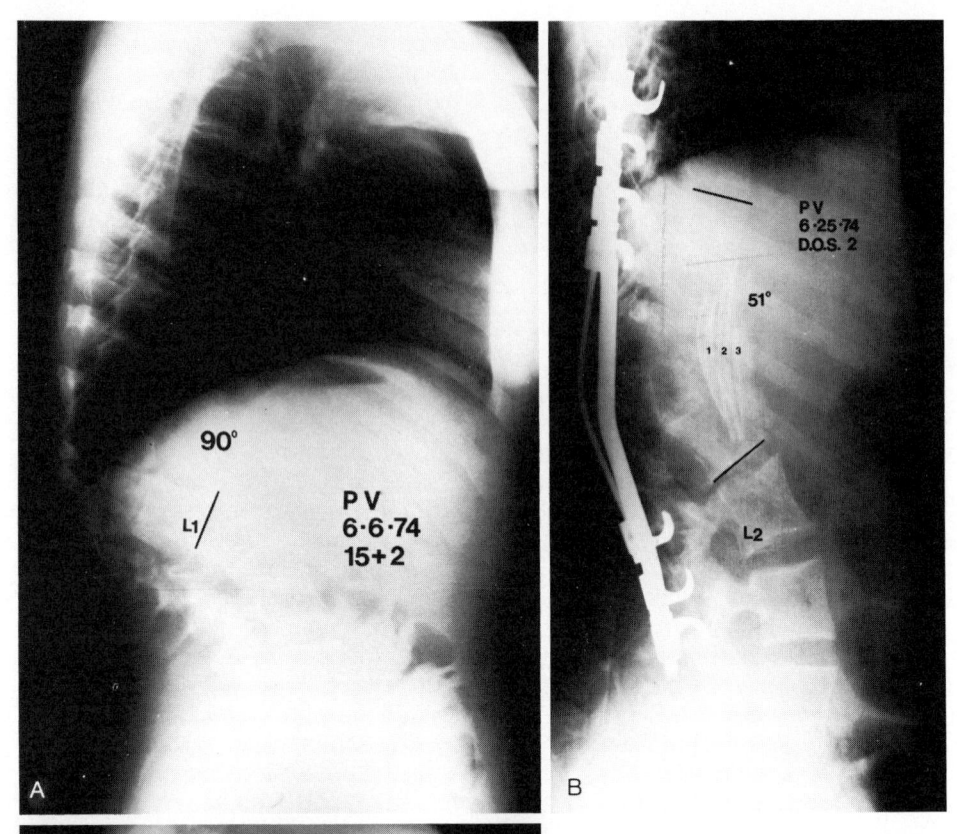

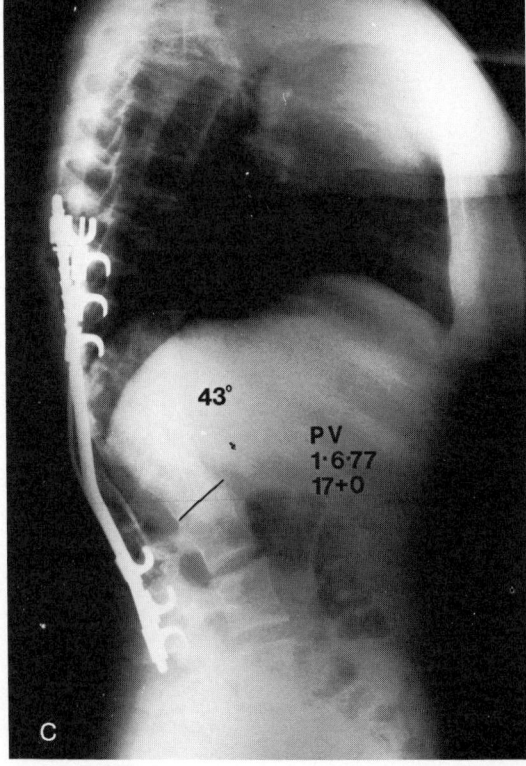

Figure 12–30. *A*, A fifteen year old girl with a sharp, angular, 90 degree congenital kyphosis due to a defect of formation. She was neurologically normal. *B*, Her first surgery was an anterior release, anterior correction, and strut grafting. One week later she had posterior fusion with Harrington rods, one compression and one bent distraction (the patient had a mild scoliosis also). *C*, At a two-year follow-up, her curve was 43 degrees, and the fusion solid. (Reprinted with permission from Winter, R. B., Moe, J. H., and Lonstein, J. E.: The surgical treatment of congenital kyphosis, a review of 94 patients age 5 or older. Spine, *10*:224–231, 1985.)

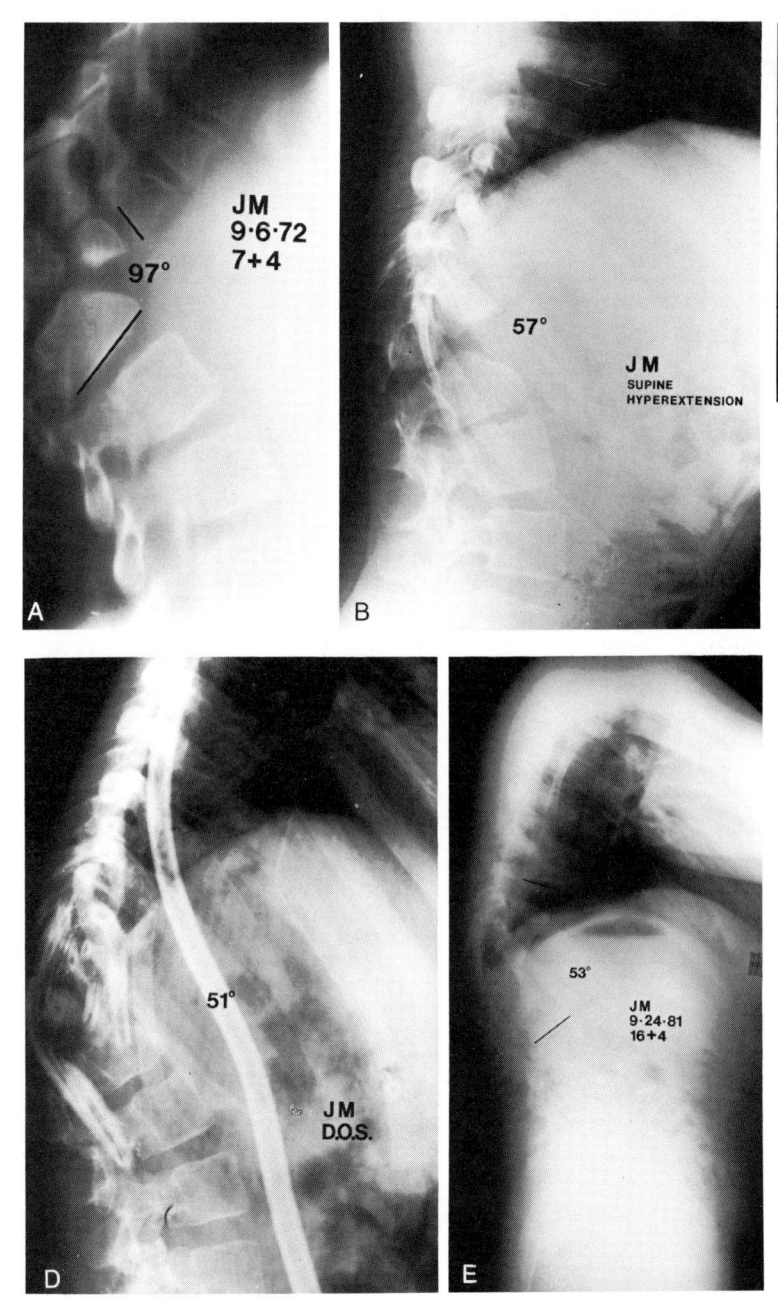

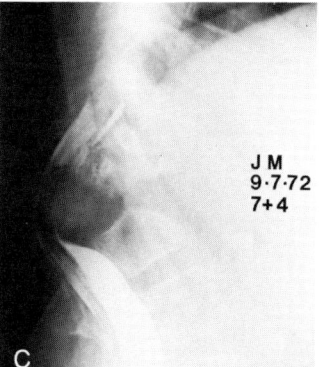

Figure 12–31. A, A seven year old boy with a 97 degree congenital kyphosis (supine tomogram) and early signs of paraparesis. There were positive Babinski reflexes and mild spasticity, but no motor weakness, sensory loss, or sphincter disturbance. B, A supine hyperextension film demonstrated remarkable flexibility for a congenital curve. C, A high volume myelogram demonstrates the marked deviation of the spinal canal around the posteriorly protruding hemivertebra. D, On the day of his first surgery, an anterior strut grafting in the corrected position was done *without* any attempt to remove the hemivertebra or expose the dura. A posterior fusion was done two weeks later. The patient was neurologically normal within one month. Postoperative treatment was six months of bedrest in a Risser cast and one year ambulatory in a Milwaukee brace. E, At a nine year follow-up, the curve is 53 degrees, no loss from the time of surgery, and the patient is neurologically normal. (Reprinted with permission from Winter, R. B.: Congenital Deformities of the Spine. New York, Thieme-Stratton, 1983.)

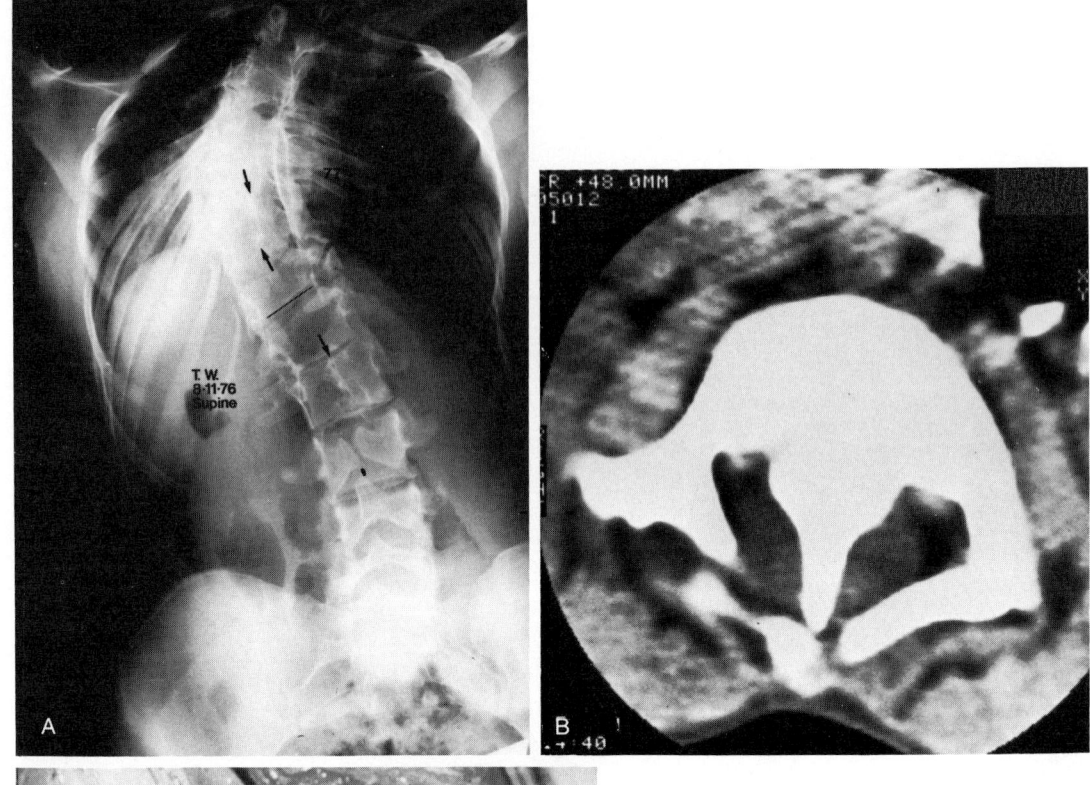

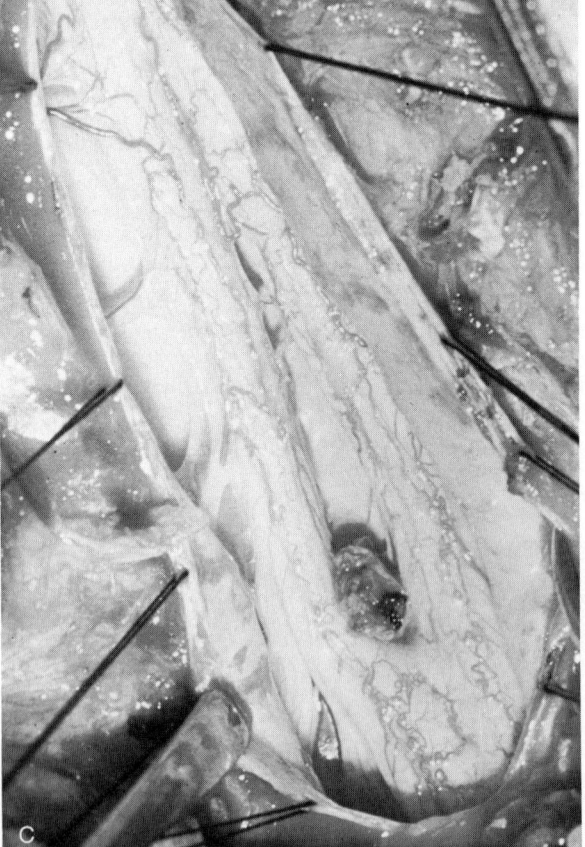

Figure 12–32. A, A 16 year old girl with a 77 degree congenital scoliosis due to a thoracic unsegmented bar. The upper two arrows indicate a thoracic diastematomyelia, and the lower arrow a lumbar diastematomyelia. She was neurologically normal. B, A CT scan of a diastematomyelia (not the same patient as in Fig. 12–32A). C, A diastematomyelia as seen at laminectomy. The spinal cord comes together just below the bony spur and is tightly pulled against it. (Note: The laminectomy is inappropriately large just to remove this spur. It made fusion of this patient somewhat difficult.) (A and C reprinted with permission from Winter, R. B.: Congenital Deformities of the Spine. New York, Thieme-Stratton, 1983.)

growth does not necessarily solve the problem. We have seen several adults with symptoms beginning anywhere from age 20 to age 65.

If these lesions are to be removed, it should be done by a neurosurgeon skilled in such procedures. The use of delicacy, microscopes, bipolar cautery, and neurologic monitoring makes the removal of most of these lesions safe. Complex lipomas with intermingled nerve tissue are not always surgically removable.

In our personal experience at our center, we have not seen any patient made worse by the neurosurgical removal of one of these lesions. After removal, we have been able to proceed with the scoliosis treatment at a separate surgery; the best results occur with slow and gradual correction by serial casts or halofemoral traction (see Figs. 12–21 and 12–25).[61]

Finally, it should be remembered that it is often safer to shorten the convexity of a curve than to lengthen the concavity. Thus, convex discectomy and convex wedge osteotomy (hemivertebra excision) are often the safer procedures (Fig. 12–32).

References

1. Akbarnia, B. A., Heydarian, K., and Ganjavian, M. S.: Concordant congenital spine deformity in monozygotic twins. J. Pediatr. Orthop., 3:502–504, 1983.
2. Andrew, T., and Piggott, H.: Growth arrest for progressive scoliosis: combined anterior and posterior fusion of the convexity. J. Bone Joint Surg., 67B:193–197, 1985.
3. Bonicoli, F., and Delveccio, E.: Scoliosis in monochorionic twins. Chir. Organi Mov., 57:178–186, 1968.
4. Bradford, D. S.: Partial epiphyseal arrest and supplemental fixation for progressive correction of congenital spine deformity. J. Bone Joint Surg., 64A:610–614, 1982.
5. Cantu, J. M., Urrusti, J., Rosales, G., et al.: Evidence for autosomal recessive inheritance of costovertebral dysplasia. Clin. Genet., 2:149–154, 1971.
6. Carcassone, M., Gregorie, A., and Hornung, H.: L'ablation de l'hemivertebrae "libre": traitement preventif de la scoliose congenitale. Chirurgie, 103:110–115, 1977.
7. Castroviejo, I. P., Rodriquez-Costa, T., and Costillo, F.: Spondylothoracic dysplasia in three sisters. Dev. Med. Child Neurol., 15:348–354, 1973.
8. Compere, E., L.: Excision of hemivertebrae for correction of congenital scoliosis. J. Bone Joint Surg., 14:555–562, 1932.
9. Dubousset, J., and Gonon, E. P.: Cyphoses et cypho-scolioses angulaires. Suppl. II, p. 69, Rev. Cir. Orthop., 1983.
10. Dubousset, J.: Congenital kyphosis. In Bradford, D., S., and Hensinger, R. M. (eds.): Pediatric Spine, New York, Thieme-Stratton, 1985.
11. Erickson, D. L.: Treatment of occult spinal dysraphic abnormalities. In Chou, S. N., and Seljeskog, E. L. (eds.): Spinal Deformities and Neurological Dysfunction. New York, Raven Press, pp. 201–208, 1978.
12. Goldberg, C., Fenlon, G., and Blacke, N. S.: Diastematomyelia: a critical review of the natural history and treatment. Spine, 9:367–372, 1984.
13. Gutkelch, A. N.: Diastematomyelia with median septum. Brain, 97:729–742, 1974.
14. Haffner, J.: Einige Zwillinge mit Symmetrishcher Wirbelsaulendeformitat. Keilwibel. Acta Radiol., 17:529–541, 1936.
15. Hall, J. E.: Congenital scoliosis. In Bradford, D. S., and Hensinger, R. M. (eds.): Pediatric Spine. New York, Thieme-Stratton, 1985.
16. Hall, J. E., Herndon, W. A., and Levine, C. R.: Surgical treatment of congenital scoliosis with or without Harrington instrumentation. J. Bone Joint Surg., 63A:608–619, 1981.
17. Hall, J. E., Levine, C. R., and Sudhir, K. G.: Intraoperative awakening to monitor spinal cord function during Harrington instrumentation and spine fusion. J. Bone Joint Surg., 60A:533–536, 1978.
18. Hathaway, G. L.: Congenital scoliosis in one of monozygotic twins: a case report. J. Bone Joint Surg., 59A:837–838, 1977.
19. Hensinger, R., Lang, J. E., and MacEwen, G. D.: Klippel-Feil syndrome: a constellation of associated anomalies. J. Bone Joint Surg., 56A:1246–1253, 1974.
20. Herbert, J. J.: Osteotomie Pour Cyphose Congenitale. Rev. Chir. Orthop., 37:506–508, 1951.
21. Hoffman, H. J., Hendrick, E. B., and Humphreys, R. P.: The tethered spinal cord: its protean manifestations, diagnosis, and surgical correction. Childs Brain, 2:145–155, 1976.
22. Hood, R. W., Riseborough, E., Nehme, A., et al.: Diastematomyelia and structural spinal deformities. J. Bone Joint Surg., 62A:520–528, 1980.
23. James, C. C. M., and Lassman, L. P.: Diastematomyelia and the tight filum terminale. J. Neurol. Sci., 10:193–196, 1970.
24. James, J. I. P.: Paraplegia in congenital kyphoscoliosis. J. Bone Joint Surg., 57B:261, 1975.
25. Jarcho, S., and Levin, P. M.: Hereditary malformations of the vertebral bodies. Bull. Johns Hopkins Hosp., 62:215–226, 1938.
26. Kuhns, J. E., and Hormell, R. S.: Management of congenital scoliosis. Arch. Surg., 65:250–263, 1952.
27. Langenskiold, A.: Correction of congenital scoliosis by excision of one-half of a cleft vertebra. Acta Orthop. Scand., 38:291–300, 1967.
28. Leatherman, K. D., and Dickson, R. A.: Two-stage corrective surgery for congenital deformities of the spine. J. Bone Joint Surg., 61B:324–328, 1979.
29. Letts, R. M., and Hollenberg, C.: Delayed paresis following spinal fusion with Harrington instrumentation. Clin. Orthop., 125:45–48, 1977.
30. Lonstein, J. E., Winter, R., Moe, J., et al.: Neurologic deficits secondary to spinal deformity: a review of the literature and report of 43 cases. Spine, 5:331–355, 1980.
31. MacEwen, G. D., Conway, J. J., and Miller, W. T.:

Congenital scoliosis with a unilateral bar. Radiology, 40:711–715, 1968.
32. MacEwen, G. D., Winter, R. B., and Hardy, J. H.: Evaluation of kidney anomalies in congenital scoliosis. J. Bone Joint Surg., 54A:1341–1454, 1972.
33. MacLennan, A.: Scoliosis. Br. Med. J., 2:864, 1922.
34. Mayfield, J. K., Winter, R. B., Bradford, D. S., and Moe, J. H.: Congenital kyphosis due to defects of anterior segmentation. J. Bone Joint Surg., 62A:1291–1301, 1980.
35. McMaster, M. J., and Ohtsuka, K.: The natural history of congenital scoliosis: a study of 251 patients. J. Bone Joint Surg., 64A:1128–1147, 1982.
36. McMaster, M. J.: Occult intraspinal anomalies and congenital scoliosis. J. Bone Joint Surg., 66A:588–601, 1984.
37. Mensink, J. H. A., and Rogge, C. W. L.: Congenital scoliosis. Arch. Chir. Neerl., 26:109–129, 1974.
38. Montgomery, S. P., and Hall, J. E.: Congenital kyphosis. Spine, 7:360–364, 1982.
39. Morscher, E.: Experiences with the transthoracic hemilateral epiphyseodesis in the treatment of scoliosis. In Operative Treatment of Scoliosis, 1971 Symposium, Nijmegan, Stuttgart, Georg Thieme, pp. 135–137, 1973.
40. Nasca, R. J., Stelling, F. H., and Steel, H. H.: Progression of congenital scoliosis due to hemivertebrae and hemivertebrae with bars. J. Bone Joint Surg., 57A:456–466, 1975.
41. Ominus, M., and Michel, C. R.: Problemes poses par la resection des hemivertebres lombosacrees. Chir. Pediatr., 19:119–121, 1978.
42. Peterson, H. A., and Peterson, L. F. A.: Hemivertebra in identical twins with dissimilar spinal columns. J. Bone Joint Surg., 49A:938–942, 1967.
43. Rathke, W. F., and Sun, H. Y.: Untersuchungen uber Missbildungsskoliosen. Z. Orthop., 97:173, 1963.
44. Reckles, L. H., Peterson, H. A., Bianco, A. J., and Weidman, W. H.: The association of scoliosis and congenital heart defects. J. Bone Joint Surg., 57A:449–455, 1975.
45. Rimoin, D. L., Fletcher, B. D., and McKusick, V. A.: Spondylocostal dysplasia. A dominantly inherited form of short trunked dwarfism. Am. J. Med., 45:948–953, 1968.
46. Roaf, R.: Vertebral growth and its mechanical control. J. Bone Joint Surg., 42B:40, 1960.
47. Roaf, R.: The late results of unilateral growth arrest of the spine for scoliosis. Acta Orthop. Scand., 33:393, 1963.
48. Roaf, R.: The treatment of progressive scoliosis by unilateral growth arrest. J. Bone Joint Surg., 45B:637–651, 1963.
49. Royle, N. D.: Operative removal of an accessory vertebra. Med. J. Austral., 1:467, 1928.
50. Shapiro, F., and Eyre, D.: Congenital scolioses: a histopathologic study. Spine, 6:107–117, 1981.
51. Slabaugh, P., Winter, R., Lonstein, J., and Moe, J.: A review of lumbosacral hemivertebra with excision in eight. Spine, 5:234–244, 1980.
52. Stagnara, P.: Les Deformations du Rachis. Paris, Masson, pp. 344–354, 1985.
53. Stoll, J., and Bunch, W.: Segmental spinal instrumentation for congenital scoliosis: a report of two cases. Spine, 8:43–47, 1983.
54. Touzet, P., Rigault, P., and Padovani, J. P.: Les hemivertebres: classification historie naturelle et elements de prognostic. Rev. Chir. Orthop., 65:173–186, 1979.
55. Tsou, P., Yau, A., and Hodgson, A.: Congenital spinal deformities: natural history, classification, and the role of anterior surgery. J. Bone Joint Surg., 56A:1767, 1974.
56. Van Assen, J.: Angeborene kyphose. Acta Orthop. Scand., 67:14–33, 1930.
57. Wiles, P.: Resection of dorsal vertebrae in congenital scoliosis. J. Bone Joint Surg., 33A:151–154, 1951.
58. Winter, R. B.: Congenital Deformities of the Spine. New York, Thieme-Stratton, 1983.
59. Winter, R. B.: Congenital kyphoscoliosis with paralysis following hemivertebra excision. Clin. Orthop., 119:116–125, 1976.
60. Winter, R. B.: Convex anterior and posterior hemiarthrodesis and epiphyseodesis in young children with progressive congenital scoliosis. J. Pediatr. Orthop., 1:361–366, 1981.
61. Winter, R. B., Haven, J. J., Moe, J. H., and Lagaard, S. M.: Diastematomyelia and congenital spine deformities. J. Bone Joint Surg., 56A:27–39, 1974.
62. Winter, R. B., and Moe, J. H.: The results of spinal arthrodesis for congenital spine deformity in patients younger than 5 years old. J. Bone Joint Surg., 64A:419–432, 1982.
63. Winter, R. B., Moe, J. H., and Bradford, D. S.: Congenital thoracic lordosis. J. Bone Joint Surg., 60A:806–810, 1978.
64. Winter, R. B., Moe, J. H., and Eilers, V. E.: Congenital scoliosis: a study of 234 patients treated and untreated. J. Bone Joint Surg., 50A:1–47, 1968.
65. Winter, R. B., Moe, J. H., and Lonstein, J. E.: Posterior spinal arthrodesis for congenital scoliosis. J. Bone Joint Surg., 66A:1188–1197, 1984.
66. Winter, R., B., Moe, J. H., and Lonstein, J. E.: The surgical treatment of congenital kyphosis: a review of 94 patients age 5 years or older with 2 years of more followup in 77 patients. Spine, 10:224–231, 1985.
67. Winter, R. B., Moe, J. H., MacEwen, G. D., and Peon-Vidales, H.: The Milwaukee brace in the nonoperative treatment of congenital scoliosis. Spine, 1:85–96, 1976.
68. Winter, R., B., Moe, J. H., and Wang, J. F.: Congenital kyphosis. J. Bone Joint Surg., 55A:223–256, 1973.
69. Wynne-Davies, R.: Congenital vertebral anomalies: etiology and relationship to spina bifida oystica. J. Med. Genet., 12:280–288, 1975.

13

NEUROMUSCULAR SPINAL DEFORMITY

David S. Bradford, M.D.

There are a wide variety of diseases of the neuromuscular system in which spinal deformity is a natural outcome. Regardless of the location of the neurologic lesion, the ultimate effect is on the skeletal muscle, leading to varying degrees of paralysis. Because most of these diseases occur in the perinatal period an early onset of spinal deformity is decreed. With growth and development, progression of the deformity is common. Furthermore, the primary disease may be progressive and may affect the sensory and autonomic nervous system as well as the patient's intelligence. Indeed this group of diseases poses the most difficult and challenging problems for the spinal surgeon.

CLASSIFICATION

Classification of neuromuscular spinal deformity has been developed by the Scoliosis Research Society and consists of the following:
A. Neuropathic
  1. Upper motor neuron
     a. Cerebral palsy
     b. Spinocerebellar degeneration
        i. Friedreich's ataxia
        ii. Charcot-Marie-Tooth
        iii. Roussy-Levy
     c. Syringomyelia
     d. Spinal cord tumor
     e. Spinal cord trauma
  2. Lower motor neuron
     a. Poliomyelitis
     b. Other viral myelitides
     c. Traumatic
     d. Spinal muscular atrophy
        i. Werdnig-Hoffmann
        ii. Kugelberg-Welander
     e. Dysautonomia (Riley-Day)
B. Myopathic
  1. Arthrogryposis
  2. Muscular dystrophy
     a. Duchenne (pseudohypertrophic)
     b. Limb-girdle
     c. Facioscapulohumeral
  3. Fiber type disproportion
  4. Congenital hypotonia
  5. Myotonia dystrophica

This is the most common classification currently in use, and as can be seen, it divides these deformities into neuropathic or myopathic categories, depending on whether the muscle or the nerve is the primary source of pathology. Another useful concept is that recently presented by Brown and Swank,[13] which considers the location of the lesion in the neuromuscular system to be of primary importance in the resultant abnormal muscle activity. As they note, the muscle may be either spastic, rigid, athetoid, or flaccid. Although combinations do exist, the two main categories of abnormal muscle activity that are associated with curvatures of the spine are spastic and flaccid; spasticity is produced primarily by disorders of the brain, cerebellum, and upper motor neuron, and flaccidity is produced by lesions involving the anterior horn cell or motor neuron and primary muscle diseases. By considering the type of muscle activity associated with the spinal deformity, a more logical treatment plan may be constructed.

GENERAL PRINCIPLES[11, 13, 35, 53, 81]

Patients with neuromuscular scoliosis present with significantly different and more complicated problems than those with idiopathic scoliosis. Progression is much more common than in idiopathic scoliosis, and the progression usually begins with the onset of the disease. This occurs not infrequently in the perinatal or childhood period, and therefore the magnitude of the deformity eventually attained without treatment may be much greater. Furthermore, these deformities are capable of increasing even after maturity is reached. Those at greatest risk for developing greater degrees of deformity are those with a high level of paralysis, asymmetrical paralysis, or as mentioned, deformity appearing during growth child.

Untreated, these curvatures will have a much greater adverse affect on the patient's activities of daily living. In a patient who is severely incapacitated because of generalized neuromuscular dysfunction, a progressive spinal curvature that interferes with balance may convert the patient from an independent household ambulator to wheelchair ambulation. In those who are already wheelchair ambulators, progressive deformity may severely limit upper extremity function, sitting balance, and head control (Fig. 13–1).

Pulmonary dysfunction in this group of patients is usually greater in severity and more frequent than in patients with idiopathic scoliosis. Associated intercostal paralysis may cause a significant decrease in pulmonary function in the absence of a curvature. A small curvature with loss of thoracic kyphosis may severely limit vital capacity and interfere with functional independence.

Other organ systems may be affected as a result of the neuromuscular process. This includes a cardiomyopathy in Duchenne's or Friedreich's ataxia, hydrocephalus and urinary tract disease in myelodysplasia and

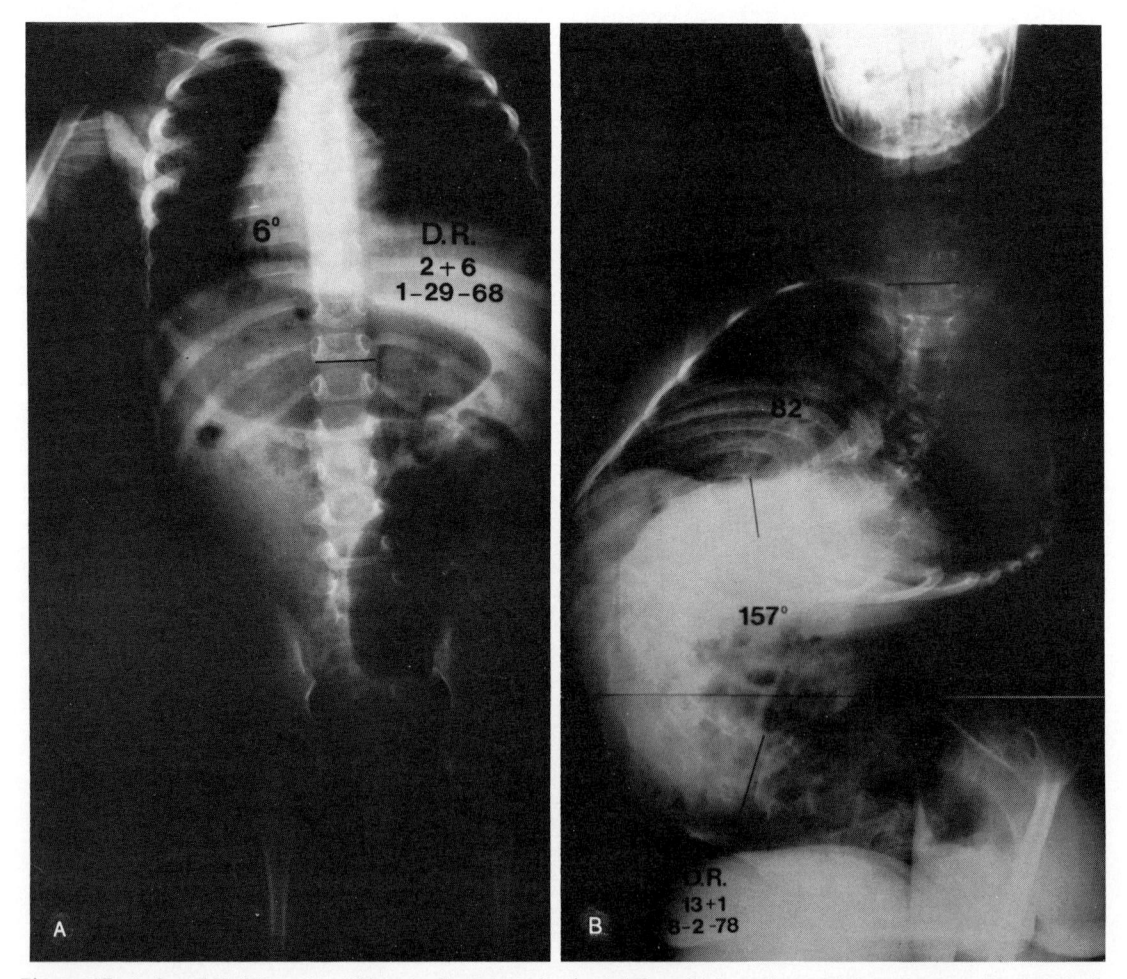

Figure 13–1. A and B, The natural history of untreated spinal deformity in patients with neuromuscular scoliosis. This female patient presented at age 2+6 years with spinal muscle atrophy. Early brace treatment was recommended but refused by the family. Surgery likewise was recommended but was refused.

traumatic paraplegia, pressure sores in patients with absent sensation, and hip dislocation in patients with muscle imbalance with or without pelvic obliquity.

Furthermore, the management of these patients by surgical means may be associated with a much greater risk. The bone is osteoporotic, metallic implants may dislodge, there is a high risk of pseudarthrosis, postoperative external supports are not well tolerated, absent or poor skin sensation may lead to pressure ulcerations, decreased pulmonary function may necessitate postoperative ventilatory support, and spastic muscle activity along with decreased intelligence may complicate postoperative management. It should be appreciated that these problems and many others that we will discuss make the management of this group of patients the most difficult and complicated of all spinal disorders.

One may then ask, Why treat patients with progressive neuromuscular disease who may have shortened life expectancies, poor intellectual capacity, and careers that may prove less than productive by our standards? Untreated, these deformities will usually progress even in the adult period, and this progression can be halted by surgery. By maintaining the patients at functional levels, and at times even improving their function, prevention of future neurologic problems is possible if the disease process is static. By treatment one may prevent progressive deterioration of pulmonary function, and free the upper extremities for activities of daily living. Nursing care may be eased, and prevention of back pain possible. Many of these patients will have productive lives. We feel an aggressive therapeutic approach should always be considered.

EVALUATION OF THE PATIENT

Evaluation of the patient with spinal deformity has been presented in detail in Chapter 5. For patients with neuromuscular disease, a few points should be stressed. The correct diagnosis of the patient's disease process should be substantiated beyond reasonable doubt if at all possible. A competent neurologist may prove of great assistance in determining the correct diagnosis and prognosis of the patient. A rapidly progressive neuromuscular disease and a poor prognosis would certainly have an impact on the type of treatment planned for the patient with spinal deformity. In examination of the patient particular attention should be directed toward the type of curvature, the location, and the collapsing nature of the spine. For instance, does the patient have trunk support or is the patient totally flaccid and unable to sit upright without arm support. Associated contractures should be determined and pelvic obliquity, with or without iliotibial band contractures or hip flexion contractures, should be evaluated. It may prove necessary to release contractures about the pelvis prior to undertaking corrective surgery on the spine, depending upon the type of deformity and the type of neuromuscular disease. Pulmonary function should be carefully evaluated as well. We have found it desirable to have patients with decreased pulmonary function seen in consultation and evaluated by an internist or pediatrician with expertise in pulmonary medicine. Following major spinal surgery, prolonged ventilatory support may be necessary, and assistance by a specialist competent in this area is immensely beneficial.

Routine radiographs as previously described are helpful. Standing films may be useful in patients able to stand; however, one should make certain that if standing films are obtained, the patient is not using support to maintain the standing posture. Otherwise, the magnitude of the curvature recorded may be less than its true value. Often, sitting films are much more helpful, showing the true magnitude of the spinal deformity while eliminating the suspension effect of crutches and the effects of contractures about the hip and pelvis. Distraction x-rays taken on a Risser frame may be more beneficial than bending films, although neither may prove particularly helpful in patients with severe spasticity or rigidity.

Patients with neuromuscular spinal deformity undergoing surgery will need a careful evaluation of pulmonary function. Nickel and Perry[84, 85] have stated that patients with vital capacities of less than 30 per cent require respiratory support postoperatively. These authors as well as Brown and Swank[13] have recommended a tracheostomy in patients without a voluntary or cough reflex and a vital capacity of below 30 per cent. At our institution, we have not had to perform a tracheotomy on any patient undergoing corrective spinal surgery in the past ten years. We have preferred to use an indwelling endotracheal tube for patients requiring postoperative respiratory assist as long as is necessary. No particular test at this time helps us to define with 100 per cent confidence which patients will need prolonged respiratory assist after surgery. Certainly, the inability to generate a cough with a vital capacity of less than 300 cc., would make such postoperative assist likely (see Chapter 22).

TREATMENT

The modalities of treatment for neuromuscular spinal deformities are similar to those of idiopathic scoliosis; observation, bracing, and spinal reconstructive surgery. Their role and indication however are different.

Observation

Observation is an important part of management of any spinal deformity. It is particularly relevant in patients with minor degrees of curvature and in those in whom the natural history of the neuromuscular process as well as the curvature have not been established. Periodic clinical and radiographic evaluation is therefore desirable. Six to eight month follow-up visits with repeat radiographs in both the coronal and sagittal planes are recommended. Any patient that has developed a curvature greater than 20 to 25 degrees secondary to neuromuscular deformity of the flaccid type and has growth remaining should be considered for treatment with an orthosis.

Orthosis

Many may question whether orthoses do indeed have a role in neuromuscular scoliosis. However, in a child with a flaccid paralysis and a deformity greater than 20 degrees, it has been shown that bracing may indeed retard the progressive nature of the curvature, allowing a longer period of spinal growth until the optimal age for surgery (approximately age ten in girls and age 12 in boys).[13, 15, 17, 35, 83] These orthoses function as purely passive body containers. The body jacket should be made of a semi-rigid synthetic material lined with a soft material such as Plastazote; pressure points over bony protuberances should be avoided.[31, 126] The chief advantage of bracing is that it provides the flaccid patient with trunk support, allowing use of upper extremities for purposeful activity. The brace, therefore, establishes a stable link between the pelvis and upper trunk. Furthermore, it may delay progression of the spinal deformity, as mentioned. It has less benefit in the patient with spasticity, although studies by Bunnell[18] and MacEwen[67] suggest that in the very mild spastic, it may occasionally stop progression and be the only treatment required. This in our experience has been unlikely, however, and at best only a delay of surgery can be anticipated.

If not carefully fitted and frequently checked, the brace may cause pressure ulcerations. It may also decrease the ambulatory level of patients who may be heading toward a wheelchair status. In athetoid patients, it has a most limited role. In the flaccid patient, a snug fitting brace may decrease chest expansion, resulting in decreased pulmonary function.

Specialized seating systems may prove particularly beneficial (Fig. 13–2).[19, 40] These devices may facilitate support of the trunk while the patient is in a wheelchair, and they allow accommodation of a pelvic obliquity, proper distribution of forces, and prevention of pressure ulcerations. At our institution it has been found to be most useful in patients with severe cerebral palsy, spinal muscle atrophy, or advanced muscular dystrophy. Specially designed outriggers to the brace may provide additional support for the head.

Electrospinal stimulation in patients with neuromuscular spinal deformity would in our opinion be without use or benefit, although Swank and Brown have suggested that it may be beneficial in patients with normal lower motor neuron function without spasticity, i.e., spinal cord injured children.[117]

Surgery

The surgical approach to patients with neuromuscular spinal deformity may prove a major undertaking, as previously mentioned. Preoperative evaluation should be extensive, and the patient's course during and after surgery should be carefully monitored. Preoperative halo traction has not proven to be beneficial in obtaining greater correction or in the intraoperative management of the deformity. However, in patients with severe cardiopulmonary dysfunction, it may be of

Figure 13–2. A and B, The usefulness of a sitting orthosis for a patient with collapsing type spinal deformity is shown. Although the curvature may not be controlled with this device, the patient can maintain a more functional sitting posture, facilitating nursing care and decreasing the incidence of pressure sores.

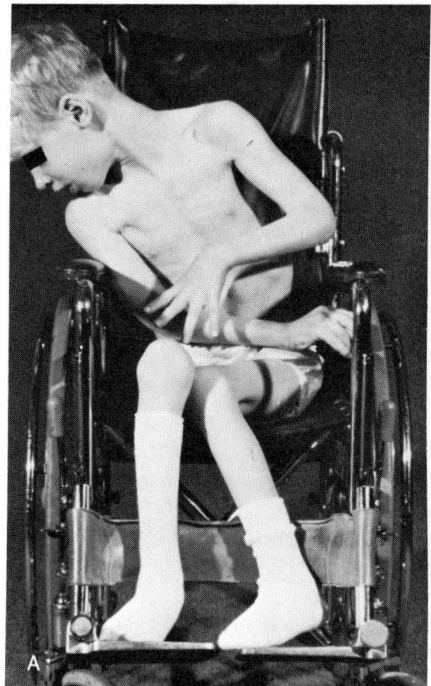

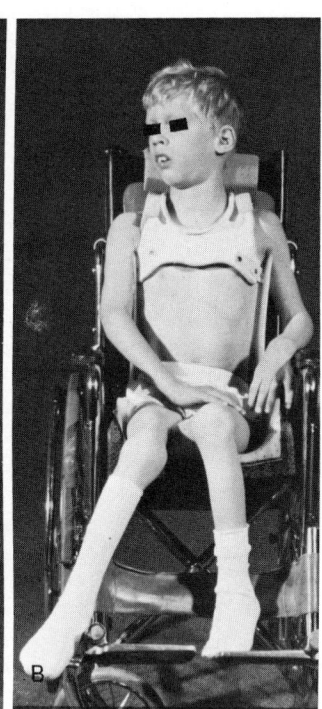

assistance in evaluating possible reversability of the dysfunction, particularly in the postpolio patient.[119] If a two-stage procedure is planned, the halo may be beneficial in mobilizing the patient between surgery, (i.e., in a halo wheelchair). In patients with spinal muscle atrophy, the use of the halo is ill advised. The presence of severe hip flexion contractures may necessitate release before spinal surgery to allow optimal positioning of the patient on the operating table, particularly if lumbar hyperlordosis is to be corrected.

Prior to induction of anesthesia, we have favored insertion of an arterial line, a urinary catheter, and a rectal probe to monitor temperature. Arterial hypotension during surgery is useful to minimize blood loss. A blood warmer, heating blanket, and cell saver are all useful modalities. We have found a bone bank of great benefit in providing a ready source of allograft bone to augment local or deficient quantities of iliac bone.

Surgical techniques are similar to those previously described in the Techniques of Surgery section. Blood loss, however, is expected to be more extensive. The bone is osteoporotic, and easily fractures if too rigorous elevation of the soft tissue is attempted. Thrombin-soaked Gelfoam along with topical collagen (Avitene) is most beneficial in controlling local bleeding. Bone wax may be used as liberally as necessary.

The methods and techniques of surgical fusion have varied considerably over the past 30 years. With the advent of better fusion techniques and more secure internal fixation systems,[1, 63, 116, 120] improved correction and decreased pseudarthrosis have been evident. Posterior surgery with the use of a variety of available implants remains the mainstay of treatment for the majority of these patients. In very young patients (<10 years), instrumentation without fusion is a preliminary procedure to the eventual arthrodesis. In the past ten years a general tendency to manage more severe rigid deformities with combined surgery coupled with anterior segmental implants (Dwyer or Zielke) and/or the use of a posterior segmental implant (Luque) has resulted in superior correction (50 to 60 per cent) and a decreased pseudarthrosis rate to less than 7 per cent.[27, 58] These combined techniques have for the most part resulted in a significant correction of pelvic obliquity (60 to 80 per cent).[27, 33, 71, 88, 89, 90] If residual pelvic obliquity remains and poses a functional disability, then a transiliac lengthening procedure as described by Millis and Hall might be considered.[78]

The more recently developed techniques of combined anterior and posterior surgery with segmental instrumentation may be equally applicable to flaccid as well as spastic paralysis. We have found the combined approach to be most beneficial in the more severe curvatures (>80 degrees) with limited flexibility (<50 per cent) and in lumbar curvatures associated with a fixed pelvic obliquity or all obliquity that remains uncorrectable even with traction.

POLIOMYELITIS

It is of interest historically that many of the current concepts in managing spinal deformities grew out of or were a direct result of the experience gained through management of spinal problems associated with poliomyelitis.[37, 38, 81] Efforts at spinal stabilization initiated by Cobb,[20] Garrett,[37, 38] Moe,[80] and others[42] provided a vast background of experience that ultimately proved useful in the management of idiopathic spinal deformity. The evolution of these treatment methods at Rancho Los Amigos over a 16 year period from 1954 through 1970 as described by Bonnett and associates[11] is indeed interesting reading. Coincident with the evolution of increased fixation and improved fusion techniques, correction improved from 20 to 57 per cent, although the incidence of pseudarthrosis remained approximately 30 per cent.

A discussion of poliomyelitis would be incomplete without mentioning the classical papers of Colonna and Vomsaal,[21] Steindler,[114] James,[53] and Roaf.[99] These papers are certainly worthwhile reading for those interested in the historical aspects of poliomyelitis spinal deformity. Although poliomyelitis has been virtually eradicated in North America and indeed in most parts of the world, much of the stigmata in terms of residual spinal deformity remains. In fact at our Center we are still treating adult patients now presenting with significant curvatures secondary to poliomyelitis in childhood.

The incidence of scoliosis developing in a patient afflicted with poliomyelitis is approximately 30 per cent.[21] Prognosis of deformity is again related to the age of onset of the curvature and the degree of muscle imbalance rather than the site of the primary curve.[53] The curves may follow one of four patterns. The most common are long, sweeping thoracolumbar C-shaped curves in patients with only slight paralysis or the generalized collapsing type of deformity, presenting as a combined thoracic and lumbar curve with extensive spinal weakness. Two other types of curvatures may be present, the lumbar curve with varying degrees of pelvic obliquity and muscle imbalance in the trunk musculature, and a primary thoracic curve often associated with weakness of the scapular muscles. Usually the most severe curves that we have seen have been those associated with untreated spinal deformities secondary to polio in the childhood period. The most cosmetically unacceptable deformities are those that involve the upper thoracic cervical junction and result in marked shoulder and neck deformity with trunk collapse. Curvatures that involve the thoracic area are usually associated with severe vertebral rotation, rib hump deformity, intercostal paralysis, and pulmonary dysfunction. Lower curvatures involving the lumbar spine and associated with pelvic obliquity may severely compromise the patient's ambulation and sitting balance.

Non-operative Treatment

Curvatures secondary to poliomyelitis are best managed by surgery. Bracing, however, is a useful modality in delaying fusion until a more optimal age (pre-puberty or puberty), allowing maximum spinal growth. Occasionally, curvatures have been managed successfully by bracing alone, but this is uncommon and should not be an expected result. Any curvature progressing to 20 degrees in a growing child should be braced. Continued progression warrants a surgical approach. Hip flexion contractures and iliotibial band contractures should be released as these procedures may facilitate bracing in maintaining a level pelvis. Great caution should be exercised in preventing chest compromise by a Milwaukee or an underarm orthosis (Fig. 13–3). Earlier surgery is preferable to increasing chest wall deformity with an externally applied orthosis.

Surgical Treatment

Management of patients with polio by surgical means is not greatly different from that of other patients with spinal deformities secondary to neuromuscular disease.[43, 59, 63, 72, 92] Timing of surgery should be based on the magnitude of the deformity and the age of the patient. If the curvature can be controlled, then surgery should be delayed until the beginning of the adolescent growth spurt, since this is the period during which

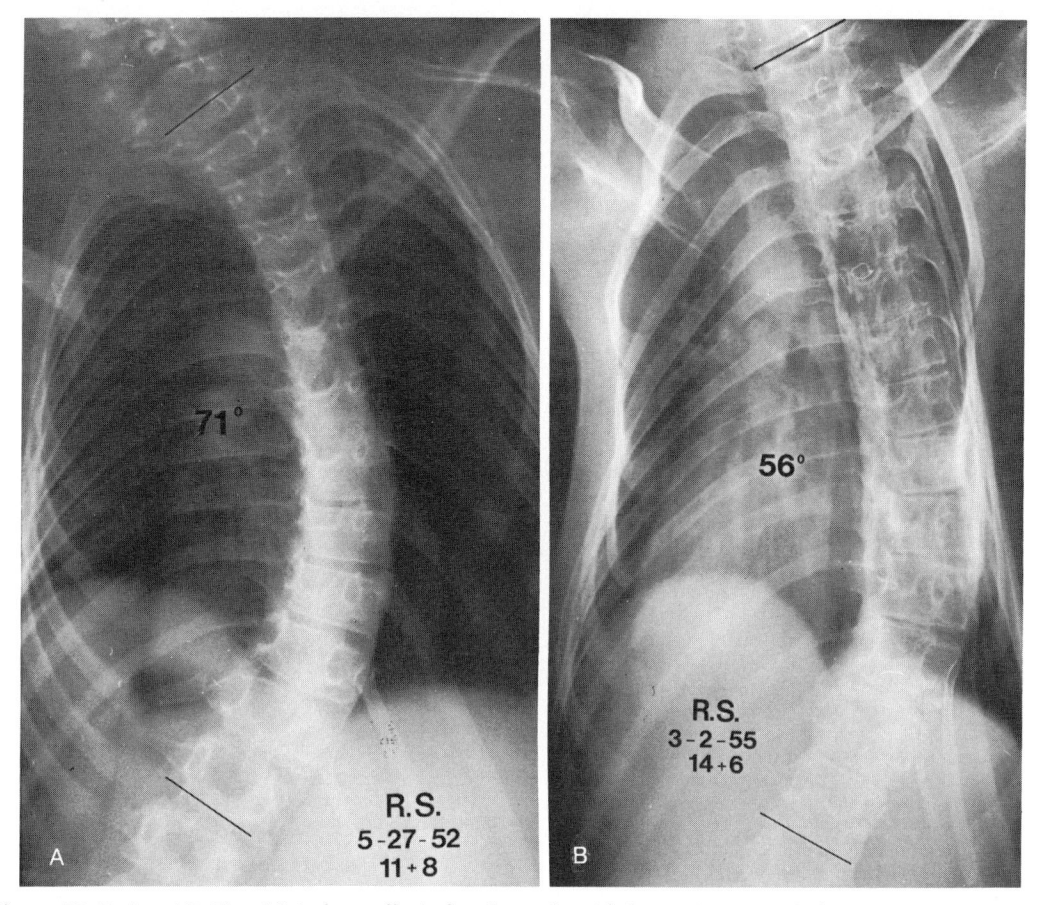

Figure 13-3. A and B, The deleterious effect of prolonged restrictive casts on producing chest wall deformity in patients with paralytic scoliosis is shown. Restrictive body braces may likewise have a deleterious effect and one should keep this in mind when using a brace while attempting to hold a curve until a more optimal time for surgical arthrodesis.

more severe progression of the curve develops and bracing tends to fail (Fig. 13-4). On the other hand, if the curvature cannot be controlled and progresses beyond 40 to 50 degrees in the brace, then earlier surgical treatment will be necessary. Again, it is important to remember, "better a slightly shortened straight spine than a very very short crooked one." Surgery should not be delayed until the end of growth.

Once the decision is made to proceed with surgery, the level of fusion is carefully determined preoperatively. Poliomyelitis patients with spinal curvatures will require a longer fusion than patients with idiopathic scoliosis. The collapsing nature of the deformity, the severe degree of vertebral rotation, and the lack of normal muscle function impact on this decision. Furthermore, these patients may have a component of true sagittal plane deformity and a fusion in such cases must encompass the anteroposterior and lateral deformities as well. All rotated vertebrae should be fused, and the fusion should extend to the first non-rotated vertebra as well. Occasionally, this may require fusion into the cervical spine.[94] The top and the bottom of the fusion area should lie directly over the center of the sacrum, similarly to the arrangement described by Harrington as a "stable zone." If there is pelvic obliquity and the sacrum is part of the curvature and the lumbar musculature is weak and deficient, the fusion should extend to the sacrum.[43] If on the other hand the obliquity is not part of the curvature and is caused by iliotibial band contractures, then the contractures should be released and the fusion stopped at L4 or L5. Independent ambulation and mobility in these patients is facilitated by a flexible lumbosacral joint, and every attempt should be made to maintain this mobility if feasible.

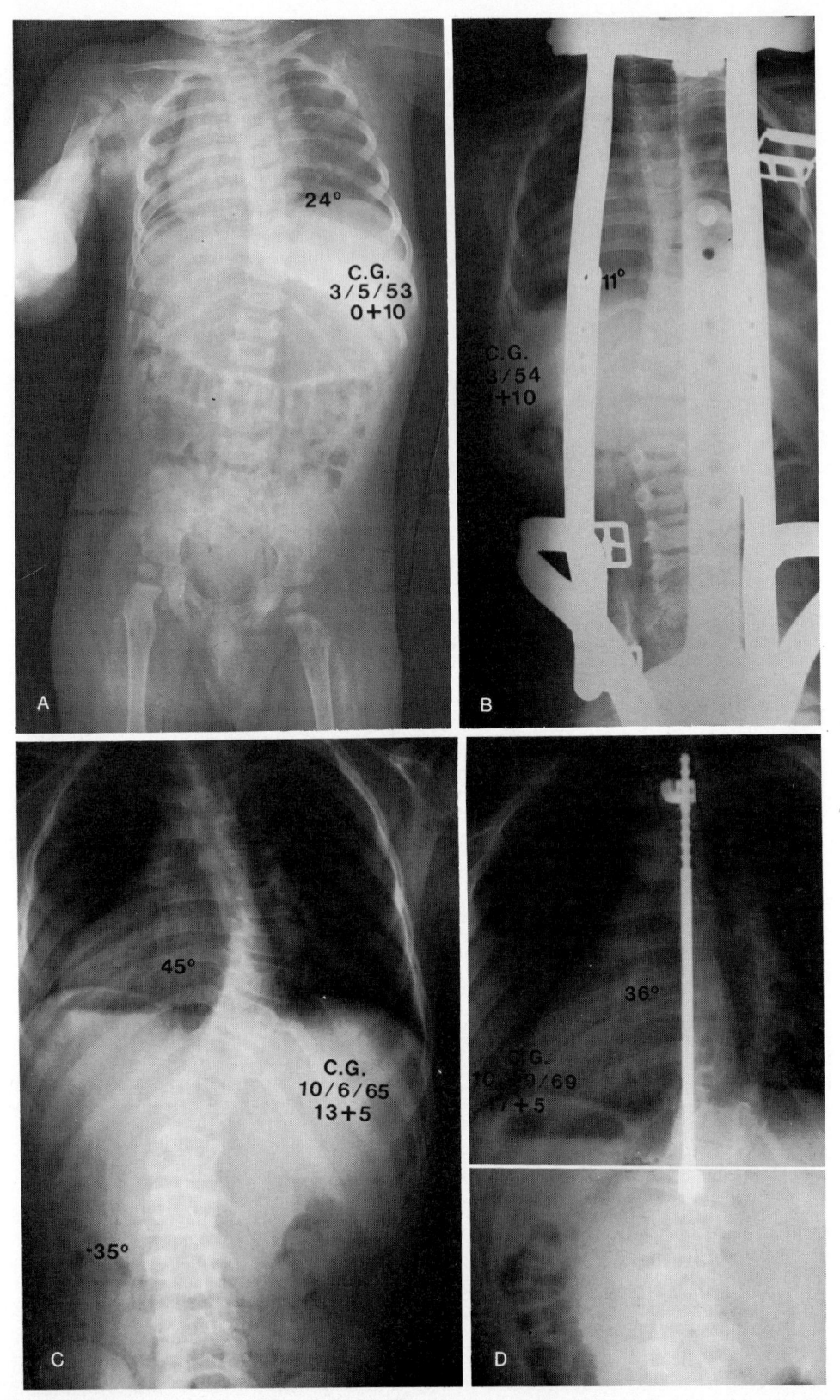

Figure 13–4. *A*, The x-rays of a 10 month old child with polio first seen in 1953. *B*, Treatment was begun shortly thereafter with a brace. The curvature was improved to 11 degrees. *C*, The patient was continued in the brace until the adolescent growth spurt, when curvature control was no longer possible. *D*, Surgical arthrodesis was carried out to satisfactory outcome.

ILIOTIBIAL BAND CONTRACTURES

Yount[129] and Irwin[51] described with a great degree of clarity the presentation and the problems relating to iliotibial band contractures. The contraction of the iliotibial band unilaterally may contribute directly or indirectly to: (1) flexion and abduction of the contractures of the hip, (2) external rotation contractures of the hip, (3) genu valgum, (4) knee flexion deformity, and (5) external torsion of the tibia. Furthermore, it may lead to severe pelvic obliquity and to an exaggerated lumbar lordosis when flexion contractures are present on both sides. The relationship of pelvic obliquity to the curvature, therefore, must be carefully considered. Pelvic obliquity can be caused in part by factors above the pelvis (scoliosis), or by factors below the pelvis (iliotibial band contractures), or a combination of both. To confirm the presence of a contracture, a level pelvis can be produced by flexing, abducting, and externally rotating the extremity. If the pelvic obliquity is corrected by this maneuver, treatment of the iliotibial band contracture is desirable. A complete surgical release, proximally as well as distally, followed by traction or casting would be indicated. Traction on the well leg has proven useful,[81] and the application of halofemoral pin traction is equally effective. One may then proceed to treat the scoliosis in the presence of a more level pelvis (Fig. 13-5). If surgery is necessary for the curvature, extension of the fusion to the sacrum may usually be avoided. This evaluation and contracture release is most useful in younger patients with more flexible deformities. Older patients presenting with fixed lumbar curvatures with extreme degrees of pelvic obliquity where the sacrum is part of the curvature are best managed by combined anterior and posterior surgery with fusion to the sacrum.[58, 89, 90]

PREOPERATIVE TRACTION

As a general rule, preoperative traction in neuromuscular scoliosis is neither helpful nor indicated. In the past we have advocated preoperative traction to reduce the curvature and improve it over the preoperative bending films to facilitate better correction at the time of surgery. However, such traction has not improved the degree of correction we have ultimately obtained with the use of internal fixation devices, has inordinately prolonged the patient's hospital stay, has not proven cost effective, and has not decreased the risk of neurologic complications. It only promotes more severe degrees of osteopenia or osteoporosis and may result in a greater incidence of thromboembolic disease. Halopelvic traction at our institution has not been used for the past ten years. We would disagree with the work of Leong and coworkers,[58] therefore, that traction of curvatures of greater than 100 degrees is beneficial. Granted, the percentage of correction with distraction by this type of traction is greater than that which would be obtained on side bending, but it is not greater than that which could be obtained with instrumentation. However, there is one exception to this and that is in regards to the patient with limited pulmonary function.

MANAGEMENT OF THE POLIO PATIENT WITH PULMONARY INSUFFICIENCY

In polio patients presenting with severe spinal deformity and impending cor pulmonale or overt right heart failure, preoperative traction is a useful adjunct in their management. Swank and associates[119] reported on a series of 20 patients from our Center with cor pulmonale due to scoliosis and associated spinal deformities and curvatures ranging from 90 to 200 degrees. Of these, 15 were placed in halo traction, and nine went on to surgical stabilization. The best results were in post poliomyelitis patients who had an average increase in vital capacity from 595 to 1071 cc. The average PaO_2 increased in this group of patients from 55 to 64 mm. Hg, whereas the pCO_2 decreased in this group of patients from 52 to 43 mm. Hg. Preliminary halo traction facilitates evaluating the reversability of pulmonary dysfunction and improving the patient's general cardiopulmonary status prior to surgery. We have also felt that cardiac catheterization could give additional information in assessing the possible reversability of pulmonary hypertension in these patients.

Halo traction may also be of benefit in patients with limited pulmonary function in whom combined procedures are planned. Following anterior surgery, mobilization of the patient in a halo wheelchair may facilitate pulmonary rehabilitation. Concerning the indications for a tracheostomy in this group of patients, we have not found it useful or beneficial, and in fact have not done a tracheostomy at our institution in the past ten

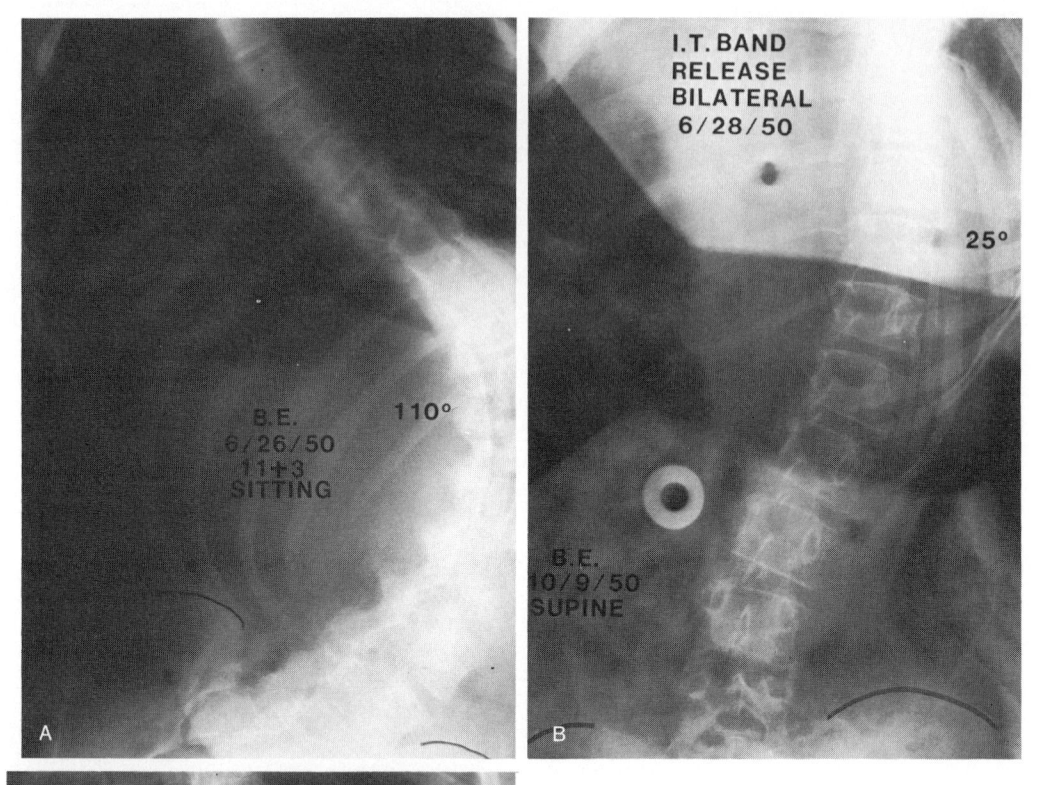

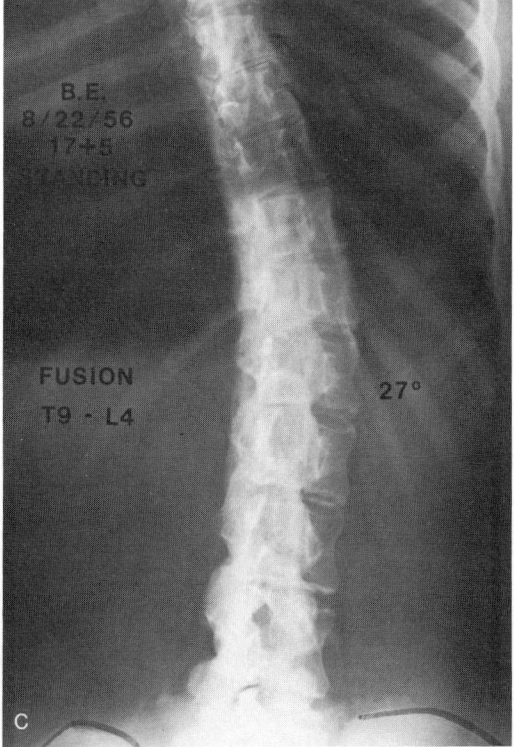

Figure 13–5. A, The preoperative x-rays of an 11 year old patient with scoliosis and pelvic obliquity. The patient had ilioband contracture, which was released. B, Following traction, there is no longer a pelvic obliquity. C, Surgical arthrodesis therefore was carried down to L4 only with a satisfactory outcome, maintenance of a level pelvis, and a mobile lumbosacral joint.

years. Patients who need prolonged ventilatory assist after surgery can be safely and conveniently managed with indwelling nasotracheal tubes. We have had these in place for as long as two weeks after surgery without difficulties (see section on Pulmonary Function).

POSTERIOR SURGERY

A major improvement in surgery for the patient with poliomyelitis was brought about through the innovative work of Harrington,[46] and in fact, Harrington's original instruments were designed for poliomyelitis patients in order to overcome the catastrophic or deleterious affects from cast correction on pulmonary function. The importance of adequate fusion techniques and satisfactory and secure implants cannot be overstated. Perhaps the most revolutionary development in implants in the past ten years has occurred through the innovative work of Eduardo Luque with his development of posterior segmental instrumentation.[62, 64, 65] This concept has radically altered the treatment of patients with paralytic spinal deformities by providing more secure fixation at multiple levels. Postoperative support is no longer necessary, and the constricting effect of casts and braces with their adverse affects on pulmonary function is now hopefully a thing of the past. For most patients with collapsing scoliotic curvatures in whom the curvature remains flexible and the pelvic obliquity correctable by bending or muscle releases, posterior instrumentation with L-rods and fusion alone is the treatment of choice. For collapsing deformity extending even into the neck, it is possible to use the L-rod fixation, although this is likely to be associated with a high risk of neurologic injury. For smaller children, the ⅛ inch rod may be sufficient. However, for young adults and older patients, ¼ inch rods are more desirable in order to avoid rod bending and implant failure.

Harrington rods are still useful, particularly in the thoracic curve and in the technique of instrumentation without fusion, but they should not be used or certainly be used with extreme caution if a radical resection anteriorly has been done as a first stage. If fusion into the lumbar spine or to the sacrum is indicated, the L-rod system is preferable and is less likely to be associated with pseudarthrosis, implant failure, or loss of lordosis.[90]

ANTERIOR FUSION

The anterior approach to the spine in patients with paralytic deformity secondary to poliomyelitis may be indicated in two situations: (1) a long, C-shaped curve with fixed pelvic obliquity and (2) a rigid and severe thoracic curve (>80 to 100 degrees) in which correction is deemed advisable and is unlikely to be achieved by posterior surgery alone. It should be stressed that young patients presenting with poliomyelitis curvatures that are flexible rarely if ever need anterior surgery, and correction and stabilization can be achieved by posterior approaches alone. However, the patients we are currently seeing are mostly adults whose previous treatments have failed or whose polio was untreated who present with fixed rigid deformity and usually require combined surgery.

Curvatures that are C-shaped with fixed pelvic obliquity are best managed by combined approaches. The correction of the pelvic obliquity is often complete, the stability of correction is excellent, and pseudarthrosis significantly reduced. O'Brien and coworkers[90] presented 39 cases with poliomyelitis scoliosis and pelvic obliquity, demonstrating that superb correction of obliquity is possible with the combined anterior approach with Dwyer instrumentation followed by posterior fusion and instrumentation. Recently, Leong and associates[58] have confirmed these results and noted a marked decrease in the pseudarthrosis rate from 25 to 7 per cent by combined surgery.

With the improvements in implants over the past five years, we are no longer using Dwyer instrumentation, and in cases in which anterior implants are felt desirable or useful, we have preferred the Zielke for its derotational and superior stabilizing qualities. On the other hand, in patients with long C-curves and fixed pelvic obliquity, we have favored a first stage anterior approach with complete discectomies and fusion to the sacrum without instrumentation followed by a second stage posterior approach, L-rod instrumentation to the pelvis with the Galveston technique, and posterior fusion. The use of anterior implants in the first stage may be difficult because the bone is often osteoporotic. If there is a pelvic obliquity in association with the fixed curvature, the sacrum itself is not part of the curvature, and it is anticipated that correction of the lumbar curve alone may lead to reasonable alignment of the sacrum, then it may be preferable to use the anterior Zielke implant followed by posterior L-rod instrumentation to L4 or L5. This allows a mobile lumbosacral articulation and will facilitate the patient's ambulation.

In those cases with fixed, thoracic curvatures greater than 80 to 100 degrees in which correction is felt desirable, a first stage anterior approach with discectomies and/or vertebrectomies followed by second stage posterior instrumentation with the L-rod system would be a useful alternative (Fig. 13–6). Distraction implants may be used in the second stage posterior approach if discectomies alone have been done, but if total vertebrectomies have been done anteriorly, distraction implants during the second stage posterior procedure would be undesirable and likely would be associated with an increased risk of neurologic impairment from distraction of the spinal cord.

POSTOPERATIVE IMMOBILIZATION

A wide variety of postoperative devices is available for this group of patients, including the Milwaukee brace, underarm orthoses (TLSO), a halo cast, or halo braces. With the use of segmental instrumentation casts are usually not necessary, and braces only rarely so. For patients who have undergone extensive resections, postoperative braces of a light plastic material (polypropylene) that are well padded and maximally open in the front to allow chest expansion are desirable.

Results of Treatment

Results of treatment in patients with collapsing curves secondary to poliomyelitis have changed tremendously over the past 15 to 20 years. With combined surgery, correction of lumbar curvatures from 60 to 80 per cent is likely,[90] and correction of pelvic obliquity of 92 per cent,[89] ranging from 33 to 100 per cent,[58] is possible. Anterior release and fusion followed by second stage posterior fusion with L-rod instrumentation has given an average correction of 63 per cent of the lumbar curvature and 67 per cent of the pelvic obliquity.[33] The extent of pelvic obliquity correction is related in part to the adequacy of discectomy, the extent of the posterior release, and the technique of instrumentation. Maximum correction is assured by total discectomy to the sacrum as a first stage, complete release of the contracted fascia and muscles of the contracted iliac crest during the posterior procedure, and secure fixation of L-rods into the pelvis with derotation of the pelvis to a neutral position (Galveston technique).

SPINAL MUSCLE ATROPHY

Spinal muscle atrophy refers to a variety of disease entities characterized by a disorder of the anterior horn cell. These entities have been classified as Werdnig-Hoffmann disease, Kugelberg-Welander disease, amyotonia congenita, and so forth.[32, 107] The term spinal muscle atrophy comprises a spectrum of diseases caused by degeneration or deficiency of the anterior horn cells of the spinal cord in childhood and resulting in symmetrical muscle paralysis of the trunk and proximal musculature.[82] The spectrum of disease processes has been commented on by Dubowitz,[29] who likewise has noted that over 80 per cent of patients survive into adulthood and achieve sitting ability. Children affected with spinal muscle atrophy have normal intelligence yet may show atrophy of the tongue and skeletal muscles and coarse tremors of the extremities. Normal serum enzymes of creatinine phosphokinase and aldolase differentiate this disease process from the primary myopathies. Signs of denervation such as atrophy and decreased motor unit potentials are always present.[82] Muscle atrophy is common histologically but biopsy is not helpful prognostically.[29]

Many well-defined syndromes are included in the diagnosis of spinal muscle atrophy and have been described as a dominant type scapuloperoneal syndrome, distal type hereditary motor neuron disease.[93] Genetic studies have also shown three different autosomal recessive forms of the disease: an infantile form of Werdnig-Hoffmann disease, a classic form with slow progression and early death, type 2 Werdnig-Hoffmann disease, with later onset, and a type 3 spinal muscle atrophy, usually a more chronic type that develops between ages 2 and 17.[2]

Spinal deformity is extremely common in these patients and virtually all have significant muscle involvement.[7] Schwentker and Gibson[107] reported that scoliosis was the most severe problem in those patients who survived. Its onset is variable and usually related to the onset of the disease process and the

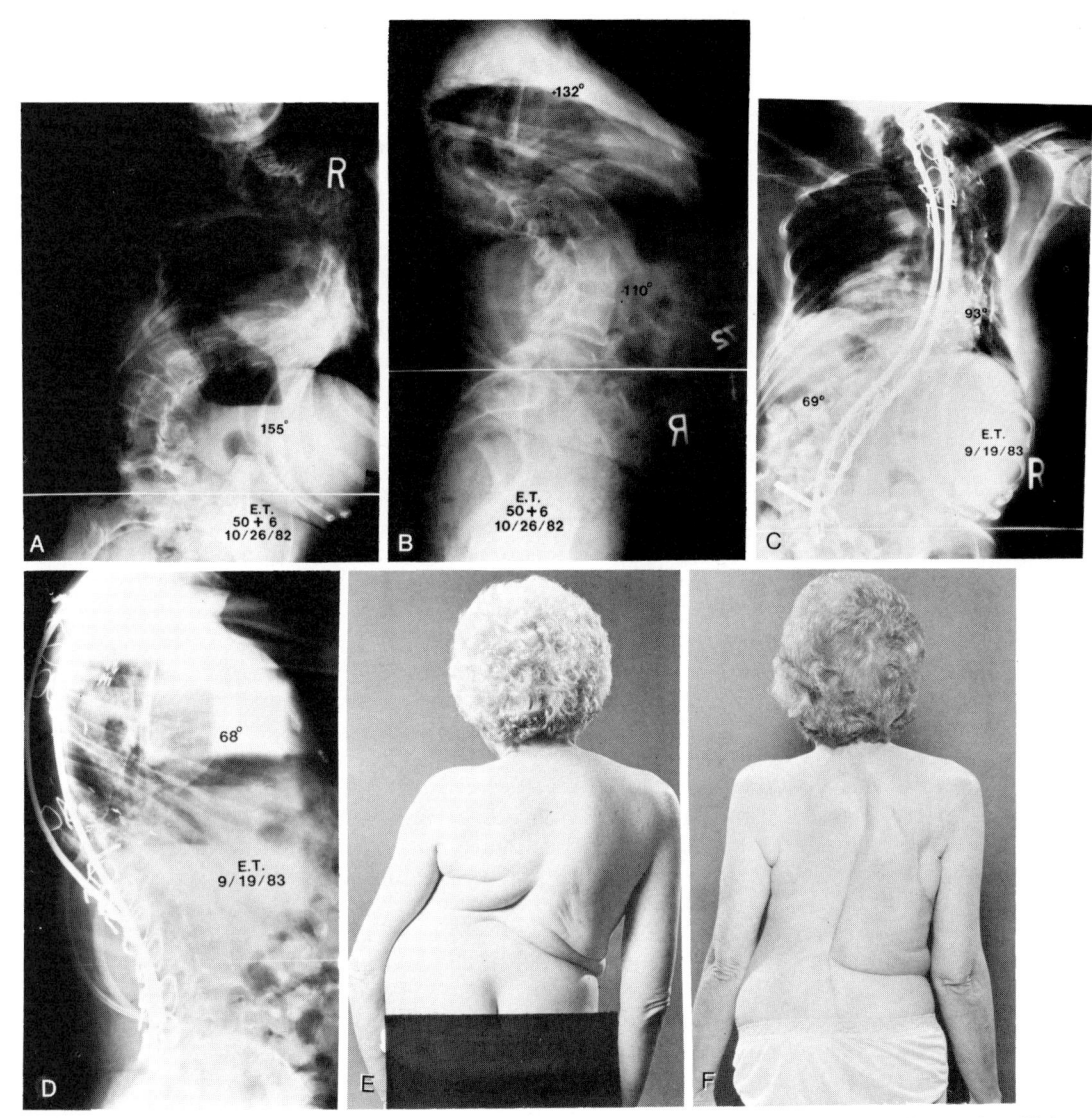

Figure 13-6. The preoperative AP (A) and lateral (B) x-rays of a 50 year old patient with respiratory insufficiency, back pain, and thoracic deformity secondary to poliomyelitis. The curvatures had undergone an autofusion and no correction was possible with either traction or side bending. C and D, A two stage anterior and posterior resection and fusion was carried out using L-rod fixation. The patient tolerated the procedure quite well and obtained a substantial improvement in her deformity and relief of her back pain. One year following surgery her lung volumes, pO_2 and pCO_2 had likewise improved. Her pre- (E) and post-operative (F) clinical appearance is noted.

magnitude of muscle involvement. It is invariably progressive, and surgery is the treatment of choice. These authors also felt that the incidence of scoliosis was higher in non-walkers than those who could walk and that the onset of scoliosis was earlier in non-walkers. However, in a recent report by Aprin,[2] no difference in onset of scoliosis between non-walkers and those who could walk was demonstrated. In fact, the average age at onset of scoliosis in the series reported by Aprin was 7 years, and in this series, likewise, the scoliosis was always progressive.

Schwentker and Gibson[107] felt that braces did slow the progression of the curvature and allowed sitting for more prolonged periods of time. A similar finding was noted by Riddick and coworkers[96] who also stressed the importance of collapsing kyphosis and its management by three-point support orthosis.

Posterior spinal fusion has been reported to give excellent results in selected cases.[23, 109] Aprin felt that posterior fusions could be performed in patients with curvatures of more than 120 degrees and a vital capacity of 25 to 30 per cent of normal. Makley and coworkers[70] felt that there was no significant improvement in pulmonary function in their series; however, four of the 13 patients in Aprin's series[2] did show an average increase in vital capacity of 35 per cent, whereas the remaining nine showed an average reduction of 22 per cent. They also felt that pulmonary function deteriorates with time and spinal fusion does not stop that progress. These authors also noted that occasionally a two stage procedure was necessary. In a series reported by Dorr and coworkers,[28] reviewing 34 patients treated surgically they also noted that occasionally an anterior approach was helpful, particularly for lumbar lordoscoliosis. The most common complications in these patients are pneumonitis and atelectasis.

Treatment Recommendations

Scoliosis or kyphosis in these patients invariably progresses and therefore requires treatment. For curvatures over 20 to 30 degrees, two options are available: no treatment and continued observation or bracing in order to delay the inevitable progression. In patients in whom progression is inevitable and bracing may not be tolerated, one could wait until the patient had developed a more significant curve (over 40 degrees) and then proceed with surgical arthrodesis at that time. This treatment protocol recognizes, as stated, that the curves are invariably progressive, bracing will not stop the progression, and braces are poorly tolerated and may lead to chest restriction and deformity in their own right. On the other hand, a logical avenue of treatment in these patients would also be bracing and attempting to slow the curve progression, allowing more spinal growth and delaying the inevitable surgical procedure.

Both options are certainly viable and depend in part on the patient's age at presentation of the deformity, the magnitude of the initial deformity, and the reception of the patient and the parent to an operative approach. If a patient is seen at an early age, for instance, 7 to 8 years, with a significant curve (>40 degrees) that nevertheless demonstrates some flexibility and the parents are reluctant to consider an operative approach, bracing with careful follow-up at six month intervals, and trying to delay surgery for two to three years is reasonable. If the curvature is too severe to adequately brace (>70 degrees) or if progression continues in spite of bracing, instrumentation without fusion that allows further spinal growth should be considered (see Techniques of Surgery, Chapter 10).[62] On the other hand, if the patient presents at age ten with a curvature that is already 50 degrees, little would be accomplished by delay, and surgery with fusion would be indicated (Fig. 13–7).

Surgery remains the definitive treatment of choice in these patients. Preoperative assessment of pulmonary function as previously stated is essential in this group for invariably decreased pulmonary function is present and postoperative ventilatory assist may be necessary. The vast majority of these patients may be managed by the posterior approach alone, and segmental instrumentation is the treatment of choice. Local bone as a graft may be deficient, and the availability of allograft bone from a bone bank is most desirable. These patients will require fusion to the pelvis, and the L-rod system and intra-iliac fixation as described by Allen and Ferguson[1] appears at this time to be the optimal fixation available. Postoperative immobilization in a brace is generally not necessary but if implant fixation is precarious, a

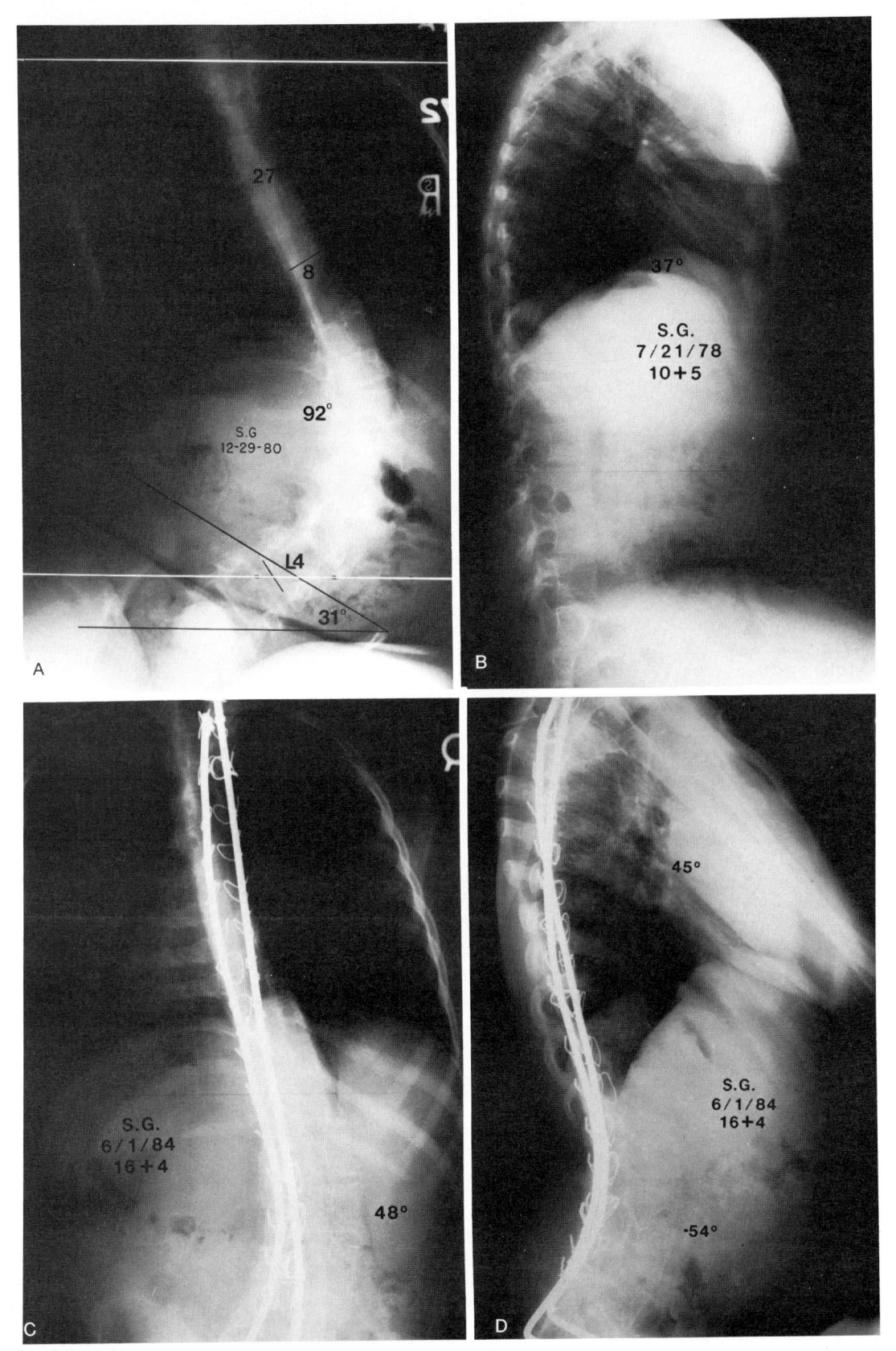

Figure 13–7. The preoperative AP (A) and lateral (B) x-rays of a 10 year old patient with spinal muscle atrophy. C and D, Three and a half years following surgery the patient has maintained this correction and improved sitting balance. Preoperative pelvic obliquity of 31 degrees has been corrected to 8 degrees.

285

polypropylene body jacket may provide a useful adjunct. Anterior surgery combined with posterior surgery may be necessary in patients presenting with severe, fixed lumbar curves with pelvic obliquity (Fig. 13-8).

Complications are frequent in this group of patients and, as previously stated, pulmonary problems are foremost. A tracheostomy has not been necessary in our experience and we have operated on a patient with a vital capacity as low as 16 per cent of normal with a satisfactory outcome. With a vigorous pre- and postoperative program of physical therapy, loss of strength can be avoided.[47] We would not favor using traction in these patients and encourage early ambulation or sitting after surgery to avoid further muscle atrophy and loss of function.

CORD INJURY

Paraplegia in children is a devastating problem.[12, 69, 77, 91] The prognosis and orthopaedic complications have been well summarized by Norton and Foley over 25 years ago.[87] Kilfoyle in 1965,[54] undertook a study to determine the natural history of spine and pelvic deformities in childhood paraplegia. Out of 104 patients, 73 were associated with a congenital paralysis, (i. e., myelomeningocele) and 31 were acquired. Ninety-seven patients developed significant spine and pelvic deformity, lordosis was most common, scoliosis occurred in 36 patients, and kyphosis in 14. Many had mixed deformities. Lordosis was attributed to the combined effects of paralysis and the position of the trunk and the upright posture. All deformities tended to become worse during growth unless arrested surgically. Harrington instrumentation and spinal fusion, including the sacrum, was found to be the most effective means of controlling the spine and pelvic deformity.

Wedge and Gillespie in 1975,[123] reported on 20 children with paraplegia who were treated surgically. In only five of their patients was the paraplegia due to trauma, spinal meningitis or spinal teratoma. The remaining cases were secondary to myelomeningocele. It was their conclusion that patients with early-presenting curvatures that were fully corrected should be fused from the high thorax to the sacrum and that patients with pelvic obliquity should not be fused unless the pelvic obliquity could be overcome completely and a solid fusion to the sacrum achieved.

Lancourt[56] in a more recent publication stated that all juveniles under age 11 sustaining paralysis, partial or complete, above T10 will inevitably develop scoliosis with a true lordosis component. The likelihood of scoliosis developing in these patients is also supported by the work of Jackson,[52] Von Bazan,[121] Leidholt,[57] and Bedbrook.[6] The problems in the management of kyphosis in the paralytic spine have been well summarized by Bunch and coworkers.[17]

Mayfield and coworkers[73] reviewed 40 children who had incurred spinal cord injury between birth and age 18. In all the patients who were injured prior to the adolescent growth spurt, paralytic spinal deformity developed and in 96 per cent it was progressive. Scoliosis developed in 23, kyphosis in 16, and lordosis in five. Management by bracing was difficult, and 17 of the patients required fusion, usually to the sacrum. Complications were frequent. Progressive paralytic deformity was uncommon in the post-adolescent patient.

Non-Operative Treatment

Children rendered paraplegic prior to the adolescent growth spurt will usually, if not invariably, develop a spinal deformity. In those patients developing paralysis prior to puberty, a brace is recommended in order to prevent deformity from occurring.[95] The brace should be well cushioned and snug fitting, and it should be well open in the front to allow maximum chest expansion. It may be removed when the patient is prone or supine and may be off at night when the patient is sleeping. It is possible that such treatment may prevent deformity from developing. In those patients who do develop a progressive deformity, surgery is the treatment of choice.

Surgical Treatment

The development of a spinal curvature in any patient with paraplegia prior to the adolescent growth spurt should alert the physician that surgery will almost invariably be necessary. The presence of a structural curve, the loss of sitting balance because of the

Figure 13–8. The x-rays of a 27 year old patient with spinal muscle atrophy. Progression of her deformity with back pain necessitated surgery. *A* and *B*, The preoperative x-rays show significant scoliosis with severe kyphosis. *C*, The traction film shows minimal correctability with distraction. A combined anterior and posterior approach, therefore, was felt indicated. *D* and *E*, Her result is noted. Pelvic obliquity measuring 42 degrees preoperatively was corrected to 19 degrees postoperatively. Improvement of obliquity would have been enhanced if the anterior arthrodesis had been extended to the L5-S1 articulation.

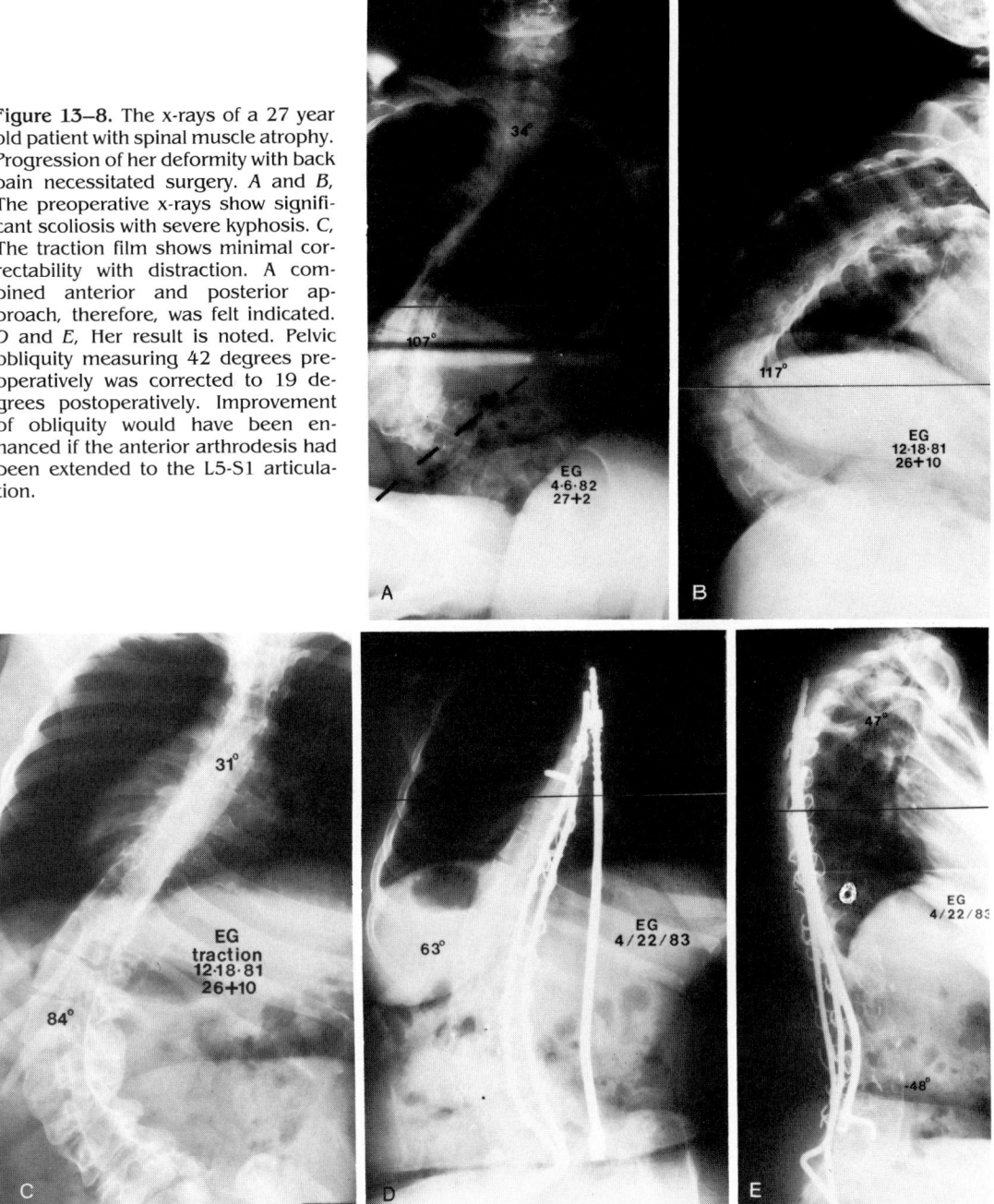

curvature, the development of pelvic obliquity, or the progression of deformity while under brace treatment would all be indications for spinal fusion. For those patients with collapsing type curvatures, we would favor posterior segmental instrumentation with L-rods to the pelvis. The fusion usually must extend from the upper thoracic area to the sacrum. Combined anterior/posterior approaches may be necessary in the presence of a fixed pelvic obliquity. Postoperative immobilization is generally not necessary (Fig. 13–9).

FAMILIAL DYSAUTONOMIA

Familial dysautonomia is an uncommon genetic disease found almost exclusively in Jews of Ashkenazi descent. There are over

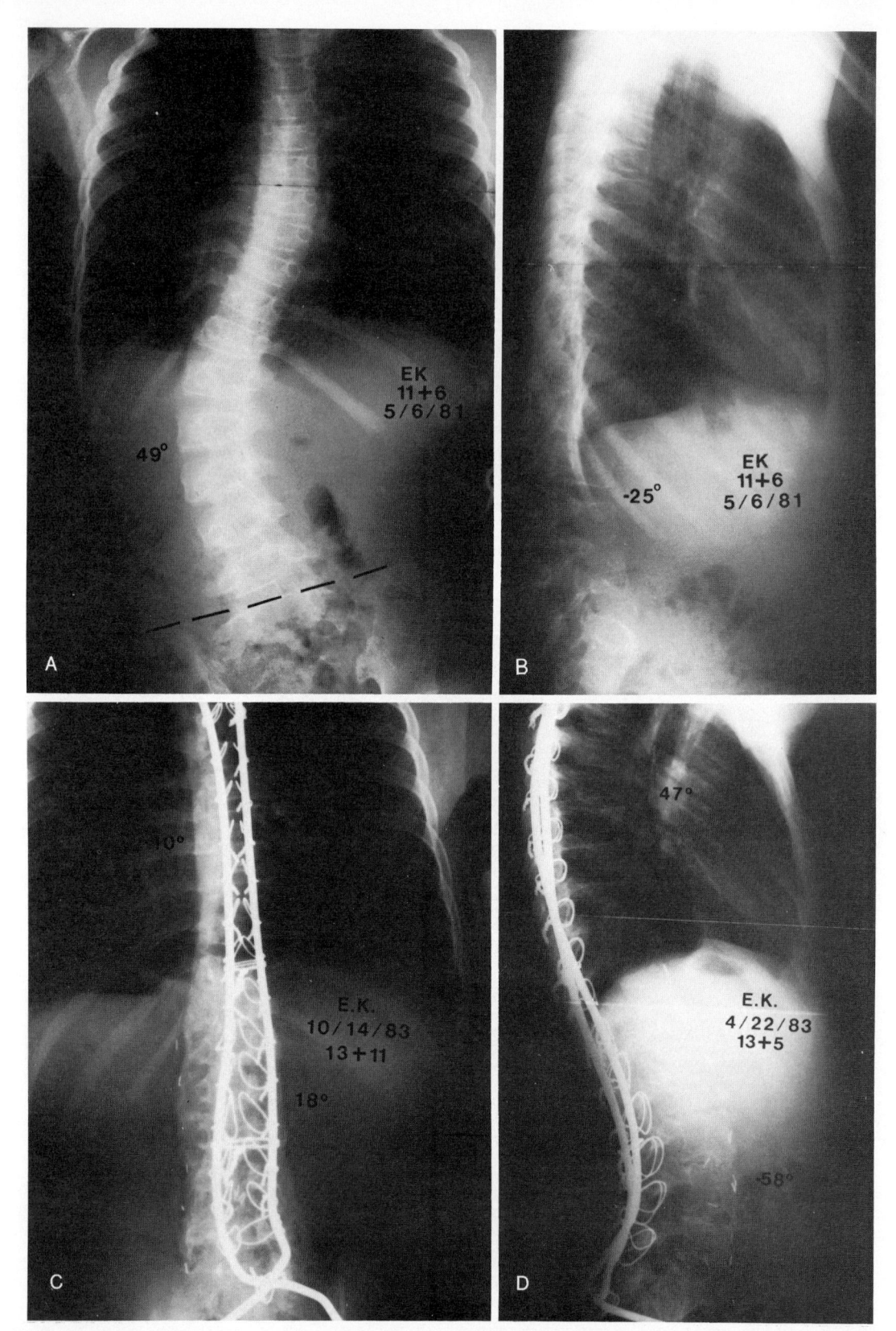

Figure 13–9. The x-rays of an 11 year old patient who presented with paraplegia secondary to a cord injury at birth. Progressive deformity necessitated surgical stabilization. With the use of L-rods contoured to produce lordosis, excellent correction of both the scoliosis and sagittal plane deformity were produced. Although a combined approach was carried out, it is highly possible that an equally satisfactory result could have been obtained with a single stage posterior L-rod instrumentation and fusion.

300 known cases in the United States and about 50 in Israel. The disease was first described by Riley and Day and their colleagues in 1949.[98] It has now been shown that over 90 per cent of patients suffering from this disease will show a spinal curvature, most commonly scoliosis, at some time in their life. The scoliosis is truly a kyphoscoliosis and thoracic lordosis is generally not a component. It usually begins during the first decade of life. McKusick[74] has noted that by 8 years of age most of the patients have already developed a curvature. Goldstein[41] first reported on the treatment of scoliosis in this disease in 1968. It has been established that these curvatures are always progressive, are usually thoracic, and kyphosis is a major component of the problem.[8, 128]

These patients present major treatment problems.[60] First of all, life expectancy is not good, few patients survive longer than the early twenties,[74] and the numerous symptoms of the disease make treatment extremely difficult. The disease is a neurologic one and the basic defect is a reduction in the number of neurons in the posterior root ganglion, in the sympathetic ganglion, and in the lateral columns of the spinal cord.[3] These patients have vasomotor instability, excessive sweating, erratic temperature control, hypothermia, hypoesthesia, relative indifference to pain, episodic hypertension and postural hypotension, vomiting, absent gag reflex, frequent aspiration, pneumonia, ataxia, emotional lability, psychomotor retardation, delayed sexual maturation, and spinal deformity, to mention but a few of the symptoms.[100] Respiratory control is also abnormal.[26]

Robin has recently reported experience on management of six patients with this disorder and outlined in some detail the intraoperative problems that are possible and how they might be avoided.[100]

Spinal fusion has been performed in a few of these patients at our institution. The risks and complications are high and should be well appreciated prior to undertaking any surgical correction.[115]

DUCHENNE MUSCULAR DYSTROPHY

Spinal deformities in patients with Duchenne muscular dystrophy pose a difficult dilemma. Markedly shortened life expectancy, progressive deterioration of pulmonary function, and the rapidly progressive nature of the curvature once the patient loses the ability to walk, complicate treatment decisions and present difficult options. Every patient eventually subsides into a wheelchair status, in which he spends approximately the last half of his life. Eighty per cent of the children will develop a collapsing type scoliosis,[40] and once the scoliosis becomes established it will progress relentlessly in almost all cases. The discomfort, aching, progressive loss of sitting balance, and fatigue may prove so disabling that patients may choose to stay home in bed rather than sit in their chair. In short, the management of the spinal deformity is the most difficult and major problem in the post-ambulatory patient with Duchenne muscular dystrophy.

The majority of Duchenne muscular dystrophy cases are inherited as a sex-linked recessive form. This implies that 50 per cent of all males will receive the defective gene and become involved. The mutation rate is high and perhaps as many as one third of all cases occur in this fashion.[16] In approximately 10 per cent of the cases the disorder is inherited as an autosomal recessive, explaining the occasional occurrence of this disease in a girl. The progressive form of muscular dystrophy, Duchenne's, is by far the most common of all types of dystrophies. The incidence rate is 275 males per million male births. The onset is usually before the fifth year of life, and frequently during the second. The earliest symptoms include clumsiness and a tendency to fall frequently. As the disease progresses, difficulty in walking becomes apparent, and the development of a lumbar lordosis inevitable. Because of weak hip extensor musculature, the child must hyperextend the spine in order to maintain his weight in line with his hips. Progressive weakness of the quadriceps muscles forces the child to maintain the weightline in front of the knees. This is made increasingly difficult by hip flexion contractures. As the disease progresses, because of progressive weakness of the hip abductor musculature, the patient has difficulty clearing the floor during the swing phase of the gait. During the second decade the child usually becomes confined to a wheelchair, developing progressive contractures of the leg musculature and the almost inevitable occurrence of spinal deformity. Near the end of the second decade most patients die from either respiratory infections or cardiac involvement. A very small percentage of patients will live until the fourth or fifth decade.

Bunch[16] has described two patterns of scoliosis. One develops just before the patient stops walking, progresses very slowly, and then once the patient is confined to a wheelchair, rapid progression follows. The other type of curve pattern, which is much less common, develops after the patient has been confined to a wheelchair for some time; this is only slowly progressive and may not require treatment. Siegel[111, 112] has stated that scoliosis in ambulatory Duchenne muscular dystrophy patients rarely occurs; if it does occur, it is usually with pelvic or intrapelvic obliquity secondary to uncorrected lower extremity contractures. He has stated that the lordosis tendency of these patients secondary to muscle weakness literally locks in the lumbar and lumbosacral facets, giving some stability in the coronal plane However, once the patient becomes wheelchair-bound, the patient tends to lean to the dominant side, bringing the dominant extremity to more functional use. Spinal extension is often lost, and progressive deformity occurs. Dubowitz[30] has also noted the tendency for scoliosis to develop in patients primarily after they become wheelchair-bound.

The rapid progressive nature of these curvatures has been outlined by Robin,[101, 102] who noted that in patients with progressive curves, 15 to 30 degrees of progression per year was usual. Curvatures were typically long, thoracolumbar in type, with pelvic obliquity an associated component. Wilkins and Gibson[124] in a report in 1976 outlined five different curve patterns—Group 1 has early straight spine, Group 2 has kyphosis, Group 3 has kyphosis combined with a lateral curve, Group 4 has severe lateral curve without kyphosis, and Group 5 has an extended spine. They felt that the Group 4 patients ended up with the most severe deformities, whereas the Group 5 patients developed little deformity. They suggested that attempts should be made to develop an extended spine position, in this way perhaps avoiding a progressive tendency. They felt that a lumbar curve of 35 degrees or more with rotation of 15 degrees at the apex prognosticated the progressive deformity in nearly all cases. Hsu[48] noted in a brief series that all patients with curvatures greater than 40 degrees progressed.

Orthotic devices in this group of patients may have a limited benefit. There is no proof that these devices prevent progression of the degree of scoliosis.[101] Seeger and coworkers,[108] in a more recent report (1984), have also found that spinal support systems in Duchenne muscular dystrophy failed to keep the spine straight and progression of the deformity continued unabated. On the other hand, Siegel[111, 112] feels that orthotic devices that maintain the spine in an extended position may slow the development of scoliosis.

Prevention of progression is only provided by surgery, and the indication for surgery remains a difficult treatment decision. It is apparent that over the past five years an increasing trend has developed toward surgical stabilization of these curvatures once the patients become wheelchair bound. The monitoring of pulmonary function and specifically vital capacity may prove most beneficial in deciding if and when surgery should be carried out. There is general agreement that once the vital capacity falls below 30 to 35 per cent, surgery may be associated with pulmonary failure.[40, 101]

More recently, Rideau and coworkers[97] have suggested three profiles of clinical severity, identified on the basis of the restrictive pulmonary disease, in Duchenne muscular dystrophy patients. They found that every Duchenne muscular dystrophy patient has an absolute vital capacity, which stabilizes at a maximum plateau phase before progressively decreasing. The determination of this plateau vital capacity occurs generally between ages 10 to 12 in their experience and permits prognosis of the restrictive pulmonary syndrome. In Type 1 patients, the plateau existed at a maximum absolute value lower than 1200 cc. vital capacity. This occurred in 30 per cent of the patients. This group was most homogeneous and had the poorest prognosis, with the patients being confined to a wheelchair before age ten and dying at an average age of 17. Type 2 cases, consisting of 40 per cent of their Duchenne muscular dystrophy patients, have plateaued vital capacities between 1200 and 1700 cc. and lost the ability to walk at about 10 years of age. Their Type 3 cases have average plateau vital capacities greater than 1700 cc., and their life expectancy was greater than Types 1 and 2. It was their contention that once the vital capacity had decreased to less than 40 per cent of the predicted normal and the scoliotic curve passed to greater than 23 degrees, surgery should be carried out, otherwise rapid deterioration of vital capacity would contraindicate the procedure.

Sakai and associates[105] felt that prophylactic tracheostomy should be done for patients with vital capacities below 40 per cent of normal or for a poor functional cough as this prevented pulmonary complications after surgery. However, if vital capacity decreased below 25 per cent they felt surgery was contraindicated. Once these patients were tracheostomized they were permanently dependent on the respirator. Inkley[50] has also presented data to suggest that the reduction in lung volume increases as the disease advances, and the changes in lung volume and flow rates parallel the loss of muscle strength. The loss of pulmonary function, therefore, does appear to be a good way to monitor deterioration and progression of the disease process. Milne and Rosales[79] also use pulmonary function tests in assessing the risk and survival of patients following surgery; the range of 30 per cent vital capacity would appear to be adequate in patients with muscular dystrophy requiring fusion, in their experience. If surgery is felt indicated and pulmonary function appears adequate, the technique of choice appears to be a long posterior spinal fusion using segmental instrumentation to the pelvis. Any associated kyphosis should also be appreciated and corrected as well.

Whether surgery should or should not be undertaken in these patients is dependent upon the progressive nature of the deformity, symptoms of the patient, presence of wheelchair confinement, and the general pulmonary capacity of the patient.[118] It is our feeling that provided the patient's pulmonary function is satisfactory, he is wheelchair bound and is symptomatic or losing sitting balance because of the progressive nature of the curvature, surgical stabilization is a valid and useful procedure; L-rod instrumentation we feel is the preferred technique at this time (Fig. 13–10).

LIMB-GIRDLE DYSTROPHY, FACIOSCAPULOHUMERAL DYSTROPHY, AND DYSTROPHIA MYOTONICA

Patients with facioscapulohumeral dystrophy are often complicated by scoliosis, and on the other hand, patients with dystrophia myotonica and limb-girdle dystrophy seldom develop structural scoliosis.[111] Our experience with these conditions is limited. In a recent review consisting of 11 patients having surgical treatment at the Twin Cities Scoliosis Center, the spinal curvatures were found to be slowly progressive and non-operative treatment was usually not effective. Posterior spinal fusion produced a satisfactory result. None of our patients had pelvic obliquity yet thoracic lordosis was a frequent accompaniment, leading to decreased vital capacity and shortness of breath.

ARTHROGRYPOSIS SCOLIOSIS

See Chapter 22 for a discussion of arthrogryposis scoliosis.

CEREBRAL PALSY

Patients presenting with a delay in motor development and neurologic signs consisting of abnormal muscle tone, spasticity, and hyperreflexia are classified as having cerebral palsy. This may or may not be accompanied by mental retardation. The development of scoliosis associated with cerebral palsy may add a major functional disability to otherwise handicapped individuals. A walker may now become a sitter. A patient who would have been a sitter may become bedridden by virtue of decompensation with the associated pelvic obliquity. Presence of a curvature in a minimally involved patient with cerebral palsy may produce severe psychological problems.[18] The prevalence of scoliosis in cerebral palsy patients has been shown to vary between 5 and 64 per cent.[5, 67, 68, 103, 104, 106] Scoliosis was most common in spastics, but the highest incidence was in spastic quadriplegics (Fig. 13–11). The incidence paralleled the severity of the neurologic deficit and also appeared to be aggravated by the effects of gravity when individuals were artificially placed in sitting positions. The presence of spasticity and the severity of neurologic deficit were the most important factors in predicting the presence of scoliotic deformity.

Postural deformity, especially kyphosis, is very common in this group of patients and, in our experience, is most likely to develop in those patients with mental retardation and delayed development of trunk extensor musculature.

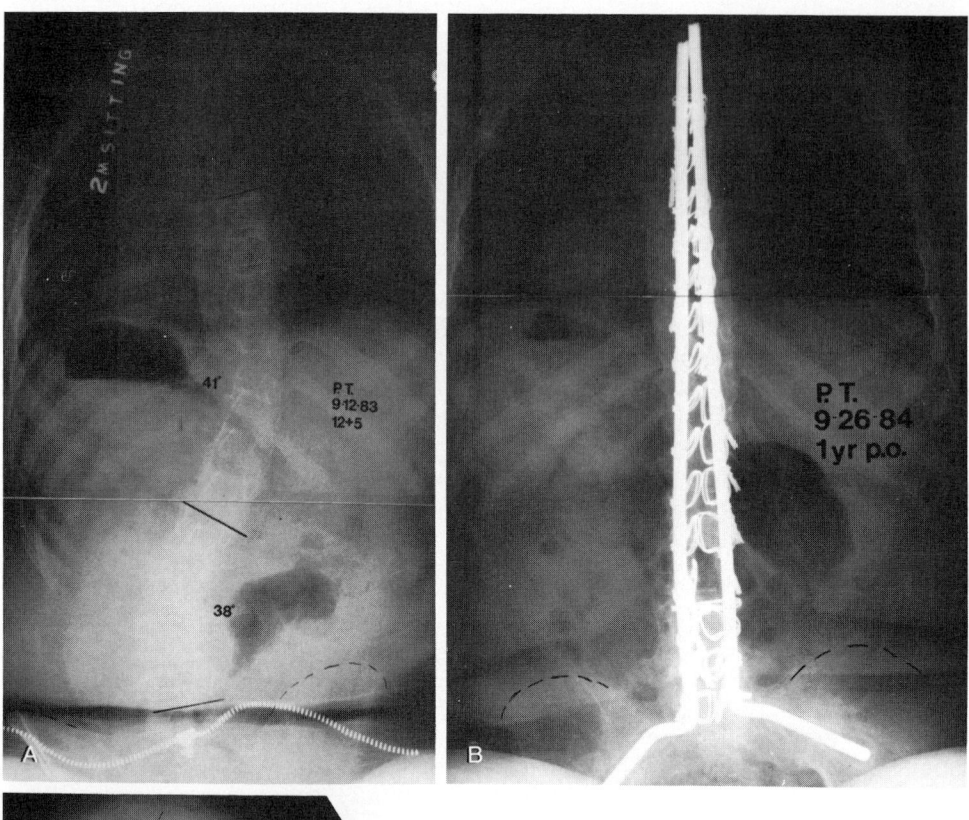

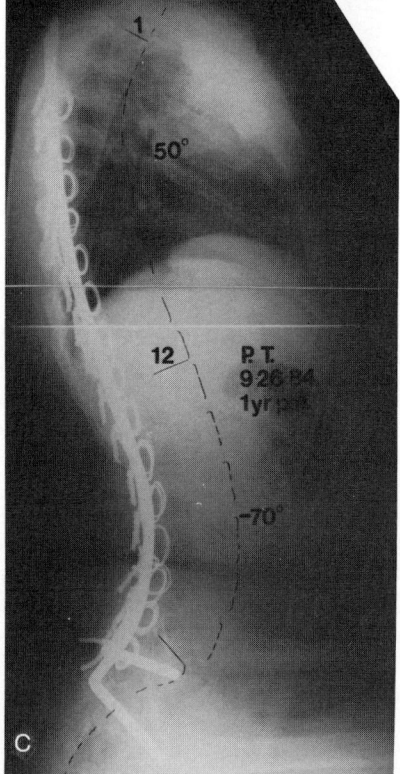

Figure 13–10. A, Preoperative x-ray of a Duchenne muscular dystrophy patient, aged 12+5, presenting with progressive spinal deformity and pelvic obliquity. A single stage posterior approach with segmental instrumentation was carried, carefully contouring the rods to maintain lordosis. An excellent correction, seen in both the AP (B) and sagittal (C) views, was obtained.

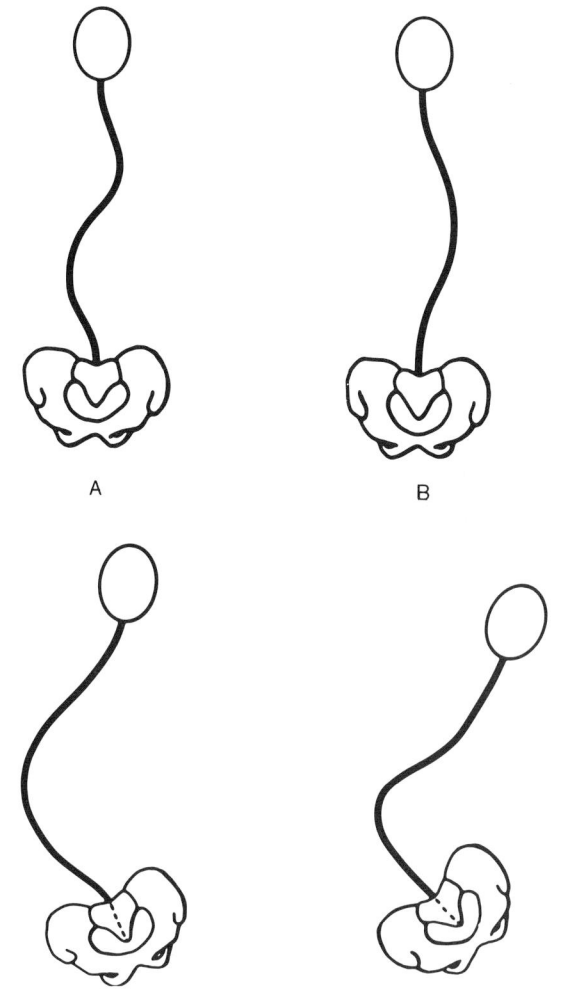

Figure 13–11. Examples of curve patterns seen in cerebral palsy. Group I (A and B) curves consist of double curves with thoracic and lumbar components and little, if any, pelvic obliquity. Group II curves present with lumbar or thoracolumbar curvatures associated with pelvic obliquity. In those patients in whom the pelvic obliquity is part of the curvature, the obliquity is greater and the incidence of spastic quadriplegia and dislocation of the hips is higher. (Reprinted with permission from Lonstein, J. E., and Akbarnia, B. A.: Operative treatment of spinal deformities in patients with cerebral palsy or mental retardation. An analysis of 107 cases. J. Bone Joint Surg., 65A:43–55, 1983.)

Spinal deformities in this group of patients may often be progressive and frequently disabling. The indications for treatment may be controversial and problematic. The vagaries of determining improved self-image in a patient with mental retardation, improved functional capacity in a spastic athetoid who is unable to feed himself, or improved nursing care and decreased medical cost when controlled studies have not been carried out make the indications for surgery less than precise. On the other hand, when patients present with a painful progressive pelvic obliquity, inability to sit without pain and fatigue, inability to use their upper extremities for useful activities because they are needed to maintain trunk balance, and progressive loss of pulmonary function associated with progressive curvature, surgical correction of the deformity is a valid option. At our institution surgery is more frequently being undertaken in this group of patients, and it is our perception that the functional improvement obtained has justified this more aggressive surgical approach.[61, 113]

Non-Operative Treatment

Long-term results from brace treatment of patients with cerebral palsy are not available.[67] Bunnell and MacEwen[18] in a study of 48 patients with cerebral palsy treated for short periods of time from nine to 60 months, felt that conservative treatment of scoliosis was certainly feasible. They used a removable plastic jacket, and in 35 of their patients the curvature was held within 5 degrees of the initial curvature. In three patients the curve had progressed more than 5 degrees, and in three patients improvement had occurred greater than 5 degrees. It is to be stressed, however, that this was a short term study and follow-up data was not given. It is our contention that it would be unlikely that any of these curvatures that were progressive would be held through the adolescent growth period by this type of orthotic device. In more flexible collapsing type curvatures, the brace may again prove helpful as a temporary assist allowing more spinal growth prior to eventual arthrodesis (Fig. 13–12). Bleck[9] has reported no decrease in spinal curvature in three of his patients treated with a brace. On the other hand, sitting orthoses (SSO) have proven of benefit in maintaining sitting balance, head control, and pressure distribution.[19]

Surgical Treatment

One of the earliest discussions on treatment for spinal deformity in cerebral palsy was presented by Haas in 1942.[44] He described correction of a 45 degree lumbar curve in a 13 year old girl by extensive muscle

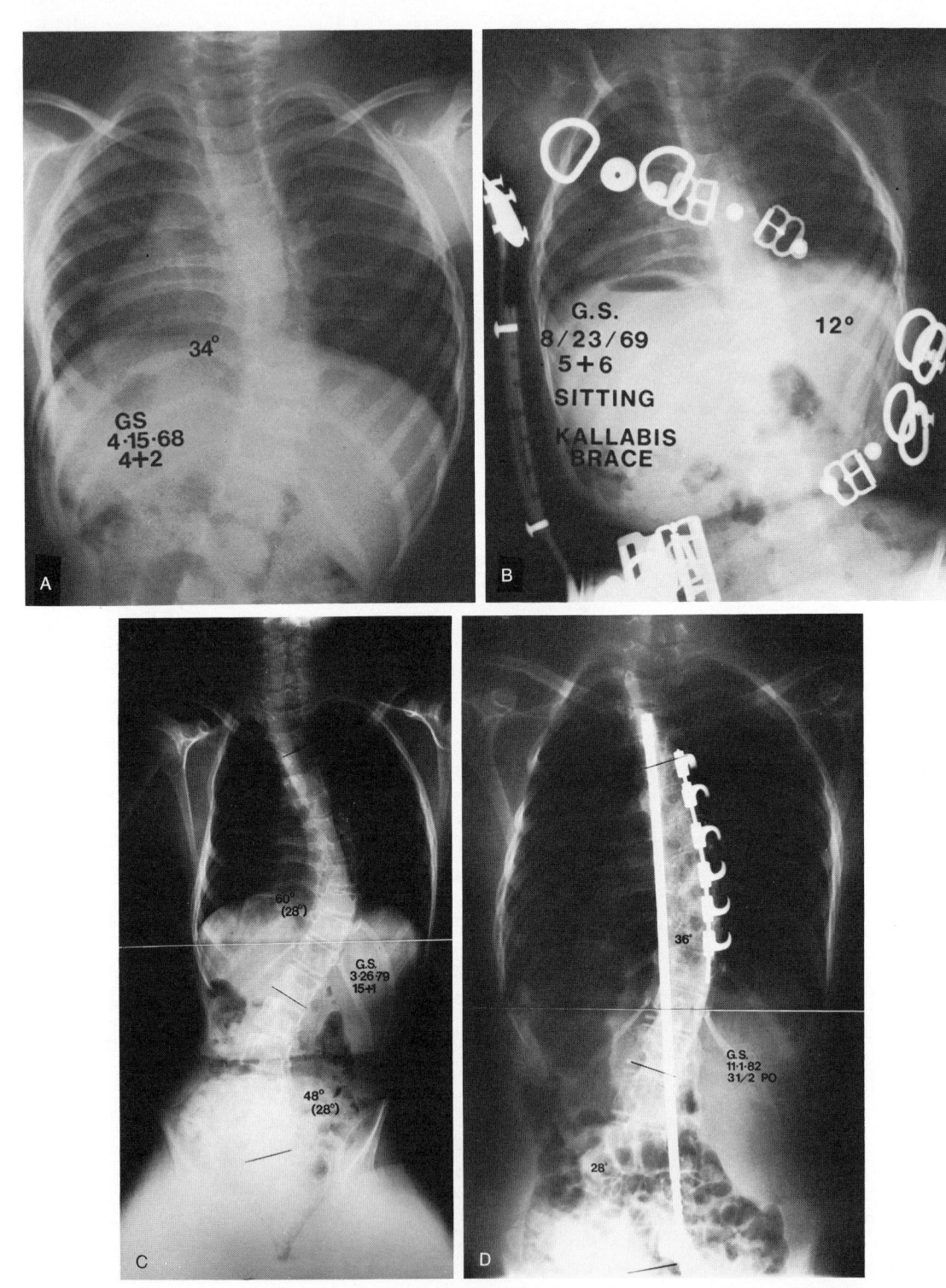

Figure 13–12. *A*, X-ray of a 4 year old female with spastic quadriparesis secondary to cerebral palsy. *B*, A three-point brace (Kallabis) was used as an assist to maintain the spine in a corrected position. *C* and *D*, At age 15, having been in a brace for 11 years, she underwent a spinal fusion and Harrington instrumentation, with a satisfactory outcome.

releases and transfers. MacEwen, in 1972,[66] reported on the operative treatment of 16 patients with cerebral palsy by posterior fusion and Harrington instrumentation. The average correction was 50 per cent with an average loss of 14 per cent. Two patients had poor results, with one showing total loss of correction. The pseudarthrosis rate was 20 per cent. Bonnett, Brown, and Growe,[10] in 1976, reviewed 294 patients with cerebral palsy seen from 1960 to 1972. Thirty-three were treated by spinal fusion, five by a combined two stage anterior and posterior fusion. They concluded that only the combined procedure appeared to give adequate correction and a low incidence of pseudarthrosis. Of particular interest were their results in terms of patient function. Over half of the patients (17 of 33) with preoperative back pain were relieved of it, and sitting tolerance and balance were noticeably improved in 17 of the 33 patients. The requirements for attendant nursing care were unaltered in 27 of 33 patients. Equipment needs remain unchanged in 23 patients, and eating patterns were unchanged in 30 and improved in only 2 patients. It should be remembered that their series was associated with a high degree of complications and only five of their patients underwent the combined procedures, which clearly produce the best results. Brown, Swank, and Specht[14] recently reviewed 17 cerebral palsy patients managed by combined anterior and posterior fusions. Curve correction averaged 16 per cent and the pseudarthrosis rate was 18 per cent—lower than that for the previously reported patients with anterior or posterior fusions alone from the Rancho Los Amigos group. Instrumentation complications occurred in 50 per cent of the patients with athetosis, while only 12 per cent of patients with spasticity had similar problems. The most extensive experience reported to date was that by Lonstein and Akbarnia[61] who reviewed the experience at our Center consisting of 77 patients with cerebral palsy and 32 with mental retardation. The indications for surgery were curve progression in 63 per cent, loss of function in 35 per cent, and the magnitude of the curve in 77 per cent. Functionally, one patient was worse after surgery, 82 showed no change, and 24 showed improvement. The scoliosis correction averaged 63 per cent and pseudarthrosis occurred in 17 per cent of patients. The authors found it useful to divide the curvatures into those with and without pelvic obliquity and stressed that Type II curves (curve with pelvic obliquity) did much better with combined procedures.

Recommended Approach

Patients presenting with spinal deformities secondary to cerebral palsy should be treated provided the indications as previously described are present. If there is a gray zone we would favor erring on the side of treating the deformity rather than not treating it at all. Bracing in our experience has not proven useful in athetoid or severely spastic patients but may prove somewhat helpful as a temporary holding device in curvatures less than 40 degrees in patients presenting prior to the adolescent growth spurt. Progression of the deformity or inability to tolerate a brace would necessitate operative intervention.

Preoperative halo traction has not proven useful and is not recommended. In athetoid or combative patients, halofemoral traction may prove helpful in allowing better control of the patient, preventing him from getting out of bed and so forth. Patients presenting with primarily Type I curvatures, that is, right thoracic or right thoracic/left lumbar curvatures without pelvic obliquity may be managed by posterior instrumentation and fusion alone (Fig. 13–13).[61] If the lumbar curve is much over 70 degrees and the patient is skeletally mature, a combined approach is desirable. L-rod instrumentation at the second stage has furnished superior fixation and may allow the patients to go without a postoperative orthosis. In Type II curvatures associated with pelvic obliquity, a combined anterior and posterior approach is usually the treatment of choice (Fig. 13–14).[61] If a balanced spine and level pelvis can be obtained on a traction film, a posterior approach alone should be sufficient. For the combined approach we have generally found anterior release and interbody fusion without instrumentation followed by second stage posterior instrumentation and fusion to the pelvis with L-rods to be preferable. On the other hand, anterior instrumentation at the first stage may be useful in patients with severe spasticity and athetosis. Hip and abduction/flexion contractures in the presence of severe lordosis may rarely require release as a first stage, or between the anterior and posterior procedure. In lumbar lordoscoliosis

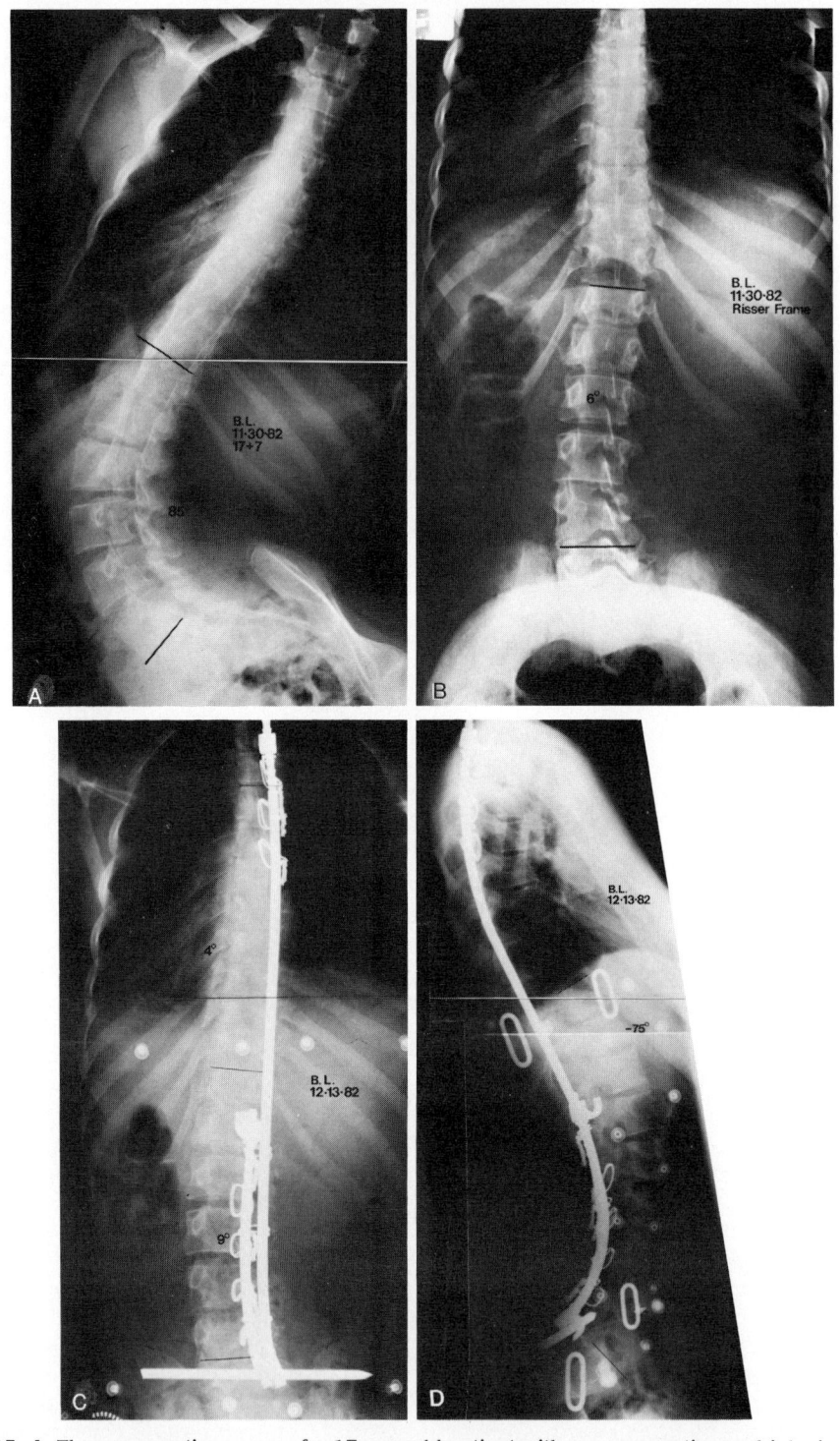

Figure 13–13. A, The preoperative x-rays of a 17 year old patient with severe spastic quadriplegia (A). She had been seen at age 12 with a 5 degree curve, progressing to an 85 degree curve at age 17. After being placed on a Risser table (B) her pelvic obliquity was completely correctable. Surgery therefore consisted of a posterior spinal fusion only with a complete release of the right paraspinal and sacrospinalis musculature from the right iliac crest. Posterior instrumentation with contoured Harrington rods and sublaminar wires produced a satisfactory result in the AP (C) and lateral plane (D). Note contoured Harrington rods and their importance in maintaining sagittal plane curvatures.

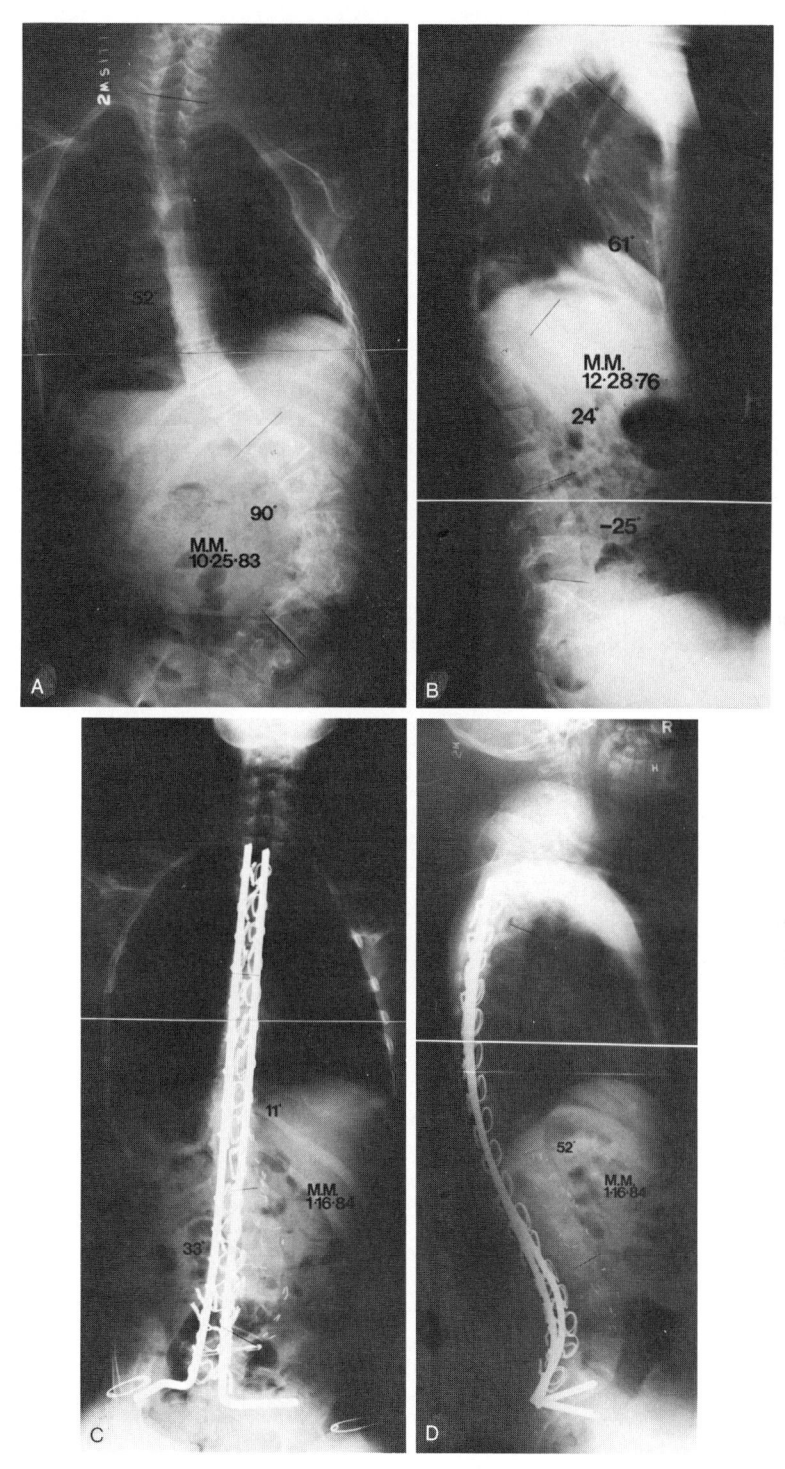

Figure 13–14. In the presence of a fixed pelvic obliquity and a right structural major lumbar curvature (greater than 60 to 70 degrees), a combined approach is useful. The preoperative AP (A) and lateral (B) x-rays of a patient with spastic quadriplegia are demonstrated. Following combined anterior and posterior surgery with L-rod instrumentation and fusion to the pelvis (C and D), excellent correction of obliquity with production of lumbar lordosis and normal thoracic kyphosis has been achieved.

with flexion contractures, further loss of lordosis will increase the degree of flexion contracture and make positioning on the operative table more difficult. Complete release of the musculature inserting onto the elevated iliac crest in the presence of pelvic obliquity is desirable in order to facilitate maximum correction of the obliquity.

SPINOCEREBELLAR DEGENERATIVE DISEASES

Spinocerebellar degenerative diseases most likely to be associated with spinal deformity are Friedreich's ataxia and Charcot-Marie-Tooth disease.

Friedreich's Ataxia

Geoffrey's[39] criteria for a clinical diagnosis of typical Friedreich's ataxia consists of the following: onset before age 20, ataxia of gait, progression of ataxia, dysarthria, decrease in position and/or vibratory sense, muscle weakness, and deep tendon areflexia. The secondary symptoms and signs consist of a positive Babinski reflex, pes cavus, scoliosis, and cardiomyopathy. The etiology of the disease is unknown. It is definitely hereditary and is usually transmitted as an autosomal recessive gene. The main symptoms begin with clumsiness of the hands, dysarthria, and nystagmus. Affected children frequently become wheelchair bound during the second and third decades of life.[110] Scoliosis has ranged from an incidence of 75 to 100 per cent in reported series. Labelle and coworkers,[55] in a review of 56 patients with typical Friedreich's ataxia, noted that 55 (98 per cent) presented with scoliosis greater than 10 degrees. An associated kyphosis greater than 40 degrees was present in 66 per cent. The most common curve pattern was a combined thoracic and lumbar curve, occurring in 57 per cent of their population. They noted that the majority of patients with progressive curvatures had the onset of scoliosis before 15 years of age, whereas the majority of patients with non-progressive curves had the onset of scoliosis after 15 years of age. Treatment of progressive curvatures with bracing has generally been a failure in the series reported to date. From the experience of Labelle and coworkers,[55] all 12 of their patients treated conservatively with braces showed continued progression of the curvature, progression occurred as well in the three treated by electrical stimulation. These authors conclude that bracing is not indicated for progressive curvatures, and surgery is the treatment of choice. Furthermore, the authors postulated that the etiology of scoliosis was due to the ataxia and not from muscle weakness. Results from large numbers of patients treated for spinal deformity have not been reported. Hensinger[47] described three cases, with death in one from cardiomyopathy three years postoperatively.

At our institution,[24] 12 patients have undergone surgery at an average age of 18 years, range 14 to 29 years. All have undergone a single stage posterior fusion and instrumentation. Three patients had increased loss of function following surgery, one after being supine for five months and two owing to the weight of the external support. One patient had cardiac failure after surgery that was successfully treated. The last patient had a posterior fusion that was too short, and a kyphosis developed above the fused area. He became wheelchair bound four years after surgery and died a year later from a cardiomyopathy.

It is our current recommendation that patients with progressive spinal deformity from Friedreich's ataxia whose cardiac status is stable or satisfactory are best managed by spinal fusion. We have favored segmental instrumentation with early ambulation without external support. Braces are poorly tolerated and do not control progressive curvatures.

Charcot-Marie-Tooth Disease

Charcot-Marie-Tooth disease is a demyelinating neuropathy, which is inherited as an autosomal dominant train with variable expressivity. Hensinger and associates[47] reported 69 patients with Charcot-Marie-Tooth disease in whom seven had kyphoscoliosis (10 per cent). Two of their patients had mild to moderate degrees of curvature that did not require treatment, four were treated in a Milwaukee brace, which was successful in two. Three patients underwent a posterior spinal fusion with instrumentation. They were immobilized in a corrective cast, kept recumbent for six months, and then ambulated in a cast for an additional four months. There were no postoperative complications.

We have treated three patients with Charcot-Marie-Tooth disease non-operatively; one patient is still under care, one showed increase in the curvature in the brace, and the third patient had the curve controlled by the Milwaukee brace.[25] Surgery has been carried out in five patients; one patient developed a superior mesenteric artery syndrome and there were two pseudarthroses. It is our feeling in support of Hensinger and MacEwen's series[47] that these patients with spinal deformity may be managed with the same techniques used for idiopathic scoliosis, including bracing and surgery. If surgery is felt indicated, we would prefer segmental instrumentation without postoperative support.

SYRINGOMYELIA

Syringomyelia is a term used to define a tubular cavity containing fluid within the spinal cord.[34, 127] Williams[125] suggested that syringomyelia patients were best divided into two groups, those in whom the cord cavity was flaccid and contained cerebrospinal fluid and communication existed between the cavity and posterior fossa, and those in whom a non-communicating syringomyelia secondary to tumor or traumatic paraplegia existed. In this second group the cyst was tense, containing fluid under pressure without any functional communication between the syrinx and the fourth ventricle. Presenting features of patients with syringomyelia consist of pain, headache, neck ache, and at times, pain within any part of the body. In this latter situation the presentation may be most confusing, and patients may go for years without a proper diagnosis being made. Patients may also present with joint pain, which may mask as a type of osteoarthritis or rheumatoid disease.[75] Williams[125] has well outlined the clinical features of patients presenting with syringomyelia. Suffice it to say that the presentation is at times confusing, obscure, and a diagnosis initially may be most difficult.

Scoliosis may be the first manifestation of a syringomyelia.[4, 34, 36, 122] McRae and Standen,[76] in 1966, reported 43 patients with syringomyelia of whom 27 had scoliosis. Of all the patients with symptoms presenting with syringomyelia before the age of 16 years, 87 per cent had scoliosis. Williams[125] reviewed the experience at Midland Centre for Neurosurgery and Neurology and found 52 out of 73 men with syringomyelia had a scoliosis of 6 degrees or more, and 56 out of 75 women likewise had a scoliosis of 6 degrees or greater. Huebert and MacKinnon[49] reviewed 43 patients with syringomyelia and noted that 27 (63 per cent) had evidence of scoliosis; 15 had mild curves of 0 to 25 degrees, five had moderate curves of 25 to 50 degrees, and seven had severe curves greater than 50 degrees.

Certain physical findings may lead one to suspect a syringomyelia in association with scoliosis. Hall[45] has noted the association of a developmental scoliosis with myelodysplasia, and its cause is almost always due to syringomyelia. Nordwall[86] has pointed out that abnormal neurologic findings that may or may not be present should lead one to suspect a syringomyelia. Coonrad has recently noted the high incidence of syringomyelia associated with left thoracic curvatures.[22]

The most important radiographic finding is widening of the diameter of the cervical spinal canal. Williams[125] has given data to suggest that if the ratio of the canal to the vertebral body size is greater than 1.5 cm., that is if the canal is more than half as big as the vertebral body, then intrinsic pathology is to be expected. In his experience only 0.5 per cent of normal patients exceed this ratio. The definitive study consists of metrizamide myelography with delayed CT scanning. Cystic dilatation of the spinal cord with delayed dye uptake in the central canal is characteristic. MRI (magnetic resonance imaging) appears at the time of this writing to be the optimal study (Fig. 13–15).

The treatment of scoliosis associated with syringomyelia may pose considerable hazards, yet there is only limited information available in the literature on the results from surgical treatment. Huebert and MacKinnon[49] reported two patients who developed paraplegia during fusion even though Harrington rods were not used. Nordwall and Wikkelso[86] noted delayed onset of paraplegia in a 15 year old male treated for scoliosis with Harrington rod instrumentation. Ten days after surgery the patient complained of difficulty in voiding, and six days later spastic paraparesis had developed. The syringomyelia was aspirated 17 days after surgery, and the patient subsequently showed marked improvement, although residual weakness and atrophy remained at follow-up. It is our opinion that scoliosis in

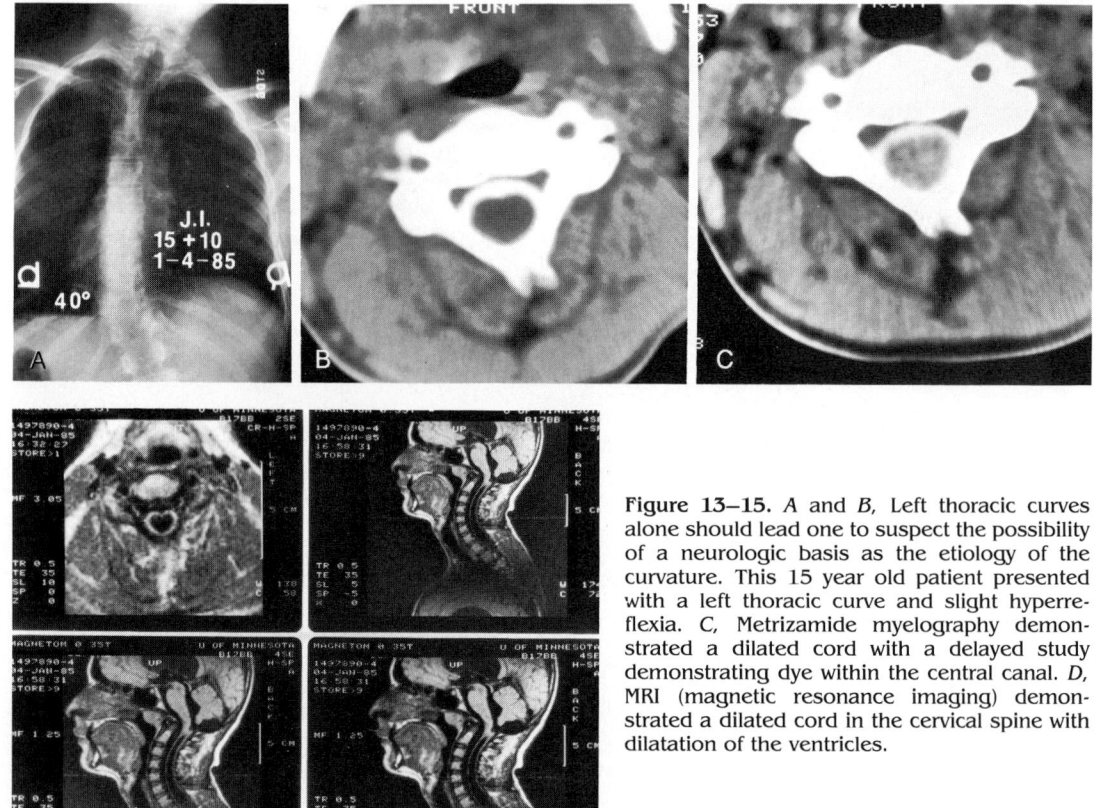

Figure 13–15. *A* and *B*, Left thoracic curves alone should lead one to suspect the possibility of a neurologic basis as the etiology of the curvature. This 15 year old patient presented with a left thoracic curve and slight hyperreflexia. *C*, Metrizamide myelography demonstrated a dilated cord with a delayed study demonstrating dye within the central canal. *D*, MRI (magnetic resonance imaging) demonstrated a dilated cord in the cervical spine with dilatation of the ventricles.

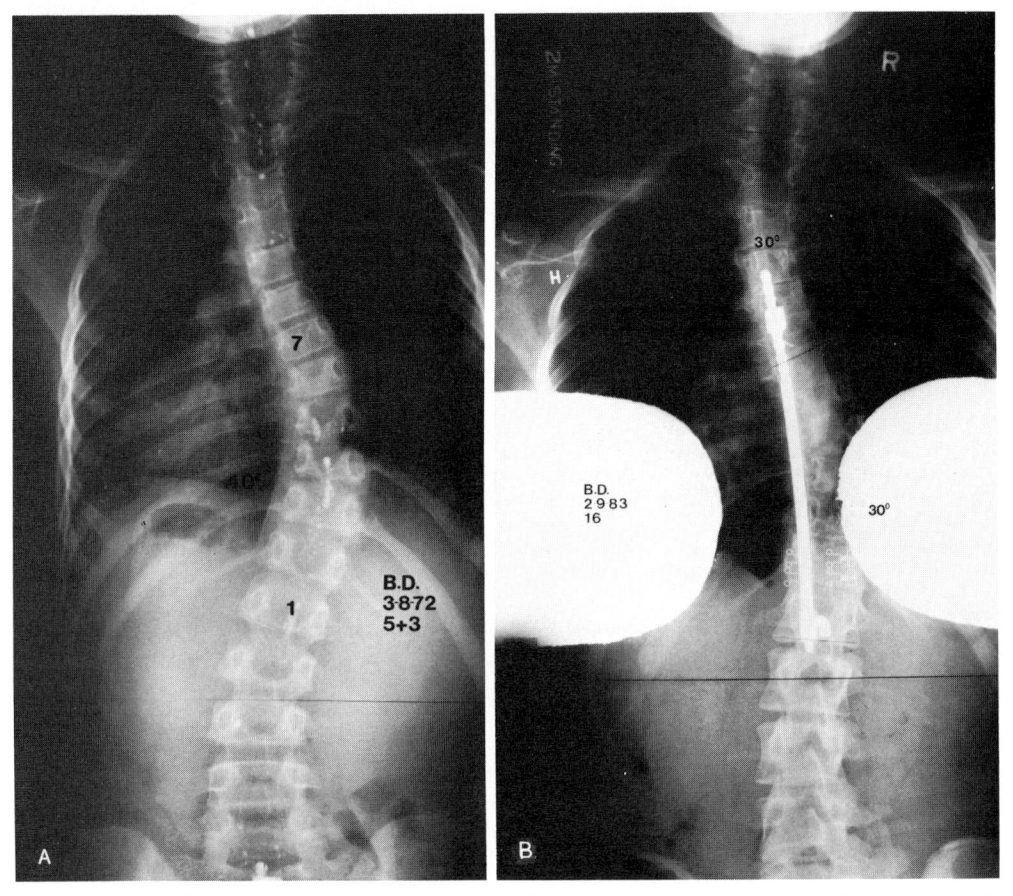

Figure 13–16. This patient presented at age 5 with a scoliosis secondary to a cervical syringomyelia. Following laminectomy with shunting of the syrinx, the patient made a satisfactory neurologic recovery. B, The Milwaukee brace did not control the curvature, so the patient was subsequently treated with a spine fusion and Harrington rod instrumentation, with a satisfactory outcome.

the presence of syringomyelia may be managed successfully and surgical treatment is not as hazardous as the literature would suggest provided certain safeguards are observed. Treatment initially should consist of drainage of the cyst followed by observation to determine the subsequent curve status. If the curvature progresses, surgical stabilization and fusion should be carried out. Although we have no data, sublaminar wiring would appear to pose a greater risk in the presence of a dilated spinal cord, and it would certainly be more troublesome if subsequent repeat laminectomy is necessary. We would favor the use of Harrington instrumentation alone with intraoperative monitoring by the somatosensory evoked potentials or the wake-up test (Fig. 13–16).

In summary then, in dealing with patients with rapidly progressing curvatures, any abnormality of neurologic function, an unusual curve with a high thoracic location, bony anomalies of the upper cervical spine, and increased diameter of the cervical spinal canal should lead one to suspect syringomyelia. Correction of these patients by surgical means appears to be risky and if it is felt indicated, the syrinx should no doubt be drained prior to surgical correction.

References

1. Allen, B. L., and Ferguson, R. L.: L-rod instrumentation for scoliosis in cerebral palsy. J. Pediatr. Orthop., 2:87–96, 1982.
2. Aprin, H., Bowen, J. R., MacEwen, G. D., and Hall, J. E.: Spine fusion in patients with spinal muscular atrophy. J. Bone Joint Surg., 64A:1179–1187, 1982.
3. Axelrod, F. B., Iyer, K., and Fish, I.: Progressive sensory loss in familial dysautonomia. Pediatrics, 67:517–522, 1981.
4. Baker, A. S., and Dove, J.: Progressive scoliosis as the first presenting sign of syringomyelia:

report of a case. J. Bone Joint Surg., 65B:472–473, 1983.
5. Balmer, G. A., and MacEwen, G. D.: The incidence and treatment of scoliosis in cerebral palsy. J. Bone Joint Surg., 52B:134–137, 1970.
6. Bedbrook, G. M.: Correction of scoliosis due to paraplegia sustained in paediatric age group. Paraplegia, 15:90–96, 1977–1978.
7. Benady, S. G.: Spinal muscle atrophy in childhood: review of 50 cases. Devel. Med. Child. Neurol., 20:746, 1978.
8. Bethea, J. S., III, and Doherty, J. H.: Scoliosis and dysautonomia. J. Bone Joint Surg., 52A:409, 1971.
9. Bleck, E. E.: Deformities of the spine and pelvis in cerebral palsy. In Samilson, R. L. (ed.): Orthopaedic Aspects of Cerebral Palsy. Philadelphia, JB Lippincott, pp. 124–144, 1975.
10. Bonnett, C. A., Brown, J. C., and Grow, T.: Thoracolumbar scoliosis in cerebral palsy. Results of surgical treatment. J. Bone Joint Surg., 58A:328–336, 1976.
11. Bonnett, C., Brown, J., Perry, J., et al.: The evolution of treatment of paralytic scoliosis at Rancho Los Amigos Hospital. J. Bone Joint Surg., 57A:206–215, 1975.
12. Bonnett, C. A., Metani, M., and Guess, V.: Spinal cord injury. In Lovell, W. W., and Winter, R. B. (eds.): Pediatric Orthopaedics. Philadelphia, J. B. Lippincott Co., pp. 495–531, 1978.
13. Brown, J. C., and Swank, S. M.: Paralytic spine deformity. In Bradford, D. S., and Hensinger, R. (eds.): The Pediatric Spine. New York, Thieme and Stratton, pp. 251–272, 1985.
14. Brown, J. C., Swank, S. M., and Specht, L.: Combined anterior and posterior spine fusion in cerebral palsy. Spine, 7:570–573, 1982.
15. Bunch, W. H.: The Milwaukee brace in paralytic scoliosis. Clin. Orthop., 110:63–68, 1975.
16. Bunch, W. H.: Muscular dystrophy. In Hardy, J. H. (ed.): Spinal Deformity in Neurological and Muscular Disorders. St. Louis, C. V. Mosby Co., 1974.
17. Bunch, W. H., Smith, D., and Hakala, M.: Kyphosis in the paralytic spine. Clin. Orthop. Rel. Res., 128:107–112, 1977.
18. Bunnell, W. P., MacEwen, G. D.: Nonoperative treatment of scoliosis in cerebral palsy. Preliminary report on the use of a plastic jacket. Devel. Med. Child Neurol., 19:45–49, 1977.
19. Carlson, J. M., and Winter, R. B.: The "Gillette" sitting support orthosis for non-ambulatory children with severe cerebral palsy or advanced muscular dystrophy. Minn. Med., 61:469–473, 1978.
20. Cobb, J. R.: Technique, after-treatment, and results of spine fusion for scoliosis. In the American Academy of Orthopaedic Surgeons. Instructional Course Lectures, Vol. 9, pp. 65–70, St. Louis, C. V. Mosby, Co., 1952.
21. Colonna, P. C., and Vom Saal, F.: A study of paralytic scoliosis based on 500 cases of poliomyelitis. J. Bone Joint Surg., 23:335, 1941.
22. Coonrad, R. W., Richardson, W. J., and Oakes, W. J.: Left thoracic curves can be different. Presented at the 19th annual meeting of the Scoliosis Research Society, Orlando, Florida, 1984.
23. Daher, Y. H., Lonstein, J. E., Winter, R. B., and Bradford, D. S.: Spinal surgery in spinal muscular atrophy. J. Pediatr. Orthop., 5:391–395, 1985.
24. Daher, Y. H., Winter, R. B., Lonstein, J. E., and Bradford, D. S.: Spinal deformities in patients with Friedreich's ataxia: a review of 19 patients. J. Pediatr. Orthop., 5:553–557, 1985.
25. Daher, Y. H., Winter, R. B., Lonstein, J. E., and Bradford, D. S.: Spinal deformities in patients with Charcot-Marie-Tooth: a review of 12 patients. Clin. Orthop. Rel. Res., 202:219–222, 1986.
26. Dancis, J., and Smith, A. A.: Current concepts in familial dysautonomia. New Engl. J. Med., 274:207–209, 1966.
27. DeWald, R. L., and Faut, M. M.: Anterior and posterior spinal fusion for paralytic scoliosis. Spine, 4:401–409, 1979.
28. Dorr, J., Brown, J., and Perry, J.: Results of posterior spine fusion in patients with spinal muscle atrophy—A review of 25 cases. J. Bone Joint Surg., 55A:436–437, 1973.
29. Dubowitz, V.: Benign infantile spinal muscular atrophy. Devel. Med. Child Neurol., 16:672–675, 1974.
30. Dubowitz, V.: Progressive muscular dystrophy: prevention of deformities. Clin. Pediatr., 3:323–328, 1964.
31. Duval-Beaupere, G., Poiffaut, A., Bovier, C. L., et al.: Plexidur jackets for correction of paralytic scoliosis. Results after seven years. Acta. Orthop. Belg., 41:652, 1975.
32. Evans, G. A., Drennan, J. C., and Russman, B. S.: Functional classification and orthopaedic management of spinal muscular atrophy. J. Bone Joint Surg., 63B:516–522, 1981.
33. Ferguson, R. L., and Allen, B. L.: Staged correction of neuromuscular scoliosis. J. Pediatr. Orthop., 3:555–562, 1983.
34. Finlayson, A. I.: Syringomyelia and related conditions. In Baker, A. B. (ed.): Clinical Neurology, 2nd ed. New York, Harper and Brothers, p. 1571, 1962.
35. Fisk, J. R., and Bunch, W. H.: Scoliosis in neuromuscular disease. Orthop. Clin. North Am., 10:863–875, 1979.
36. Gardner, W. J., and Collis, J. S.: Skeletal anomalies associated with syringomyelia, diastematomyelia and myelomeningocele. J. Bone Joint Surg., 42A:1265, 1960.
37. Garrett, A. L., Perry, J., and Nickel, V. L.: Paralytic scoliosis. Clin. Orthop., 21:117, 1961.
38. Garrett, A. L., Perry, J., and Nickel, V. L.: Stabilization of the collapsing spine. J. Bone Joint Surg., 43A:474, 1961.
39. Geoffrey, G., Barbeau, A., Breton, G., et al.: Classifical description and roentgenologic evaluation of patients with Friedreich's ataxia. Can. J. Neurol. Sci., 3:279, 1976.
40. Gibson, D. A., Koreska, J., Robertson, D., et al.: The management of spinal deformity in Duchenne's muscular dystrophy. Orthop. Clinics North Am., 9:437–450, 1978.
41. Goldstein, L. A., Fuller, J., Haake, P., and Crumline, R.: Surgical treatment of thoracic scoliosis in patients with familial dysautonomia. J. Bone Joint Surg., 51A:205, 1969.
42. Gucker, T.: Experience in poliomyelitic scoliosis after correction and fusion. J. Bone Joint Surg., 38A:1281, 1956.
43. Gui, L., Savini, R., Vicenzi, G., and Ponzo, L.:

Surgical treatment of poliomyelitic scoliosis. Ital. J. Orthop. Traumat., 2:191–205, 1976.
44. Haas, S. L.: Spastic scoliosis and obliquity of the pelvis. J. Bone Joint Surg., 24:774–780, 1942.
45. Hall, P. V., Lindseth, R. E., Campbell, R. L., and Kalsbeck, J. E.: Myelodysplasia and developmental scoliosis. Spine, 1:48–56, 1976.
46. Harrington, P. R.: Treatment of scoliosis: correction and internal fixation by spine instrumentation. J. Bone Joint Surg., 44A:591–610, 1962.
47. Hensinger, R. N., and MacEwen, G. D.: Spinal deformity associated with heritable neurological conditions: spinal muscle atrophy, Friedreich's ataxia, familial dysautonomia, and Charcot-Marie-Tooth disease. J. Bone Joint Surg., 58A:13–24, 1976.
48. Hsu, J. D.: The natural history of spine curvature progression in the nonambulator Duchenne muscular dystrophy patient. Spine, 8:771–775, 1983.
49. Huebert, H. T., and MacKinnon, W. B.: Syringomyelia and scoliosis. J. Bone Joint Surg., 51B:338–343, 1969.
50. Inkley, S. R., Oldenburg, F. C., and Vignos, P. J., Jr.: Pulmonary function in Duchenne muscular dystrophy related to stage of disease. Am. J. Med., 56:297–306, 1974.
51. Irwin, C. E.: The iliotibial band: its role in producing deformity in poliomyelitis. J. Bone Joint Surg., 31A:141–146, 1949.
52. Jackson, R. W.: Surgical stabilization of the spine. Int. J. Paraplegia, 13:71–74, 1975.
53. James, J. I. P.: Paralytic scoliosis. J. Bone Joint Surg., 38B:660–685, 1956.
54. Kilfoyle, R. M., Foley, J. J., and Norton, P. L.: Spine and pelvic deformity in childhood and adolescent paraplegia—a study of 104 cases. J. Bone Joint Surg., 47A:659–682, 1965.
55. LaBelle, H., Tohme, S., Duhaime, M., and Allard, P.: Natural history of scoliosis in Friedreich's ataxia. Presented at the 19th Annual Meeting of the Scoliosis Research Society, Orlando, Florida, 1984.
56. Lancourt, J. C., Dickson, J. H., and Carter, R. E.: Paralytic spinal deformity following traumatic spinal cord injury in children and adolescents. J. Bone Joint Surg., 63A:47–53, 1981.
57. Leidholt, J. D.: Evaluation of late spinal deformities with fracture dislocations of the dorsal and lumbar spine in paraplegics. Paraplegia, 7:16–28, 1969.
58. Leong, J. C. Y., Wilding, K., Mok, C. D., et al.: Surgical treatment of scoliosis following poliomyelitis: a review of 100 cases. J. Bone Joint Surg., 63A:726–740, 1981.
59. Levine, D. B.: Poliomyelitis. In Hardy, J. H. (ed.): Spinal Deformity in Neurological and Muscular Disorders. St. Louis, C. V. Mosby, pp. 111–139, 1974.
60. Levine, D. B.: Orthopaedic aspects of familial dysautonomia. In Zorab, P. A. (ed.): Scoliosis and Muscle. Philadelphia, J. B. Lippincott, pp. 143–150, 1974.
61. Lonstein, J. E., and Akbarnia, B. A.: Operative treatment of spinal deformities in patients with cerebral palsy or mental retardation. An analysis of 107 cases. J. Bone Joint Surg., 65A:43–55, 1983.
62. Luque, E. R.: Paralytic scoliosis in growing children. Clin. Orthop., 163:202–209, 1982.
63. Luque, E. R.: Segmental spinal instrumentation for correction of scoliosis. Clin. Orthop., 163:192–198, 1982.
64. Luque, E. R.: The anatomic basis and development of segmental spinal instrumentation. Spine, 7:256–259, 1982.
65. Luque, E. R.: The correction of postural curves of the spine. Spine, 7:270–275, 1982.
66. MacEwen, G. D.: Operative treatment of scoliosis in cerebral palsy. Reconstr. Surg. Traumatol., 13:58, 1972.
67. MacEwen, G. D.: Cerebral palsy and scoliosis. In Hardy, J. H. (ed.): Spinal Deformity in Neurological and Muscular Disorders. St. Louis, C. V. Mosby, pp. 191–199, 1974.
68. Madigan, R. R., and Wallace, S. L.: Scoliosis in the institutionalized cerebral palsy population. Spine, 6:583–590, 1981.
69. Makin, M.: Spinal problems of childhood paraplegia. Isr. J. Med. Sci., 9:732, 1973.
70. Makley, J., Herndon, C., Inkley, S., et al.: Pulmonary function in paralytic and non-paralytic scoliosis, before and after treatment: a study of 63 cases. J. Bone Joint Surg., 50A:1379–1390, 1968.
71. Mayer, L.: Further studies of fixed paralytic pelvic obliquity. J. Bone Joint Surg., 18:87–100, 1936.
72. Mayer, P. J., Dove, J., Ditmanson, M., and Shen, Y.: Post-poliomyelitis paralytic scoliosis. Spine, 6:573–582, 1981.
73. Mayfield, J. K., Erkkila, J. D., and Winter, R. B.: Spine deformity subsequent to acquired childhood spinal cord injury. J. Bone Joint Surg., 63A:1401–1413, 1981.
74. McKusick, V. A., Norum, R. A., Farkas, H. J., et al: The Riley-Day syndrome: observations on genetics and survivorship (an interim report). Isr. J. Med. Sci., 3:372–379, 1967.
75. McIlroy, W. J., and Richardson, J. C.: Syringomyelia: a clinical review of 75 cases. Can. Med. Assoc. J., 93:731, 1965.
76. McRae, D. L., and Standen, J.: Roentgenologic findings in syringomyelia and hydromyelia. Am. J. Roentgenol., 98:695–703, 1966.
77. McSweeny, T.: Spinal deformity after spinal cord injury. Paraplegia, 6:212, 1969.
78. Millis, M. B., and Hall, J. E.: Transiliac lengthening of the lower extremity; a modified innominate osteotomy for the treatment of postural imbalance. J. Bone Joint Surg., 61A:1182–1194, 1979.
79. Milne, B., and Rosales, J. K.: Anaesthetic considerations in patients with muscular dystrophy undergoing spinal fusion and Harrington rod insertion. Can. Anaesth. Soc. J., 29(3):250–254, 1982.
80. Moe, J. H.: A critical analysis of methods of fusion for scoliosis. Evaluation of 266 patients. J. Bone Joint Surg., 40A:529–554, 1958.
81. Moe, J. H.: The management of paralytic scoliosis. South. Med. J., 50:67–81, 1957.
82. Namba, T., Aberfeld, D. C., and Grob, D.: Chronic proximal spinal muscular atrophy. J. Neurol. Sci., 11:401–423, 1970.
83. Nash, C. L.: Current concepts review: scoliosis bracing. J. Bone Joint Surg., 62A:848–852, 1980.
84. Nickel, V., Perry, J., Affeldt, J., and Dail, C.: Elective surgery on patients with respiratory paralysis. J. Bone Joint Surg., 39A:989, 1957.

85. Nickel, V., and Perry, J.: Respiratory evaluation of patients for major surgery. In The American Academy of Orthopaedic Surgeons Instructional Course Lectures, Vol. XVIII, St. Louis, C. V. Mosby, 1961.
86. Nordwall, A., and Wikkelso, C.: A late neurologic complication of scoliosis surgery in connection with syringomyelia. Acta Orthop. Scand., 50(4):407–410, 1979.
87. Norton, P. L., and Foley, J. J.: Paraplegia in children. J. Bone Joint Surg., 41A:1291–1309, 1959.
88. O'Brien, J. P., and Yau, A. C.: Anterior and posterior correction and fusion for paralytic scoliosis. Clin. Orthop., 86:151–153, 1972.
89. O'Brien, J. P., Dwyer, A. P., and Hodgson, A. R.: Paralytic pelvic obliquity—its prognosis and management and the development of a technique for full correction of the deformity. J. Bone Joint Surg., 57A:626–631, 1975.
90. O'Brien, J. P., Yau, A. C., Gertzbein, S., and Hodgson, A. R.: Combined staged anterior and posterior correction and fusion of the spine in scoliosis following poliomyelitis. Clin. Orthop., 110:81–89, 1975.
91. Odom, J., and Jackson, R. W.: Scoliosis in paraplegia. Int. J. Paraplegia, 11:290–292, 1974.
92. Pavon, S. J., and Manning, C.: Posterior spine fusion for scoliosis due to anterior poliomyelitis. J. Bone Joint Surg., 52A:420–431, 1970.
93. Pearn, J. H.: Scoliosis in the spinal muscular atrophies of childhood. In Zorab, P. A. (ed.): Scoliosis and Muscle. Philadelphia, J. B. Lippincott, pp. 135–142, 1974.
94. Perry, J., and Nickel, V. L.: Total cervical spine fusion for neck paralysis. J. Bone Joint Surg., 41A:37, 1959.
95. Renshaw, T. S.: Paralysis in the child—orthopaedic management. In Bradford, D. S., and Hensinger, R. (eds.): The Pediatric Spine. New York, Thieme and Stratton, pp. 118–130, 1985.
96. Riddick, M., Winter, R. B., and Lutter, L: Spinal deformities in patients with spinal muscle atrophy. Spine, 8:476–483, 1982.
97. Rideau, Y., Glorion, B., Delaubier, A., et al.: The treatment of scoliosis in Duchenne muscular dystrophy. Muscle Nerve, 7:281–286, 1984.
98. Riley, C. M., Day, R. L., Greeley, D. M., and Langford, W. S.: Central autonomic dysfunction with defective lachrymation: report of five cases. Pediatrics, 3:468–478, 1949.
99. Roaf, R.: Paralytic scoliosis. J. Bone Joint Surg., 38B:640, 1956.
100. Robin, G. C.: Scoliosis in familial dysautonomia. Bull. Hosp. for Joint Dis. Orthop. Inst., 44(1):16–26, 1984.
101. Robin, G. D.: Scoliosis in Duchenne muscular dystrophy. Isr. J. Med. Soc., 13(2):203–206, 1977.
102. Robin, G. C., and Brief, L. P.: Scoliosis in childhood muscular dystrophy. J. Bone Joint Surg., 53A:466–476, 1971.
103. Robson, P.: The prevalence of scoliosis in adolescents and young adults with cerebral palsy. Dev. Med. Child Neurol., 10:447–452, 1968.
104. Rosenthal, R. K., Levine, D. B., and McCarver, C. L.: The occurrence of scoliosis in cerebral palsy. Dev. Med. Child Neurol., 16:664–667, 1974.
105. Sakai, D. N., Hsu, J. D., Bonnett, C. A., and Brown, J. C.: Stabilization of the collapsing spine in Duchenne muscular dystrophy. Clin. Orthop. Rel. Res., 128:256–260, 1977.
106. Samilson, R., and Bechard, R.: Scoliosis in cerebral palsy: incidence, distribution of curve patterns, natural history, and thoughts on etiology. Curr. Pract. Orthop. Surg., 5:183–205, 1973.
107. Schwentker, E. P., and Gibson, D. A.: The orthopaedic apsects of spinal muscular atrophy. J. Bone Joint Surg., 58A:32–38, 1976.
108. Seeger, B. R., Sutherland, A. D., and Clard, M. S.: Orthotic management of scoliosis in Duchenne muscular dystrophy. Arch. Phys. Med. Rehabil., 65:83–86, 1984.
109. Shapiro, F., and Bresnan, M. J.: Current concepts review. Management of childhood neuromuscular disease. Part I: Spinal muscular atrophy. J. Bone Joint Surg., 64A:785–798, 1982.
110. Shapiro, F., and Bresnan, M. J.: Current concepts review. Orthopaedic Management of Childhood Neuromuscular Disease. Part 2: Peripheral neuropathies, Friedreich's ataxia and arthrygryposis multiplex congenita. J. Bone Joint Surg., 64A:949–953, 1982.
111. Siegel, I. M.: Scoliosis in muscular dystrophy. Clin. Orthop., 93:235–238, 1973.
112. Siegel, I. M.: Spinal stabilization in Duchenne muscular dystrophy: rationale and method. Muscle Nerve, 5:417–418, 1982.
113. Stanitski, C. L., Micheli, L. J., Hall, J. D., and Rosenthal, R. K.: Surgical correction of spinal deformity in cerebral palsy. Spine, 7:563–569, 1982.
114. Steindler, A.: Diseases and Deformities of the Spine and Thorax. St. Louis, C. V. Mosby Co., 1929.
115. Stenquist, O., and Sigurdson, J.: The anaesthetic management of a patient with familial dysautonomia. Anaesthesia, 37:929–932, 1982.
116. Sullivan, J. A., and Conner, S. B.: Comparison of Harrington instrumentation and segmental spinal instrumentation in the management of neuromuscular spinal deformity. Spine, 7:299–304, 1982.
117. Swank, S. M., and Brown, J. C.: Electrical stimulation in the management of spinal deformities—present update. In Bradford, D. S., and Dickson, R. (eds.): Management of Spinal Deformities. London, Butterworth's Ltd., pp. 145–161, 1984.
118. Swank, S. M., Brown, J. C., and Perry, R. E.: Spinal fusion in Duchenne's muscular dystrophy. Spine, 7:484–491, 1982.
119. Swank, S. M., Winter, R. B., and Moe, J. H.: Scoliosis and cor pulmonale. Spine, 7:343, 1982.
120. Taddonio, R. F.: Segmental spinal instrumentation in the management of neuromuscular spinal deformity. Spine, 7:305–311, 1982.
121. Von Bazan, U. K. B., and Paeslack, V.: Scoliotic growth in children with acquired paraplegia. Paraplegia, 15:65–73, 1977–1978.
122. Weber, F. A.: The association of syringomyelia and scoliosis. J. Bone Joint Surg., 56B:589, 1974.
123. Wedge, J. H., and Gillespie, R.: The problems of scoliosis surgery in paraplegic children. J. Bone Joint Surg., 57B:536, 1975.

124. Wilkins, K. E., and Gibson, D. A.: The patterns of spinal deformity in Duchenne muscular dystrophy. J. Bone Joint Surg., *58A*:24–34, 1976.
125. Williams, B.: Orthopaedic features in the presentation of syringomyelia. J. Bone Joint Surg., *61B*:314–323, 1979.
126. Winter, R. B., and Carlson, J. M.: Modern orthotics for spinal deformities. Clin. Orthop., *23*:74–86, 1977.
127. Woods, W. W., and Pimenta, A. M.: Intramedullary lesions of the spinal cord. Arch. Neurol. Psych., *52*:383, 1944.
128. Yoslow, W., Becker, M. H., Bartels, J., and Thomson, W.: Orthopaedic defects in familial dysautonomia: a review of 65 cases. J. Bone Joint Surg., *53A*:1541–1550, 1971.
129. Yount, C. C.: The role of the tensor fascia femoris in certain deformities of the lower extremities. J. Bone Joint Surg., *8*:171, 1926.

14

MYELOMENINGOCOELE
Robert B. Winter, M.D.

INTRODUCTION

Of all the causes of spinal deformity, myelomeningocoele is probably the most difficult to treat. The advances in neurosurgery with early sac closure and effective shunting of hydrocephalus, coupled with urologic advances in management of the paralytic bladder, have led to an increased survival rate for affected children. As they mature, spinal deformity becomes in increasingly prominent problem. If neglected, the spinal deformity may become so severe as to destroy all previous rehabilitative efforts.

The treatment of these difficult deformities is now possible. These children are best managed in centers accustomed to and competent in the general care of the child with myelomeningocoele. Their spine deformities cannot be cared for in isolation from their other problems.

The surgeon responsible for the treatment of the spinal deformity must not only be skilled in the treatment of idiopathic scoliosis, but very experienced in the treatment of neuromuscular spine deformities of other causes.

NATURAL HISTORY

Raycroft and Curtis[39] reviewed the natural history of spinal deformities in 130 children with myelomeningocoele at Newington Children's Hospital. They distinguished two types of deformities, the developmental (paralytic) and the congenital (with anomalous vertebrae). These were further subdivided into scoliosis, lordosis, and kyphosis.

Of the 103 patients without congenital anomalies other than spina bifida, 53 had spine deformity. Of these, 41 had scoliosis, 30 had lordosis, and 12 had kyphosis; most patients had mixed deformity. All 27 of the congenitally anomalous spines had spinal deformity, 21 with scoliosis and 6 with kyphosis.

The children with congenital anomalies usually had some deformity at birth, but the children with the developmental type did not. The age at curve onset in the developmental type was 0 to 5 years in 33 patients, 6 to 10 years in 18 patients, and 11 to 15 years in 2 patients. The researchers also noted that the higher the level of paralysis, the greater the likelihood of spinal deformity.

Hall and Martin,[18] in an unpublished report, analyzed a group of 130 myelomeningocoele patients, all of whom had finished growth. Seventy-eight per cent of these had obvious spinal deformity.

Mackel and Lindseth[29] reported on 82 patients age 10 or older. Of these, 54 had spinal deformity, 42 developmental and 12 congenital. Of those with a T12 level paralysis, 100 per cent had deformity. All curves progressed relentlessly once they appeared.

Roth[41] reviewed 149 patients, 26 per cent with congenital anomalies other than the spina bifida. Of the 149, 29 had scoliosis, 32 had kyphosis, and 13 had lordosis. The higher the level of paralysis, the more likely was a spinal deformity.

Banta and coworkers[2] reviewed 268 patients followed for at least four years. Sixteen per cent had scoliosis by age 4, 35 per cent by age 9, and 52 per cent by age 15. With a lesion at T12 or higher, 100 per cent had scoliosis, and of four non-functional ambulators, 80 per cent had scoliosis.

Shurtleff and associates[42] analyzed a large number of patients as to the level of the lesion and age of development of "significant" (30 degrees or more) scoliosis and kyphosis. At age one only 3 per cent had scoliosis. By age 10, 33 per cent of the T12 level patients, 22 per cent of the L1-L2 level patients, 18 per cent of the L3-L5 level patients, and 3 per cent of the S1 level patients had scoliosis. By the end of growth, 88 per cent of the thoracic level patients, 63 per cent of the L1-L2 level patients, 23 per cent of the L3-L5 level patients, and 9 per cent of the S1 level patients had significant scoliosis. Kyphosis was a problem predominantly of the thoracic level patients.

Piggott[36] reviewed 250 patients with myelodysplasia and found scoliosis in 90 per cent of those over age 10, kyphosis and lordosis being less common.

Hall and associates from Indiana[21, 22] have stressed the importance of evaluating progressive curves for hydromyelia. They found 14 of 15 patients with progressive developmental scoliosis to have a communicating hydrosyringomyelia. Eight of these were also noted to have progressive extremity paralysis. Ventricular shunting improved neurologic deficits and stabilized some of the scolioses. Their findings have been confirmed by Bunch.[8, 9]

These appear to be accurate and consistent reports and indicate the very severe nature of the problem. In summary, spinal deformity is very common in patients with myelomeningocoele, may be either paralytic or congenital (or both), and may be scoliotic, kyphotic, or lordotic. The higher the level of paralysis, the more common is spinal deformity (Figs. 14–1 to 14–3).

PATIENT EVALUATION

History

The physician should first ask about the general health of the child, and then ask questions specific to the spine. In terms of the general status, one needs to know about the child's mental capacity, school level, presence or absence of hydrocephalus, any surgical procedures for shunting of the hydrocephalus, bladder and bowel function, urinary tract infection, use of indwelling or intermittent catheterization, urinary diversion procedure, urinary medications, arm and hand function, quality of ambulation, use of ambulatory aids (wheelchair, crutches, braces), pressure sores, and socialization level and skills.

With regard to the spine, questions are asked about the level of nerve function, the onset of the curve, curve progression, previous spinal surgery, previous bracing attempts, and functional problems related to the curve (e.g., pain, decreased sitting balance, ischial pressure sores, breathing problems, and loss of neurologic function).[10]

Physical Examination

The examination must be complete, paying attention to the whole child. The head is examined for hydrocephalus, the presence of a shunt, abnormal eye motion, blindness, and the quality of cerebral function. The chest is examined for deformity, breathing quality, and any sign of pneumonia. The abdomen is examined for shunt surgery, renal surgery, or bladder surgery. The breasts and genitalia are examined for their status of maturity.

The hips are examined for dislocation, subluxation, or contractures. Contractures may be in any area including flexors, extensors, abductors, or adductors. The iliotibial bands are especially prone to contracture. The quality of active muscle power about the hips must also be noted.

The knees are examined for contractures, varus or valgus deformity, and for active motor function. The feet are examined for pressure sores, varus or valgus deformity, dorsiflexion or plantar flexion deformity, and active motor strength.

The upper extremities should be examined for subtle paralysis, as hydromyelia may extend into the cervical spine even with a lumbar myelomeningocoele.[6]

The neurologic examination should also include areas of sensory deficit and reflex changes. Some children with myelomeningocoele have spastic lower extremities, which greatly compounds their problems. The neurologic pattern may be different in the two lower extremities, even to the point of total paralysis of one lower extremity and total normalcy of the other, a condition called hemimyelodysplasia.[31]

The spine is examined for the precise pattern of deformity. Is there scoliosis, lordosis, kyphosis, or a combination thereof? Are the absent laminar levels palpable? What is the quality of the skin over the spine? The ischiae must be examined for pressure sores. What is the quality of skin sensation around the hips? This can be of great importance when considering bracing, either as part of nonoperative treatment or following surgery.

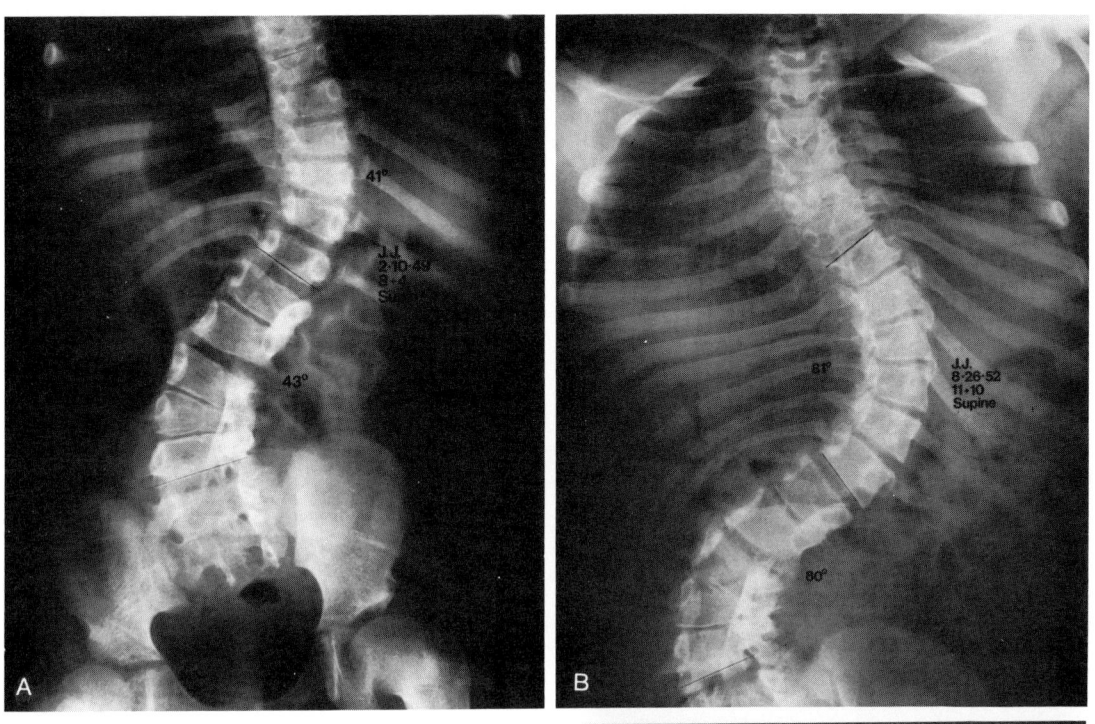

Figure 14–1. *A*, An eight year old girl with an L1 neurologic level myelomeningocoele and a left lumbar scoliosis due to a congenital defect of segmentation at L1-L2 and L3-L4-L5 on the right. She also has bilateral segmentation defects of the upper thoracic spine. She had no treatment. *B*, Three years later, her curves had increased to 81 degrees and 80 degrees. *C*, A follow-up at age 30 showed the curves at 93 degrees and 86 degrees. When last seen in 1984 at age 35, the curves remained unchanged, but the patient was bothered by a tendency to fall to one side in her wheelchair.

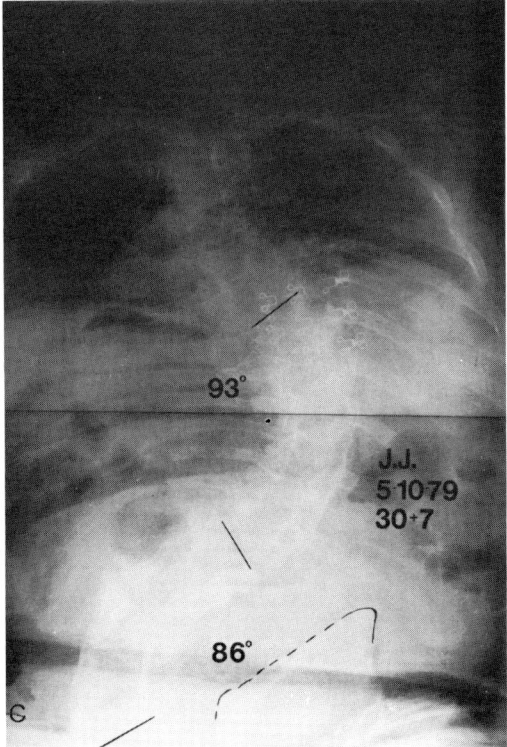

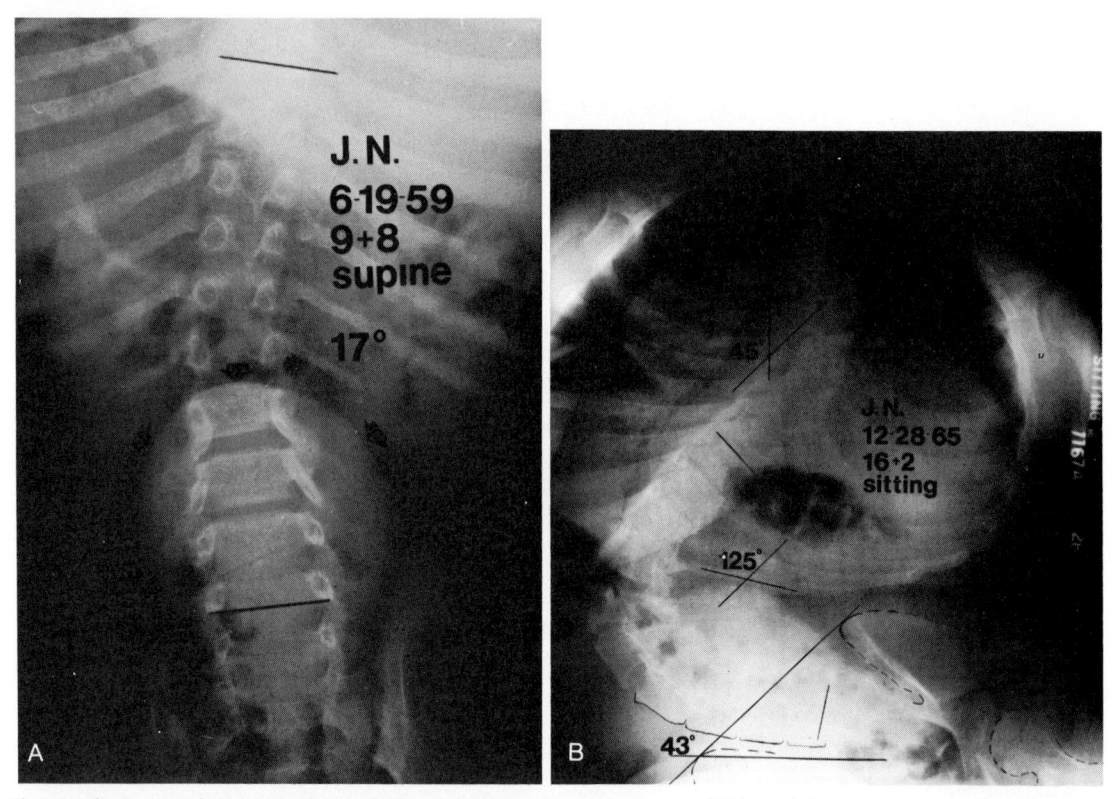

Figure 14–2. *A*, This 9+8 year old girl is seen here with a 14 degree, T8 to pelvis curve on a supine film. She had an L1 neurologic level. No treatment was given. *B*, The same patient at age 16, seen here sitting, with a 125 degree scoliosis and a 43 degree pelvic obliquity. She had lost all sitting ability and had pressure sores on the left ischium and trochanter.

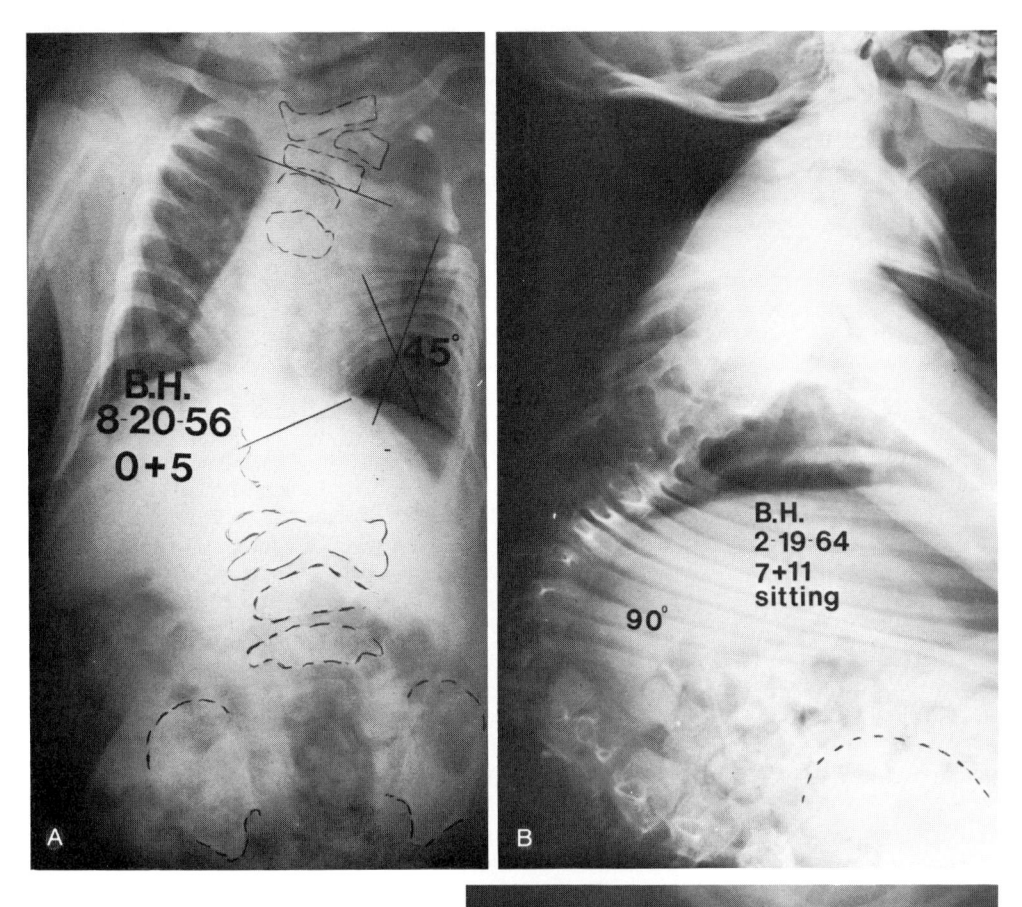

Figure 14–3. *A*, A 5 month old boy with a 45 degree congenital scoliosis. *B*, A lateral x-ray at age eight shows a 90 degree kyphosis. *C*, Both the scoliosis and kyphosis progressed, and the patient presented at age 14 in terminal cor pulmonale with severe sores over the apex of the kyphosis and osteomyelitis.

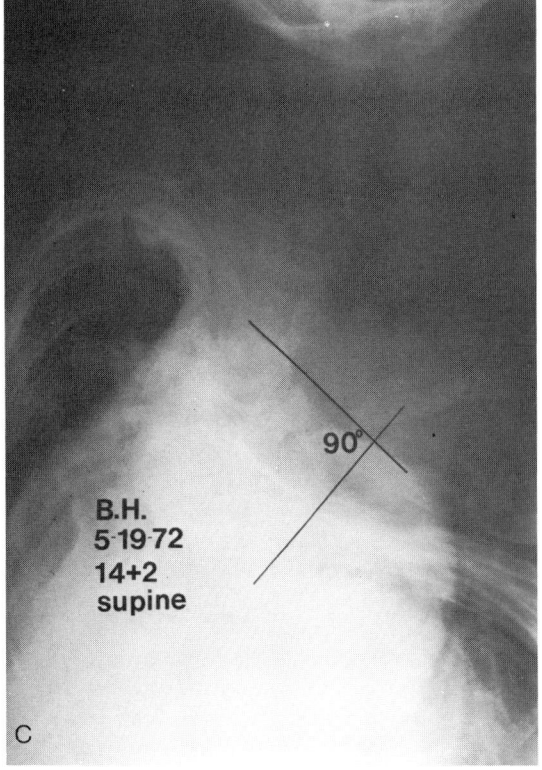

Radiologic Examination

Many of the customary radiographs taken for the patient with idiopathic scoliosis are not applicable for the patient with myelomeningocoele. Upright films, both anteroposterior and lateral, should be taken standing if the patient can walk, but sitting if the patient is a wheelchair ambulator. Supine films, both anteroposterior and lateral are also taken, and these should be done with the hips flexed at least 45 degrees and abducted at least 30 degrees. This hip position eliminates the effect of hip contractures on the spine, and the supine position eliminates the effect of gravity. Thus one can see the spine's true character, unaffected by these external elements. The supine films also provide better bone detail, allowing one to better determine the presence or absence of congenital defects and to assess the extent and character of the spina bifida.

The rigidity and flexibility of the curvature are determined best by radiographs in firm traction. Active supine bending films, useful for the idiopathic patient, are worthless for the paralytic patient. When there is pelvic obliquity, there should be head traction and traction on the leg of the "high" side to see the correctibility of the pelvic obliquity.

Lordosis correctibility is best determined by a forced flexion lateral radiograph, whereas kyphosis correctibility is best seen by forced extension or a traction lateral view (see Chapter 5, p. 64).

Specialized radiologic techniques may occasionally be necessary. Metrizamide myelography is being increasingly used to examine the neural axis for hydromyelia as well as for tethering lesions that may be responsible for continued neurologic deterioration.[8, 21, 22] In looking for hydromyelia, the contrast medium should be carried all the way up to the foramen magnum (to look for cervical syringomyelia as well as Arnold-Chiari malformation) and computerized tomography of the myelogram should also be done to examine the spinal cord diameter and shape, and a late (3 to 4 hour) examination to see if the dye concentrates in the center of the cord (see Chapter 5, p. 80).

Computerized tomography can also be used in the lumbar spine to better evaluate the extent of the spina bifida and to evaluate the quality of the vertebrae in preparation for surgical fixation.

Intravenous pyelography should be done at regular intervals to be sure there is no obstructive uropathy or other pathology that might need treatment prior to the surgery for spine deformity (Fig. 14–4).

GENERAL PRINCIPLES AND GOALS

In dealing with neuromuscular problems, in general, the physician should strive toward certain goals. These include preservation of respiratory function, maintenance of sitting stability, obtaining maximal torso length, and the removal of unsightly prominences. Although cosmetic aspects are secondary to functional goals, it must be remembered that neuromuscular patients, even those with myelomeningocoele, have valid concepts of self-image. It is far better to be sitting straight and tall in a wheelchair than to be sitting shrunken and deformed.

Hip subluxation and dislocation are common to all neuromuscular problems, and especially so in myelomeningocoele. It is helpful for hip stability if the pelvis is level. Thus, one of the prime goals of spinal treatment is the maintenance of a level pelvis. This is also important for the prevention of ischial pressure sores.

Maintenance of trunk growth and thus the achievement of adequate trunk length are also very important. Many years ago, we did extensive spine fusions at an early age in patients with myelomeningocoele. These patients are now mature, and their very short torsos are displeasing to them and also cause considerable functional problems due to the crowding of thoracic and abdominal contents.

Congenital curves, whether kyphotic or scoliotic, become rigid early in life, have no potential for vertical growth, and require early arthrodesis. The paralytic component should preferably be done later.

NON-OPERATIVE TREATMENT

Non-operative treatment of neuromuscular scolioses is difficult, especially in myelomeningocoele patients. Some surgeons are so pessimistic about the chance of controlling the curve that they do not try, a defeatist attitude that is not justifiable. At the same time, it would be foolish to suggest that the treatment is easy and that "most patients do well."

MYELOMENINGOCOELE

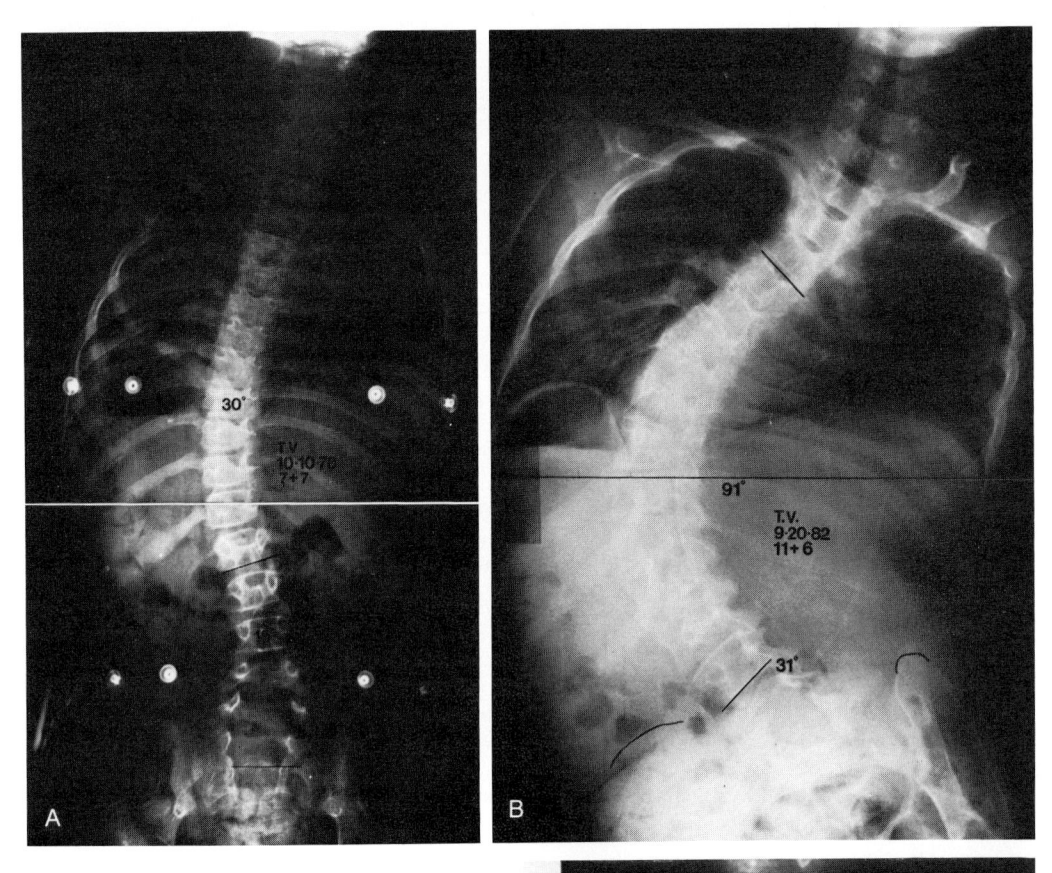

Figure 14–4. *A*, A 7 year old girl with a 30 degree scoliosis, spina bifida of L3, L4, L5, and the sacrum, and an L1 neurologic level. *B*, When seen at age 11, her curve had progressed to 91 degrees. Surgery was obviously needed, but did she need both anterior and posterior fusion, or was she flexible enough to do only a posterior fusion? *C*, A radiograph in traction on the Risser table showed correction to 52 degrees and excellent balance of the torso over the pelvis. Successful treatment was achieved by posterior fusion only.

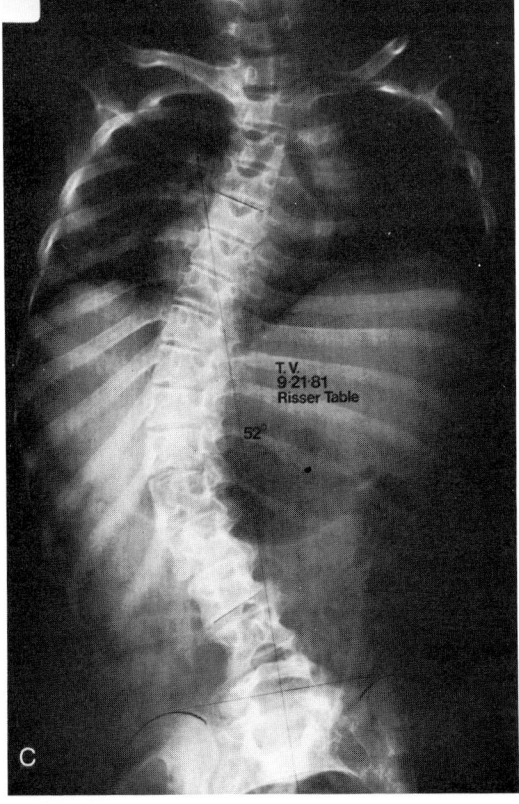

The goal of non-operative treatment is to *delay* spine fusion until adequate spinal growth has occurred, not to prevent spine fusion. At the same time, the curve must be kept under control, that is, progression must be halted and the scoliosis maintained below 50 degrees.

One should *never* delay surgery until all growth has ceased, as irretrievable progression will have taken place. The realities would seem to indicate that bracing can succeed in scoliosis control during the relatively quiet growth years prior to the adolescent growth spurt, but when accelerated growth occurs, the ability to control the curve without surgery is lost. This means that most scolioses surgeries will be done between ages 10 and 12 in females and 12 and 14 in males.

The only form of non-operative treatment with any chance of success is bracing. In general, the Milwaukee brace has not worked well, and thus most surgeons use carefully molded, custom-fitted body jackets. These can be either one-piece or two-piece, are usually padded, and require very diligent fabrication and fitting. Once fitted, great care must be taken to observe the skin frequently for pressure areas. The brace should be promptly adjusted before skin necrosis occurs.[13]

Angular kyphotic deformities cannot be controlled by bracing, and usually require early surgery (see p. 327).

The indications for brace treatment are neuromuscular (developmental) curves, either scoliosis, kyphosis, or lordosis. Congenital deformities do not respond to brace treatment. In general, scolioses of less than 20 degrees are merely observed, but progressive curves of 20 to 50 degrees in growing children are braced. Flexible curves can respond to braces but rigid ones cannot, and thus a supine bending or traction radiograph will help to determine whether a curve has adequate flexibility for treatment.

The indications for cessation of brace treatment can be (1) the attainment of an adequate age for fusion, (2) failure of the curve to respond to bracing, or (3) skin problems making bracing impossible. The results of brace treatment have been analyzed by Bunch[7] and by Johnston and associates,[25] who reviewed 15 myelomeningocoele patients having an average pre-bracing scoliosis of 43 degrees. They had an average curve of 26 degrees in the brace and 39 degrees at the most recent follow-up. The average duration of bracing was 4.5 years, and no brace was discontinued because of sores (Figs. 14–5 and 14–6).

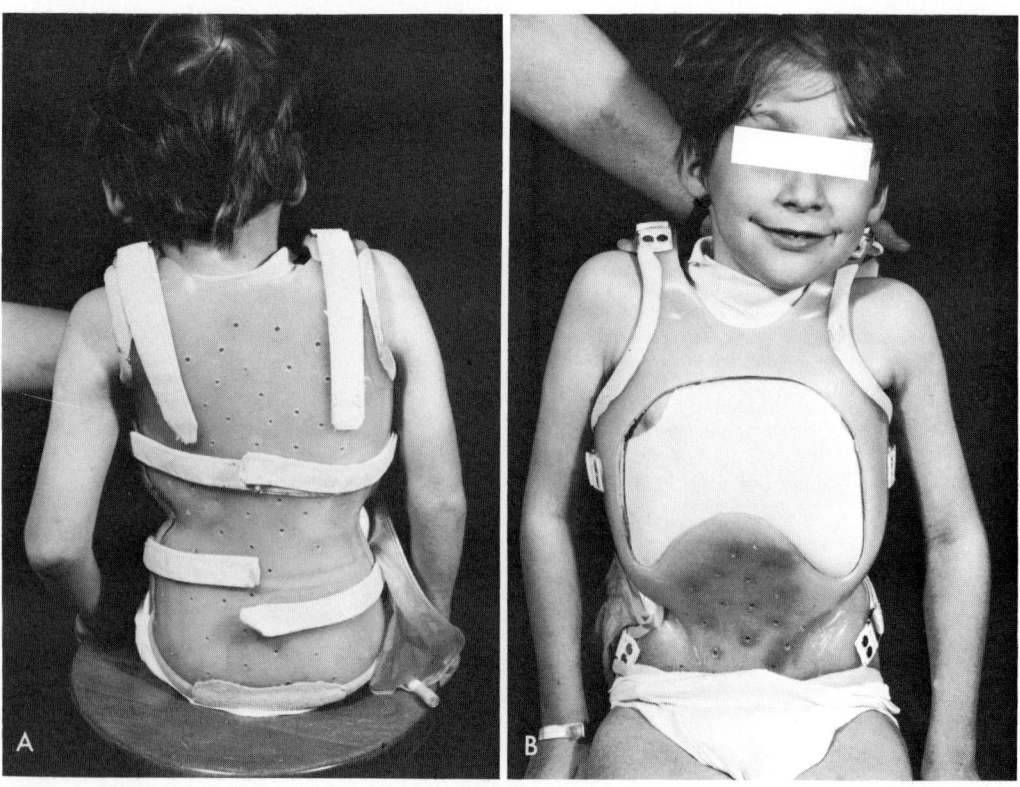

Figure 14–5. Views of a bivalved polypropylene body jacket. *A*, PA view. *B*, AP view.

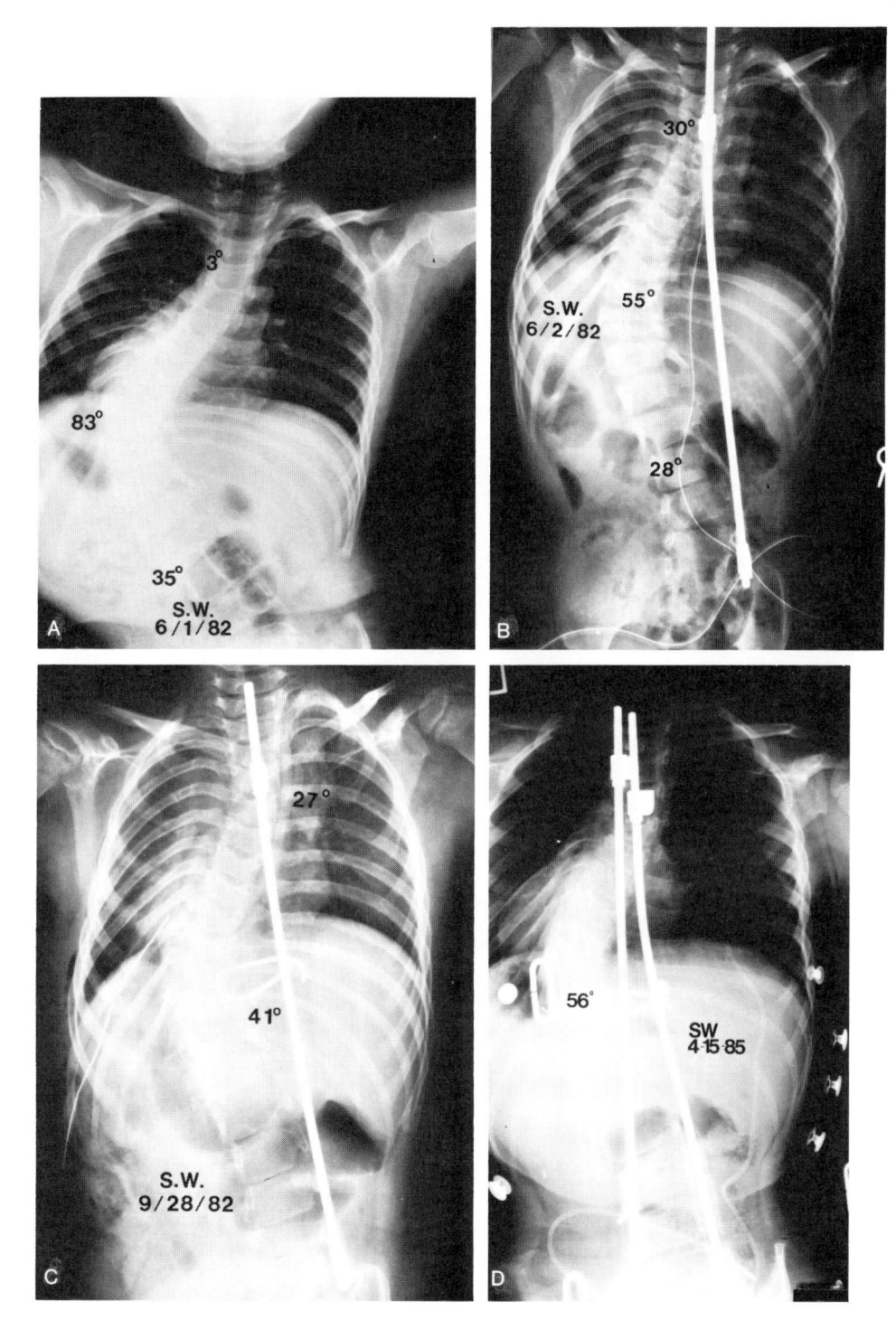

Figure 14–6. A, This 6 year old female had a progressive developmental scoliosis of 83 degrees. This amount of curvature is beyond brace treatment. A fusion at this age would result in excessive stunting of trunk length. B, A subcutaneous rod was inserted, the upper hook under the lamina of T3 and the lower hook on the ala of the sacrum. The pelvic obliquity was slightly overcorrected (as planned). The curve was corrected to 55 degrees. Only a minimal amount of force can be placed on these soft, small bones. C, Three months after the first procedure, the rod was lengthened, an apical sublaminar wire added, and an anterior convex epiphyseodesis-arthrodesis was done at the apex of the curve in order to slow down the excessive convex growth (and to help a developing thoracic lordosis). D, At her most recent follow-up, the curve is being successfully controlled at 56 degrees. A second subcutaneous rod has been added for greater internal support. She uses an underarm orthosis during all upright activities.

RODDING WITHOUT FUSION

What should be done for the child with a paralytic curve that is progressing despite brace treatment? If it has not already been done, Metrizamide myelography should be done to rule out a hydromyelia. If the child is only 7 or 8 years old, it is best to delay fusion by utilizing rodding without fusion combined with continued brace support. Preliminary placement of bone grafts at the site of future hook placement is often desireable because of the soft bone and hypoplastic alar development (Fig. 14–7).

OPERATIVE TREATMENT

Preoperative Evaluation

Once the decision has been made that surgery is indicated, it is imperative that a general evaluation be made concerning the patient's ability to successfully tolerate the procedure. The critical areas are (1) the hydrocephalus and shunt function, (2) the presence or absence of urinary tract infection, and (3) the quality of the skin in the areas of intended surgery.

Any hydrocephalus should be stable or well controlled by shunting. The urinary tract should be free of obstructive uropathy, and ideally the urine should be sterile. Often one has to operate even though the urinary tract is infected, but the organism should be known, and adequate control achieved with appropriate antibiotics. The surgery must be done with antibiotic prophylaxis, and the antibiotic selected must be demonstrated by appropriate sensitivity tests to be bacteriocidal for the organism present. Failure to adequately protect the urinary tract can lead to a disastrous infection rate.[24]

If the skin is contaminated in the area of intended surgery (the greatest danger is an old, scarred sac), appropriate plastic skin procedures should be done first in order to have clean skin of good quality.

Selection of the Fusion Area (Paralytic Deformities)

The area of fusion should be determined prior to surgery; selection is based on both clinical and radiologic criteria. Most patients with paralytic deformities require fusion from the upper thorax (T2) to the sacrum.[6] As stated previously, the goal is to achieve *a vertical torso centered over a level pelvis.*[26, 33] There are occasional patients with good muscular control of the thorax who require a lesser fusion, but these are the exceptions.

Selection of the Fusion Area (Congenital Scoliosis)

This is discussed in Chapter 12, pp. 233–269, the chapter on congenital spine deformities. The neuromuscular component of the curvature is fused according to the rules listed there.

Selection of the Operative Technique (Paralytic Scoliosis and Lordoscoliosis)

It is difficult to be dogmatic on this subject, since there are many different forms and severities of the deformity as well as different forms of treatment.[3, 11, 14, 45] In a major paper reviewing the surgical treatment of paralytic scoliosis in myelomeningocoele, Osebold and coworkers[34] found the best results to be in those patients who had both anterior and posterior fusion combined with both anterior and posterior instrumentation. These patients had the best amount of correction achieved, the best maintenance of correction, the best correction of pelvic obliquity, and the least percentage of pseudarthrosis (it was still 23 per cent!). The posterior instrumentation in this series was all with Harrington rods, and the anterior fixation with either Dwyer or Zielke devices. Almost all of the pseudarthroses were at the lumbosacral (L4-L5 or L5-S1) level.

Because of the high incidence of pseudarthrosis at the lumbosacral level, others have suggested modifications of technique in order to conquer this problem. The first alteration is the extension of the anterior fusion down to S1, removing both the L4-L5 and the L5-S1 discs, packing them with autogenous bone grafts, and if possible extending the anterior fixation to the sacrum. This is not always possible, since the great vessels may lie directly on the screw heads, and eventually the vessel walls may erode (death from vascular erosion at this site has been reported).

Second is the attempt to achieve better

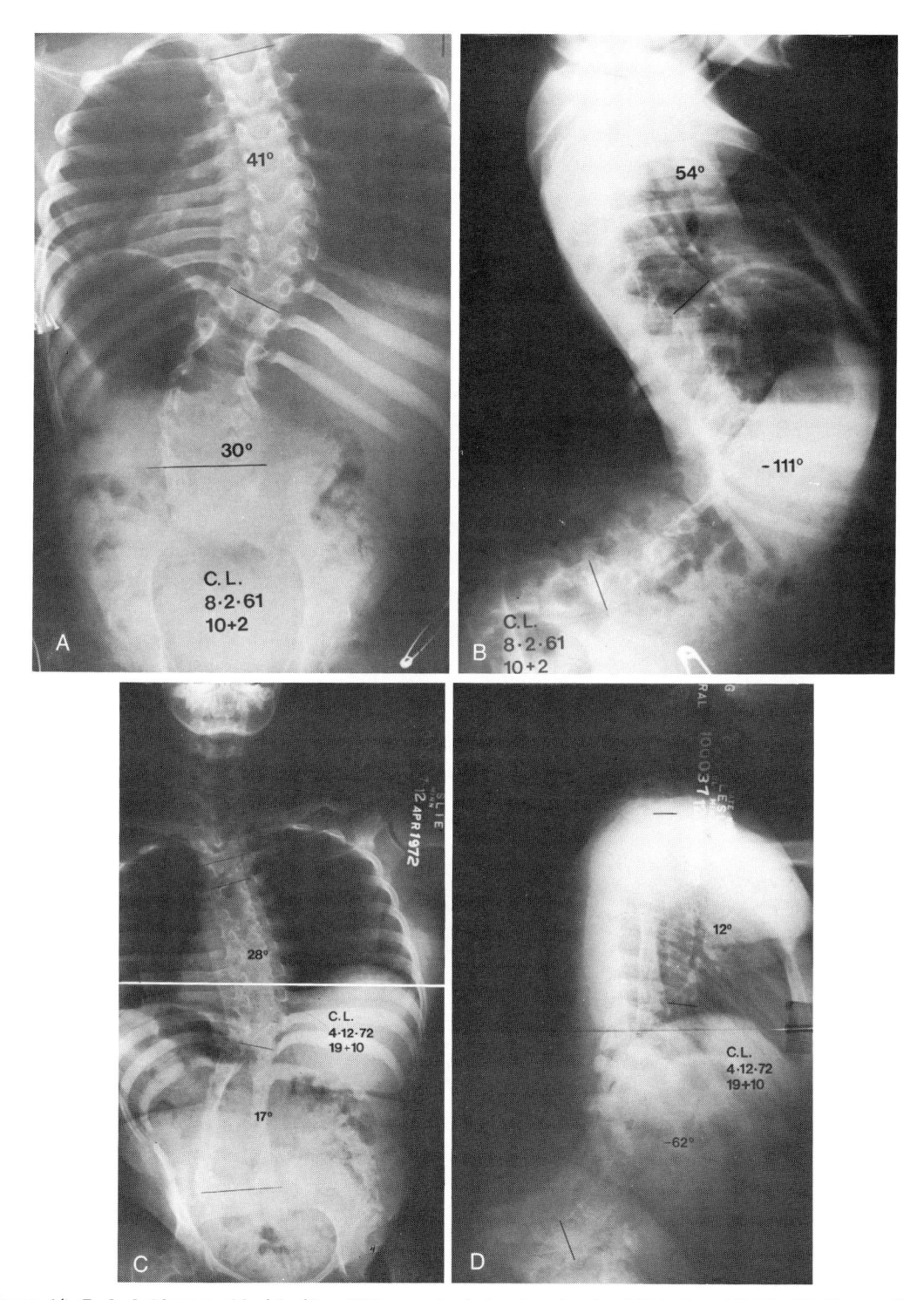

Figure 14–7. *A*, A 10 year old girl with a T11 neurologic level and spina bifida from T11 to S2. Her scolioses were 41 degrees at T2 to T11, and 30 degrees at T11 to L5. Despite the high neurologic lesion, she had never had hydrocephalus and had a normal I.Q. *B*, Although her scolioses were significant, her primary clinical deformity was this −111 degree thoracolumbar lordosis. She was fused in 1961 from T2 to the sacrum with cast correction. *C*, At a nine year follow-up, her fusion is solid and the scolioses are 28 degrees and 17 degrees. The thoracic fusion was in the midline, and the lumbar spine by transverse process fusions were done through separate incisions one month apart. No instrumentation was used. *D*, A lateral view at age 19 shows the residual −62 degree thoracolumbar lordosis. She is still alive and with a solid fusion at age 34 (1986).

fixation to the pelvis. Even in patients with normal bone development (e.g., poliomyelitis, cerebral palsy) fusion to the sacrum is difficult. The spina bifida patient with a hypoplastic sacrum and hypoplastic iliac crests has a uniquely challenging fixation problem. Most experts in the field would probably agree that the ideal fixation method is yet to be discovered.

The development of the Galveston technique of insertion of Luque rods into the pelvis has provided a form of fixation superior to a single Harrington rod and sacral alar hook (see Chapter 10, p. 153). This technique was developed by Allen and Ferguson, and their first six myelomeningocoele patients were reported in 1979.[1]

With the development of Luque rods, it has become less important to use anterior fixation, unless the spina bifida extends through the entire lumbar spine. The anterior fusion is still very important, both for its arthrodesis effect as well as for its ability to make the curve more flexible.

The major problem with the Luque procedure appears to be the hypoplasia and osteoporosis of the iliac wings. The rods can migrate in the bone and even break through the thin cortices. The second problem is the difficulty obtaining secure wire fixation to the lower lumbar vertebrae when the laminae are absent.

Dunn[15] has suggested a modification of the Luque technique in which the lower end of the Luque rod is pre-bent to curve over the sacral alae and then pass downward either within or anterior to the sacrum.

If laminae are present, sublaminar wiring can be done in the usual manner. If the only laminae absent are those at L4, L5, and S1, wiring of these levels can be ignored. If virtually all of the lumbar laminae are absent, some attempt is usually made to achieve segmental fixation. A wire can be passed around a pedicle, twisted on itself, and then twisted around the rod. If the pedicle is large enough, a screw can be passed down the pedicle into the vertebral body (remember the oblique path of these pedicles) and the wire twisted around the screw head and the rod (Figs. 14–8 to Fig. 14–10).

Selection of Surgical Technique (Congenital Scoliosis)

Most patients with congenital scoliosis in addition to the paralaytic scoliosis will require early fusion of the congenital deformity

Text continued on page 327

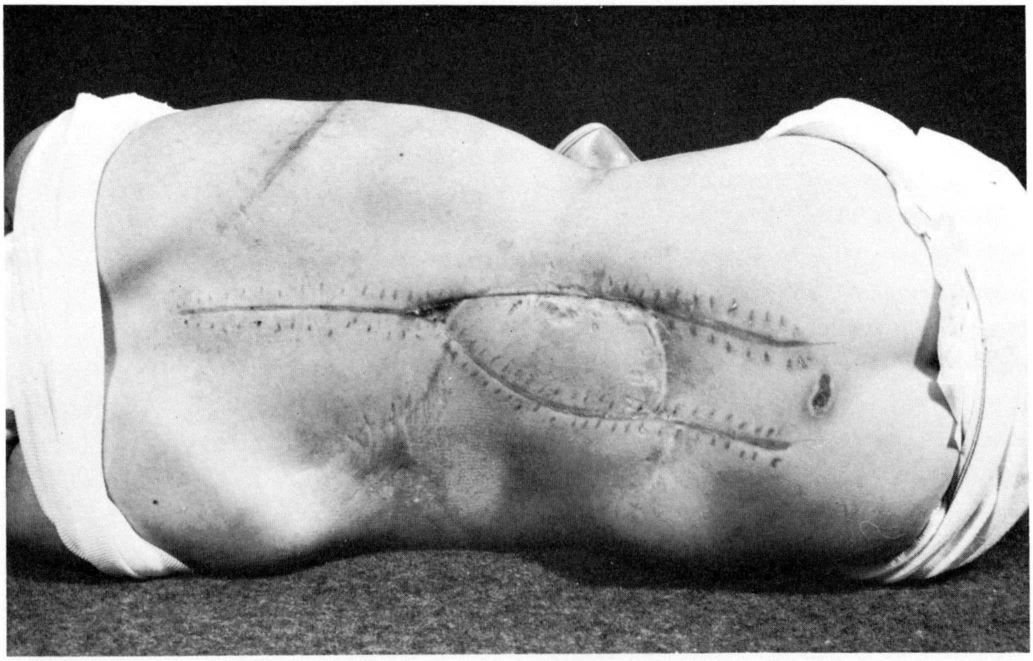

Figure 14–8. Posterior photograph of a patient three weeks following posterior spine fusion with instrumentation from T3 to the sacrum. An anterior fusion of the thoracic spine had been done two weeks previously. This "inverted Y" incision has been useful in approaching the transverse processes and avoiding the midline sac area. The midline lumbar area is not undermined.

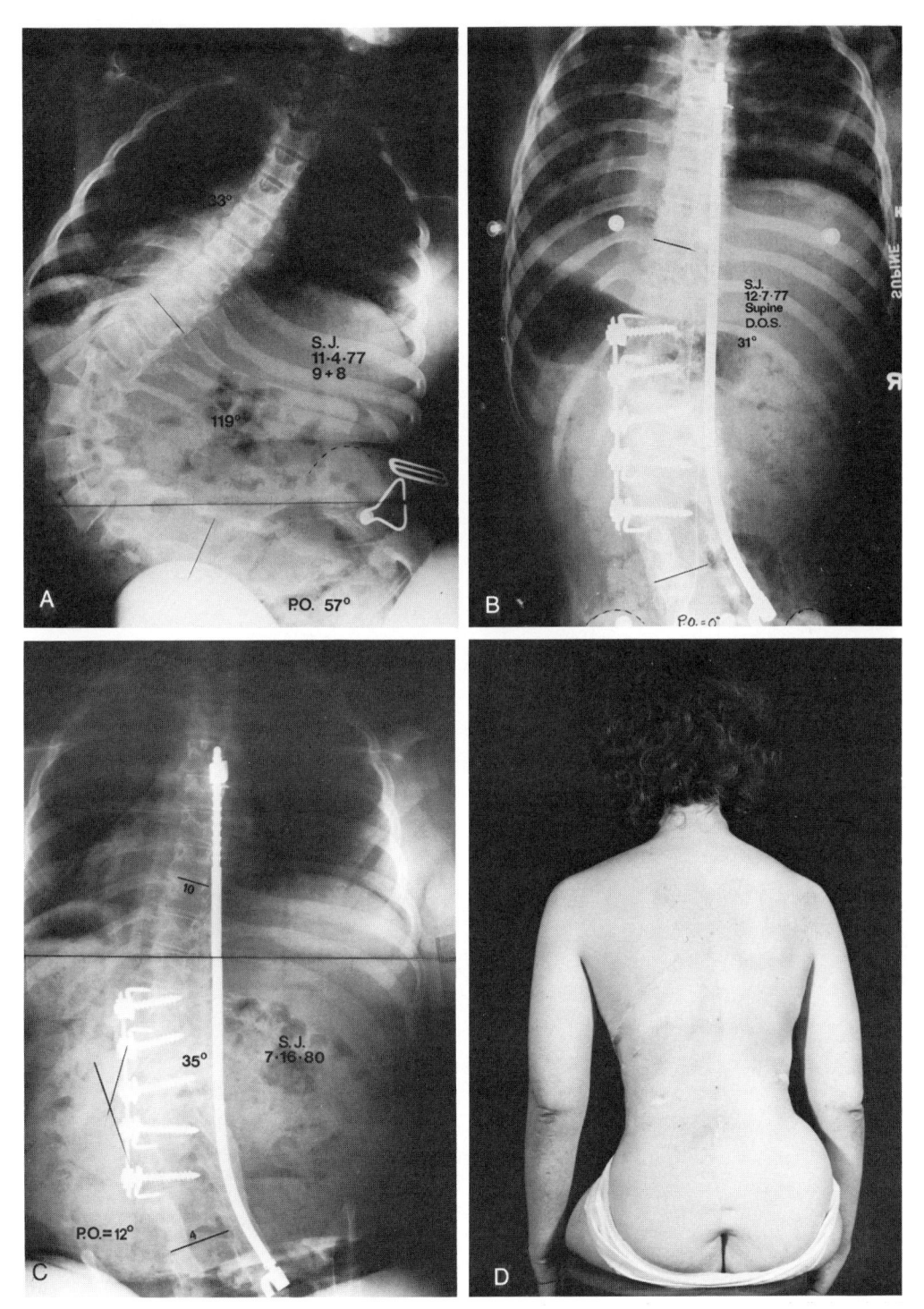

Figure 14–9. *A*, A 9+8 year old girl (bone age 12) with a rapidly progressive curve of 119 degrees. Note the lack of wedging of the vertebral bodies and that all the deformity is in the disc spaces. Her pelvic obliquity is 57 degrees. Combined anterior and posterior surgery is mandatory in such a case. *B*, She underwent a five level Zielke procedure (a screw could not be placed in a more distal vertebra owing to an abnormally placed common iliac vein), and two weeks later a Harrington procedure. The scoliosis was corrected to 31 degrees and the pelvic obliquity to zero. *C*, At a three year follow-up, the scoliosis was 35 degrees, the pelvic obliquity 12 degrees, and the fusion solid. *D*, A photograph at follow-up showing the excellent torso balance. She can now sit without using her arms or hands for balance. (Reprinted with permission from Osebold, W., et al.: Surgical treatment of paralytic scoliosis in myelomeningocoele. J. Bone Joint Surg., *64A*:841–856, 1982.)

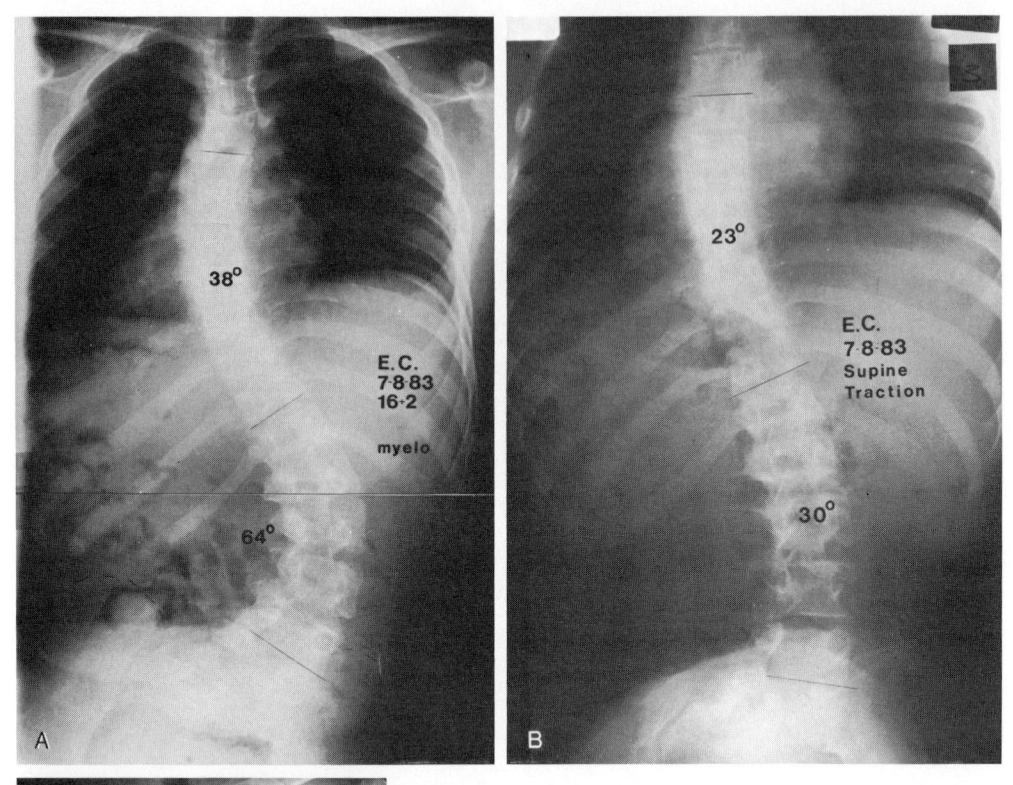

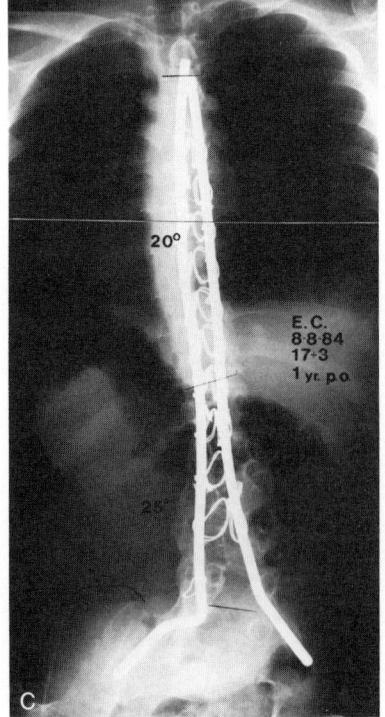

Figure 14–10. A, This 16 year old male presented with an increasing scoliosis, now measuring 64 degrees. There was a 38 degree compensatory scoliosis of the thoracic spine and a significant pelvic obliquity, the left side being higher. B, A traction film on the Risser table showed correction of the two curves to 23 degrees and 30 degrees. A slight pelvic obliquity remained. Laminae were absent at L4, L5, S1, and S2. Surgery consisted of anterior discectomy and fusion from T12 to S1 and two weeks later a posterior fusion from T3 to the sacrum with Luque rods. Bank bone was used for grafting. A plastic body jacket was worn for nine months. C, At a one year follow-up, the curves are 20 degrees and 25 degrees, the pelvis is level, and the fusion is solid.

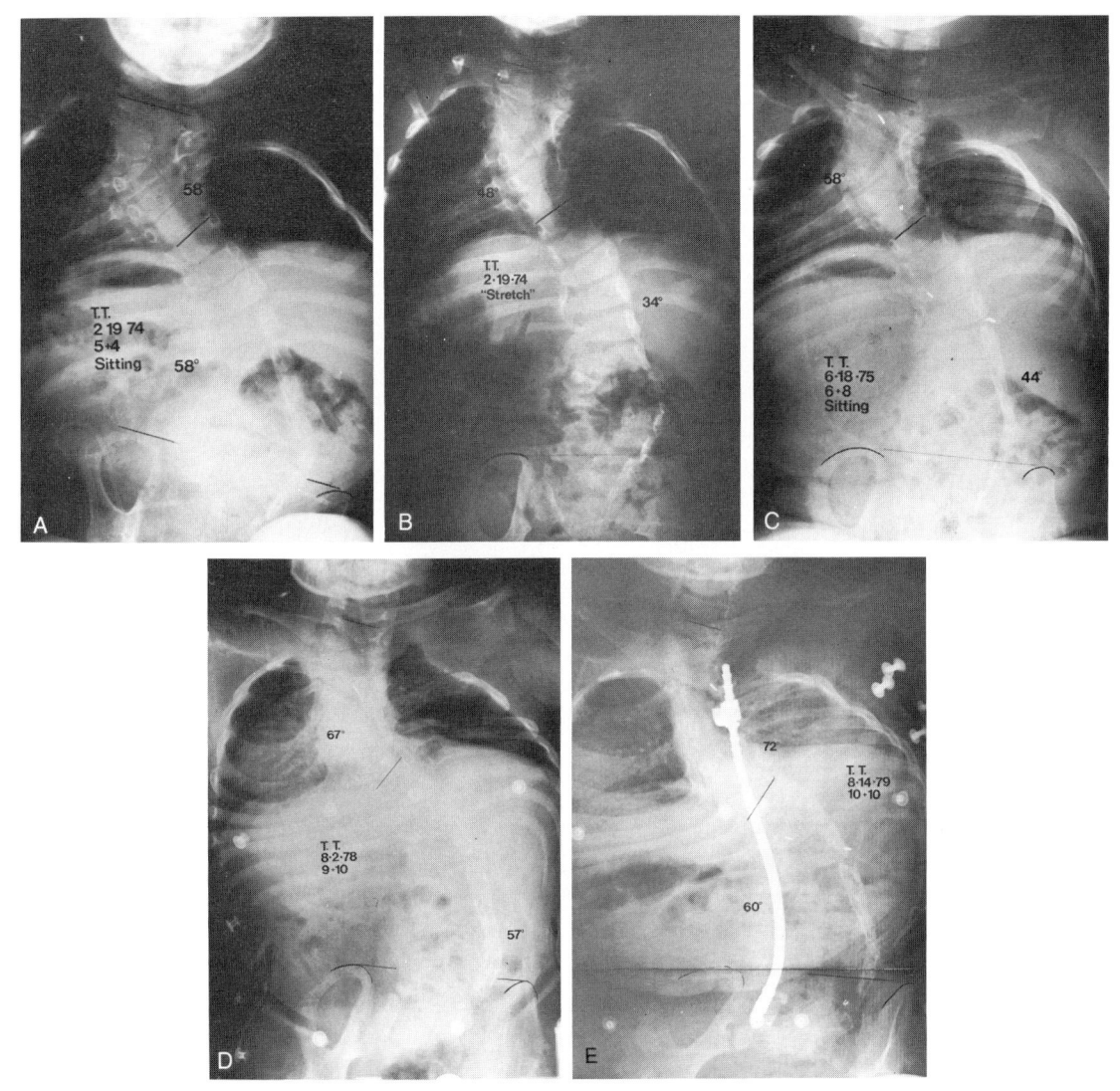

Figure 14–11. *A*, A 5-year old girl with myelomeningocoele and congenital scoliosis. She had two 58 degree congenital curves, one in the upper thoracic area with a unilateral unsegmented bar, and one in the lumbar spine with a hemivertebra. *B*, A supine "stretch" (traction) radiograph shows the greater rigidity of the upper curve and shows the lumbar congenital defects better. The curves are 48 degrees and 34 degrees. The patient underwent posterior fusion of the T1-T7 area and anterior and posterior fusion of the T11-S1 area with cast immobilization. *C*, One year after surgery, the curves are 58 degrees and 44 degrees. The fusions appear solid. *D*, This radiograph at age 9+10 shows the curves were increasing, the deformity occurring primarily in the unfused segments between the two fused areas. Additional surgery to correct and connect the two fusions was planned. *E*, One year later the curves are 72 degrees and 60 degrees; the upper curve was increasing because of extension into the cervical spine. This case demonstrates well the ongoing and difficult challenges of the myelomeningocoele spine, especially in those with congenital anomalies. (Reprinted with permission from Winter, R. B.: Congenital Deformities of the Spine. New York, Thieme-Stratton, 1983.)

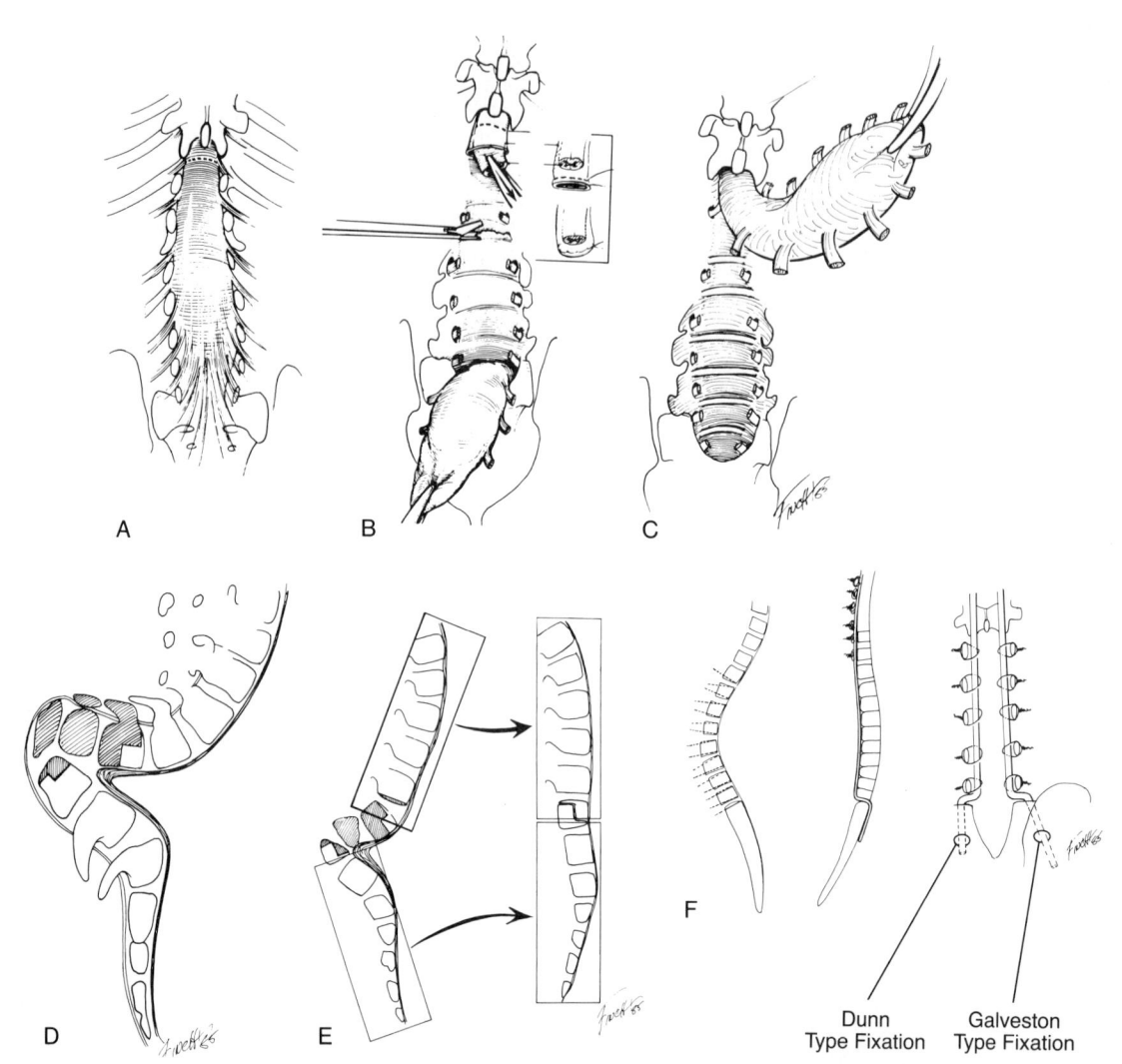

Figure 14–12. *A*, A typical total spina bifida of the lumbar spine as seen in a kyphotic patient. The dotted line shows the level of dural transection. *B*, The non-functional cord is transected and the dura is sutured *distal* to the cord transection. The central canal of the cord must be left open to communicate with the subdural space. The nerve roots are transected at each foramen. The discs are removed from behind. *C*, An alternative technique is the distal detachment of the neural sac and progressive upward dissection with division of the nerve roots at the level of the foramen. The sac is not entered, and the cord is not transected. The risks of acute hydrocephalus are reduced and the sac is laid down over the instrumentation, providing better coverage. *D*, A typical rigid myelomeningocoele kyphosis. The hatched area represents the vertebrae to be resected, always the ones between the apex of the kyphosis and the apex of the lordosis. *E*, The general principle is to relate the distal segment (the sacrum and lower lumbar vertebrae) to the proximal segment (the thorax) so that the two are in a stable vertical relationship. The anterior longitudinal ligament is preserved as the hinge upon which the segments are aligned. *F*, In the more flexible types of kyphosis, the discs are removed along with a thin wedge of bone from the adjacent vertebral bodies. Every effort should be made to achieve normal sagittal alignment. The type of instrumentation varies greatly, and is dependent on local anatomy problems.

MYELOMENINGOCOELE

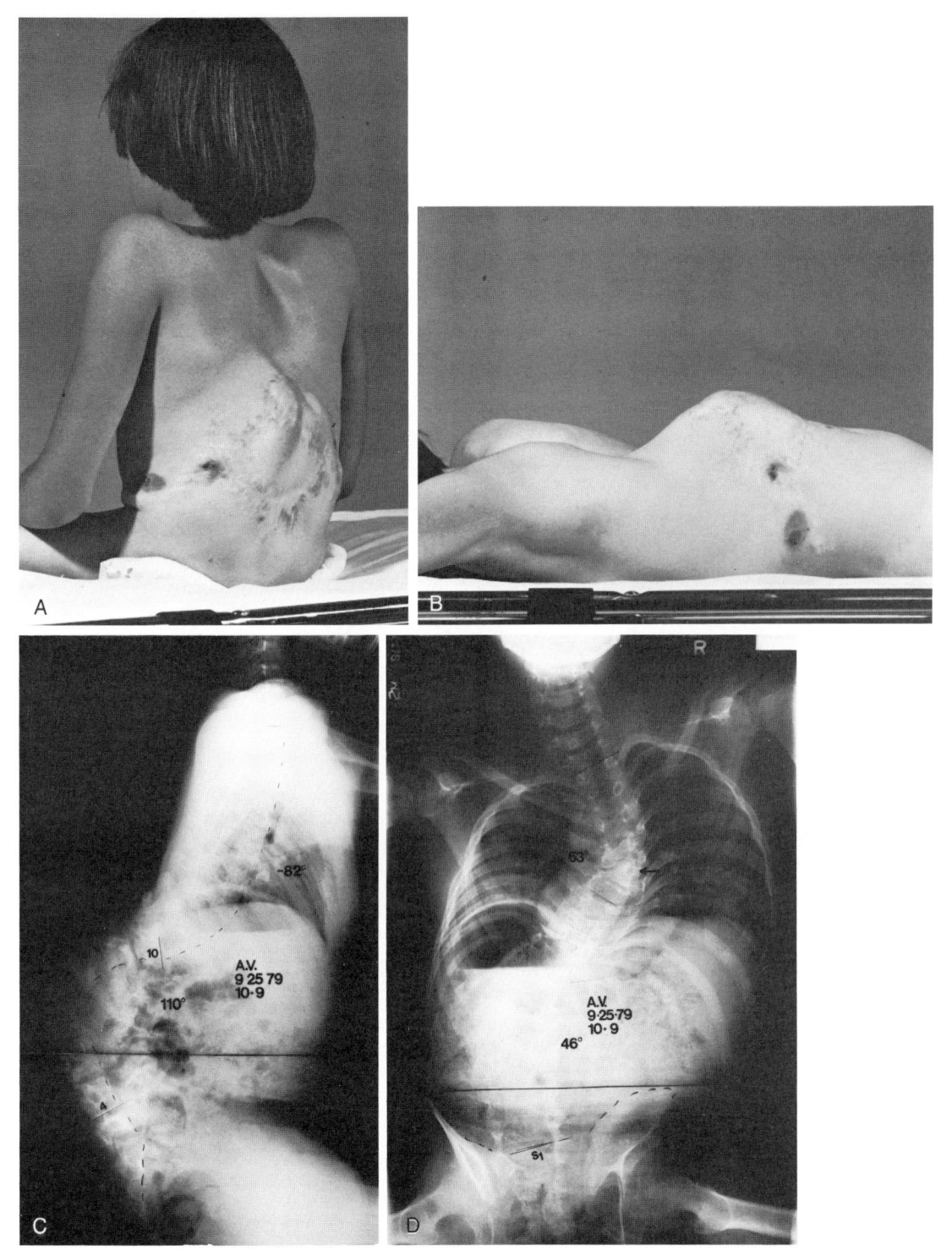

Figure 14–13. *A* A posterior oblique photograph of a 10+9 year old girl with a T12 level neurologic defect, a severe upper lumbar kyphosis, and severe thoracic lordosis. She had a normal I.Q. and attended regular school. *B*, A prone view shows the severe kyphosis and its clinical rigidity. *C*, Her lateral sitting x-ray shows a 110 degree thoracolumbar kyphosis and a −82 degree thoracic lordosis. The horizontally oriented vertebrae are T10, T11, and T12. *D*, Her AP sitting x-ray revealed a hemivertebra on the right at T5 with a 63 degree thoracic scoliosis and a 46 degree thoracolumbar scoliosis.

Illustration continued on following page

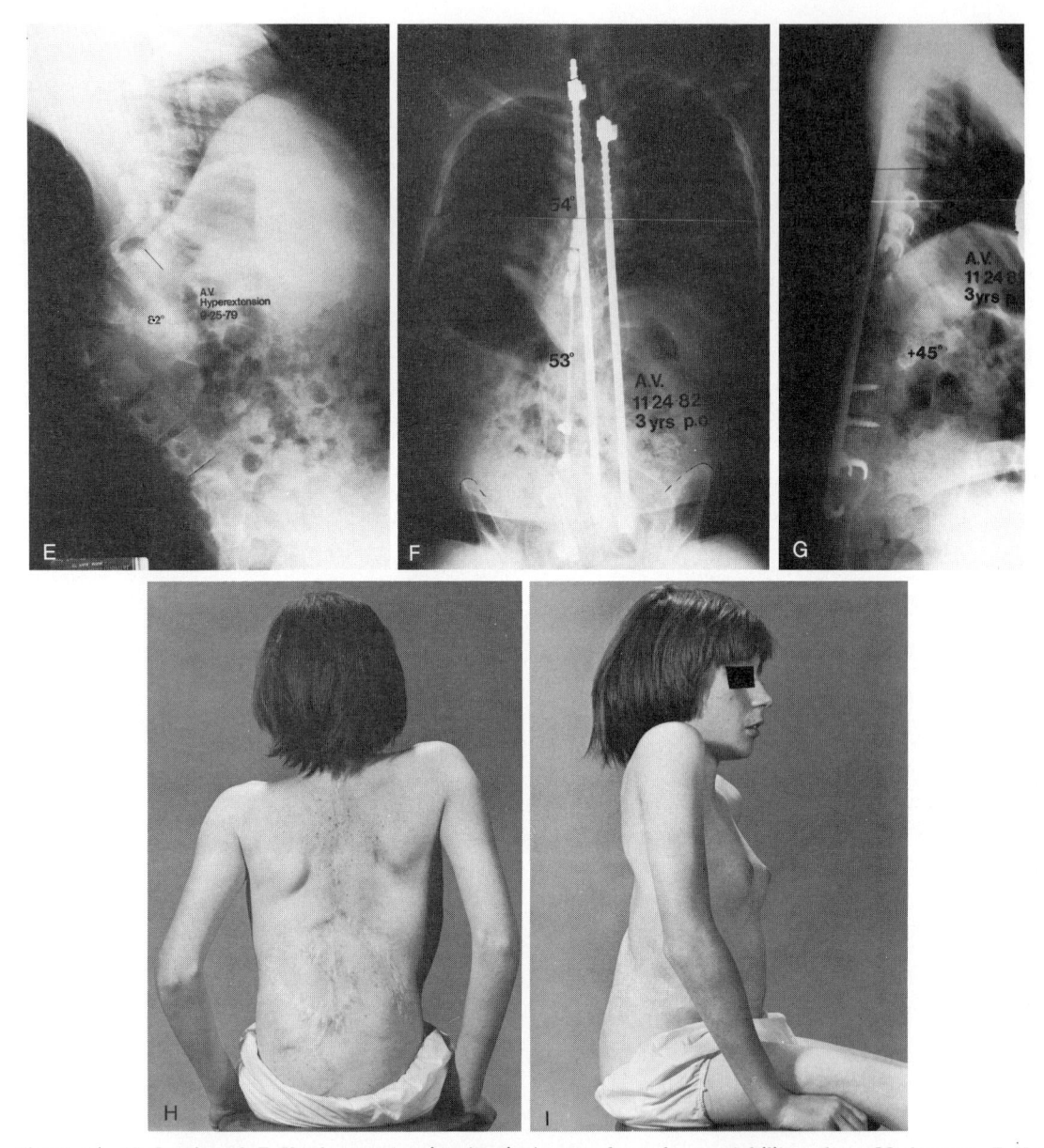

Figure 14–13 *Continued.* *E,* Her hyperextension (supine) x-ray showed correctability only to 82 degrees. *F,* Her surgery was done in one stage, and consisted of making a long posterior incision, resection of the non-functional dural sac, division of the cord proximal to the dural suture, excision of T11 and T12, and insertion of a posterior compression system using hooks (Titanium) and a Dwyer cable, two long distraction rods (T1 to L5 and T2 to S1), and a short compression rod (L5 to S1). This film is at the three-year follow-up. *G,* A lateral film three years post-surgery shows a balanced spine, with −62 degrees thoracic lordosis and +45 degrees lumbar kyphosis. If I were to do this case now (1986), a preliminary removal of the thoracic discs would be added, plus sublaminar wiring in the thoracic spine in order to obtain better correction of the thoracic lordosis. *H,* A posterior photograph one year after surgery. *I,* A lateral photograph one year after surgery.

MYELOMENINGOCOELE

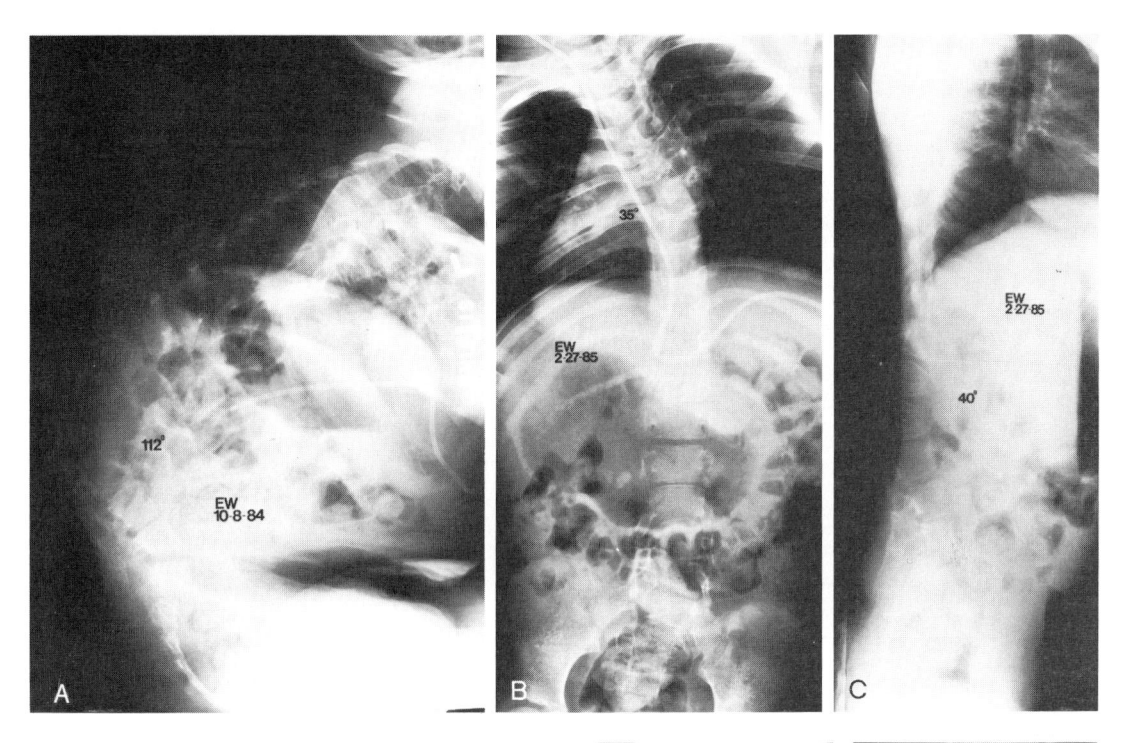

Figure 14–14. *A*, An 8 year old female with a severe 112 degree thoracolumbar kyphosis. *B*, An AP radiograph showing a 35 degree congenital thoracic scoliosis, no lumbar scoliosis, and a mild pelvic obliquity. *C*, A hyperextension radiograph demonstrates a relatively flexible kyphosis of 40 degrees. With this amount of flexibility, excision of whole vertebrae is not necessary, but rather excision of the discs along with a small wedge of bone above and below the discs is sufficient. *D*, At surgery, the sac was excised, the discs and wedges of bone removed, and internal fixation accomplished with Luque rods and Dunn type distal rod placement. *E*, An AP view at surgery shows the Luque rods, the distal rod bending to fit over the sacral alae, and the lumbar segmental fixation with wires around the pedicles.

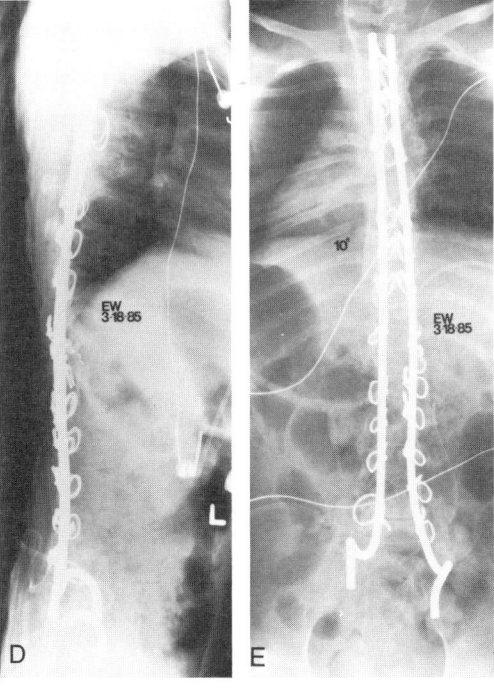

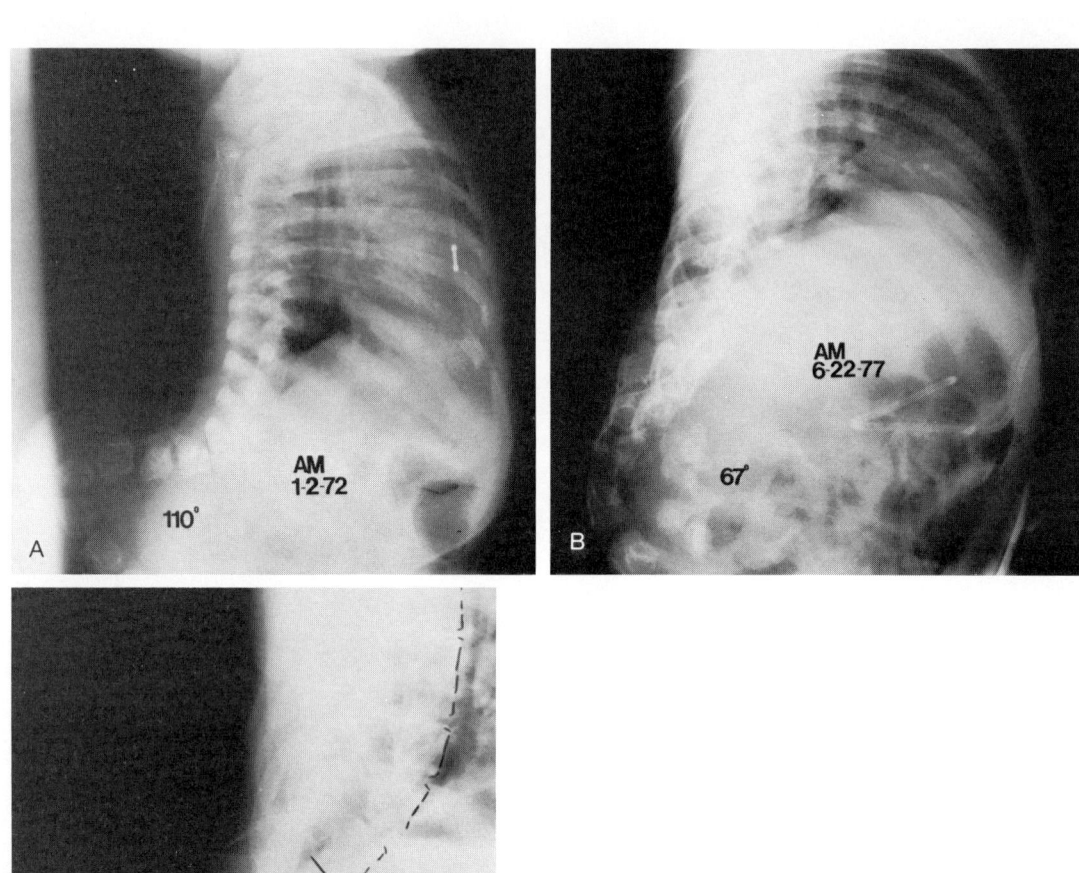

Figure 14–15. *A,* Preoperative photograph. *B,* Immediate postoperative photograph. *C,* Follow-up photograph. (Courtesy of Dr. Richard Lindseth.)

and late fusion of the paralytic deformity. If there is a lumbar hemivertebra accentuating the paralytic pelvis obliquity, hemivertebra resection is important in order to achieve a level pelvis (Fig. 14–11).

Postoperative Management

Plaster casts are difficult to apply, prevent adequate skin observation, and are too heavy for these handicapped children. Thus, plastic body jackets, identical to those used for nonoperative treatment, are used following surgery. Because of the problems of pseudarthrosis at the lumbosacral area, the brace should be built very low, covering the buttocks, symphysis pubis, and trochanters, but cut adequately in front of the thighs to allow 90 degrees of hip flexion for adequate sitting. We have often attached thigh cuffs with hip joints to the spinal orthosis in order to add more pelvic stabilization.

Some authors have attempted to treat these patients without external protection when using Luque fixation. As yet there is no documentation that this is effective in a significant series of patients.

Selection of Operative Technique (Kyphosis)

If the treatment of myelomeningocoele scoliosis is difficult, the treatment of myelomeningocoele kyphosis is the ultimate challenge to the spinal surgeon. Most of the patients have high level (T12 or higher) neurologic deficits, very major deformities, rigid deformities, and very little good bone with which to work.[4, 12, 17, 23, 40]

Lindseth and Stelzer reported in 1979 a procedure for the younger child with significant and progressive kyphosis.[28] A limited excision of the apical vertebra is performed, along with positions of the adjacent two vertebrae, and the gap is closed by wiring together the pedicles. The anteriorly displaced erector spinae muscles are sutured more posteriorly after resecting the flared-out laminae.

In the first 30 patients treated by this technique (average follow-up 6 years), only 10 have progressed more than 10 degrees, and only three of these 10 have required additional surgery.[27, 28] Those done before age 2½ have had the best results, none requiring further surgery. The worst results were those done in the teenage years. The youngest done was at age 14 months. The procedure works best if there is a severe lordotic curve just above the kyphosis.

The older child with a major deformity requires a complex reconstruction in which the deformed area is radically resected and the proximal and distal segments of the spine are reconnected with metallic implants. To accomplish this, the non-functional spinal cord and dural sac remnants are resected or reflected, allowing circumferential exposure of the spine from posteriorly. Acute hydrocephalus is a possible complication of this technique.[44] It is tempting to consider lengthening of the front of the spine rather than shortening posteriorly, but often the congenitally short and bowstringed aorta prevents this.[35] McKay[32] has reported a small series of patients treated with anterior ligament release, anterior discectomy and fusion, a large anterior plate, and bolts coming from posteriorly to the plate to pull the spine to the plate. The author has had no experience with this technique.

Most authors have favored the posterior approach with preservation of the anterior longitudinal ligament as the "hinge" on which the spine is corrected. Fusion to the sacrum is mandatory. Various forms of internal fixation have been devised, including Harrington compression rods,[19, 20, 37, 38] compression hooks on Dwyer cables[30] and Luque rods,[5, 15] (Figs. 14–12 to 14–15).

References

1. Allen, B., and Ferguson, R.: Operative treatment of myelomeningocoele spinal deformities. Orthop. Clin. North Am., 10:845–862, 1979.
2. Banta, J. V., Whiteman, S., Dyck, P. M., et al.: Fifteen year review of myelodysplasia. J. Bone Joint Surg., 58A:726, 1976.
3. Banta, J., and Park, S. M.: Improvement in pulmonary function in patients having combined anterior and posterior spine fusion for myelomeningocoele scoliosis. Spine, 8:766–770, 1983.
4. Barson, A. J.: Radiological studies of spina bifida cystica: the phenomenon of congenital lumbar kyphosis. Br. J. Radiol., 38:294–300, 1065.
5. Bodel, J. G., and Stephane, J. P.: Luque rods in the treatment of kyphosis in myelomeningocoele. J. Bone Joint Surg., 65B:98, 1983.
6. Brown, H. P.: Management of spinal deformity in myelomeningocoele. Orthop. Clin. North Am., 9:391–402, 1978.

7. Bunch, W. H.: The Milwaukee brace in paralytic scoliosis. Clin. Orthop., *110*:63–68, 1975.
8. Bunch, W. H.: Myelomeningocoele patients should not lose function. Orthop. Trans., *3*:444, 1981.
9. Bunch, W. H.: Myelomeningocoele. In Loell, O., and Winter, R. B. (eds.): Pediatric Orthopaedics, 2nd Ed., Philadelphia, J. B. Lippincott, 1986.
10. Charney, E. B., McMorron, M., and Bruce, D. A.: Assessment of spinal deformities in children with myelomeningocoele. Orthop. Trans., *8*:116, 1984.
11. Dickens, D. V. R.: The surgery of scoliosis and spina bifida. J. Bone Joint Surg., *61B*:386, 1979.
12. Drennan, J. C.: The role of muscle in the development of human lumbar kyphosis. Devel. Med. Child. Neurol., *12*:33–38, 1970.
13. Drennan, J. C.: Orthotic management of the myelomeningocoele spine. Dev. Med. Child. Neurol. (Suppl.), *37*:97, 1976.
14. Drummond, D. S., Morear, M., and Cruess, R. L.: The results and complications of surgery for the paralytic hip and spine in myelomeningocoele. J. Bone Joint Surg., *62B*:49, 1980.
15. Dunn, H. K.: Kyphosis of myelodysplasia, operative treatment based on pathophysiology. Orthop. Trans., *7*:19–20, 1983.
16. Emergy, J. L., and Lendon, R. G.: Clinical implications of cord lesions in neurospinal dysraphism. Develop. Med. Child. Neurol., *14*:45–51, 1972.
17. Gillespie, R., Torode, I., and van Olm, R. S. Jr.: Myelomeningocoele kyphosis fixed by kypectomy and segmental spinal instrumentation. Orthop. Trans., *8*:162–163, 1984.
18. Hall, J. E., and Martin, R.: The natural history of spine deformity in myelomeningocoele. A study of 130 patients. Presented to the Canadian Orthopaedic Association, Bermuda, June 1970.
19. Hall, J. E., and Bobechko, W. P.: Advances in the management of spinal deformities in myelodysplasia. Clin. Neurosurg., *20*:164–173, 1973.
20. Hall, J. E., and Poitras, B.: The management of kyphosis in patients with myelomeningocoele. Clin. Orthop., *128*:33, 1977.
21. Hall, P. V., Lindseth, R. E., Campbell, R., L., and Kalsbeck, J. E.: Myelodysplasia and developmental scoliosis, a manifestation of syringomyelia. Spine, *1*:48–56, 1976.
22. Hall, P. V., Lindseth, R. E., Campbell, R., et al.: Scoliosis and hydrocephalus in myelocoele patients: the effect of ventricular shunting. J. Neurosurg., *50*:174–178, 1979.
23. Hoppenfeld, S.: Congenital kyphosis in myelomeningocoele. J. Bone Joint Surg., *49B*:276–280, 1967.
24. Hull, W. J., Moe, J. H., and Winter, R. B.: Spinal deformity in myelomeningocoele: natural history, evaluation, and treatment. J. Bone Joint Surg., *56A*:1767, 1974.
25. Johnston, C. E., 3, Hakala, M. W., and Rosenberg, R.: Paralytic spinal deformity: orthotic treatment in spinal discontinuity syndromes. J. Pediatr. Orthop., *2*:233–241, 1982.
26. Kilfoyle, R. M., Foley, J. J., and Norton, P. L.: Spine and pelvic deformity in childhood and adolescent paraplegia: a study of 104 cases. J. Bone Joint Surg., *47A*:659–682, 1976.
27. Lindseth, R.: Personal communication. 1985.
28. Lindseth, R. E., and Selzer, L: Vertebral excision of kyphosis in myelomeningocoele. J. Bone Joint Surg., *61A*:699–704, 1979.
29. Mackel, J. L., and Lindseth, R. E.: Scoliosis in myelodysoplasia. J. Bone Joint Surg., *57A*:1031, 1975.
30. Mayfield, J. K.: Severe spine deformity in myelodysplasia and sacral agenesis: an aggressive surgical approach. Spine, *6*:498–509, 1981.
31. McGuire, C. D., Winter, R. B., Mayfield, J. K., and Erickson, D. L.: Hemimyelodysplasia: a report of ten cases. J. Pediatr. Orthop. *2*:9–14, 1982.
32. McKay, D. A.: The McKay plate for kyphosis of the spine. Presented at the Annual Meeting of the Scoliosis Research Society, Louisville, September, 1975.
33. Menelaus, M. B.: Orthopaedic management of children with myelomeningocoele: a plea for realistic goals. Dev. Med. Child. Neurol., *18* (Suppl. 37):3–11, 1976.
34. Osebold, W., Mayfield, J. K., Winter, R. B., and Moe, J. H.: Surgical treatment of paralytic scoliosis in myelomeningocoele. J. Bone Joint Surg., *64A*:841–856, 1982.
35. Park, W. M., and Watt, I.: The preoperative aortographic assessment of children with spina bifida cystica and severe kyphosis. J. Bone Joint Surg., *57B*:112, 1975.
36. Piggott, H.: The natural history of scoliosis in myelodysplasia. J. Bone Joint Surg., *61B*:122, 1979.
37. Poitras, B., and Hall, J. E.: The management of kyphosis in patients with myelomeningocoele. Clin. Orthop., *128*:33–40, 1977.
38. Poitras, B., Rivard, C., Duhaime, M., et al.: Correction of the kyphosis in myelomeningocoele patients by both anterior and posterior stabilization procedure. Orthop. Trans., *7*:432, 1983.
39. Raycroft, J. F., and Curtis, B. H.: Spinal curvature in myelomeningocoele. Am. Acad. Orthop. Surg. Symposium on Myelomeningocoele, St. Louis, C. V., Mosby Co., 1972.
40. Rose, G. K., Owen, R., and Sanderson, J. M.: Transposition of rib and blood supply for stabilization of spinal kyphosis. J. Bone Joint Surg., *57B*:112, 1975.
41. Roth, K.: Spinal deformities in myelomeningocoele: a radiologic assessment. Harrington, P. R. (ed.): Scoliosis. pp. 1–29, 1971.
42. Shurtleff, D. B., Goiney, R., Gordon, L. H., and Livermore, N.: Myelodysplasia: the natural history of kyphosis and scoliosis. Develop. Med. Child. Neurol., *18* (Suppl. 37):126–133, 1976.
43. Sriram, K., Bobechko, W. P., and Hall, J. E.: Surgical management of spinal deformities in spina bifida. J. Bone Joint Surg., *54B*:666–676, 1972.
44. Winston, K., Hall, J. E., Johnson, D., and Micheli, L.: Acute elevation of intracranial pressure following transection of non-functional spinal cord. Clin. Orthop., *128*:41–44, 1977.

15

NEUROFIBROMATOSIS
John H. Moe, M.D.
Bruce E. van Dam, M.D.

INTRODUCTION

Neurofibromatosis is a genetically transmitted disease that results in a number of skeletal deformities of interest to the orthopaedic surgeon. Deformity of the spine is common with this diagnosis and may present a therapeutic challenge, especially when dystrophic bony change is present. Although the association of neurofibromatosis and spine deformity has been recognized since 1921, the treatment until recently was not well defined. Refinements of treatment will occur with further experience. Nevertheless, we believe that a successful outcome from operative and non-operative care of these spine deformities should now be common.

HISTORY

Wilhelm G. Telesius von Tilenau, in 1793, submitted the earliest clinical description of neurofibromatosis.[55] In addition to the cutaneous manifestations of the disease, his drawings also demonstrated a spinal deformity in the patient. Virchow described neurofibromatosis among members of the same family in 1847. Later, in 1863, he described in detail the pathology of the peripheral nerve tumors found in neurofibromatosis.[11] In 1849, R. W. Smith, Professor of Surgery at the Dublin Medical School, reported necropsy findings in two individuals with neurofibromatosis.[16] However, Frederick Daniel von Recklinghausen is given credit for first recognizing the essentials of this disease as a clinical entity. In 1882, he published his book "Ueber die multiplen Fibrome der Haut und ihre Beziehung zu den multiplen Neuromen" and introduced the term neurofibromatosis.[56] Von Recklinghausen recognized the hereditary nature of the disease and its variable expression. He demonstrated that in each instance where a cutaneous tumor was present a corresponding cutaneous nerve communicated with the tumor. Curiously, he made no mention of the presence of café-au-lait spots. However, he did note that others had mentioned skin pigmentation changes.[11] In 1909, Thomson also noted the hereditary pattern of the disease,[54] and in 1918, Preiser and Davenport described the heredity of the disease as being consistent with an autosomal dominant trait.[43]

In 1921, Weiss, a dermatologist, reported 15 cases of lateral curvature of the spine associated with neurofibromatosis. He gave credit to Engman, a fellow dermatologist, for pointing out this association. He stated in his article, "I merely wish to call attention to this observation, as its constant occurrence appears to be of some clinical significance. It seems to be a part of the syndrome in this peculiar disease." Three years later Brooks and Lehman published a comprehensive description of the skeletal deformities associated with neurofibromatosis. All seven of their cases had scoliosis.[4] Indeed, as multiple clinical studies have subsequently documented, abnormal spinal curvature is the most common skeletal abnormality in neurofibromatosis.[5, 17, 21, 25, 34, 48]

INCIDENCE

The incidence of neurofibromatosis in the general population is estimated to be 1:3,000.[45] It is as common in the general population as either cystic fibrosis or trisomy 21 and is more than twice as common as muscular dystrophy.[21] In a patient population of 10,000 with spinal deformity, the Twin Cities Scoliosis Center reported 102 patients having neurofibromatosis.[60] Out of 3,209 cases of scoliosis, Rezaian reported 98 patients with a diagnosis of neurofibromatosis.[44] Cotrel found neurofibromatosis in 65 patients during a review of 3,000 scoliosis cases.[10] In a group of 46 patients with the diagnosis of neurofibromatosis, McCarroll reported 19 with scoliosis.[34] Chaglassian reported 37 of 141 patients with a diagnosis of neurofibromatosis having scoliosis.[7] Other reports have documented the frequent association of scoliosis and kyphoscoliosis with neurofibromatosis.[4, 5, 17, 21, 25, 41, 47] Although it is an infrequent cause of spine deformity, neurofibromatosis is not a rare clinical entity. Moreover, in individuals having the diagnosis of neurofibromatosis, the occurrence of spine deformity is common.

PATHOGENESIS

Holt has defined neurofibromatosis as a hereditary, hamartomatous disorder, probably of neural crest origin, involving not only neuroectoderm and mesoderm but also endoderm, with the potential of appearing in any organ system of the body.[21] Moreover, all the cellular elements of the peripheral nerve have been demonstrated to play a part in the formation of the tumors found in neurofibromatosis.[28] However, an abnormality of the neural crest as the only embryologic explanation for neurofibromatosis has recently been questioned. Riccardi relates that, although neurofibromatosis appears to be a neurocristopathy, the primary problem may not be intrinsic to the neural crest alone. In order to explain the multiple findings in neurofibromatosis, one must postulate some interaction, either chemical or cellular, between the neural crest cells and cells of mesodermal and endodermal origin.[45] At present the etiology of neurofibromatosis remains to be defined.

GENETICS

The genetic mode of inheritance of neurofibromatosis has classically been stated to be consistent with an autosomal dominant trait having variable penetrance. A spontaneous mutation rate has been said to account for 50 per cent of cases.[21] However, this has recently been challenged by Steg and coworkers. Their discovery of abnormal dermatologic findings in the parents of those patients previously thought to be spontaneous mutants contradicts this rather high reported rate of spontaneous mutation.[52]

Clinically, the expression of this genetic disease is found in three basic forms. The first is classical neurofibromatosis with the typical neurofibromas and café-au-lait spots associated with other common features of the disease. The second is acoustic neurofibromatosis (neuroma of cranial nerve VIII) which, in contradistinction to classical neurofibromatosis, demonstrates a paucity of café-au-lait spots and cutaneous neurofibromas. Crowe and Schull and Eldridge have commented on this.[12, 15] A third entity is segmental neurofibromatosis, which is characterized by café-au-lait spots and cutaneous neurofibromas usually confined to an upper body segment, including the ipsilateral upper extremity.[45]

DIAGNOSIS

The diagnosis of neurofibromatosis rests on the documentation of certain characteristic lesions and some associated lesions that are common to patients with this disease. A family history will naturally alert the clinician to the possibility of neurofibromatosis. However, as indicated previously, the expression of this genetic disease is highly variable, and a positive family history may not be readily elicited.

The lesions that typically characterize neurofibromatosis are café-au-lait spots (Fig. 15–1), multiple neurofibromas (Fig. 15–2), and Lisch nodules of the iris (Fig. 15–3). Two studies have helped to define the presence of café-au-lait spots as a criterion for making the diagnosis of neurofibromatosis.[21] In the adult, an individual with six or more café-au-lait spots measuring 1.5 cm. or greater in diameter should be considered to have neurofibromatosis unless proven otherwise.[12] A child, 5 years old or younger, having five or more café-au-lait spots measuring .5 cm. or greater in diameter should also be considered to have neurofibromatosis unless proven otherwise.[59] Axillary freckling can be an associated finding. Freckling may also be found on the neck and the perineum.[21, 45]

The presence of neurofibromas, multiple in number, is a classic feature of this disease. Subcutaneous as well as pedunculated and sessile neurofibromas of varying sizes are typical. Neurofibromas are not always pres-

NEUROFIBROMATOSIS

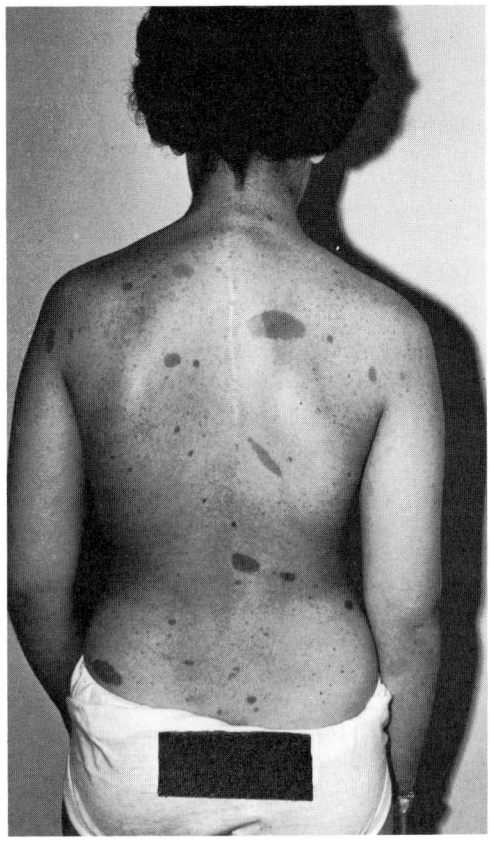

Figure 15–1. This 12 year old female required surgical stabilization of a thoracic curve. She has multiple café-au-lait spots on her trunk and limbs.

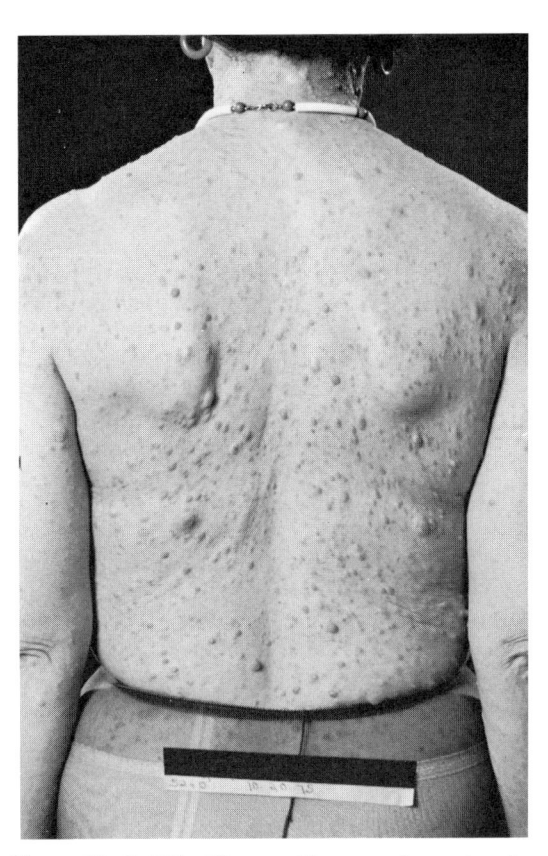

Figure 15–2. This 32 year old woman has extensive neurofibroma involvement of her skin.

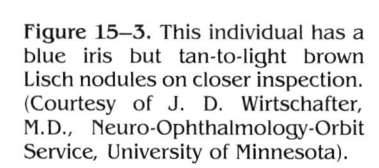

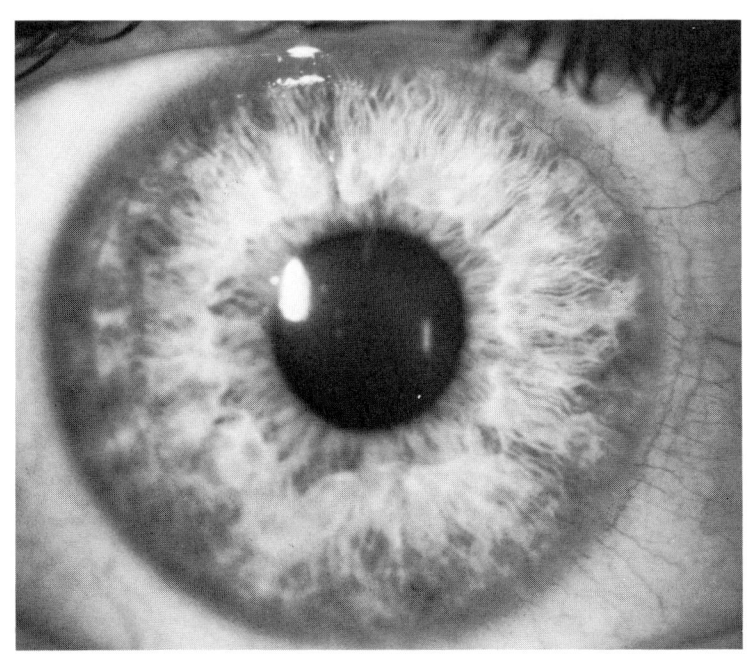

Figure 15–3. This individual has a blue iris but tan-to-light brown Lisch nodules on closer inspection. (Courtesy of J. D. Wirtschafter, M.D., Neuro-Ophthalmology-Orbit Service, University of Minnesota).

ent in early childhood and may not appear until the second decade of life. They are frequently found to increase in size and number during puberty and pregnancy.[17, 45, 53] The routine biopsy of these lesions has not been recommended, as they demonstrate no pathognomic histologic features.[45]

Lisch nodules are a more subtle finding, which has not been as widely recognized for its diagnostic importance.[30] These nodules are pigmented hamartomas of the iris. They are present in 94 per cent of patients with neurofibromatosis who are six years old or older. They are found in 28 per cent of patients with neurofibromatosis who are younger than six years.[29] Lisch nodules are not found in normal individuals and they do not correlate with the degree of severity of neurofibromatosis or any other manifestations of the disease. Of interest is their absence in those individuals with acoustic neurofibromatosis.[45]

A number of other clinical entities are common to patients with neurofibromatosis, particularly skeletal deformities (Fig. 15–4), and have been extensively reviewed by Holt and Riccardi. Associated spinal deformities include cervical kyphosis, scoliosis, kyphoscoliosis, lordoscoliosis and spondylolisthesis.[4, 7, 17, 19, 21, 25, 33, 41, 45, 47, 48, 60, 61, 62, 64]

ROENTGENOGRAPHIC CHANGES OF THE SPINE

The dystrophic bony changes found in neurofibromatosis were documented early in the century by Gould and later by Brooks and Lehman.[4, 18] The radiographic appearance of these dystrophic changes has subsequently been documented by a number of authors.[17, 19, 21, 25, 46, 48] The typical radiographic deformities seen in the spine with neurofibromatosis are scalloping of the vertebral bodies, sharpening of the vertebral margins, severe rotation of apical vertebrae, widening of the spinal canal, widening of the intervertebral foramina, "penciling" of the ribs, and a spindled appearance of the transverse processes (Fig. 15–5). The exact cause of these changes has been a point of some controversy. It has been well documented that these changes may occur in the absence of any adjacent tumor.[17, 19, 21, 46] Vertebral scalloping in neurofibromatosis can be seen in the absence of scoliosis,[6] with dural ectasia often noted as the apparent cause.[38, 46] Myelography has demonstrated ectasia of the dura with corresponding deformity in the vertebral body (Fig. 15–6). Large meningoceles have also been described, some extending into the thorax, resulting in compression of the lung, trachea, and esophagus.[40, 42, 63]

The typical appearance of scoliosis associated with neurofibromatosis is said to be a short, sharp curve involving approximately six vertebral bodies or less. Holt feels this appearance is virtually diagnostic of neurofibromatosis.[21] Heard has described dystrophic changes in cervical kyphosis progressing to a degree that results in a gross distortion of the vertebrae.[19] In the case of spondylolisthesis in the lumbar spine, a pseudarthrosis of the pedicles has been implicated as the etiology rather than a defect in the pars interarticularis.[17, 32, 61]

NATURAL HISTORY

Although the expression of this genetic disease is variable, all neurofibromatosis pa-

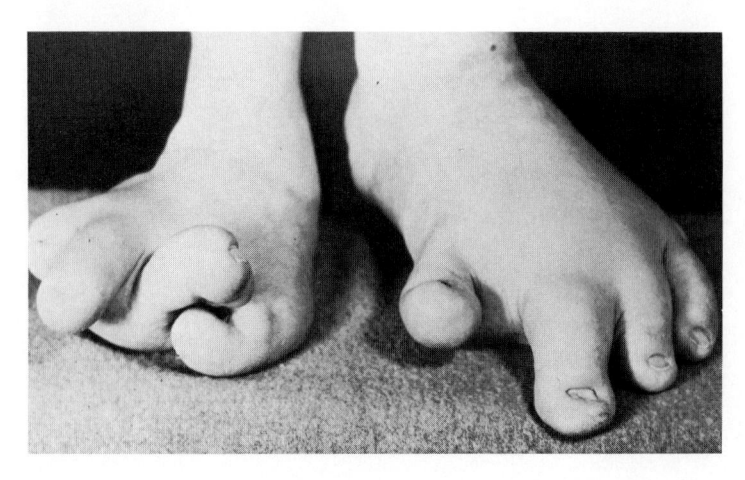

Figure 15–4. This patient with neurofibromatosis and scoliosis also has gigantism of his feet.

NEUROFIBROMATOSIS

Figure 15–5. The radiographic appearance of the spine of this 12+2 year old female demonstrates the typical findings of dystrophic change. She also has extensive neurofibroma involvement in the mediastinum and paraspinal musculature.

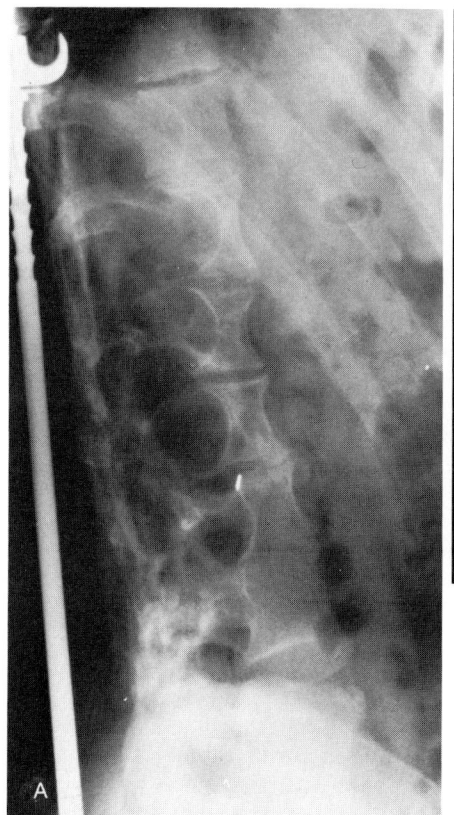

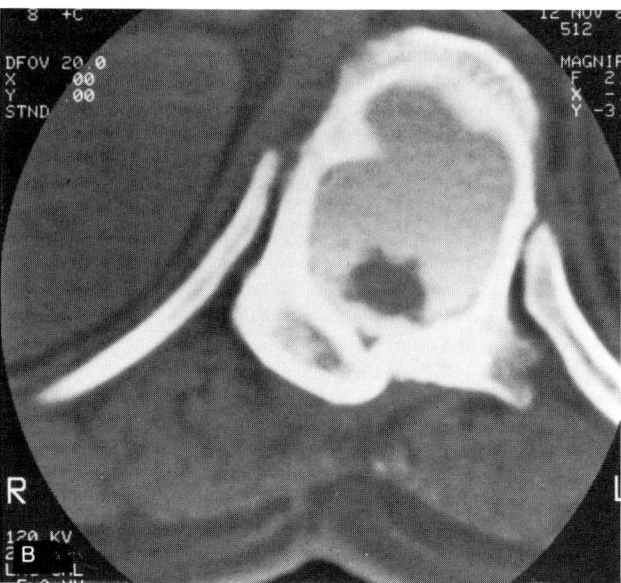

Figure 15–6. *A*, This adolescent male was referred following a posterior spinal fusion. Marked scalloping of the vertebrae is evident. *B*, A metrizamide computed tomogram in the thoracic spine demonstrates dural ectasia. (Courtesy of Robert C. Zuege, M.D., Milwaukee, Wisconsin)

tients have one thing in common—progression of their disease. An increase in the number and size of pigmentary changes in the skin occurs throughout the patient's life. These pigmentary changes are frequently apparent at birth. Neurofibromas, on the other hand, may not become apparent until the latter half of the second decade of life. At the time of puberty or pregnancy, the number and size of neurofibromas tends to increase. The malignant degeneration of a neurofibroma or the sudden appearance of a malignancy in the absence of a pre-existing lesion is an ever-present possibility.[1, 14, 22, 23, 27, 35, 37, 51, 57]

However, an immediate problem is the high incidence of skeletal deformity, particularly of the spine. Two forms of scoliosis have been recognized to occur in association with neurofibromatosis. Specifically, scoliosis may occur with or without dystrophic bony change. Scoliosis in the presence of dystrophic bony change is almost always progressive (Fig. 15–7). However, in the absence of dystrophic change, the curve behaves in a manner consistent with the course of idiopathic scoliosis.[60] No doubt it is possible that idiopathic scoliosis occurs in patients with all the features of neurofibromatosis, thereby accounting for the appearance of non-dystrophic curves. An exception to this has been reported by Biot, who has described patients with neurofibromatosis having non-dystrophic curves that behave like idiopathic scoliosis initially. As adults their vertebrae become dystrophic and the curves progress.[2]

Cobb recognized the implications of the dystrophic versus non-dystrophic curve. In the case of the dystrophic curve, he noted that almost all patients needed early fusion if a progressive deformity was to be avoided.[8, 9] This observation has been documented by the natural history of 145 neurofibromatosis curves reported by Bunyatov in the Soviet Union (Fig. 15–8). In the absence of surgical stabilization, an unremitting progression of deformity that is unresponsive to bracing frequently occurs.[20, 49, 60] Catastrophic neurologic consequences have been well documented.[5, 13, 26, 31, 49, 60]

TREATMENT

As mentioned previously, it is important to distinguish between the dystrophic and the non-dystrophic curve. The remainder of this chapter will deal with the dystrophic spine deformity only. The non-dystrophic curve may be treated like an idiopathic curve. It is the dystrophic spine deformity that exhibits an unremitting progression with non-operative care and must be dealt with surgically. Despite meticulous technique pseudarthrosis is common. Persistence may be necessary in some cases to achieve a solid arthrodesis.

Cervical Spine

Judging from the literature, there has been a paucity of experience in the management of cervical spine deformity in neurofibromatosis. Yong-Hing has pointed out that the incidence of cervical spine abnormalities correlates directly with the severity of spine deformity elsewhere. In his group of patients with scoliosis and kyphoscoliosis, 44 per cent had cervical lesions.[64] In Curtis' series, four of eight patients had paraplegia secondary to deformities of the cervical spine.[13]

Frequently, however, abnormalities of the cervical spine may be concealed, and deformity is not apparent on physical examination. Consequently, it is recommended that patients with scoliosis and kyphoscoliosis exhibiting dystrophic change have periodic cervical spine radiographs. Indications for surgical stabilization of the cervical spine include dystrophic change with instability or symptoms of neurologic compromise (Fig. 15–9).

SCOLIOSIS

Cervical scoliosis usually responds well to posterior fusion alone. A single procedure without subsequent exploration of the fusion mass may be sufficient. Postoperative halo immobilization is recommended. If instability is present, as evidenced by translation of one vertebra on another, anterior and posterior fusion may be needed to assure stabilization. A two-stage posterior fusion with bone graft reinforcement at six months is an alternative to anterior and posterior fusion.

KYPHOSIS

Kyphotic deformity of the cervical spine is usually seen in concert with advancing dystrophic change of the vertebrae. Anterior and posterior fusion or a two-stage posterior fu-

NEUROFIBROMATOSIS

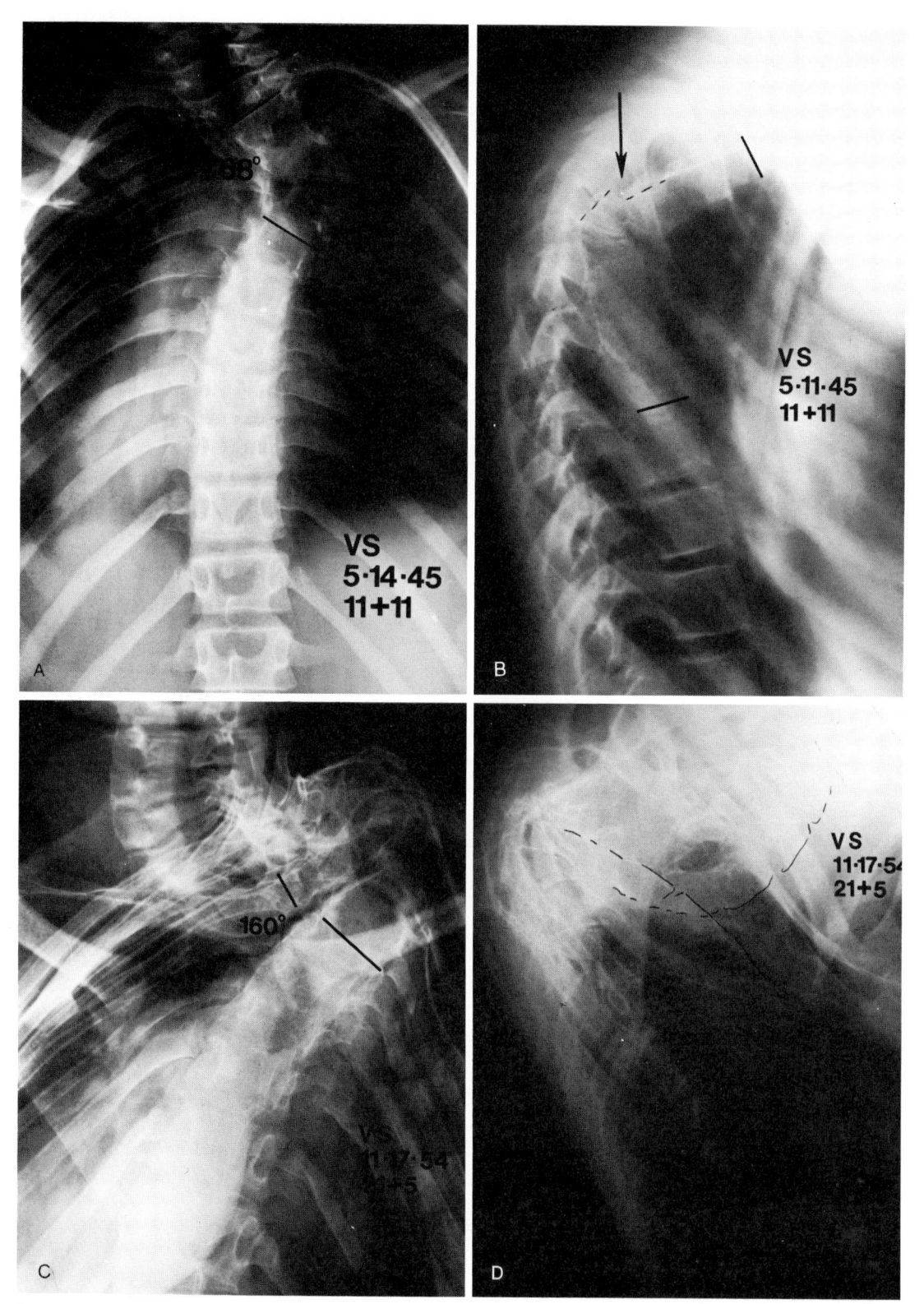

Figure 15–7. *A* and *B*, This female patient presented at age 11 + 11 with a sharp kyphoscoliosis of the thoracic spine. She received no treatment. *C* and *D*, Nearly 10 years later she had progressed to a grossly deformed state. Surprisingly, she had no neurologic deficit.

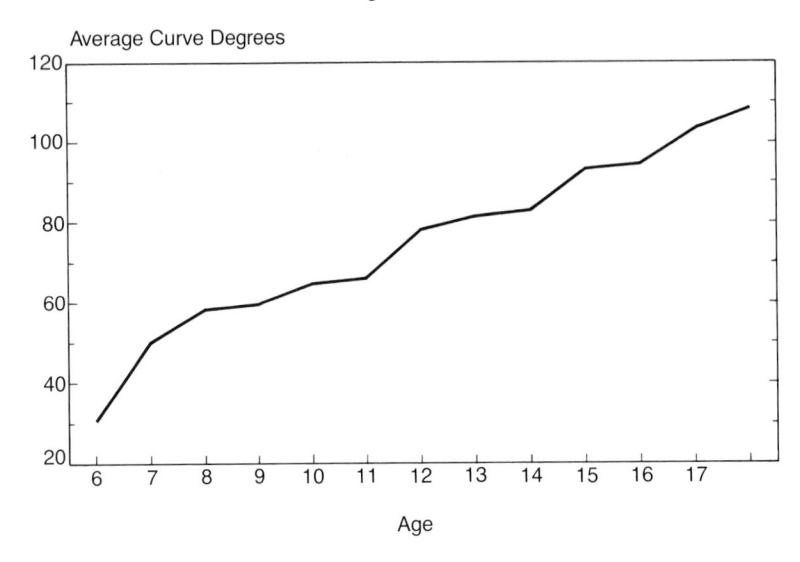

Figure 15–8. Progression of dystrophic scoliosis. (Data extracted from Bunyatov, R.: Clinical roentgenographic characteristics of scoliosis in neurofibromatosis. Pediatrics [USSR] 5:49–51, 1983.)

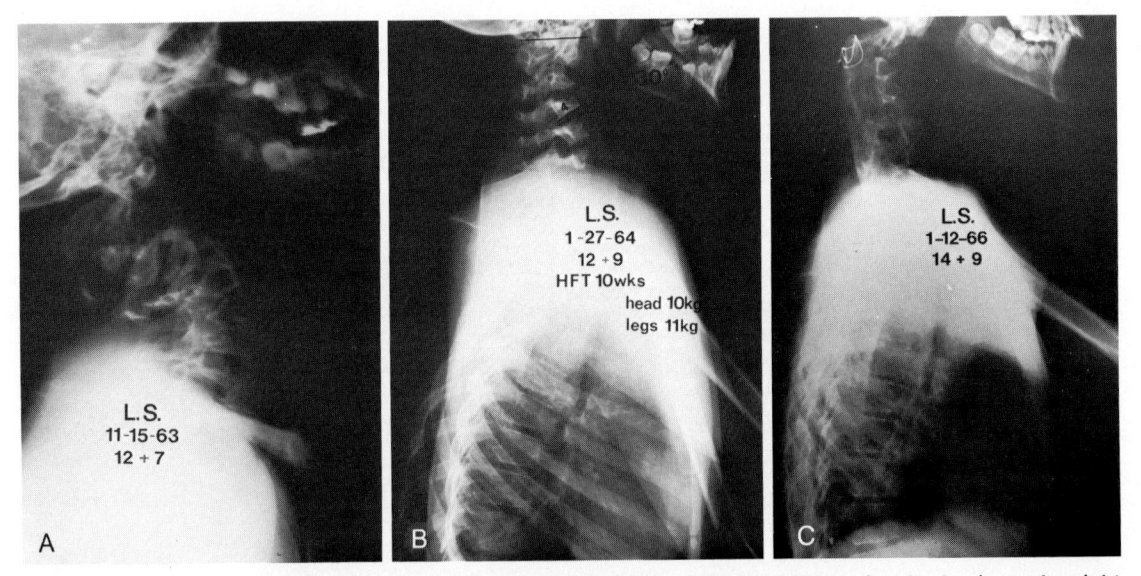

Figure 15–9. *A,* This 12 year old male presented with cervicothoracic scoliosis, cervical kyphosis, and a right paracervical mass. An extradural neurofibroma was excised. His cervical spine demonstrated instability. *B,* He was initially placed in halofemoral traction, which rapidly reduced the kyphosis. *C,* A posterior fusion was performed in a halo cast following halofemoral traction. Follow-up two years postoperatively.

sion is recommended. Postoperative halo immobilization is preferred.

Kyphosis of the cervical spine may result in spinal cord compression. When this occurs a course of gentle halo traction is warranted. Mild neurologic symptoms will frequently respond to this form of treatment. When successful, traction may then be followed by fusion as outlined before. If prolonged, gentle traction fails to relieve neurologic symptoms, anterior decompression accompanied by anterior and posterior fusion is necessary.

It should be emphasized that the area of spinal cord compromise in kyphosis is anterior and must be dealt with anteriorly. Laminectomy as a treatment for spinal cord compression secondary to kyphosis is contraindicated. Laminectomy will result in a rapid progression of the kyphosis with increased paralysis.

It should be emphasized that before halo traction is implemented a high-volume, total spinal myelogram is needed in addition to evaluation of the cervical spine. Failure to appreciate an intraspinal tumor may result in paralysis with traction.

Thoracic Spine

The majority of spine deformities in neurofibromatosis occur in the thoracic spine.[7, 33, 48, 60] In this area it is important to distinguish not only dystrophic from nondystrophic scoliosis but, when dystrophy is present, to determine the degree of kyphosis as well. As the Twin Cities Scoliosis Center study and subsequently Savini have indicated, the treatment of kyphosis, when present, falls into three categories.[48, 60] These three categories are dystrophic scoliosis with kyphosis less than 50 degrees, dystrophic scoliosis with kyphosis greater than 50 degrees, and dystrophic scoliosis with spinal cord compression secondary to kyphosis (see section on Spinal Cord Compression).

SCOLIOSIS WITH KYPHOSIS LESS THAN 50 DEGREES

Treatment of dystrophic scoliosis should be very aggressive. Attempting brace treatment is an exercise in futility and will not halt progression of the deformity. As previous work from the Twin Cities Scoliosis Center has emphasized, there is no justification for passive observation of a progressive spine deformity.[60] The curve with documented progression but having less than 50 degrees of kyphosis has the best chance of stabilization with posterior fusion alone. Therefore, once a dystrophic scoliosis has been recognized, surgical stabilization should be carried out immediately (Fig. 15-10). The use of Harrington instrumentation with autogenous bone graft is the recommended surgical treatment. Postoperatively, the patient should be placed in a Risser-Cotrel cast. If greater than mild dystrophy of the bony elements exist, a reinforcement of the graft at six months should be performed. This form of treatment has been employed successfully in individuals as young as 4 years of age.[60] Trunk height may be diminished as a result of this treatment; however, it should be pointed out that there is very poor vertical growth potential in the involved vertebrae. Moreover, early fusion will cause minimal shortening of the trunk as the curves being fused are short because of their very nature. Finally, the loss of height resulting from an early fusion should be less than if the curve were allowed to progress. Although our experience is limited, there is a role for subcutaneous rod treatment in young children.[39]

SCOLIOSIS WITH KYPHOSIS GREATER THAN 50 DEGREES

Once kyphosis exceeds 50 degrees, the treatment of dystrophic kyphoscoliosis changes. It becomes necessary to perform an anterior fusion in addition to a posterior fusion. Furthermore, in these individuals preoperative halo-femoral or halo wheelchair traction is of benefit. This is particularly true if the patient has flexibility of the kyphosis, pulmonary compromise secondary to thoracic deformity, or spinal cord compression secondary to the kyphosis. Frequently, individuals with compromised pulmonary status are able to improve their pulmonary volume and arterial blood gases preoperatively with the use of halo traction. However, it is emphasized again that evaluation of the cervical spine and a high volume myelogram of the entire spine is necessary prior to instituting traction. If it is possible by traction or extension alone to correct the kyphosis to 50 degrees or less, a posterior spinal fusion with instrumentation followed by anterior spinal fusion and strut graft should be considered. In this instance, the first-stage posterior fusion and instrumentation will pro-

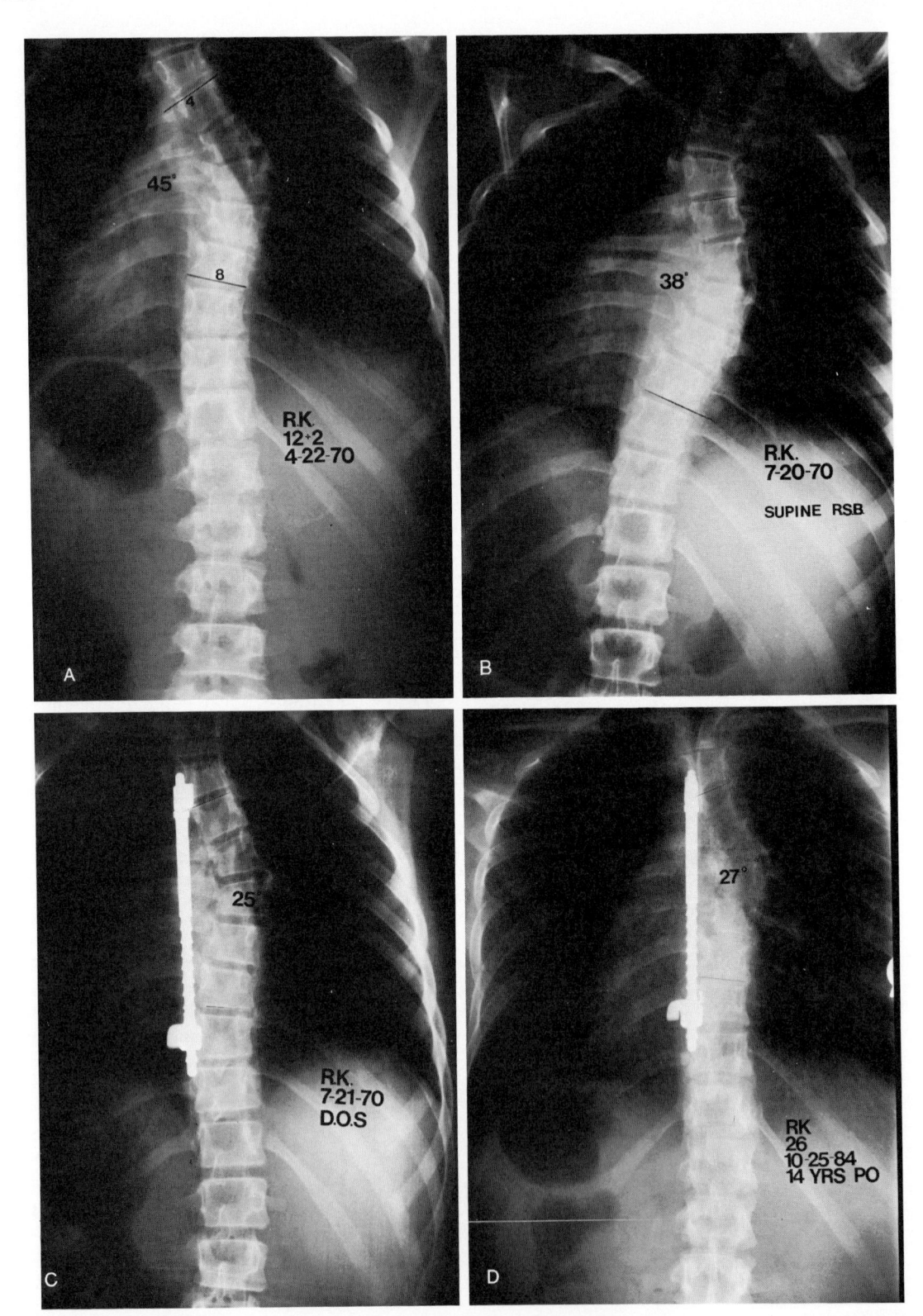

Figure 15–10. *A*, This 12+2 year old female presented with a right thoracic curve of 45 degrees, involving five vertebrae. *B*, A preoperative supine side bending radiograph demonstrated correction to 38 degrees. *C*, The immediate postoperative film. *D*, 14 years postoperative. An aggressive surgical approach is necessary and successful in managing the dystrophic curve.

vide stability and preclude the possible event of a second-stage anterior strut graft dislodgement.

When the kyphotic deformity is rigid, optimal correction will result by performing the anterior procedure first. The entire structural area of the deformity should be fused with complete disc excision and placement of a strut graft, preferably from the fibula. Augmentation of the graft with iliac and rib bone is usually necessary. The strut graft must make contact with the additional bone graft material and the vertebral bodies in continuity. Any interruption of the graft with interposed soft tissue will result in resorption of the graft in its mid-portion. Following the anterior fusion, a posterior fusion with instrumentation should be performed (Fig. 15–11). Individuals with large kyphotic deformities are routinely treated in a halo cast postoperatively. After six to nine months, a Milwaukee brace may be worn while the graft matures. Brace wear should continue until trabeculation of the graft is evident. This usually requires 18 months. Failure of this form of treatment has been reported;[24] however, the necessity of fusing the entire structural portion of the kyphosis and not the apex alone must be stressed.[50, 60]

LORDOSCOLIOSIS

The incidence of thoracic lordoscoliosis in neurofibromatosis compared to the occurrence of scoliosis and kyphoscoliosis is very low. In 1979, the Twin Cities Scoliosis Center reported five cases in a group of 102 patients with neurofibromatosis and spinal deformity. Recently, Winter reported on two cases treated with posterior fusion, Harrington distraction instrumentation, and sublaminar wiring.[62]

Although our experience is limited, we are unaware of any other reports specifically addressing the treatment of this entity in neurofibromatosis. Our recommendation for surgical treatment is posterior spinal fusion with Harrington instrumentation and sublaminar wiring. A square-ended Moe rod and lower hook will allow contouring of the rod to provide sagittal plane correction (Fig. 15–12). The use of sublaminar wires in the face of dystrophic laminae has not been a problem. However, the surgeon must use prudence. The use of ¼ inch contoured Luque rods may also provide satisfactory instrumentation.

Spondylolisthesis

Spondylolisthesis, like thoracic lordoscoliosis, is an unusual spine deformity in neurofibromatosis. With only ten reported cases, the experience in the treatment of this problem is scant (McCarroll, Hunt, Mandell, Winter). However, the deformity is known to result from dystrophic change in the pedicles and not just the pars interarticularis, although it too may evidence lysis.[61]

In 1981, Winter described the treatment of an adolescent male with an L5 spondylolisthesis. Preoperative halofemoral traction as described by Bradford[3] and McPhee and O'Brien[36] was used. A Gill procedure along with posterior spinal fusion and Harrington instrumentation was performed. Postoperative immobilization in a double pantaloon cast with the hips in extension was continued for six months, with the patient on bedrest. At that time, the Harrington rods were removed and the fusion was explored and found to be solid (Fig. 15–13).

Spinal Cord Compression

KYPHOSCOLIOSIS WITH SPINAL CORD COMPRESSION

When spinal cord compression results from kyphoscoliosis, the treatment as outlined previously should be employed. In conjunction with an anterior arthrodesis, anterior decompression of the cord may rarely be required. As in the case of cervical kyphosis, a trial of gentle halo traction is worthwhile when neurologic symptoms are present. Cast correction may also provide relief. If this treatment is successful, anterior and posterior fusion can be carried out without having to decompress the spinal cord.

INTRASPINAL NEUROFIBROMA AND POST LAMINECTOMY KYPHOSIS

Neurofibromatosis may exist in the paraspinal musculature, the intervertebral foramina, or the spinal canal. Intraspinal neurofibromas may produce a neurologic deficit (Fig. 15–14).

When spinal cord compression occurs secondary to a neurofibroma but in the presence of dystrophic bony change, a fusion must accompany the decompression and laminec-

Text continued on page 344

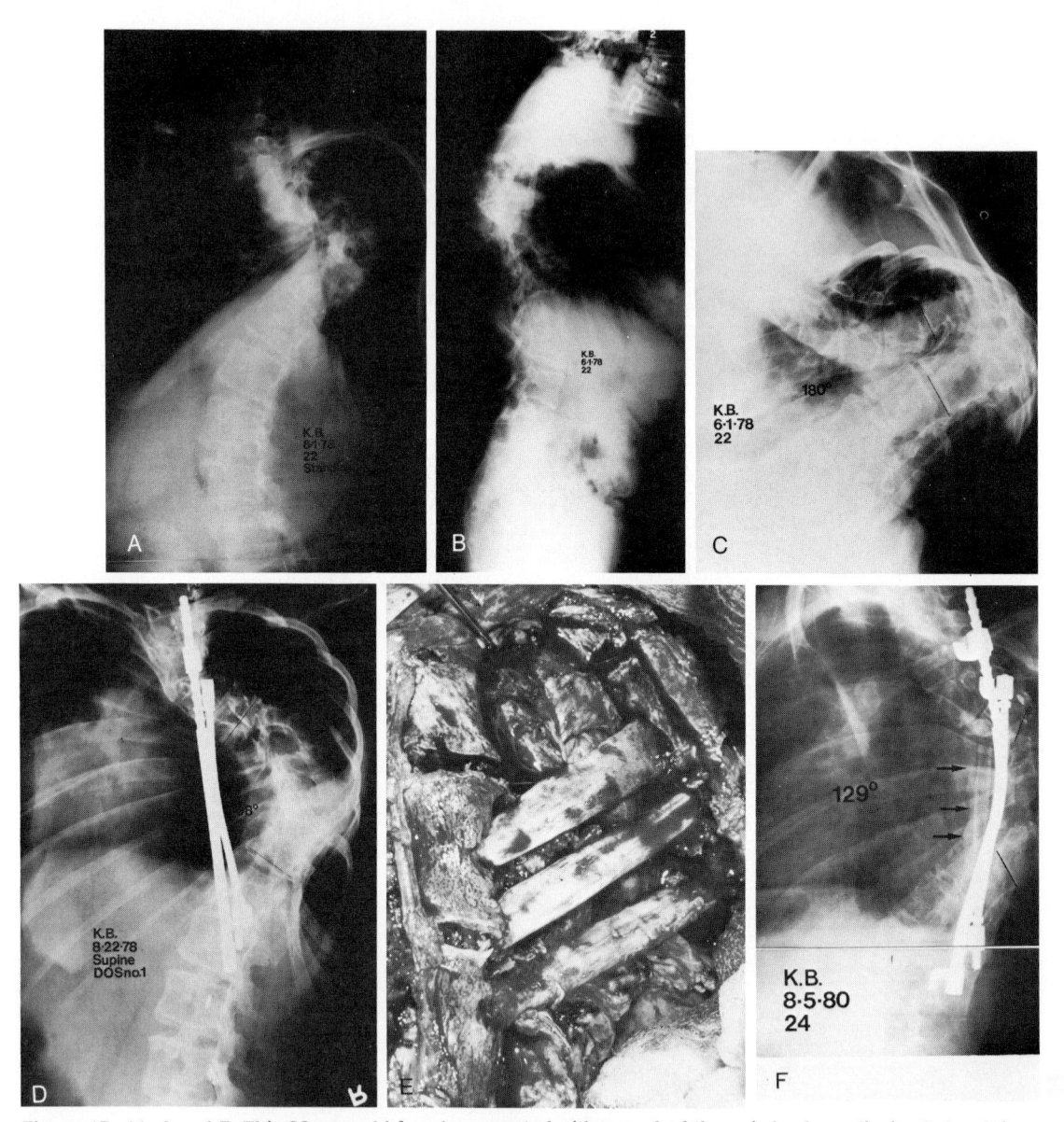

Figure 15–11. *A* and *B*, This 22 year old female presented with a marked thoracic kyphoscoliosis. *C*, An oblique view of the thoracic spine demonstrates the true magnitude of the kyphosis. *D*, A posterior spinal fusion with Harrington instrumentation was performed first. *E*, Appearance of the rib struts at the time of anterior fusion. Later, all the intervening space to the apex of the kyphosis was filled with bone graft. *F*, An oblique radiograph two years postoperatively demonstrates the anterior strut grafts and posterior instrumentation.

Illustration continued on opposite page

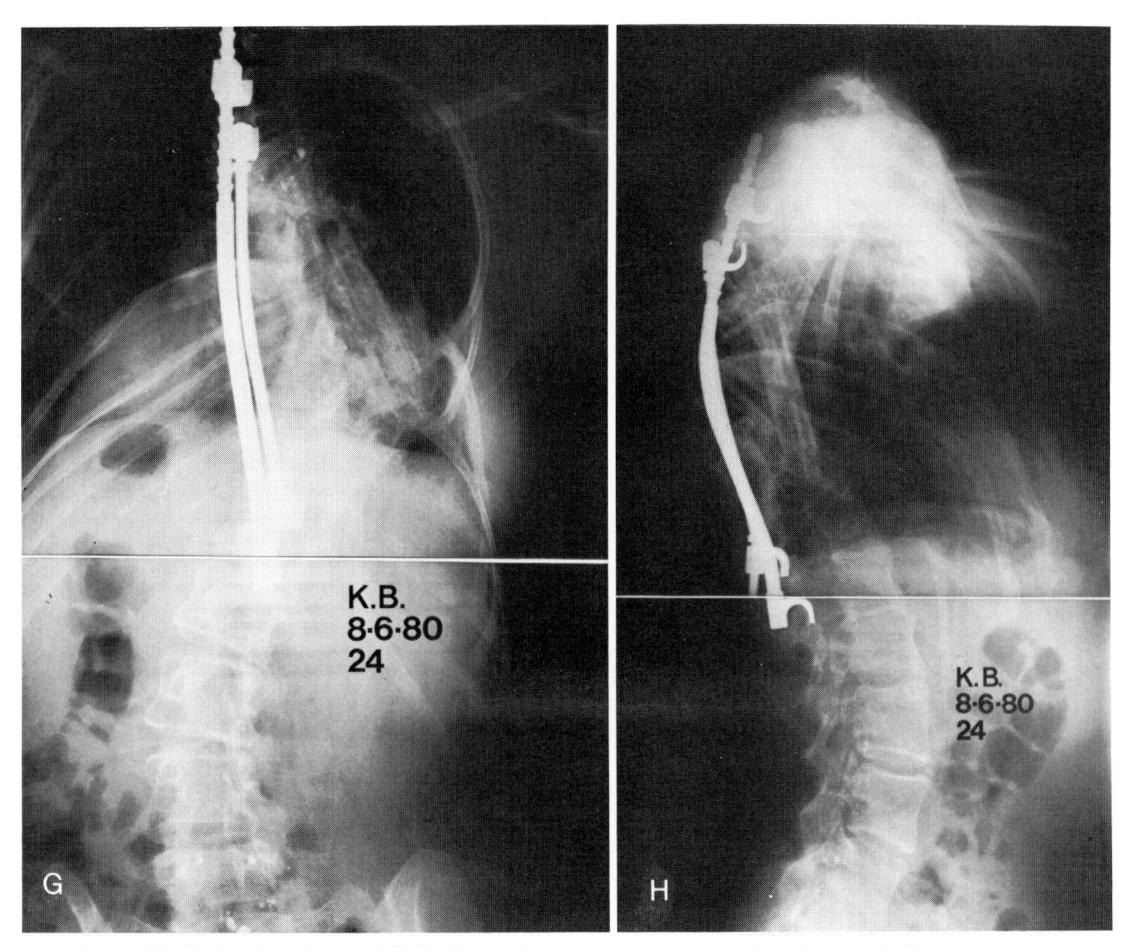

Figure 15–11 *Continued. G* and *H,* Radiographs two years postoperative. No pseudarthrosis occurred.

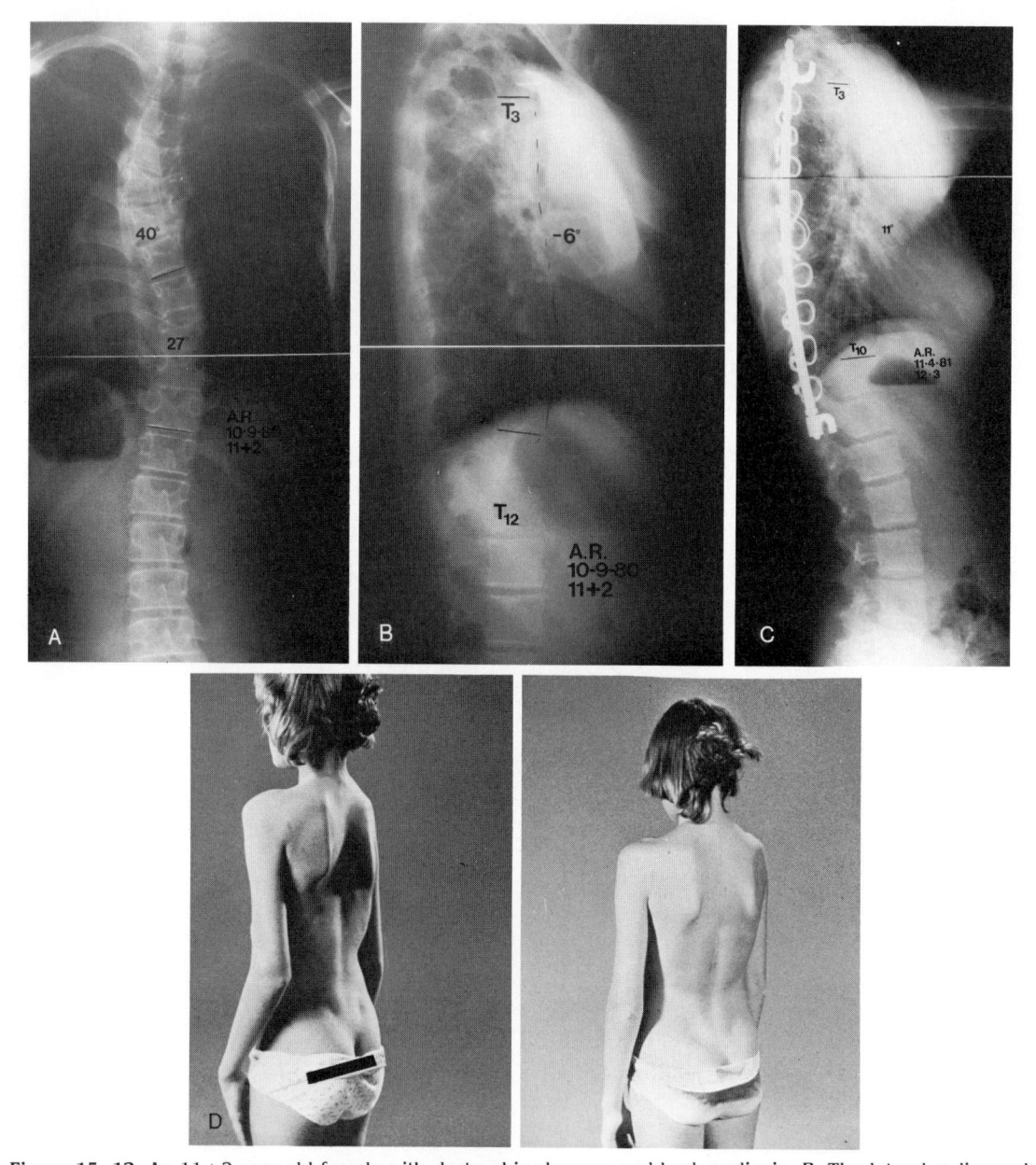

Figure 15–12. An 11+2 year old female with dystrophic changes and lordoscoliosis. *B,* The lateral radiograph shows a lordosis of −6 degrees. *C,* The lateral radiograph one year postoperative. Posterior fusion with a Harrington distraction rod and sublaminar wiring resulted in a thoracic kyphosis of 11 degrees. *D,* The patient preoperatively (left) and postoperatively.

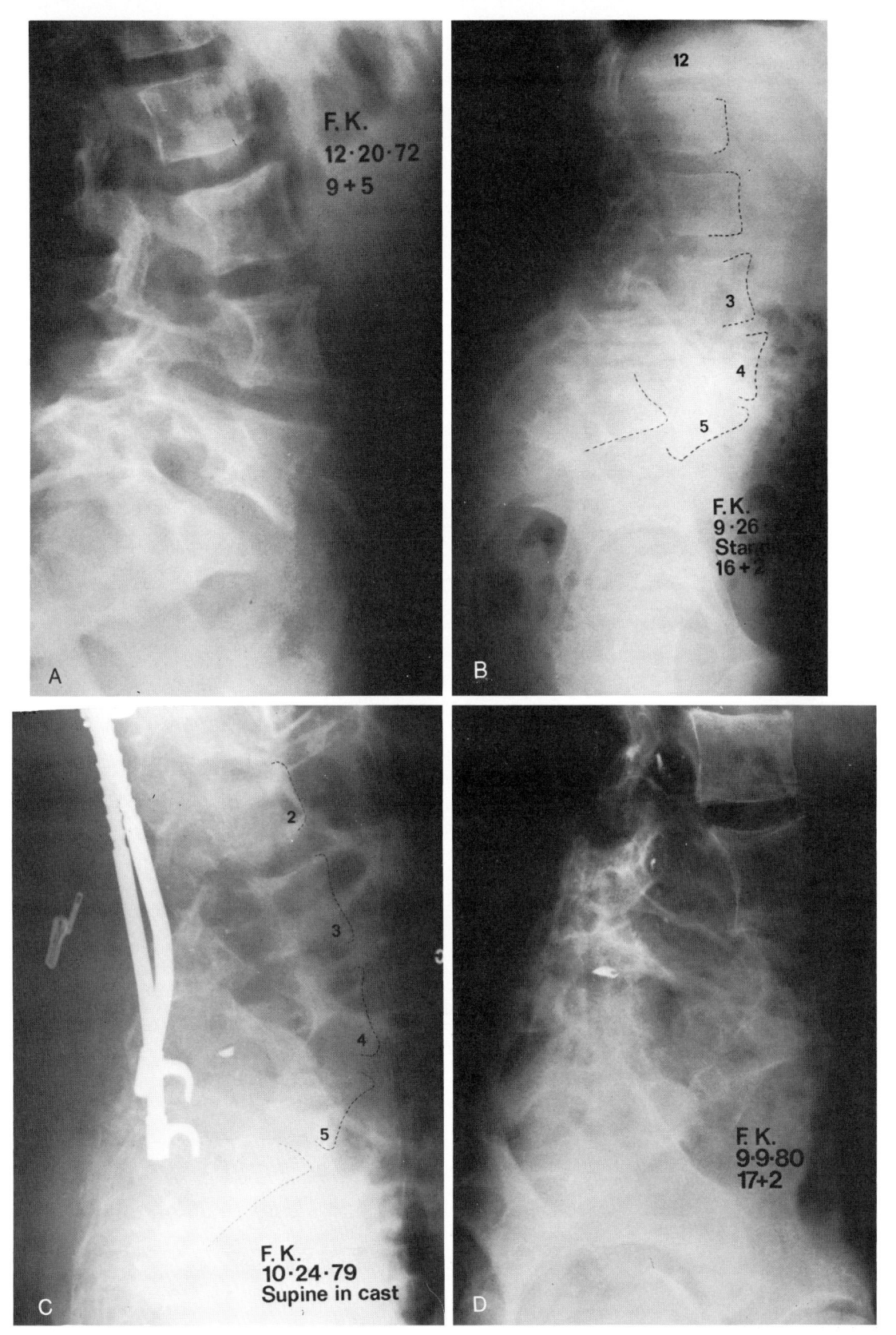

Figure 15–13. *A*, A 9+5 year old male with dystrophic change of the lumbosacral spine. This is spondylolysis of one L5 pedicle. *B*, At age 16+2 years, spondylolisthesis has occurred. *C*, The lateral postoperative radiograph with the patient in a cast. Note reduction of the slip of L5. *D*, One year postoperatively, following removal of instrumentation and exploration of the fusion.

343

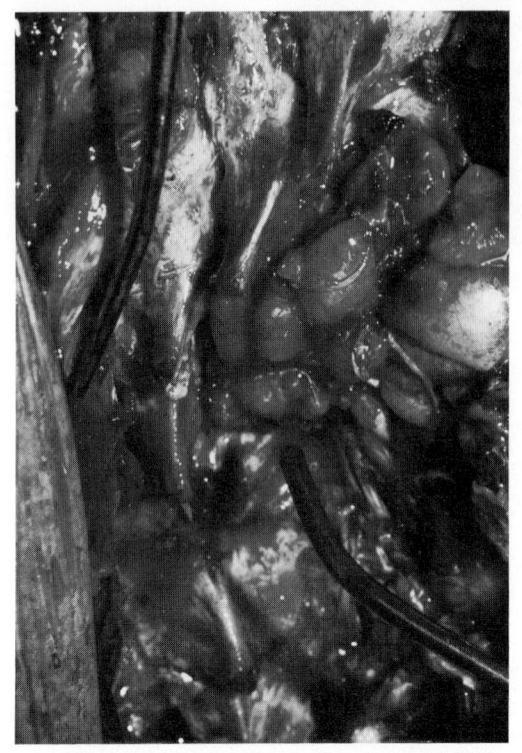

Figure 15–14. These grape-like neurofibromas produced a paraparesis in a 14+6 year old male. Preoperatively a myelogram demonstrated a complete block. Laminectomy decompressed the thoracic spinal cord and revealed the tumors. A posterior fusion and Harrington instrumentation were also performed.

tomy. Failure to perform a fusion in conjunction with the laminectomy will lead to catastrophic kyphotic deformity and neurologic injury. The results of laminectomy in neurofibromatosis without fusion are well described by Cobb who stated, "The spinal deformity resulting from neurofibromatosis may be horrible, but laminectomy without stabilization will make it a nightmare."[8]

SUMMARY

Although an infrequent overall cause of spinal deformity, neurofibromatosis is a common cause of spinal deformity in those individuals with the disease. It is important to recognize the dystrophic spine deformity because of its great predilection for progression. Passive observation of a progressive deformity is not justified. An aggressive surgical approach to a progressive deformity is warranted since brace treatment is without benefit. This requires prompt posterior fusion for those with scoliosis and mild kyphosis and combined anterior and posterior fusion for those with kyphosis greater than 50 degrees. Prolonged postoperative support is needed.

Evaluation of the cervical spine and high-volume myelography of the entire spine are required before instituting traction or surgical treatment. Laminectomy without surgical stabilization has no place in the treatment of these patients.

References

1. Bader, J., and Miller, R.: Neurofibromatosis and childhood leukemia. J. Pediatr., 92:925–929, 1978.
2. Biot, B., Fauchet, R., and Stagnara, P.: Les lesions vertebrales de la neurofibromatose. Revue Chir. Orthop., 60:607–621, 1974.
3. Bradford, D.: Treatment of severe spondylolisthesis: a combined approach for reduction and stabilization. Spine, 4:423–429, 1979.
4. Brooks, B., and Lehman, E.: The bone changes in Recklinghausen's neurofibromatosis. Surg. Gynecol. Obstet., 38:587–595, 1924.
5. Bunyatov, R.: Clinical roentgenographic characteristics of scoliosis in neurofibromatosis. Pediatrics (USSR), 5:49–51, 1983.
6. Casselman, E., and Mandell, G.: Vertebral scalloping in neurofibromatosis. Radiology, 131:89–94, 1979.
7. Chaglassian, J., Riseborough, E., and Hall, J.: Neurofibromatosis. J. Bone Joint Surg., 58A:695–702, 1976.
8. Cobb, J.: Discussion of McCarroll, H., "Clinical manifestations of congenital neurofibromatosis." J. Bone Joint Surg., 32A:617, 1950.
9. Cobb, J: Outline for the study of scoliosis. Am. Acad. Orthop. Surg. Instructional Course Lecture, 5:261–275, 1948.
10. Cotrel, Y.: La scoliose dans la maladie de Recklinghausen. Groupe d'etudes de la scoliose. Lyon, Reunion de Lyon, C. R. F. Massues, 1970.
11. Crawford, A.: Neurofibromatosis. In Lovell, W., and Winter, R. B. (eds.): Pediatric Orthopaedics. Philadelphia, J. B. Lippincott, 1985.
12. Crowe, F., and Schull, W.: Diagnostic importance of café-au-lait spot in neurofibromatosis. Arch. Intern. Med., 91:758–766, 1953.
13. Curtis, B., Fisher, R., Butterfield, W., and Saunders, F.: Neurofibromatosis with paraplegia. J. Bone Joint Surg., 51A:843–861, 1969.
14. D'Agostino, A., Soule, E., and Miller, R.: Sarcoma of the peripheral nerves and somatic soft tissues associated with multiple neurofibromatosis (Von Recklinghausen's disease). Cancer, 16:1015–1027, 1963.
15. Eldridge, R.: Central neurofibromatosis with bilateral acoustic neuroma. Adv. Neurol., 29:57–65, 1981.
16. Fulton, J.: Robert W. Smith's description of generalized neurofibromatosis (1849). New Engl. J. Med., 200:1315–1317, 1929.

17. Goel, M.: Osseous lesions in neurofibromatosis. Lecture, Columbia Presbyterian Hospital, New York, 1973.
18. Gould, E.: The bone changes in Von Recklinghausen's disease. Q. J. Med., 11:221–230, 1918.
19. Heard, G., Holt, J., and Naylor, B.: Cervical vertebral deformity in Von Recklinghausen's disease of the nervous system. J. Bone Joint Surg., 44B:880–885, 1962.
20. Hensinger, R.: Kyphosis secondary to skeletal dysplasias and metabolic disease. Clin. Orthop., 128:113–128, 1977.
21. Holt, J.: Neurofibromatosis in children. Am. J. Roentgenol., 130:615–639, 1978.
22. Hope, D., and Mulvihill, J.: Malignancy in neurofibromatosis. Adv. Neurol., 29:33–56, 1981.
23. Hosoi, K: Multiple neurofibromatosis (Von Recklinghausen's disease). Arch. Surg., 22:258–281, 1931.
24. Hsu, L., Lee, P., and Leong, J.: Dystrophic spinal deformities in neurofibromatosis. J. Bone Joint Surg., 66B:495–499, 1984.
25. Hunt, J., and Pugh, D.: Skeletal lesions in neurofibromatosis. Radiology, 76:1–19, 1961.
26. Hvorslev, V., and Reiter, S.: A case of neurofibromatosis with severe osseous disease of the thoracic spine. Pediatr. Radiol., 8:251–253, 1979.
27. Knight, W., Murphy, W., and Gottlieb, J.: Neurofibromatosis associated with malignant neurofibromas. Arch. Dermatol., 107:747–750, 1973.
28. Lassman, H., Jurecka, W., and Gebhart, W.: Some electron microscope and autoradiographic results concerning cutaneous neurofibromas in Von Recklinghausen's disease. Arch. Dermatol. Res., 255:69–81, 1976.
29. Lewis, R., and Riccardi, V.: Von Recklinghausen neurofibromatosis: incidence of iris hamartomata. Ophthalmology, 88:348–354, 1981.
30. Lisch, K.: Ueber Beteiligung der Augen, insbesonderedas Vorkommen von Irisknoetchen bei der Neurofibromatose (Recklinghausen). Z. Augenheilkd., 93:137–143, 1937.
31. Lonstein, J., Winter, R., Moe, J., et at.: Neurologic deficits secondary to spinal deformity. Spine, 5:331–355, 1980.
32. Mandell, G.: The Pedicle in neurofibromatosis. Am. J. Roentgenol., 130:675–678, 1978.
33. Marchetti, P.: Le scoliosi. Rome, Aulo Gaggi, 1968.
34. McCarroll, H.: Clinical manifestations of congenital neurofibromatosis. J. Bone Joint Surg., 32A:601–617, 1950.
35. McKeen, E., Bodurtha, J., Meadows, A., et al.: Rhabdomyosarcoma complicating multiple neurofibromatosis. J. Pediatr., 93:992–993, 1978.
36. McPhee, I., and O'Brien, J.: Reduction of severe spondylolisthesis: a preliminary report. Spine, 4:430–434, 1979.
37. Miller, A.: Neurofibromatosis—with reference to skeletal changes, compression myelitis and malignant degeneration. Arch. Surg., 32:109–122, 1936.
38. Mitchell, G., Lourie, H., and Berne, A.: The various causes of scalloped vertebrae with notes on their pathogenesis. Radiology, 89:67–74, 1967.
39. Moe, J., Kharrat, K., Winter, R., and Cummine, J.: Harrington instrumentation without fusion plus external orthotic support for the treatment of difficult curvature problems in young children. Clin. Orthop., 185:35–45, 1984.
40. Nanson, E.: Thoracic meningocele associated with neurofibromatosis. J. Thorac. Surg., 33:650–662, 1967.
41. Perricone, G., and Giulani, G.: Scoliosi in neurofibromatosi de Von Recklinghausen. Chir. Organi Mov., 59:45–56, 1970.
42. Pohl, R.: Meningokele in brustraum unter dem bilde eines intrathorakalen rundschattens. Roentgenpraxis, 5:747–749, 1933.
43. Preiser, S., and Davenport, C.: Multiple neurofibromatosis (Von Recklinghausen's disease) and its inheritance: with description of a case. Am. J. Med. Sci., 156:507–540, 1918.
44. Rezaian, S.: The incidence of scoliosis due to neurofibromatosis. Acta Orthop. Scand., 47:534–539, 1976.
45. Riccardi, V.: Von Recklinghausen neurofibromatosis. New Engl. J. Med., 305:1617–1627, 1981.
46. Salerno, N., and Edigken, J.: Vertebral scalloping in neurofibromatosis. Radiology, 97:509–510, 1970.
47. Savini, R., Parisini, P., and Bartolozzi, M: Cifosi neurofibromatosica: evoluzione e trattamento. In: Le Cifosi, Bologna, Aulo Gaggi, 1982.
48. Savini, R., and Vicenzi, G.: Le deformita del rachide nella neurofibromatosi. Ital. J. Orthop. Traumatol., 2:37–50, 1976.
49. Savine, R., Parisini, P., Cervellati, S., and Gualdrini, G.: Surgical treatment of vertebral deformities in neurofibromatosis. Ital. J. Orthop. Traumatol., 9:13–24, 1983.
50. Stagnara, P., Biot, B., and Fauchet, R.: Evaluation critique due traitement chirurgical des lesions vertebrales de la neurofibromatose. Revue Chir. Orthop., 61:17–38, 1975.
51. Stay, E., and Vawter, G.: The relationship between nephroblastoma and neurofibromatosis (Von Recklinghausen's disease). Cancer, 39:2550–2555, 1977.
52. Steg, N., Wong, A., Vogel, M., et al.: The potential of computerized dermatoglyphic analysis as demonstrated through studies of patients with meningomyelocele and neurofibromatosis. In Bergsma, D. (ed.): Numerical Taxonomy of Birth Defects and Polygenic Disorders. March of Dimes, White Plains, N.Y., pp. 158–159, 1977.
53. Swapp, G., and Main, K.: Neurofibromatosis in pregnancy. Br. J. Dermatol., 80:431–435, 1973.
54. Thomson, A.: On neuroma and neurofibromatosis. Edinburgh, Turnbull and Spears, 1900.
55. Tilesius Von Tilenau, W.: Historia Pathologica Singularis Cutis Trupitudinus. Jo Godogredi Rheinhardi Viri 50 annorum, Leipzig, S. L. Crusins, 1793.
56. von Recklinghausen, F.: Ueber die multiplen Fibrome der Haut und ihre Beziehung zu den multiplen Neuromen. Festschrift dur Rudolph Virchow, Berlin, August Hirschwald, 1882.
57. Walden, P., Johnson, A., and Bagshawe, K.: Wilms's tumor and neurofibromatosis. Br. Med. J., 1:813, 1977.
58, Weiss, R.: (A) Von Recklinghausen's disease in the negro; (B) Curvature of the spine in Von Recklinghausen's disease. Arch. Derm., 3:144–151, 1921.
59. Whitehouse, D.: Diagnostic value of the café-au-

lait spot in children. Arch. Dis. Child., *41*:316–319, 1966.
60. Winter, R., Moe, J., Bradford, D., et al.: Spine deformity in neurofibromatosis. J. Bone Joint Surg., *61A*:677–694, 1979.
61. Winter, R., and Edwards, W.: Neurofibromatosis with lumbosacral spondylolisthesis. J. Pediatr. Orthop., *1*:91–96, 1981.
62. Winter, R.: Thoracic lordoscoliosis in neurofibromatosis—treatment by a Harrington rod with sublaminar wiring. J. Bone Joint Surg., *66A*:1102–1106, 1984.
63. Yaghoobian, J.: Intrathoracic mass in a young woman with skin lesions. JAMA, *242*:2007–2008, 1979.
64. Yong-Hing, K., Kalamchi, A., and MacEwen, D.: Cervical spine abnormalities in neurofibromatosis. J. Bone Joint Surg., *61A*:695–699, 1979.

16

JUVENILE KYPHOSIS

David S. Bradford, M.D.

INTRODUCTION

Of the deformities that may develop during childhood and adolescence, kyphosis remains one of the most frequently neglected. Parents and even physicians may recognize that a child has a minimal roundback deformity of the spine and diagnose it as a problem of poor posture. This may indeed prove to be correct but more often than not, the "poor posture" is a manifestation of severe structural alteration of the vertebral column. Early recognition and treatment of patients with roundback deformity may produce a satisfactory result in the correction of the deformity as well as the alleviation of back complaints.

Juvenile kyphosis was a recognized entity long before the advent of x-rays. Schanz[96] first suspected that the posterior curvature developing in children was not necessarily due to poor posture in school, as was previously believed, but rather was a result of heavy work and strenuous demands on the back. He had earlier coined the term "apprentice kyphosis" to describe this condition.[95] After the advent of x-rays, Holger Scheuermann, in 1920,[97] first outlined the radiographic manifestations of this deformity (Fig. 16–1). He noted that the deformity was caused by wedging of the vertebral bodies, and he also outlined characteristic vertebral body changes associated with the vertebral wedging. In 1964, K. Harry Sorenson[108] further categorized the disease process and suggested that the definition of Scheuermann's disease should be a kyphosis including three central adjacent vertebra with wedging of five or more degrees. This definition has been further complicated by the realization that Sorenson was describing two forms of kyphosis, not only thoracic but also lumbar, and that normal ranges of kyphosis had not been described. Furthermore, the more recent realization that atypical forms of Scheuermann's disease (i.e., non-flexible, thoracic hyperkyphosis without vertebral wedging and vertebral body changes without wedging) may exist in patients with symptoms and findings not dissimilar to classic Scheuermann's disease[19, 111] has further clouded the issue.

"NORMAL" THORACIC KYPHOSIS

Although the normal ranges of thoracic kyphosis remain arbitrary and imprecise, studies over the past 20 years have been of assistance in further narrowing the range between normal and abnormal degrees of thoracic sagittal curvature. Roaf,[88] in 1960, stated that the normal thoracic kyphosis ranged between 20 and 40 degrees. Rocher and Perez-Case[89] found that the normal adult thoracic kyphosis measured 35 degrees. Stagnara,[110] in 1982, found that the variations in normal kyphoses were quite extensive and concluded that average values could not be used. He felt that the range of normal kyphosis was 30 to 50 degrees. Fon, Pit, and Thies[39] reviewed 316 normal chest x-rays, attempting to establish normal ranges for thoracic kyphosis according to age. They found that with increasing age there was an increase in kyphosis. Males and females were similar up to the age of 40 after which females exhibited a significantly larger kyphosis. In males from 2 to 9 years of age, they found a mean kyphosis of 20.8 degrees (range 5 to 40 degrees). Females the same age had a mean thoracic kyphosis of 23.8 degrees (range 8 to 36 degrees). In the 10 to 19 year old age group, males had a mean kyphosis of 25 degrees (range 8 to 39 degrees) and females a mean thoracic kyphosis of 26 degrees (range 11 to 41 degrees).

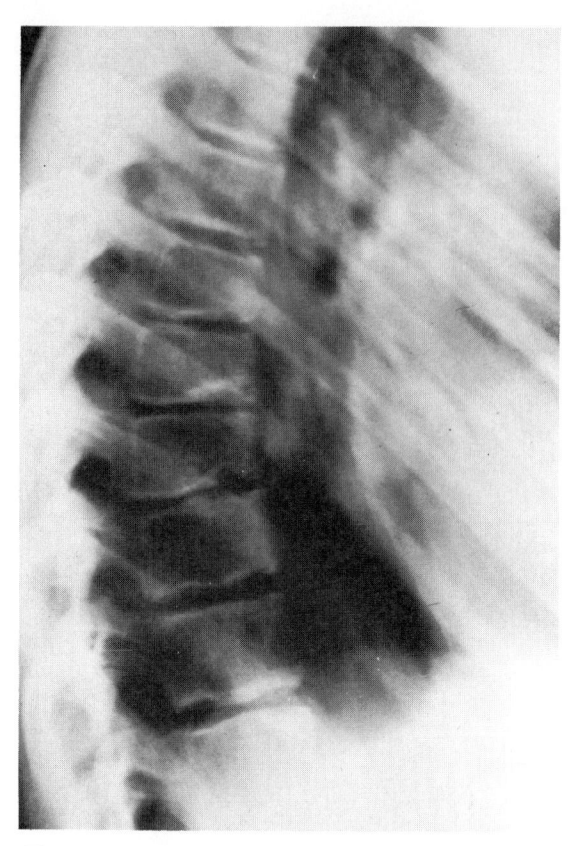

Figure 16–1. A classical x-ray appearance of the spine in a patient with Scheuermann's disease. Note the wedged vertebra, Schmorl's nodules, and marked irregularity of the vertebral endplates.

From these studies and our own experience, we have felt that a range of thoracic kyphosis from 20 to 45 degrees in a growing child is normal and that one above 45 to 50 degrees should be considered excessive. Any kyphosis at the thoracolumbar junction or in the lumbar spine is abnormal.

ETIOLOGY AND PATHOGENESIS[14–16, 35]

The etiology of Scheuermann's disease remains unknown. Scheuermann, in 1920, first proposed that the disease process was caused by avascular necrosis of the cartilage ring apophysis of the vertebral body.[97] With the onset of avascular necrosis of the rings, growth inhibition occurred, and subsequently kyphosis developed. However, this theory has never been verified. Bick and Copel[16, 17] noted that the limbus or ring apophysis was not connected to the growth plate and therefore contributed nothing to the longitudinal growth of the vertebra. Any changes or alterations that occur in the limbus, therefore, would not necessarily alter the growth potential of the vertebral body.[56, 63, 66, 103, 104] We and others have failed to demonstrate evidence of avascular necrosis in histologic material.[21, 55, 101]

Schmorl, in 1930, suggested that herniation of the intervertebral disc material through the growth plate produced kyphosis.[101, 102] He believed that changes first started as bulging of the disc material in the area of the nucleus pulposus, presumably because of developmental disturbances. Through congenital or traumatic tears in the endplates, part of the disc material was then forced into the bony spongiosum, resulting in diminished height of the intervertebral disc. Disturbed enchondral growth ultimately produced the kyphosis. Recently, Ippolito and Ponseti[55] have noted on histologic material an abnormality in the cartilage of the vertebra and growth plates. The intervertebral disc material was normal histologically. Whether these changes are primary or secondary, of course, could not be substantiated. It is known, however, that disc protrusions may occur outside the area of kyphosis in patients with Scheuermann's disease.[80] In addition, patients who have no evidence of Scheuermann's disease may have Schmorl's nodules, which may be noticed as an incidental finding on chest x-rays.

Mechanical factors have been implicated in the development of kyphosis. Scheuermann[97, 98] noted that the disease, in his experience, occurred most often in young agricultural workers who were involved in heavy labor. This mechanical factor has been stressed by numerous authors.[95, 96, 119] Micheli,[70] in 1979, found lumbar changes to be common in young rowers and suggested the etiology of stress injury to the vertebral growth plates of the thoracolumbar junction. Hensinger[51] and Kehl[58] have also stressed the mechanical theory of the etiology of thoracolumbar and lumbar kyphoses.

Muscle contractures are occasionally noted in patients with Scheuermann's disease. Lambrinudi,[65] in 1934, noted tight hamstrings in many patients and felt that this was of significance in the development of the deformity. Michelle[69] believed that contractures of the iliopsoas muscle were instrumental in producing this disease process. Although these findings are of interest, they are not present in all patients with Scheuermann's disease, and their significance consequently remains unknown. Muscle weakness[85] and an infectious process[109] have both been suggested, but proof is lacking.

A familial occurrence of Scheuermann's disease has been described in the past.[108] It has not been established whether this observation is of genetic or environmental importance. This familial occurrence has also been reported by Haggen,[47] Halal,[48] and Rathke.[86] We have noted many families in which a very high incidence of Scheuermann's disease has occurred, but we have also seen patients in whom there is no family history of roundback deformity or even scoliosis.

Of particular interest are the questions raised in the past concerning the relationship of Scheuermann's disease to endocrine or nutritional abnormalities[67] or to other disease processes.[61] In 1969, Muller and Gschwend[75] noted that of 22 patients with Turner's syndrome, 11 demonstrated radiographic changes of Scheuermann's disease. Patients with Turner's syndrome are known to have severe osteoporosis, not unlike that developing in the postmenopausal female (Fig. 16–2).[30] Simon[105] has suggested that vitamin deficiency is instrumental in the onset of Scheuermann's disease, and Kemp and coworkers[59, 60] have noted an association between malnutrition and the onset of kyphosis during growth. Muhlback and associates[74] and Gardenmin and Herbst[40] have published work to suggest that patients with Scheuermann's disease may show alterations in bone metabolism.

Recent work in our department has suggested that many of these patients may indeed have a mild form of juvenile osteoporosis.[25] A dietary analysis suggested that a deficiency of calcium may be a common finding in these patients. Furthermore, we have been impressed with the clinical and radiologic similarity between Scheuermann's disease and kyphosis in children secondary to malabsorption diseases such as non-tropical sprue and cystic fibrosis. Thus it would seem that kyphosis may occur in the adolescent period as a consequence of deficient skeletal mass, much as one would see in the adult patient, although the x-ray changes are not entirely similar.

Anthropometric and hormonal studies carried out by Ascani and coworkers[5, 6] have suggested that there is an increase in growth hormone levels in patients with juvenile ky-

Figure 16–2. A relationship may exist between Scheuermann's disease and certain endocrine and metabolic disturbances. A high incidence of kyphosis is found in A, Turner's syndrome and B, cystic fibrosis.

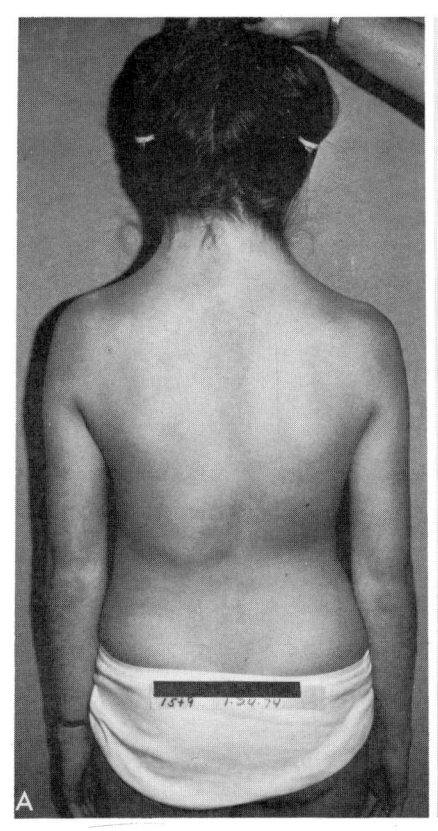

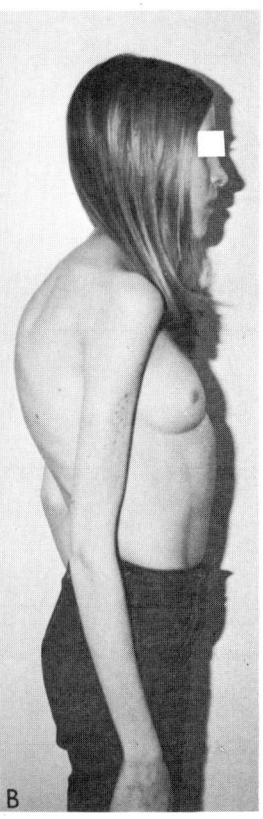

phosis. Their patients were taller than average, and the degree of skeletal maturity was advanced beyond the chronological age.

Gross and microscopic findings from pathologic material from patients with Scheuermann's disease are of interest (Fig. 16–3).[21] Grossly, at the time of surgery one will often find a thickened anterior longitudinal ligament that, in affect, acts as a bow-string across the kyphosis, serving to maintain the relative inflexibility of the deformity. The width of the intervertebral disc is normal or narrowed, and the vertebral body is wedge-shaped anteriorly. Histologic studies[11, 12, 55] have demonstrated abnormalities in the endplate growth cartilage with stunted ossification at the sites of the abnormal cartilage. Histological and histochemical abnormalities of the intervertebral disc have not been observed by Ippolito and Ponseti.[55] Furthermore, they did not note osteoporosis of the vertebra as postulated by Bradford and associates, but they did note abnormal bone in the vertebral rings and under the defective growth plate. Histologic and histochemical studies carried out by Ascani and workers[6, 9] likewise have not demonstrated necrosis of the ring apophysis nor abnormalities of the intervertebral disc. They have noted, however, an increase in the collagen-proteoglycan ratio in the matrix of the vertebra and growth plate cartilages.

In summary, the etiology remains obscure. Abnormalities have been identified histologically. Whether they are primary or secondary to altered mechanics, or secondary to repeated stress or trauma, is unknown.

CLINICAL DESCRIPTION

The prevalence of Scheuermann's disease varies from 0.4 to 8.3 per cent of the general population, depending upon whether the diagnosis is based on radiographic or clinical criteria.[108] From a review of 1338 cases reported in the literature, the male-to-female ratio appeared to be equally divided. From school screening programs started in 1972,

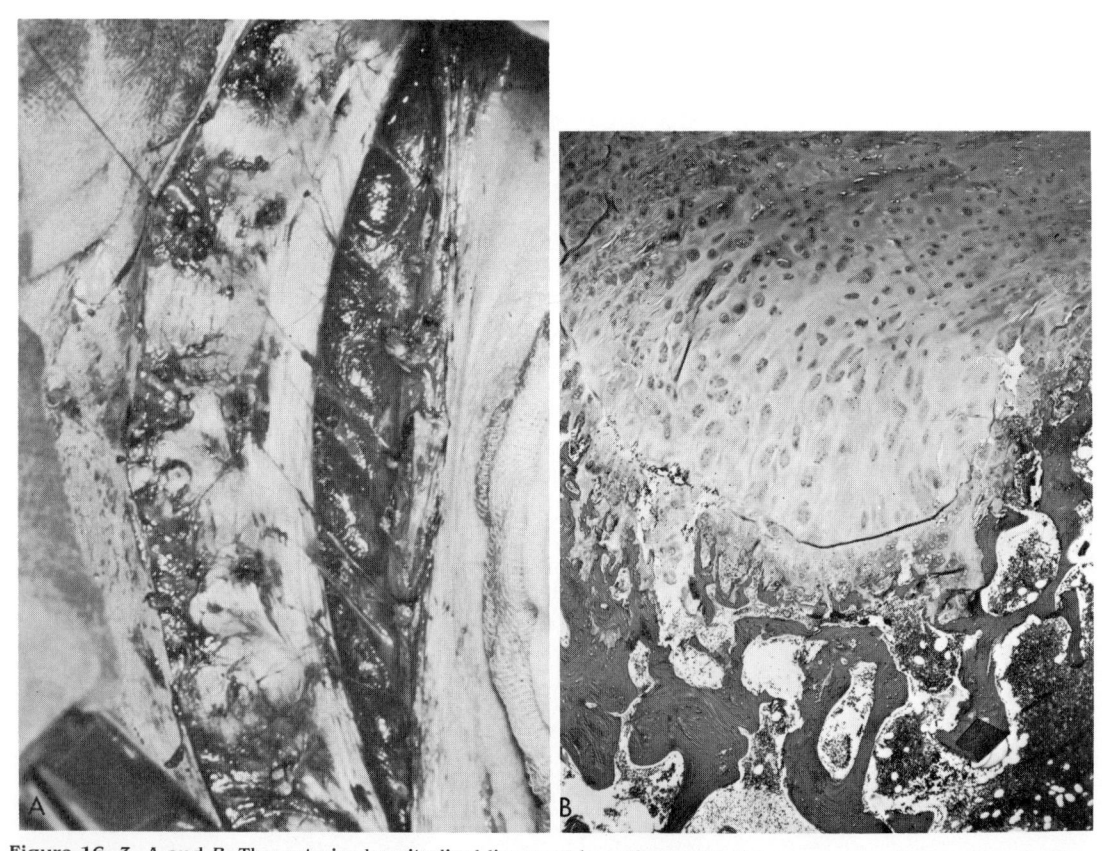

Figure 16–3. *A* and *B*, The anterior longitudinal ligament in patients with Scheuermann's disease is quite tight and thickened. Histologically, nuclear material can be seen disrupting the endplate and lying in the bony spongiosum. (Reprinted with permission from Bradford, D. S., and Moe, J. H.: Scheuermann's juvenile kyphosis—a histologic study. Clin. Orthop., *11*:45, 1975.)

Ascani and workers[7, 10] found a prevalence rate approaching 1 per cent. Their female-to-male ratio was 1.4:1. In recent studies in our department, we have found a female-to-male ratio approaching 2:1.[23] The age of the onset of the disease is difficult to establish because radiographic changes typical of Scheuermann's disease are rarely demonstrable prior to age 10 or 11. However, by age 12 to 13 years, typical vertebral changes along with wedging and kyphosis are usually present.

Symptoms

Initial complaints usually relate to the deformity and to its location. Most patients presenting with thoracic Scheuermann's disease do so because of a deformity. Albanese[3] and Guntz[44, 45] have noted pain in only 20 per cent of their patients, whereas Scheuermann,[98] and Nathan and Kuhns[76] reported an incidence greater than 60 per cent. Sorenson[108] has noted that pain is infrequent in the early stages of the deformity but when the patient is in the early teens, when the more florid stage of the disease is apparent, the incidence of pain rapidly increases. In his 103 patients, he found that pain was present in over 50 per cent. Furthermore, the incidence of pain was much higher in patients with a kyphosis involving the first or second lumbar vertebra (78 per cent). These are similar statistics to those presented by Hensinger, Greene, and Hunter.[51] They found that pain was the dominant complaint in patients presenting with thoracolumbar kyphosis. The pain is usually intermittent and aching rather than constant and incapacitating. It is usually localized over the involved area of the kyphosis and is non-radiating. Often a definite history of injury coincident with the onset can be elicited.

Physical Examination (Fig. 16–4)

On examination, an increase in normal thoracic kyphosis and lumbar lordosis is readily apparent.[22, 33, 72, 79, 119] The kyphosis will appear rather fixed and will not fully correct when the patient attempts thoracic hyperextension in the prone position. The lumbar lordosis is usually not structural except in rare circumstances and is readily correctible on forward bending. The thoracic hump may be increased with forward bending as seen in the lateral view.

Thoracolumbar or lumbar kyphosis is not easily visible; it may be noticed by slight prominence of the spinous processes over the thoracolumbar or lumbar junction.

A minimal scoliosis of the spine may be noticed on forward bending. Direct tenderness with muscle spasm may be elicited over the kyphosis, be it thoracic or lumbar. Muscle tightness and apparent contractures, particularly of the hamstrings, are common. Patients should be examined carefully neurologically to rule out a spastic paraparesis manifested by ataxia and hyperreflexia, which may present on rare occasions secondary to spinal cord compression (see Complications of Scheuermann's Disease).

Radiographic Findings

For the radiographic evaluation of the patient with Scheuermann's disease, several views are desirable (see Chapter 22). A lateral 2-meter standing film of the spine with the arms held parallel to the floor and the hands resting on a support is most helpful in evaluating the kyphosis. The patient should be instructed to hold his or her head erect. A standing 2-meter anterior-posterior x-ray is also taken to rule out an associated scoliosis. A hyperextension lateral x-ray of the spine is taken using a polyurethane plastic wedge placed at the apex of the curvature. Skeletal maturation may be assessed by noting the status of the iliac crest apophyses and the vertebral ring apophyses. The angles of kyphosis and lordosis are outlined by marking the end vertebrae, which are maximally tilted into the concavity of the curve. The angle from the endplates of the end vertebrae is considered to be the kyphotic angle. The sacrum is considered to be the end vertebra for the measurement of lordosis. Vertebral wedging is outlined in a similar fashion, marking lines parallel to the endplates and measuring the angle thus created.

Characteristic changes of the vertebral bodies secondary to Scheuermann's disease include vertebral wedging, Schmorl's nodules, and irregular endplates. A mild scoliosis (10 to 20 degrees) with or without vertebral rotation is seen in 20 to 30 per cent of patients.[23] Persistent vascular grooves, if present, appear to be more related to the immaturity of the vertebral body and do not have an etio-

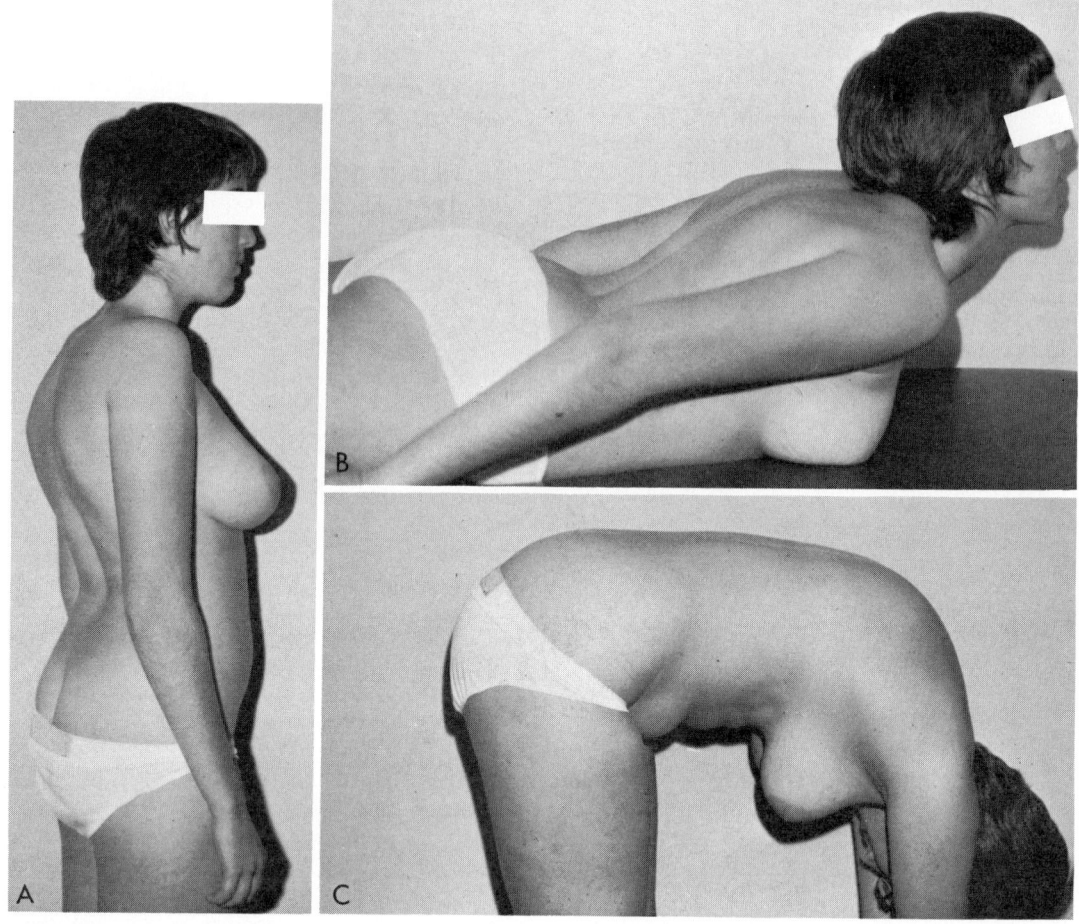

Figure 16–4. A, On physical examination, a definite increase in thoracic kyphosis and lumbar lordosis is visualized. B, The thoracic kyphosis does not fully correct on thoracic extension. C, The lumbar lordosis, on the other hand, usually corrects on forward bending.

logic or prognostic value. Late radiographic changes in patients over age 40 include those associated with degenerative arthritis of the spine, such as osteophyte formation anteriorly and degenerative facet changes posteriorly. The AP x-ray of the spine should be carefully evaluated for evidence of increased interpedicular distance, which may be seen in association with spinal epidural cysts.[31] The changes in the lumbar spine have been outlined by Hafner[46] and Hensinger.[51] It is important to realize that these changes are not caused by infection, and vertebral body biopsy is not necessary or indicated.

We have found that the best radiographic criteria for the diagnosis of classic Scheuermann's disease are (1) irregular vertebral endplates, (2) apparent narrowing of the intervertebral disc space, (3) one or more vertebrae wedged five or more degrees, and (4) an increase in normal thoracic kyphosis above 45 degrees.

RELATIONSHIP BETWEEN POSTURAL ROUNDBACK, SCHEUERMANN'S DISEASE (CLASSIC), AND ATYPICAL SCHEUERMANN'S DISEASE

Scheuermann's disease should be distinguished from postural roundback deformity. Children with postural roundback have only a slight to modest increase in thoracic kyphosis (40 to 60 degrees) and an accentuated lumbar lordosis (Fig. 16–5). Although the kyphosis may rarely be greater, clinically it is quite mobile, easily and voluntarily correctable, and unassociated with muscle contractures. X-rays show normal vertebral body contours without vertebral wedging or endplate irregularity. Since radiographic changes of Scheuermann's disease may not be apparent until age 10 to 12 years, it is possible that early Scheuermann's disease could be incorrectly diagnosed as a postural roundback deformity. It is also possible that a severe

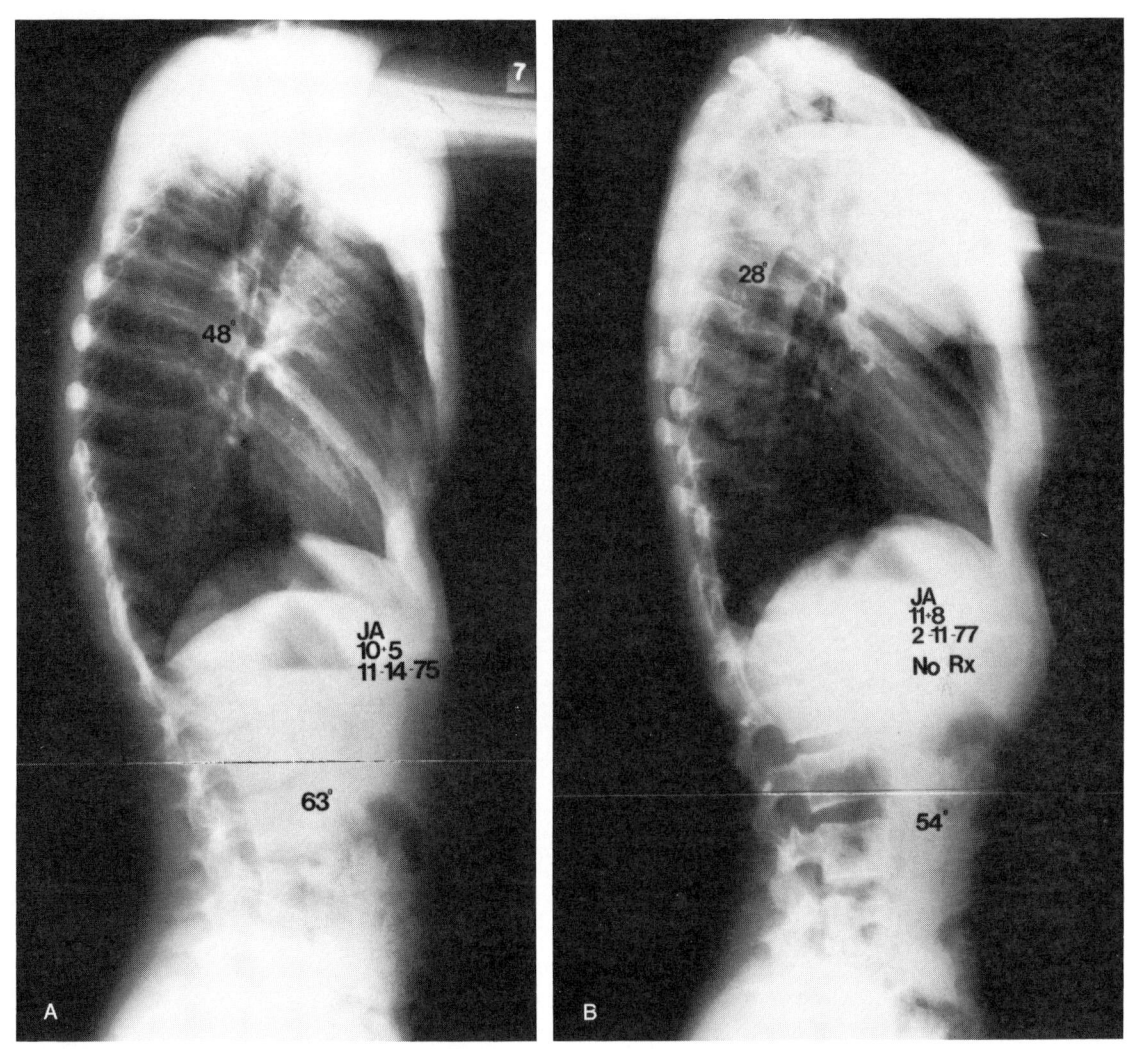

Figure 16–5. A, A 10 year old patient with postural roundback. Note mild kyphosis with absence of vertebral body changes. B, No treatment was prescribed and a year and a half later the kyphosis is noted to have improved considerably.

untreated postural roundback might progress into Scheuermann's disease with vertebral wedging. Finally, there is an atypical form of Scheuermann's disease that may present in two fashions: (1) vertebral body changes without wedging or increased kyphosis, or (2) increased kyphosis without vertebral body changes. In the former case, patients often have back pain and spasm with radiographic changes of endplate irregularity, disc space narrowing, and Schmorl's nodules. These changes may be completely confined to the thoracolumbar spine, even resulting in a minimal thoracolumbar kyphosis (less than 40 degrees).[35, 46, 97] In the other situation, we may see a structural kyphosis in a teenager without radiographic changes of endplate irregularity or vertebral wedging. This is not common but may present a clinical appearance of classic Scheuermann's disease. The relationship of these kyphoses to each other as well as to Scheuermann's disease is unknown. We feel that they are variations or perhaps subtypes of the same pathophysiologic condition (Fig. 16–6).

Differential Diagnosis

Besides differentiating Scheuermann's disease from its atypical forms and from postural roundback, other types of kyphosis should be considered.[22, 30, 108, 121]

Many authors have emphasized the prob-

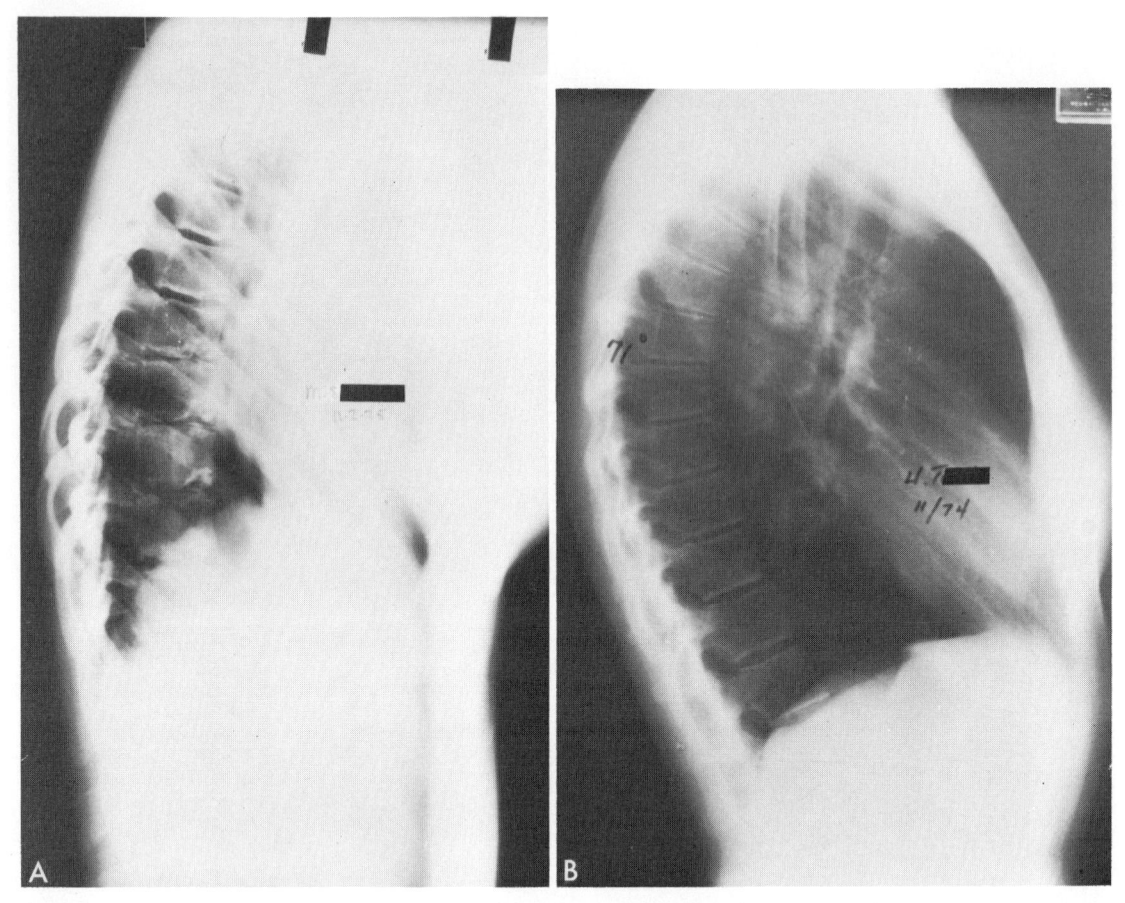

Figure 16–6. Atypical forms of Scheuermann's disease. A, Vertebral body abnormalities without kyphosis. B, Increased kyphosis without vertebral changes.

lems occasionally encountered in differentiating Scheuermann's disease from infectious spondylitis. However, with a thorough clinical and laboratory evaluation, as well as tomography and bone scans of the spine, a true diagnosis should be readily established. Traumatic injuries to the spine occasionally present a confusing picture, but in these cases, usually only one vertebra is involved, while in Scheuermann's disease, often more than one vertebra is affected. Multiple compression fractures of the spine can arise from severe flexion injuries, and after healing, differentiation from Scheuermann's disease may be extremely difficult, if not impossible. Osteochondrodystrophies, such as Morquio's disease and Hurler's disease, as well as postlaminectomy kyphosis, tumors, and congenital deformities of the spine, may be considered in the differential diagnosis of this group.

Type 2 congenital kyphosis may be mistaken for Scheuermann's disease (Fig. 16–7). In this type of kyphosis, however, anterior interbody fusion develops spontaneously, whereas in Scheuermann's disease it does not. Osteophytes may form anteriorly, but bony bridging across the disc space does not develop even in the untreated adult. Lumbosacral anomalies should always be ruled out. Spondylolisthesis at L5-S1 can produce a severe lumbar lordosis and consequently a compensatory thoracic kyphosis. These patients will be completely asymptomatic except for a roundback deformity. They usually do not show the radiographic changes of the vertebrae that are characteristic of Scheuermann's disease. Finally, ankylosing spondylitis should be ruled out in the male; if the clinical and x-ray evaluations do not furnish a reliable differentiation, HL-A tissue typing will prove helpful. Ninety-seven per cent of patients with ankylosing spondylitis will be B-27 positive.

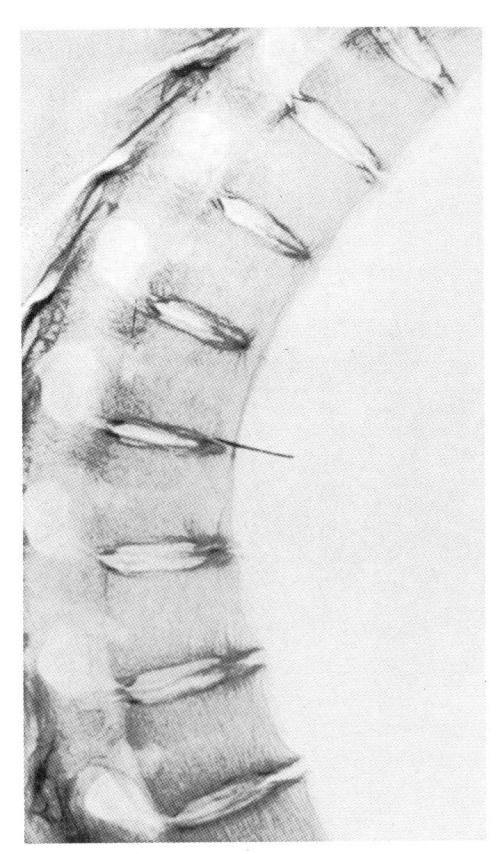

Figure 16–7. A Type II congenital kyphosis, which may be mistaken for Scheuermann's disease. In this type of congenital deformity, spontaneous interbody fusion may develop after birth, whereas in Scheuermann's disease this does not occur, although osteophytes may arise anteriorly as a late sequela. (Reprinted with permission from Schmorl, G., and Junghanns, H.: Deformities of the Spine. New York, Grune & Stratton, 1959.)

COMPLICATIONS OF SCHEUERMANN'S DISEASE

A kyphosis of less than 45 degrees in the thoracic spine is rarely, if ever, of cosmetic significance. Deformities above 65 or 70 degrees are noticeable, and because of an increased compensatory lumbar lordosis and cervical lordosis, the cosmetically objectionable appearance may be apparent. Curves of this magnitude certainly may increase even after skeletal maturation is complete, although the frequency with which this occurs is not known. Small degrees of kyphosis in the lumbar and thoracolumbar spine may be more readily apparent as a greater distortion of sagittal contours at this level is more obvious (Fig. 16–8).

Back pain, when present in a growing child with Scheuermann's disease, may be transient with or without treatment.[108] The incidence of thoracic pain in the untreated adult has ranged from 10 to 42 per cent of patients in reported series.[44, 53, 54] Low back pain developing in Scheuermann's disease after the completion of growth appears to be much more common. Guntz[44] noted that 42 per cent of 50 patients with this disease had low back pain after they reached skeletal maturity. He stated that from the fourth decade on, Scheuermann's disease predisposed to low back pain and disc degeneration. Sanders and Inman[94] and Schlegel[100] supported this concept.

Dittmar[34] reported that pain in the low back as well as thoracic spine was found in 89 per cent of his 36 patients. Patients with a herniated disc would likewise be expected to have a higher incidence of Scheuermann's disease than is present in the general population. Soderberg and Andren[106] found that of 106 patients with back pain and sciatica, 46 per cent had Scheuermann's disease, whereas a control series showed only 13 per cent had Scheuermann's disease. Sorenson,[108] in reviewing long-term follow-up on 239 patients, noted that one half had back pain at the site of the kyphosis before they reached the age of 20. After the age of 20, the incidence fell to one fourth of the patients. The pain did not influence the patient's working ability and only occasionally required treatment. On the other hand, he found that low back pain was no more frequent in these patients than in the normal population except in those with the long or low kyphosis involving the first and second lumbar vertebrae. Nearly all of these patients had complaints of low back pain. Of interest is the work of Niethard,[77] who recently noted an increased incidence of spondylolysis in patients with Scheuermann's disease. Hensinger and workers[51, 62] have also noticed this finding and reported that 32 per cent of their patients with thoracolumbar or lumbar Scheuermann's disease had spondylolysis or spondylolisthesis.

Neurologic complications in Scheuermann's disease, although rare, have been outlined in the past. (Fig. 16–9).[25] Cord compression presenting as a spastic paraparesis may develop secondary to the angular deformity alone, or in association with a herniated thoracic intervertebral disc at the apex of the curvature. Ryan and Taylor[92] have suggested that males between the ages of 14

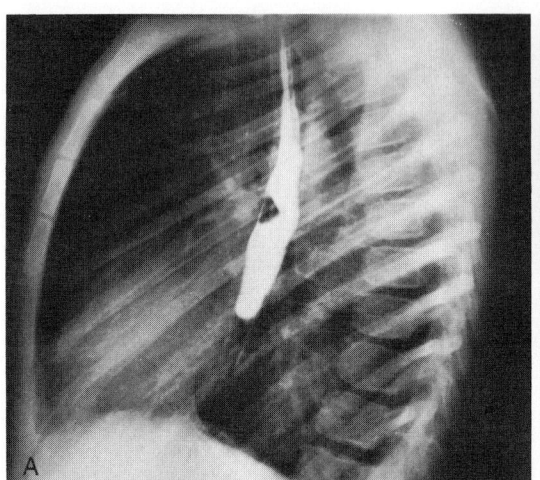

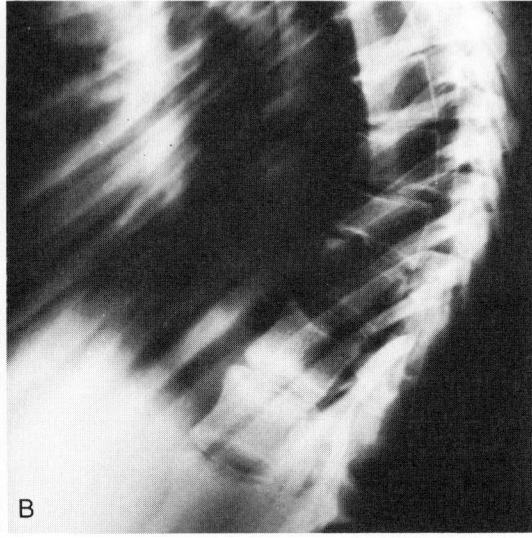

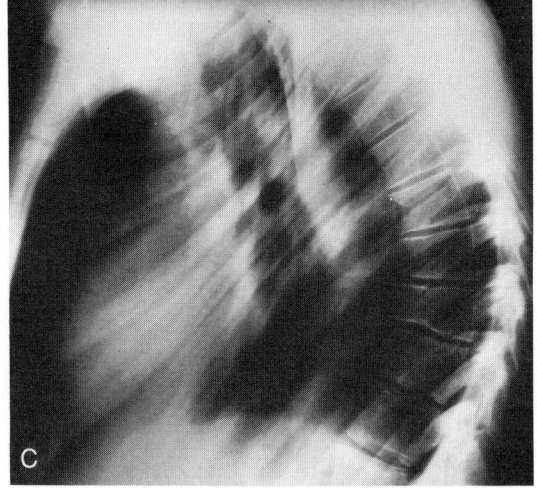

Figure 16–8. *A, B,* and *C,* Untreated Scheuermann's disease may progress severely during the adolescent period. This series demonstrates a marked progression of the kyphosis over a 10-year period. (Reprinted with permission from Rothman, R. H., and Simeone, F. A.: The Spine, Vol. I, 2nd ed. Philadelphia, W. B. Saunders Co., 1982.)

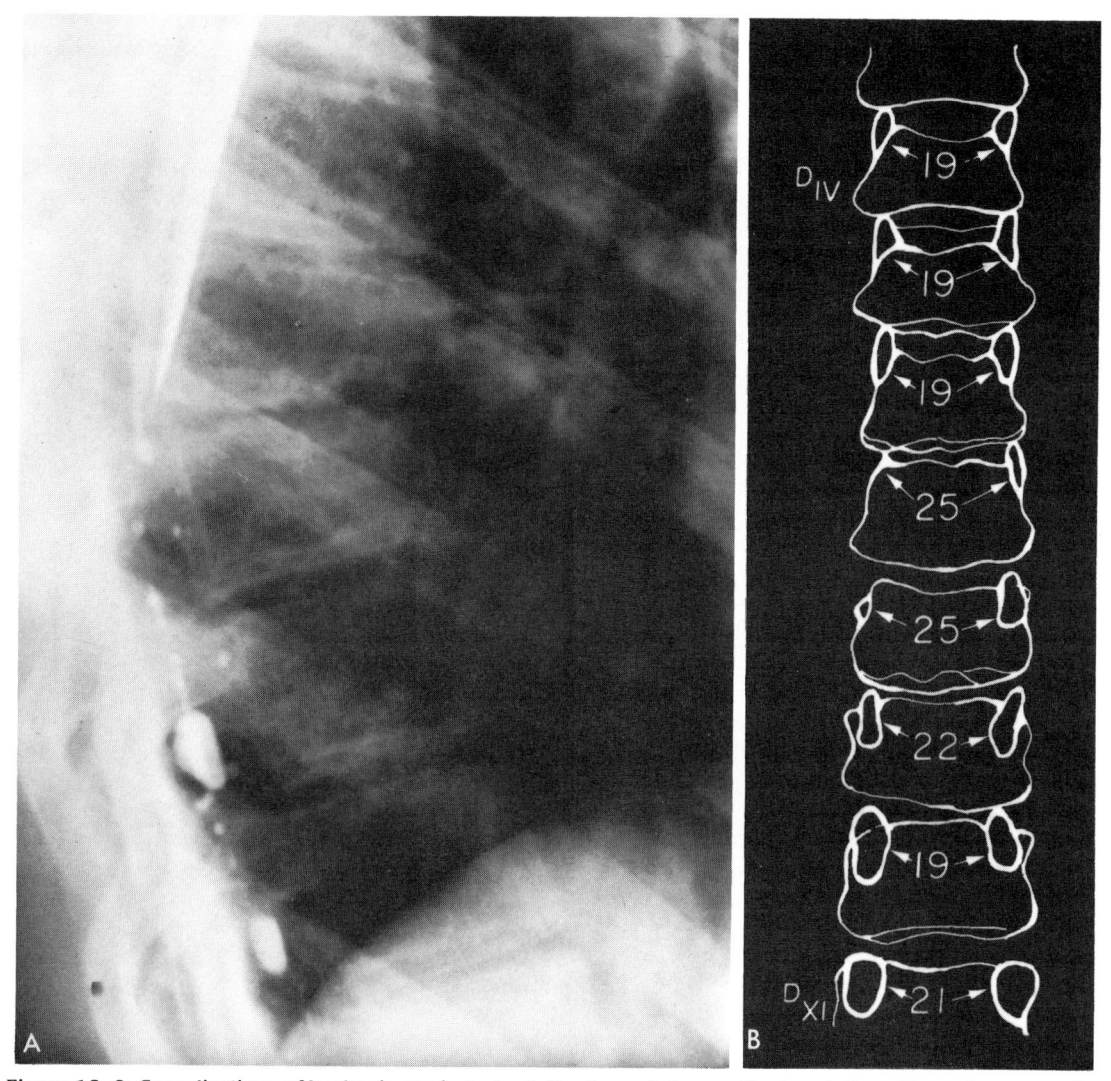

Figure 16–9. Complications of kyphosis can include: A, Cord angulation or disc herniation with cord compression at the apex of the curvature; B, A kyphosis associated with spinal epidural cysts. In the latter instance, the diagnosis may be suspected by the presence of a widened interpedicular space. (Reprinted with permission from Rothman, R. H., and Simeone, F. A.: The Spine, vol. I., 2nd ed. Philadelphia, W. B. Saunders Co., 1982.)

and 20 years seem to be at greatest risk for development of herniated disc in the thoracic spine with neurologic compromise. One should always examine carefully the anterior-posterior x-ray of the thoracolumbar spine in patients with Scheuermann's disease to be sure that widening of the interpedicular space is not present. A spinal epidural cyst may be associated with classic radiographic changes of Scheuermann's disease and present on x-ray with widening of the interpedicular space.[1, 31, 36]

INDICATIONS FOR TREATMENT

The difficulty in determining whether treatment should or should not be undertaken in juvenile kyphosis revolves around several considerations: (1) the lack of a clear, concise, definitive study on whether treatment in the juvenile period decreases the incidence of back pain in the adult period, (2) the lack of a clear, concise, long-term study until recently on the natural history of untreated juvenile kyphosis, and (3) whether or not any correction from treatment obtained in the childhood or juvenile period is maintained throughout the adult period.

Sorenson[108] has suggested that if Scheuermann's disease is confined to the thoracic spine the prognosis is favorable, and no treatment need be prescribed. Such an outcome has not been our experience. Adult patients frequently present to us with untreated thoracic kyphosis that is not only a psychological handicap but also a source of significant and disabling thoracic back pain. The pain alone is at times difficult to manage except by spinal fusion. Rarely, the kyphosis may be a cause of paraplegia developing in late adolescence or the early adult years.

Travaglini[117] has recently published work to suggest that patients with juvenile kyphosis followed for 25 years or more do show a significant increase in their deformity. In 50 cases of kyphosis followed for up to 25 years, he showed that 80 per cent of thoracic forms that exceeded 40 to 45 degrees worsened in the adult period. This is as one would expect from the study of Fon and associates[39] who noted that on the average the kyphosis was greater in the adult in normal controls than in children. Finally, whether orthotic treatment and the correction obtained in the childhood and juvenile period is maintained in the adult period has not been clearly determined. Recent work from our department[93] has determined that although some correction has been lost in patients followed five or more years after completion of brace treatment, over 60 per cent of the patients maintain their improvement.

We feel, therefore, that the treatment of kyphosis in the growing child is worthwhile not only to correct the cosmetic deformity and to prevent the possibility of progression of the deformity during the treatment phase, but also to alleviate present symptoms and hopefully to prevent future problems from developing. It is recognized that some loss of correction will occur, but at the present time we feel that the increase in deformity is less than that that would have occurred from the natural evolution.

TREATMENT

Non-operative Methods

Numerous methods of treatment have been described in the past. Exercises alone have been suggested,[76, 105] but definitive evidence of improvement has been noted only rarely. Indeed, one study has shown that although the kyphosis improved slightly, vertebral wedging actually increased.[22] Exercise as a supplement to other forms of treatment,[26, 115] however, has been found to be beneficial and may furnish a means of correcting tightness of the hamstrings and pectoral musculature.

Bedrest, the use of a plaster shell or body jacket, and hyperextension treatment on a Bradford frame have been recommended.[36, 37, 56, 76, 105, 113, 120] Such combined methods of treatment have been advocated by many authors.[40, 76, 99, 115]

A hyperextension cast applied in one or two stages has also proven to be effective as a method of treatment. With a two-stage technique,[3, 36, 43, 87, 114] the lordosis is corrected first by having the patient bend forward while the cast is applied over the lumbar spine, and then as a second stage, the plaster is extended up to the upper part of the trunk, correcting the kyphosis. The cast is changed every three months for approximately one year, a technique described by Stagnara and Perdriolle.[112] Other authors have found bracing and casting techniques to be effective in the correction of kyphosis.[42, 78, 86, 90, 91, 111] Ponte has recently reported excellent results with cast treatment alone.[83]

The use of the Milwaukee brace in the nonoperative treatment of scoliosis was first reported by Blount[18] in 1958. Moe,[71] in 1965, reported successful results in correcting the deformity of juvenile kyphosis by using the Milwaukee brace. Bradford and coworkers[23] reported in 1974, on 75 patients who had completed Milwaukee brace treatment. Although only 19 patients had a follow-up of greater than 18 months, their results showed that the vertebral wedging and kyphosis improved by 40 per cent and the lumbar lordosis improved by 36 per cent. More severe degrees of kyphosis (greater than 75 degrees), skeletal maturity, or increased vertebral wedging, averaging greater than 10 degrees were factors that limited the degree of correction (Fig. 16–10). Montgomery and Irwin[73] studied 21 patients treated with the Milwaukee brace for Scheuermann's disease,

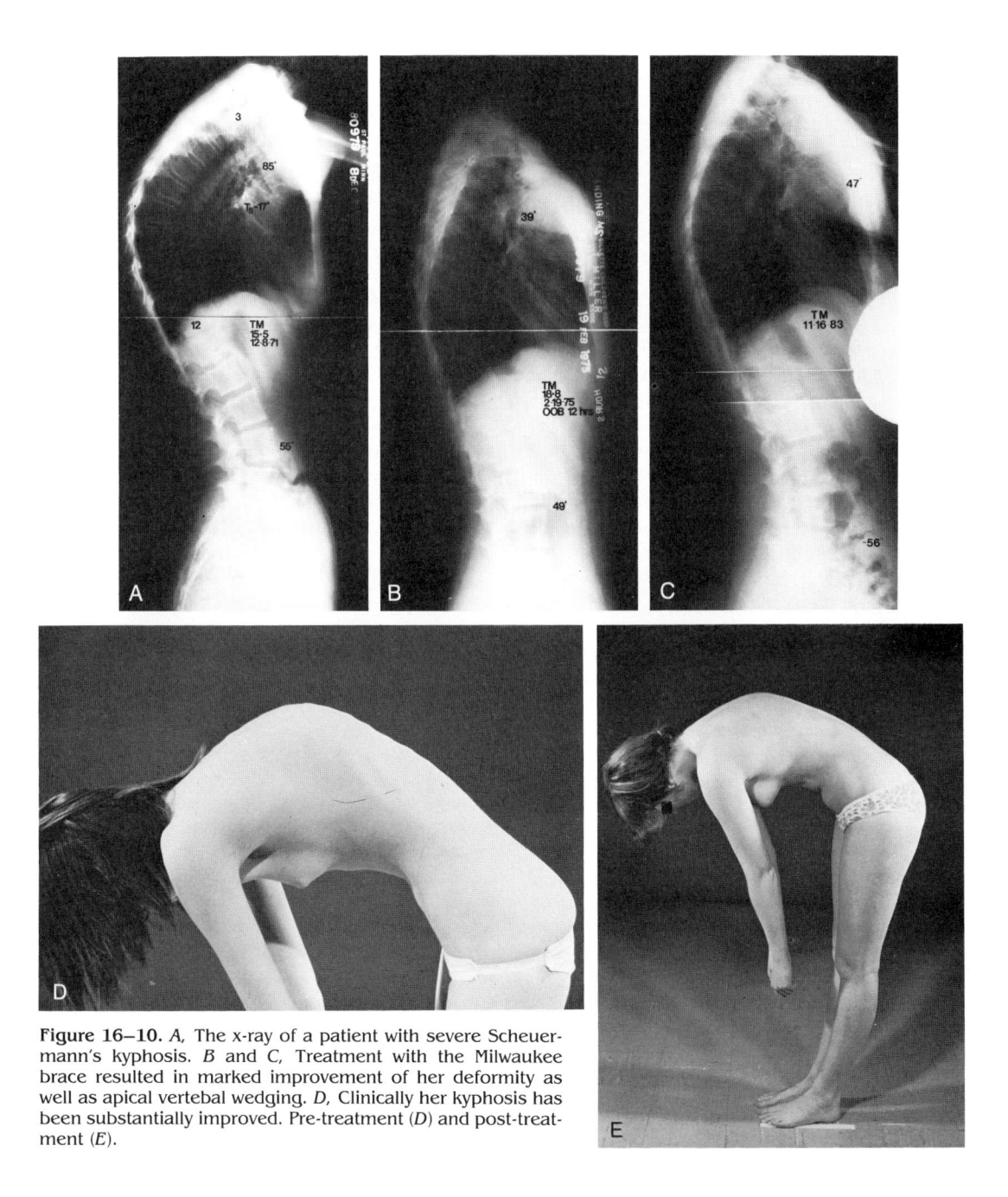

Figure 16–10. *A*, The x-ray of a patient with severe Scheuermann's kyphosis. *B* and *C*, Treatment with the Milwaukee brace resulted in marked improvement of her deformity as well as apical vertebal wedging. *D*, Clinically her kyphosis has been substantially improved. Pre-treatment (*D*) and post-treatment (*E*).

followed for more than 18 months after completion of treatment. They noted that although the initial curve improved from an average of 62 to 41 degrees, loss of correction averaging 15 degrees developed. They recommended that in order to avoid this loss of correction the endpoint of brace wear should occur when vertebral wedging is approximately five degrees or less. They felt that the majority of patients should wear the brace longer than 18 months in order to obtain an optimal result.

The Lyonaise method of treatment as proposed by Stagnara[111, 112] involves antigravity casting followed by a plexidur brace. The early results from this treatment program appear similar to those results reported in America from the use of the Milwaukee brace.

Longer follow-ups, however, are now available, and the loss of correction has been disturbing. In fact, in the cases presented by Mauroy and Stagnara,[68] a 60 per cent loss of correction over a 15 year period after treatment was terminated has been reported. Pratelli and Bartolozzi[84] also evaluated 74 cases 15 years following treatment with the antigravity plaster cast. They reported a total loss of correction. They attributed this, in part, to a reduced period of treatment that averaged nine months. We have recently reviewed our results on 122 patients with Scheuermann's disease treated with a Milwaukee brace in which a minimum five year follow-up was available.[93] Ten patients were inconsistent brace wearers: two of the ten had improvement of the kyphosis, five worsened, and three went on to surgical arthrodesis. Of the remaining 110 patients, nine ultimately required surgery. Kyphoses were evaluated in four subgroups: Group I were 45 to 54 degrees, Group II were 55 to 64 degrees, Group III were 65 to 74 degrees, and Group IV were greater than 75 degrees. The average initial kyphosis for each group was 50 degrees, 58 degrees, 67 degrees, and 81 degrees, respectively. The kyphosis at the end of brace treatment for each group was 36 degrees, 38 degrees, 43 degrees, and 49 degrees, respectively. At five years or more of follow-up, the kyphosis averaged 45 degrees, 51 degrees, 54 degrees, and 62 degrees, respectively. It appeared that the amount of correction obtained for each group was similar, and the patients with more severe degrees of kyphosis, Group IV, had less favorable final results (Fig. 16–11).

PLAN OF PATIENT MANAGEMENT

Following complete and thorough history and physical examination along with x-ray evaluation as previously outlined, the patient is fitted for a Milwaukee brace. If the curve is quite rigid, demonstrating less than 15 to 20 degrees of mobility on the hyperextension x-ray, it may prove worthwhile to initiate treatment by applying a hyperextension Risser antigravity cast that includes the neck. The cast may be changed two or three times over the next three to four months in order to obtain more correction. A Milwaukee brace may be fabricated during this period. Once the brace is ready, it is applied and a specific exercise program in the brace as well as out of the brace is initiated by the physical therapist. This includes pelvic tilting exercises to decrease lumbar lordosis, muscle stretching exercises designed to overcome contractures, and thoracic extension exercises to build up the thoracic extensor muscle group. The patients are allowed to be out of the brace at least one hour per day for personal hygiene and bathing. In patients who are active in sports, it may also prove desirable to allow them out of the brace for two to four hour periods necessary to participate in athletics. We have found that brace acceptability is increased markedly by allowing patients this diversion. In our experience, kyphosis and vertebral wedging are generally corrected within one year and once these are corrected a slow weaning process may be begun. Patients may not necessarily require full-time bracing until skeletal maturation or closure of the vertebral ring apophyses. The total time in the brace has generally averaged from two to three years, with at least one year of full-time wear, but there are obvious individual variations that are dependent upon the response to the brace, the age of the patient, and the magnitude of the deformity.

It should be appreciated that more severe curvatures are less likely to obtain full correction to physiologic ranges of normal kyphosis. As stated above, although we have found that improvement occurs even in the more severe degrees of kyphosis, the final result at least at five year follow-up is unlikely to be in the normal ranges of a desired physiologic kyphosis, i.e., less than 45 degrees. Therefore, if a patient is approaching skeletal maturity with a 70+ degree range of kyphosis, it would be more reasonable to consider surgical correction if correction is

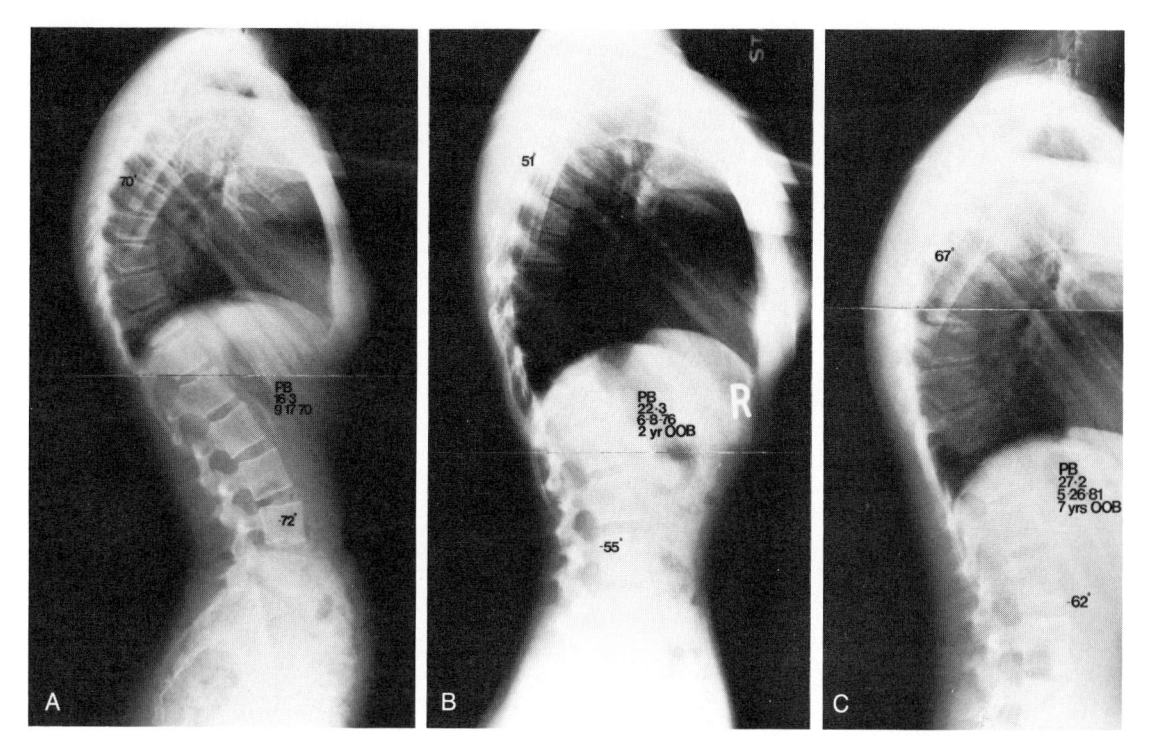

Figure 16–11. A kyphosis of 70 degrees in a skeletally immature female. Although initial response to the brace was satisfactory, and correction appeared to be maintained reasonably well, two years out of the brace (B), and seven years out of the brace (C) the curvature is almost the same as before treatment. Severe degrees of kyphosis greater than 75 degrees have a less favorable final result on longterm follow-up.

deemed advisable or no treatment at all other than continued observation. Finally, it should be remembered that correction is still possible in the older patient even though the iliac apophysis may be closed. As long as the ring apophyses of the vertebral bodies are open, some skeletal remodeling potential is still possible. However, it is unlikely that the results from this older group of patients will be as good as those that are obtained in patients who are physiologically immature.

COMMENTS ON POSTURAL ROUNDBACK

The management of patients with postural roundback may follow the same principles as outlined for Scheuermann's disease. If the child is a young, preadolescent individual with a supple kyphosis, exercises alone may prove sufficient. If progression of the kyphosis is noted or the patient develops radiographic evidence of vertebral wedging or other changes of Scheuermann's disease, we would recommend institution of brace treatment. Exercises alone are usually adequate for managing postural roundback or postural increased lumbar lordosis. We have not favored bracing for a purely postural problem.

UNDERARM BRACES AND ELECTRICAL STIMULATION

Underarm braces may be effective in the correction of thoracic kyphosis and, in fact, this is the type brace described by the Lyonaise treatment program. We have found it more useful in a kyphosis with an apex below T9, and particularly useful for the thoracolumbar or lumbar kyphosis. With a kyphosis in the mid-thoracic spine, we continue to favor the Milwaukee brace (Fig. 16–12).

Electrical stimulation as a treatment program for managing thoracic Scheuermann's disease has been described by Axelgaard, Brown, and Swank.[13] They have reported minimal experience with this technique, and the early results of eight patients showed an average decrease in the kyphosis from 51 degrees at the start of treatment to 46 degrees at one year, and 42 degrees at one and a half years. Further follow-up with larger numbers of patients are necessary before the role of this mode of treatment can be fully evaluated.

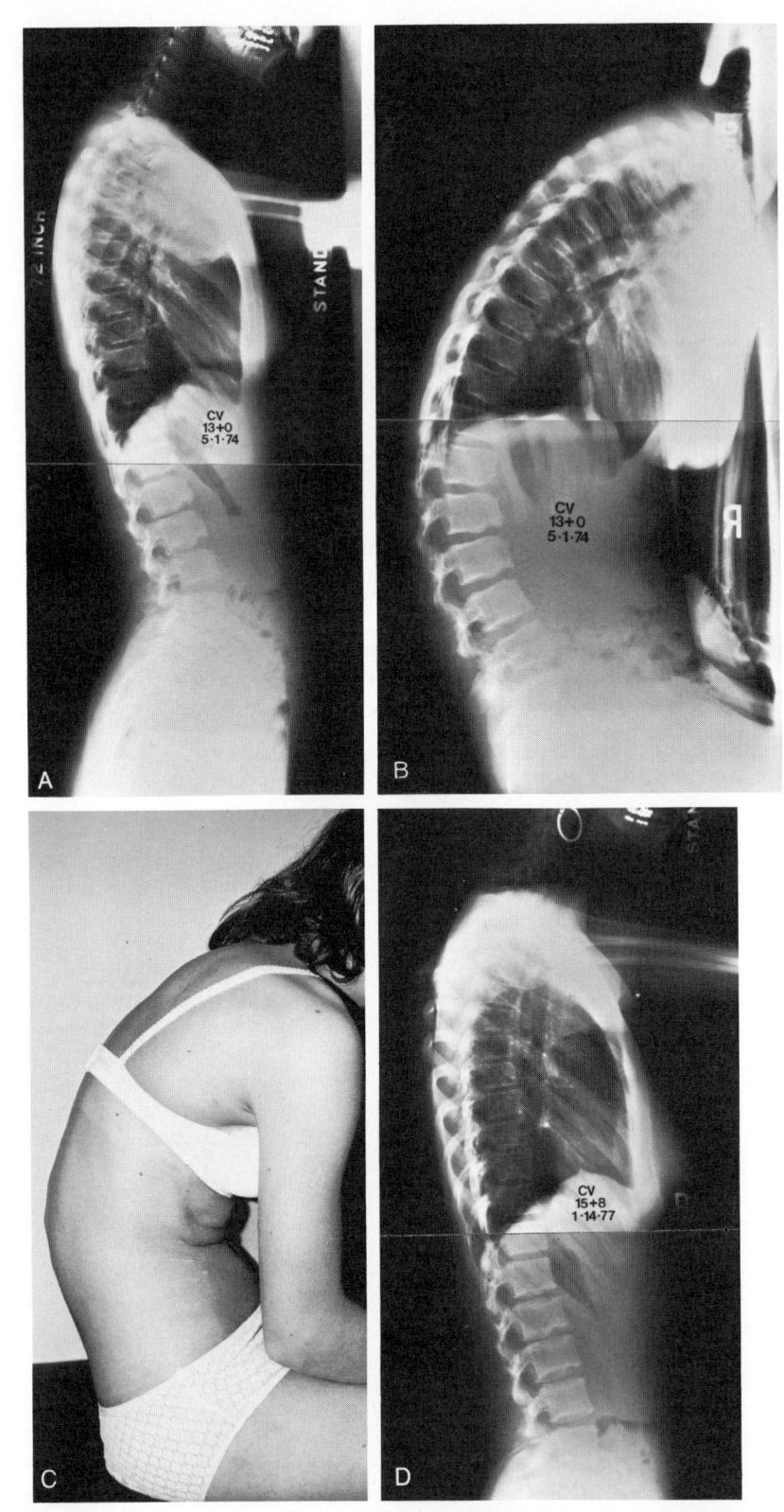

Figure 16–12. Thoracolumbar kyphosis as demonstrated in a standing view (*A*) and better in the flexion view (*B*) may be well managed with an underarm brace. *C*, The clinically apparent thoracolumbar kyphus can be seen. At follow-up three years later, the vertebral body has partially filled in (*D*) and the patient's back discomfort has been greater relieved.

Operative Treatment

Surgery for juvenile kyphosis may be indicated in those patients who present with significant deformity that is symptomatic and who are poor candidates for brace treatment, or in adults who present with residual deformity, or continued back pain uncontrolled by conservative management.

Spinal fusion for the treatment of juvenile kyphosis has until recently only received scant attention in the literature.[4, 14, 15, 107, 112, 118] Ferguson[37] suggested that fusion may be occasionally indicated, but Hallock and associates[49] felt that posterior spine fusion alone would not correct a kyphosis unless the fusion was done over an extensive area. Roaf[88] noted that posterior fusion could be advantageous in correcting the deformity from continued growth anteriorly. Moe,[71] in 1965, presented early experience with posterior fusion alone for the management of kyphosis. Bradford and coworkers[24] reporting on results in 22 patients in 1975, noted that although posterior fusion alone could substantially correct a deformity, loss of correction averaged 15 degrees at follow-up. They commented on the problems inherent in obtaining a solid posterior arthrodesis over a kyphosis in which the fusion mass was under tension rather than compression. They recommended a combined approach for a kyphosis greater than 65 degrees. Kostuik[64] also found a high percentage of pseudarthrosis from posterior arthrodesis alone. The loss of correction through the posterior approach could be lessened by a stronger and modified compression system, as reported by Cotrel.[32] Re-exploration and augmentation of the posterior fusion in four to five months, as reported by Ponte[81, 82] or positioning the upper Harrington hooks underneath the lamina rather than the transverse processes as described by Taylor and workers[116] appears useful.

We, however, have favored a combined approach for the majority of these patients, especially for those with curvatures greater than 70 degrees in whom surgical correction is deemed advisable.[20] In a review of 24 patients treated by the combined approach, the average loss of correction was only 6 degrees. The average kyphosis preoperatively was 77 degrees and postoperatively, 41 degrees.[20] This report is similar to the results reported by Herndon and coworkers in 1981.[52]

It should be appreciated that surgery is only rarely necessary in these patients, and the need for two operations with inherent complications in each procedure should be well appreciated.

PLAN OF PATIENT MANAGEMENT

If surgery is felt indicated for the reasons previously stated, we favor a first stage anterior transthoracic spine fusion,[19] completely removing the intervertebral disc, dividing the anterior longitudinal ligament over the apical six to seven interspaces, and bridging the intervertebral disc space with rib or iliac bone graft (Fig. 16–13) (see Techniques of Spinal Surgery). One to two weeks after the anterior procedure, a posterior spinal fusion, using either a Harrington compression device with the larger compression rods, ¼ inch (6.4 mm.) L-rods, or CD instrumentation, is carried out. If Harrington compression rods are used, we have found it preferable to extend the fusion up to T2, placing the compression assembly over the transverse processes of the upper thoracic vertebra. If these are deficient, the hooks should be placed on the lamina, although this does require a more substantial laminotomy. The compression hooks distal to the apex of the kyphosis are placed underneath the lamina. We prefer to instrument as many levels as possible and to use, as mentioned, the larger compression assembly. L-rods may prove advantageous, but it is more difficult to titrate the correctability with SSI than with posterior Harrington compression instrumentation (Fig. 16–14).

If compression rods have been used, we favor the use of a postoperative brace or cast, including the neck. If L-rods or the CD system has been used, no postoperative support is applied.

Is posterior instrumentation alone ever considered? In the more flexible degrees of kyphosis or in the adolescent patient with growth remaining anteriorly, and if the magnitude of deformity is less than 70 degrees, we will consider posterior instrumentation alone with posterior spine fusion (Fig. 16–15). With greater degrees of deformities or in adult patients we feel the combined approach gives the best result.

Is halo traction beneficial? The halo may be useful to mobilize adult patients between procedures in a halo wheelchair, and it may assist in positioning the patient for the second stage procedure. We are now more in-

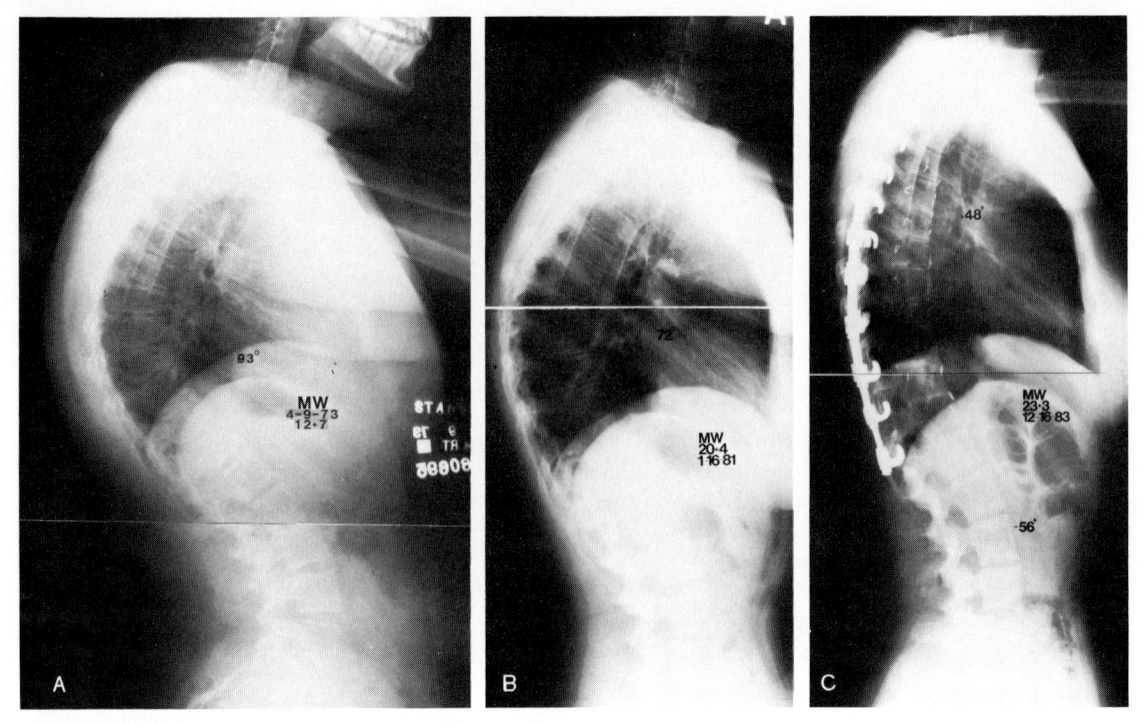

Figure 16–13. A, At age 12, M. W. was treated with a brace with only modest improvement. B, Because of continued pain and deformity at age 20, combined anterior and posterior fusion and instrumentation was done. C, At follow-up correction has been maintained and her pain has been relieved.

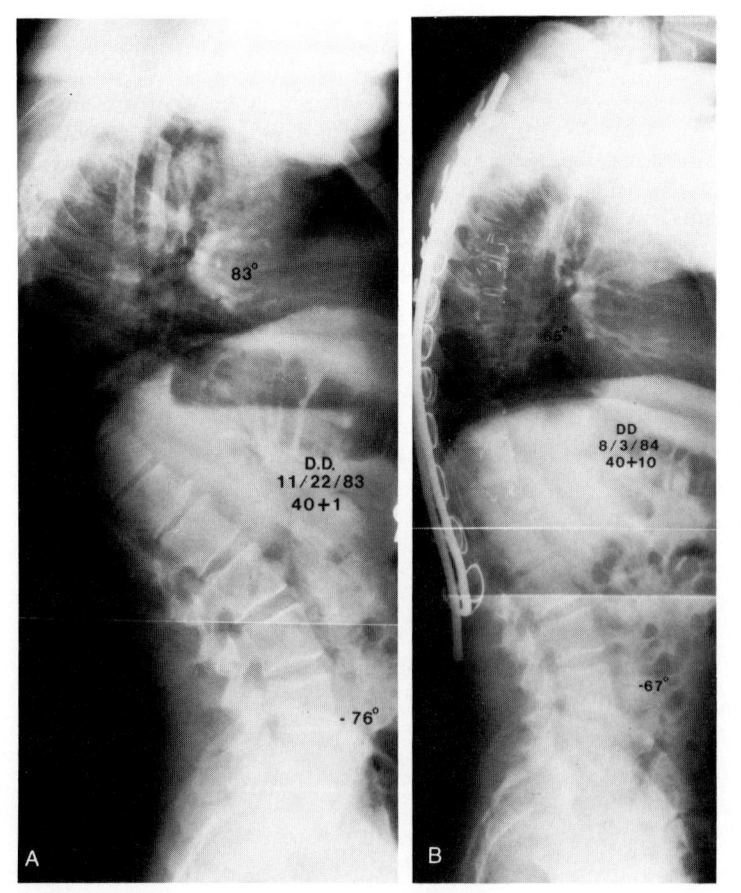

Figure 16–14. L-rod instrumentation may be a useful technique for posterior instrumentation in combined procedures. Determining the amount of rod bend to produce the desired correctability, however, is more difficult than compression instrumentation.

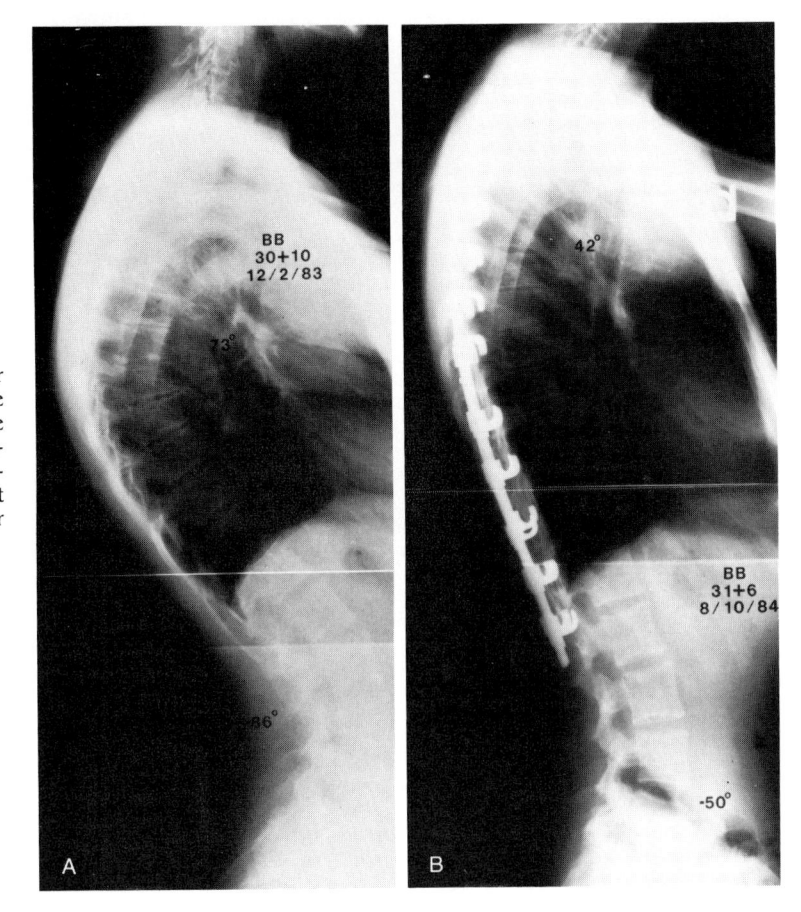

Figure 16–15. *A* and *B*, Posterior instrumentation and fusion alone may be a satisfactory procedure for correcting kyphosis and maintaining the correction in deformities less than 70 degrees that show flexibility to 45 degrees or less.

clined to mobilize the patients between procedures without a halo and to perform the second stage posterior procedure without traction. The results at this time appear satisfactory. If the halo is needed only for positioning for the second stage posterior procedure, it may be applied following induction of anesthesia and then removed at the completion of the posterior surgery.

References

1. Adelstein, L. J.: Spinal extradural cyst associated with kyphosis dorsalis juvenilis. J. Bone Joint Surg., 23A:93, 1941.
2. Agostini, S., Ferraro, C., Mammano, S., et al.: La scoliosi nella malattia de Scheuermann. Morfogenesi delle curve di compenso. Progressi in patologia vertebrale. In Gaggi, A. (ed.): Le cifosi. Bologna, 5:265, 1982.
3. Albanese, A.: Le cifosi dell'adolescenze. Arch. Orthop., 52:189, 1936.
4. Allal, M., Scheiner, J. P., Sedat, P., and Bergoin, M.: Le traitement chirurgical des formes graves de la maladie de Scheuermann de l'adulte jeune. Reunion de groupe d'etude de la scoliose, Aix Provence, 1:82, 1978.
5. Ascani, E., Borelli, P., La Rosa, G., et al.: Malattia de Scheuermann. I: Studio ormonale Progressi in patologia vertebrale. In Gaggi, A. (ed.): Le cifosi. Bologna, 5:97, 1982.
6. Ascani, E., Ippolito, E., and Montanaro, A.: Scheuermann's kyphosis: histological, histochemical and ultrastructural studies. Orthop. Trans., 7:28, 1982.
7. Ascani, E., Giglio, G., and Salsano, V.: Scoliosis screening in Rome. In Zorab, P. A., and Siegler, D. (eds.): Scoliosis 1979. London, Academic Press, p. 39, 1979.
8. Acani, E., and Montanaro, A.: Scheuermann's disease. In Bradford, D. S., and Hensinger, R. (eds.): The Pediatric Spine. New York, Thieme and Stratton, pp. 307–324, 1985.
9. Ascani, E., Montanara, A., La Rosa, G., and Crostelli, M.: Malattia di Scheuermann II: Studio istologico, istochimico e ultrastrutturale. Progressi in patologia vertebrale. In Gaggi, A. (ed.): Le cifosi. Bologna, 5:105, 1982.
10. Ascani, E., Salsano, V., and Giglio, G.: The incidence and early detection of spinal deformities. J. It. Ortop. 3:1977.
11. Aufdermaur, M.: Zur Pathogenese der Scheuermannschen Krankeit. Deutsche Med. Wochenshr., 89:73, 1964.
12. Aufdermaur, M.: Juvenile kyphosis (Scheuermann's disease): radiography, histology and pathogenesis. Clin. Orthop., 154:166, 1981.
13. Axelgaard, J., Brown, J. C., and Swank, S. M.:

Kyphosis treatment by electrical surface stimulation. Orthop. Trans., 6:1, 1982.
14. Becker, K. J.: Uber die Behandlung jugendlicher Kyphosen mit einem aktiven bzw. einem kombinierten zweiteiligen akitz-passiven Reklinationshkosett. Z. Orthop., 89:464, 1958.
15. Berg, A.: Contribution to the technique in fusion operations on the spine. Acta Orthop. Scand., 17:1, 1948.
16. Bick, E. M., and Copel, J. W.: Longitudinal growth of the human vertebra; contribution to human osteogeny. J. Bone Joint Surg., 32A:803, 1950.
17. Bick, E. M., and Copel, J. W.: Ring apophysis of human vertebra; contribution to human osteogeny. J. Bone Joint Surg., 33A:783, 1951.
18. Blount, W. P., Schmidt, A. C., and Bidwell, R. G.: Making the Milwaukee brace. J. Bone Joint Surg., 40A:523, 1958.
19. Bradford, D. S.: Juvenile kyphosis. Clin. Orthop. 128:45, 1977.
20. Bradford, D. D., Khalid, B. A., Moe, J. H., et al.: /The surgical management of patients with Scheuermann's disease. A review of 24 cases managed by combined anterior and posterior spine fusion. J. Bone Joint Surg., 62A:705, 1980.
21. Bradford, D. S., Moe, J. H.: Scheuermann's juvenile kyphosis: A histologic study. Clin. Orthop., 110:45, 1975.
22. Bradford, D. S., Moe, J. H., and Winter, R. B.: Kyphosis and postural roundback deformity in children and adolescents. Minn. Med., 56:114, 1973.
23. Bradford, D. S., Moe, J. H., Montalvo, F. J., and Winter, R. B.: Scheuermann's kyphosis and roundback deformity, results of Milwaukee brace treatment. J. Bone Joint Surg., 56A:749, 1974.
24. Bradford, D. S., Moe, J. H., Montalvo, F. J., and Winter, R. B.: Scheuermann's kyphosis: results of surgical treatment in 22 patients. J. Bone Joint Surg., 57A:439, 1975.
25. Bradford, D. S., Brown, D. M., Moe, J. H., et al.: Scheuermann's kyphosis, a form of juvenile osteoporosis? Clin. Orthop., 118:10, 1976.
26. Bradford, D. S.: Neurological complications in Scheuermann's disease. J. Bone Joint Surg., 51A:657, 1969.
27. Brocher, J. E. W.: Die Prognose der Wibelsaulenleiden. Stuttgart, G. Thieme, 1957.
28. Brocher, J. E. W.: Die Scheuermannsche Krankheit und ihre Differential diagnose. Basel, B. Schwabe and Co., 1946.
29. Brocher, J. E. W.: Die Wirbelsaulentuber Kulose und ihre Differential diagnose. Stuttgart, G. Thieme, 1953.
30. Brown, D. M., Jowsey, J., and Bradford, D. S.: Osteoporosis in ovarian dysgenesis. J. Pediatr., 84:816, 1974.
31. Cloward, R. B., and Bucy, P. C.: Spinal extradural cyst and kyphosis dorsalis juvenilis. Am. J. Roentgenol., 38:681, 1937.
32. Cotrel, Y., and Paluszak, M.: Resultats du traitement chirurgical par voie posterieure d'une serie de cyphose regulieres pendant la periode de croissance. Reunion de Groupe d'etudes de la Scoliose. Aix en Provence, 1:78, 1978.
33. Dameron, T. B., and Gulledge, W. H.: Adolescent kyphosis. U. S. Armed Forces Med. J., 4:871, 1953.
34. Dittmar, O.: Die rundruckenbildung der Jugendilcher (Kyphosis juvenilis). Med. Klin., 35:1203, 1939.
35. Edgren, W.: Osteochondrosis juvenilis lumbalis. Acta Chir. Scand., Suppl. 227:1, 1957.
36. Elsberg, C. A., Dike, C. G., and Brewer, E. D.: The symptoms and diagnosis of extradural cysts. Bull. Neurol. Inst., 3:395, 1934.
37. Ferguson, A. B., Jr.: Etiology of pre-adolescent kyphosis. J. Bone Joint Surg., 38A:149, 1956.
38. Ferguson, A. B., Jr.: Roundback in children. J. Med. Assoc. Ga., 45:458, 1956.
39. Fon, G. T., Pitt, M. J., and Thies, A. C.: Thoracic kyphosis: range in normal subjects. Am. J. Roentengol., 134:979, 1980.
40. Gardemin, H., and Herbst, W.: Wirbeldeformierung bie der Adoleszentenkyphose und Osteoporose. Arch. Orthop. Unfallchir., 59:134, 1966.
41. Gonon, G., DeMauroy, J. C., and Stagnara, P.: Resultats a long terme du traitement chirurgical des cyphoses regulieres. Reunion du groupe d'etude de la Scoliose. Aix en Provence, 1:91, 1978.
42. Grospic, F.: Kyphosis dorsalis adolescentium. Zentralbl. Chir., 55(1):61, 1928.
43. Gschwend, N., and Muller, G. P.: Egebnisse einer aktivpassiven Behandlungsmethode fixierter juveniler Thorakalkyphosen. Arch. Orthop. Unfallchir., 61:55, 1967.
44. Guntz, E.: Kyphosis juvenilis sive adolescentium. Z. Orthop., 65:53, 1937.
45. Guntz, E.: Gedanken zur Begutachtung von Wirgelsaulenschaden nach orthopadischen Gesichtspunkten. Arch. Orthop. Unfallchir., 47:558, 1955.
46. Hafner, R. H.: Localized osteochondritis. Scheuermann's disease. J. Bone Joint Surg., 34B:38, 1952.
47. Hagen, U. H.: Erbbiologische untersuchungen Bei der Scheurmannschen Krankheit. These, Gottingen, 1951.
48. Halal, F. Gledhill, R. B., and Fraser, F. C.: Dominant inheritance of Scheuermann's juvenile kyphosis. Am. J. Dis. Child., 132:1105, 1978.
49. Hallock, H., Francis, K. D., and Jones, J. B.: Spine fusion in young children. A long-term end-result study with particular reference to growth effects. J. Bone Joint Surg., 39A:481, 1957.
50. Harrington, P. R.: Treatment of scoliosis. Correction and internal fixation by spine instrumentation. J. Bone Joint Surg., 44A:591, 1962.
51. Hensinger, R. N., Greene, T. L., and Hunter, L. Y.: Back pain and vertebral changes simulating Scheuermann's kyphosis. Spine, 6:341–342, 1982.
52. Herndon, W. A., Emans, J. B., Micheli, L. J., and Hall, J. E.: Combined anterior and posterior fusion for Scheuermann's kyphosis. Spine, 6:125, 1981.
53. Hodgen, J. T., and Frantz, C. H.: Juvenile kyphosis. Surg. Gynecol. Obstet., 72:798, 1941.
54. Hult, L.: Cervical dorsal and lumbar spinal syndromes. Acta Orthop. Scand., 24:174, 1954.
55. Ippilito, E., and Ponsetti, I.: Juvenile kyphosis. Histological and histochemical studies. J. Bone Joint Surg., 63A:175, 1981.
56. Jaffe, H. L.: Metabolic, Degenerative and Inflammatory Diseases of Bones and Joints. Philadelphia, Lea & Febiger, 1972.
57. Junghanns, H.: Fur Atiologic, Prognose und

Therapie des M. Scheuermann. Medizinische, 1:300, 1955.
58. Kehl, D., Lovell, W. W., and MacEwen, G. D.: Scheuermann's disease of the lumbar spine. Orthop. Trans., 6:342, 1982.
59. Kemp, F. H., and Wilson, D. C.: Some factors in the aetiology of osteochondritis of the spine. Br. J. Radiol., 20:410, 1947.
60. Kemp, F. H., Wilson, D. C., and Emrys-Roberts, E.: Social and nutritional factors in adolescent osteochondritis of the spine. Br. J. Soc. Med., 2:66, 1948.
61. Kewalramani, L. S., Riggins, R. S., and Fowler, W. M.: Scheuermann's kyphoscoliosis associated with Charcot-Marie-Tooth Syndrome. Arch. Phys. Med. Rehabil., 57:391–397, 1976.
62. Kling, T. F., and Hensinger, R. H.: Scheuermann's disease: natural history, current concepts, and management. In Dickson, R. A., and Bradford, D. S. (eds.): Management of Spinal Deformities. London, Butterworths International Medical Reviews, pp. 252–274, 1984.
63. Knutson, F.: Observations of the growth of the vertebral body in Scheuermann's disease. Acta Radiol., 30:97, 1948.
64. Kostuik, J., and Lorenz, M.: Longterm follow-up of surgical management in adult Scheuermann's kyphosis. Orthop. Trans., 7:28, 1983.
65. Lambrinudi, L.: Adolescent and senile kyphosis. Br. Med. J., 2:800, 1934.
66. Larsen, E. H., and Nordentaft, E. L.: Growth of the epiphyses and vertebrae. Acta Orthop. Scand., 32:210, 1962.
67. Lyon, M.: Krankheiten der wirbelkorperepiphyse. Fortschr. Geb. Rontgenstr. Nuklear Med., 44:498, 1931.
68. Mauroy, J. C., and Stagnara, P.: Resultats a long terme du traitement orthopedique. Reunion du groupe d'etude de la Scoliose. Aix en Provence, 1:60, 1978.
69. Michelle, A. A.: Osteochondrosis deformans juvenilis dorsi. N. Y. J. Med., 61:98, 1961.
70. Micheli, L. J.: Low back pain in adolescents: differential diagnosis. Am J. Sport Med., 7:362, 1979.
71. Moe, J. H.: Treatment of adolescent kyphosis by nonoperative and operative methods. Manitoba Med. Rev., 45:481, 1965.
72. Monnet, J. C.: Osteochondritis deformans. J. Okla. State Med. Assoc., 52:376, 1959.
73. Montgomery, S. P., and Erwin, W. E.: Scheuermann's kyphosis. Long term results of Milwaukee brace treatment. Spine, 6:5, 1978.
74. Muhlbach, von R., Hahnel, H., and Cohn, H.: Zur Bedeutung biochemischer Parameter bei der Beurteilung der Scheuermannschen Krankheit. Medizin und Sport, 10:331, 1970.
75. Muller, G., and Gschwend, N.: Endokrine Storungen und Morbus Scheuermann. Arch. Orthop. Unfallchir., 65:357, 1969.
76. Nathan, L., and Kuhns, J. G.: Epiphysitis of the spine. J. Bone Joint Surg., 22:55–62, 1940.
77. Neithard, F. V.: Scheuermann's disease and spondylolysis. Orthop. Trans., 7:103, 1983.
78. Nicod, L.: Traitement de la maladie de Scheuermann et des dystrophies rachidiennes de croissance. Praxis, 46:1619, 1968.
79. Outland, T., and Snedden, H. E.: Juvenile dorsal kyphosis. Clin. Orthop., 5:155, 1955.
80. Overgaard, K.: Prolapses of nucleus pulposus and Scheuermann's disease. Nord. Med., 5:593, 1940.
81. Ponte, A., and Siccardi, G. L.: Surgical treatment of Scheuermann's hyperkyphosis. Presented at the 19th Annual Meeting of the Scoliosis Research Society, Sept. 19–22, 1984, Orlando, Florida.
82. Ponte, A., Vero, B., and Siccardi, G. L.: Il trattamento chirurgico delle iperdifosi osteocondritiche. Progressi in patologia vertebrale. In Gaggi, A. (ed.): Le cifosi. Bologna, 5:181, 1982.
83. Ponte, A., Gebbia, F., and Eliseo, F.: Nonoperative treatment of adolescent hyperkyphosis. Orthop. Trans., 9:108, 1985.
84. Pratelli, R., Bartolozzi, P., Allegra, M., and Gatti, U.: Valutazione dei risultati a distanza del trattamento del dorso curvo osteocondritico mediante apparecchi gessati in reclinazione tipo Risser. Progressi in patologia vertebrale. In Gaggi, A. (ed.): Le cifosi, Bologna, 5:157, 1982.
85. Raisman, V.: Adolescent round back deformity — a late result of poliomyelitis. Bull. Hosp. Dis., 16:94, 1955.
86. Rathke, F. W.: Pathogenese und Therapie der juvenilen Kyphose. Z. Orthop., 102:16, 1966.
87. Risser, J. C., Lauder, C. H., Norquist, D. M., and Craig, W. A.: Three types of body casts. In The American Academy of Orthopaedic Surgeons: Instructional Course Lectures, Vol. 10, pp. 131–142. Ann Arbor, Minn., J. W. Edwards, Inc. 1953.
88. Roaf, R.: Vertebral growth and its mechanical control. J. Bone Joint Surg., 42B:40, 1960.
89. Rocher, Y. R., and Perez-Casas, A.: Anatomia Funcional del Aparato Locomotor de la Inervacion Periferica. Madrid, Casa Editorial Bailly-Bailliere, 1965.
90. Romer, U.: Behandlung des Morbus Scheuermann. Schweiz. Med. Wochenschr., 97:1615, 1967.
91. Rutt, A.: Zur Therapie der Scheuermannschen Krankheit. Beitr. Orthop., 13:731, 1966.
92. Ryan, M. D., and Taylor, T. K. F.: Acute spinal cord compression in Scheuermann's disease. J. Bone Joint Surg., 64B:409, 1982.
93. Sachs, B. L., Bradford, D. S., Winter, R. B., et al.: Scheuermann's kyphosis: longterm results of Milwaukee brace treatment. Orthop. Trans., 9:108, 1985.
94. Saunders, J. B. de C. M., and Inman, V. T.: Intervertebral disc; critical and collective review. Int. Abs. Surg., 69:14, 1939.
95. Schanz, A.: Berl. Klin. Wochenschr., 44:986, 1907.
96. Schanz, A.: Schule und Skoliose. Jagrb. f. Kinderh., 73:1, 1911.
97. Scheuermann, H. W.: Kyfosis dorsalis juvenilis. Ugeskr. Laeger, 82:385, 1920.
98. Scheuermann, H. W.: Kyphosis juvenilis (Scheuermann's krankheit). Fortschr. Geb. Rontgenstrahlen, 53:1, 1936.
99. Schildbach, J.: die Entwicklung der juvenilen Kyphose. Zentralbl. Chir., 64:2086, 1937.
100. Schlegel, K. F.: Die biologische Bedeutung der jungendlichen Kyphosen. Med. Klin., 48:917, 1953.
101. Schmorl, G.: Die Pathogenese der juvenilen Kyphose. Fortschr. Geb. Roentgenstr. Nuklearmed., 41:359, 1930.
102. Schmorl, G.: The Human Spine in Health and Disease. New York, Grune and Stratton, 1971.

103. Scholder, P.: Aspect morphologique des dystrophies rachidiennes de croissance de type Scheuermann. Praxis, 46:1608, 1968.
104. Scholder, P., and Basti, H.: Vers une meilleure comprehension des lesions de Scheuermann. Schwiez. Med. Wochenschr., 50:1979, 1968.
105. Simon, R. S.: The diagnosis and treatment of kyphosis dorsalis juvenilis (Scheuermann's kyphosis) in the early stage. J. Bone Joint Surg., 24:681, 1942.
106. Soderberg, L., and Andren, L.: Disc degeneration and lumbago-ischias. Acta Orthop. Scand., 25:137, 1955.
107. Soeur, R.: A propos de la pathogenie et du traitement du dos rond de l'adolescent. Acta Orthop. Belg., 24:146, 1958.
108. Sorenson, K. H.: Scheuermann's Juvenile Kyphosis. Copenhagen, Munksgaard, 1964.
109. Sorrel, E., and Delahaye, A.: Growing pains simulating Pott's disease. Presse Med., 32:737, 1924.
110. Stagnara, P., DeMauroy, J. C., Dran, G., et al.: Reciprocal angulation of the vertebral bodies in the sagittal plane: approach to references for the evaluation of kyphosis and lordosis. Spine, 7:335, 1982.
111. Stagnara, P., DuPelou, J., and Fauchet, R.: Traitement orthopedique ambulatoire de la maladie de Scheuermann en periode d'evolution. Rev. Chir. Orthop., 52:585, 1966.
112. Stagnara, P., and Perdriolle, R.: Elongation vertebrale continue par platre a tendeurs. Possibilites therapeutiques. Rev. Chir. Orthop., 44:57, 1958.
113. Stein, H., and Zahn, von L.: Zur Pathogenese, Fruhdiagnose und Prophylaxe des Morbus Scheuermann. Dtsch. Med. Wochenschr., 81:200, 1965.
114. Steindler, A.: Post-Graduate Lectures on Orthopedic Diagnosis and Indications. Springfield, Ill, Charles C Thomas, 1952.
115. Stracker, O.: Zur Behandlung der Kyphosis adolescentium-Scheuermann. Wien. Med. Wochenschr., 99:48, 1949.
116. Taylor, T. C., Wenter, D. R., Stephen, J., et al.: Surgical management of thoracic kyphosis in adolescents. J. Bone Joint Surg., 61A:496, 1979.
117. Travaglini, F., and Conte, M.: Cifosi 25 anni dopo. Progressi in patologia vertebrale. In Gaggi, A. (ed.): Le cifosi. Bologna, 5:163, 1982.
118. Vidal-Naquet, G.: Un cas de resection des apophyses epineuses pour une cyphose dorsal douloureuse. Bull. Mem. Soc. Chir. Paris, 27:571, 1935.
119. Wassman, K.: Kyphosis juvenilis Scheuermann. Acta Orthop. Scand., 21:65, 1951.
120. Watermann, H.: Die Kyphosis Adolescentium und die Notwendigkeit ihrer Erkenntis in der Unfallbegutachtung. Arch. Orthop. Unfallchir., 24:179, 1927.
121. Williams, E. R.: Observations on the differential diagnosis and sequelae of juvenile vertebral osteochondrosis. Acta Radiol., Suppl. 116:293, 1954.

17
ADULT SCOLIOSIS

John E. Lonstein, M.D.

INTRODUCTION

The number of adults presenting to the physician with scoliosis is increasing. This is due to a greater awareness of scoliosis in the community and the knowledge that adult scoliosis can be effectively treated. The improved ability to operate on adults and the availability of orthopaedic surgeons trained to treat spine deformities also contribute to the increase in the number of adult scoliosis patients seen.

PREVALENCE

The first question in determining prevalence rates is, What constitutes an adult? An adult is an individual who has completed growth and whose growth centers have fused. In the spine, this means that the iliac epiphysis has fused (Risser 5)[54] and the vertebral ring apophyses have fused. An arbitrary age is not applicable, as a large number of people reach adulthood at age 18, whereas others show growth activity into their early twenties. Most studies on adult scoliosis arbitrarily define an adult as chronologic age 20, or older.

Exact prevalence studies on adult scoliosis are not available. It can be estimated by extrapolating from statistics in the adolescent that the number of adults with scoliosis over 30 degrees is 450,000 to 500,000 in the United States. The percentage of these adults that present to the physician with clinical complaints is low. Studies have shown that curves can progress in adulthood and that curves can arise de novo in the adult.[1, 4, 6, 11, 16, 17, 20, 21, 24, 26, 31, 42, 45, 52, 53, 55, 56, 73, 74, 75] Robin showed that scolioses of minor degree arise de novo in the sixth and seventh decades and may progress at this age. He found no relationship between scoliosis, osteoporosis, or back pain, and radiographic signs of degeneration in the spine.[56]

The only study of the prevalence of scoliosis in adults is that of Kostuik and Bentivoglio.[37] They studied the intravenous pyelograms of 5000 patients in their sixth to eighth decades. On these supine views they found a 3.9 incidence of lumbar curves over 10 degrees with 59 per cent of these patients having back pain. The pain was unrelated to age or occupation, but was more common in curves over 45 degrees and in those curves showing facet sclerosis radiographically.

NATURAL HISTORY

Scoliosis in adults usually begins in childhood or adolescence. Some lumbar curves arise de novo in adults because of disc degeneration and collapse of the intervertebral space.[4, 45, 56] If this process is more severe at one space, lateral or rotatory subluxation can occur. The relationship between osteoporosis and the de novo development of curves or the progression of curves in adults is controversial.

The long-term effects of untreated scoliosis, cardiopulmonary problems, disability, pain, and progression, are well known and are discussed in Chapter 4.[3, 5, 7, 10, 14, 33, 39, 40, 41, 44, 46, 47, 49, 61, 70, 76] Weinstein and Ponsetti[74] and Ascani and coworkers[1] have shown in a 40 year follow-up that the average curve increase was 14 degrees, their average curve being 54 degrees. The curves most likely to have progressed were thoracic curves of 50 to 80 degrees at skeletal maturity and the lumbar component of double thoracic and lumbar curves that were 50 to 74 degrees at skeletal maturity. Curves under 30 degrees rarely progressed. Currently, no factors are known that will help predict exactly which of these curves will progress and which will not.

Adults who were treated with the Milwaukee brace during adolescence tend to lose correction after brace discontinuance, so the curve 10 years later approximately equals the original curve. Some curves stabilize by age 20, whereas others stabilize when the patient is in the twenties or perhaps even in the thirties. A study by Nachemson suggests that in brace-treated patients multiple pregnancies before age 23 may be associated with an increased likelihood of curve progression.[48] In untreated adults pregnancy has no direct effect on curve progression; the curves that increase during pregnancy were progressing anyway.[8] In addition, even when severe, the scoliosis has no effect on the pregnancy and does not lead to increased cardiorespiratory problems.[59]

Long term follow-up of patients fused without instrumentation indicates less low back pain than in the general population (or in patients with unfused scoliosis) but increased degenerative disease in the lumbosacral area as demonstrated by radiographic narrowing of the L5-S1 disc, and L5-S1 facet sclerosis. These radiographic changes did *not* correlate with low back pain or the lower limit of the fusion.[44] A study of patients fused with instrumentation to the lumbar area showed an increasing incidence of back pain the closer the fusion is to the sacrum, that is, the fewer disc spaces that remain. The incidence of low back pain was greater than the control population only with fusion to L5, leaving one motion segment not fused.[15]

Two broad groups of adults with scoliosis present for treatment, those who have not had previous surgery and those who have had previous surgical treatment. The adult who has not had surgical treatment is discussed here; adults with previous surgery needing re-operation are discussed in Chapter 18.

PRESENTATION

In our experience, adult patients presenting for treatment are of all ages, with a larger number of elderly patients presenting now than in years past. The majority of patients are aged 20 to 40 and are mainly women, matching the greater incidence of curves requiring treatment in adolescence.

In the adult, the presenting complaints are pain, deformity (with or without curve progression), cardiopulmonary problems, functional loss in neuromuscular curves, and on rare occasions neurologic problems.

Pain

In all the studies on adult scoliosis treatment[9, 11, 19, 27, 29, 30, 34–36, 38, 39, 41–43, 51, 53, 57, 58, 61, 62, 65, 69, 76, 77] and those of treatment of curves over 90 or 100 degrees,[18, 50, 63, 64, 66] pain is the most common presenting symptom. The pain occurs alone or in combination with deformity as the presenting problem. Pain is rare in thoracic scoliosis, and is much more frequent in lumbar or thoracolumbar curves. The pain is usually in the curve, either on the concave or convex side, or it may be outside the curve at the lumbosacral area or at the junction of two curves. Rarely is the pain of a radicular nature.

Early in the symptomatic phase the pain tends to be on the convexity of the curve and of muscular origin; ache and fatigue characterize it. The pain is not present on arising but occurs and increases as the day progresses, and with activities. On lying down the pain rapidly disappears, and it is also relieved by heat and analgesics. With the passage of time the pain tends to concentrate on the concavity of the curve as the facet joints undergo arthritic changes. The pain becomes more severe, occurs more frequently, and less upright activity is necessary to aggravate the pain. The pain may decrease the patient's activities and markedly change the lifestyle. Certain activities cannot be performed, and daily periods of rest are required because of the pain. Analgesics, which once helped control the pain, are now ineffective. The exact cause of the back pain in scoliosis is probably a combination of muscular pain, facet joint arthrosis, and disc degeneration.

On rare occasions true radicular pain occurs. The degenerative facet joint disease causes facet hypertrophy. This facet hypertrophy, combined with spur formation, encroaches on the intervertebral foramen and causes radicular symptoms. This commonly occurs in the concavity of the fractional lumbosacral curve below a lumbar scoliosis, or it may occur at the apex of a lumbar curve when marked degenerative changes are present. These radicular symptoms may exist alone, but are more commonly associated with lumbar curve pain or lumbosacral pain.

Deformity

Adults commonly present because of the deformity, which may or may not be accompanied by pain. When the deformity alone is the reason for presentation, the patient is concerned with the rotational prominence, waist line changes, decompensation, and thoracic rotation. These cosmetic changes often affect the patient more than the treating physician realizes. The treating physician, once he gets to know the patient (often after surgical treatment), appreciates the psychologic effect of the pre-existing deformity. More attention needs to be paid to the psychologic effect of the curve.

Progression of the deformity is a common presenting symptom, with or without pain (Fig. 17–1). The patient may have had previous non-operative therapy and has noted a gradual loss in height with an increase in the deformity. The waistline difference and decompensation increase as does the rotational prominence. This prominence in the thoracic, thoracolumbar, or lumbar area appears to be an increasing kyphotic deformity. This is *not* true kyphosis but is due to rotation of the vertebrae and is termed kyphosing scoliosis (scolioses cyphosantes) by Stagnara.[62]

In addition to the changes noted by the patient, serial radiographs will show curve progression. The adult may have had previous bracing as an adolescent, or prior x-rays as an adult may be available. These x-rays should be obtained for comparison to document progression. As curves progress slowly in adulthood (at an average of 1 degree per year), x-rays over a number of years are necessary to show true curve increase. These x-rays are combined with a measurement of the patient's height at each visit.

Often an asymptomatic adult comes for evaluation when in the thirties with a previous x-ray taken when in the early twenties. A current x-ray shows that the curve has progressed in the intervening years, but it does not show whether the curve is *currently* progressing. Only if the patient has noted recent increase in deformity or a subsequent x-ray shows progression, can this curve be diagnosed as currently progressing.

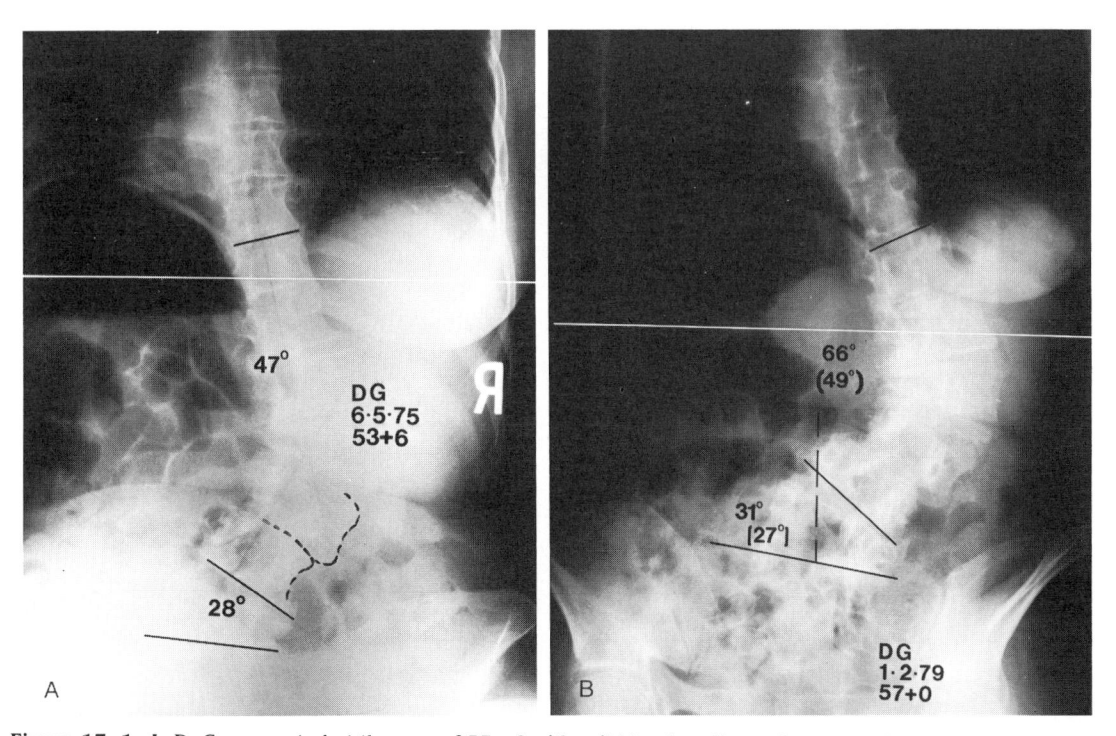

Figure 17–1. *A*, D. G. presented at the age of 53+6 with mild lumbar discomfort and a 47 degree right lumbar curve secondary to a congenital wedge vertebra at L5. *B*, Three and a half years later the curve had progressed to 66 degrees. Note the rotatory subluxation of L3 on L4.

Cardiopulmonary Decompensation

The reason for correcting and stabilizing thoracic curvatures is the prevention of pulmonary compromise and subsequent cardiac failure. This is rarely the reason for presentation and treatment.[70]

Patients often present with symptoms of fatigue, tiredness, and dyspnea with exertion. These often accompany a painful curve that is decreasing the patient's activities. In addition, a patient's activities and exercising tend to decrease with increasing age. With these thoracic curves, pulmonary function testing is important (see Chapter 22). Baseline pulmonary function testing is necessary, and if there is a decrease in the pulmonary function with time, an indication for surgical stabilization is present. This is a rare occurrance.

Rarely is cardiopulmonary failure the main indication for surgery. In these cases, surgical correction may cause an increase in the volumetric studies, as well as an increase in the arterial partial pressure of oxygen (PaO_2) due to decreased arteriovenous shunting as a result of straightening of the curve.[79] If cor pulmonale is present, a decrease in pulmonary artery pressure may follow straightening of the curve by traction and stabilization by fusion. Careful evaluation of these patients is essential (see Chapter 22).

Functional Loss

In neuromuscular curves, an increase in the curve (either scoliosis or kyphosis) results in a change in the center of gravity and an alteration in the functional level. This loss of functional ability is often the presenting complaint in neuromuscular curves and represents curve progression. This is discussed fully in Chapter 13.

Neurologic Problems

The presenting neurologic problem can be paraparesis or paraplegia or radiculopathy.[4,22,23] Cord compression with paraparesis or paraplegia does not occur in idiopathic scoliosis but can be seen with congenital kyphosis, neurofibromatosis, or after trauma, and is discussed in Chapters 12, 15, and 20.

Radiculopathy with pain and/or weakness accompanies the foraminal encroachment on the concavity of the lumbar curve that occurs in the lumbar area or the compensatory lumbosacral curve below. The pain is typically radicular in radiation and is increased by the upright position and activities. As stated, it is often accompanied by curve or lumbosacral pain.

PATIENT EVALUATION

In adults, the main indications for surgery are pain and progressive curvature. The evaluation must assess these two areas fully.

History

Why is the adult seeking evaluation? If there is pain, What is the nature of the pain? What is its site, severity, and radiation? What activities aggravate the pain and what must be done to relieve the pain? Are analgesics necessary and if so, what type and how often? Is daily rest necessary to help cope with the pain? What activities have been restricted because of the pain? Has the pain affected the patient's ability to be employed? The aim is to determine how the pain has affected the patient's activities and lifestyle, and if these changes are progressive.

Has any increase in the deformity been noted? Has there been recent or progressive loss of height? Have changes in the waistline, decompensation, or rotational prominence been noted? Are there any previous x-rays available for comparison? The comparison of current with prior x-rays is the only valid method of documenting progression, and thus these x-rays should be obtained for comparison whenever possible.

The symptoms of cardiorespiratory dysfunction must be documented. Symptoms of tiredness, dyspnea, tachycardia, and palpitations with effort are important. Some of these symptoms normally accompany increasing age. It is important to document whether these symptoms are static or progressive, showing deterioration in respiratory or cardiac function.

The evaluation of the patient as outlined in Chapter 3, is carried out. In the adult, this evaluation is expanded. A full history of pain is obtained with its occurrence, aggravating and relieving factors, and its effect on the patient's activities and lifestyle. In addition, a full history of previous spine treatment and surgery is important. A full general health history is essential.

The physical examination of the spine is outlined in Chapter 3. In addition, localization of the pain and its cause is carried out. The patient should point out the area of pain. In the prone position, the back is carefully palpated to accurately localize areas of tenderness. Is this in the muscles or over the spine? Is it in the curve or at the lumbosacral area? Is the tender area on the concavity or convexity of the curve? Using slow, careful palpation the area of pain can be accurately localized clinically, giving a guide to an area that may require special radiologic evaluation.

Radiographs

Radiographs are obtained as described in Chapter 3. Curves in adults tend to be large, often over 100 degrees. They are more rigid, as shown by less correction on side bending or traction evaluation. The facet joints show enlargement and sclerosis on the curve concavity due to the facet arthrosis, or they may show spontaneous fusion. In addition, in the lumbar curve, these changes may be accompanied by rotatory subluxation at or below the apex of the curve (Fig. 17–2).

The lateral view is important, as an apparent clinical kyphotic deformity accompanies the scoliosis. The amount of vertebral rotation must be assessed in the frontal and sagittal planes. What appears as kyphosis clinically is not due to a posterior angulation of the vertebrae in the sagittal plane, but is due to extreme vertebral rotation. In larger curves (over 90 degrees) a derotated view of Stagnara is useful (see Chapter 3). This will show the true magnitude of the scoliosis and in addition the vertebral anatomy, allowing identification of any congenital anomalies.

Pulmonary function tests are important in the assessment of the effects of a thoracic curve. In thoracic curves in which there is no clear cut indication for surgery, the pulmonary function tests may demonstrate the harmful effects of the curve. With significant reduction in pulmonary function, or where serial tests show progressive deterioration, an indication for surgery is present.

When a decision to operate on a lumbar or thoracolumbar curve has been made, discography is often useful.[28, 34] Lumbosacral pain in these cases can be referred from the curve above, or can be caused by disc or facet degeneration in the lumbosacral area. Discograms of the lumbosacral area are performed. If on discography the patient's typical pain is reproduced in character and radiation, that disc level may need to be included in the fusion. The radiographic appearance on discography is *not* as important owing to the high incidence of disc degeneration in the adult population. This evaluation is used with other tests in patient evaluation to help in the decision making process (Fig. 17–2c).[28, 34]

Metrizamide myelography is used with radicular pain to differentiate disc herniation from the more common root compression of scoliosis. The source of root compression, either the enlarged facet or the pedicle, can be visualized. With the distortion of the anatomy present, careful oblique views are necessary to accurately visualize the nerve roots and determine the compressing pathology. In some cases the myelographic information can be augmented by computerized tomography (Fig. 17–2B).

In cases with unusual pain patterns, facet blocks are sometimes useful in decision making. Under radiographic control, a combination of local anesthetic and steroid is injected *into* the facet joints in the area of pain. With relief of the pain after injection, the facet joint is shown to be the source of the pain, and thus fusion will most likely relieve the pain.

TREATMENT

The indications for treatment of an adult who has not had prior surgery and who presents with a spine deformity are mainly pain and deformity; rarely are neurologic problems or cardiorespiratory failure indications for treatment. The choices for treatment are non-operative or operative. The first decision to be made is not What surgical technique should be used in this case? Rather it is, Is surgery the best treatment in this case?

Non-operative Treatment

Non-operative treatment is used for (1) mild to moderate complaints of pain, (2) older adults with pain, or (3) atypical pain patterns. In an adult presenting with back pain and scoliosis, the pain may be unrelated

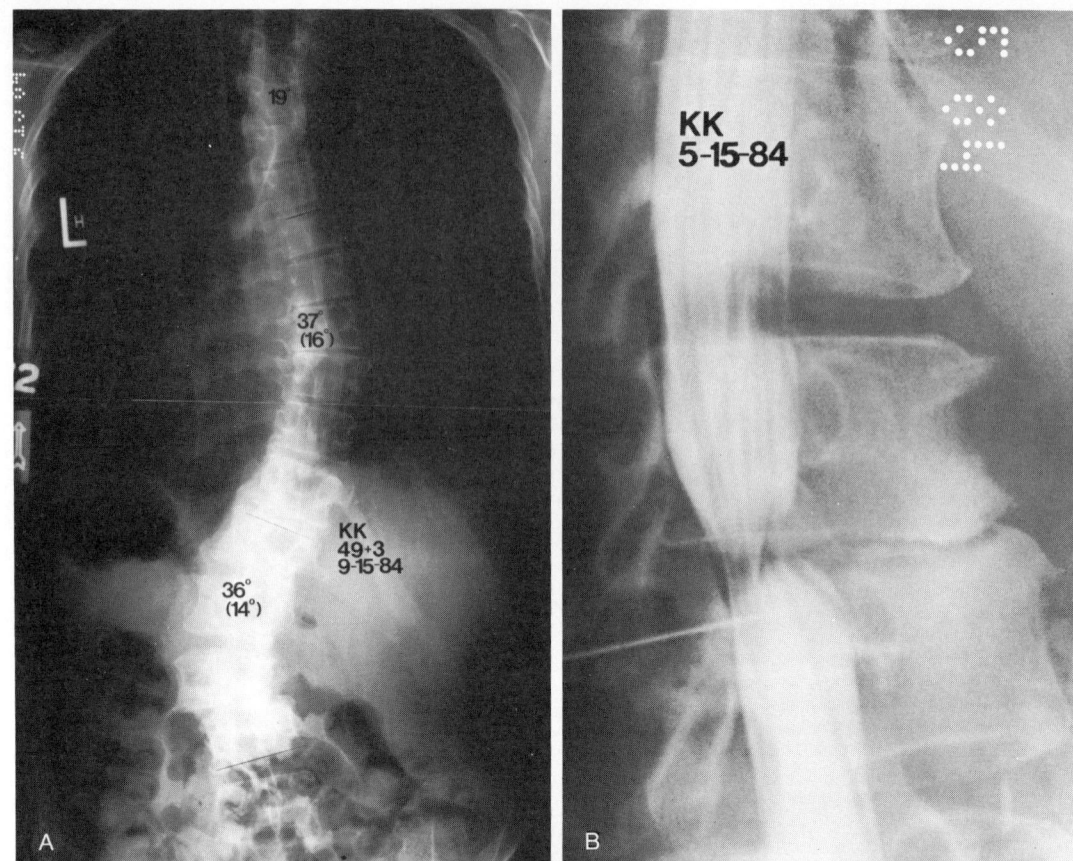

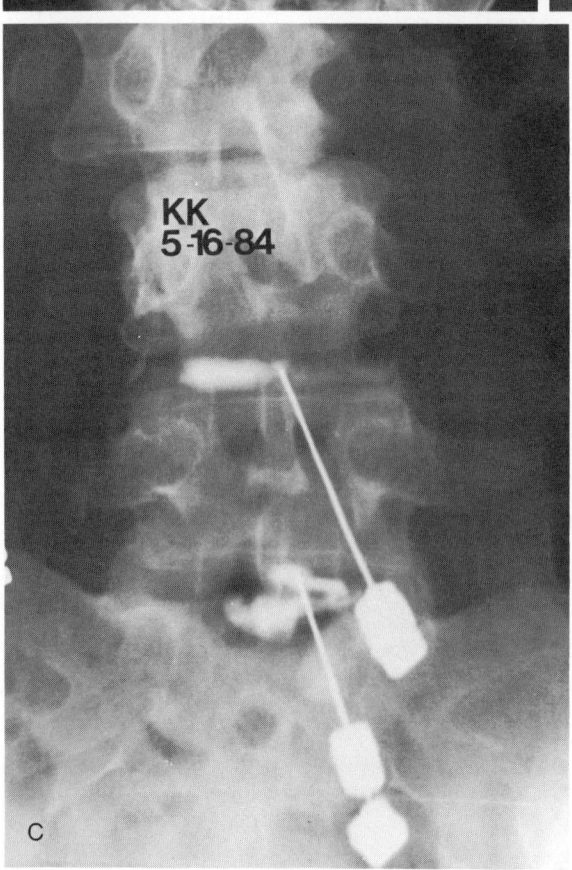

Figure 17–2. *A*, K. K. presented at the age of 49 + 3 with a double curve idiopathic scoliosis associated with low back pain and right thigh and leg pain. A standing posteroanterior radiograph showed the double curve and rotatory subluxation of L3 on L4. *B*, A lumbar myelogram showed the encroachment of the dye column at L3-L4. *C*, A discogram at L4-L5 and L5-S1 did not reproduce her pain pattern and demonstrated normal discs radiographically.

to the scoliosis or caused by the scoliosis. Therefore, in the evaluation all other possible causes of back pain must be excluded before it can be ascribed to the scoliosis.

The initial treatment is the same as for low back pain in general, involving analgesics, anti-inflammatory medications, and instruction for back care, posture, and back use. In a high percentage of cases this treatment is successful.[41] If only one or two facet joints are highly symptomatic, injection with local anesthetic and steroids can give significant relief. These injections are performed under fluoroscopic control so that precise placement of the needle and medications in and around the facet joints is possible.

Muscle strengthening exercises play a role in rehabilitation of the patients. The exercises and activities are for muscle toning and strengthening and *not* to encourage motion of the spine. Motion is usually detrimental to arthritic facet joints, rest being required to relieve pain. In many cases an external support is used for this purpose, combined with muscle strengthening. In mild curves with minimal deformity, commercial supports, for example, orthosis with metal supports or corsets with metal stays, are applicable. In cases with more severe deformities, these off-the-shelf models will not fit. In these cases a custom made orthosis to support and immobilize the spine is prescribed (Fig. 17–3). The manufacture of these orthoses requires the expertise of an orthotic facility well versed in fabricating supports for the deformed spine. The support is worn when the patient is upright and active but is not worn at night or at rest. With the support provided by the orthosis, the pain is markedly reduced and surgery avoided. In younger patients these orthoses are *not* meant for long term use, but rather for a period of time during an acutely painful period. In the elderly, an orthosis may be used for a long period of time to give pain relief because the orthosis is preferable to surgery at this age.

Operative Treatment

Before discussing the approaches available in the adult with spine deformities, a note about decision making and principles is important. All studies on adult scoliosis show that the morbidity and mortality rates after surgery are significantly higher than in adolescents.[19, 29, 38, 50, 51, 61, 66, 77] The incidence of neurologic problems, pseudarthrosis, wound infection, urinary tract infection, instrumentation problems, and psychologic problems is higher than in adolescents. The healing is more prolonged and thus immobilization is longer. Immobilization (casts and braces) is not tolerated as well, as it interferes with normal activities and a normal sex life.

Decision Making

The two key decisions in the treatment of the adult with spine deformities are: Is surgical treatment necessary? and What technique of surgery is best? The main surgical objectives are pain relief and curve stabilization; curve correction is secondary. In some cases curve correction is necessary to help rebalance the spine.

An adult presenting with a spine deformity may have pain or be pain-free. The adult under age 25 should be evaluated and treated using criteria similar to those in the older adolescent. In general, we have recommended that patients with thoracic curves over 60 degrees be treated surgically, as well as patients with single lumbar or thoracolumbar curves of over 50 degrees, or with double curves of over 55 to 60 degrees. Curves under these limits are followed with yearly x-rays to see whether they are progressive or not. Any progressive curve at this age should be treated surgically. If there is marked concern on the patient's part regarding the cosmetic deformity, especially in decompensated lumbar and thoracolumbar curves, surgery should be considered.

Asymptomatic curves in patients over age 25 present a problem in decision making. In the thoracic area pulmonary function tests are important. In all curves evidence of curve progression by radiographic analysis is important. An additional factor is the patient's attitude about the deformity. If there are markedly reduced or deteriorating pulmonary functions, or the curve is progressing, or the curve has a marked psychologic effect on the patient, surgical stabilization is indicated. Note that the amount of the curvature is not considered as the main factor. If a patient has a thoracic curve of 90 degrees with stable pulmonary functions, no curve progression, and no psychologic effects from the deformity, there is no indication for surgical intervention. This scoliosis is followed

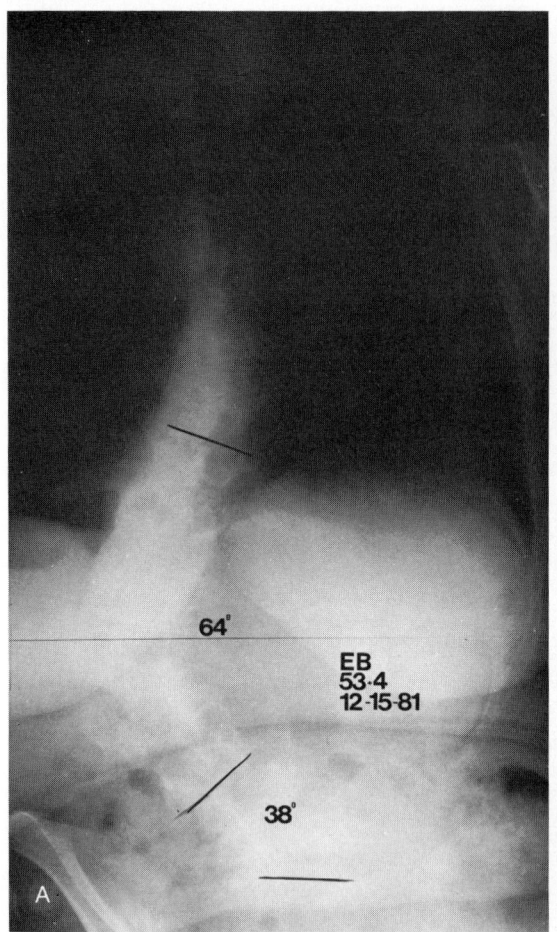

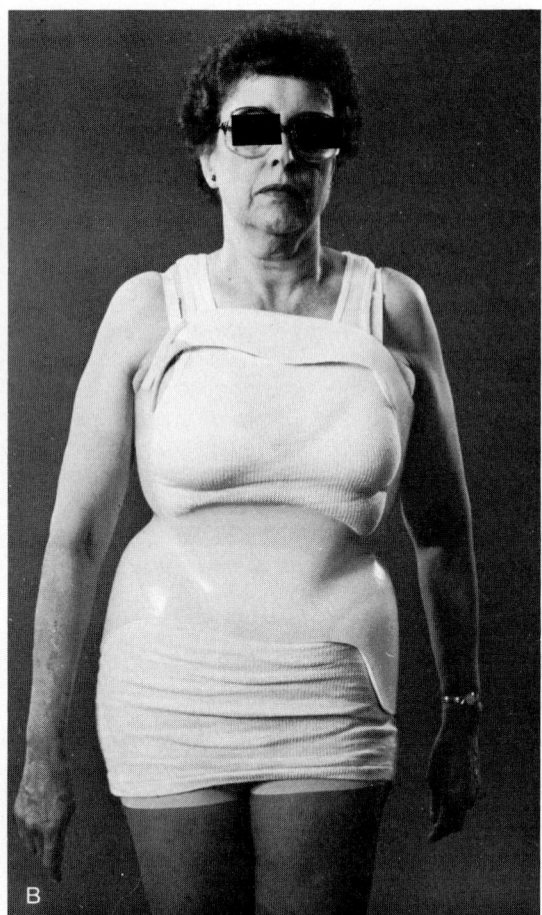

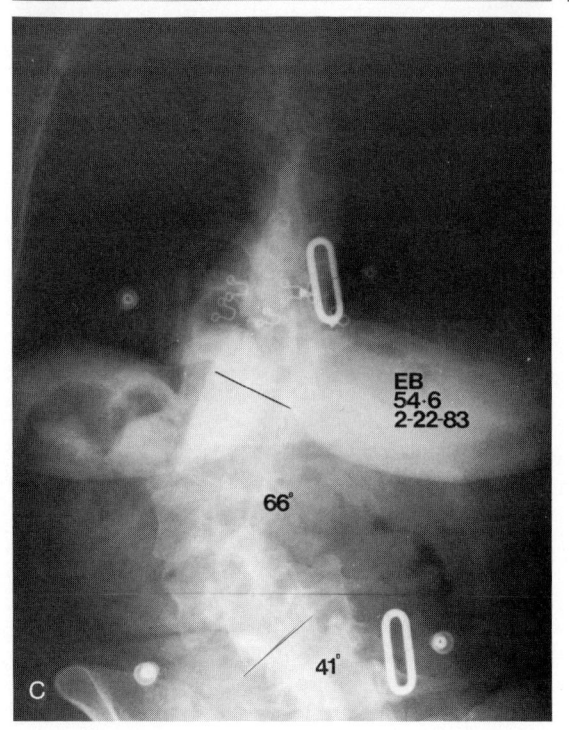

Figure 17–3. *A*, E. B., a 53+4 year old female presented with a 64 degree left lumbar curve and incapacitating lumbar back pain. *B*, A one-piece back opening TLSO was fitted and was worn when she was up and active. *C*, The TLSO gave relief of her symptoms, the curve remaining stable a year later.

with yearly x-rays and pulmonary function tests.

The symptomatic adult with pain and/or progressive deformity usually presents a clear cut problem in decision making. When pain alone is present, the patient is the one who must decide whether the pain is severe enough and modifies his or her lifestyle enough to consider surgical treatment. This decision must be made with a full knowledge of the dangers and possible complications of surgery. In many cases yearly re-evaluation is important. It the interim the pain may increase or the patient may decide that the restrictions imposed by the pain are too great. Other adults, on the other hand, may wish to live with their pain, and as long as the pain is tolerable and the curve is stable, periodic re-evaluations at yearly or bi-yearly intervals are continued.

In cases in which the pain pattern is unusual or the decision making difficult, additional tests are of benefit. Discograms, myelograms, and facet blocks will help localize the source of the pain. In some cases a trial of immobilization in either a cast or brace will help show that immobilization (and thus surgical stabilization) will partially or completely relieve the pain.

Principles

Certain differences exist in the treatment of spine deformities in adults as compared with the adolescent. Pain relief and curve stabilization are the prime surgical aims. The pseudarthrosis rate is higher in adults and, in general, immobilization is less well tolerated. Thus techniques are used that minimize the pseudarthrosis rate and the period of immobilization. These techniques include the use of additional instrumentation to stabilize the spine internally and the use of homologous banked bone if the autologous iliac bone is insufficient. In addition, a two-stage anterior and posterior fusion is often performed with lumbar or thoracolumbar curves to help reduce the pseudarthrosis rate and improve the result.

Surgery in adults is technically more difficult than in children and adolescents. The periosteum is thin and the exposure takes longer. The curves are more rigid and correction is correspondingly less. True kyphosis and rotatory "kyphosis" are common, and the instrumentation must be contoured to fit the curve. Contouring is especially important in the lumbar spine to maintain a normal lordosis. With the use of distraction there is a tendency toward flattening of the lumbar spine with elimination of the normal lordosis (see Chapter 21). The lateral x-ray must thus be carefully studied and appropriate steps taken to treat kyphosis and preserve lordosis. When instrumenting lumbar or thoracolumbar curves posteriorly, care must be taken *not* to stop at the apex of the thoracic kyphosis above, but to include the whole kyphosis in the fusion.

When instrumenting large thoracic curves, the ribs on the concavity are often deformed and obstruct rod insertion. In these cases, ribs are removed subperiosteally to allow as straight a distraction rod as possible to be inserted, maximizing the safe distractive force. The bone in adults is more osteopenic and thus the distribution of forces over multiple sites is beneficial to maintain stable internal fixation. This is achieved with the use of multiple distraction rods, combined distraction and compression rods, or with the use of sublaminar wires.

The advent of sublaminar wires with Luque rods or Harrington distraction rods has resulted in the ability to obtain more secure internal stabilization. This is because of the segmentally stabilized fixation with sublaminar wires at each level. An alternate method of segmental fixation is a Harrington compression rod with hooks at every level of the curve.

Some surgeons are now using the Luque technique for the majority of fusions. Certain curve types require distraction for correction and stabilization; this force is not supplied by the Luque technique (see Biomechanics, Chapter 2). In addition the Luque technique has not proven to obviate the need for external support in the healing phase. Preliminary studies of this technique in idiopathic scoliosis have shown a higher pseudarthrosis rate and greater loss of correction when no external support (cast or brace) is used.[12, 71]

The choice of fusion levels in the adult follows the principles discussed in the adolescent (see Chapter 11).[32] Attention must be paid to the lateral x-ray so that the deformity is appreciated in three dimensions and the fusion does not end at the apex of a kyphotic deformity—a situation doomed to failure owing to increase in the kyphosis.

An important question in decision making is whether fusion to the sacrum is necessary.

This decision occurs in single lumbar curves and in double curves with a lumbar component. Fusion to the sacrum is necessary if there is lumbosacral pain with pain coming from the degenerative lumbosacral discs or from the lumbosacral facets. The use of discography and facet blocks may help determine these cases. With lumbosacral pathology producing pain, the fusion must include the pathologic motion segment. Another indication to extend the fusion to the sacrum depends on the rigidity of the fractional lumbosacral curve. If, on the bending x-ray, the decompensation corrects with a correction of the L4-S1 curve, then fusion to the sacrum is not necessary to restore spine balance. If, on the other hand, the fractional lumbosacral curve is rigid with persisting decompensation and significant tilt of L4, then fusion to the sacrum is indicated. Fusion to the sacrum must not be undertaken lightly because of the problems of obtaining a solid fusion at the lumbosacral area[2, 67] and of altering the lumbar lordosis (see Chapter 21).

Techniques

The techniques applicable for the care of adult scoliosis with no prior surgery include: (1) one-stage posterior fusion and instrumentation, (2) anterior fusion and instrumentation, (3) combined anterior and posterior fusion, and (4) nerve root decompression. The instrumentations available are many, and the role of each will be discussed.

In general there is *no* place for routine preoperative halo or femoral traction. The use of traction does *not* increase the correction over that obtained on a bending or traction x-ray (see Chapter 3). In addition there are many complications of traction including thrombophlebitis, pulmonary emboli, atelectasis, and osteoporosis. With the exception of patients in cardiopulmonary failure in whom traction improves their health preoperatively, we follow the principle of Harrington and Dickson. They stated that the patient is healthiest on admission and any bedrest places him or her in a less optimal condition.

The use of posterior facetectomies, traction, and then a second stage posterior fusion has proven to be ineffective in obtaining increased correction.[69] In these cases the best way to obtain improved correction and to improve balancing and stabilization is to use the anterior approach. Anterior releases and fusion with wedge excision at each disc space or with wedge vertebrectomies shorten the curve convexity and allow correction to be obtained with a second stage posterior approach.

Monitoring of spinal cord function is desirable in all cases of posterior surgery. This is performed using the wake-up test, with or without electronic monitoring (see Chapter 22).

In general, in adults the treatment plan is as follows. A full preoperative evaluation is performed, the extent depending on the age and health of the patient. Pulmonary function tests, electrocardiogram, serum electrolytes, and a medical consultation are obtained when necessary. In multiple stage procedures, one week is necessary between the stages to allow the patient to recover from the first surgery. This period was previously 14 days, but with intensive preoperative evaluation, nursing experience, and improved surgical care, it has been reduced to 7 days in the majority of patients.

Five to seven days after the posterior procedure, a model for a postoperative TLSO is taken. This model is taken in the standing position whenever possible. The patient is allowed to stand, use a commode or the bathroom and ambulate short distances from the fourth day when good internal fixation is present. The TLSO is fitted and worn full-time, with time allowed out only for showering. Care is taken that no twisting or bending occurs in the shower.

Immobilization is continued until oblique x-rays show a solid arthrodesis, which takes from 6 to 12 months. At this time the TLSO is discontinued. Occasionally in older patients or in those with a long history of pain, weaning from the TLSO over a few months is necessary. In the TLSO, activities are encouraged, and the patient is encouraged to be active and start a walking program, aiming at a minimum of a mile (1500 meters) per day.

SINGLE THORACIC CURVE

A posterior fusion with Harrington instrumentation is the most common procedure performed, as the majority of the curves in this group are less than 90 degrees and still have sufficient flexibility to allow a balanced spine to be obtained with the thorax positioned over the pelvis. One or more distraction rods are used, depending on the magnitude of the curve, with the addition of a Harrington compression rod if there is kyphosis. To increase the stability of instrumentation, segmental sublaminar wires or a compression rod can be added, the latter is secured to the distraction rod using a transverse force with transverse fixation devices or wires (Fig. 17–4). See Chapter 10.

In larger or more rigid curves in which achieving correction is important, a two stage approach is preferable. The anterior approach is to the convexity of the curve. Five to seven discs are excised over the apex of the curve, and correction is augmented by wedge excision of bone at each level before the interbody fusion is performed. To allow greater correction the apical vertebra or vertebrae can be excised. The second stage involves facetectomies and often osteotomies through spontaneously fused facet joints. If a vertebrectomy has been performed anteriorly, a similar wedge of bone is removed posteriorly. Spine stabilization is obtained using a combination of Harrington distraction and compression instrumentation or Luque rods and sublaminar wires. The ribs on the concavity often need to be removed in the path of the distraction instrumentation, and the ribs on the convexity are either osteotomized or removed in the area of the rib prominence. Rib removal also supplies bone graft material and helps improve the cosmetic result (Fig. 17–5).

In cases presenting with cardiopulmonary symptoms, halo traction is beneficial. Previously halofemoral traction was the routine, but this has been replaced by halo gravity traction with an inclined bed at night and a halo wheelchair during the day. The use of the traction is not to improve the correction but to obtain a healthier, more functional patient. The traction is continued as long as improvement in pulmonary function occurs. If there is no improvement in cardiopulmonary function in traction, surgery is impossible because of the severe anesthetic risks in such a patient. The results have shown that cardiopulmonary failure in neuromuscular scoliosis responds better to this program compared with idiopathic or congenital scoliosis (Fig. 17–6).[70] Treatment is more effective and safer if performed prior to frank

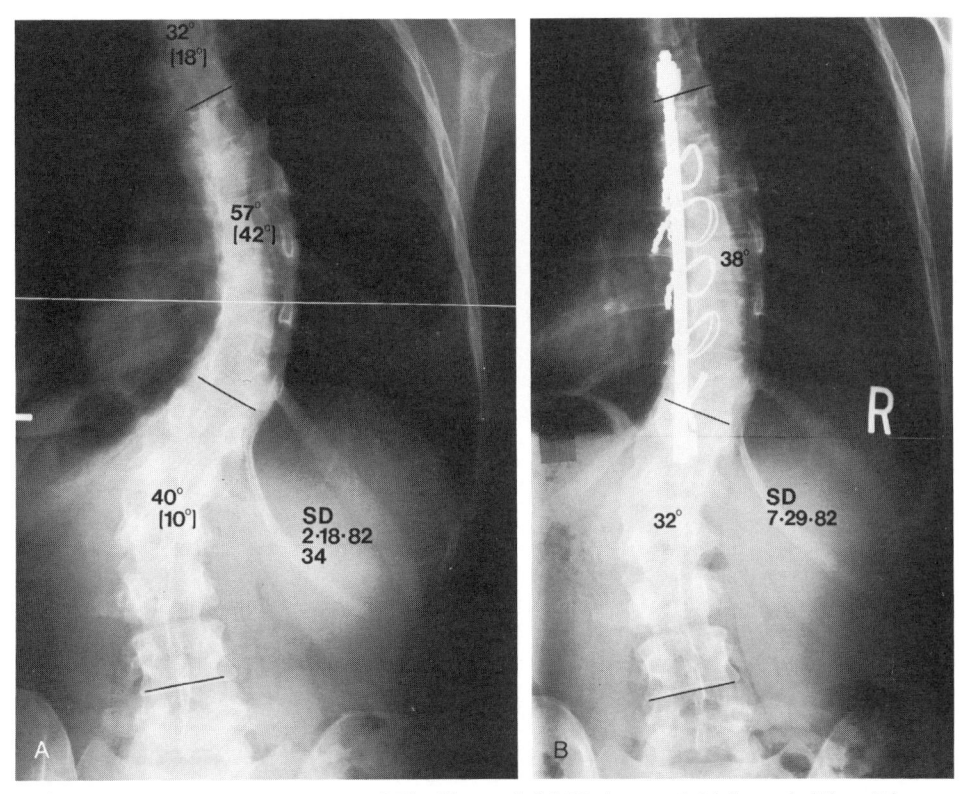

Figure 17–4. *A*, S. D. presented at the age of 34 with a painful 57 degree right thoracic idiopathic curve, which was flexible to 42 degrees on side bending. Stabilization and pain relief were the goals of surgery. A large amount of correction was *not* necessary. *B*, A posterior fusion with a Harrington rod and sublaminar wires was performed. Five months later the fusion was solid, with a 38 degree curve, one degree loss since the day of surgery, and the pain was completely relieved.

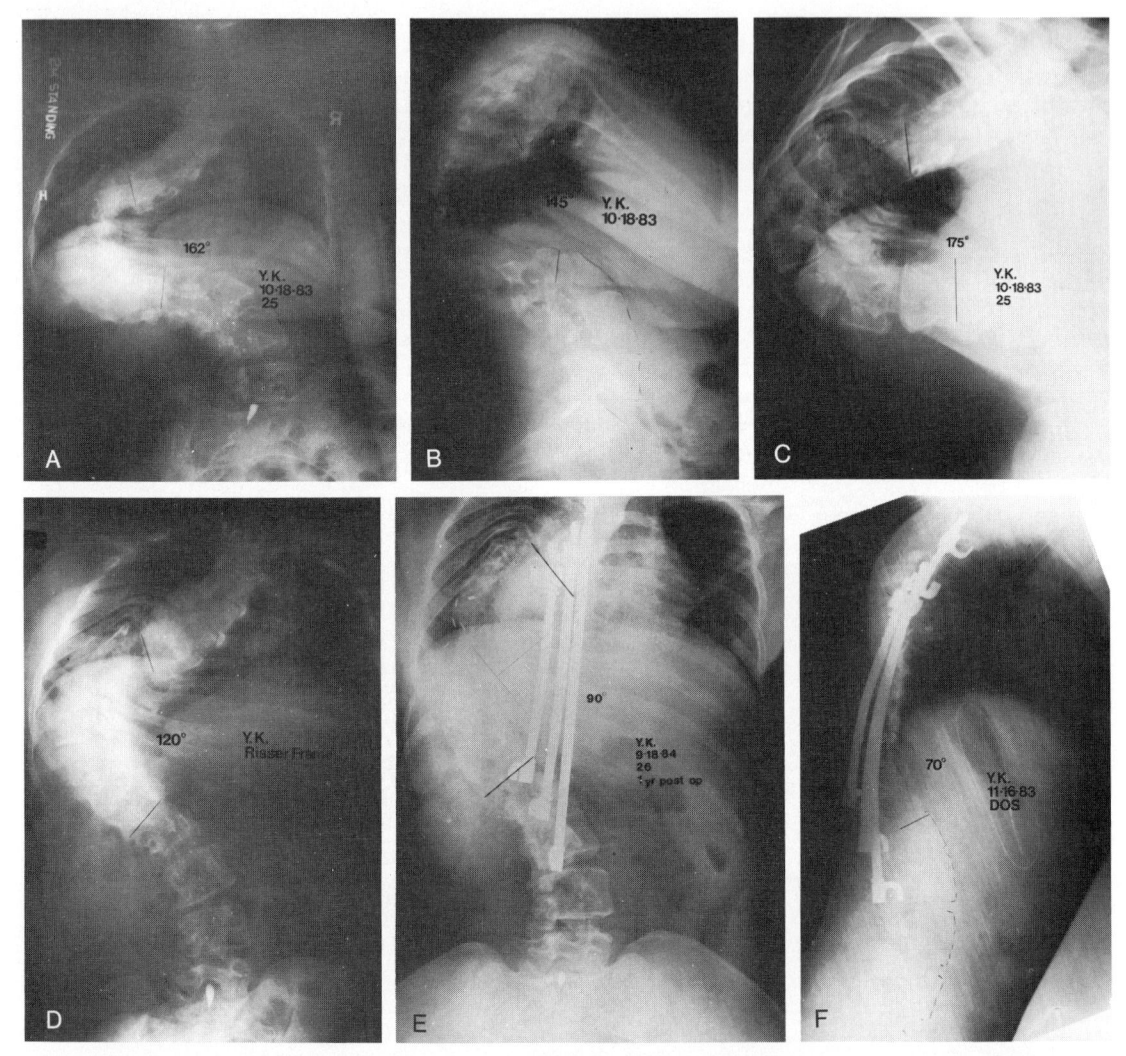

Figure 17–5. Y. K. presented at the age of 25 with untreated infantile idiopathic scoliosis and a 162 degree left thoracic scoliosis (A) and 145 degrees of thoracic kyphosis (B). C, The true magnitude of this kyphosing scoliosis is seen on the Stagnara view, which shows a curve of 175 degrees. D, Correction of the scoliosis to 120 degrees is seen on a traction radiograph taken on the Risser frame. E, An anterior fusion with discectomies and apical vertebrectomy was performed, followed by a posterior fusion with three Harrington distraction rods. A year later the fusion is solid, with correction of the scoliosis to 90 degrees. F, The kyphosing component was corrected to 70 degrees.

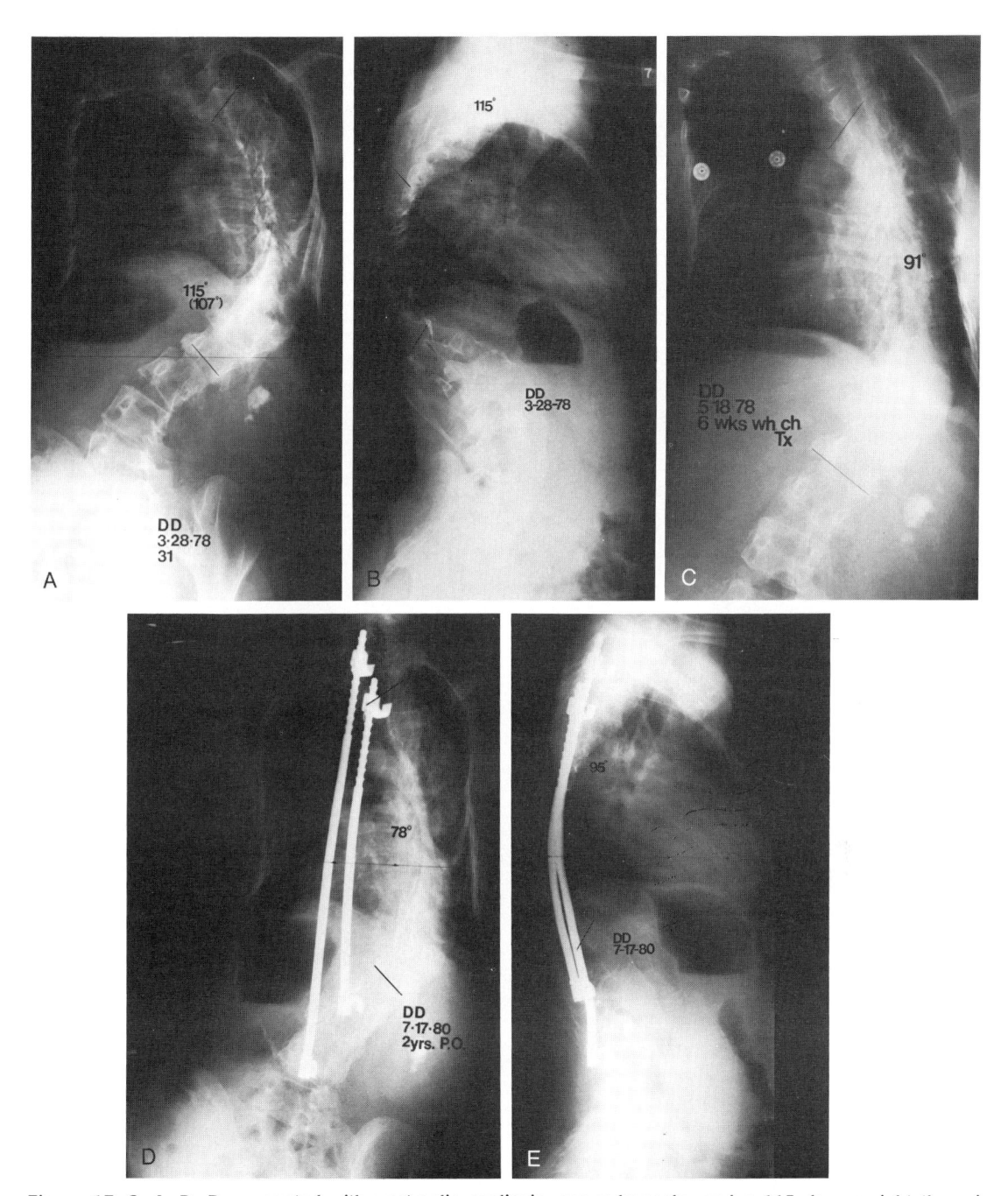

Figure 17–6. A, D. D. presented with post-polio scoliosis, cor pulmonale, and a 115 degree right thoracic scoliosis. B, She also had a 115 degree thoracic kyphosis. Her pulmonary functions were: vital capacity of 600 cc., PaO_2 of 47 mm. Hg, and $PaCO_2$ of 61 mm. Hg. C, After six weeks of halo wheelchair traction with correction of her curve to 91 degrees, her pulmonary functions had improved to a vital capacity of 900 cc., a PaO_2 of 66 mm. Hg, and a $PaCO_2$ of 51 mm. Hg. She was now operable. D, She underwent a posterior fusion with Harrington instrumentation. Two years later the scoliosis was 78 degrees. E, The kyphosis was 95 degrees. Her pulmonary functions 6½ years postoperative were stable with a vital capacity of 1200 cc., PaO_2 of 91 mm. Hg, and $PaCO_2$ of 41 mm. Hg. She was fully employed as a school teacher and taking no cardiac medications.

cardiopulmonary failure. In patients with marked cardiopulmonary compromise, traction is useful between stages (when a two stage procedure is performed) to allow upright positioning of the patient and allow better postoperative pulmonary care.

SINGLE THORACOLUMBAR OR LUMBAR CURVE

This curve pattern is unusual in adults, there commonly being a thoracic curve above. As pain is a common surgical indication in these cases, the lumbosacral area is carefully assessed by history, physical examination, and if necessary with discography and facet blocks.

In a single curve with no lumbosacral pathology and a smaller thoracic curve, fusion can be limited to the thoracolumbar or lumbar curve. The choice is between a posterior or an anterior fusion. In this area the sagittal contour is important. The lumbar lordosis must be maintained and not reduced. In the posterior approach the use of a bent square-ended distraction rod with or without the addition of a compression rod will maintain the lumbar lordosis.[25] Segmental sublaminar wires help stabilize the spine. An alternative is the use of Luque instrumentation contoured to maintain the lordosis. In the posterior approach, the lateral view must be studied to ensure that the upper end of the fusion does not end at the apex of the thoracic kyphosis. The distraction force exerted by the distraction rod will push the thoracic spine forward over the upper end of the fusion. This results in forward tilt of the torso with increased kyphosis and back pain. To prevent this the fusion must extend cephalad to include the kyphosis.

The anterior approach with Zielke instrumentation offers definite advantages,[27, 30, 43, 68, 77] and is preferred by the authors. The fusion is shorter, leaving more motion segments unfused. By careful screw insertion as far posteriorly as possible and by the use of bone blocks anteriorly, the kyphosing tendency of this instrumentation is prevented, and the lordosis is maintained. Derotation is superior to the posterior approach, and correction is also better (Fig. 17–7). (See Chapter 10.)

The anterior approach can only be used if on a side bending of the lumbosacral curve the lower vertebra of the proposed fusion area is nearly parallel to the upper margin of S1. If this vertebra is not parallel, then a longer fusion to the parallel vertebra *or* a posterior procedure is performed.

The anterior approach, as it shortens the convexity of the curve, results in correction greater than that on a side bending x-ray. Care must be taken not to correct the instrumented curve more than the ability of the thoracic curve above to compensate. This ability is shown on the side bending correction of the thoracic curve, the lumbar curve being corrected to near this flexibility. If necessary, an x-ray is taken during the surgery to monitor this correction. If there is a rigid lumbosacral curve, too much correction of the lumbar or thoracolumbar curve will result in tilting of the whole spine to the side; an anterior fusion is contraindicated in this situation. It is seen that the spine balance is important in this case, the thoracic curve above and the lumbosacral curve below must be evaluated as well as the sagittal contours appreciated.

The instrumentation used anteriorly can either be the Dwyer of Zielke. We prefer the Zielke because of its ability to allow gradual correction and to better avoid lumbar kyphosis.

If there is lumbosacral pain or a rigid lumbosacral curve, fusion must extend to the sacrum. This condition is unusual with a single curve, but it is more common with the more common double curve pattern. Extension of the fusion to the sacrum is discussed below.

NERVE ROOT DECOMPRESSION

When there is radiculopathy its site is important. Root compression on the concavity of the lumbar curve is treated by root explortaion and decompression.[22, 23] The accompanying lumbar curve is treated, depending on the symptoms present. With no back pain or curve progression, arthrodesis is usually unnecessary. If decompression is substantial or if the patient has a symptomatic curve, arthrodesis should accompany the root decompression. In some cases, if cast or brace immobilization eliminates the radicular pain, curve correction without nerve root exploration is possible. The root is "decompressed" by correction of the curve.

Nerve root decompression in the concavity of the fractional lumbosacral curve is treated one of two ways. If mild, straightening of the lumbar curve will open the nerve root

ADULT SCOLIOSIS

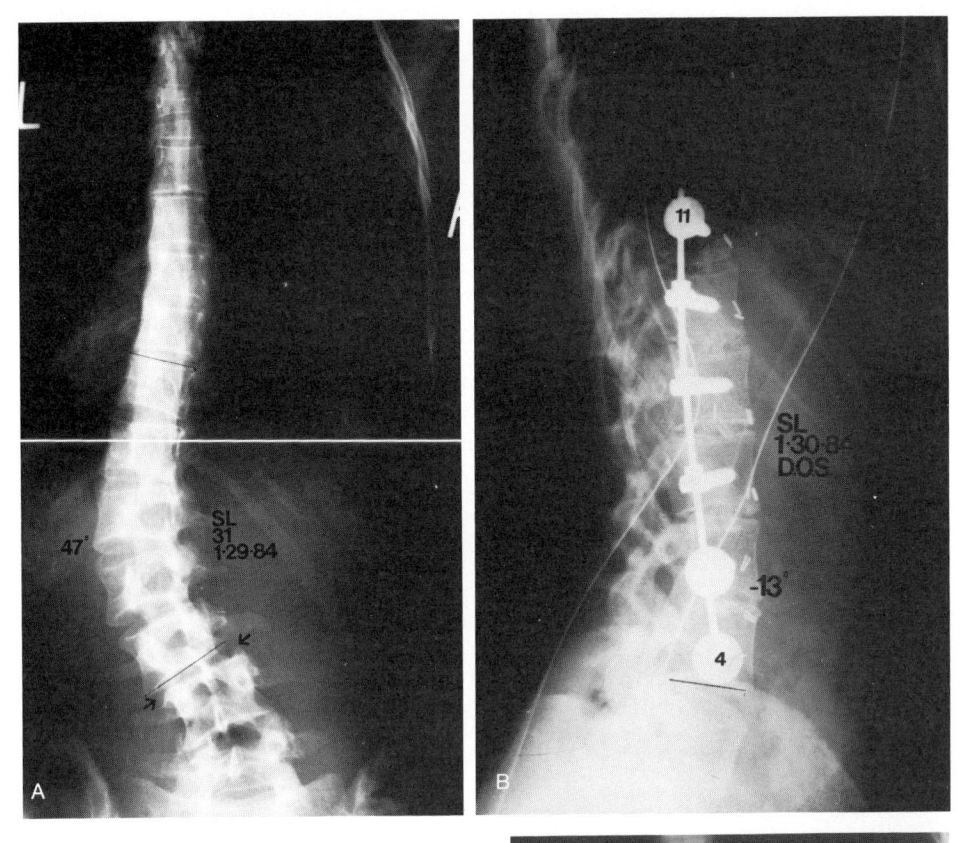

Figure 17–7. *A*, S. L. presented at age 31 with a 47 degree left thoracolumbar idiopathic scoliosis and curve pain that was progressive. Rotatory subluxation at L3-L4 was present. *B*, She underwent an anterior fusion with Zielke instrumentation, care being taken in screw placement to maintain lumbar lordosis. *C*, Seven months postoperative the curve was 16 degrees—a two degree loss since the day of surgery. The fusion was solid and the pain relieved.

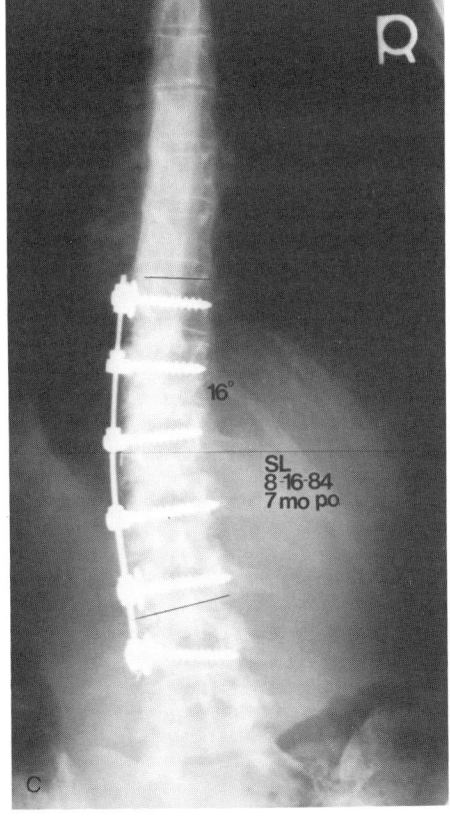

foramen and thus decompress the root. This technique, with flexible lumbar and lumbosacral areas and anterior fusion and instrumentation of the lumbar curve, gives good results.[60] If the compression is severe or the curves are rigid, root decompression is the treatment of choice. The symptoms present and the spinal stability will determine whether an arthrodesis must accompany the decompression (Fig. 17–8).

DOUBLE THORACIC AND LUMBAR CURVES

Fusion in these patients involves both curves. The technique depends on the magnitude of the curves. In moderate, balanced curves a posterior fusion and instrumentation is the procedure of choice. The instrumentation choices are a single Harrington distraction rod, distraction plus compression rods, a distraction rod plus sublaminar wires, and the Luque system. The instrumentation chosen depends on the balance, the sagittal curve (thoracic kyphosis or lordosis), and the surgeon's preference and expertise. Care must be taken to contour the instrumentation to maintain lumbar lordosis and prevent forward tilting of the spine.

In an unbalanced deformity in which the lower curve is larger or more rigid, a two-stage procedure is preferred. The lumbar or thoracolumbar area is approached anteriorly, the discs and anterior longitudinal ligament excised, and an anterior fusion performed. Rib bone is used; it is augmented by iliac or banked bone when additional graft is required. No instrumentation is added. A second stage posterior fusion and instrumentation of both curves is performed a week later. The anterior fusion allows correction, reduces the rotational deformity, reduces the pseudarthrosis rate, and allows the spine to be balanced. This combined approach has proven to give an improved result with rapid incorporation of bone graft and solid fusion, with a lower pseudarthrosis rate and better spine balancing in the coronal and sagittal planes (Fig. 17–9).[13, 72]

Fusion of scoliosis to the sacrum in the adult is associated with a high complication rate. The most important of these are pseudarthrosis, decompensation, loss of lumbar lordosis, and instrument failure.[2, 67] Fusion to the sacrum should be performed only if absoutely necessary, that is, the lumbosacral area is part of the pain complex on history or with discograms and facet blocks *or* there is a very rigid lumbosacral curve with L4 not correcting over the sacrum on side bending of the lumbosacral curve. If at all possible, the fusion should end at L4.

When fusion to the sacrum is necessary there are two choices of technique. The approach can be posteriorly with fusion and instrumentation and possible reinforcement of the fusion six months later, with continued immobilization for an additional four to six months. In our experience, the use of the Harrington rod alone has been accompanied by a high incidence of pseudarthroses as well as post-surgical loss of lordosis, and thus the Luque technique is currently used. In the Luque technique, dual ¼ inch rods are used with sacral fixation using the Galveston tech-

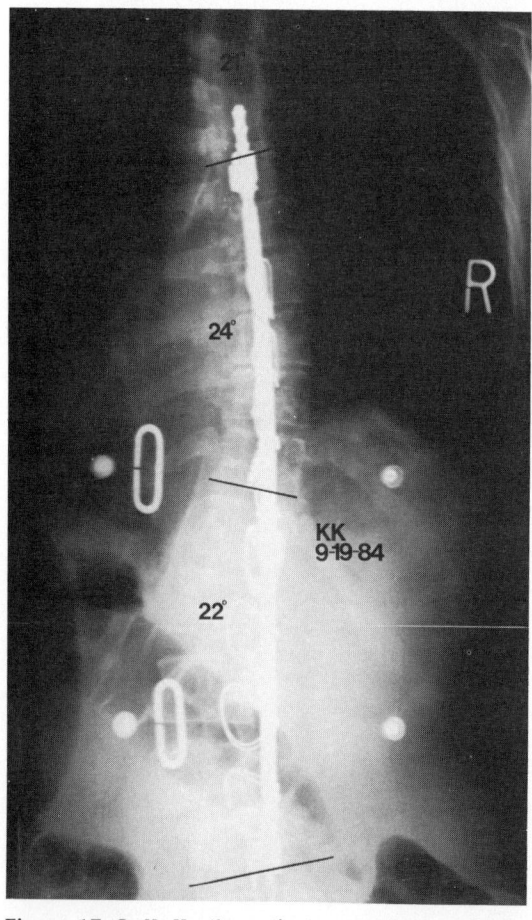

Figure 17–8. K. K., the patient presented previously in Figure 17–2, underwent a nerve root decompression at L3-L4 on the right plus a posterior fusion with Harrington instrumentation and segmental sublaminar wires. The fusion extended to L4, the lower discs being normal on discography, with no pain reproduction with this test.

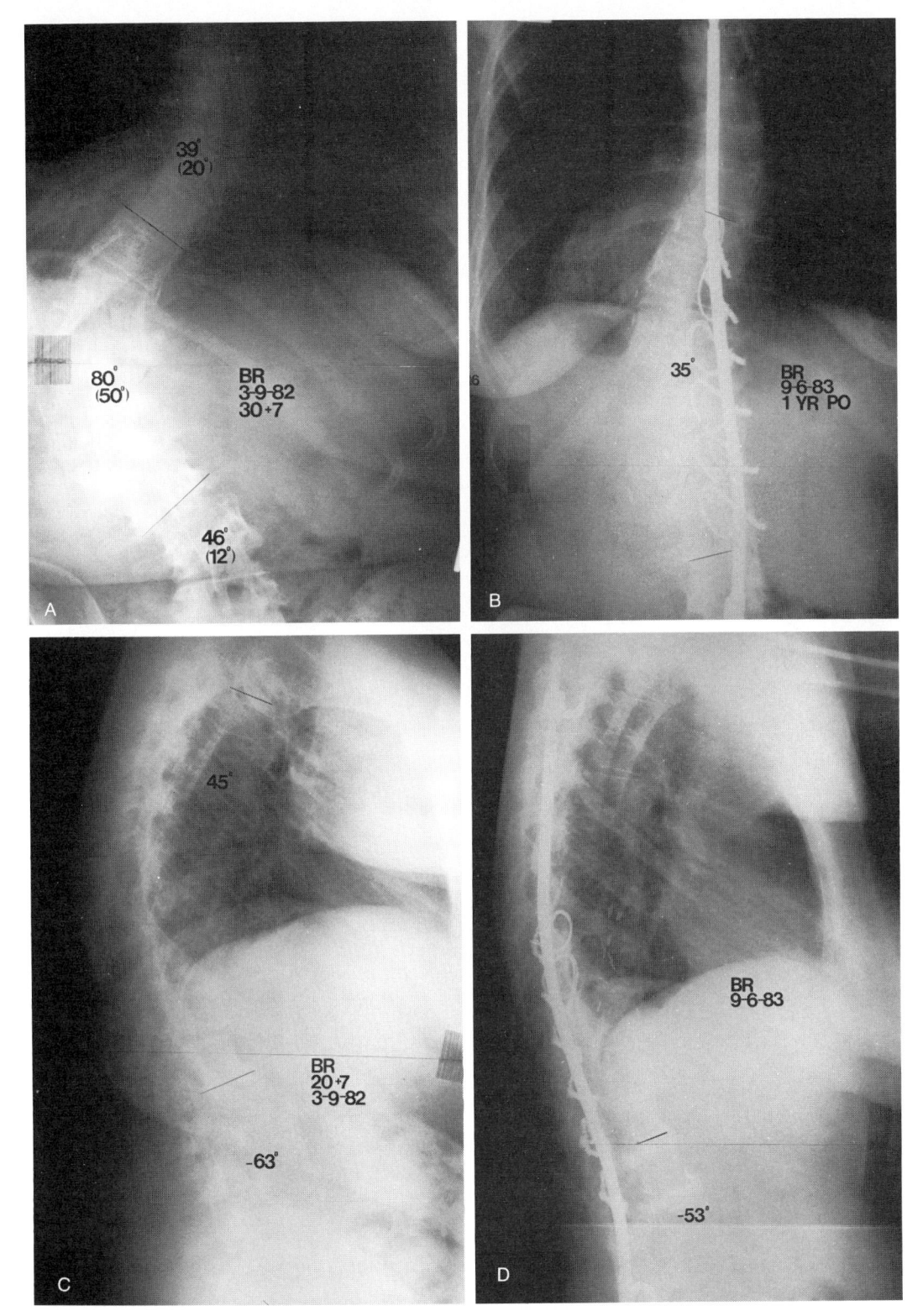

Figure 17–9. *A*, B. R. presented with a progressive left thoracolumbar idiopathic scoliosis associated with progressive curve pain. The 80 degree thoracolumbar curve was fairly rigid, only correcting to 50 degrees, while the fractional lumbosacral curve was flexible, correcting from 46 degrees to 12 degrees. *B*, As there was no lumbosacral pain and the lumbosacral curve was flexible, fusion to the sacrum was not necessary. She underwent a two-stage procedure, consisting of an anterior discectomy and fusion from T10 to L4 and posterior fusion with a Harrington rod and segmental sublaminar wires from T5 to L4. A year later the fusion was solid, and she was pain-free. The lateral preoperative view (*C*) and the lateral postoperative view (*D*) show the rod contours and maintenance of the lumbar lordosis. Additional sublaminar wires should have been added in the thoracic area to increase the stability of the fixation.

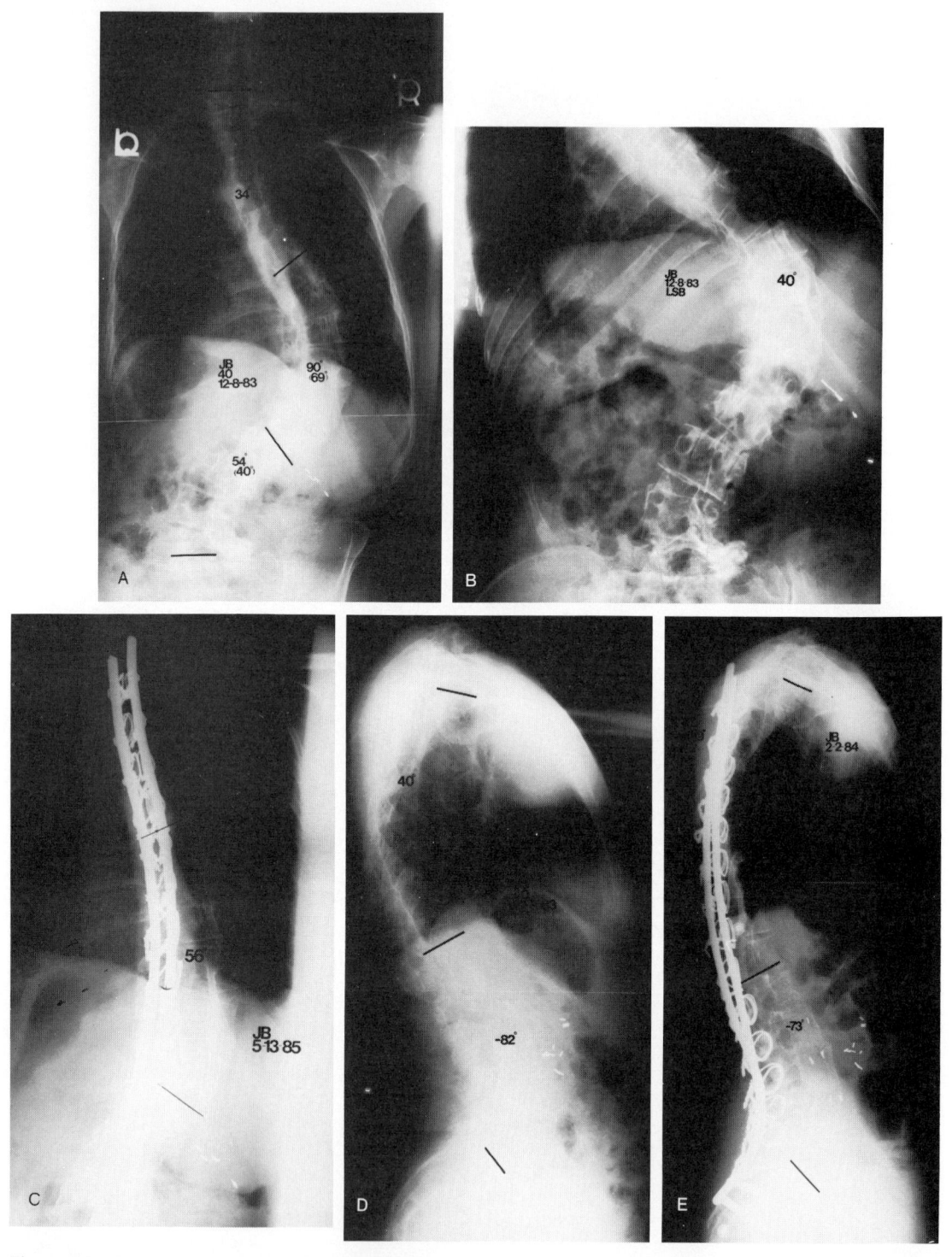

Figure 17–10. *A*, J. B. presented with a progressive and painful idiopathic scoliosis with curve and lumbosacral pain, a 90 degree right thoracolumbar curve, and a 54 degree fractional lower lumbar curve, both curves being minimally flexible on side bending. Note the decompensation of the thorax to the right. *B*, The stiffness of the lower lumbar curve did not allow the spine to be corrected over the sacrum on the left bending view. Because of this stiff curve and the lumbosacral pain, fusion to the sacrum is necessary, and because of this stiffness, an anterior discectomy and fusion was first performed from L2 to the sacrum using a *left* flank approach. *C*, A posterior fusion with Luque instrumentation and Galveston pelvic fixation was performed. Eighteen months postoperatively the fusion was solid, the patient pain-free, and the thorax in balance over the pelvis. The lateral preoperative view (*D*) and the lateral postoperative view (*E*) show the contouring of the Luque rods and maintenance of the lumbar lordosis.

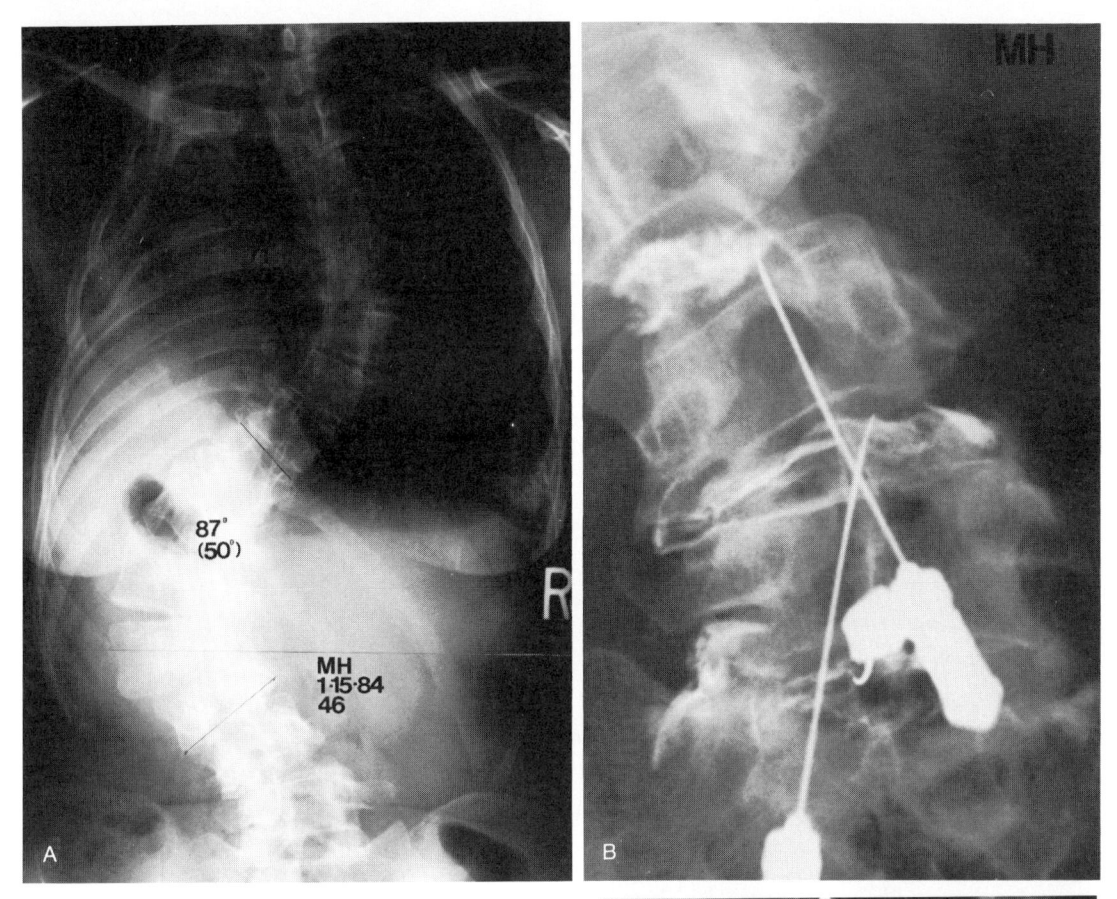

Figure 17–11. *A*, M. H. presented at age 46 with progressive, painful idiopathic thoracolumbar scoliosis. The pain was in the curve as well as in the lumbosacral area, and there was L5 root distribution pain. *B*, A myelogram confirmed the L5 root compression and the discogram reproduced her lumbosacral pain, showing degeneration at L4-L5 and at L5-S1. Fusion to the sacrum was thus necessary. *C*, She underwent anterior discectomy and fusion of the left thoracolumbar curve, the fusion extending to the sacrum. At the second stage the L5 nerve root was decompressed and fusion performed, using Luque instrumentation with Galveston pelvic fixation. The fusion is solid with maintenance of the correction and she was pain-free a year postoperatively.

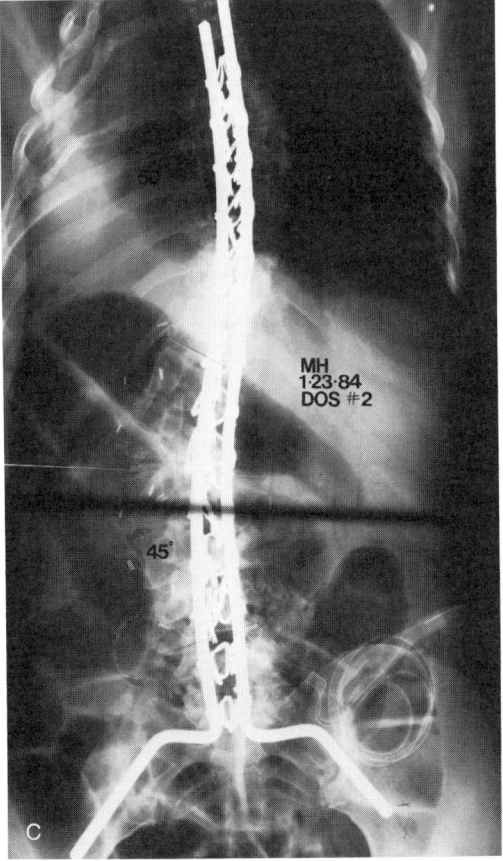

nique (see Chapter 10). Iliac bone graft is taken and augmented with banked bone when the graft is insufficient or iliac bone cannot be taken, for example, in the Luque technique to the sacrum.

The current alternative and the preferred technique is a two-stage anterior and posterior fusion. The anterior fusion is of the entire lumbar curve and extends to the sacrum. A second stage posterior correction and stabilization is performed using Luque rods and the Galveston pelvic fixation technique. Sagittal bending of the rods is essential to maintain the normal contours of the spine (Figs. 17–10 and 17–11). The two-stage approach or the posterior approach with a six month reinforcement has given a lower pseudarthrosis rate.[2]

After fusion and stabilization posteriorly, the patient is kept on bedrest for four to five days, at which time, if the internal fixation is secure, ambulation is started. When the general condition and abdominal distension allow, a standing model for a one-piece postoperative TLSO is taken (see Chapter 7). In cases in which fusion to the sacrum is performed, the orthosis is fabricated with bilateral trochanteric extensions. Once the orthosis is fitted and comfortable, the patient is discharged, usually 10 to 14 days following surgery. The orthosis is worn full-time, except for a short period for showers. At this time no bending, stooping or twisting is allowed. Immobilization is continued until a solid fusion is seen on oblique x-rays, which takes 6 to 12 months. Occasionally, if the fusion mass is continuous but immature, sleeping out of the orthosis is allowed, usually about six months postoperatively. Activities are encouraged in the orthosis. The patient usually returns to work two to three months postoperatively. Daily exercising by brisk walking is encouraged, the aim being to walk one mile daily by two to three months after surgery. Occasionally, once the fusion is solid, weaning from the orthosis is necessary, gradually increasing the time out of the orthosis. Generally, once the fusion is solid, abrupt cessation of external immobilization is possible.

SUMMARY

As can be seen, scoliosis in adults poses many problems in patient evaluation, decision making, and the choice of surgical techniques. In the whole adult population with scoliosis, problems and treatment are actually uncommon. On the other hand, once symptoms or problems are sufficient to warrant seeking care, the need for active intervention increases. With careful patient evaluation, careful patient selection for surgery, and the use of newer techniques that give improved fixation and improved fusion rates, successful surgery in adults is possible.

In the decision making process, the risk/benefit ratio is important. Complications are common in adults;[2, 18, 19, 29, 38, 42, 43, 51, 69] the most common are pseudarthroses, instrumentation failure, and loss of correction. Although uncommon, death and paralysis are both more frequent in adults than adolescents (see Chapter 21). The possibility and severity of these complications must always be considered and weighed against the possible benefits of surgery to the patients.

References

1. Ascani, E., Bartolozzi, P., Logroscino, C. A., et al.: Natural history of untreated scoliosis after skeletal maturity. Presented at a Symposium on Epidemiology, Natural History and Non-Operative Treatment of Idiopathic Scoliosis at the Annual Meeting of the Scoliosis Research Society, Orlando, Florida, September, 1984.
2. Balderston, R., Winter, R. B., Moe, J. H., et al.: Fusion to the sacrum for non-paralytic scoliosis in the adult. Orthop. Trans., 8:170, 1984.
3. Benetsson, F., Fallstrom, D., Jansson, F., and Nachemson, A.: A psychological and psychiatric investigation of the adjustment of female scoliosis. Acta Psychiatr. Scand., 50:50, 1974.
4. Benner, B., and Ehni, G.: Degenerative lumbar scoliosis. Spine, 4:548–552, 1979.
5. Bergofsky, E. H., Turino, G. M., and Fishman, A. P.: Cardiorespiratory failure in kyphoscoliosis. Medicine, 38:263–317, 1959.
6. Bjerkreim, E., and Hassan, I.: Progression in untreated idiopathic scoliosis after end of growth. Acta Orthop. Scand., 53:897–900, 1982.
7. Bjure, J., and Nachemson, A.: Non-treated scoliosis. Clin. Orthop., 93:44–52, 1973.
8. Blount, W. P., and Mellencamp, D. D.: The effect of pregnancy on idiopathic scoliosis. J. Bone Joint Surg., 62A:1083–1087, 1980.
9. Bonnett, C., Brown, J. C., Cross, B., and Barron, R.: Posterior spinal fusion with Harrington rod instrumentation in 100 consecutive patients. Contemp. Orthop., 2:396–399, 1980.
10. Boyer, A.: Etude de la restriction ventilatoire des scolioses adultes avant et apres traitment chirurgical. Doctoral thesis, University of Claude Bernard, Lyon, 1973.
11. Briard, J. L., Jegou, D., and Cauchoix, J.: Adult lumbar scoliosis. Spine, 4:526–532, 1979.
12. Broadstone, P., Johnson, J. R., and Leatherman, K. D.: Consider post-operative immobilization of

double L-rod SSI patients. Orthop. Trans., 8:171, 1984.
13. Byrd, J. A., Winter, R. B., Bradford, D. S., et al.: Adult idiopathic scoliosis treated by anterior and posterior spinal fusion. Presented at the Annual Meeting of the Scoliosis Research Society, San Diego, CA., September 1985.
14. Chapman, E. H., Dill, B. D., and Graybiel, A.: The decrease in functional capacity of the lungs and heart resulting from deformities of the chest pulmocardiac failure. Medicine, 18:167–202, 1939.
15. Cochran, R., Irstam, L., and Nachemson, A.: Long term anatomic and functional changes in patients with adolescent idiopathic scoliosis treated by Harrington rod fusion. Spine, 8:576–584, 1983.
16. Collis, D. K., and Ponsetti, I. V.: Long term followup of patients with idiopathic scoliosis not treated surgically. J. Bone Joint Surg., 51A:425–445, 1969.
17. Coonrad, R. W., and Feierstein, M. S.: Progression of scoliosis in the adult. J. Bone Joint Surg., 58A:156, 1976.
18. Curtis, R. S., Dickson, J. H., Harrington, P. R., and Erwin, W. D.: Results of Harrington instrumentation in the treatment for severe scoliosis. Clin. Orthop., 144:128–134, 1979.
19. Dawson, E. G., Moe, J. H., and Caron, A.: Surgical management of scoliosis in the adult. J. Bone Joint Surg., 55A:437, 1973.
20. Drummond, D. S., Fowles, J. V., Ecoyer, S., et al.: Untreated scoliosis in the adult. J. Bone Joint Surg., 58A:156, 1976.
21. Duriez, J.: Evolution de la scoliose idiopathique chez l'adulte. Acta Ortho. Belg., 33:547–550, 1967.
22. Epstein, J. A., Epstein, B. S., and Lavine, L. S.: Surgical treatment of nerve root compression caused by scoliosis of the lumbar spine. J. Neurosurg., 41:449–454, 1974.
23. Epstein, J. A., Epstein, B. S., and Jones, M. D.: Symptomatic lumbar scoliosis and degenerative changes in the elderly. Spine, 4:542–547, 1979.
24. Fowles, J. V., Drummond, D. S., L'Ecuzer, S., et al.: The prognosis and management of untreated scoliosis in the adult. Presented at the Annual Meeting of the Scoliosis Reesearch Society, Louisville, Kentucky, 1973.
25. Gaines, R. W., and Leatherman, K. D.: Benefits of the Harrington compression system in lumbar and thoracolumbar idiopathic scoliosis in adolescents and adults. Spine, 6:483–488, 1981.
26. Ghavamian, T.: Future of minor scoliotic curves of the spine. Exhibit, Am. Acad. Orthop. Surg., Washington, D. C., 1972.
27. Griss, P., and Jentschura, G.: Early results of operative treatment of scoliosis using the anterior derotation spondylodesis technique (VDS-Zielke). Z. Orthop., 119:115–122, 1981.
28. Grubb, S. S., Lipscomp, H. J., and Brashear, H. R.: Relative value of lumbar x-rays, metrizamide myelography and discography in assessment of patients with chronic low back pain. Orthop. Trans., 4:199, 1980.
29. Gui, L., and Savini, R.: The surgical treatment of scoliosis in the adult. Ital. J. Orthop. Traum., 1:191–208, 1975.
30. Hall, J. E.: Dwyer instrumentation in anterior fusion of the spine. J. Bone Joint Surg., 63A:1188–1190, 1981.
31. Keim, H. A.: Scoliosis can progress in the adult. Orthop. Rev., 3:23–28, 1974.
32. King, H. A., Moe, J. H., Bradford, D. S., and Winter, R. B.: The selection of fusion levels in thoracic idiopathic scoliosis. J. Bone Joint Surg., 65A:1302, 1983.
33. Kolind-Sorenson, V.: A followup study of patients with idiopathic scoliosis. Acta Orthop. Scand., 44:98, 1973.
34. Kostuik, J. P.: Decision making in adult scoliosis. Spine, 4:521–525, 1979.
35. Kostuik, J.: Halo-pelvic traction in the surgical management of adult scoliosis. J. Bone Joint Surg., 55B:232, 1973.
36. Kostuik, J. P.: Recent advances in the treatment of painful adult scoliosis. Clin. Orthop., 147:238–252, 1980.
37. Kostuik, J. P., and Bentivoglio, J.: The incidence of low back pain in adult scoliosis. Spine, 6:268–273, 1981.
38. Kostuik, J. P., Israel, J., and Hall, J. E.: Scoliosis surgery in adults. Clin. Orthop., 93:225–234, 1973.
39. Leidholt, J., and Ballard, A.: The disability of lumbar curves in adulthood. J. Bone Joint Surg., 56A:444, 1974.
40. Marchetti, P. G.: Le Scoliosi. Bologna, Aulo Gaggi, 1968.
41. McKinley, L. M., Gaines, R. W., and Leatherman, K. D.: Adult scoliosis: recognition and treatment. Kentucky Medical Assoc., 75:235–238, 1977.
42. Micheli, L. J., Riseborough, E. J., and Hall, J. E.: Scoliosis in the adult. Orthop. Rev., 6:27–39, 1977.
43. Moe, J. H., Purcell, G. A., and Bradford, D. S.: Zielke instrumentation (VDS) for the correction of spinal curvature—analysis of results in 66 patients. Clin. Orthop. 180:133–153, 1983.
44. Moskowitz, A., Moe, J. H., Winter, R. B., and Binner, H.: Long term followup of scoliosis fusion. J. Bone Joint Surg., 62A:364–376, 1980.
45. Nachemson, A.: Adult scoliosis and back pain. Spine, 4:512–517, 1979.
46. Nachemson, A.: A long term followup study of non-treated scoliosis. J. Bone Joint Surg., 50A:203, 1969.
47. Nachemson, A.: A long term followup study of non-treated scoliosis. Acta Orthop. Scand., 39:466–476, 1968.
48. Nachemson, A., Cochran, R. P., Irstram, L., and Fallstrom, K.: Pregnancy after scoliosis treatment. Orthop. Trans., 6:5, 1982.
49. Nilsonne, U., and Lundgren, K. D.: Long term prognosis in idiopathic scoliosis. Acta Orthop. Scand., 39:456–465, 1968.
50. Pellin, B., and Zielke, K.: Scolioses severes de l'adulte et du grand adolescent—41 cas operes. Rev. Chir. Orthop., 60:623–633, 1974.
51. Ponder, R. C., Dickson, J. H., Harrington, P. R., and Erwin, W. D.: Results of Harrington instrumentation and fusion in the adult scoliosis patient. J. Bone Joint Surg., 57A:797–801, 1975.
52. Ponseti, I. V.: The pathogenesis of adult scoliosis. In Zorab, P. A. (ed.): Proceedings of Second Symposium on Scoliosis Causation. Edinburgh, E&S Livingstone, 1968.
53. Riseborough, E. J.: Scoliosis in adults. Cur. Pract. Orthop. Surg., 7:36–55, 1977.
54. Risser, J. C.: The iliac apophysis: an invaluable

sign in the management of scoliosis. Clin. Orthop., *11*:111–119, 1958.
55. Risser, J. C., Igbal, Q. M., and Nagata, K.: Scoliosis after termination of vertebral growth. Ann. R. Coll. Surg., *59*:119–123, 1977.
56. Robin, G. C., Span, Y., Steinberg, R., et al.: Scoliosis in the elderly—a followup study. Spine, 7:355–359, 1982.
57. Sicard, A., Lavarde, G., and Chaleil, B.: La greffe vertebrale dans les scolioses de l'adulte. J. Chir. (Paris), *93*:517–526, 1967.
58. Sicard, A., Lavarde, G., and Chaleil, B.: Seventy instances of adult scoliosis treated with spinal fusion. Surg. Gynecol. Obstet., *126*:682, 1968.
59. Siegler, D., and Zorab, P. A.: Pregnancy in thoracic scoliosis. Br. J. Dis. Chest, 75:367–370, 1981.
60. Simmonds, E. H., and Jackson, R. P.: The management of nerve root entrapment syndromes associated with the collapsing scoliosis of idiopathic lumbar and thoracolumbar curves. Spine 4:533–541, 1979.
61. Stagnara, P.: Scoliosis in adults. Surgical treatment of severe forms. Excerpts Med. Found. International Congress Series No. 192, 1969.
62. Stagnara, P.: Traitement chirugical des scoliosis cyphosantes ches l'adulte. Acta Orthop. Belg., 47:721–739, 1981.
63. Stagnara, P., Jouvinroux, P., Pelous, J., et al.: Cyphoscolioses essentielles de l'adulte. Formes severes de plus de 100°. Redressement partial et arthrodese. XI Sicot Congress, 206–233, Mexico City, 1969.
64. Stagnara, P., Fleury, D., Pauchet, R., et al.: Scolioses majeures de l'adulte superieures a 100°—183 cas traites chirurgicalement. Rev. Chir. Orthop., *61*:101–122, 1975.
65. Stagnara, P.: Scoliose de l'Adulte chirurgie du rhumatisme. *In* D'Aubigne, R. M. (ed): Chirurgie du Rhumatisme. Paris, Masson et Cie, 1971.
66. Stagnara, P.: Utilization of Harrington's device in the treatment of adult kyphoscoliosis above 100 degrees. Fourth International Symposium, 1971. Nijmegen. Stuttgart, Georg Thieme Verlag, 1973.
67. Steenaert, B. A.: Posterior spinal fusion including the sacrum in scoliosis. J. Bone Joint Surg., *63B*:289–290, 1981.
68. Swank, S. M., Brown, J. C., Williams, L., and Stark E.: Spinal fusion using Zielke instrumentation. Orthopaedics, 5:1172–1182, 1982.
69. Swank, S. M., Lonstein, J. E., Moe, J. H., et al.: Surgical treatment of adult scoliosis—a review of 220 cases. J. Bone Joint Surg., *63A*:268–287, 1981.
70. Swank, S., Winter, R. B., and Moe, J. H.: Scoliosis and cor pulmonale. Spine, 7:343–354, 1982.
71. Taddonio, R. F., Weller, K., and Appel, M.: A comparison of patients with idiopathic scoliosis managed with and without postoperative immobilization following segmental spinal instrumentation with Luque rods. Orthop. Trans., *8*:172, 1984.
72. Van Dam, B. E., Bradford, D. S., Lonstein, J. E., et al.: Adult idiopathic scoliosis treated by posterior spinal fusion and instrumentation. Presented at Annual Meeting of the Scoliosis Research Society, San Diego, CA., September, 1985.
73. Vanderpool, D. W., James, J. I. P., and Wynne-Davies, R.: Scoliosis in the elderly. J. Bone Joint Surg., *51A*:446–455, 1969.
74. Weinstein, S. L., and Ponsetti, I. V.: Curve progression in idiopathic scoliosis. J. Bone Joint Surg., *65A*:447, 1983.
75. Weinstein, S. L., Zavala, D. C., and Ponseit, I. V.: Idiopathic scoliosis—long term followup and prognosis in untreated patients. J. Bone Joint Surg., *63A*:702–711, 1981.
76. Winter, R. B.: Treatment of the adult with scoliosis. Minn. Med., 67:25–29, 1984.
77. Zielke, K., and Pellin, B.: Ergebnisse Operativer Skoliosen-und Kyphoskoliosen-benhandlung beim Adoleszenten Uber 18 jahre and Beim Erwachsenen. S. Orthop., *113*:157–174, 1975.

18

SALVAGE AND RECONSTRUCTIVE SURGERY

John E. Lonstein, M.D.

Reconstructive, recorrective, or salvage surgery are the terms applied to the additional surgical procedure or procedures necessary to achieve a solid, balanced fusion in a patient who has had previous surgery for the treatment of a spinal deformity. This term applies to children and adults, the latter having undergone the initial fusion either as a child or as an adult.

The patients most commonly requiring reconstructive surgery are those with idiopathic scoliosis or neuromuscular spine deformities. These patients account for 31 per cent of Kostuik's series of 107 patients.[8] Eleven of the 132 adult cases reported by Ponder and coworkers had had previous spine fusions[17] as had 29 of Stagnara's series of 183 patients,[20] 8 of Pellin and Zielke's 41 cases[15] and all of Cummine and associates' series of 59 patients.[1]

PRESENTATION

Reconstructive surgery may be required for one or more of the following reasons: pseudarthrosis, curve progression, too short a fusion, loss of lumbar lordosis, or persistent lateral decompensation.

Pseudarthrosis

Single or multiple pseudarthroses, alone or in combination with one of the foregoing problems, constitute the most common problem. The diagnosis can be made preoperatively on finding localized tenderness of the fusion mass, loss of correction with or without fracture of the instrumentation and a visible defect in the fusion mass. The defect is seen on careful inspection of the anteroposterior, lateral, and oblique radiographs of the fusion mass, and is more common in the thoracolumbar or lumbosacral areas. The serpentine nature of the pseudarthrosis often makes it difficult to identify.

Early detection of the pseudarthrosis *before* loss of correction or failure of the instrumentation is the ideal. Careful evaluation of the aforementioned views at the time of discontinuance of immobilization and at subsequent follow-up visits will allow an early diagnosis to be made.

Curve Progression

Curve progression indicates an increase in the spinal deformity, scoliosis, kyphosis, or rarely lordosis. It can result from a pseudarthrosis of the fusion or from "bending" of the fusion. Bending of the fusion may occur in a child who was fused at an early age and in whom, with bone growth and remodeling, the curve has increased, but the fusion length has remained unchanged.[10] It is important to remember that the loss of correction can be in three dimensions, and thus two views of the spine are necessary. In some patients who present with loss of height there is no change in the scoliosis; only the lateral view shows that the deformity is an increasing kyphosis. Another type of increased deformity can occur in fusions performed in the juvenile or early adolescent years. In the presence of a solid posterior fusion, there is continued anterior growth with resultant increasing rotational deformity.

Too Short a Fusion

Some patients present for reconstructive surgery with a fused area that is shorter than the presenting curve. This occurs for one of two reasons. Perhaps the initial fusion involved the whole major curve, but with the passage of time the curve became longer with the addition of vertebrae that were initially not part of the curve (adding on). This occurs most commonly in children fused at a young age; the adding on is usually caudad. In some cases, when the presurgical film is reviewed, a number of parallel end vertebrae are present. If the fusion extends to the one closest to the curve apex, the additional parallel vertebrae will bend at the end of the fused area.

Lack of appreciation of the sagittal curves of the spine can result in fusion proximally that does not include the whole kyphotic thoracic spine when hyperkyphosis is present. The unfused kyphosis will increase by bending over the top of the fused spine.

Loss of Lumbar Lordosis[7, 10, 14]

Distraction instrumentation in the lumbar spine may lead to flattening of the lumbar lordosis. This loss of lordosis occurs in fusions to the sacrum in which a straight Harrington distraction rod was used. It is often accompanied by a pseudarthrosis in the lumbosacral area, which adds to the deformity. An unappreciated thoracic kyphosis above the fusion also adds to the deformity, increasing the forward stoop. The result is a tilting forward of the whole trunk. The patient attempts to compensate with hyperextension of the hips or by standing with hips and knees flexed (Fig. 18–1). In post poliomyelitis patients with hip flexion contractures or weak hip extensors these compensatory methods are impossible, and the patient leans forward.

Appreciation of this potential complication is important. A lateral view of the spine is essential in all cases of scoliosis so that the spine can be visualized in three dimensions. For fusions extending to the lower lumbar area or sacrum, the normal lumbar lordosis must be maintained. Contouring of the Harrington distraction rod and the use of the special Moe square-ended rod will help maintain lordosis, as will adequate contouring of the Luque system when this is used. Another method for maintaining lordosis is the use of a compression rod on the convexity of the lumbar curve.[4] In addition, the normal lordosis must be created by positioning the patient on the operating table with hips *extended*, not flexed.

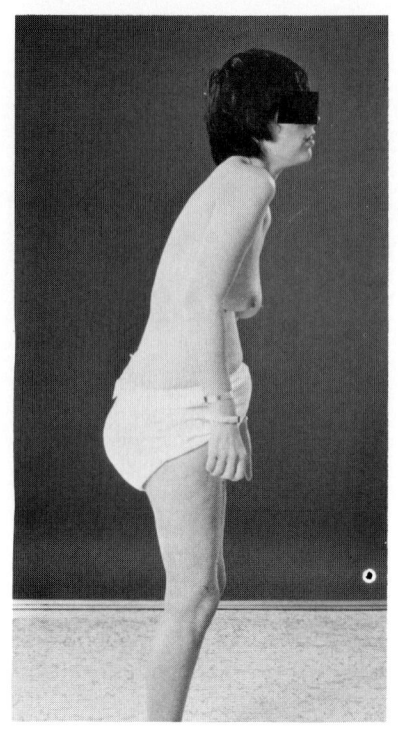

Figure 18–1. Posture of a 36 year old patient with post-polio scoliosis treated two years prior to admission with a fusion from T4 to the sacrum. She felt stooped forward, the stoop increasing in the evening. There was aching that got worse as day progressed. This side view shows the marked forward stooping posture. The knees are bent to allow a more upright posture.

PRESENTING SYMPTOMS

The presenting symptoms are pain, progression of deformity, or dyspnea. These symptoms usually occur in combination, but may occur alone.[1, 2, 8, 10]

Pain

The most common site of pain is in the area of the pseudarthrosis, or below a previous fusion that is too short. The pain is of a mechanical nature; it is relieved by bedrest and aggravated by the upright position, and it increases in intensity the longer the patient is up. The pain tends to be progressive and is often associated with loss of correction and a change in the patient's functional abilities.

A second type of pain is found in patients with loss of lordosis. In the morning the patient is usually pain-free and able to stand erect. As the day progresses a forward stoop develops, which gets worse as the day progresses. This posture is accompanied by an aching muscular fatigue in the back, thighs, and cervical area as the muscles try to maintain an upright position. The pain caused by fatigue is often accompanied by pain due to a lumbosacral pseudarthrosis.

A third type of pain occurs below or above a previous fusion and is due to facet arthrosis or disc degeneration. This problem can often be treated non-operatively, but extension of the fusion is occasionally necessary.

On rare occasions the pain may be radicular in nature. The fibrocartilaginous tissue of the pseudarthrosis or the degenerative changes below a previous fusion can result in localized spinal stenosis and nerve root compression.

Increasing Deformity

The patient may notice an increasing deformity, loss of height, or increasing rotational prominence. Serial radiographs will document the increasing scoliosis or kyphosis; the latter is easily missed if the scoliosis is treated and follow-up lateral views are not taken. It is imperative to compare the current views with the x-rays taken after the surgical procedure. This comparison is invaluable to document the source of increase, for example, increase at a pseudarthrosis, bending of the fusion, bending above or below the fusion, or development of kyphosis.

Dyspnea

Occasionally the presenting complaint is dyspnea, or rarely cardiopulmonary failure, usually occurring in conjunction with progression of deformity. As the curve progresses, there is reduction of cardiopulmonary function and dyspnea. In post poliomyelitis patients with pre-existing intercostal paralysis and pulmonary compromise, any reduction due to the scoliosis is readily appreciated by the patient.

RADIOGRAPHIC EVALUATION

The patient evaluation is the same as that described in Chapter 3. Upright (sitting or standing) posteroanterior and lateral views give an appreciation of the spine deformity in three dimensions. With loss of lordosis or marked lateral decompensation, the patient compensates by standing with one or both knees flexed. The upright radiographs must be taken with the knees extended to adequately represent the deformity without compensation. The area of the fusion and the integrity of the fusion mass are seen with the aid of supine oblique views. Careful inspection of the oblique views will show the presence of a pseudarthrosis.

The flexibility of the unfused portions of the curve is seen on side bending views for scoliosis, a hyperextension view for kyphosis, and a hyperflexion film for lordosis. A derotation view (Stagnara's "plan d'election") is obtained when there is marked rotation.[19] This view defines the vertebral bodies and demonstrates if there is any spontaneous anterior interbody fusion, and whether the disc spaces are of near normal height or narrowed. Early fusions in childhood lead to changes in anterior vertebral growth with loss of disc height as the vertebral endplates grow at the expense of the adjacent disc space. In these patients a persistent wide disc space points to the presence of a pseudarthrosis in that area.

TREATMENT

The treatment plan depends on the problem or problems identified on evaluation of the patient and radiographs. The aim is to obtain a solid, pain-free fusion with the head balanced over the sacrum in both the coronal and sagittal planes. This can be achieved with a single procedure or by a staged correction with fusion mass osteotomies. A one-stage reconstruction is performed when a single problem is present, and it is possible to obtain a balanced spine in one operation (e.g., pseudarthrosis repair alone, extension of fusion alone, or loss of lumbar lordosis). A staged reconstruction is usually necessary to correct multiple problems.

Pseudarthrosis Repair

When only a pseudarthrosis is present with minimal or no loss of correction, a one-stage repair is the planned approach. Often the fusion defect is found in conjunction with a short fusion and marked loss of correction, and in these cases a staged correction is necessary. In cases of persistent pseudarthroses, the addition of an anterior fusion may aid in healing of the pseudarthrosis.

The exposure of the fusion mass is the same in all types of reconstructive surgery. Anesthetic administration and positioning are described in Chapters 10 and 22. The skin incision follows the scar of the previous procedure; the skin scar is excised when it is widened. Infiltration of the subcutaneous tissue is difficult because of the dense tissue present. The incision is deepened by cutting through the scar tissue to the fusion mass. This tissue can be very tough, and bleeding can be excessive. Careful dissection using new sharp scalpels or a cutting electrocautery knife will aid in this procedure. The periosteum is stripped off the fusion using a Cobb periosteal elevator. The periosteum is thick and can usually be easily stripped off the fusion mass except at the pseudarthrosis site. Sharp dissection is used when stripping of the periosteum is difficult.

The fusion mass is exposed completely from its proximal to distal limits and laterally on both sides. Only with this exposure can the integrity of the whole fusion mass be visualized. Normal body landmarks are absent, but the remnants of the previous spinous processes are often present. The transverse processes in the thoracic area and facet joints in the lumbar area give the sides of the fusion mass an irregular contour. Any excessive fibrous tissue is removed using a sharp curette, and any instrumentation is completely removed.

The area of the pseudarthrosis is identified using two clues. The periosteum is adherent in the area of the defect and there is a line of fibrous tissue crossing the fusion mass. The line of fibrous tissue often crosses the fusion obliquely in an irregular serpentine fashion. The pseudarthrosis is usually between two unfused facet joints. The fibrous tissue is removed, the unfused facets exposed, and any remaining articular cartilage removed. It is important to remove all the fibrocartilage of the defect into the depths of the pseudarthrosis; care should be taken since the dura is often adherent to this fibrous tissue.

After complete exposure, instrumentation is inserted. As with fractured long bones, compression aids in healing. Whenever possible two or three parallel compression rods are placed across the defect, with two hooks above and two below. The large 4.8 mm. rods are used whenever possible. If there is loss of correction, a distraction rod is used on the concavity, with one (or two) compression rods added. It is possible to use more than two rods when the fusion mass is wide.

The hooks are inserted into the fusion mass, which, when mature, consists of a thick dorsal cortex and a thin inner cortex with cancellous bone between the cortices. When the fusion mass is thin, the inner cortex is removed and the hook firmly seated around the whole thickness of the fusion.

Once the compression has been applied, the fusion mass is decorticated and local bone, with the addition of autologous iliac bone, placed in this area.

An anterior fusion plays an important role in pseudarthrosis repair. When an adequate previous pseudarthrosis repair has been unsuccessful, an anterior interbody fusion is used in conjunction with the posterior repair. The disc at the level of the pseudarthrosis is removed and the disc space packed with autologous iliac bone. The other role of an anterior fusion is in the low lumbar or lumbosacral pseudarthrosis. There is a solid fusion above and a mobile pelvis below. Because of the difficulty in obtaining a successful result with a posterior approach alone, an anterior interbody fusion increases the success rate. Posteriorly, multiple compression rods are used, the number (3 or 4) depending on the width of the fusion mass. The fusion mass over the sacrum is thick, and the insertion of two hooks on a rod below the pseudarthrosis is usually possible. In some of these problem cases, the use of a body cast with unilateral thigh extension will help immobilize the lumbosacral area postoperatively (Fig. 18-2).

Extension of Fusion

When the previous fusion is to be extended, the fusion mass plus the appropriate proximal or distal spine is exposed. Instrumentation, usually a combination of Harrington compression and distraction rods, is in-

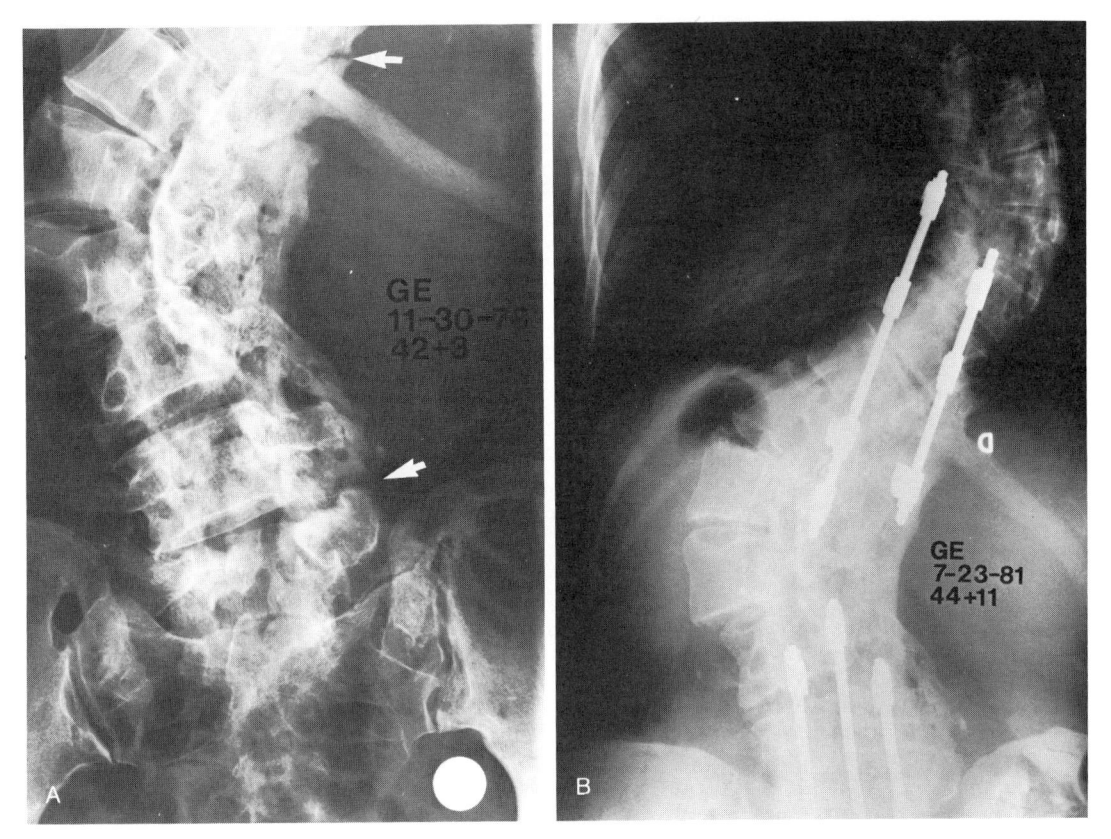

Figure 18–2. A, This 42 year old female with idiopathic scoliosis had a spinal fusion at age 19 and six subsequent procedures, three for pseudoarthrosis repairs and three for re-insertion of hooks. She presented with severe back pain, the pain being in the thoracolumbar and lumbosacral areas. A supine radiograph shows the pseudarthroses at these two areas (arrows). B, She underwent a posterior pseudarthrosis repair with the insertion of multiple large compression rods and the use of local and banked autologous bone. Postoperatively, she was placed in a body cast with a leg extension and ambulated. The cast was changed after four months to one without a leg extension, and the spine was kept immobilized for an additional eight months. Two years postoperatively the fusion is solid and she is completely pain free.

serted. The additional spine is fused in a routine manner with facet excision and packing, decortication, and the addition of local autologous iliac bone. If the fusion is extended to the sacrum, Luque rods with Galveston pelvic fixation are used with a compression rod added centrally to stabilize the lumbosacral area. In these cases in addition, an anterior lumbosacral fusion is performed to help obtain a solid fusion.

Loss of Lumbar Lordosis

This syndrome, as described previously, is frequently accompanied by a pseudarthrosis at the lumbosacral area.[6, 7, 10, 13, 14] This is treated with a posterior closing wedge lumbar osteotomy.[10] The osteotomy is performed in the mid-lumbar area as described in Chapter 10. The osteotomy is fashioned so that a trapezoid of bone is removed, with the apex of the wedge falling in the posterior third of the intervertebral disc. All the deep cortex is removed, and the deep edges of the osteotomy are undercut to prevent pinching of the dura during closure of the osteotomy. Care must be taken at the sides of the osteotomy to adequately undercut the fusion in the area of the nerve roots in order to prevent trapping the nerve as the osteotomy is closed. The edges of the osteotomy are parallel, unless some correction of lateral tilt is also desired, and the osteotomy is wider posteriorly. Two large (4.8 mm.) compression rods are used with the hooks inserted into the fusion mass; two hooks above and two below the osteotomy on each rod is the minimum. If there is a coexisting pseudarthrosis, this is widened, the compression rods cross both the osteotomy and pseudarthrosis, and some additional correction occurs through the pseudarthrosis site. The osteotomy is closed completely so that good bone to bone contact is obtained. The fusion is decorticated and autologous iliac bone added to supplement the local bone graft.

We have found at follow-up that there is often a significant loss of correction following the posterior closing wedge osteotomy. To prevent this, and also to allow adequate correction to occur, we currently perform multiple level anterior interbody releases and fusion. This is usually performed first in the mid-lumbar area with removal of the discs and packing of the disc spaces with autologous iliac bone. If there is a pseudarthrosis, the disc at that level is also fused. Rarely, the posterior procedure is performed first, the interbody fusion being performed at a second stage a week later (Fig. 18-3).

Progressive Rotation

Posterior fusions performed in the juvenile or early adolescent years are sometimes complicated by an increasing rotational deformity in the presence of a solid posterior fusion. This is because continued anterior growth lengthens the anterior aspect of the spine and causes the spine to rotate around the posterior fusion mass. This rotation may be accompanied by bending of the solid posterior fusion with an increasing coronal measurement.

The progressive rotation is treated by eliminating the anterior growth with an anterior interbody fusion, approaching the spine on the side of the convexity of the scoliosis. If there is an accompanying bending of the fusion mass, a second posterior stage is added. The fusion mass is osteotomized at the apex of the deformity, and the osteotomy is stabilized with compression and distraction instrumentation. Bone graft is added to increase the bulk of the posterior fusion mass. If the rib prominence is significant, a thoracoplasty is added to reduce it.

Staged Reconstruction

A staged reconstruction is necessary to treat multiple problems, usually a pseudarthrosis combined with a fusion that is short and has lost correction. The objective is to realign the spine so that it is balanced in the sagittal and coronal planes with the head and thorax aligned over the sacrum. This involves fusion mass osteotomy, usually multiple, combined with extension of the fusion and pseudarthrosis repair. The reconstruction is staged, consisting of anterior and posterior stages or two posterior stages.

The choice of the staging depends on the problems present (i.e., increasing scoliosis, kyphosis, lordosis, the loss of lumbar lordosis, or severe decompensation). Our current choice is the two-stage anterior-posterior approach, with the two-stage posterior approach reserved for special cases. The advantage of the latter approach is that correction is achieved with the patient awake, allowing neurologic monitoring. Intraoperative spinal cord monitoring using the wake-up test with or without electronic monitoring has allowed safe intraoperative osteotomies and correction at one stage.

ANTERIOR-POSTERIOR RECONSTRUCTION

After analyzing the reconstruction problem, the spine is approached anteriorly on the convexity of the scoliosis in the two stage anterior-posterior reconstruction. The disc spaces are often narrow; after the disc is

---

Figure 18-3. A, F. D., a female, had a fusion for low back pain at age 57 and three subsequent procedures for instrumentation dislodgement. She presented at age 58 + 8 with severe incapacitating back pain and the clinical picture of loss of lumbar lordosis. This lateral x-ray shows the loss of lumbar lordosis, with kyphosis extending into the thoracic area. Multiple areas of pseudarthroses in the lumbar area were seen on the supine oblique views. B, She underwent an anterior spinal fusion from T10 to L4, and a week later a posterior pseudarthrosis repair and extension of the fusion to the upper thoracic area were done. Three heavy compression rods were used in the lumbosacral area and two small rods to correct the thoracic area. This x-ray shows the correction of the lateral deformity. C, A year later there was recurrence of the thoracolumbar pain and the stooping posture. The lateral view shows the recurrence of the kyphosis and apical pseudarthrosis (*arrow*). D, The anteroposterior view shows breakage of both small compression rods (*arrows*). E, The pseudarthrosis was repaired with a staged anterior and posterior approach with insertion of large compression rods, two extending from the upper thoracic area to the sacrum and one from the thoracolumbar area to the sacrum. This lateral x-ray shows restoration of the lateral contour. The fusion is now solid, and she is pain free.

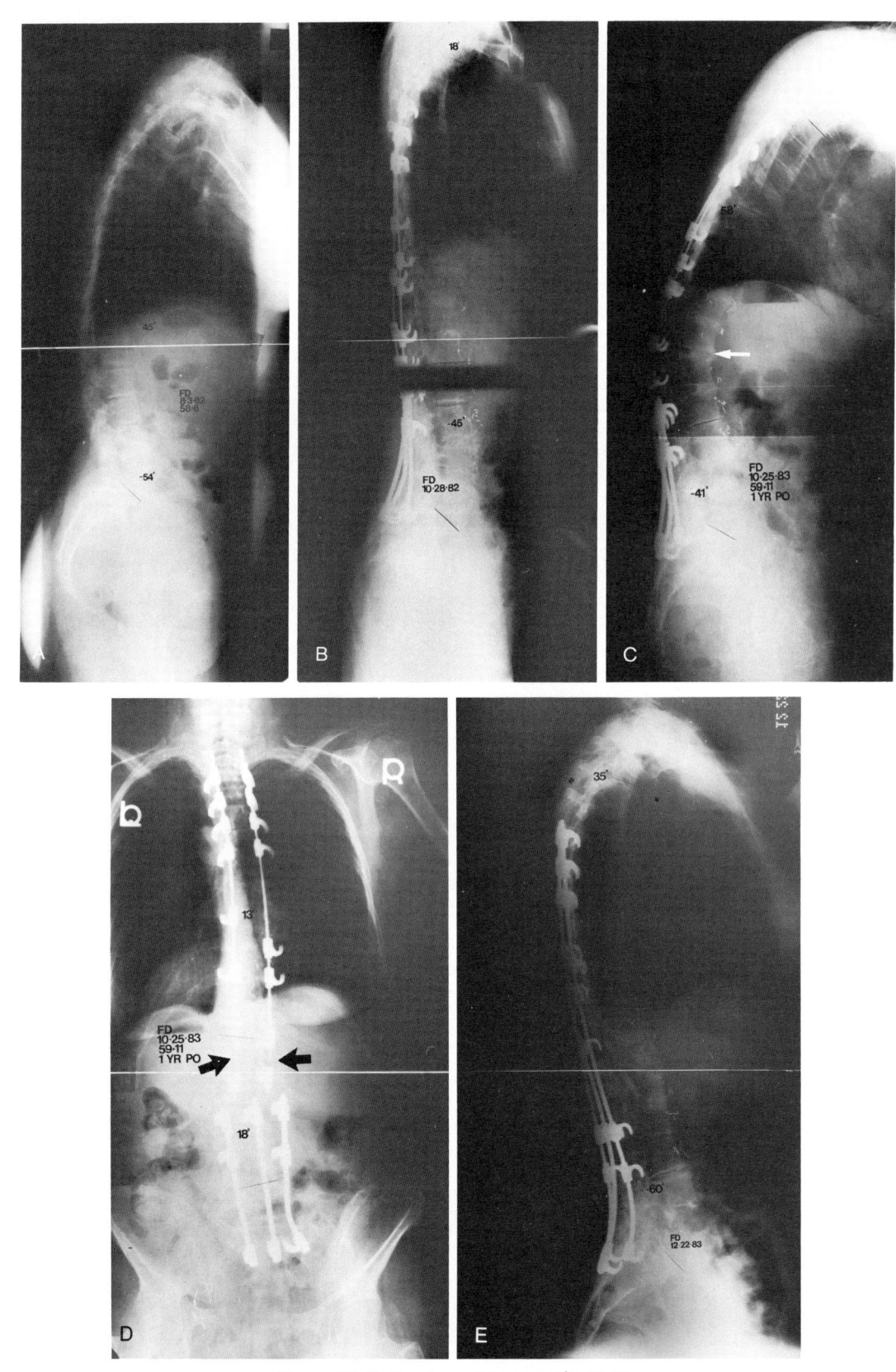

Figure 18–3. *See legend on opposite page*

excised, an additional wedge of endplate is removed to aid in the correction. All the discs in the area of the deformity are removed and endplate and rib bone is packed into the disc spaces for the fusion. In very angular deformities, multiple large wedges at each disc space or an apical vertebrectomy is performed to allow correction. If a pseudarthrosis is present, the disc at that level must be excised and fused. The posterior stage is usually performed a week later.

The spine and any additional vertebrae to be fused are exposed as described before. When a pseudarthrosis is present, it is widened and used as an additional area to gain correction. Osteotomies are performed using the technique described in Chapter 10.[3, 4, 5, 9, 11, 12, 16, 18] The first osteotomy is performed at the apex of the deformity, with additional osteotomies performed at every level or at alternate segments, obtaining good mobility at each level. The indication for the osteotomy will determine the planning of the bone excision. When multiple osteotomies are performed for recorrection of scoliosis, the bone removal is wide on both sides. When kyphosis (true or rotational) is present, the osteotomies are wider posteriorly. With a significant lateral shift of the trunk, the osteotomy is wider on the convexity. The bone must be removed completely from the depths of the osteotomy, and the edges undercut so that no bone can impinge on the dura during correction. When the previous fusion has extended onto the ribs, rib osteotomy or a partial rib resection is necessary to obtain mobility.

If a vertebrectomy has been performed anteriorly, the same wedge of bone is removed posteriorly, ensuring adequate bone removal in the area of the nerve roots. These releases anteriorly and posteriorly have made the spine more mobile and allow correction. Correction and stabilization are now carried out using either the Luque system or a combination of Harrington compression and distraction instrumentation. The Luque system, using the concave technique, is usually performed because it approximates the spine to the instrumentation and prevents distraction. If the Harrington system is used, the compression rod is usually inserted first so that overdistraction is prevented. Neurologic monitoring with repeated wake-up tests if necessary is used to ensure safe correction.

The wires or hooks are passed between the cortices when the fusion mass is thick and strong. With a thin fusion mass, careful placement in the canal is necessary. The facets in any non-fused spine that is added to the fusion area are excised and packed. The spine is decorticated, and the local bone is augmented by autologous iliac bone, which is packed around the osteotomies, pseudarthrosis, and in the area of extension of the fusion. If the iliac bone is insufficient, homologous banked bone is added (Fig. 18–4).

POSTERIOR-POSTERIOR RECONSTRUCTION

In cases in which a two-stage posterior approach is planned, the initial stage is exposure and osteotomies as described before. The excised bone is placed in the distal portion of the wound and is used at the second stage. Clips are placed to mark the area of extension of the fusion so the extent of the exposure can be confirmed on the postoperative x-ray.

Correction is obtained in traction, usually halo gravity (halo wheelchair). The halo is applied while the patient is under the same anesthetic, prior to performing the osteotomies. Weights are gradually added and the patient's neurologic status is carefully monitored. All the correction is obtained in traction, which allows careful spinal cord monitoring during the distraction and correction because the patient is awake. The second-stage procedure stabilizes the spine in the corrected position; no additional correction is usually obtained. If pelvic obliquity is present, halofemoral traction is used with a femoral pin on the high side.

At the second stage, the previous incision is opened and the spine exposed. The spine is stabilized in the corrected position using multiple rods, usually a combination of compression and distraction rods,[15] or the Luque system. The fusion is performed as described above.

When significant kyphosis is present owing to bending of the fusion into kyphosis or bending of the unfused spine over the fusion mass, an anterior fusion is necessary to rebalance the spine; a three-stage procedure is sometimes necessary. At the first stage, posterior osteotomies are performed. A week or two later after a period of hyperextension traction, an anterior release and strut graft fusion is performed to correct and fuse the kyphosis. A week later the spine is instrumented and fused using compression rods;

SALVAGE AND RECONSTRUCTIVE SURGERY 399

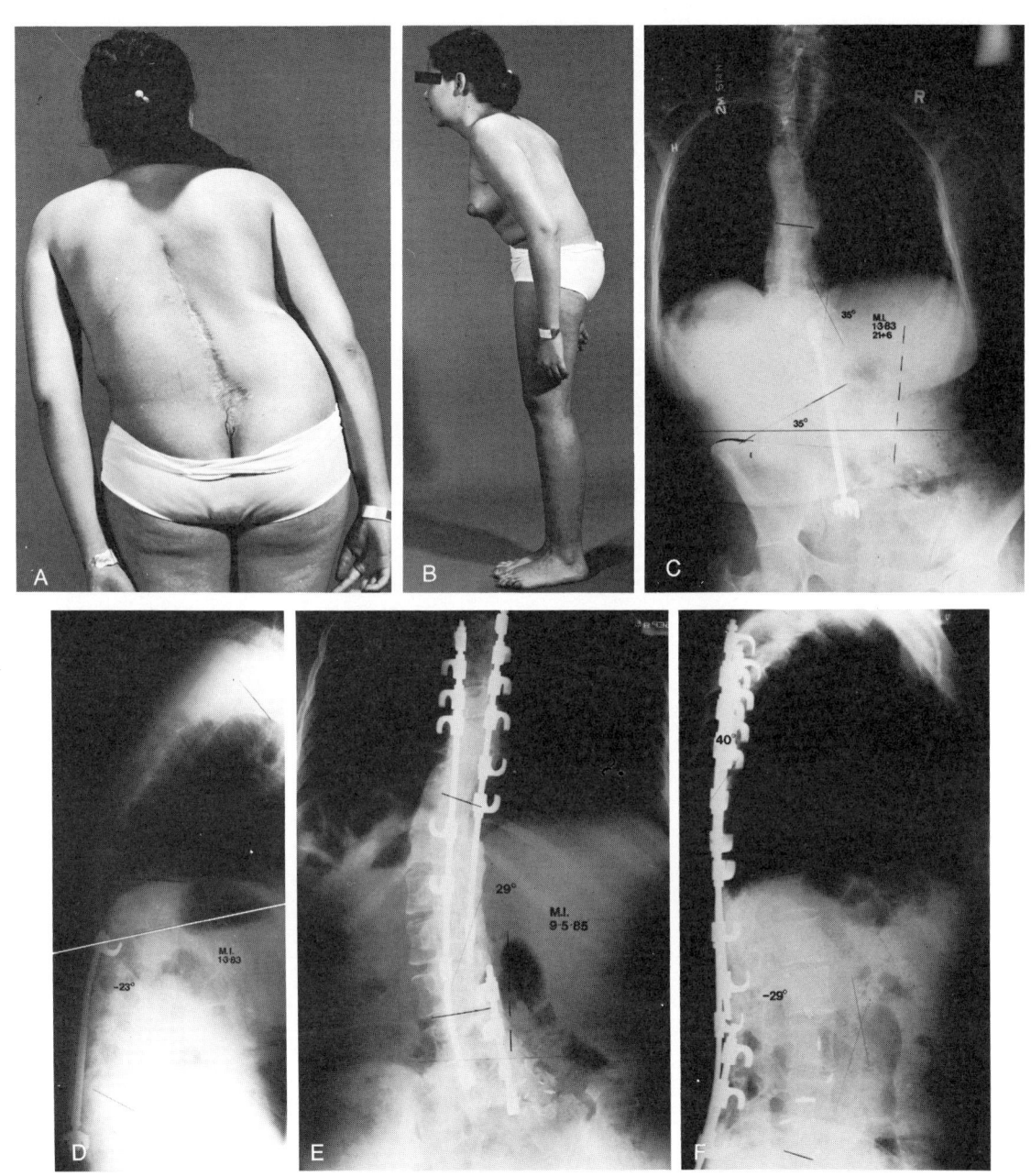

Figure 18–4. M. I., a female with a congenital lumbosacral hemivertebra, had four previous procedures, two for fusion and two for hemivertebra excision in this area. *A* and *B*, She presented at the age of 21+6 with back pain, leaning to the right and a forward stooping posture. *C*, Anteroposterior x-ray showing the marked shift of the trunk to the left due to the lumbosacral hemivertebra on the right. *D*, The flattening of the lumbar lordosis and the forward tilt of the trunk are seen in the lateral x-ray. *E*, The patient underwent an anterior lumbosacral wedge excision and a posterior wedge excision with insertion of large compression rods, the short right lumbosacral rod being inserted first. This anteroposterior view two and a half years postoperatively shows correction of the lateral shift and a solid fusion. *F*, A lateral x-ray shows restoration of the sagittal contour and the solid fusion.

Illustration continued on following page

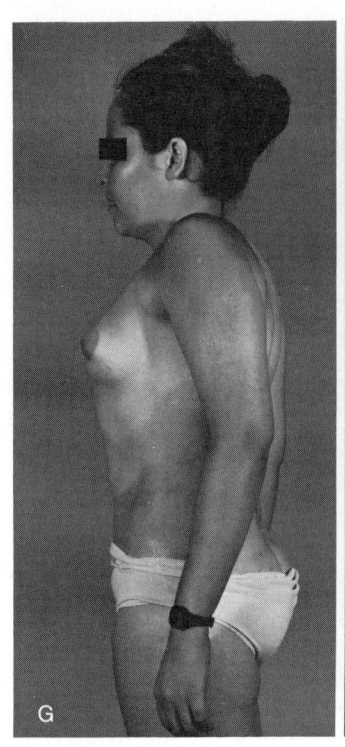

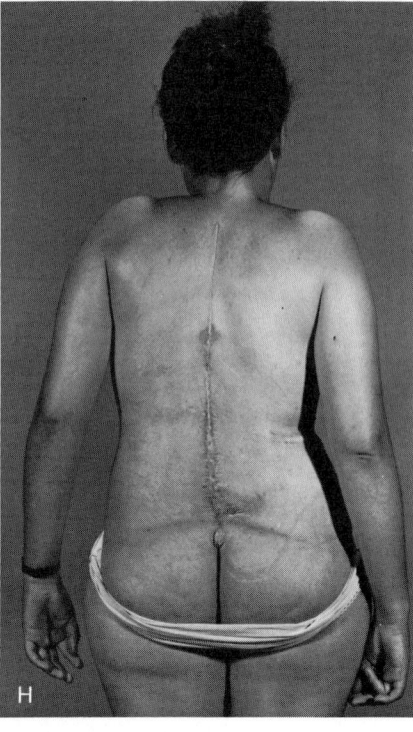

Figure 18–4 *Continued. G, H,* Postoperative clinical photographs show cosmetic improvement.

the larger 4.8 mm. rods are used whenever possible (Fig. 18–5).

IMMOBILIZATION

Four to seven days postoperatively the patient is placed in a one-piece TLSO. If the internal stabilization is secure, ambulation is even allowed prior to fitting of the orthosis. This permits adequate resolution of the postoperative ileus and abdominal distension. A standing mold for the orthosis is taken, which in adults gives a far superior fit. Rarely, in cases of fusions to the upper thoracic area or in which the instrumentation is not secure, a halo cast is used to provide additional stabilization.

Total immobilization time varies and depends on the problem treated and the age of the patient. With a single problem treated or the use of an anterior arthrosis, the fusion is solid in six to nine months. Often the fusion mass is continuous but immature and additional immobilization is necessary for adequate consolidation of the fusion. Here the orthosis is not used at night (usually after five to six months postoperatively) and is only used during the day until the oblique x-rays show a fusion of sufficient maturity with trabeculation.

COMPLICATIONS

The complication rate in these patients is high. A review of adults undergoing reconstructive surgery revealed a total complication rate of 71 per cent.[1] The most frequent complications were pseudarthrosis (17 per cent), wound infection (17 per cent), and wound hematoma (12 per cent). Less frequent complications were urinary tract infections, loss of lumbar lordosis, and pressure sore, all occurring in an incidence of 8 per cent. Changes in technique have reduced many of these complications. The greater use of heavy compression rods and Luque instrumentation combined with anterior fusion all have reduced the pseudarthrosis rate. The routine use of prophylactic antibiotics has reduced the infection rate to 2 per cent.[21] With the recognition of the syndrome of loss of lumbar lordosis, this syndrome as a complication of reconstructive surgery *or* after the initial surgical procedure has become less common.

Figure 18–5. D. C., a female, had Wilms' tumor treated at the age of 10 months with a right nephrectomy and irradiation. She developed a post-irradiation kyphosis and had a posterior fusion at age 11; the procedure was complicated by a wound infection. She presented at age 14 + 4 with marked decompensation to the right and a thoracolumbar kyphosis. *A,* This anteroposterior x-ray shows the decompensation and a 75 degree right thoracic and 76 degree left lumbar curve. *B,* The lateral x-ray shows a T11 to L3 kyphosis of 85 degrees. *C,* She underwent multiple posterior osteotomies of the previous fusion (*arrows*) and was placed in halofemoral traction. This x-ray in traction shows correction of the scoliosis, and the lumbar osteotomies are well seen. *D,* An anterior fusion was performed in the area of kyphosis and a posterior fusion with compression, and distraction Harrington instrumentation was done a week later. This anteroposterior x-ray taken three and a half years postoperatively shows a solid fusion with correction of the scoliosis to 31 degrees and 35 degrees. *E,* The lateral x-ray shows correction of the kyphosis to 34 degrees. A solid anterior fusion is well demonstrated.

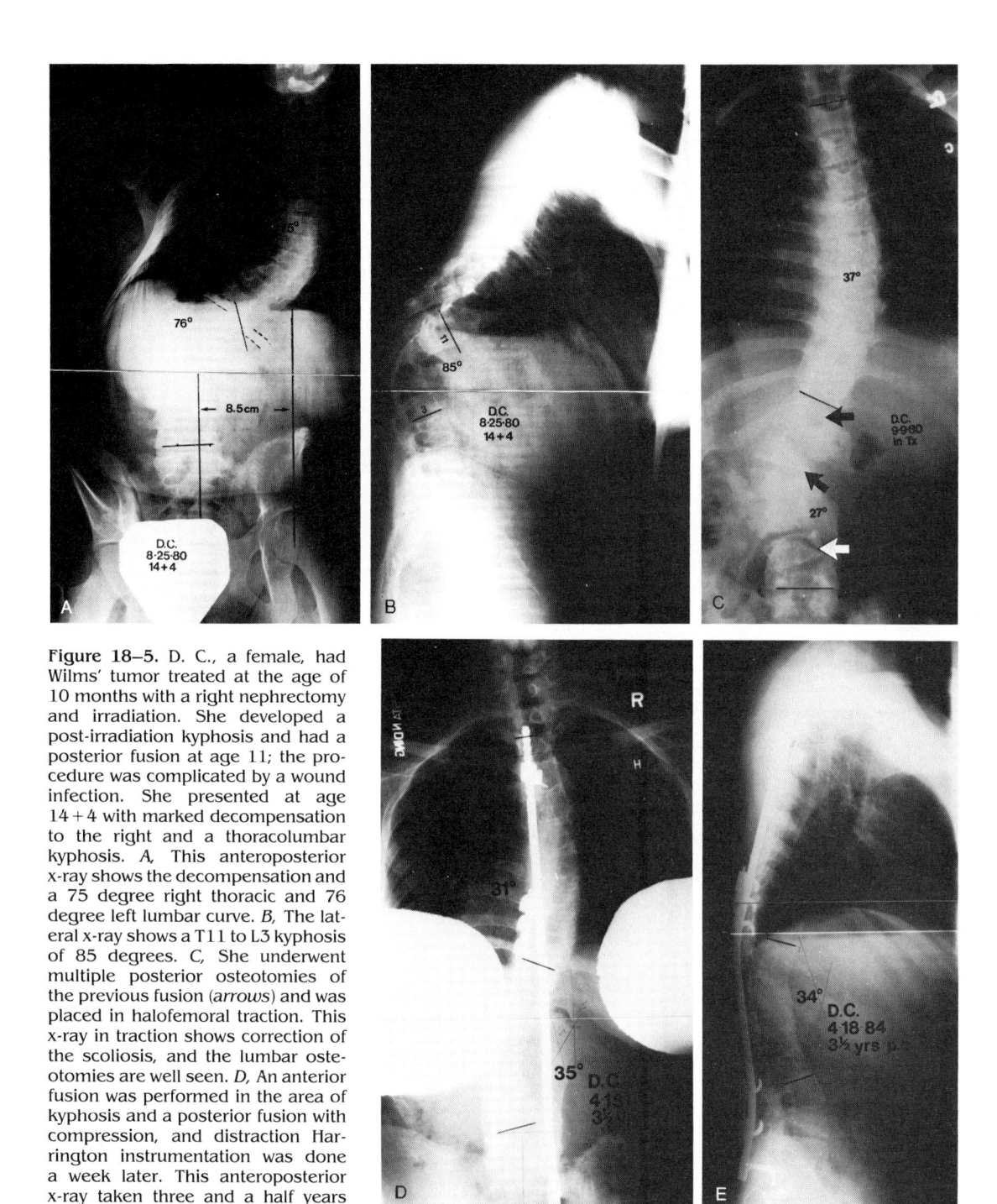

SUMMARY

Reconstructive spinal surgery is becoming more common as a large number of patients undergo spinal fusion. Pseudarthrosis, loss of correction, adding on, and loss of lordosis are the most common presenting problems. Appreciation of the deformity in three dimensions is essential for the evaluation of the spine and to enable formation of a successful surgical plan.

References

1. Cummine, J. L., Lonstein, J. E., and Moe, J. H. et al.: Reconstructive surgery in the adult for failed scoliosis fusion. J. Bone Joint Surg., *61A*: 1151–1161, 1979.
2. Dawson, E. G., Moe, J. H., and Caron, A.: Surgical management of scoliosis in the adult. Scoliosis J. Bone Joint Surg., *55A*:437, 1973.
3. Doherty, J.: Complications of fusion in lumbar scoliosis. Presented at the annual meeting of the Scoliosis Research Society, Wilmington, Delaware, 1972.
4. Floman, Y., Penny, J., Micheli, L., et al.: Osteotomy of the fusion mass in scoliosis. J. Bone Joint Surg., *64A*:1307–1316, 1982.
5. Gaines, R. W., and Leatherman, K. D.: Benefits of the Harrington compression system in lumbar and thoracolumbar idiopathic scoliosis in adolescents and adults. Spine, *6*:483–488, 1981.
6. Herbert, J. J.: Vertebral osteotomy. Technique, indications and results. J. Bone Joint Surg., *30A*:680–689, 1948.
7. Kostuik, J.: Halo-pelvic traction in the surgical management of adult scoliosis. J. Bone Joint Surg., *55B*:232, 1973.
8. Kostuik, J. P., and Gross, M.: Correction of iatrogenic lumbar kyphosis—flat back syndrome. Orthop. Trans., *6*:27, 1982.
9. Kostuik, J. P., Israel, J., and Hall, J. E.: Scoliosis surgery in adults. Clin. Orthop., *93*:225–234, 1973.
10. Law, W. A.: Osteotomy of the spine. J. Bone Joint Surg., *44A*:1199–1206, 1962.
11. Lonstein, J. E.: Reconstructive surgery for spinal deformities. Orthop. Clin. North Am., *10*:905–917, 1979.
12. Meiss, W. C.: Spinal osteotomy following fusion for paralytic scoliosis. J. Bone Joint Surg., *37A*:73–77, 1955.
13. Moe, J. H., and Denis, F.: Iatrogenic loss of lumbar lordosis. Orthop. Trans., *1*:131, 1977.
14. Moe, J., and Welch, J. A.: Post fusion spinal osteotomy. Presented at Gillette Children's Hospital, December 18, 1971.
15. Pellin, B., and Zielke, K.: Scolioses severes de l'adulte et du grand adolescent—41 cas operes. Rev. Chir. Orthop., *60*:623–633, 1974.
16. Ponder, R. C., Dickson, J. H., Harrington, P. R., and Erwin, W. D.: Results of Harrington instrumentation and spinal fusion in the adult idiopathic scoliosis patient. Presented to the Am. Acad. Orthop. Surg., San Francisco, March, 1975.
17. Ponder, R. C., Dickson, J. H., Harrington, P. R., and Erwin, W. D.: Results of Harrington instrumentation and fusion in the adult scoliosis patient. J. Bone Joint Surg., *57A*:797–801, 1975.
18. Schmidt, A. C.: Osteotomy of the fused scoliotic spine and use of halo traction apparatus. *In* Symposium on the Spine. St. Louis, C. V. Mosby Co., pp. 265–282, 1969.
19. Smith-Peterson, M. N., Larson, C. B., and Aufrand, O. E.: Osteotomy of the spine for correction of flexion deformity in rheumatoid arthritis. J. Bone Joint Surg., *27*:1-11, 1945.
20. Stagnara, P., Fleury, D., Fauchet, R., et al.: Scolioses majeures de l'adulte superieures a 100–183 cas traites chirurgicalement. Rev. Chir. Orthop., *61*:101–122, 1975.
21. Transfeldt, E., Lonstein, J. E., Winter, R. B., et al.: Infection in spine fusions. Orthop. Trans., *9*:128–129, 1985.
22. Von Lackum, W. H., and Smith, A.: Removal of vertebral bodies in the treatment of scoliosis. Surg. Gynecol. Obstet., *57*:250, 1933.

19

SPONDYLOLYSIS AND SPONDYLOLISTHESIS

David S. Bradford, M.D.

Spondylolisthesis is defined as a slipping forward of one vertebra on another; the origin of the word is from the Greek derivatives "spondylos" meaning vertebra and "olisthesis" meaning to slip. Herbiniaux, a Belgian obstetrician, is credited with first describing this condition.[59] In 1782, he reported a complete dislocation of the L5 vertebral body in front of the sacrum with narrowing of the birth canal and resultant problems in delivery. Kilian,[71] in 1854, coined the term spondylolisthesis and proposed that the slippage occurred gradually, secondary to body weight and subluxation of the lumbosacral facets.

In 1855, Robert[177] reported on anatomic studies involving the neural arch. By removing all soft tissue from the lumbosacral junction, he demonstrated that the vertebra would not sublux as long as the arch was intact. After a defect was made, the vertebra was free to sublux. In 1858, Lambl[76] proved the existence of a neural arch defect in cadaver specimens. The fact that these defects were not always found in anatomic specimens was resolved by Neugebauer's scholarly work published in 1888.[102] He concluded that spondylolisthesis might arise from a lysis of the pars interarticularis or from elongation of the neural arch.

It is actually only in the last 20 years that attention has again focused on the various etiologic considerations in spondylolisthesis and that a workable classification has been established.[103, 105, 157]

CLASSIFICATION (Fig. 19–1)

One of the more useful classifications of spondylolysis and spondylolisthesis appears to be that compiled by Wiltse, Newman, and Macnab.[157]

Type 1. *Dysplastic*. A congenital deficiency of the superior sacral facet or the arch of L5 that allows a forward slippage of L5 on S1 to occur.

Type 2. *Isthmic*. The lesion is located in the pars interarticularis, permitting L5 forward slippage on S1 with the inferior lumbar and superior sacral facet maintaining a normal relationship.

1. A lytic fracture of the pars (stress fracture)
2. An elongated but intact pars interarticularis
3. An acute pars fracture

Type 3. *Degenerative*. Secondary to long-standing degenerative arthritis and intersegmental instability of the facet joints[106] as well as disc degeneration.

Type 4. *Traumatic*. Acute fracture in areas other than the pars interarticularis, for example, pedicle, laminae, or facet.

Type 5. *Pathologic*. Attenuation of the pedicle secondary to generalized bone disease, for example, osteogenesis imperfecta, Paget's disease, and so forth.

For the purpose of this chapter, discussion will be focused primarily on the isthmic, dysplastic, and degenerative types. It should be well recognized and appreciated that the symptom complex and natural history of spondylolisthesis in children and adults is different[25, 53, 58, 79, 103] as is the response to treatment.[51]

ETIOLOGY

The etiology of the majority of cases of spondylolysis and spondylolisthesis remains

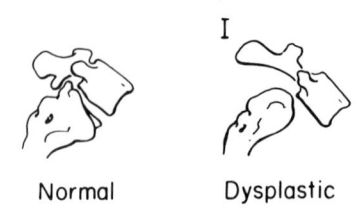

Spondylolisthesis

Figure 19–1. Classification of spondylolisthesis.

I Normal
Dysplastic
II-A Break in pars interarticularis
II-B Elongated but intact pars
II-C Acute fracture
III Degenerative
IV Fracture other than pars
V Pathological

confusing and arbitrary. The current concepts have focused on congenital and traumatic etiologies but it is well known that no patient has yet been identified at birth with spondylolisthesis or spondylolysis and that it is not uncommon for a patient to present with back pain and spondylolysis without any history or antecedent trauma. Furthermore, x-ray evaluation in cases with more severe degrees of slippage may show a combination of pathologies, for example, a pars elongation with lysis. Does this represent Type 1 dysplastic (congenital) with lysis or Type 2 lysis with elongated pars? To explain these apparent discrepancies a brief review of the studies and work published to date might prove helpful.

Incidence

The incidence of spondylolysis in adult caucasian males is reported to be 5 to 6 per cent.[124] In females it is reported to be 2 to 3 per cent.[3] The incidence varies between races; in Eskimos it is reported to be 50 per cent[70, 138] and in blacks, less than 3 per cent.[124]

Growth

That growth and age may indeed play some role is suggested by the finding that spondylolisthesis rarely occurs in children before age five and more commonly occurs between the ages of seven to ten years.[3, 124, 154, 156] Borokow and Kleiger described the case of a four month old, the youngest patient reported.[8] Several other children younger than five years have been reported in a recent review by Wertzberger and Peterson, but spondylolisthesis in young children is indeed rare.[151] The incidence increases with age until approximately 20, then appears to remain the same as the general population.[3, 75, 77, 81, 151–154, 158]

Trauma

Trauma has been suggested by many authors to be instrumental in producing a pars defect. Hitchcock[60] was able to produce neural arch defects in dissected fetal specimens by hyperflexion. However, Rowe and Roche were unable to reproduce Hitchcock's results even with vigorous flexion and extension.[124] It is well known that a specific antecedent traumatic event is difficult to ascertain in many cases and if a history of trauma is elicited, the injury rarely would be classified as severe.[9, 25, 58, 89, 144] The onset of symptoms appears to coincide with the adolescent growth spurt and an increased level of physical activity.[5, 57-59, 144] Wiltse[158] has felt that spondylolysis represents a "stress" or fatigue fracture; although a severe traumatic episode can lead to an acute fracture,[73] repeated stress is the usual mechanism of injury. Athletes appear to have a higher incidence of spondylolysis,[64] especially gymnasts,[47, 66] new Army recruits or soldiers performing exercises to which they are unaccustomed,[158] weight lifters,[12] and college football linemen.[36] On the other hand, spondylolysis or spondylolisthesis does not appear to occur in adults who have never walked or in animals other than man.[122, 129, 155]

Hereditary Factors

It has been noted by many authors that spondylolisthesis frequently occurs in members of the same family.[41, 109, 161] Shahriaree and Harkness have described a family of four with spondylolisthesis.[131] Fraternal[6] and identical twins[142, 150] with spondylolisthesis have been reported. The incidence in near relatives has ranged from 27 to 69 per cent versus the expected range of 4 to 8 per cent in the general population.[41, 56, 70, 79] Wynne-Davies and Scott in a recent radiographic survey have noted that patients with dysplastic lesions had a higher proportion of affected relatives (33 per cent) than those with isthmic type lesions (15 per cent).[160] Sacral spina bifida is more common in individuals with spondylolysis (28 to 42 per cent) as is deficient development of the proximal sacrum and superior facets.[25, 160] Posterior arch defects at L5 and S1 have been reported in 94 per cent of dysplastic cases, and they are more common in isthmic cases (32 per cent) than in the general population.[24, 160]

Biomechanical Considerations

Biomechanical considerations are of great importance in explaining the development of pars defects and their progression. The presence of a lumbar lordosis and upright posture in man and not other species has been felt relevant in explaining the presence of the defect in man only.[122, 153, 155] Under stress analysis with polarized light, the greatest stress concentration occurs at the pars interarticularis.[111, 128] Marked lordosis and rotational stresses have been suggested recently by Neithard as having etiologic importance.[101] He noted that patients with Scheuermann's disease have a higher incidence of spondylolisthesis or spondylolysis, and an increase in lordotic angle is associated with a higher incidence of spondylolysis. Farfan[35] has described the three mechanisms that may result in failure of the neural arch with or without vertebral body displacement: flexion overload, unbalanced shear forces, and forced rotation with flexion. Troup[143] felt that a combination of fatigue-failure and high strain rate of forces induced in the extended position was the most likely cause of the defect. This has also been supported from work by Munster.[98]

Although it is apparent that the etiology may easily be considered multifactorial, a congenital predisposition on a hereditary basis associated with repeated stress to the pars interarticularis has received the most support in the literature.[97] The term "congenital" has now been replaced by dysplastic in order to include those cases that have a "congenital" predisposition to develop a slippage as noted by abnormalities in the lumbosacral articulation. Although a higher incidence of spina bifida occulta is noted in these dysplastic cases, one must appreciate that dysplastic Type 1 is a diagnosis made after the fact and that the associated sacral facet abnormalities may be developmental and secondary to altered mechanics brought about by L5-S1 slippage in a growing spine. In this case, therefore, the differentiation between Type 1 dysplastic with lysis in the pars and Type 2 elongation with lysis is of academic interest only and could in effect be more of a manifestation of the age at which slippage first occurred. This could explain the "dysplastic" type predisposition to be associated with a greater degree of slippage, and to the greater likelihood of this group requiring surgical stabilization. On the other hand, those patients presenting with pure isthmic spondylolisthesis without evidence of elongation or sacral dysplasia are extremely unlikely to show further progression during growth. In the recent report by Fredrickson and coworkers, only seven of their 30 patients followed from childhood through the completion of growth showed any increase in the percentage of slippage, and all of these were less than 30 per cent.[39] No patient in this series developed spondylolisthesis. It is important to note, however, that in this series standing x-rays were not taken and this could prejudice the results in terms of magnitude of progression.

CLINICAL FINDINGS

Spondylolysis and spondylolisthesis present different problems for the child and for the adult. Symptoms are relatively uncommon in children. In LaFond's series, 23 per cent or 415 patients with spondylolisthesis or spondylolysis had the onset of complaints before age 20 but only 9 per cent had sought medical attention during childhood or adolescence.[75] The onset of complaints when they do occur is usually during the adolescent growth spurt.[10, 57, 58]

If children do present with pain, two types of patterns emerge. One, usually associated with spondylolysis or mild degrees of slippage, is described as mild low back pain or aching, occasionally radiating into the buttocks and thighs. The discomfort is related to a high activity level or competitive sports. The symptoms will usually decrease with restriction of activities.[56, 93] The pain in the back is often secondary to instability of the affected segment. Disc herniation is uncommon. The second type of pain is localized to the back with a significant radicular component to the posterior thighs. Pain radiating to the foot or calf is rarely felt.[57, 58] Back and radicular pain is more often, in my experience, associated with high degrees of slippage (grade 3 to 4).[12, 14, 15]

The magnitude of the pain cannot always be correlated with the severity of the deformity.[85] Patients presenting with grade 4 spondylolisthesis may be asymptomatic even though their posture is markedly distorted. The back pain, as mentioned, may be secondary to mechanical instability, whereas the radicular pain may arise from foraminal stenosis at the site of the pars defect, fibrocartilaginous callus that is found at the fractured pars site,[97] sacral root compression at the dome of the sacrum secondary to L5 forward displacement, or hypertrophy of the ligamentum flavum and associated disc herniation.[1, 70, 87, 140]

The physical findings may correlate to some extent with the degree of slippage (Fig. 19–2). If the child has a minimal slip, grade 1 to 2, and few if any symptoms, little restriction of motion may be apparent and the gait is essentially normal. With more significant slippage, a visible and palpable step-off at the lumbosacral junction will be readily noticeable. There may be some splinting and guarding with restricted motion of the lumbar spine and hamstring tightness as noted by the patient's inability to flex the hips with the knees fully extended.[3, 10, 105, 132] Paraspinal spasm with trunk deviation on forward bending is common. With progressive and continuous slippage, compensating mechanisms are brought into play and produce significant deformity.[55] For instance, as L5 begins to slip further forward it leaves the lamina, spinous processes, and inferior articular facet behind. The body's center of gravity is displaced anteriorly, and to compensate for this marked displacement, the lumbar spine above the lesion becomes hyperextended and the upper part of the trunk is thrown backward. This creates, in effect, a lordosis extending into the upper thoracic spine. As the slippage becomes greater and the kyphosis increased at the lumbosacral joint, the pelvis becomes more retroverted or rotated about its transverse axis so that the sacrum becomes vertical. One can see this more clearly by noting that the anterior superior spine rises to the same level or even becomes higher than the posterior superior spine. The buttocks appear "heart-shaped" secondary to the sacral prominence. The hip joint rotates with the tilted pelvis until the thigh, even in the extreme degree of full extension, is unable to place the knee joint vertically underneath the trunk. The patient can do so only by allowing the upper trunk to tilt forward to an extreme degree. To maintain an upright posture, on the other hand, the patient must stand with the knees partially flexed and the thoracic and upper lumbar spine in a hyperlordotic posture. As the slip becomes even greater, the trunk is severely shortened, so there is complete absence of the waistline and the rib cage abuts on the iliac crest. It is useful to think of this extreme degree of deformity as a kyphosis of the lumbosacral articulation.[125, 126]

The abnormal gait in these patients can be explained by two factors: (1) hamstring tightness, the so-called Phalen-Dixon sign (Fig. 19–3)[110] and (2) lumbosacral kyphosis.

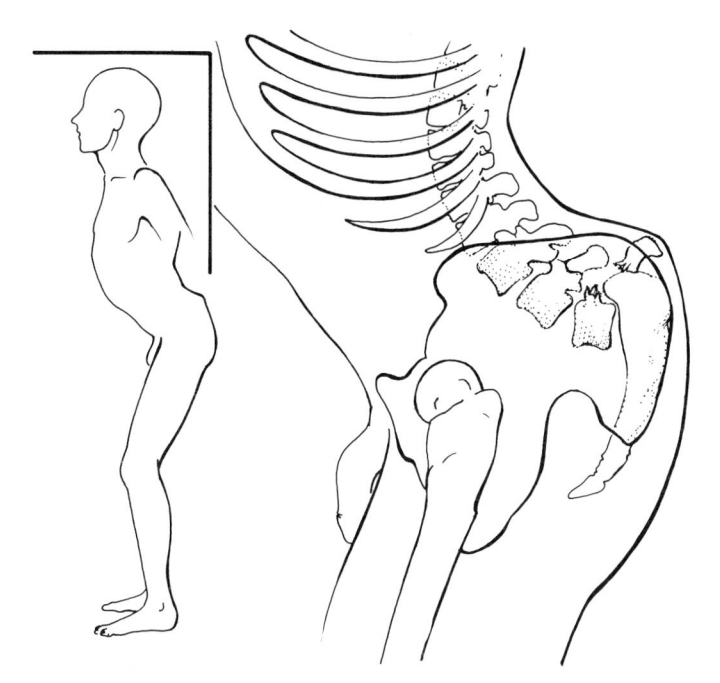

Figure 19–2. The characteristic posture of a patient with spondyloptosis or a high degree of slippage. (Redrawn from Harris, R. J.: Spondylolisthesis. Ann. R. Coll. Surg. Engl., 8:259, 1951.)

Hamstring tightness may vary between patients, and the severity does not necessarily appear to be related to the magnitude of the deformity. It is thought by some to be a sign of nerve root irritation;[144] however, there is no evidence to support this contention.[3, 110] Hamstring tightness is not necessarily accompanied by neurologic signs, and its mechanism is not well understood.[3, 10, 58] It may, however, be associated with a very bizarre gait pattern, the Phalen-Dixon sign, which may or may not be associated with pain and may indeed be the primary reason for the patient's referral to the orthopaedic surgeon. The gait pattern is described as a pelvic waddle by Newman;[105] it is associated with a rather stiff-legged, short-strided gait similar to a child walking in a humped position. In more significant degrees of spondylolisthesis, grades 4 and 5, associated with marked increase in lumbosacral kyphosis, the abnormal gait pattern may be related to the altered pelvic orientation and anatomy from the extreme degree of slippage.[11, 12, 55]

Neurologic evaluation may reveal motor, sensory, or reflex changes. Turner and Bianco[144] reported only four of their 173 pediatric patients demonstrated a neurologic deficit. In our experience, in patients who demonstrated a 50 per cent slippage or greater, 35 per cent demonstrated neurologic abnormalities.[10]

Scoliosis may be associated with spondylolisthesis.[9, 10, 37, 58, 79] Generally, it is not a structural curve, and in our experience and that reported by Hensinger[58] and Risser,[116] the curvature resolves with recumbency and/or the relief of symptoms. Occasionally the curvature will become structural and require treatment.[11, 14, 87] Tojner has described an olisthetic scoliosis that is characterized as a minimal lateral curvature, but the lumbar spine may show significant rotation.[141] Spondylolysis and spina bifida appear to occur with the same frequency in patients with scoliosis as in the general population.[37]

RADIOGRAPHIC FINDINGS
(Fig. 19–4)

Routine X-rays

Radiographic evaluation of the lumbosacral spine in children suspected of having pathology should include anteroposterior, lateral, and oblique x-rays. If there is spondylolisthesis, a routine lateral x-ray will show the defect, but if there is spondylolysis only, the pars defect can best be seen with oblique x-rays. It is important to remember that unilateral defects may occur in 20 per cent of patients, making the visualization quite difficult without adequate x-rays.[29, 74, 99, 112, 143] teoma will show increased uptake as will the reactive sclerosis of an impending stress fracture of the pars interarticularis.[43]

As the slippage progresses, it will be possible to see the pathology and make a diagnosis on a routine lateral x-ray. The oblique x-rays will show the defect in the pars interarticularis, an elongation of the pars interarticularis, or a defect with elongation. With slippage greater than 25 to 30 per cent, elongation of the pars or lysis of the pars must occur, otherwise cauda equina paralysis will result.[157]

In calculating as accurately as possible the magnitude of the deformity in cases of spondylolisthesis, it is important to establish reproducible techniques for evaluating patients over a period of time. From a review of the literature, it is apparent that there are numerous methods for measuring the deformity associated with spondylolisthesis[10, 25, 79, 92, 105, 139] and that no one technique is entirely satisfactory. It is important, however, to stress that x-rays should be taken in a standing position, since significant variations in magnitude of deformity not only in percentage of slippage but also in slip angle may be seen between standing and supine x-rays.[83]

Deformity results from translational or tangential displacement of L5 on S1 (percentage of slippage) as well as angular displacement of L5 on S1, which is referred to as a lumbosacral kyphosis. These two measurements have proven to be extremely helpful in following a patient with spondylolisthesis and in determining the natural history and the results of treatment (Fig. 19–5).

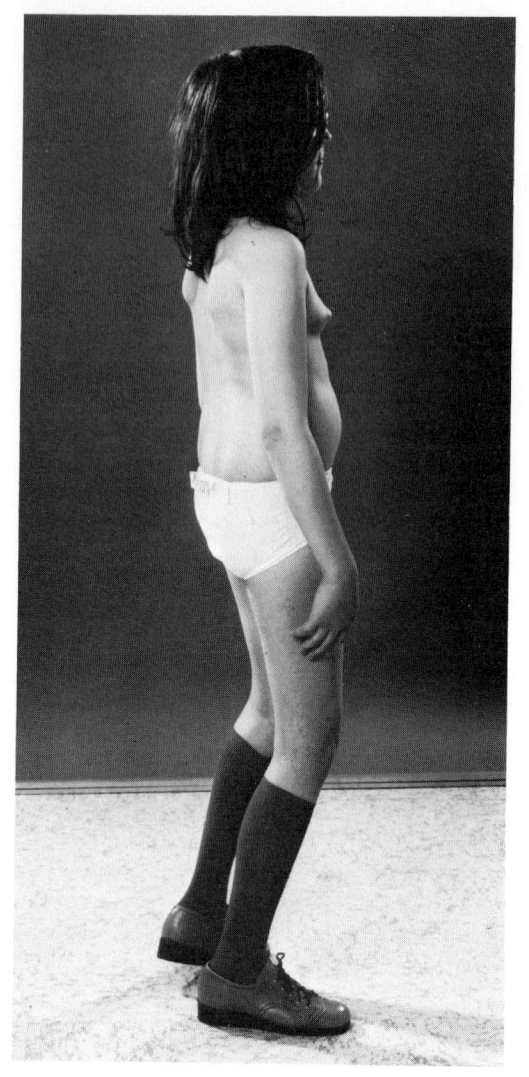

Figure 19–3. A patient with spondyloptosis with the characteristic posture and tight hamstrings, producing the so-called Phalen-Dixon sign on ambulation.

Spondylolysis should be suspected clinically if there is asymmetry of the neural arch and unilateral wedging of the vertebral body. Sclerosis of the opposite pars interarticularis or lamina may facilitate the diagnosis. If a defect is suspected but cannot be confirmed, oblique tomograms or a radioactive bone scan have proven very useful in our experience. Sherman and associates[133] have also noticed the presence of unilateral spondylolysis with reactive sclerosis on the other side. Radiographically this may be confused with an osteoid osteoma. Tomography or CT scanning may be of benefit in these cases.[88] A bone scan will not differentiate these, because the reactive nidus of an osteoid os-

Translational or Tangential Displacement (Percentage of Slippage)

Meyerding[92] described a grading system for classifying the percentage of slippage. In this system Grade 1 is slippage of 0 to 25 per cent, Grade 2 is slippage of 25 to 50 per cent, Grade 3 is slippage of 50 to 75 per cent, and Grade 4 is slippage greater than 75 per cent.

Taillard[139] measured the displacement of the olisthetic vertebra over the sacrum and expressed this result as a percentage. We use a similar technique with a slight modification. A line is drawn along the posterior aspect of the body of the first sacral vertebra for reference. This is a consistent reproducible line and serves as a reference point for all future

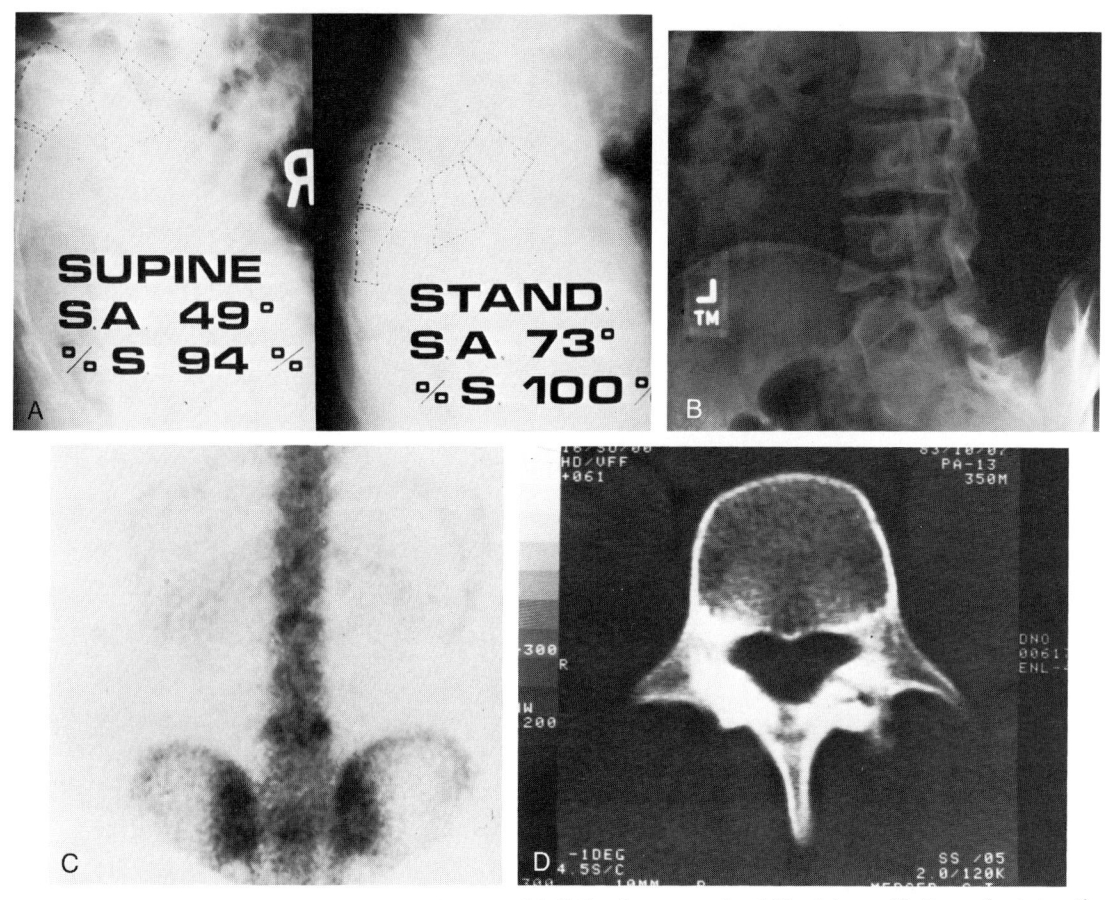

Figure 19–4. A, In evaluating the patient with spondylolisthesis, x-rays should be taken with the patient standing. Otherwise, the true magnitude of slip angle may not be apparent. B, Oblique x-rays are most helpful in demonstrating the defect. C, Tomography may demonstrate unilateral increased bone activity, which may be confused with the radiographic findings of an osteoid osteoma. D, A CT scan may help confirm the presence of a unilateral defect and an impending stress fracture of the opposite pars, which will demonstrate a hot spot on the bone scan (CT scan courtesy of William Carr, M.D.).

measurements. The width of the sacrum is calculated at its widest dimension to give the denominator. A perpendicular line from the posterior inferior cortex of L5 is drawn; the amount of displacement in comparison to sacral width gives the percentage of slippage.

Slip angle or the angle of lumbosacral kyphosis is calculated by first drawing a line perpendicular to the reference line and then drawing a second line parallel to the endplate of the L5 vertebral body. One may use the upper or the lower endplate. The upper plate will not reflect the true magnitude of slip angle in cases of spondylolisthesis in which the vertebral body is juxtapositioned against the anterior sacrum. On the other hand, the lower plate line may become distorted or difficult to visualize following arthrodesis. I favor using the lower endplate, whereas some of the other members of our group use the upper. Again, this calculation must be made from an x-ray taken with the patient standing. Normally, the slip angle should be 0 degrees or less.

Sacral inclination is calculated, again on the standing x-ray, by a line drawn perpendicular to the floor and the angle formed from this line to the reference line along the posterior sacral vertebra. Based on experience alone, we feel the sacral inclination angle should be greater than 30 degrees. Lumbar lordosis is calculated on the angle formed from a line parallel to the upper or lower endplate of L5 and the uppermost lumbar or lower thoracic vertebra maximally tilted into the lordotic curvature.

The S1 contour of the sacrum is noted, although it is not measured. Reproducible

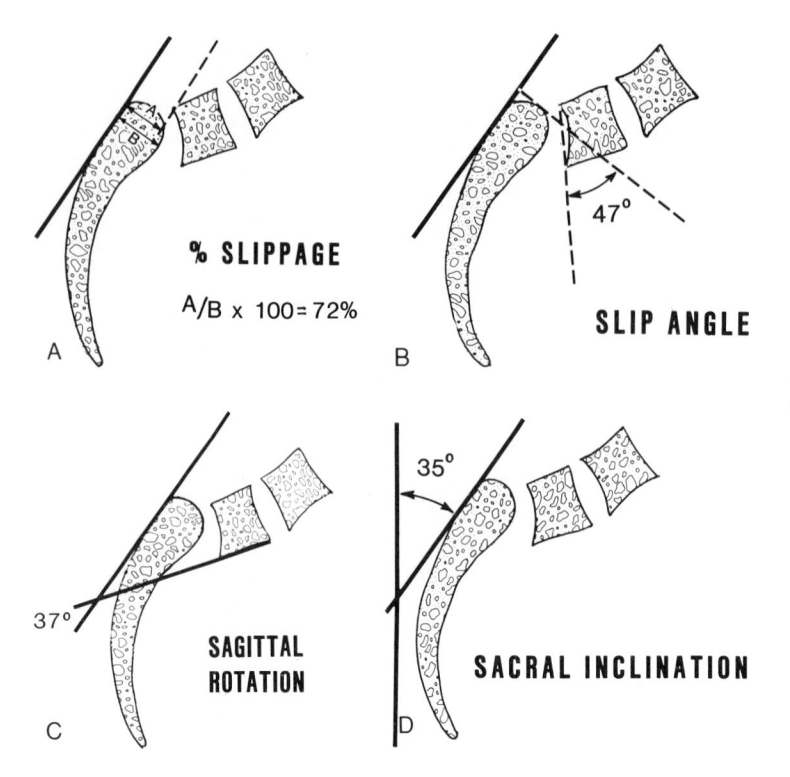

Figure 19–5. Techniques of measuring translational or tangential displacement (see text for details).

measurements are difficult. Similarly, the lumbar index is no longer used as it has not been found to be as important in prognosis as the percentage of slip or slip angle in my experience.

Stress X-rays

Supine hyperextension or hyperflexion x-rays are quite useful in determining mobility of the lumbosacral slippage. Traction x-rays in a hyperextension traction frame likewise are useful to determine the mobility of L5 on S1.

Myelographic Evaluation. Routine myelography on children presenting with symptomatic spondylolysis is generally not necessary.[10, 11, 14, 58, 154, 156] Even in patients presenting with mild degrees of spondylolisthesis in the absence of neurologic findings, we have not recommended routine myelography. Disc protrusion in these patients is extremely uncommon.[78] Bosworth[9] and Adkins[1] have each reported two cases of disc protrusion in their series, and Meyerding[91] reported seven prolapses in 143 operative cases (5.5 per cent). The incidence ranges from 0 to 6 per cent. Disc protrusion, therefore, may be the reason for sciatica in spondylolisthesis, but it is rare.[1, 9, 46] Certainly, one could not argue about performing routine myelography on patients with spondylolisthesis. Myelography can rule out other causes of back pain in children and adolescents, especially tumors. It would appear advisable in cases in which the pain is inconsistent or out of proportion to the radiographic manifestations of the defect, if neurologic signs or symptoms are present, or if sciatica dominates the patient's presenting complaint.[78, 160] Finally, if reduction is planned, we favor myelography.

CT scanning for suspected spondylolysis that is not well visualized on routine x-rays has proven very useful. This has recently been noted by Grogan and coworkers,[49] who have described various abnormalities present in an intact pars, which they feel may represent variants or stages in the development or healing of pars defects. McAfee and Yuan have felt that CT scans may be useful in determining which cases would warrant decompression in addition to fusion. As they noted, myelography alone was of limited use in some patients because a complete block of contrast material did occur but the etiology of the nerve root compression was not visualized. Metrizamide-enhanced CT scanning, in their study, provided optimal diagnostic capability.[88]

TREATMENT OF SPONDYLOLYSIS

Non-operative

It is noted from the previous paragraphs that adolescents with spondylolysis are rarely symptomatic. Those who do become symptomatic and continue to have complaints may be managed successfully with bedrest, traction, restriction of activities, and a body brace. If symptoms improve, progressive activities are permitted.[94] If the patient remains asymptomatic, there is no need to restrict the patient's activities, and contact sports are permissible. In cases in which there is an acute onset of symptoms associated with a definite history of trauma and radiographic evidence of acute spondylolysis, treatment with a cast or brace may result in healing of the pars defect.[93, 103, 119, 158] However, in my experience and that reported by others,[160] not all of these patients go on to heal their defects. Interestingly enough, even though the defect may still be present, the patient's symptoms will usually subside. A bone scan may be helpful to determine the age of the lesion and its healing status. Hamstring tightness is also an excellent clinical tool to determine the level of healing and the success or failure of the treatment program.[58] As mentioned earlier, if the patient remains asymptomatic, there is no need to restrict the patient's activities, and I favor allowing the patient to return to all sports activities, including contact sports. Similar opinions have been expressed by Wiltse[154, 157] and Hensinger.[57] In this regard, it is important to remember that 5 to 8 per cent of the American population have spondylolysis,[95] and symptomatic spondylolysis is indeed quite uncommon. A negative lumbosacral radiograph does not rule out a developing pars defect. A bone scan may reveal an early stress fracture, and a CT scan may show defects in the pars not visualized on other radiographic techniques. If a bone scan does reveal an early impending stress fracture without a radiographic lytic defect, some authors have suggested that the athlete or patient restrict activities or use a brace with activity restriction. These lesions will usually heal without progressing to a detectable spondylolysis.[66]

Operative

FUSION

If surgery is undertaken and posterior lateral fusion is done, postoperative immobilization may or may not be carried out, depending upon the wish of the surgeon. Surgeons have reported good results with no immobilization,[120, 158] with immobilization in a corset,[9, 100] and with immobilization in a cast.[144] We generally prefer a brace or a body cast postoperatively in these patients. Leg immobilization is not necessary. Although the rates of spinal fusion for spondylolysis, as differentiated from spondylolisthesis, in children managed by posterior lateral L5 to sacral fusion with iliac bone grafting are not well discussed in the literature, from the work presented by Turner and Bianco[144] and that reported by Rombold[120] as well as my experience, a fusion rate of 90 per cent or better may be expected. This has likewise been Nachemson's[100] experience, except that there was a minor modification of the technique, the addition of iliac bone graft to the defect. Relief of symptoms likewise may be expected in a similar percentage of patients.[9, 58, 83]

REPAIR OF DEFECT

Techniques for direct repair of the defect in spondylolysis either by screw fixation across the fracture of the pars[18] or lumbosacral fusion with the addition of iliac bone grafting across the defect[100] have been described. The technique first described by Buck is indeed appealing because the pathology alone is treated and fusion across the normal joints does not occur. The technique, however, is difficult, and possible neurologic and mechanical problems associated with screw fixation across the defect are readily apparent. Wire fixation of the transverse process to the spinous process with iliac crest bone grafting spanning the defect appears to offer an attractive alternative (the technique described by James Scott). The author has now performed this procedure on 22 patients, with ages ranging from 16 to 41 years. All patients under 18 have gone on to heal their defects.[13] This procedure appears most useful in lesions of L1 to L4 in patients under 30 and in the presence of a symptomatic defect without significant slippage (Fig. 19–6).

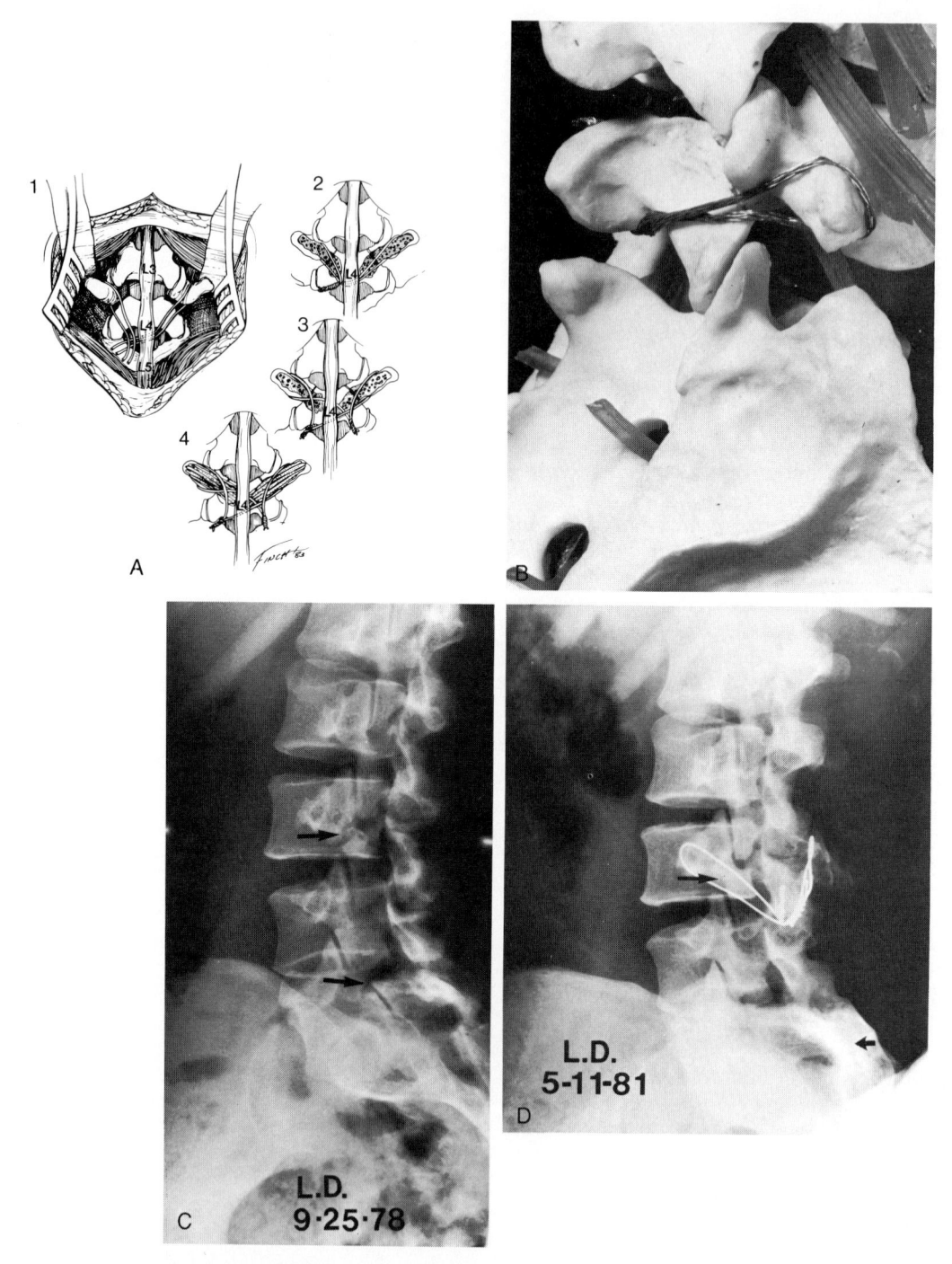

Figure 19–6. *A* and *B,* The technique of circlage wire fixation and repair of the defect. *C,* The patient, L. D., presented with spondylolysis that was symptomatic of L3 and L5. *D,* Following successful lumbosacral fusion her symptoms continued. Repair of the defect at L3 alone without extension of the fusion to the sacrum resulted in relief of back as well as leg pain.

TREATMENT OF SPONDYLOLISTHESIS

Asymptomatic

The management of asymptomatic children and adolescents with spondylolisthesis may pose a difficult problem. Clinically the long-term results of untreated patients are not well known. Recent work by Fredrickson and coworkers[39] suggests that patients with isthmic spondylolisthesis are unlikely to show progression of deformity and they never show progression after skeletal maturity. Only seven of their 30 patients with spondylolysis showed progression, and it was never over a 30 per cent slippage. It should be noted, however, that none of their patients had standing x-rays taken and this could certainly prejudice their conclusions. Harris and Weinstein reported a small series of 12 patients presenting between ages ten and 24 years with a greater than 50 per cent slippage and followed for 11 to 25 years.[54] Although they concluded that the patients functioned well, 42 per cent showed increase in the deformity and 25 per cent showed increase in symptoms. Three patients ultimately came to surgery because of increased symptoms. In our experience of well over 50 patients presenting to our center with grade 4 spondylolisthesis or spondylolysis, disabling back and leg pain was the most common presenting complaint. Symptoms of spinal stenosis were common as was progression of the deformity after skeletal maturity. It is appreciated that this experience may not reflect the true natural history of this condition because only symptomatic patients were, for the most part, referred to our center. However, it is apparent that high degrees of slippage may increase significantly in some patients, resulting in spondylolysis even in the patient who is skeletally mature. The degree of deformity may or may not be associated with major symptoms.

With a careful review of the literature as has been well summarized by Hensinger,[57] it is felt that certain clinical and radiographic factors appeared to increase the probability of progression of the slippage or of back pain in patients presenting with radiographic deformity.

CLINICAL RISK FACTORS

Age of Patient. Progression of spondylolisthesis occurs primarily during the adolescent growth spurt;[10, 25, 46, 79] it is most uncommon in the adult, and it occasionally develops in the older patient if extensive laminectomy has been carried out.[12]

Sex. Females appear to be at a much greater risk for developing further slippage of a severe degree and having changes suggestive of dysplastic type defects.[10, 25, 132]

Symptoms. Children and young adolescents who have had one episode of back pain related to the spondylolisthesis of any grade have a higher incidence of recurrent episodes.[145]

RADIOGRAPHIC RISK FACTORS

Type of Slippage. Children with dysplastic lesions (Type 1) are more likely to have progressive slippage than those with isthmic defects (Type 2).[25, 58] Hensinger has noted that teenagers with Type 2 lesions comprise 40 per cent of the group requiring surgery and only 15 per cent of the non-operative group.[58]

Stability. Children presenting with a dome-shaped sacrum and a corresponding trapezoidal 5th lumbar vertebral body have a greater likelihood of further slippage.[10, 57] Once disc narrowing occurs and a sclerotic buttress of the anterior lip of the sacrum appears, further slippage is less likely.[139]

Degree of Slippage. Children with 50 per cent slippage or more appear at a higher risk for developing further progression and increased deformity.[3, 10, 58] Indeed, it is our feeling and that of others[57, 80, 100, 104, 157] that surgical stabilization is indicated in the child with a 50 per cent or more slippage even if no symptoms are present.

Slip Angle. We have previously stressed the importance of the angle of slip and have found that this angle is often of greater help in determining further progression of the deformity than the percentage of slippage.[10] A high degree of slip angle, over 40 to 50 degrees, in a growing child is likely to be associated in my experience with further progression of the deformity.

Dynamic Views. Standing x-rays rather than supine or flexion-extension x-rays of the lumbosacral spine may demonstrate considerable mobility in terms of percentage of slippage or more importantly, in terms of a slip angle. Mobility of this deformity indicates continued instability and, in all probability, further progression if untreated.

In children or adolescents with a slippage of less than 50 per cent who remain asymptomatic, what should be the proper course of treatment, if any? This remains somewhat controversial. Wiltse[53] suggested that with slips of less than 25 per cent, activities need not be limited, but with slips greater than 25 per cent, contact sports should be avoided and activities restricted. At our center we have generally recommended repeat x-rays every six months to one year until completion of the adolescent growth spurt. We have not favored restriction of activities in these patients unless they become symptomatic. If their symptoms persist in spite of conservative management, or if their degree of slippage either in percentage of slippage or slip angle increases during the growth period, we would favor surgical stabilization. Surgical stabilization of the lumbosacral area is also favored in children and adolescent patients who present with greater than 30 to 40 per cent slippage even if asymptomatic. Although Weinstein has noted in his series that many untreated patients (with asymptomatic severe slips) may remain asymptomatic in adulthood, it is readily apparent that some patients do develop problems apart from progression of the slippage. Neurogenic intermittent claudication associated with severe spondylolisthesis during the adult period,[38] autoamputation of the first sacral nerve root,[44] and disabling back pain[12, 14] have been reported in these patients.

SYMPTOMATIC

The treatment of the child with spondylolisthesis depends on the severity of symptoms and the degree of slippage. As noted previously, if the symptoms are minimal and the slippage is less than 30 per cent, conservative treatment consisting of restricted activities and the temporary use of a lumbosacral corset or a plastic brace may prove beneficial. Once the symptoms subside, the patients should be allowed to progress their activities accordingly. Persistent symptoms that are unresponsive to conservative management and interfering with normal activities necessitate surgical management.[11, 14, 58] More important in this regard is the measurement of the lumbosacral kyphosis. With a 30 to 50 per cent slippage, the kyphosis usually becomes more apparent and progression of the deformity more likely.[11, 14]

Spinal fusion for spondylolisthesis may be carried out with or without decompression by laminectomy.[45] Laminectomy (Gill procedure) as an isolated technique in a growing child is contraindicated.[27, 156] In fact, it should be remembered that Gill cautioned against the use of this procedure in young patients.[46] Further slippage will occur in a high percentage of these cases. Some doubt has been expressed as to whether decompression with removal of the loose posterior element of L5 should ever be done in children, irrespective of the signs and symptoms of neurologic compromise.[10, 154, 156] Wiltse believes that severely tight hamstrings, decreased Achilles reflexes, and even foot drop will recover after solid arthrodesis.[156] Furthermore, it should be remembered that a nerve can function normally and still be reduced by compression to 25 per cent of its normal size if the compression occurs slowly. But beyond that constriction, some reflex and sensory change is likely to occur.[31] Although one cannot argue with those who do posterior decompressions with fusion for symptomatic spondylolisthesis, it should be stressed that spine stabilization by fusion is the most important part of the procedure and decompression with or without the fusion increases the risk of further slippage. Furthermore, merely removing the loose posterior arch does not furnish an adequate decompression. Frequently, the attenuated pars interarticularis shows a laminated type defect from aborted attempts at repair. Merely taking off the posterior arch may leave portions of this laminated bone and fibrocartilaginous debris within the neural canal next to the fifth root. For decompression to be thorough, complete removal of all offending bone and cartilage from the pars at its junction with the base of the pedicle and the transverse process is necessary. This may also require partial removal of the pedicle and transverse process for higher degrees of slip and removal of the disc underneath and inferior to the root.

The most effective treatment for spondylolisthesis is lumbosacral fusion with extension to L4 if the slippage is greater than 50 per cent (Fig. 19–7). The fusion should be done posterolaterally. It may be done through a midline incision, through a paraspinal approach splitting the sacrospinalis muscle about two finger-breadths lateral to the midline, or through an approach lateral to the paraspinal muscles. Fusion should extend to the tips of the transverse process from L4 to the sacral ala using autogenous

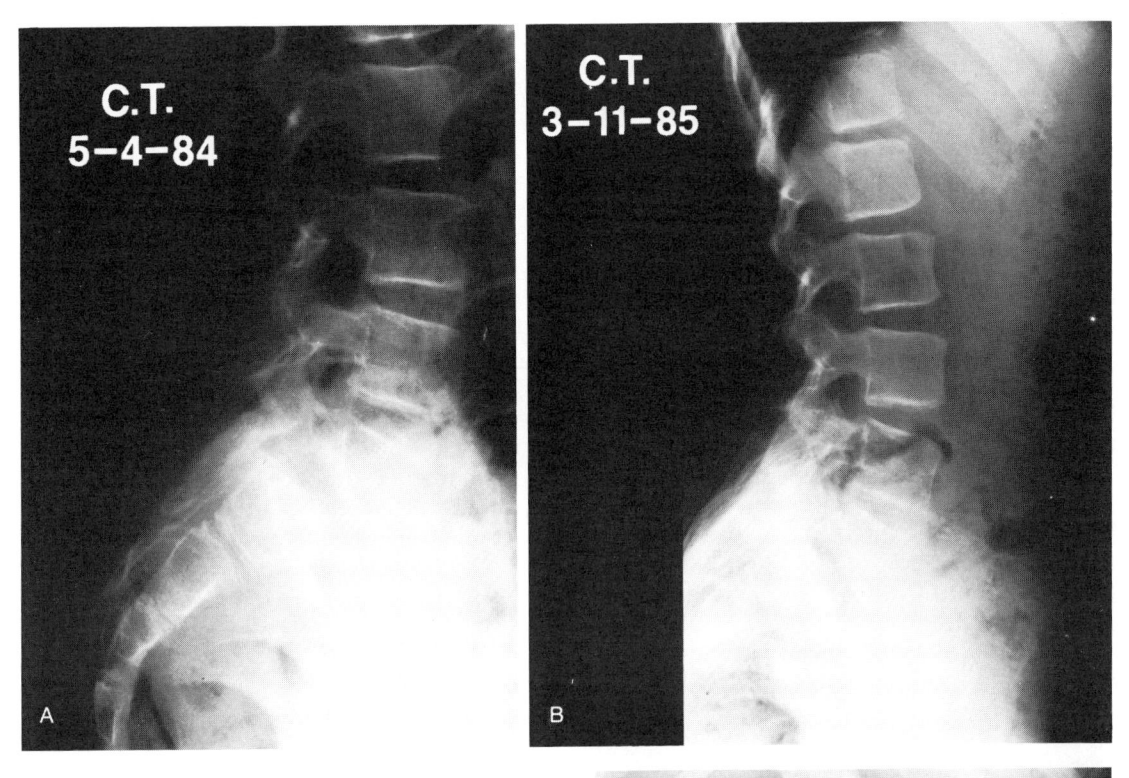

Figure 19–7. A, The x-ray of a 13 year old girl with a 40 per cent slippage, without any significant slip angle. Persistent symptoms with evidence of progression necessitated surgery. B and C, An L4 to sacral fusion was carried out with complete relief of her symptoms.

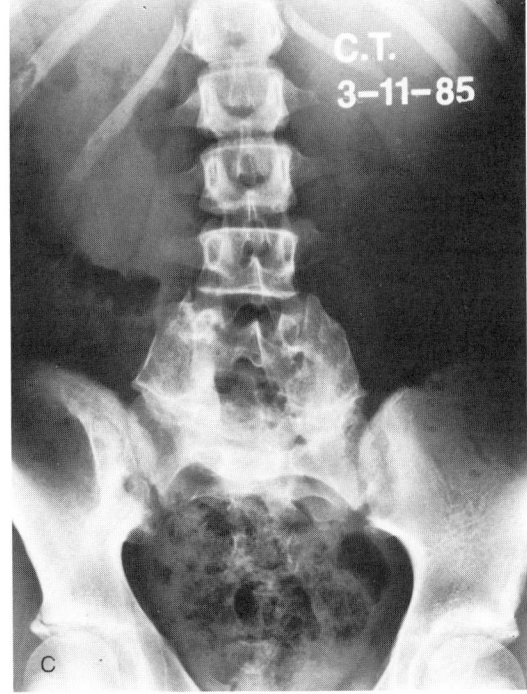

iliac bone for grafting. It may be helpful to countersink a cortical strut graft into a hole made into the sacral ala and extend the strut to the transverse process of L4.[58] The capsule of the articular joints of L4 and L5 and S1 should be removed. Facet joint fusion is elective; there is no evidence that it increases the success of arthrodesis. Postoperative management depends on the age of the patient, the severity of the slip, the procedure performed, and the desire of the operating surgeon. If the slip is less than 50 per cent and laminectomy has not been done, ambulation may be encouraged shortly after surgery. A corset, brace, or cast may be used, but it is not essential.[120] I feel that if laminectomy has been done or the slip is greater than 50 per cent, it is best to use a body cast, including one thigh with the hips in hyperextension. If there is any evidence of loss of correction or increased deformity on ambulation, the patient should be kept supine for approximately three to four months. This is more important in those patients who demonstrate a high slip angle (greater than 45 degrees) and instability as noted in the lumbar spine flexion/extension x-rays. Following the initial three to four month immobilization, the patient may be up in a body cast with or without leg extension or a brace, depending on the radiographic quality of the fusion, for an additional two to four months until the fusion is solid. Hensinger recommends similar immobilization,[58] whereas Wiltse prefers no immobilization,[154] Nachemson recommends only a lumbosacral corset,[100] and Turner prefers a cast (Fig. 19–8).[144]

It should be stressed that further slippage may occur after spinal fusion,[80, 114] even if the patient is kept supine.[10, 25, 58] Progressive slippage appears more likely to occur in those patients who have a Gill procedure along with the posterolateral fusion.[9] Wiltse believes that the use of the midline posterior approach may increase the instability and permit further slippage. If the posterolateral approach is used without removing the loose lamina, further slippage, he feels, is less likely.[156] Boxall and coworkers,[10] on the other hand, have noted that in patients with a slip greater than 55 degrees and with a slippage greater than 50 per cent, progression of the

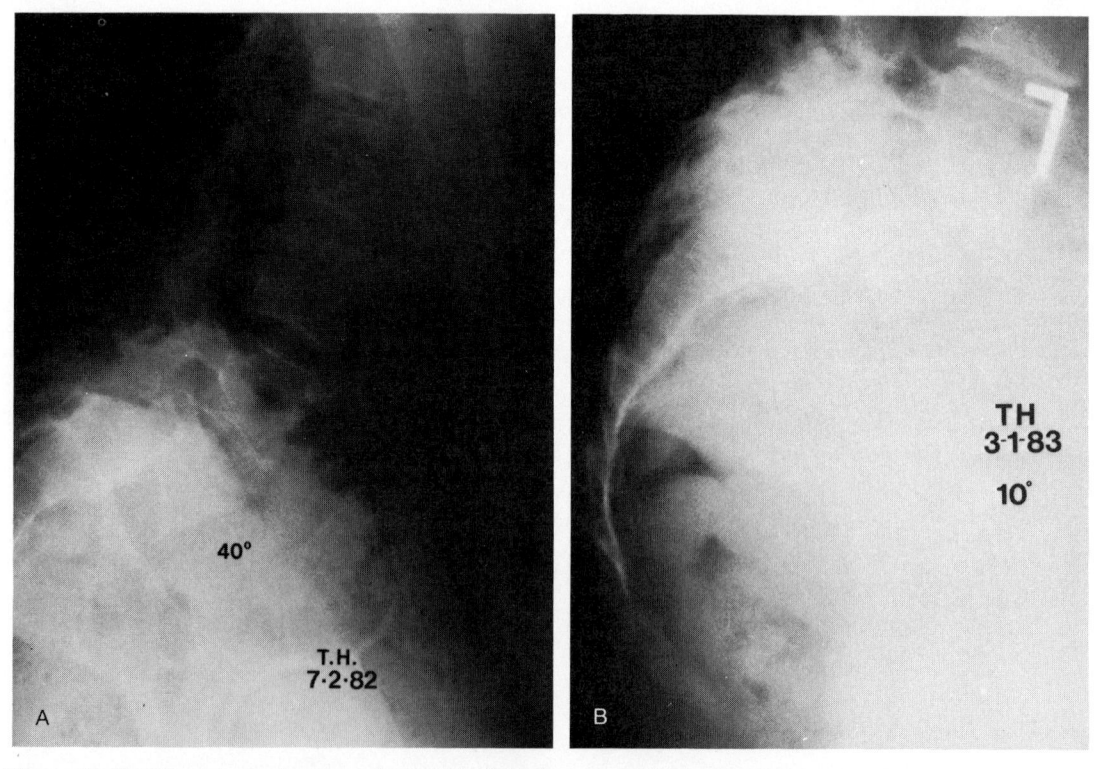

Figure 19–8. More severe degrees of spondylolisthesis may still be managed successfully by posterolateral fusion. To prevent increased kyphosis with further displacement, however, a laminectomy is best avoided if possible. Cast reduction of the kyphosis, incorporating one thigh and keeping the patient supine for several months, may be necessary to achieve fusion without loss of correction. A, Preoperative roentgenogram. B, Post arthrodesis with cast reduction.

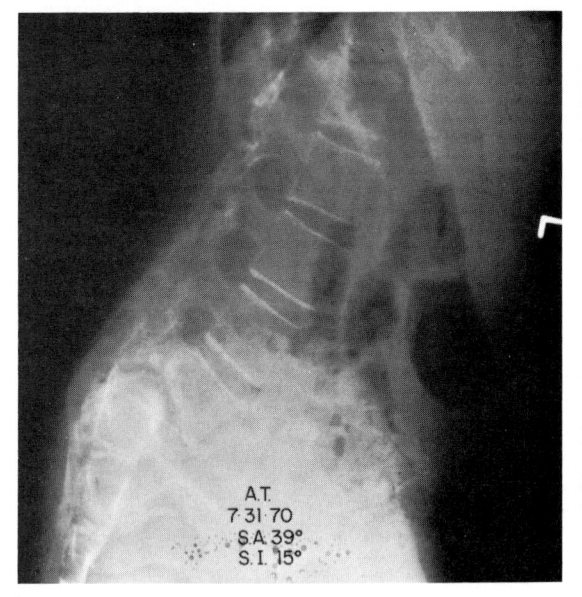

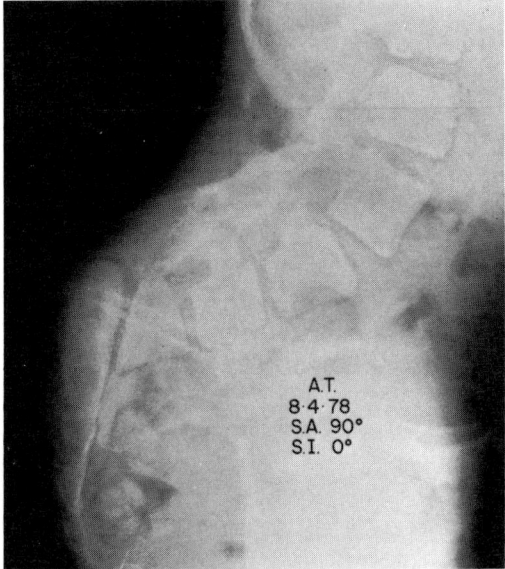

Figure 19–9. Progression of a grade III spondylolisthesis to total spondyloptosis following lumbosacral fusion with laminectomy. Progression of the slippage may occur in the presence of a solid arthrodesis, especially with high degrees of slippage and lumbosacral kyphosis.

deformity may continue even in the presence of a solid arthrodesis. This is comparable to kyphosis progression in a growing child in the presence of a solid posterior arthrodesis, which is under tension and subjected, therefore, to distraction forces (Fig. 19–9).

Pseudarthrosis ranged from 0 per cent to 25 per cent in Boxall's series.[10] It appears that children with higher degrees of slippage treated by posterolateral arthrodesis with iliac bone grafting are not likely to achieve the highest rate of successful arthrodesis (Fig. 19–9).[51] (See Reduction following.) Relief of symptoms does not necessarily correlate with a successful fusion,[10] but symptomatic relief in 75 per cent or more patients is expected.[10, 58, 104, 120, 132, 139, 144, 146]

ANTERIOR FUSIONS IN SITU

Anterior fusion was first suggested for spondylolysis or spondylolisthesis by Capener in 1932.[20] In 1933, Burns[19] performed the first anterior operation through a transperitoneal approach. Hodgson has extensively reviewed the history of anterior approaches to the lumbosacral spine and it will not be discussed further here.[61] In the series presented by Freebody in 1971,[40] 84 per cent of 252 patients operated on through a transperitoneal approach achieved a solid arthrodesis.

The results on clinical grounds showed that 92 per cent of results were rated excellent or good. The retroperitoneal approach appears equally effective. Results reported by Sevastikoylov in 10 cases of patients aged 12 to 17 years were excellent, all were relieved of their pain and all had a solid arthrodesis 2 to 14 years later.[130] Van Rens and Van Horn reported 21 of 24 patients had pain relief, while one had a pseudarthrosis. Although some adults were reported in their series, all patients were followed for greater than ten years.[145] Verbiest also has described an anterior fusion technique for in situ stabilization for spondylolisthesis that appears useful.[147]

Sterility secondary to retrograde ejaculation has been reported by the anterior approach,[68] but awareness of the presacral sympathetic nervus plexus and avoiding damage to it may decrease this unlikely complication. A solid anterior arthrodesis may not completely relieve the symptoms referable to root entrapment by a loose posterior element.

Anterior interbody fusion through the posterior approach has been reported by Cloward[23] to be highly successful. Bohlman[7] has described two patients treated by posterior decompression and posterior lateral fusion along with posterior interbody fusion with good results in pain relief. I have had no experience with either technique in patients with spondylolisthesis.

REDUCTION OF SPONDYLOLISTHESIS (Fig. 19–10)

In the past several years increasing attention has been given to the reduction of spondylolisthesis by traction or casting and then performing a surgical arthrodesis, either posteriorly, anteriorly, or by both approaches. Reduction of spondylolisthesis was first described by Scherb in 1921.[127] The first description in the English literature was by Jenkins in 1936.[67] R. I. Harris, in 1951,[55] demonstrated that skeletal traction could reduce spondylolisthesis. Work by Taillard,[139, 140] Newman in 1965,[105] Lance in 1966,[77] Harrington and Tullos in 1971,[53] Del Torto,[28] and Harrington and Dickinson[52] have all demonstrated techniques for reduction and arthrodesis by posterior approaches. Other authors have developed alternative and promising procedures for reducing spondylolisthesis by combined anterior and posterior procedures.[12, 30, 82, 90, 107, 135, 136] One of the most appealing methods for reducing spondylolisthesis is the cast technique described by Scaglietti, Frontino, and Bartolozzi.[125, 126] In this technique, the patient is placed on a fracture table. Following longitudinal distraction, the hips are hyperextended, reducing the slippage and the angulation and correcting the abnormal forward pelvic inclination. A plaster cast is then applied (Fig. 19–11). A posterolateral fusion is necessary in order to maintain the reduction. This technique is particularly useful in unstable spondylolisthesis with an increased

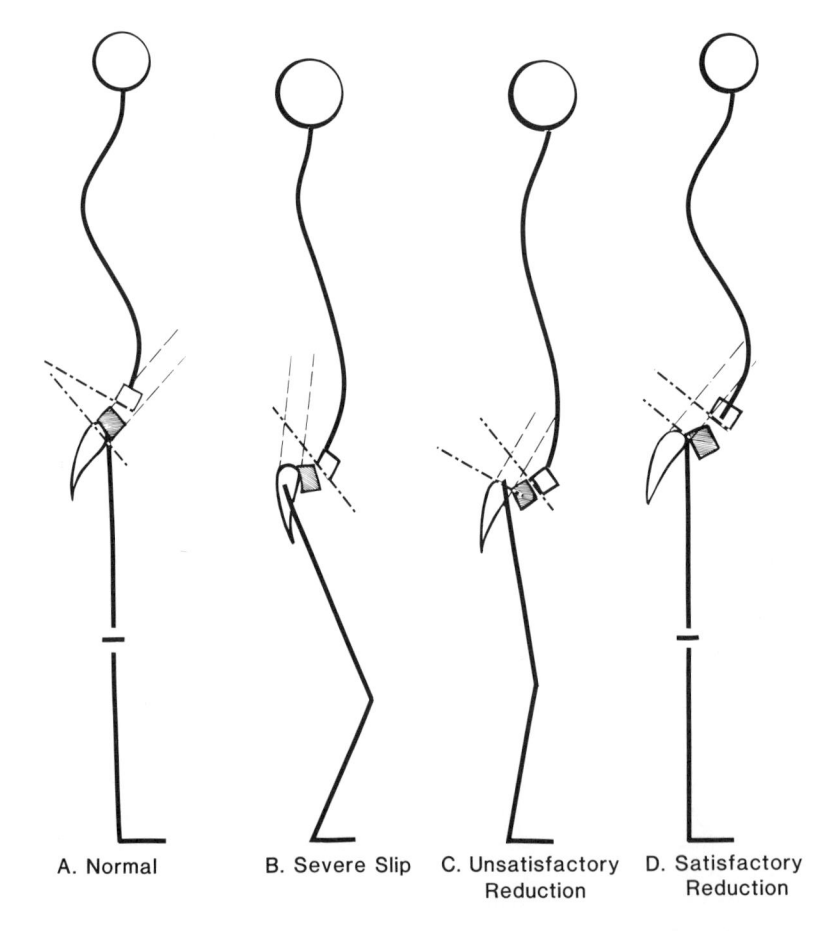

Figure 19–10. A, Normal sagittal plane spinal alignment. B, Loss of alignment can be visualized following a severe L5 spondylolisthesis. The sacrum becomes vertical and the resultant lumbosacral kyphosis "pushes" the lumbar spine forward. C, An unsatisfactory reduction occurs when L5 has little mobility and L4 lays anterior to the "anatomic zone" and kyphotic in relation to the sacrum. The fusion in this case will be under tension and less likely to hold. D, A satisfactory reduction occurs when L4 can be placed in the "anatomic zone" and oriented lordotic in relation to the sacrum. E, The more L4 can be positioned over the sacrum the greater posterior compressive forces will be directed across the fusion. In this position also sagittal plane alignment and hence deformity will be corrected.

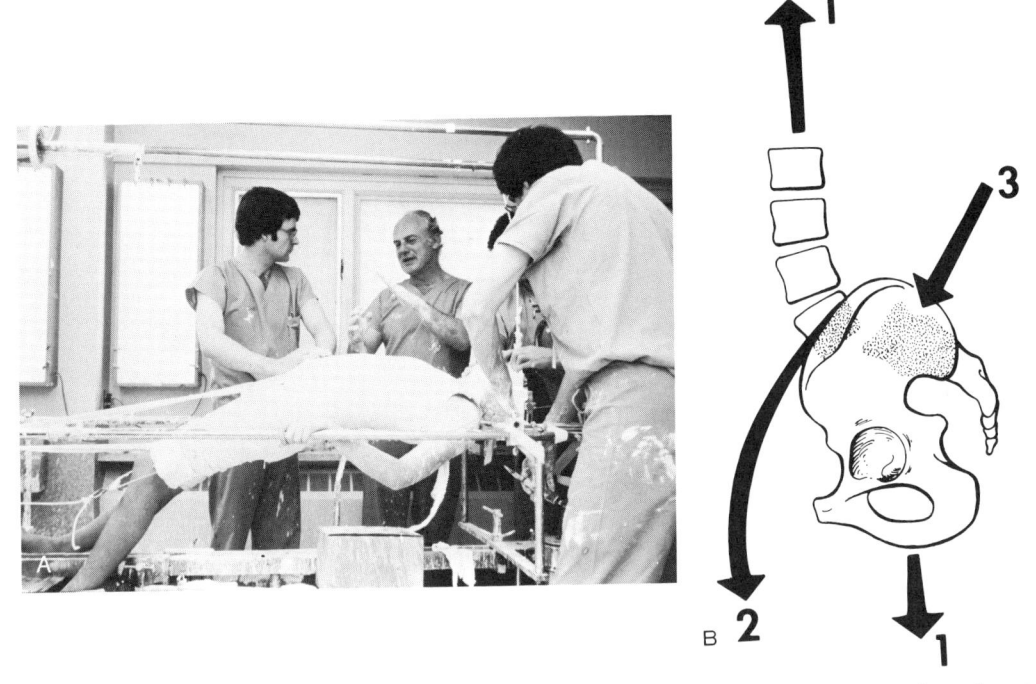

Figure 19–11. A, A cast reduction technique for spondylolisthesis. B, A diagram of the mechanism of applying forces.

lumbosacral kyphosis that is partially correctable as demonstrated on flexion and extension x-rays. At our center we favor doing the cast reduction seven to ten days after the posterolateral fusion rather than operating through a cast. The technique is advantageous for it may significantly reduce the slip angle and reduce the translational displacement. With lumbosacral extension the posterior fusion mass is placed under compression, and the growth plate of the anterior sacral cortex is in effect "decompressed." Sacral remodeling thus is effected (provided there is remaining sacral epiphyseal growth potential) with the result of a more stable sacral buttress (Figs. 19–11 and 19–12). In cases in which there are more severe degrees of spondylolisthesis, however, and in those associated with elongation of the pars interarticularis, significant reduction by the casting technique may not always be possible.[12] Posterolateral fusion in situ in these cases, especially in the growing teenager, may lead to variable degrees of increased slippage and/or increased angulation. This has been reported to occur in 20 to 30 per cent of patients.[9, 10, 25, 80] Furthermore, the magnitude of this deformity, particularly in grade 4 slippage, may prove unacceptable. Increased attempts in this country as well as in Europe, Japan, and South America have been made in the past ten years to achieve a more stable fusion as well as reduction of severe spondylolisthesis. The question must be continually asked, however, whether these techniques are safe, are they desirable, what is the indication, and is the risk/reward ratio appropriate?

The goals of treatment should be (1) to prevent progression, (2) to relieve pain, (3) to reverse neurologic deficit, and (4) to improve function. The correction of deformity, radiographic as well as clinical, would be an indication for surgery only if it impacts favorably on these goals. For instance, posterolateral fusion alone is an acceptable and appropriate treatment in the young, skeletally immature patient with symptomatic grade 1 to 3 spondylolisthesis with no clinical sagittal plane malalignment and a lumbosacral kyphosis of less than 25 degrees. In these cases the deformity is insignificant and is not associated with any sagittal plane malalignment, and progressive slippage with successful arthrodesis posteriorly is unlikely to occur.

Several techniques of reduction and their indications will be discussed.

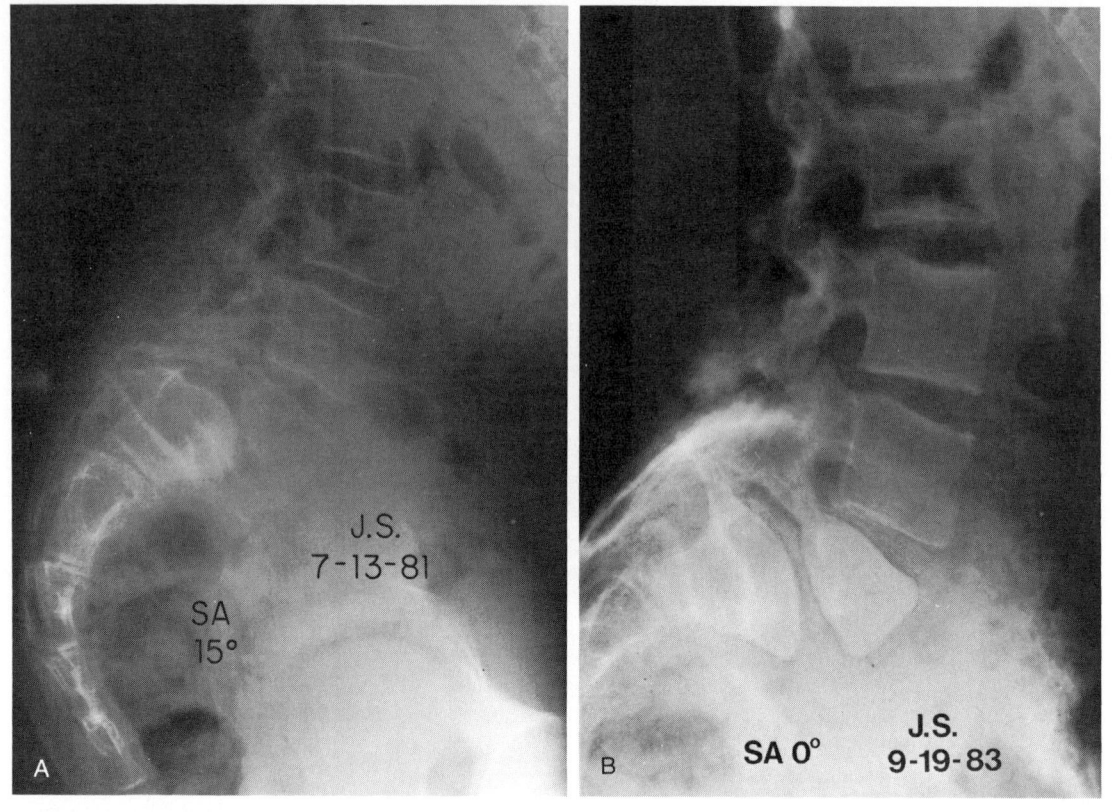

Figure 19–12. Pre- (A) and postoperative (B) radiographs of a patient with a high degree of slippage treated by posterolateral fusion from L4 to the sacrum and cast reduction. Note the sacral remodeling that has occurred two years after the posterior fusion.

Cast Techniques

Skeletally immature patients with high degrees of slippage (high grade 3 or grade 4) and clinically evident sagittal plane malalignment with increased lumbosacral kyphosis should be considered for cast reduction with posterolateral fusion of L4 to the sacrum. The total sagittal alignment of the spine and the relationship of L4 to the sacrum are important determinants in this treatment plan. In the normal spine, L4 is lordotic to the sacrum and the L4 vertebral body is dorsal or posterior to a line continuous with the anterior cortex of the sacrum (see Fig. 19–10). In severe spondylolisthesis, L4 as well as L5 is kyphotic in relation to the sacrum, and L4 lies well anterior to the sacrum. An optimal reduction would place L4 parallel or lordotic in relation to the sacrum and within, or posterior to, the "anatomic zone" created by an imaginary extension of the sacrum (see Fig. 19–10). If L4 can be held within this zone and parallel or lordotic to the sacrum, the fusion would be under compression. An unsatisfactory reduction would leave L4 displaced forward and kyphotic in relation to the sacrum, and the posterolateral fusion would be under tension.

To facilitate a satisfactory reduction and fusion a single pantaloon cast is sufficient. The patient is generally kept supine or semi-reclined in a wheelchair for three to four months and then ambulated in an extension body jacket for an additional three to four months.

If the deformity is rigid, skeletal traction followed by Gill decompression and L4-sacral fusion with percutaneous spinous process wiring of L2, L3, and L4 might be considered. This is particularly helpful in the skeletally immature patient (Fig. 19–13).[4] This technique is completed by applying a reduction cast one week after surgery, incorporating the Hoffman pelvic pins into the cast, and attaching the percutaneous wires to an outrigger attached to the cast. Tightening the wires can further correct the translational displacement and provide increased stability. Again, the patient is kept supine for three to

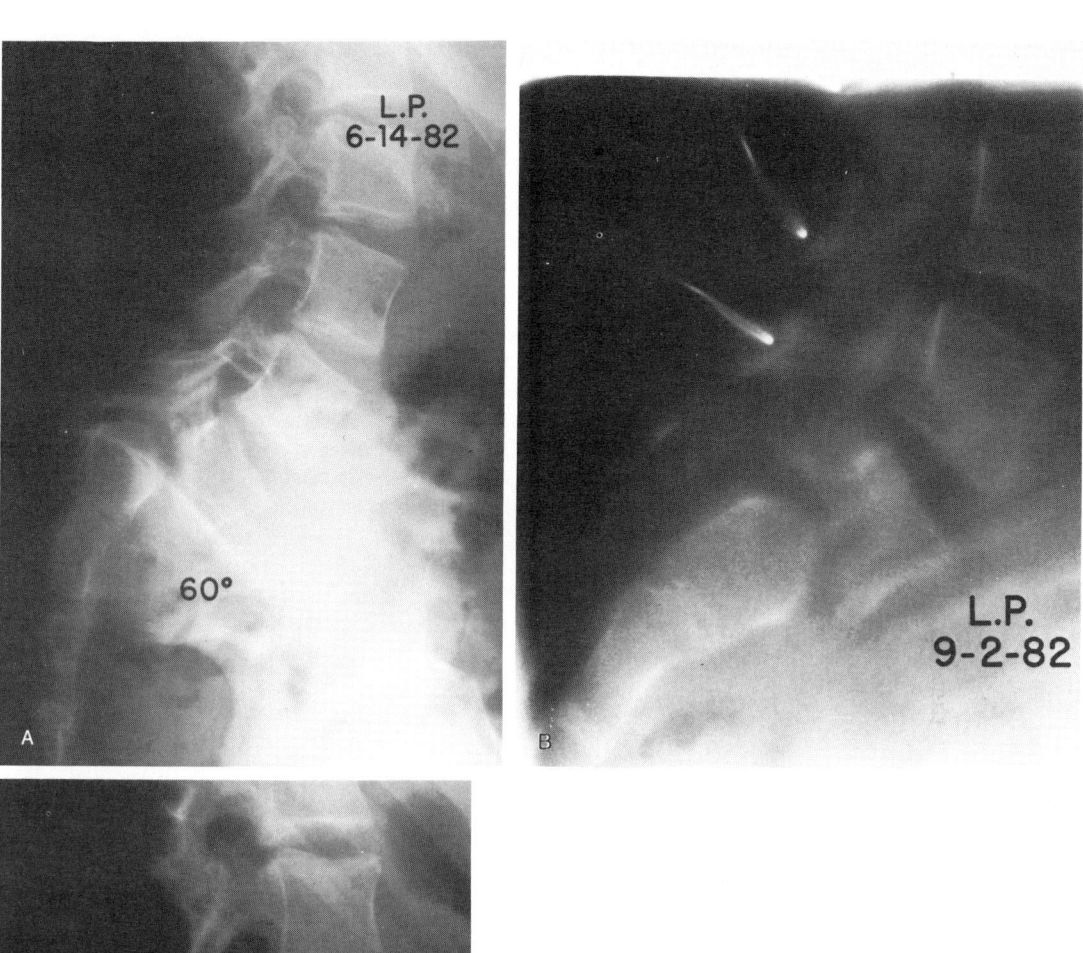

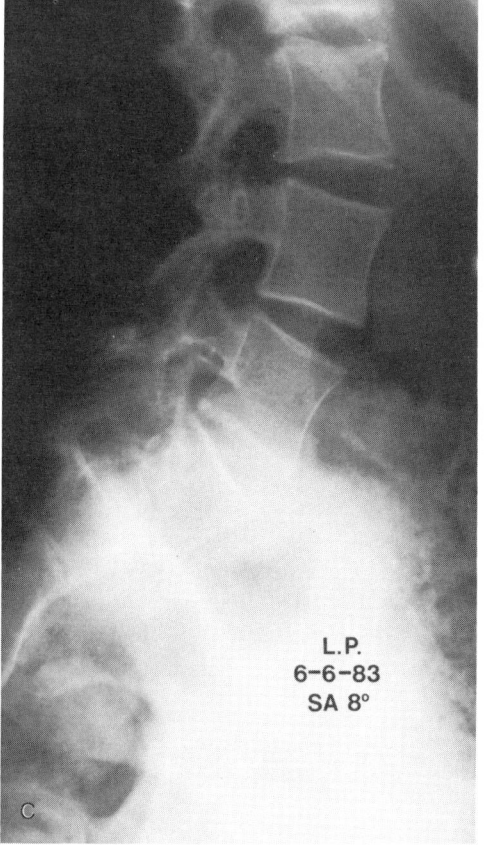

Figure 19–13. A, Preoperative x-ray of an adolescent patient with a high degree of slip and severe back and leg pain. B, Decompression, posterolateral fusion was carried out along with application of a halo-Hoffman traction. Spinous process wires at L2, L3, and L4, applied at the time of surgery, were brought up through the skin and subsequently attached to the plaster cast. Total reduction of the slippage was carried out. C, At follow-up she has gone on to a solid fusion with complete relief of her pain and maintenance of her correction.

four months. The wires and Hoffman pins and plaster are then removed and the patient ambulated in a body extension brace for an additional three to four months.

Posterior Implants

Reduction by posterior distraction forces such as Harrington or Knodt rods has achieved some popularity.[28, 30, 52, 53, 149] We have noted, however, that although the percentage of slip may be somewhat improved and a partial reduction of the slip angle may be obtained, the vertical orientation of the sacrum is in fact aggravated. This occurs, as one would expect, since the distraction force is placed at the apex of the kyphosis. If the technique is combined with an anterior fusion through a second stage anterior transperitoneal approach, increased stability and successful arthrodesis are possible. It should be noted, however, that loss of lumbar lordosis is usual with any distraction implant over the lumbar spine and this loss results in a major disability for patients with severe spondylolisthesis. In this group, sagittal plane alignment approaching normalcy can only be achieved by correcting the deformity or promoting lordosis above the slippage. If lumbar lordosis is lost for any reason and the deformity of lumbosacral kyphosis remains, sagittal plane malalignment is further aggravated and the patient's disability is increased. Even instrumenting long (T12-sacrum) and fusing short (L4-sacrum) may put L4-sacrum alignment in a flexion rather than an extension mode and may be associated with permanent facet degenerative changes even if the distraction implant is ultimately removed (Fig. 19–14).[69] Reduction with transpedicular screws and plate fixation appears to offer major advantages in that the fixation is superior and a more anatomic reduction is possible.[82]

Combined Approaches

Combined anterior and posterior reduction techniques for spondylolisthesis might be considered only in those cases in which (1) the patient presents with severe back and/or sciatic pain with major disability, (2) the percentage of slippage is greater than 75 to 80 per cent and the slip angle is 45 degrees or more, (3) the patient is approaching skeletal maturity or is skeletally mature, and (4) the patient has a rigid deformity with significant loss of sagittal plane alignment that interferes with function and is uncorrectable by closed reduction techniques. By the combined technique reported,[12, 16] a 40 to 50 per cent correction in the slippage has been achieved along with almost total correction of the slip angle (<10 degrees) and restoration of sagittal alignment in 32 patients operated on by the author with at least a one year follow-up (Fig. 19–15). The preoperative percentage of slippage averaged 100 per cent and the slip angle >75 degrees. Complications are frequent and should be stressed. Ten patients have developed a postoperative neurapraxia (usually L5); it has resolved in eight. One has residual loss of effective anterior tibialis muscle function unilaterally. The patient walks without a significant limp. Pseudarthrosis has occurred in one patient, graft slippage in three, partial loss of correction in seven, fibula graft fracture in one, and delayed healing in three. Seven patients have required third stage augmentation of their fusions. All patients have been relieved of pain and deformity. The procedure is a formidable one and should not be undertaken lightly.

An alternative technique of reduction consists of L5 vertebral body resection. This was first proposed to the author by MacEwen in 1979 and has been described recently by Huizenga[63] and Gaines.[42] The author has performed six cases of vertebrectomy (with at least a one year follow-up) for grade 5 symptomatic spondylolisthesis. One patient had had a previously unsuccessful combined anterior and posterior surgery. Two of the six developed a neurapraxia postoperatively: one recovered in four months and one has improved but not recovered at one year following surgery. Although the procedure appears advantageous since it is a spinal shortening procedure, it is highly risky, and I feel that it is rarely, if ever, indicated. It may have some merit in the very occasional patient with disabling stenosis, who is skeletally mature, is unresponsive to conservative management, and has a total spondylolisthesis (Fig. 19–16).

It is important to remember, however, that the main cause of the deformity is not the percentage of slippage, but the lumbosacral kyphosis. The kyphosis is responsible for the deformity with its tendency toward progression with or without laminectomy. Correct-

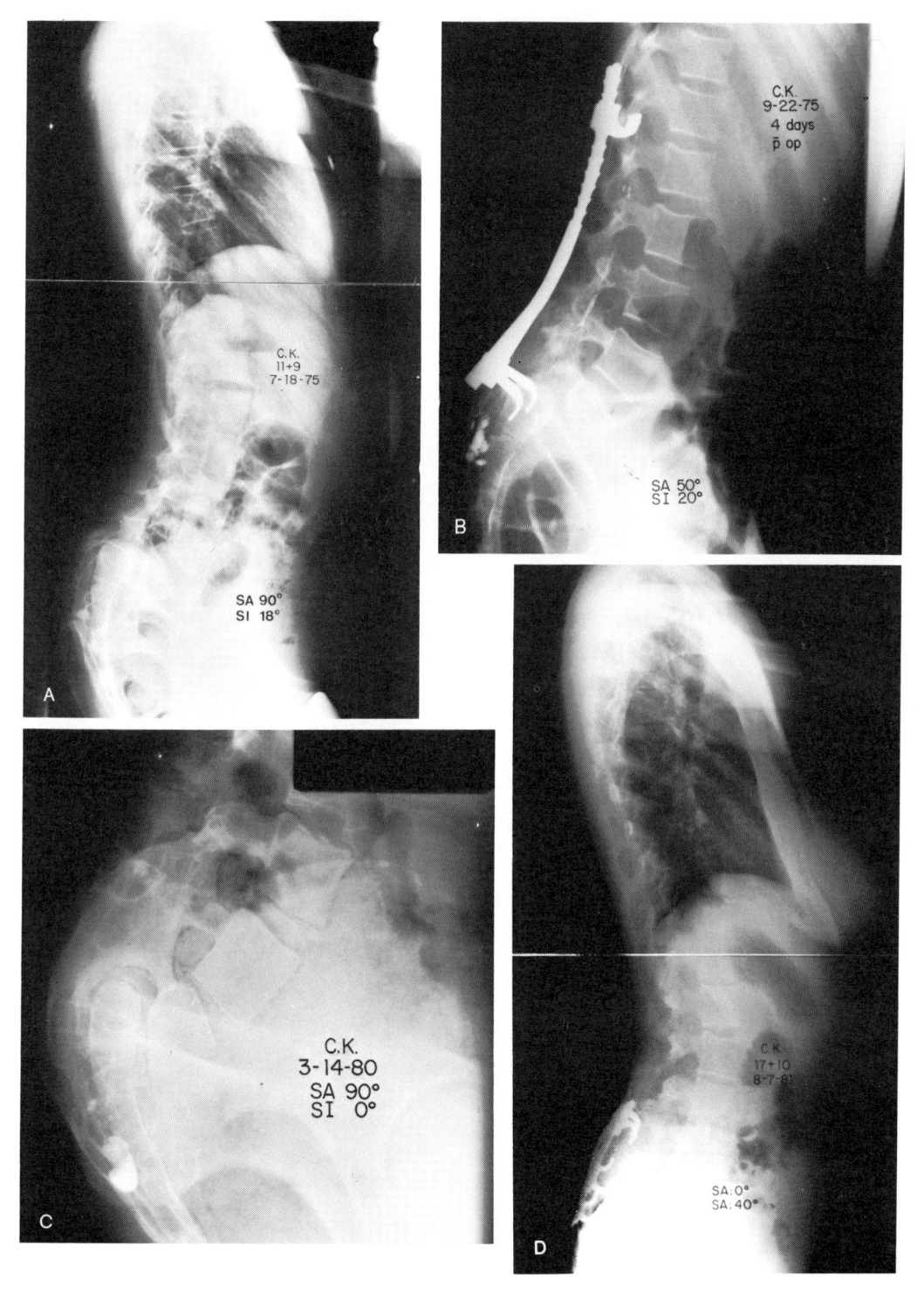

Figure 19–14. A, The preoperative x-ray demonstrates spondyloptosis in an 11 year old female. B, Because of intractable pain, posterior distraction with correction was carried out with a Gill procedure and arthrodesis from L4 to the sacrum. One and a half years later the rod was removed and the fusion looked satisfactory. C, Progressive loss of correction to complete spondyloptosis was noted over the subsequent four years. D, Because of significant disability, staged correction was carried out with satisfactory clinical and radiographic outcomes.

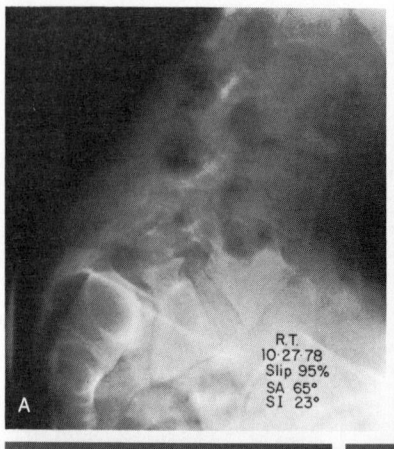

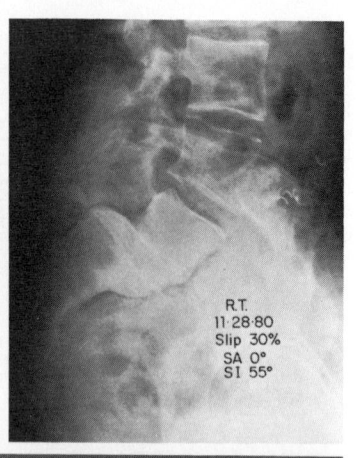

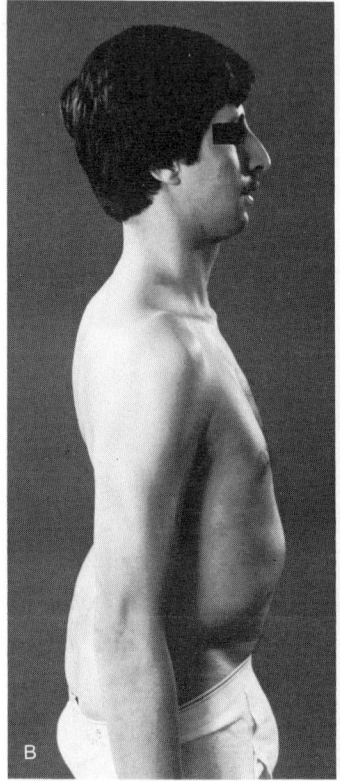

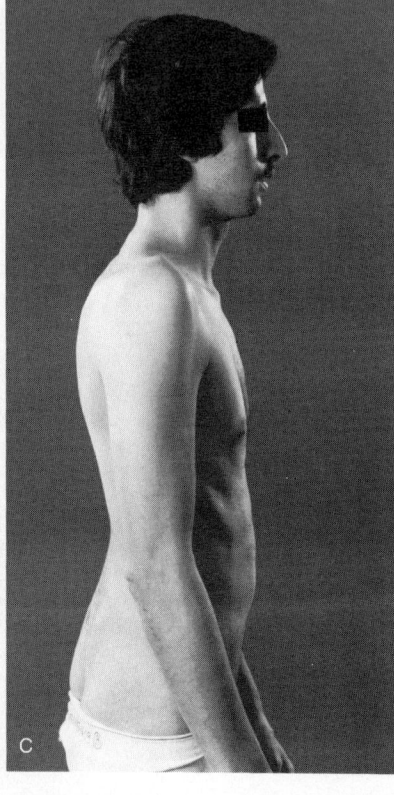

Figure 19–15. A, The pre- (left) and postoperative (right) radiography of a patient who had previously undergone unsuccessful fusion, developed progressive deformity, and presented with intractable pain and an inability to stand upright with the legs extended. Two-stage surgical correction resulted in a satisfactory result. B, Preoperative clinical photograph. C, Postoperative clinical photograph.

ing the kyphosis and promoting lumbar hyperlordosis will restore sagittal plane alignment. Surgical reduction techniques should not be undertaken lightly. Complications are frequent and the risk is greater than fusion in situ. Damage to presacral plexus may lead to retrograde ejaculation in males.[32, 68] This has not occurred in the author's series of patients.

SCOLIOSIS ASSOCIATED WITH SPONDYLOLISTHESIS (Fig. 19–17)

Since both idiopathic scoliosis and spondylolisthesis are relatively common problems, it is quite possible for both to exist in the same person. In a study of 500 consecutive patients with idiopathic scoliosis who had routine oblique x-rays of the lumbosacral area, Fisk and coworkers[37] found the incidence of pars defects to be 6.2 per cent. This corresponds to the incidence reported in the general population as noted by Roche and Rowe[119] and Moreton.[96] On the other hand, scoliosis may be related to the spondylolisthesis or may be totally separate from it. The characteristic curvature in a patient with severe spondylolisthesis is that marked by a long sweeping curve that frequently begins at the level of the slippage.[57] The curvature

SPONDYLOLYSIS AND SPONDYLOLISTHESIS 425

Figure 19–16. A, Intractable pain and inability to stand upright may pose a formidable problem in a patient with this degree of spondyloptosis. B, A spinal shortening procedure with vertebrectomy was carried out with a satisfactory outcome in terms of pain relief and body posture. This procedure may rarely have merit in such cases. Transpedicular fixation may prove preferable in assuring a patent foramina from L4 to S1.

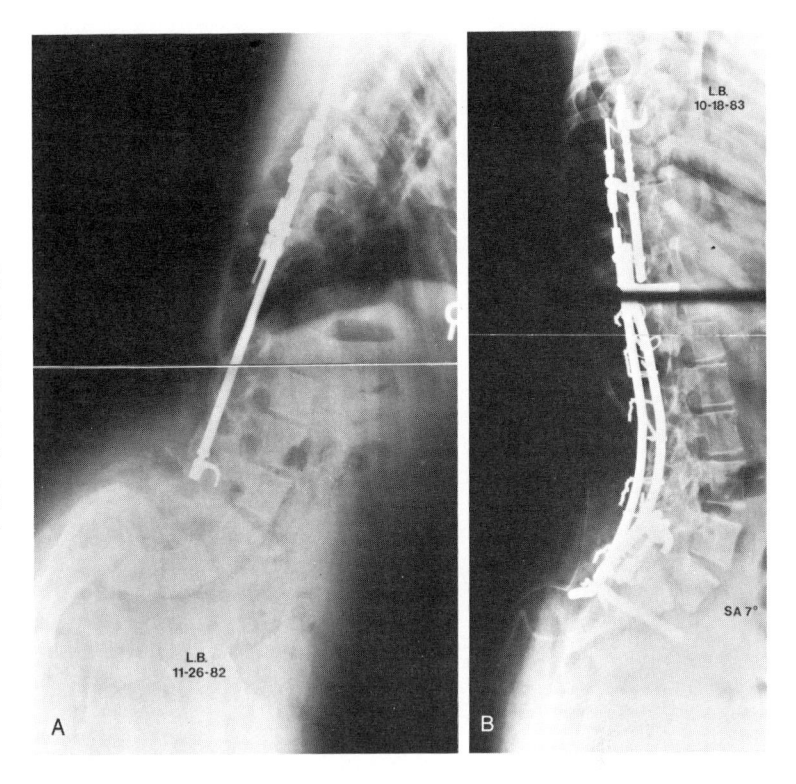

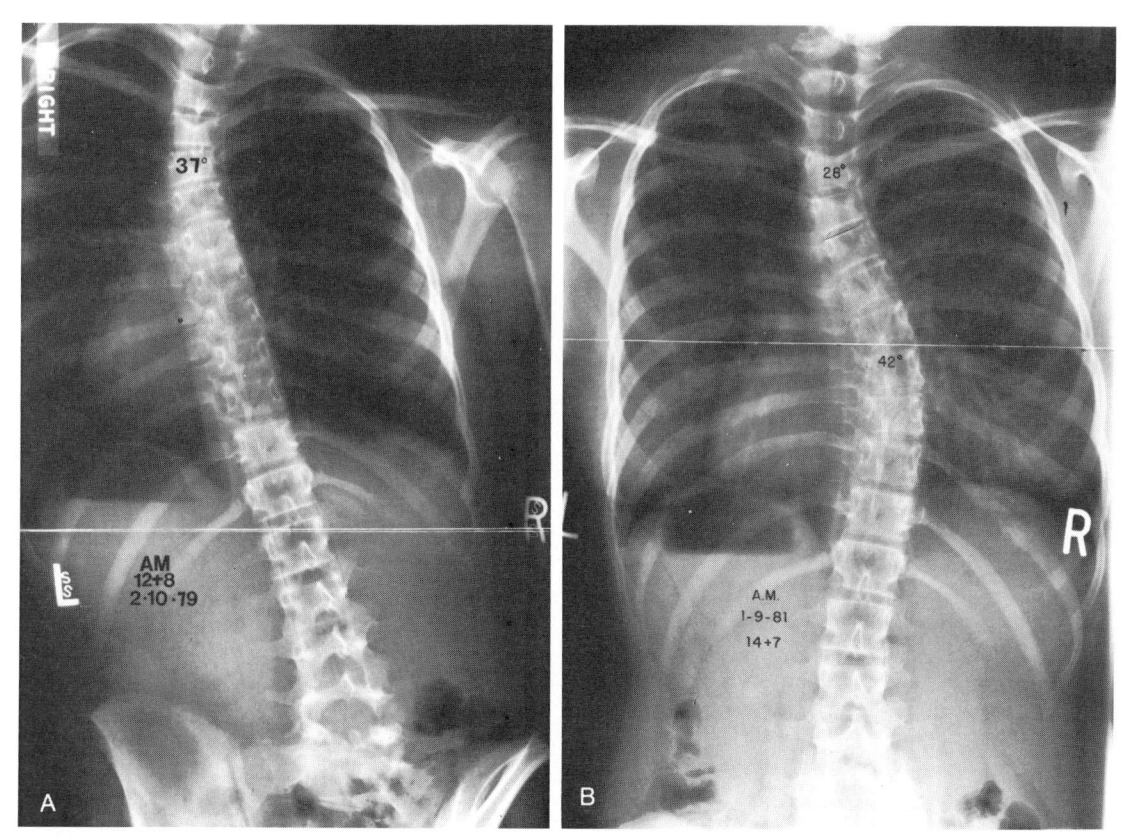

Figure 19–17. A, Scoliosis associated with spondylolisthesis may be secondary to severe spasm, as seen on this x-ray. B, Following successful lumbosacral fusion, an idiopathic type curvature emerged that has not progressed or required treatment.

may be associated with some rotation, but it is not a prominent component of the scoliosis. The curve essentially disappears in the relaxed supine position, and it will correct following successful lumbosacral fusion. Occasionally, if the spasm type curvature persists for many years, it may develop structural components and require treatment in its own right.[48]

On the other hand, if the patient presents with a characteristic idiopathic type curvature and spondylolisthesis, problems should be managed independently. If the spondylolisthesis needs fusion, it should be managed accordingly. If the scoliosis needs fusion, this likewise should be managed accordingly. There appears to be no concrete evidence that a long fusion of L4 increases the tendency for an L5 spondylolisthesis to progress. The spondylolisthesis may progress in its own right because of the natural history based on the risk factors previously outlined. If the spondylolisthesis is of low grade, less than 30 per cent in a growing child, and is essentially asymptomatic and if the child has an associated scoliosis extending to L4, I would favor managing the scoliosis with surgical arthrodesis and instrumentation to L4 only and continuing to observe the L5-S1 articulation until the completion of growth. If a Zielke anterior approach could save a level, that approach would be a desirable alternative.

DEGENERATIVE SPONDYLOLISTHESIS

The management of Type 1 or Type 2 spondylolisthesis in the adult is similar to that in the adolescent. Persistent pain that is unresponsive to conservative management for at least six months may warrant surgical treatment. Myelography with CT scanning should be done in adult patients to rule out disc herniation, generalized or localized lateral recessed stenosis, or intrinsic neuropathology. Surgical treatment should consist of stabilization by arthrodesis, decompression, or a combination of both, depending on the symptoms, the presence or absence of instability, and the age of the patient.

Degenerative spondylolisthesis results from a forward slippage of one vertebra on the other, usually combined with persistent rotatory deformity.[34, 35, 117] The deformity usually occurs at the L4-L5 level, and it occurs more frequently in females. The L5 vertebral body is often wedge-shaped rather than square, is frequently sacralized, and the sacral-horizontal angle (i.e., the angle between the top of S1 and the horizontal to the floor in the standing position) is usually reduced, resulting in loss of lumbar lordosis. The body of L5 rides more cephalad between the iliae than normal. Wiltse has stated that the L4-L5 disc falls at or caudal to the intercrestal line, the line drawn across the top of the iliac crests, in 70 per cent or more of the cases.[115] Degenerative spondylolisthesis occurs about ten times more often at L4-L5 than at L5-S1, and as mentioned, is six times more common at L5 than the normal population, and it appears to be more common in black females than in caucasians; it does not occur in patients below the age of 40, and in women past 70 it is by far the most common type of spondylolisthesis presented for treatment.

The etiology is unknown.[35, 72, 121] The degeneration of the intervertebral disc along with degenerative osteoarthritis of the articulating facets and hypertrophic osteophytes is a characteristic finding. The event leading to degeneration at this level and forward slippage is not clear. Suffice it to say that the changes are quite similar to degenerative osteoarthritis of any joint in the body.

Signs and Symptoms[33, 121, 123, 134, 147, 148]

Patients presenting with degenerative spondylolisthesis usually do so after the fifth or sixth decade and primarily present with back ache with or without sciatica. The presenting complaint of back ache may persist for years, and leg pain may never develop. Leg pain may be unilateral or bilateral. The pain may be similar to radicular pain from disc herniation, or be the sciatic or the claudicant type pain. The sciatic type pain symptoms are quite similar to those of a herniated disc. These patients may have few organic findings in contradistinction to those with disc herniation. Often the patients can bend normally, are able to hold their leg straight and raise it normally, and have a negative neurologic examination. Wiltse has stated that the sciatic type pain is at least twice as common as the claudicant type pain. This type of pain is experienced while ambulating and is completely relieved while sitting or lying supine. This pain appears to be caused by the spinal nerves becoming progressively entrapped in the smaller and smaller interforaminal space. With ambulation there is minimal excursion of the spinal nerves because of entrapment. Edema and ischemia result because of compromise of the vasonervosum, and the claudication type symptoms then develop. The symptoms may be precipitated by assuming a lordotic stance and may be abolished by lumbar flexion. The posture symptom relationship is well demonstrated with the Van Gelderen bicycle test.[134] In this test, the patient leans forward on a stable bicycle without symptoms developing. However, as the patient cycles in the erect posture with narrowing of the lumbar foramen in extension, the claudication type symptoms rapidly appear.

X-ray Evaluation

Routine standing AP and lateral x-rays of the spine will reveal the pathology of the degenerative spondylolisthesis quite readily. A transitional L5 vertebral body should lead one to a high index of suspicion on a routine AP x-ray. CT scanning with metrizamide myelography and sagittal reconstruction is of great benefit. CT scanning will show marked abnormality of the canal, which assumes a trefoil shape. Facet overgrowth and lateral recessed stenosis may be readily demonstrated.

Treatment

By far the vast majority of patients with degenerative spondylolisthesis should be treated non-operatively.[135] Back exercises (flexion type), anti-inflammatory medications, and body braces, particularly the plastic TLSO, have proven of great benefit at our center. Facet joint injections and epidural blocks may likewise be beneficial, although the benefit may be temporary.[121, 123, 134]

Pain remains the primary indication for surgery. Surgical treatment in these patients consists of stabilization by arthrodesis, decompression, or a combination of both. Results of decompression in relieving pain, first described by Gill,[46] have continued to appear satisfactory in the experience of many authors.[121, 123] These reports and others, especially when compared with the high rate of pseudarthrosis[22, 50, 62] that occurs in lumbosacral fusions, have made the decompression procedure quite attractive in some circles. However, longer follow-ups have demonstrated that decompression may not always relieve symptoms in the adult and that unsatisfactory results following decompression alone in adults have varied between 30 and 42 per cent (Fig. 19–18).[2, 25, 26, 78, 108] For instance, in Cedell's report,[21] none of the patients were symptom-free. Furthermore, progressive slippage following decompression has been reported in adults, ranging from 15 to 42 per cent of cases.[2, 26, 108] On the other hand, more recent reports have noted successful fusion rates in adults treated by posterolateral arthrodesis from 67 to 96 per cent,[78, 120] with relief of symptoms in 74 to 90 per cent of cases.[120, 137] It should be noted that these results were achieved without the use of internal fixation.

With the recent development of segmental instrumentation[84] and a resurgence of techniques of transpedicular fixation, improved methods of treatment are now available, and the success rate of surgical arthrodesis should be greatly enhanced (Fig. 19–19). Surgical arthrodesis may consist of bilateral transverse process fusion, anterior interbody fusion, posterior lumbar interbody fusion, a Farfan facet fusion only,[34] or a combination of these.[114] Although the anterior lumbar interbody fusion technique is attractive in that restoration of disc heights may reduce the slippage and restore the volume of the foramen,[65] my experience with this approach has not been completely satisfactory. Graft collapse with partial loss of correction has been common. We have not had sufficient experience with posterior interbody fusion technique for this condition to give an opinion. We have been impressed, however, with the number of patients referred to our center who have undergone this technique that present with continued symptoms of pseudarthrosis and disability.

My preferred technique, once the decision for surgery has been made, is a posterior approach. If the slippage with stenosis is confined to the L4-L5 level, removal of a portion of the inferior lamina of L4 and the superior lamina of L5 is carried out (Fig. 19–20). The lateral recesses are completely decompressed, undercutting the inferior facet of L4 as well as L5. Attention is directed particularly to the fifth root, as this is the one that is usually trapped by the inferior articular facet of L4 against the posterior portion of the body of L5. The L4 root exits

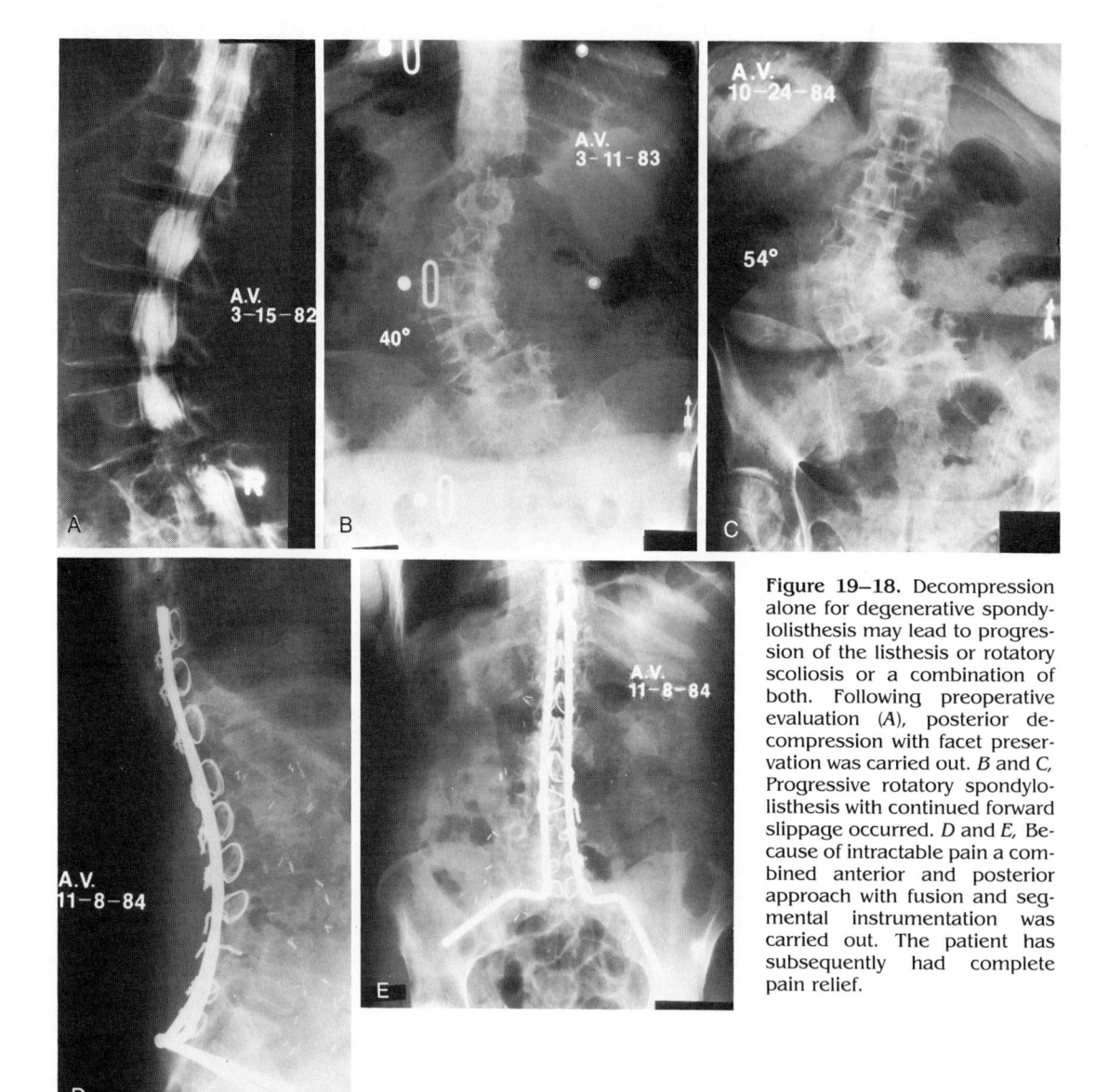

Figure 19–18. Decompression alone for degenerative spondylolisthesis may lead to progression of the listhesis or rotatory scoliosis or a combination of both. Following preoperative evaluation (*A*), posterior decompression with facet preservation was carried out. *B* and *C*, Progressive rotatory spondylolisthesis with continued forward slippage occurred. *D* and *E*, Because of intractable pain a combined anterior and posterior approach with fusion and segmental instrumentation was carried out. The patient has subsequently had complete pain relief.

SPONDYLOLYSIS AND SPONDYLOLISTHESIS

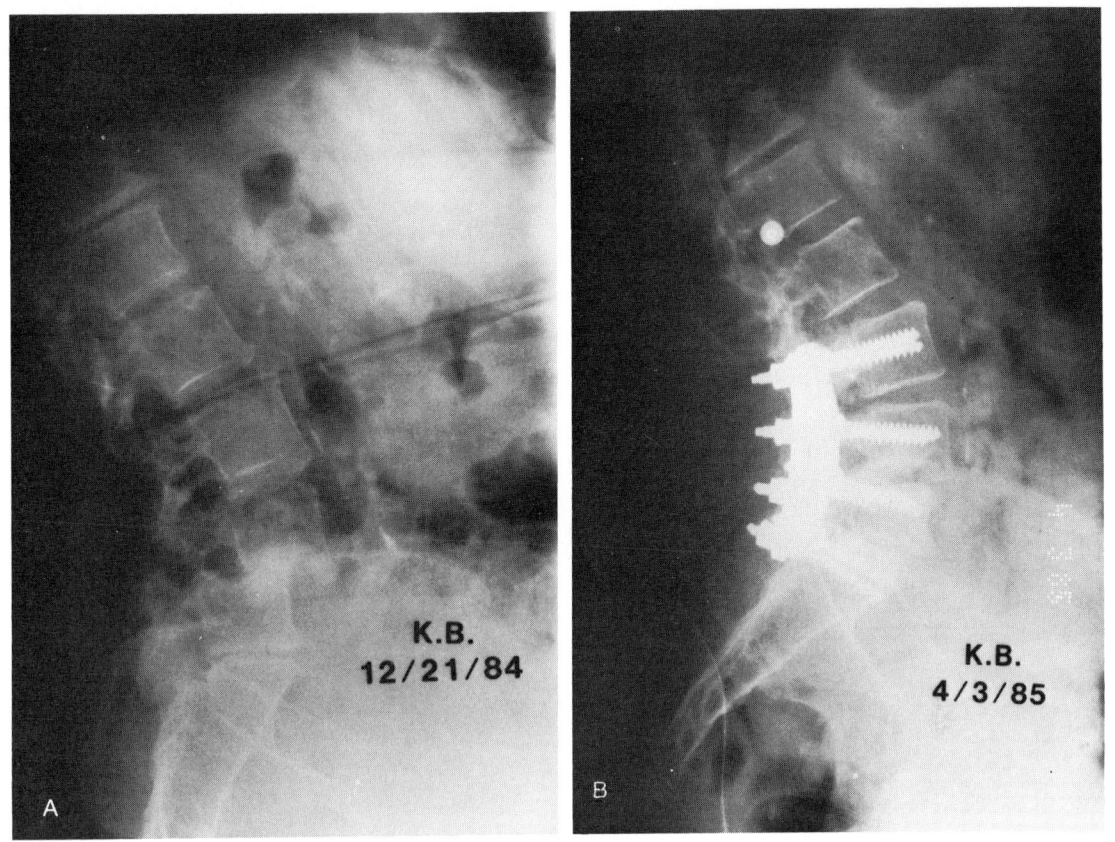

Figure 19–19. Pre- (*A*) and postoperative (*B*) lateral radiographs. Severe segmental instability in the presence of a previously total laminectomy and progressive degenerative spondylolisthesis may pose a difficult treatment problem. Segmental instrumentation with transpedicular fixation and bilateral fusion may provide significant correction of deformity as well as pain relief.

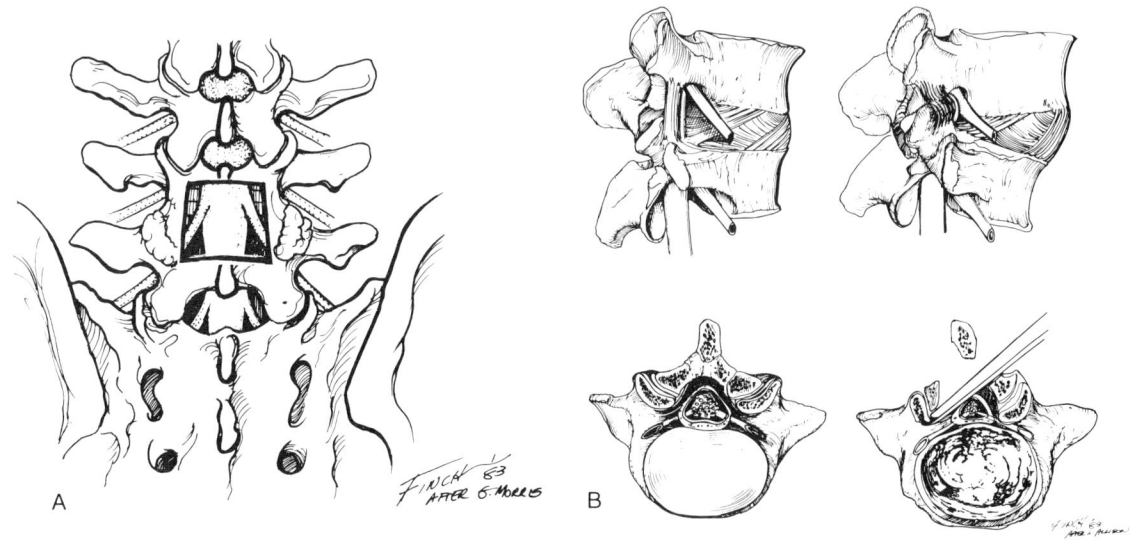

Figure 19–20. *A,* Decompression for degenerative spondylolisthesis may be carried out by removal of a portion of the inferior lamina of L4 and the superior lamina of L5, preserving the facet joints but completely decompressing the lateral recesses. This may be better seen in *B,* where the inferior facet must be undercut in order to relieve the pressure on the emerging nerve root.

above this level and is not likely to be involved, unless there is an associated pars interarticularis fracture or the osteophytes from the superior facet are unusually large. If decompression is difficult, then it is desirable to remove the whole lamina of L4, taking care to preserve the inferior and superior articulating facets as well as the pars interarticularis. Spinal fusion and segmental instrumentation are then carried out. We have found the Luque ring helpful. Fixation at the site of the laminectomy may be achieved by wiring the transverse process to the O-ring or by passing a wire carefully through the foramen, facilitating pars fixation to the O-ring. Transpedicular fixation appears to offer improved and more stable fixation and may be preferable, especially if a laminectomy has been done.

References

1. Adkins, E. W. O.: Spondylolisthesis. J. Bone Joint Surg., 37B:48, 1955.
2. Amuso, S. J., Neff, R. S., Coulson, D. B., and Laing, P. G.: The surgical treatment of spondylolisthesis by posterior element resection. J. Bone Joint Surg., 52A:529, 1970.
3. Baker, D. R., and McHollick, W.: Spondylolysis and spondylolisthesis in children. Proceedings of the American Academy of Orthopaedic Surgeons. J. Bone Joint Surg., 38A:933, 1956.
4. Balderston, R., and Bradford, D. S.: Technique for achievement and maintenance of reduction for severe spondylolisthesis using spinous process traction wiring and external fixation of the pelvis. Spine, 10:376, 1985.
5. Barash, H. L., Galante, J. O., Lambert, C. N., and Ray, R. D.: Spondylolisthesis and tight hamstrings. J. Bone Joint Surg., 52A:1319, 1970.
6. Berquet, K. H.: Konkordanz des 5. Lendenwirbelkorpers bei Zwillingen. Z Orthop., 99: 260–262, 1964.
7. Bohlman, H. H., and Cook, S. S.: One-stage decompression and posterolateral and interbody fusion for lumbosacral spondyloptosis through a posterior approach. J. Bone Joint Surg., 62A:3, 415–418, 1982.
8. Borokow, S. E., and Kleiger, B.: Spondylolisthesis in the newborn. Clin. Orthop., 81:73, 1971.
9. Bosworth, D. M., Fielding, J. W., Demarest, L., and Bonaquist, M.: Spondylolisthesis: a critical review of a consecutive series of cases treated by arthrodesis. J. Bone Joint Surg., 37A:767, 1955.
10. Boxall, D., Bradford, D. S., Winter, R. B., and Moe, J. H.: Management of severe spondylolisthesis in children and adolescents. J. Bone Joint Surg., 61A:479, 1979.
11. Bradford, D. S.: Spondylolysis and spondylolisthesis. Curr. Pract. Orthop. Surg., 8:12, 1979.
12. Bradford, D. S.: Treatment of severe spondylolisthesis: a combined approach for reduction and stabilization. Spine, 4:423, 1979.
13. Bradford, D. S.: Repair of spondylolysis or minimal degrees of spondylolisthesis by segmental wire fixation and bone grafting. Orthop. Trans., 6:1, 2, 1982.
14. Bradford, D. S.: Spondylolysis and spondylolisthesis. In Chou, I. S. N., and Seljeskog, E. L. (eds.): Spinal Deformity and Neurologic Dysfunction. New York, Raven Press, 1978.
15. Bradford, D. S.: Management of spondylolysis and spondylolisthesis. In Evarts, C. M. (ed.): Instructional Course Lectures, American Academy of Orthopaedic Surgeons. Vol. 32. St Louis, C. V. Mosby Co., p. 151, 1983.
16. Bradford, D. S.: Treatment of severe spondylolisthesis, a combined approach for reduction and stabilization. Orthop. Trans., 5:3, 410, 1981.
17. Bradford, D. S.: Spondylolysis and spondylolisthesis in children and adolescents. In Bradford, D. S. and Hensinger, R. N. (eds.): Pediatric Spine. New York, Thieme and Stratton, 1985.
18. Buck, J. E.: Direct repair of the defect in spondylolisthesis. J. Bone Joint Surg., 61A:479, 1979.
19. Burns, B. H.: An operation for spondylolisthesis. Lancet, 1:1233, 1933.
20. Capener, N.: Spondylolisthesis. Br. J. Surg., 19:374, 1932.
21. Cedell, C., and Wiberg, G.: Longterm results of laminectomy in spondylolisthesis. Acta Orthop. Scand., 40:773, 1970.
22. Cleveland, M., Bosworth, D. M., and Thompson, F. R.: Pseudarthrosis in the lumbosacral spine. J. Bone Joint Surg., 20A:302, 1948.
23. Cloward, R. B.: Spondylolisthesis: treatment by laminectomy and posterior interbody fusion. Clin. Orthop., 154:74–82, 1981.
24. Cowell, M. J., and Cowell, H. R.: The incidence of spina bifida occulta in idiopathic scoliosis. Clin. Orthop., 118:16, 1976.
25. Dandy, D. J., and Shannon, M. J.: Lumbosacral subluxation (group 1 spondylolisthesis). J. Bone Joint Surg., 53B:578, 1971.
26. Davis, I. S., and Bailey, R. W.: Spondylolisthesis. Long-term follow-up study of treatment with total laminectomy. Clin. Ortho. Rel. Res., 88:46, 1972.
27. David, I. S., and Bailey, R. W.: Spondylolisthesis: indications for lumbar nerve root decompression and operative technique. Clin Orthop., 117:129, 1976.
28. Del Torto, U.: Surgical reduction and stabilization of spondylolisthesis. Clin. Orthop., 75:281, 1971.
29. Devas, M. B.: Stress fractures in children. J. Bone Joint Surg., 45B:528–41, 1963.
30. DeWald, R. L., Faut, M., Taddonio, R. F., and Neuwirth, M. G.: Severe lumbosacral spondylolisthesis in adolescents and children: reduction and stage circumferential fusion. J. Bone Joint Surg., 63A:619, 1981.
31. Duncan, D.: Alterations in the structure of the nerves. Neuropathol. Exp. Neurol., 7:261, 1948.
32. Duncan, H. M., and Jonch, L. M.: The presacral plexus in anterior fusion of the lumbar spine. S. Afr. J. Surg., 3:93, 1965.

33. Dyck, P., Pheasant, H. C., Doyle, J. B., and Rieder, J. J.: Intermittent cauda equina compression syndrome. Spine, 2:75, 1977.
34. Farfan, H. F.: A reorientation in the surgical approach to degenerative lumbar intervertebral joint disease. Orthop. Clin. North Am., 8:9, 1977.
35. Farfan, H. F., Osteria, V., and Lamy, C.: The mechanical etiology of spondylolysis and spondylolisthesis. Clin. Orthop., 117:40, 1976.
36. Ferguson, R. J.: Low-back pain in college football linemen. J. Bone Joint Surg., 56A:1300, 1974.
37. Fisk, J. R., Moe, J. H., and Winter, R. B.: Scoliosis, spondylolisthesis and spondylolysis: their relationship as reviewed in 539 patients. Spine, 3:234, 1978.
38. Fredricksen, A., and Mangschau, A.: Neurogenic intermittent claudication in association with spondylolisthesis. Acta Neurol. Scand., 60: 385–388, 1979.
39. Fredrickson, B. E., Baker, D., Yuan, H., and Lubicky, J.: The natural history of spondylolysis and spondylolisthesis. J. Bone Joint Surg., 66A:699, 1984.
40. Freebody, D., Bendall, R., and Taylor, R. D.: Anterior transperitoneal lumbar fusion. J. Bone Joint Surg., 53B:617, 1971.
41. Friberg, S.: Studies on spondylolisthesis. Acta Chir. Scand., Vol. 82 suppl. 56, 1939.
42. Gaines, R. W., and Nichols, W. K.: Treatment of spondyloptosis by two-stage L5 vertebrectomy and reduction of L4 onto S1. Spine 10:680–687, 1985.
43. Gelfand, M. J., Strife, J. L., and Kereiakes, S. G.: Radionuclide bone imaging in spondylolysis of the lumbar spine in children. Radiology, 140:191–195, 1981.
44. Gill, G. G., and Binder, W. F.: Autoamputation of the first sacral nerve roots in spondyloptosis. Spine, 5:3, 295–297, 1980.
45. Gill, G. G., Manning, J. G., and White, H. L.: Surgical treatment of spondylolisthesis treated by arthrodesis. JAMA, 163:175, 1957.
46. Gill, G. G., Manning, J. G., and White, H. L.: Surgical treatment of spondylolisthesis without spine fusion. J. Bone Joint Surg., 37A:493, 1955.
47. Goldberg, M. J.: Gymnastic injuries. Orthop. Clin. North Am., 11:4, 717–726, 1980.
48. Goldstein, L. A., Haake, P. W., DeVanny, J. R., and Chou, P. K.: Guidelines for the management of lumbosacral spondylolisthesis associated with scoliosis. Clin. Orthop., 117:135, 1976.
49. Grogan, J. P., Hemminghytt, S., Williams, A. L., et al.: Spondylolysis studied with computed tomography. Radiology, 145:737–742, 1982.
50. Hammond, G., Wise, R. E., and Haggart, G. E.: Review of 73 cases of spondylolisthesis treated by arthrodesis. JAMA, 163:175, 1957.
51. Haraldsson, S., and Willner, S.: A comparative study of spondylolisthesis in operations on adolescents and adults. Arch. Orthop. Trauma Surg., 101:101–105, 1983.
52. Harrington, P. R., and Dickson, J. H.: Spinal instrumentation in the treatment of severe progressive spondylolisthesis. Clin. Orthop., 117:157, 1976.
53. Harrington, P. R., and Tullos, H. S.: Spondylolisthesis in children. Observation and surgical treatment. Clin. Orthop., 79:75, 1971.
54. Harris, I., and Weinstein, S. L.: Longterm followup of spondylolisthesis 50% or greater treated with or without posterior fusion. Orthop. Trans., 8:155, 1984.
55. Harris, R. I.: Spondylolisthesis. Ann. R. Coll. Surg. Engl., 8:259, 1951.
56. Harris, R. I.: Spondylolisthesis. In Nassim, R., and Burrows, H. J. (eds.): Modern Trends in Diseases of the Vertebral Column. London, Butterworth & Co., 1959.
57. Hensinger, R. N.: Spondylolysis and spondylolisthesis in children. Instructional Course Lectures, American Academy of Orthopaedic Surgeons. Vol. 32. St. Louis, C. V. Mosby Co., p. 132, 1983.
58. Hensinger, R. N., Lang, J. R., and MacEwen, G. D.: Surgical management of the spondylolisthesis in children and adolescents. Spine, 1:207, 1976.
59. Herbiniaux, G.: Traite sur divers accouchemens laborieux et sur les polypes de la matrice. Bruxelles, J. L. DeBoubers, 1782.
60. Hitchcock, H. H.: Spondylolisthesis: observations on its development, progression and genesis. J. Bone Joint Surg., 22:1, 1940.
61. Hodgson, A. R., and Wong, S. K.: A description of a technique and evaluation of results in anterior spinal fusion for deranged intervertebral disc and spondylolisthesis. Clin. Orthop., 56:133, 1968.
62. Howorth, B.: Low backache and sciatica: results of the surgical treatment. Part 3. Surgical Treatment of Spondylolisthesis. J. Bone Joint Surg., 46A:1515, 1964.
63. Huizenga, B. A.: Reduction of spondyloptosis with two-stage vertebrectomy. Orthop. Trans., 7:1, 21, 1983.
64. Ichikawa, N., Ohara, Y., Morishita, T., et al.: An aetiological study on spondylolysis from a biomechanical aspect. Br. J. Sports Med., 16:3, 135–141, 1982.
65. Inoue, S., Minami, S., Sho, E., and Ohki, I.: The results of anterior surgery in the treatment of spondylolisthesis. Presented at the 19th Annual Meeting of the Scoliosis Research Society, Orlando, Florida, Sept. 19–22, 1984.
66. Jackson, D. W., Wiltse, L. L., and Cirincione, R. J.: Spondylolysis in the female gymnast. Clin. Orthop., 117:68, 1976.
67. Jenkins, J. A.: Spondylolisthesis. Br. J. Surg., 24:80, 1936.
68. Johnson, R. M., and McQuire, E. J.: Urogenital complications of anterior approaches to the lumbar spine. Clin. Orthop., 154:114, 1981.
69. Kahnovitz, N., Bullough, P., and Jacobs, R.: The effect of internal fixation without arthrodesis on human facet joint cartilage. Orthop. Trans., 7:14, 1983.
70. Kettlekamp, D. B., and Wright, G. D.: Spondylolysis in the Alaskan Eskimo. J. Bone Joint Surg., 53A:563, 1971.
71. Kilian, H. F.: Schilderungen neuer eckenformen und ihres verhaltens in Leven. Mannheim, Verlag von Bassermann & Mathy, 1854.
72. Kirkaldy-Willis, W. H., Wedge, J. H., Yong-Hing,

K., and Riley, J.: Pathology and pathogenesis of lumbar spondylolysis and stenosis. Spine, 3:319, 1978.
73. Klinghoffer, L., and Murdock, M. G.: Spondylolysis following trauma, a case report and review of literature. Clin. Orthop., 166:72–74, 1982.
74. Krenz, J., and Troup, J. D. G.: The structure of the pars interarticularis of the lower lumbar vertebrae and its relation to the etiology of spondylolysis, with a report of the healing fracture in the neural arch of a fourth lumbar vertebra. J. Bone Joint Surg., 55B:735–41, 1973.
75. Lafond, G.: Surgical treatment of spondylolisthesis. Clin. Orthop., 22:175, 1962.
76. Lambl, W.: Beitrage zur geburtskunde un dynackologie. von F. W. V. Scanzoni, 1858.
77. Lance, E. M.: Treatment of severe spondylolisthesis with neural involvement: a report of two cases. J. Bone Joint Surg., 48A:883, 1966.
78. Laurent, L. E.: Spondylolisthesis. Acta Orthop. Scand., Suppl. 35, 1958.
79. Laurent, L. E., and Einola, S.: Spondylolisthesis in children and adolescents. Acta Orthop. Scand., 31:45, 1961.
80. Laurent, L. E., and Osterman, K.: Operative treatment of spondylolisthesis in young patients. Clin. Orthop., 117:85, 1976.
81. Laurent, L. E., and Osterman, K.: Spondylolisthesis in children and adolescents: a study of 173 cases. Acta Orthop. Belg., 35:717, 1969.
82. Louis, R., and Maresca, C.: Stabilisation chirurgicale avec reduction des spondylolysis et des spondylolisthesis. Int. Orthop., 1:215, 1977.
83. Lowe, R. W., Hayes, T. D., Kaye, J., et al.: Standing roentgenograms in spondylolisthesis. Clin. Orthop., 117:75, 1976.
84. Luque, E. R.: Segmental spinal instrumentation: a method of rigid internal fixation of the spine to reduce arthrodesis. Orthop. Trans., 4:391, 1980.
85. Lusskin, R.: Pain patterns in spondylolisthesis: a correlation of symptoms, local pathology, and therapy. Clin. Orthop., 40:123, 1965.
86. MacNab, I.: Negative disc exploration and analysis of the causes of nerve root involvement in 68 patients. J. Bone Joint Surg., 53A:891, 1971.
87. Mau, H.: Scoliosis and spondylolysis-spondylolisthesis. Arch. Orthop. Traumat. Surg., 99:29–34, 1981.
88. McAfee, P. C., and Yuan, H. A.: Computed tomography in spondylolisthesis. Clin. Orthop., 166:62–71, 1982.
89. McKee, B. W., Alexander, W. J., and Dunbar, J. S.: Spondylolysis and spondylolisthesis in children: a review. J. Can. Assoc. Radiol., 22:100, 1971.
90. McPhee, I. B., and O'Brien, J. P.: Scoliosis in symptomatic spondylolisthesis. J. Bone Joint Surg., 62B:2, 155–157, 1980.
91. Meyerding, H. W.: Low backache and sciatic pain associated with spondylolisthesis and protruded intervertebral disc. J. Bone Joint Surg., 23:461, 1941.
92. Meyerding, H. W.: Spondylolisthesis. Surg. Gynecol. Obstet., 54:371, 1932.
93. Micheli, L. J.: Low back pain in the adolescent: differential diagnosis. Am. J. Sports Med., 7:361, 1979.
94. Monticelli, G., and Ascani, E.: Spondylolysis and spondylolisthesis. Acta Orthop. Scand., 46:498, 1975.
95. Moreton, R. D.: So-called normal backs. Indust. Med. Surg., 28:216, 1969.
96. Moreton, R. D.: Spondylolisthesis. JAMA, 195:671, 1966.
97. Mosimann, P.: Die histologie der spondylolyse. Archiv. Orthop. Unfallchir., 53:264, 1961.
98. Munster, J. K., and Troup, J. D. G.: The structure of the pars interarticularis of the lower lumbar vertebrae and its relation to the etiology of spondylolysis. J. Bone Joint Surg., 55B:735, 1973.
99. Murray, R. D., and Colwill, M. R.: Stress fractures of the pars interarticularis. Proc. R. Soc. Med., 61:555–557, 1968.
100. Nachemson, A., and Wiltse, L. L.: Editorial comment: Spondylolisthesis. Clin. Orthop., 117:4, 1976.
101. Neithard, F. B.: Scheuermann's disease and spondylolysis. Orthop. Trans., 7:1, 103, 1983.
102. Neugebauer, F. L.: A new contribution to the history and etiology of spondylolisthesis. New Syndenham Society Selected Monographs 121(3):1, 1888.
103. Newman, P. H.: The etiology of spondylolisthesis. J. Bone Joint Surg., 45B:39, 1963.
104. Newman, P. H.: Surgical treatment for derangement of the lumbar spine. J. Bone Joint Surg., 55B:7, 1973.
105. Newman, P. H.: A clinical syndrome associated with severe lumbo-sacral subluxation. J. Bone Joint Surg., 47B:472, 1965.
106. Newman, P. H., and Stone, K. H.: The etiology of spondylolisthesis, with a special investigation. J. Bone Joint Surg., 45B:39, 1963.
107. Ohki, I., Inoue, S., Murata, T., et al.: Reduction and fusion of severe spondylolisthesis using halo-pelvic traction with wire reduction device. Int. Orthop., 4:107, 1980.
108. Osterman, K., Lindholm, T. S., and Laurent, L. E.: Late results of removal of the loose posterior arch(Gill's procedure) in the treatment of lytic lumbar spondylolisthesis. Clin. Orthop., 117:121, 1976.
109. Ota, H.: Spondylolysis: familial occurrence and its genetic implications. J. Jpn. Orthop. Assoc., 41:931–941, 1967.
110. Phalen, G. S., and Dickson, J. A.: Spondylolisthesis and tight hamstrings. J. Bone Joint Surg., 43A:505, 1961.
111. Piwnica, A., and Guillo, J. L.: Contribution a l'exploration fonctionnelle du rachis (analyse des contraintes par la methode photo-elasticimetrique). Ann. Chir., 12:1111, 1958.
112. Porter, R. W., and Park, W.: Unilateral spondylolysis. J. Bone Joint Surg., 64B:3, 344–348, 1982.
113. Reynolds, J. B., and Wiltse, L.: Surgical treatment of degenerative spondylolisthesis. Spine, 4:148, 1979.
114. Riley, P., and Gillespie, R.: Severe spondylolisthesis; results of postero-lateral fusion. Presented at the 19th Annual Meeting of the Scoliosis Research Society, Orlando, Florida, Sept. 19–22, 1984.
115. Riley, P., and Gillespie, R.: Severe spondylolisthesis: results of posterolateral fusion. Orthop. Trans., 9:119, 1985.

116. Risser, J. C., and Norquist, D. M.: Sciatic scoliosis in growing children. Clin. Orthop., 21:137–154, 1961.
117. Robert: Monatsschr. Geburtskunde U. Frauenkran., 5:81, 1855.
118. Roche, M. B.: Healing of bilateral fracture of the pars interarticularis of a lumbar neural arch. J. Bone Joint Surg., 32A:428, 1950.
119. Roche, M. B., and Rowe, G. G.: The incidence of separate neural arch and coincident bone variations. Anat. Rec., 109:233, 1951.
120. Rombold, C.: Treatment of spondylolisthesis by postero-lateral fusion, resection of pars interarticularis and prompt mobilization of the patient. J. Bone Joint Surg., 48A:1282, 1966.
121. Rosenberg, N. J.: Degenerative spondylolisthesis and surgical treatment. Clin. Orthop. Rel. Res., 117:112, 1976.
122. Rosenberg, N. J., Bargar, W. L., and Friedman, B.: The incidence of spondylolysis and spondylolisthesis in nonambulatory patients. Spine, 6:35, 1981.
123. Rosomoff, H. L.: Lumbar spondylolisthesis: etiology of radiculopathy and role of the neurosurgeon. Clin. Neurosurg., 27:577, 1980.
124. Rowe, G. G., and Roche, M. B.: The etiology of separate neural arch. J. Bone Joint Surg., 35A:102, 1953.
125. Scaglietti, O., Frontino, G., and Bartolozzi, P.: Technique of anatomical reduction of lumbar spondylolisthesis and its surgical stabilization. Clin. Orthop., 117:164, 1976.
126. Scaglietti, O., Frontino, G., and Bartolozzi, P.: Tecnica della ridozione de la spondelolistesi lombare esua contenzione definitiva. Atti S.I.O.T., 292:55, 1970.
127. Scherb, R.: Zur indikation und technik der albec de quervain operation. Schweiz. Med. Wochenschr., 20:763, 1921.
128. Schluter, K.: Form und struktur des normalen und des pathologisch veranderten Wirbels. Stuttgart, Hippokrates-Verlag, 1965.
129. Schults, A.: Age changes and variability in gibbons. A morphological study on a population sample of a man-like ape. Am. J. Physic. Anthrop., 2:11, 1944.
130. Sevastikoylov, J. A., Spangfort, E., and Aaro, S.: Operative treatment of spondylolisthesis in children and adolescents with tight hamstrings syndrome. Clin. Orthop., 147:192–199, 1980.
131. Shahriaree, H., Sajadi, K., and Rooholamini, S. A.: A family with spondylolisthesis. J. Bone Joint Surg., 61A:8, 1256–1258, 1979.
132. Sherman, F. C., Rosenthal, R. K., and Hall, J. C.: Spine fusion for spondylolysis and spondylolisthesis in children. Spine 4:59, 1979.
133. Sherman, F. C., Wilkinson, R. H., and Hall, J. E.: Reactive sclerosis of a pedicle and spondylolysis in the lumbar spine. J. Bone Joint Surg., 59A:49, 1977.
134. Shiloni, E., Wald, U., Robin, G. C., and Floman, Y.: Degenerative lumbar spinal stenosis. Israel J. Med. Sci., 16:9–10, 692, 1980.
135. Sijbrandij, S.: Reduction and stabilization of severe spondylolisthesis. J. Bone Joint Surg., 65B:40, 1983.
136. Snijder, J. G. N., Seroo, J. M., Snijder, C. J., and Schijvens, A. W. M.: Therapy of spondylolisthesis by repositioning and fixation of the olisthetic vertebra. Clin. Orthop., 117:149, 1976.
137. Stauffer, R. N., and Coventry, M. B.: Posterolateral lumbar spine fusion. J. Bone Joint Surg., 54A:1195, 1955.
138. Stewart, T. D.: The age indicence of neural arch defects in Alaskan natives, considered from the standpoint of etiology. J. Bone Joint Surg., 35A:937, 1953.
139. Taillard, W.: Le spondylolisthesis chez l'enfant et l'adolescent. Acta Orthop. Scand., 24:115, 1955.
140. Taillard, W.: Les spondylolisthesis. Paris, Masson & Cie, 1957.
141. Tojner, H.: Olisthetic scoliosis. Acta Orthop. Scand., 33:291, 1963.
142. Toland, J. J.: Spondylolisthesis in identical twins. Clin. Orthop., 5:184–189, 1955.
143. Troup, J. D. G.: Mechanical factors in spondylolisthesis and spondylolysis. Clin. Orthop., 117:59–67, 1976.
144. Turner, R. H., and Bianco, A. J., Jr.: Spondylolysis and spondylolisthesis in children and teenagers. J. Bone Joint Surg., 53A:1298, 1971.
145. van Rens, J. G., and van Horn, J. R.: Longterm results in lumbosacral interbody fusion for spondylolisthesis. Acta Orthop. Scand., 53:383–392, 1982.
146. Velikas, E. P., and Blackburne, J. S.: Surgical treatment of spondylolisthesis in children and adolescents. J. Bone Joint Surg., 63B:1, 67–70, 1981.
147. Verbiest, H.: Results of surgical treatment of idiopathic developmental stenosis of the lumbar vertebral canal. A review of 27 years experience. J. Bone Joint Surg., 59B:181, 1977.
148. Verbiest, H.: The treatment of lumbar spondyloptosis or impending lumbar spondyloptosis accompanied by neurologic deficit and/or neurogenic intermittent claudication. Spine, 4:68, 1979.
149. Vidal, J., Fassio, B., Buscayret, C. H., and Allieu, Y.: Surgical reduction of spondylolisthesis using a posterior approach. Clin. Orthop., 154:156–165, 1981.
150. Villiaumey, J.: Spondylolisthesis lombaire chez des jumeaux. Rev. Thum., 35:130–133, 1968.
151. Wertzberger, K. L., and Peterson, H. A.: Acquired spondylolysis and spondylolisthesis in the young child. Spine, 5:437, 1980.
152. Willis, T. A.: The separate neural arch. J. Bone Joint Surg., 13:709–721, 1931.
153. Wiltse, L. L.: Etiology of spondylolisthesis. Clin. Orthop., 10:48, 1957.
154. Wiltse, L. L.: Spondylolisthesis in children. Clin. Orthop., 21:156, 1961.
155. Wiltse, L. L.: Spondylolisthesis: classification and etiology. In American Academy of Orthopaedic Surgeons: Symposium on the Spine. St. Louis, C. V. Mosby Co., 1969.
156. Wiltse, L. L., and Jackson, D. W.: Treatment of spondylolisthesis and spondylolysis in children. Clin. Orthop., 117:92, 1976.
157. Wiltse, L. L., Newman, P. H., and Macnab, I.: Classification of spondylolysis and spondylolisthesis. Clin. Orthop., 117:23–29, 1976.
158. Wiltse, L. L., Widell, E. H., and Jackson, D. W.: Fatigue fracture: the basic lesion in isthmic

spondylolisthesis. J. Bone Joint Surg., 57A:17, 1975.
159. Wiltse, L. L., and Winter, R. B.: Terminology and measurement of spondylolisthesis. J. Bone Joint Surg., 65A:768, 1983.
160. Wynne-Davies, R., and Scott, J. H. S.: Inheritance and spondylolisthesis: a radiographic family survey. J. Bone Joint Surg., 61B:301, 1979.
161. Yano, T., Miyagi, S., and Ikari, T.: Studies of familial incidence of spondylolysis. Singapore Med. J., 8:203–206, 1967.

20

DEFORMITIES OF THE THORACIC AND LUMBAR SPINE SECONDARY TO SPINAL INJURY

David S. Bradford, M.D.

The management of acute and chronic injuries to the thoracic and lumbar spine remains a controversial subject. Deformities to the axial skeleton following trauma have only recently begun to receive the attention they rightfully deserve. In the past decade alone, a greater awareness and appreciation of acute and chronic complications associated with spinal injuries has resulted in a more rational basis for early and long-term management. It has become increasingly apparent that proper, expeditious, and intelligent treatment of acute injuries will tend to eliminate the late development of spinal deformity. On the other hand, the development of newer, more extensive classification systems assisted by computerized axial tomography, the development of more biomechanically sound instrumentation, and the more frequent use of rigid internal fixation and decompression for incomplete spinal cord injuries have stimulated controversy and led to confusion for practicing orthopaedic and neurologic surgeons.

It is the purpose of this chapter to review the current status of management of injuries to the thoracic and lumbar spine, to outline areas in which controversy remains, to define more precise guidelines for management, and to present more recent treatment results from our experience and that reported by others.

INITIAL EVALUATION AND EARLY TREATMENT

Fractures and dislocations to the spine vary considerably in severity and in the manner of presentation. Patients with mild anterior wedge compression fractures may present days or weeks after the initial injury with few complaints other than mild backache, and they may have a normal neurologic examination. On the other hand, patients may present acutely with a complete fracture-dislocation, marked bony comminution and ligament disruption, major organ system failure, and paraplegia. The initial evaluation and emergency treatment of patients in this latter category will obviously determine the success or failure of the treatment outcome.

Patients who have sustained spinal injury should be considered similar to patients presenting with polytrauma from any cause. Associated cardiopulmonary complications have been reported to occur in 40 per cent of patients, abdominal injury in 20 per cent, thromboembolic problems in 25 per cent, head and long bone fractures in 10 to 50 per cent, and secondary or multiple spinal fractures in 20 per cent.[38, 127] The initial evaluation and management of these patients for respiratory and cardiopulmonary failure and major visceral injuries may best be managed by a multidisciplinary team. The importance of thorough general physical evaluation accompanied by detailed neurologic evaluation that stresses rectal examination and evidence of sacral root spurring, cannot be overestimated. It is surprising how frequently these details are either omitted or not recorded.

Following initial stabilization of the patient, radiographic evaluation is carried out.

RADIOGRAPHIC EVALUATION
(Fig. 20–1)[74]

The radiographic evaluation of a patient with a spinal injury should be done expeditiously and with great care. It may be desirable to have the orthopaedic or the neurologic surgeon available to assist in handling the patient during the radiographic evaluation. Constant monitoring of vital signs and emergency support systems should be available in the radiology suite. The patient should be kept supine and log-rolled when necessary for special x-rays.

Initial evaluation should include AP and cross-table lateral x-rays of the entire spine. Inferior quality x-rays should be repeated. Careful attention should be directed toward visualizing soft tissues for evidence of paraspinal hematoma, hemothorax, or pneumothorax, or intraperitoneal fluid or air. Care should be taken, particularly in examining the bony structures and the spinal alignment. It may be difficult to assess the posterior

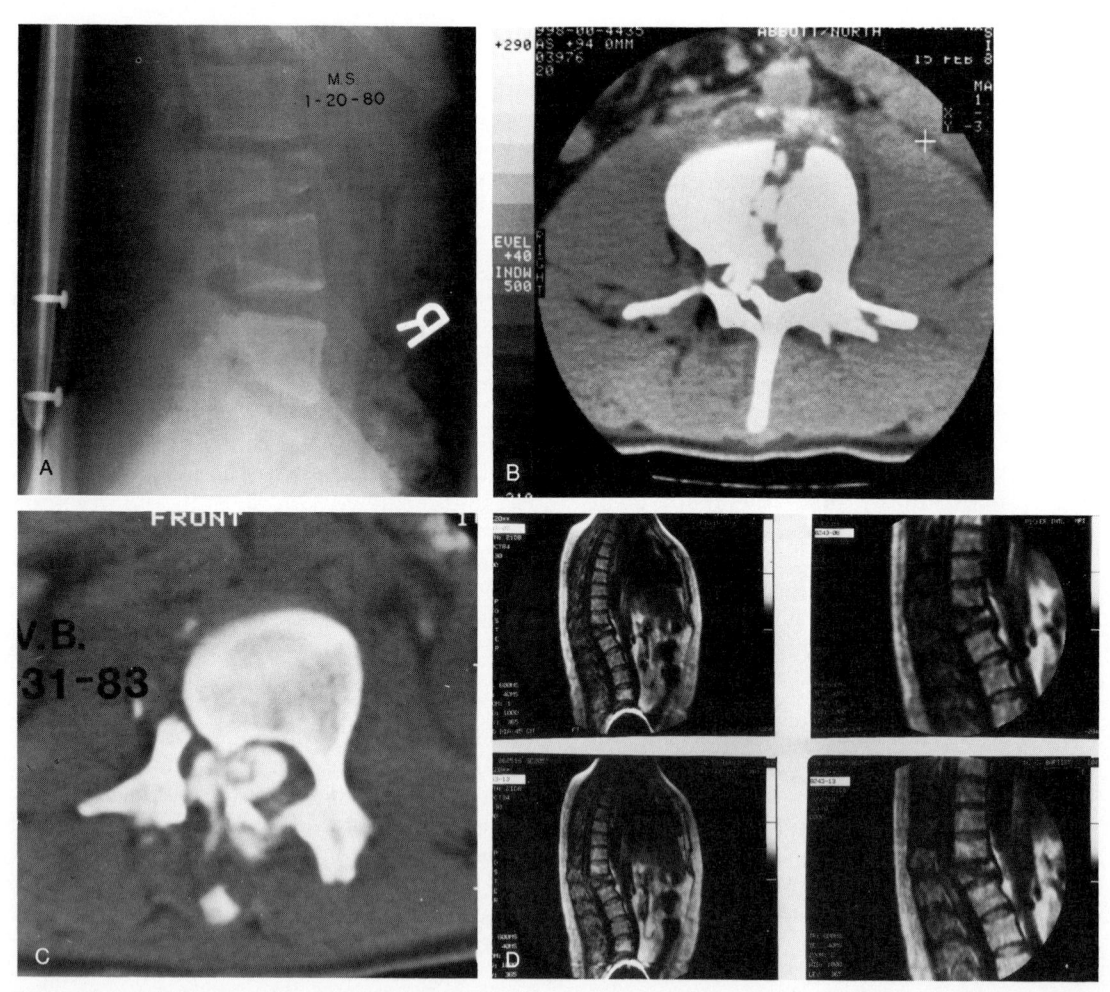

Figure 20–1. A, A burst fracture of L3 seen on routine lateral x-ray. B, The importance of CT scanning in evaluating the extent of canal encroachment and magnitude of anterior as well as posterior element injury is well demonstrated. C, A combined metrizamide CT scan is also helpful and may allow one to visualize a dural laceration. D, MRI (Magnetic Resonance Imaging) is proving increasingly useful in the initial evaluation of the patient with spinal injury.

structures because of overlying soft tissue shadows. As previously noted by Angtuaco and Binet,[1] even under the best of circumstances radiographs may underestimate the degree of injury to the spinal canal. Improper technique and poor patient positioning may lead to erroneous diagnoses.

If injury to a particular segment is suspected and cannot be well visualized, tomography may prove beneficial. Tomography can be done either in the frontal or lateral plane. During the tomographic procedure the patient must be immobilized and must hold his or her breath to facilitate a crisp, sharp image. Because of the greater detail provided, routine use of CT scans in evaluating fractures is now a common and preferable alternative.

Myelography might be considered and is preferred whenever the level of neurologic deficit does not correlate with the level of bony injury. Furthermore, if there is a suspected dural tear, myelography is extremely helpful. The use of a water-soluble agent, metrizamide, in association with CT scanning has proven extremely beneficial in the author's experience. In the acute setting, myelography may be performed through a C1 puncture or from a lumbar puncture site.

The use of computerized tomography has revolutionized the assessment and evaluation of the patient with a spinal injury.[1, 97, 105, 122] Sagittal and coronal reformatting are particularly useful when there is an associated dislocation. The advantages of CT scanning lie in its ability to totally visualize all the spinal elements and particularly the degree of retropulsion of bone into the spinal canal, the ability to reformat both in the sagittal and coronal planes, and the advantage of avoiding patient manipulation during the procedure. As pointed out by Angtuaco and Binet,[1] CT scanning is time-consuming, demands patient cooperation, and occasionally sagittal and coronal reformatting will overlook fine horizontal linear fractures of the vertebral body. Finally, soft tissue lesions within the spinal canal may be difficult to evaluate and may be assessed more accurately with interthecal contrast agents with CT scanning.[105] MRI (Magnetic Resonance Imaging) technology is so new at the time of this writing that its role in spinal injuries can not be fully assessed. Limited experience to date, however, suggests that its role will prove substantial.

Associated fractures and fracture patterns should be appreciated. Displaced sternal fractures are almost invariably associated with displaced thoracic spine fractures and failure to appreciate this may lead to further displacement and neurologic damage.[101] Three such patients with a painful thoracic kyphosis associated with a displaced spine fracture have presented to the author in the past 15 years. Although the patients were treated for the displaced sternal fracture and intrathoracic trauma, the spine fractures were not initially appreciated. Axial loading producing a burst type thoracolumbar fracture may often be associated with fractures of the os calcis and acute spondylolysis of L5. Oblique x-rays of L5 are indicated in our experience in burst injuries of the thoracolumbar spine to rule out this possibility.

MANAGEMENT OF THE NEUROLOGICALLY IMPAIRED PATIENT[4, 5, 38, 53, 54, 116]

Following initial assessment, resuscitative treatment, and radiographic evaluation of the patient with a spinal injury associated with neurologic deficit, a plan for management of the neurologic deficit and continued, ongoing care should be established. The neurologic deficit may be secondary to transection of the spinal cord or hematoma or edema in the cord, or secondary to extensive compression from bone or soft tissue, or a combination of both.[53] Although steroids, mannitol, oxygen, and spinal cord cooling have been advocated for treating these intrinsic causes,[53] there is no definite evidence that their use alters the neurologic course. On the other hand, extrinsic factors causing compression may be relieved by traction, fracture reduction, or surgical decompression. This will be discussed in a separate section. Ongoing care and prevention of complications of the respiratory, urinary, cardiovascular, digestive, and integumentary systems should be stressed, as these factors may ultimately determine the survival of the patient as well as the subsequent quality of life.[38, 111, 116]

Complications of the Respiratory System

Patients who have sustained trauma to the chest and associated spinal injury with paraplegia may be expected to have an increased incidence of atelectasis, pneumonia, and intrathoracic hemorrhage. Associated rib fractures are frequent in spinal injury patients, occurring in 25 per cent of all thoracic injuries. Increasing the risk of atelectasis and pneumonia in paraplegic patients are the following: neurologic level above T10, a history of smoking more than a pack a day for five or ten years, obesity, and recent general anesthesia. Associated rib fractures will likewise decrease the respiratory reserve and vital capacity. Respiratory dysfunction is indeed the greatest threat to survival, particularly in the patient with a high thoracic or cervical spinal cord injury. If the vital capacity drops below 1000 cc., respiratory insufficiency may be imminent.[38] A hemothorax should be evacuated, atelectasis and pneumonia treated vigorously, and fluid overload avoided.

Complications of the Cardiovascular System

Cardiac contusion and tears of the ascending aorta may be missed on initial evaluation. Subsequent widening of the mediastinum may be the first indication of a ruptured thoracic aorta. Electrocardiographic abnormalities associated with a widened mediastinum warrant an angiographic study and immediate repair of the aorta if a tear can be demonstrated. Deep venous thrombosis is not uncommon in paraplegics;[127] it has been reported in 15 per cent of these patients. It is suspected that the incidence is indeed much higher,[38] and it should be treated once the diagnosis is made.

Complications of the Genitourinary System

All patients with paralysis from spinal cord injuries should have an indwelling Foley catheter. This is important in order to monitor fluid balance and to prevent bladder distention from a paralyzed bladder. It should be remembered that spinal shock produces a sympathectomy-like effect and vasodilatation with peripheral pooling of the circulating blood volume and may result in a fall in urinary output. However, as Stauffer has pointed out, "unless there is a rapid increase in heart rate or other evidence of volume loss, continued intravenous replacement should not be administered to keep the pressure up."[116] After the third or fourth day when spinal shock effects are decreasing and the vasculature begins to regain its tone, urinary diuresis may occur. If the patient has had a fluid overload during this initial postresuscitative period, a shock-lung syndrome may develop further complicating the preexisting pulmonary insufficiency. Intermittent catheterization can begin after the diuresis occurs and the intake/output levels have stabilized. Bacterial counts greater than 100,000 colonies per cc., if developing during the acute stage, should be treated with the appropriate antibiotic.[38]

Complications of the Gastrointestinal System

Following spinal cord injury with paraplegia, a reflex ileus is common. Nasogastric drainage should be instituted, and the patient should be carefully watched for the development of gastrointestinal bleeding. This risk may be increased with the use of high dose steroids during the initial phases following injury. Under these circumstances, if steroids have been used, cimetidine should be used prophylactically and continued until the patient is on an oral diet. Antacids may likewise prove useful. Once bowel sounds have returned and the patient has started on oral supplementation, a bowel program should be begun to prevent fecal impaction. A reflex bowel evacuation program may be facilitated with the use of rectal suppositories and stimulants.

The nutritional aspects of care for spinal cord injury patients should be stressed. In those patients who have been treated acutely by rapid mobilization techniques, with or without surgery, this may not prove of great consequence. However, in those individuals who have sustained significant trauma and require repeated surgical insults for major visceral injuries, a long period of intravenous intake may result in marked weight loss and a negative caloric balance. Supplemental hyperalimentation either by nasogastric feeding or parenteral means should be initiated.

Complications of the Integumentary System

Decubital ulcers are one of the most catastrophic complications that occur in the spinal cord injured patient. Certainly, it is the most costly. Statistics have shown that it may increase the cost of hospitalization fivefold, and even in model systems, 20 per cent of all paraplegics may develop pressure ulcers. Most pressure sores occurred in spinal cord injured patients before such specialized units existed. Indeed it has been reported that patients who are referred to a spinal injury center later than six weeks after their injury had a 35 per cent incidence of pressure sores. Frequent turning of the patients, at least every two hours, especially in the first few days after injury and protecting all body prominences each time the patient is turned should prevent pressure ulcerations. This procedure is much more effective than the use of specialized beds, mattresses, or mechanical devices.[54]

CLASSIFICATION OF SPINE FRACTURES

Classification of spinal injuries has recently undergone a considerable reassessment because of the advent of computerized axial tomography. With the use of this superior technique for radiographic evaluation of the spine, it is now possible to reconstruct precisely the extent of bony and soft tissue injury. Classification schemes have expanded as a consequence,[29, 90] and the concept of stability and instability, far from being solved, has now become an increasingly complex issue. Most classification schemes have evolved from a mechanistic biomechanical comparison of possible force vectors compared with radiographic evaluation. Bohler, in 1944, identified five different mechanisms of spinal injury, and described them as: flexion, extension, rotation, shear, and axial load.[10] Nicole,[96] in 1949, classified injuries as either being stable or unstable, depending on whether the interspinous ligament was intact or ruptured. Roaf, in 1960,[109] carried out a study on the mechanics of spinal injury, noting the contribution of the intervertebral disc to the force vectors and ultimate endplate damage, and noted that the forces of rotation and compression could produce almost any type of spinal injury.

Holdsworth, in 1963,[60] defined the concept of the posterior ligament complex, consisting of interspinous and superspinous ligaments, capsules of the lateral joints, and the ligamentum flavum. He felt the integrity of this complex was essential for spinal stability. Holdsworth's classification of spinal injuries was based on the concept of stable lesions vs. unstable ones as defined by the integrity or lack thereof of the posterior ligament complex. Stable injuries were classified as simple anterior wedge fractures, burst fractures, or extension injuries, whereas unstable injuries were classified as dislocations, rotational fracture dislocations, and shear fractures.

Kelly and Whitesides[75] subsequently developed the concept of a two-column structure of the spine, an anterior column resisting compression and a posterior column resisting tensile forces. Although a mechanistic concept of fractures was not stressed, a stability concept was elucidated by this comparison. For instance, if the anterior column could not withstand compression forces and progressive kyphosis developed, or if the posterior column could not withstand tensile forces again leading to kyphosis or deformity, instability was present.

Kaufer[72] and White and Punjabi[120,121] considered the mechanisms of spinal injury by describing the relationship of one vertebral segment to another in the conventional X-Y-Z axes of three-dimensional space. This concept presupposed six degrees of freedom in spinal motion: rotation around three axes, as well as translation. Angular motion around these three axes includes flexion and extension, lateral bending, and rotation, while non-angular motion (translation) includes distraction and compression, anterior/posterior shear, and lateral shear (Fig. 20–2).

More recently, Denis[29] has proposed a three column spine concept for classifying thoracic and lumbar spinal injuries, noting as others have proposed that the posterior ligament complex alone is insufficient to create instability in flexion and extension and rotation and shear (Fig. 20–3).[106, 120] He proposed a middle column between the anterior and posterior columns that was formed by the posterior longitudinal ligament, the posterior anulus fibrosus, and the posterior wall of the vertebral body. His classification scheme is extensive and complex and contains more than 20 divisions; however, it does call important attention to retropulsion of bone, which was not well appreciated prior to CT scanning.

McAfee[89] has extended the three column concept and developed a simplified classification system based on three forces as they act to injure the middle column: axial

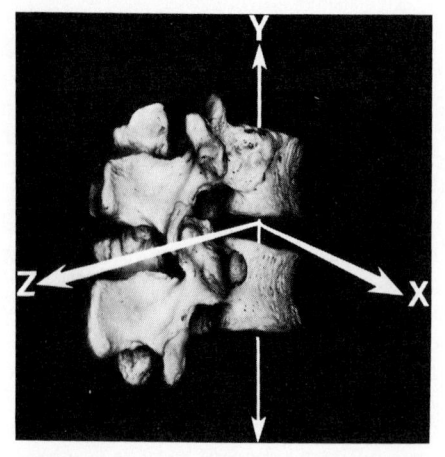

Figure 20–2. A useful technique in assessing possible mechanisms of injury and describing the relationship of one vertebral segment to the other around the conventional x, y, and z axes. This technique proposes 6 degrees of freedom in spinal motion. That is, rotation around three axes as well as translation around three axes. On viewing x-rays after injury and considering this system, a reasonable calculation of possible mechanisms involved in the injury may be deduced.

compression, axial distraction, and translation within the transverse plane. He then defined six types of fractures: compression fractures, stable burst fractures, unstable burst fractures, Chance fractures, flexion/distraction injuries, and translational injuries.

Ferguson and Allen[44] have extended these previous observations and have further refined the mechanistic classification of thoracolumbar spine fractures. They also noted that although the separation of the spinal column into three regions is useful for accurately assessing by computerized tomography the various components of injury, the three column concept is anatomically and biomechanically incorrect. They have suggested that spine fractures be classified into compressive/flexion, distractive/flexion, lateral/flexion, translation torsional flexion, vertical compression, and distractive extension injuries.

CONCEPT OF STABILITY AND INSTABILITY

Spinal instability is a loosely used term that has proven ambiguous, imprecise, and confusing.[17] In fact, because of the more extensive radiographic evaluation available with CT scanning, surgical indications are now being extended to types of fractures[30, 90] (e.g., burst fractures without neurologic deficit) not previously felt to require surgery.[61] Indeed, the term instability has implied that the fracture must be surgically stabilized,[50] and these decisions, as Gaines has summarized,[49] appear to have been based on radiographic criteria alone.[35, 45, 110] It is readily apparent that this increasing operative trend is more evident in North America than Europe.[3, 48, 56] What is also missing from these classification schemes is the element of time. This has not been considered. The fact that unstable injuries may become stable with non-operative treatment is a concept that is unfortunately too frequently forgotten.

White and Panjabi[120] have defined instability of the spine as a loss of the body's ability to maintain normal relationships between the vertebrae under physiologic loads in such a way that damage and subsequent irritation to the spinal cord or nerve roots do not occur, and in addition that incapacitating deformity or pain from structural changes does not develop. Posner and coworkers[104] have further developed a checklist for diagnosing clinical instability of the thoracic and lumbar spine. This may indeed prove helpful in more precisely defining whether a fracture is stable or not. These criteria are useful because the focus is directed toward the three major components of subsequent disability from an injury, that is, neurologic damage, pain, and deformity. It is apparent that many spinal injuries not associated with neurologic damage may subsequently develop increasing kyphosis and incapacitating pain. On the other hand, there are those lesions associated with such great instability that neurologic deficit may occur post-injury from faulty patient

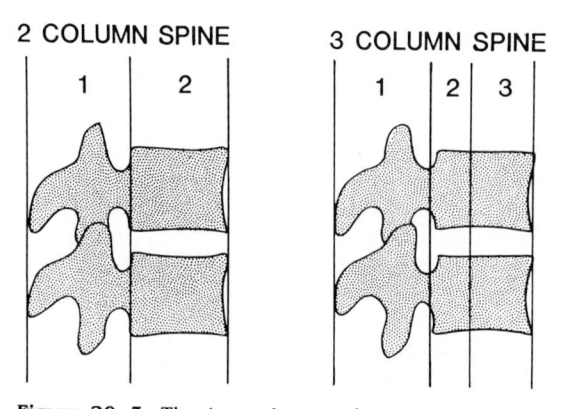

Figure 20–3. The two-column spine concept and a three-column spine concept (see text).

handling. The concept, therefore, of acute and chronic instability is worthwhile.[17] Acute instability implies a fracture that is capable of further displacement soon or immediately after injury with progressive or immediate neurologic damage. Chronic instability implies injury that may further angulate, producing greater deformity months or years after the injury. With the slow increase of deformity, progressive neurologic deterioration could occur as a result of subsequent vertebral angulation.[17, 72] In the former category, that of acute instability, would be included those fractures associated with dislocation and loss of all ligamentous support, for instance, flexion-rotation injuries or translational displacement injuries. On the other hand, burst fractures developing from axial loading with residual soft tissue support or multiple compression (anterior wedge fractures over contiguous segments) may lead to late kyphosis or further retropulsion of vertebral bone resulting in steady but progressive neurologic deterioration.[118]

It should be stressed again that stability remains a relative term and should not necessarily be equated with the indication for surgery. Careful assessment of each patient, the functional demands and rehabilitation needs, and associated injuries, plus a clear understanding of the natural history of each type of injury with or without surgical treatment, the surgical skills of the operating team, the risk benefit ratio of surgery, and the expertise of spinal injury care must all be weighed carefully in deciding the most appropriate form of treatment.

TREATMENT OF THORACIC AND LUMBAR SPINE FRACTURES

Non-operative Treatment

The past ten years have demonstrated a marked increase in the tendency for operative management of spinal fractures. What is often forgotten is that satisfactory if not good results may be obtained with non-operative treatment. As mentioned previously, instability as defined radiographically does not necessarily equate with an indication for surgery. It may be true in certain cases that stability may be furnished more rapidly with surgical treatment, but this growing tendency for operative management, particularly in North America, should not be misconstrued as a definitive statement that non-operative techniques have failed and are no longer valid. The pioneering work of Guttman,[56] Frankel,[48] and Bedbrook,[3, 7, 8] to mention a few, have demonstrated that non-operative treatment of fractures does not mean no treatment but rather that carefully carried out methods of postural reduction and intensive nursing care in sophisticated spinal injury units may lead to satisfactory results in most cases.[128] The method of postural reduction appears to have been first described by Malgaine in 1847.[86] This consists of positioning lumbar pillows to maintain lumbar lordosis and frequent turning of the patients until the fractures become stable through soft tissue and bony healing. It is noted by Bedbrook,[4] that well over 70 per cent of injuries can be functionally reduced, but the reduction must be maintained over a period of six to eight weeks. It has been pointed out as well that nursing care of the patients with these injuries is of crucial importance, and sophisticated care in centers accustomed to managing spinal injuries is essential for this success.

More recently, Burke[22] has reported experience in 115 patients with thoracic and lumbar spine injuries with neurologic involvement. Eighty-nine received conservative treatment and 26 surgical treatment. Surgery, in general, was reserved for patients with irreducible dislocations and complete neurologic lesions. Only three patients required delayed spinal fusion for suspected instability after a period of conservative treatment. Spinal pain was more common in those patients who had undergone posterior surgical procedures. They noted that neurologic recovery was not necessarily correlated with surgical stabilization but rather with the incomplete nature of the neurologic lesion with its better prognosis. Davis and associates,[28] in 1980, reviewed 34 patients treated non-operatively, noting that the neurologic recovery rate was the same in comparison with previous surgical reviews; they felt that non-operative methods were adequate in achieving reduction and maintenance of displacement. They felt surgery should be limited to those cases in which an unsuccessful reduction was obtained by conservative means, there was a dislocation with locked facets, the patient was irritable and restless and could not tolerate postural reduction methods, and the separation of the vertebral bodies was to such a degree that soft tissue in a position of non-union was likely.

What remains controversial is the optimal treatment for those patients with fractures classified as burst injuries. In the absence of neurologic deficit, McEvoy and Bradford,[92] Mino,[93] and Willen[126] have noted good results with conservative treatment, whereas Bohlman,[11] McAfee,[90] and Denis[30] have recommended surgical treatment. Of interest was the fact that in McEvoy and Bradford's series those patients treated surgically had the same incidence of pain and similar degrees of kyphosis at follow-up as those treated non-operatively.

On the other hand, Soreff,[114] in reviewing 147 thoracolumbar spine fractures, noted a high incidence of residual deformity in patients treated by conservative means who were followed more than eight years. Dorr and coworkers[39] likewise found that in flexion/rotation injuries the results were not as satisfactory at follow-up in those patients treated by non-surgical methods as in those treated surgically. The high incidence of pain in patients treated conservatively as reported by Lewis and McKibben[82] (64 per cent), Nicoll[96] (69 per cent), and Osebold[98] (71 per cent) adds further complexity to this issue.

Operative Treatment

Operative treatment of spinal fractures consists of stabilization by internal fixation and spinal fusion and/or decompression.

STABILIZATION

As previously mentioned, stabilization of radiographically determined unstable spinal injuries does not necessarily or should not necessarily equate with the insertion of a surgical implant. If the spine is properly immobilized and reduced, stabilization may occur with biological healing of the fracture. It is apparent, however, that stabilization may be more rapidly furnished with the use of an internal implant system. Although open reduction and internal fixation of fractures was proposed by Holdsworth,[62] Hardy,[57] Dick,[34] and others, the technique's development fell into dispute when Guttman[55] in 1969, reviewed over 100 patients in whom open reduction with metal plates fastened to the spinous processes had been carried out. He concluded that this particular method did not prevent redislocation regardless of what type of plate was used. Harrington developed an implant system in 1960;[58] later reports indicated that this technique of stabilization shortened the period for rehabilitation as much as 400 per cent.[45] More recently, Jacobs and associates[66, 67] showed rather conclusively, as have others, that recumbent time is decreased and rehabilitation time is shortened with the use of instrumentation. For paraplegic patients in his series the time between treatment and wheelchair immobilization was reduced from 10.5 weeks with recumbent treatment to 5.3 weeks with Harrington instrumentation. The rehabilitation time in ambulatory candidates was decreased from 7.1 weeks to 2.5 weeks. Convery also reported a 50 per cent reduction in total hospitalization cost with the use of internal fixation. The decreased hospitalization time, ease of nursing care, and early immobilization of the patient have all been stressed.[35, 45, 129]

Recent work by Lewis and McKibben[82] suggests that patients undergoing open reduction and internal fixation of unstable thoracolumbar spine fractures are also less likely to develop residual spinal deformity and subsequent serious back pain. However, increased neurologic function by internal fixation of fractures with the Harrington device has not been demonstrated.[35, 43, 115] The urgency of the surgical procedure, the type of implant, and the length of fusion remain controversial. It is apparent that if stabilization is felt indicated, earlier surgery is more likely to lead to a better reduction of the fracture.

Harrington distraction implants are the most commonly used devices.[71] They serve to lengthen the shortened spinal segments and counteract axial compression forces. The disadvantages lie in the compromised ability to counteract torsional forces with their limited usefulness in those fractures associated with posterior tension failure.[44] In fact, the author feels they are contraindicated in pure distraction seatbelt type injuries of the spine. Increased stability may be obtained in association with sublaminar wiring or spinous process wiring to the rods, and the production or maintenance of lordosis may be facilitated by using a Moe square-end hook and bending the rod into lordosis.[31, 50, 117] It should be stressed, however, that the rod is best used as a three-point fixation device and that excessive distraction should be avoided at all costs. Indeed, distraction forces alone may serve to produce cord ischemia, and this fact must be appreciated.[27, 37] To counteract overdistraction, a Harrington compression rod may be used in association with a distraction rod. Compression implants have proven particularly useful in fractures associated with tension failure. In distraction type injuries or in post traumatic kyphosis, compression implants posteriorly have been recommended.[18] They may, however, not counter axial loads on the middle element, and in the case of burst fractures their use may result in increased retropulsion of bone fragments into the spinal canal.[16, 44]

Segmental instrumentation with L-rods has been advocated in shear type fractures in which the middle element is intact.[44, 83, 119] When there is middle element failure (i.e., burst fractures), a Harrington distraction implant (with sublaminar wiring) that counteracts axial loading would prove preferable if the posterior approach is felt indicated.[9, 21]

Roy-Camille plates may be most advantageous.[112] Although they have not been used extensively in this country, they can furnish excellent stability in flexion, lateral bend, and torque and may well prove the most stable of all implant systems. However, for the uninitiated, they likewise may be the most difficult to use.[76]

Anterior spinal implants as described by Dunn,[41, 42] Kaneda,[70] Kostuick,[78, 79] and others have also been recommended for managing spinal fractures. Their major advantage lies in a direct approach to the injury and pathology, which is usually anterior.

Although it is evident that more rapid mobilization and rehabilitation may be facilitated with operative treatment of unstable spinal fractures and that a possible decreased incidence of late deformity and pain may be the result, these are by no means a foregone conclusion.[63] Complications following Harrington instrumentation and thoracolumbar fractures may be substantial. In a recent review by McAfee and Bohlman,[88] 40 of their patients undergoing 43 Harrington stabilization procedures had major complications—two patients died, one from cardiopulmonary arrest and the other from respiratory failure following progression of the neurologic deficit, 11 patients had unsuccessful reduction and spinal malalignment, and 17 patients demonstrated significant residual spinal cord impingement. It is readily apparent that the technique is exacting and should be performed only in those centers accustomed to managing spinal cord injured patients and by surgeons with demonstrated expertise in surgical treatment of spinal deformities. A good procedure poorly executed will lead to a poor result.

DECOMPRESSION

Decompression of the spinal cord or cauda equina may be accomplished by (1) reduction of the fracture and (2) anterior removal of bone in the canal. This removal of bone anteriorly may be accomplished through a posterior lateral approach,[43, 45] an extracavitary approach,[12, 81] or a formal transthoracic thoracoabdominal anterior approach.[15, 20] Since the natural history of incomplete spinal cord and cauda equina lesions is to some degree favorable, the claim that decompression by removal of bone in the spinal canal does affect a greater neurologic return has been difficult to substantiate. An increasing number of authors, however, have stated that anterior decompression does facilitate a favorable neurologic return.[12, 13, 18, 19, 44, 47, 68, 79, 81, 101, 102, 108, 125, 130] It is likewise now accepted that laminectomy alone is of no value, and it has been rightfully abandoned as a routine procedure for decompressing spinal cord injuries in which the compression is anterior.[39, 94, 95] On the other hand, spinal injury associated with post traumatic spinal epidural hematoma may well be benefited by laminectomy, especially in patients without spine fracture.[46]

The question remains, however, Does complete decompression through the anterior approach affect a more complete neurologic recovery than would be expected from natural history of incomplete neurologic lesions associated with spinal fractures in which bone is retropulsed into the spinal canal? Dolan has shown the value of decompression for acute experimental spinal cord compression injuries and has documented the deleterious effect of continued cord compression and the importance of early decompression in effecting neurologic recovery.[36] Late spinal cord decompression months and years after initial injuries in patients who remain neurologically incomplete has been shown to be advantageous in effecting neurologic improvement. This has been reported in thoracic spine fractures in which cord elements alone were involved[13, 18] as well as in cord, conus, and cauda equina lesions.[19, 84, 103] In a recent report by Maiman,[84] 17 or 20 patients treated by late anterior decompression showed improvement in neurologic function, although one patient underwent a late decompression as long as five years after the original injury and original surgery. Bradford and McBride[19] recently reported experience on 59 patients who were operatively treated for thoracic and lumbar spine fractures with incomplete neurologic deficits. Follow-up CT scans were obtained in all patients an average of 3.7 years after injury. The 20 patients who underwent initial anterior decompression showed the most complete decompression, with a more favorable neurologic return and follow-up. Eight of the patients who had undergone posterior procedures that showed residual compression of 25 per cent stenosis of the canal or more and who demonstrated a residual neurologic deficit underwent a delayed anterior decompression. (Six of the eight patients had plateaued neurologically; one patient was treated six years following his original surgery.) In spite of the time interval, all patients showed increased neurologic function following delayed anterior decompression. These authors suggested and recommended that complete decompression should be carried out in all patients with spinal fractures associated with incomplete neurologic deficits.

If incomplete neurologic deficits indeed appear to be greatly improved by complete decompression, what about complete cord injuries in the absence of neurologic transection? Conventional wisdom has stated that complete lesions are not reversible, and as a consequence decompression would not be indicated. However, it is readily apparent that in the first 24 hours following a severe injury to the spinal cord the reflex activity in the cord segments distal to the level of injury is diminished or absent all together. Consequently, the completeness of the lesion or the incompleteness thereof may not be accurately assessed in the initial period after injury. The reappearance of reflex activity in the complete absence of motor and sensory function distal to the level of injury confirms the diagnosis of a complete spinal cord lesion.[61, 116] Also, the assessment of the completeness of an injury at the thoracolumbar junction where peripheral nerve and cord elements are present is difficult if not impossible on the initial evaluation. Dunn[41] has recently reported a favorable neurologic recovery in several patients with "complete" lesions treated by early decompression. In light of these results, we feel that a reassessment of early decompression even in complete cord lesions in the absence of cord transection is certainly indicated.

Routine decompression for radiographic evidence of compression without evidence of neurologic damage appears difficult to justify. Although some authors have reported late neurologic complications from burst injuries that were initially intact neurologically,[30] this, in the author's experience, has been a most uncommon and unlikely event.[92] The author and others have found that late decompression can be performed with low risk and excellent results.[13, 19, 84] In the acute situation, on the other hand, if stabilization is felt indicated on the basis of the spinal injury and if there is radiographic evidence of compression, then decompression at the time of stabilization could be considered, particularly if the anterior approach has been elected.

AUTHOR'S PREFERRED METHOD OF TREATMENT

In order to establish a basis for operative or non-operative treatment, the fractures may be grouped into four major categories based on the radiographic appearance at the time the patient is initially evaluated. From the radiographic studies one may often establish a mechanism of injury that will facilitate a plan of management. It should be appreciated, however, that any displacement noted on x-ray may be far less than that occurring at the moment of impact,[61] and this may indeed account for the variation of neurologic deficit and the inability to correlate the amount of displaced bone with the extent of the deficit.

WEDGE COMPRESSION FRACTURES
(Figs. 20–4 and 20–5)

Anterior wedge compression fractures occur in the thoracic spine and are demonstrated radiographically by failure of the anterior column. The posterior cortical shell of the vertebral body or the middle column is visualized on lateral x-rays, lateral tomograms, or CT scans and show no evidence of bony damage. In other words, the ring surrounding the spinal cord remains intact. Radiographically these lesions rarely show greater than 50 per cent compression of the

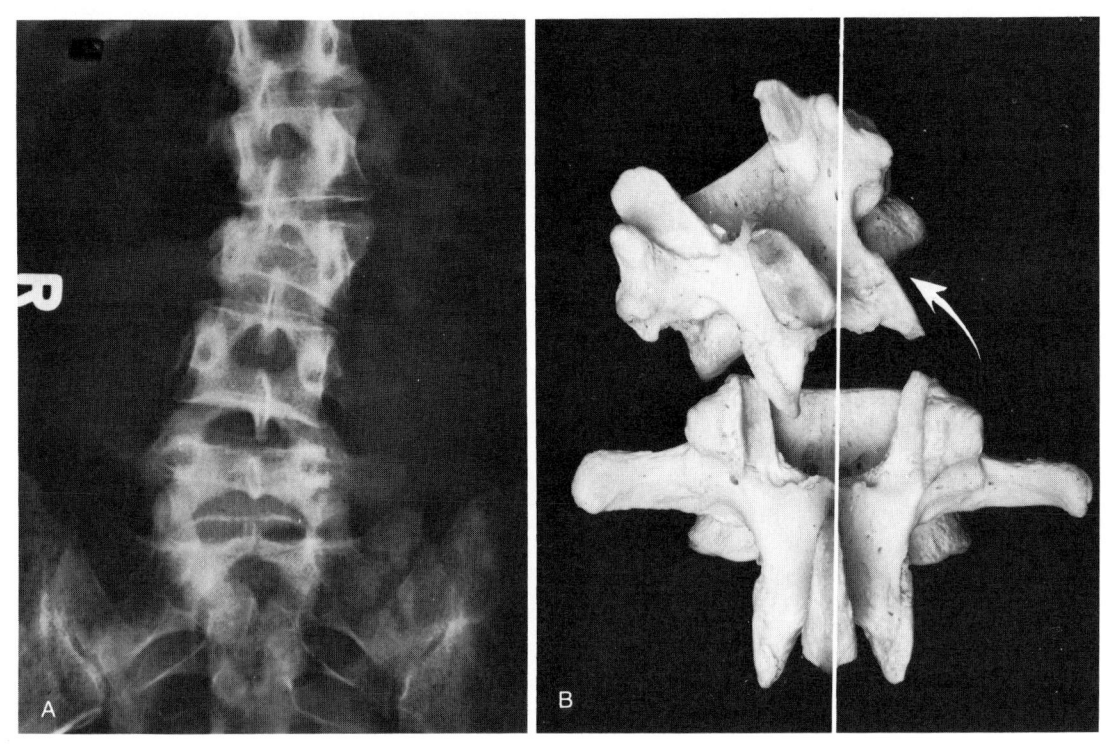

DEFORMITIES OF THE THORACIC AND LUMBAR SPINE SECONDARY TO SPINAL INJURY 445

Figure 20–4. *A* and *B*, A lateral wedge fracture and its likely mechanism of production.

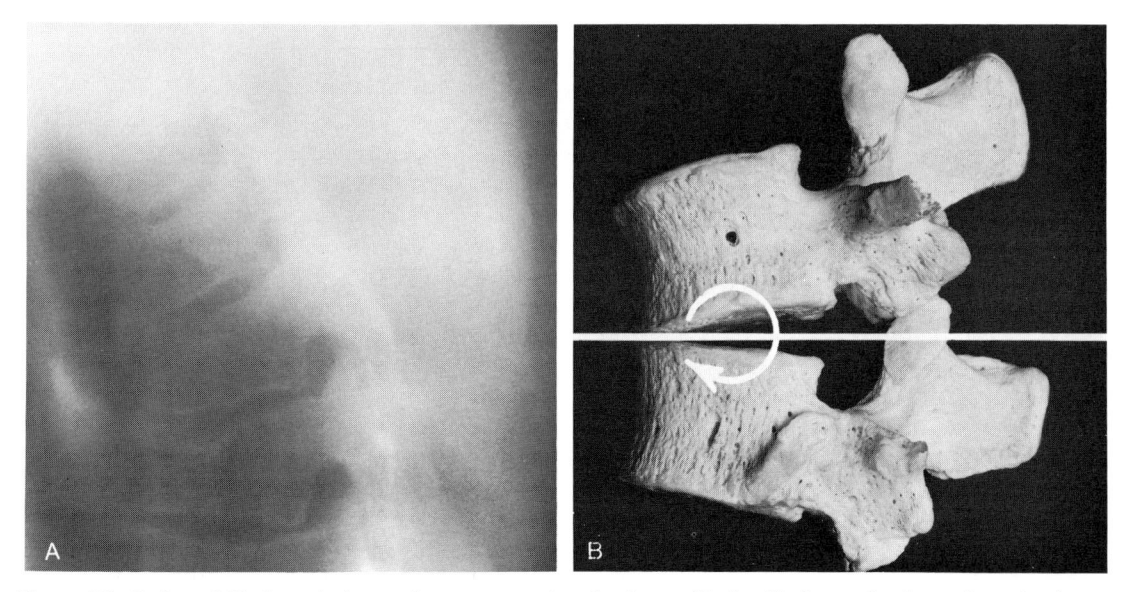

Figure 20–5. *A* and *B*, An anterior wedge compression fracture with the likely mechanism of production. It should be noticed that the posterior vertebral body height has not been compromised. With more severe degrees of wedging (more than 30 to 40 per cent) posterior column disruption is common. Lateral tomography should be obtained in all these injuries to rule out this possibility.

anterior portion of the vertebral body, infrequently collapse further, and rarely if ever cause a neurologic deficit. They may, for the most part, be virtually ignored, and the patient may be treated symptomatically and ambulated early with either an underarm brace of a plaster body jacket, depending upon the magnitude of complaints. Progressive settling may occur on occasion but this is usually in the older osteoporotic patient. Continued pain and disability lasting more than six months to one year after injury would be an indication for stabilization. In these situations, an anterior or posterior fusion in situ would be sufficient. If the patient has significant late deformity and correction is deemed advisable, a combined anterior and posterior approach may be preferred.[85]

Multiple compression fractures of the thoracic spine associated with significant kyphosis are satisfactorily managed by posterior instrumentation techniques alone. In these cases, segmental instrumentation with spinal fusion is usually adequate. Anterior fusion is generally not necessary but could be considered as well if there is marked loss of bone stock and a significant kyphosis of greater than 75 degrees.

More severe degrees of wedged compression fractures are almost invariably associated with posterior element disruption. This has been classified as a Type II compression/flexion injury by Ferguson and Allen.[44] In all patients with wedge compression fractures, careful evaluation of lateral x-rays and lateral tomography and CT scanning is necessary to rule out posterior element disruption. Although these injuries may be managed by non-operative means, the author has favored posterior reduction and stabilization with either Harrington compression rods or L-rods with sublaminar wiring, avoiding passing wires under the involved lamina. If there is impingement on neurologic tissues by the posterior element, decompression should be carried out with the stabilization procedure. As a general rule, combined anterior and posterior procedures in these cases are usually not necessary.

Lateral wedge compression fractures are not as common as anterior wedge compression injuries. These injuries result from a lateral bending force and lead to lateral compression of the vertebral body, fracture of the pedicle, and fracture of the posterior facet on the involved side. These injuries rarely require surgical treatment and can be managed by conservative methods with early ambulation. Retropulsion of bone into the spinal canal associated with the neurologic deficit is most uncommon but if present may be handled by anterior decompression followed by anterior stabilization. In these cases it is best to approach the spine on the compressed side of the deformity. If there is retropulsion of bone into the canal, the author has preferred to classify this injury as a burst fracture (described subsequently), since the management follows similar guidelines.

DISTRACTION INJURIES
(Fig. 20–6)[73, 113]

Distraction injuries of the spine are most commonly referred to as "seatbelt" injuries. They may consist of the classic Chance fracture,[25] occurring through the spinous process, pedicle, vertebral body, or through the soft tissue alone, or a combination involving bone and soft tissue. These injuries are usually associated with some degree of flexion, but the flexion axis is anterior to the anterior longitudinal ligament. If the injury occurs through the bony elements alone, casting or bracing in extension is sufficient to allow bony healing. However, if there is dislocation of the facet joints and the lesion occurs through soft tissue alone, open reduction and internal fixation through the posterior approach is the treatment of choice (Fig. 20–7). Distraction implants should be avoided in this group; the preferable implant is a Harrington compression system, which may be applied over the involved segments. If the spinous processes are adequate, following reduction, simple wiring of adjacent spinous processes may be sufficient (Fig. 20–8).

BURST FRACTURES

Perhaps no area in spinal reconstructive surgery is more controversial than the management of burst injuries. The classification, the definition of instability, and the indication for stabilization and/or decompression remain subjects of great confusion. It is apparent that the concept of burst injuries as originally described by Holdsworth[61] developed from axial loading; the ligamentous support was intact, providing a framework for long-term stability at least in shear. With

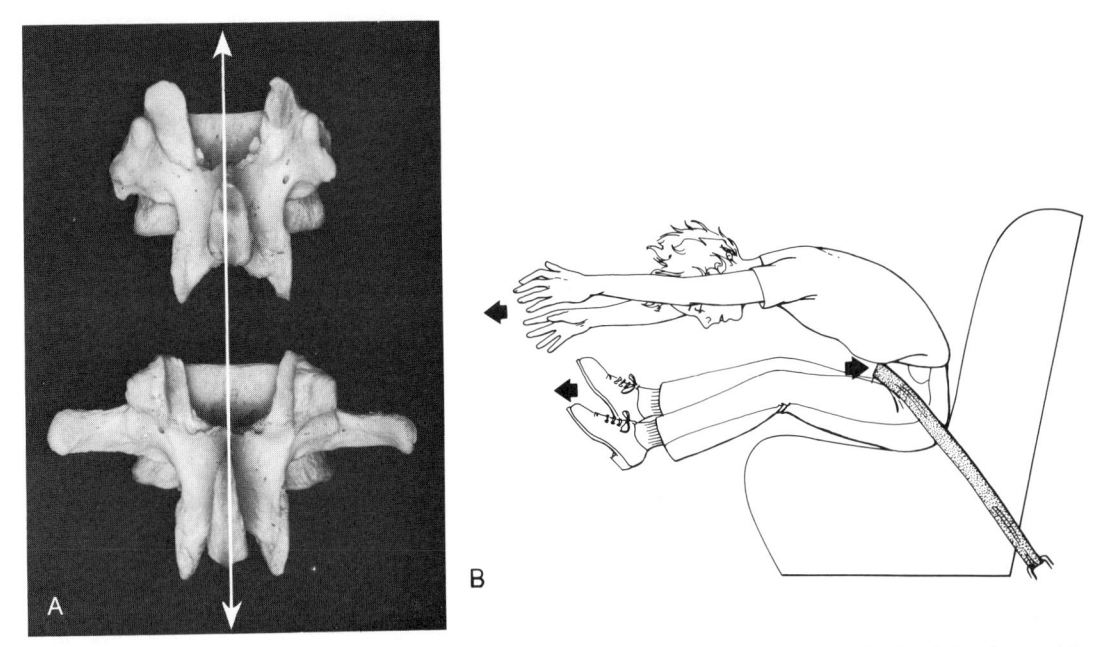

DEFORMITIES OF THE THORACIC AND LUMBAR SPINE SECONDARY TO SPINAL INJURY 447

Figure 20–6. *A,* Distraction injuries of the spine usually occur with some component of flexion following sudden deceleration where the pelvis is held fixed, such as the so-called seat belt injury (*B*).

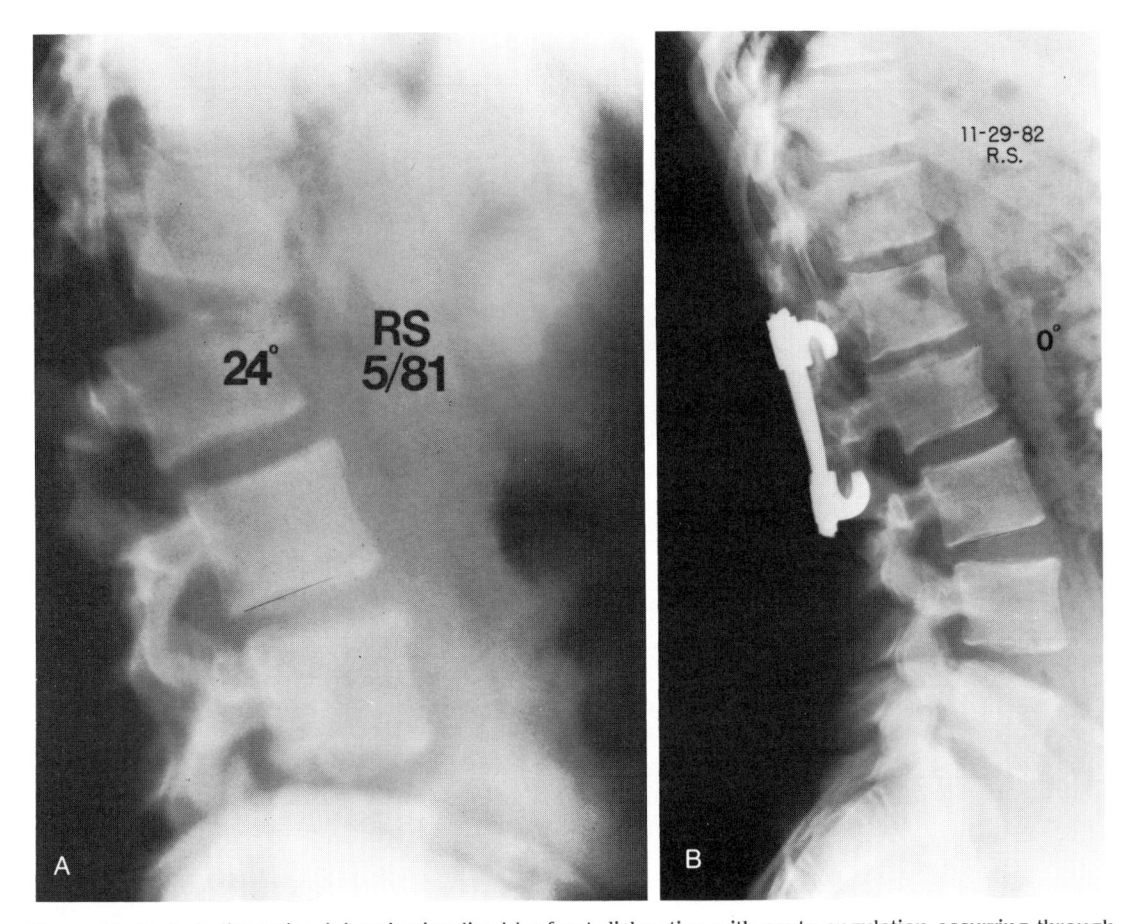

Figure 20–7. *A,* A distraction injury is visualized by facet dislocation with acute angulation occurring through the disc space. *B,* Following open reduction and compression rod instrumentation, anatomic realignment has occurred.

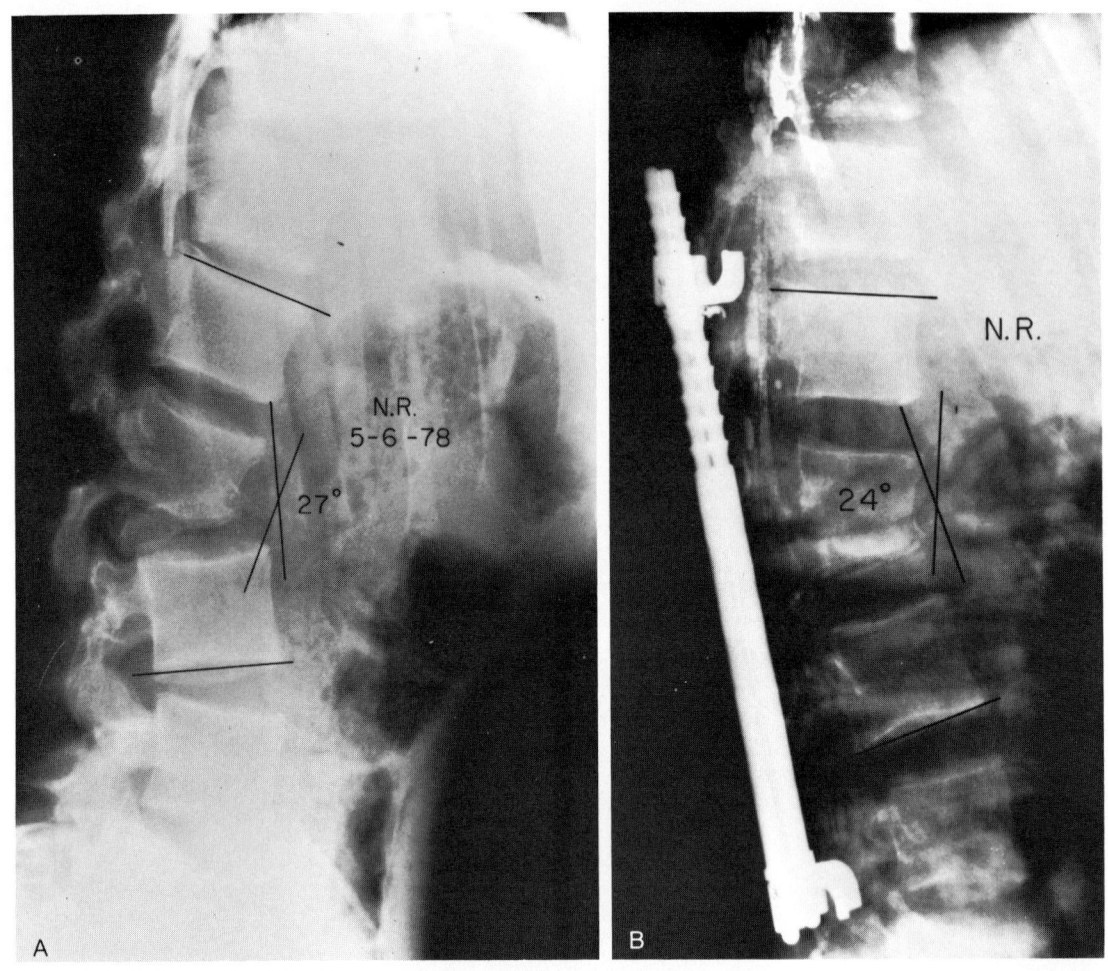

Figure 20–8. *A* and *B*, Distraction rod instrumentation should be avoided in distraction injuries. Anatomic realignment is not possible and greater risk of neurologic impairment, instability, and deformity is likely.

the advent of CT scanning and the expansion of classification of burst injuries to include stable and unstable burst fractures,[123, 124] further confusion has developed. Denis[29] has extended the classification of burst injuries into five categories. Middle column failure associated with Type A fractures of both endplates, Type B fractures of the superior endplate, and Type C fractures to the inferior endplate. The first type develops primarily from axial loading, and the second and third types develop from axial loading with some component of flexion. The Type D and E burst fractures described by Denis consist of axial loading with rotation or lateral flexion and result in more extensive ligamentous disruption and frank dislocation. These are not dissimilar to flexion/rotation injuries, as described by Holdsworth, with posterior cortical disruption of the vertebral body and retropulsion of bone into the canal. Whether this should be more appropriately referred to as an unstable burst fracture with three column failure as described by McAfee or a fracture-dislocation resulting from the combination of compression and flexion and rotational forces is of little consequence. Suffice it to say that these latter injuries may result in further translational and rotational instability, leading to further neurologic deterioration. The author prefers to include these types of injuries in the category of fracture-dislocations. All burst injuries, in the author's experience, have a linear fracture through the posterior lamina with widening of the interpedicular distance. The tendency for increased angular deformity appears to be related to the amount of posterior disruption, initial displacement of the fracture, and magnitude of bony comminution anteriorly.

The author has preferred, therefore, to define a burst fracture as an injury developing secondary to axial loading, with or without flexion. It appears radiographically as a fracture through one or both endplates. It results in loss of vertebral height, retropulsion of bone into the canal, widening of the interpedicular distance, and a linear longitudinal fracture through the lamina or the base of the spinous process. The spinal column at the fracture site shows no evidence of rotation or translation. The fracture is usually associated with a neurologic deficit. For these injuries, we favor an anterior approach consisting of vertebrectomy, anterior cord decompression, and anterior spinal fusion with a vascularized rib graft or multiple strut grafts with or without the use of an anterior implant. Combined posterior stabilization is usually not necessary. The posterior interspinous ligament complex along with the anterior longitudinal ligament and the periosteal shell surrounding the vertebra remains for the most part intact and will provide a measure of rotatory and translational stability. Patients may be ambulated within one week after surgery in an underarm brace or a plaster body jacket. If the preoperative myelogram (use water-soluble contrast material) reveals evidence of a dural leakage into or fragments in the canal posteriorly, a combined approach is preferred.

In considering the management of patients with burst injuries to the thoracolumbar spine we have found it most useful to develop our treatment program based on the presence or absence of neurologic deficit (Fig. 20–9). In the absence of neurologic deficit, stabilization as a routine procedure is not recommended. This conservative approach is based on our operative and non-operative results from treating patients with this injury. Although the author originally favored surgery by the posterior approach using Harrington distraction implants, it was apparent with longer follow-up that the results in many cases were undesirable. Using the distraction implant as recommended, two or three segments proximal and distal to the fracture site, resulted in the immobilization and fusion of a long spinal segment that was uninvolved with the injury. Loss of lumbar lordosis was a common event as was delayed collapse of the fracture anteriorly with increased kyphus and continued pain in spite of a solid posterior arthrodesis (Fig. 20–10).[59, 92] This has likewise been reported by Gertzbein and associates.[51] The disadvantage of a long fusion may be circumvented by "instrumenting long and fusing short."[33] However, this would not prevent the problem of late collapse anteriorly, and as Kahanovitz[69] has well demonstrated, internal fixation without arthrodesis in human facet joint cartilage invariably results in progressive, degenerative, osteoarthritic changes. One could certainly prevent the problem of late collapse by adding an anterior fusion to the posterior arthrodesis or doing an anterior fusion alone. However, this is a substantial amount of surgery for a fracture in the absence of a neurologic deficit that has indeed been reported to heal satisfactorily. In fact, the results from two studies have shown comparable if not better results from non-operative treatment (Fig. 20–11).[92, 93]

Should bone be removed from the canal of a patient who is neurologically intact? In the context of this particular injury as defined by the criteria given, we feel that it is not necessary to routinely remove bone in the canal in a patient who is neurologically normal. It is difficult to make a patient better than normal. In the author's series, he has not seen neurologic deterioration in patients who are neurologically intact with burst injuries.[92] This has likewise been the experience of Mino and coworkers[93] and Willen.[126] Although neurologic deterioration has been reported by other authors[11, 33] and can certainly occur, the author suspects this is more likely to occur in those burst injuries that were classified as Type D or E by Denis or in unstable burst fractures as classified by Whitesides and McAfee. However, it should be appreciated that decompressive surgery remains a major undertaking; therefore, as a general rule the author feels it is best to treat these patients non-operatively, applying a body brace one to two weeks after injury and begin slowly ambulating the patient, continuing a careful follow-up. If neurologic symptoms or findings develop, then decompression can be carried out. The results from late decompression in the author's experience[19] and in that of others[84] are sufficiently satisfactory that adopting a wait and see attitude is preferable. Symptoms and neurologic dysfunction can be treated when, and if, they develop. Continued pain more than six months after injury, progressive deformity, or the development of neurologic signs or symptoms would be an indication for surgery, and in any or all of these circumstances the anterior approach as a single stage procedure is preferred (Fig. 20–12).

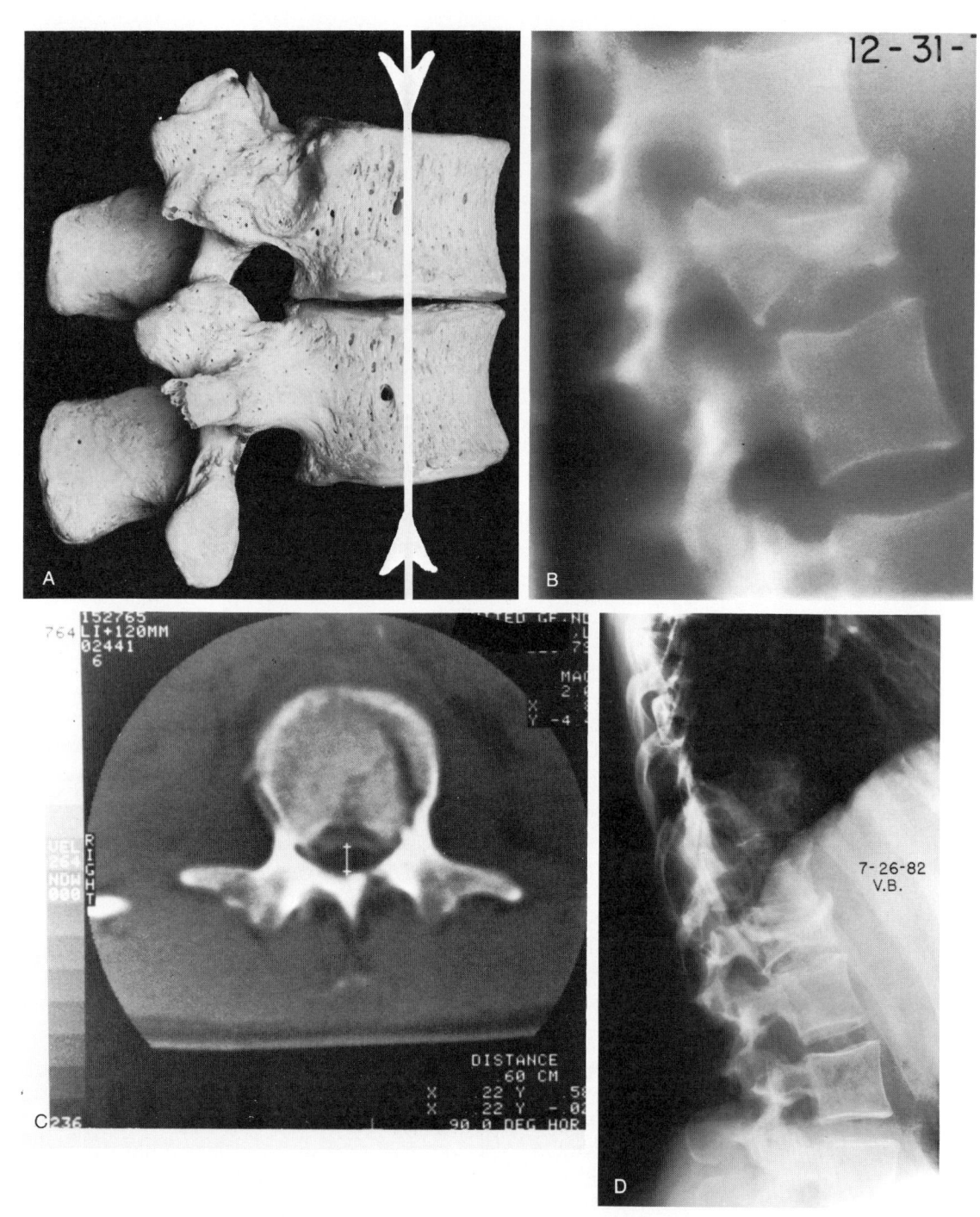

Figure 20–9. *A,* The mechanism of injury producing a burst fracture of the thoracic lumbar spine. *B,* The characteristic burst fracture deformity on the lateral tomogram. *C,* A CT scan shows significant canal compromise; however, the patient was neurologically intact. The patient was treated conservatively for four months with a brace, and has continued to function well with a minimum of discomfort and remains neurologically intact. *D,* Her x-ray two and a half years later shows no further collapse or significant angulation.

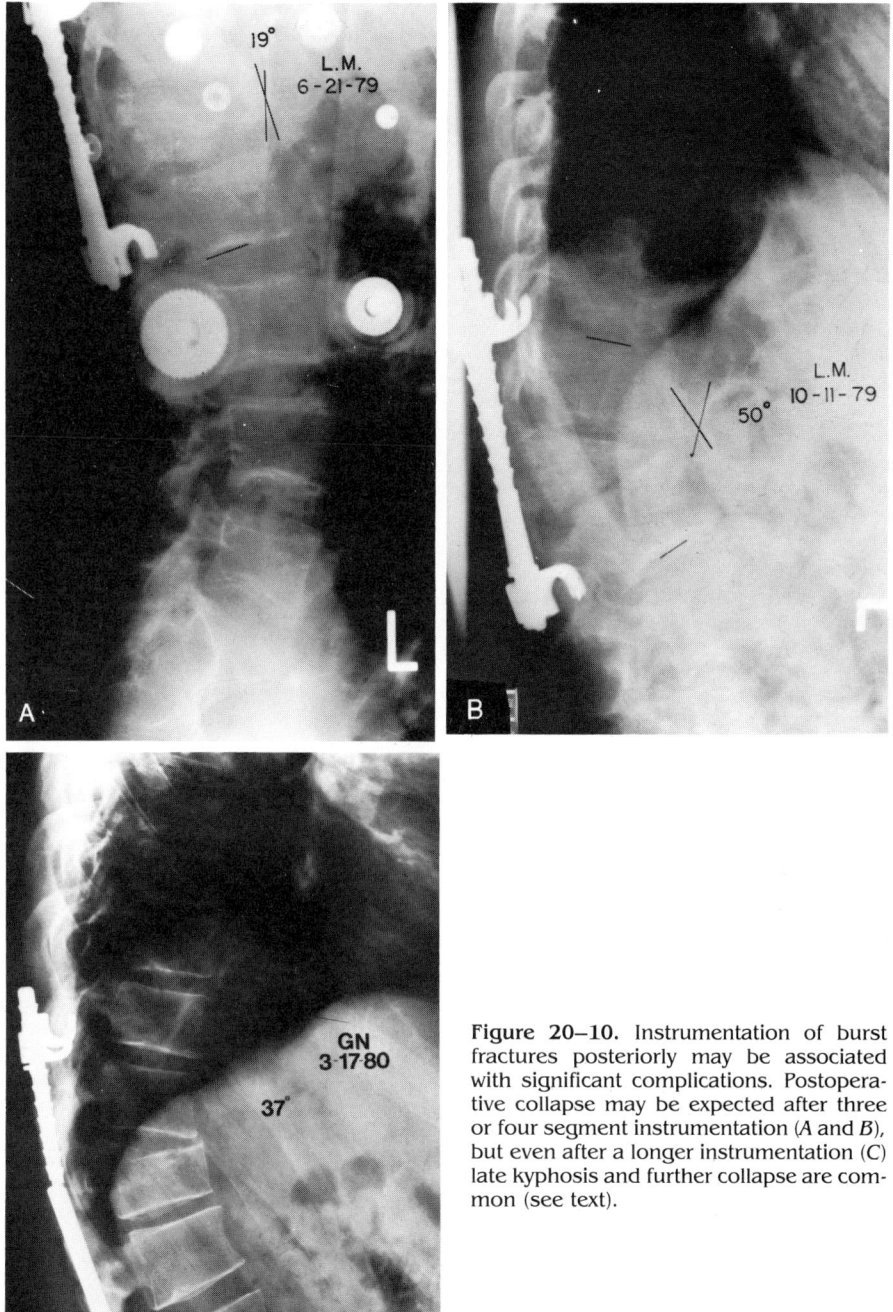

Figure 20–10. Instrumentation of burst fractures posteriorly may be associated with significant complications. Postoperative collapse may be expected after three or four segment instrumentation (A and B), but even after a longer instrumentation (C) late kyphosis and further collapse are common (see text).

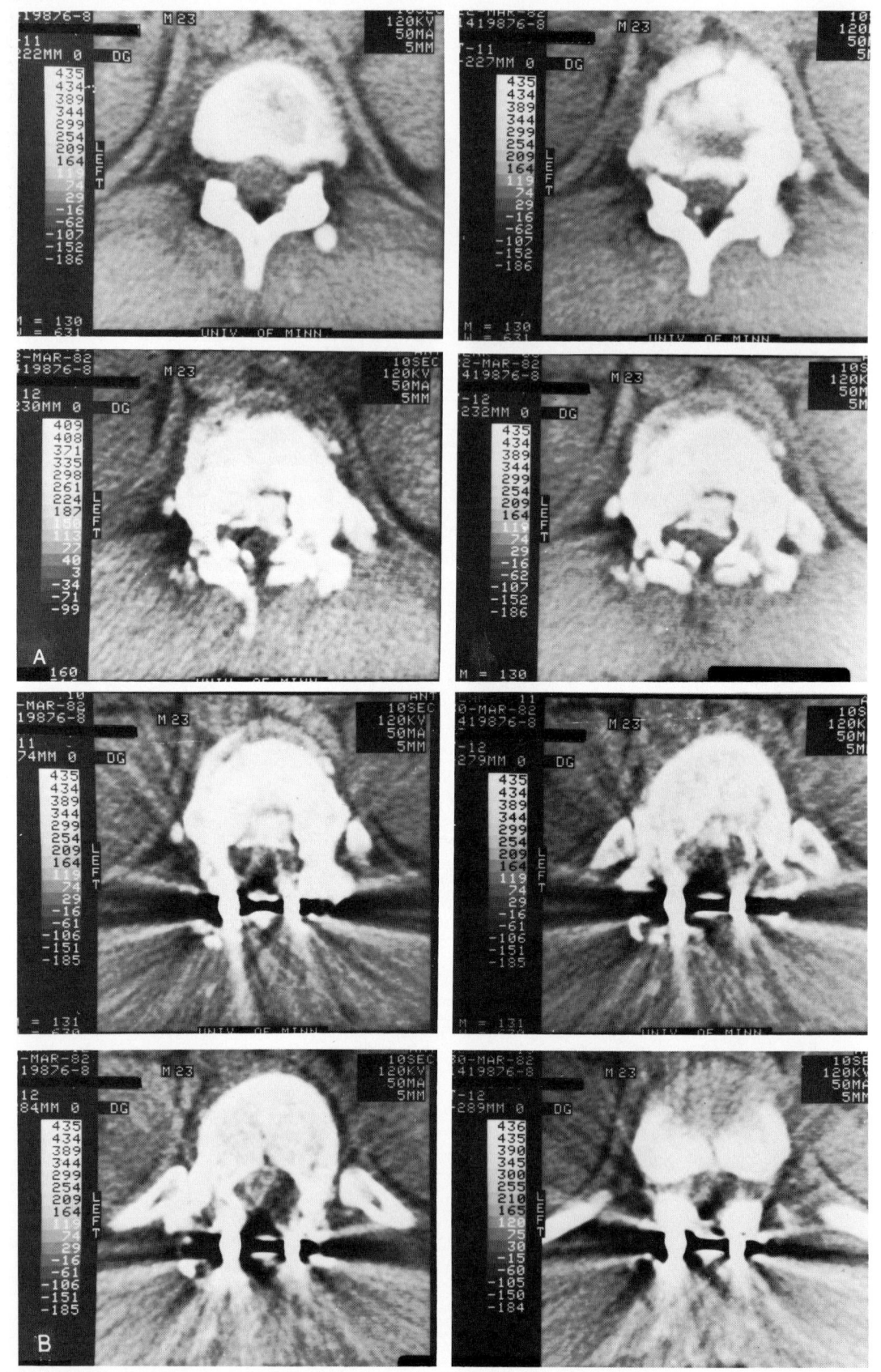

Figure 20–11. *A,* Retropulsed bone into the canal in the presence of a burst injury is not well managed by posterior approaches. *B,* In this patient following posterior instrumentation as well as posterior-lateral decompression, residual bone in the canal is readily apparent.

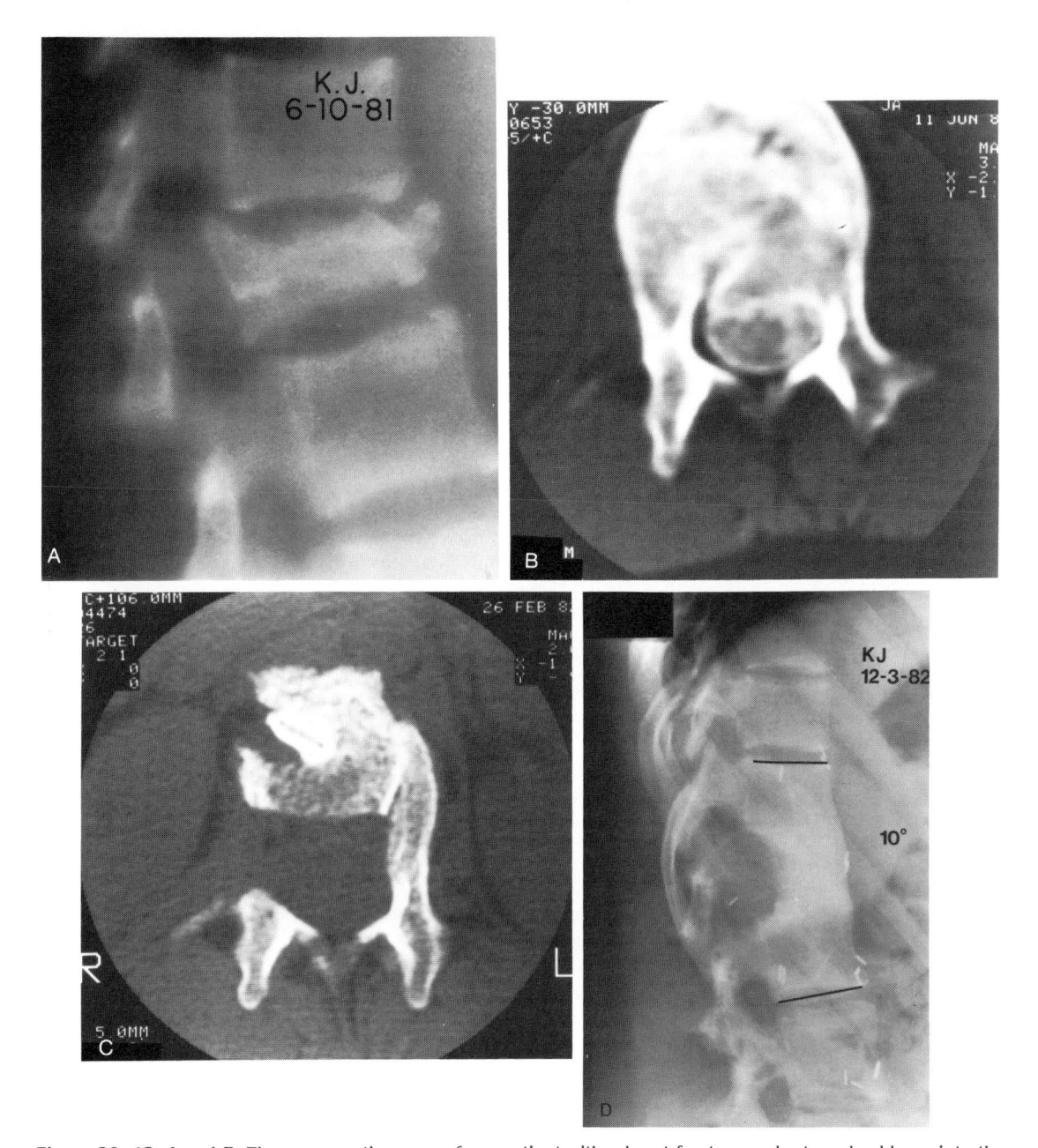

DEFORMITIES OF THE THORACIC AND LUMBAR SPINE SECONDARY TO SPINAL INJURY 453

Figure 20–12. *A* and *B,* The preoperative x-rays for a patient with a burst fracture and retropulsed bone into the canal and an incomplete neurologic deficit. *C,* Six weeks following anterior decompression with a vascularized rib graft and a femoral head allograft as a spacer one can see bone growing from the vascularized graft into the femoral head allograft. *D,* One year later excellent reconstitution is seen. The patient demonstrated one Frankel grade improvement in her neurologic deficit, although her neurologic dysfunction had plateaued prior to decompression.

Do these comments imply that surgery is never undertaken in burst injuries in the absence of neurologic deficit? Although the author has no hard data to support this contention, he suspects that patients with severe degrees of stenosis, angular deformity, and loss of bone height from vertebral comminution may not do as well in the long run. The author would therefore consider surgery acutely when there is a loss of vertebral height, canal stenosis greater than 60 to 70 per cent, or an angular deformity of greater than 30 to 40 degrees. It should be appreciated that the author uses these as general guidelines only, realizing that the definitive answer in these cases has not been forthcoming. Again, if surgery is done, it is carried out through the anterior approach.

On the other hand, in patients presenting with burst fractures seen acutely with the neurologic deficit, the author would favor immediate anterior decompression through a transthoracic or thoracoabdominal approach. There is ample evidence at the present time to suggest that increased neurologic return may be expected with anterior decompression.[19, 41, 81] Decompression should be followed with a short segment fusion consisting of a vascularized rib graft[91] or multiple strut grafts with or without the use of an anterior implant. Early ambulation or sitting is begun after fitting the patient with a polyproplyene body jacket. Combined surgery has not been necessary unless there is an associated fracture dislocation. A postoperative CT scan evaluation is carried out routinely to determine and establish the adequacy of surgical decompression.

FRACTURE-DISLOCATIONS AND TRANSLATIONAL INJURIES
(Fig. 20–13)

Translational fractures and fracture-dislocations are those injuries that are characterized by malalignment of the neural canal. All three columns have failed in shear and there is malalignment in the anteroposterior or sagittal plane. These injuries include those fractures described by Holdsworth[61] as shear injuries and rotational slice fractures along with pure dislocations and severely comminuted burst fractures associated with rotation and translational displacement. This category would also include the reverse shear fracture described by De Oliveira.[32] It is extremely important to note this latter injury, since it may appear as a benign axial compression fracture. However, it is associated with some anterior and posterior translation where the lower column is anteriorly displaced relative to the upper column (Fig. 20–14).

These injuries are usually associated with profound neurologic deficits, often complete paraplegia. It is our feeling, as has been supported by others, that these injuries are the most unstable of all spinal fractures, and we would favor surgical stabilization in order to facilitate more certain healing, earlier rehabilitation, and to shorten the hospital stay (Fig. 20–15). As a general rule the author has favored a first stage posterior approach with Harrington instrumentation and sublaminar wiring in order to realign the dislocated vertebra in the lateral and anteroposterior planes. If there is an incomplete neurologic deficit and evidence of bone comminution in the posterior or anterior column, it is removed at this time, removing the anterior bone through the posterior lateral approach and avoiding retraction of the neurologic tissue.[43, 45] If the postoperative CT scan reveals residual anterior compression in the presence of an incomplete deficit, a second stage anterior cord decompression and anterior spinal fusion is carried out (Fig. 20–16). A satisfactory alternative is a single stage anterior approach with decompression as necessary, an anterior interbody fusion, and instrumentation with a secure anterior implant such as the Dunn device.[40]

From the foregoing, it is apparent that we are now favoring an increased use of the anterior approach in fracture treatment where surgery is felt indicated.[14] Indications for anterior approaches in these fractures could be summarized accordingly: (1) when anterior decompression is felt necessary, (2) when anterior stabilization is indicated from deficient bone anteriorly, for example, burst comminuted fracture, (3) where there is deficient bone posteriorly, for example, in patients who have had a previous laminectomy, and (4) in patients presenting with late post traumatic kyphosis.[85]

FRACTURES IN CHILDREN

Fractures of the thoracic and lumbar spine in children are indeed uncommon.[65] This has been pointed out by numerous authors, and it is suggested that the incidence is only 2.5 per cent of all spinal injuries.[2] Aufdermaur has reported on 12 cases of spinal injuries in children between 0 and 18 years of age.[2] He noted that in no instance was the intervertebral disc torn, and in all cases the cartilaginous endplate was split. In the absence of a radiographic demonstration of bony injury, these fractures may be easily missed. On the other hand, in patients surviving injury, as reported by Horal and coworkers,[64] compression fractures may be visualized radiographically as quite analogous to the wedging seen in Scheuermann's kyphosis. In this latter situation, the prognosis of these wedged compression fractures appears quite good, and residual deformity and back pain are

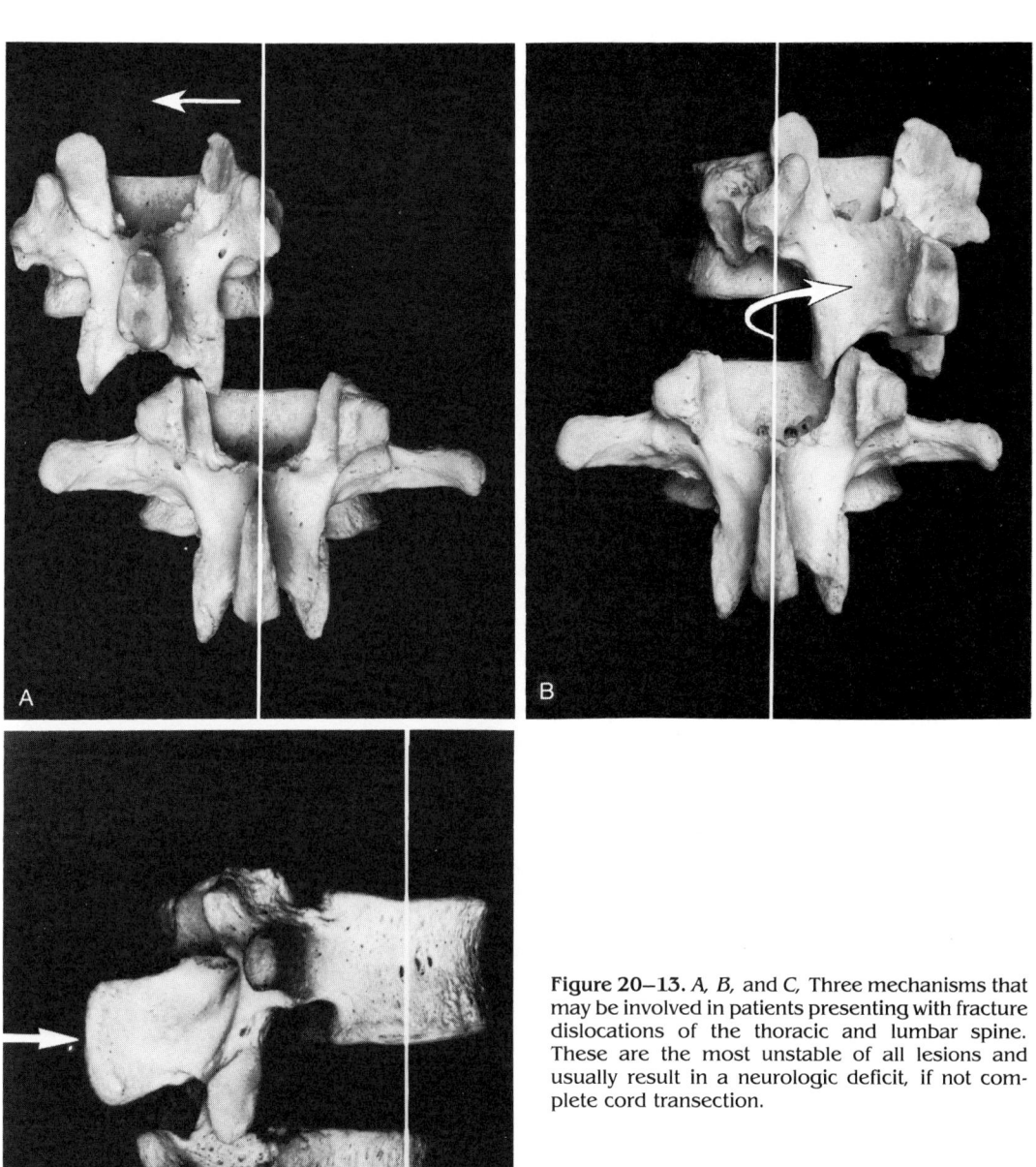

DEFORMITIES OF THE THORACIC AND LUMBAR SPINE SECONDARY TO SPINAL INJURY

Figure 20–13. A, B, and C, Three mechanisms that may be involved in patients presenting with fracture dislocations of the thoracic and lumbar spine. These are the most unstable of all lesions and usually result in a neurologic deficit, if not complete cord transection.

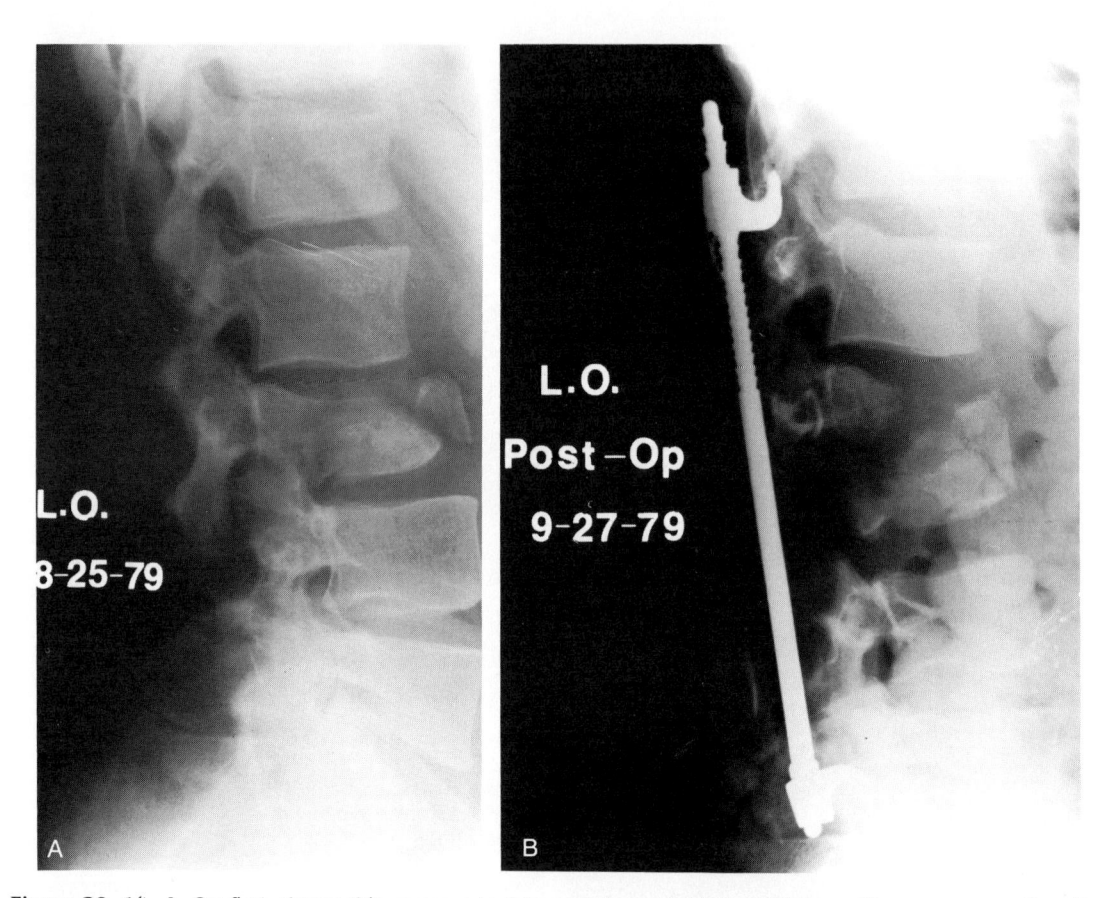

Figure 20–14. A, On first glance this appears to be a relatively stable burst injury. However, one will notice malalignment in the sagittal plane. This is the reverse shear fracture described by DeOliveira. B, This is a most unstable lesion, and distraction as a method of reduction is contraindicated.

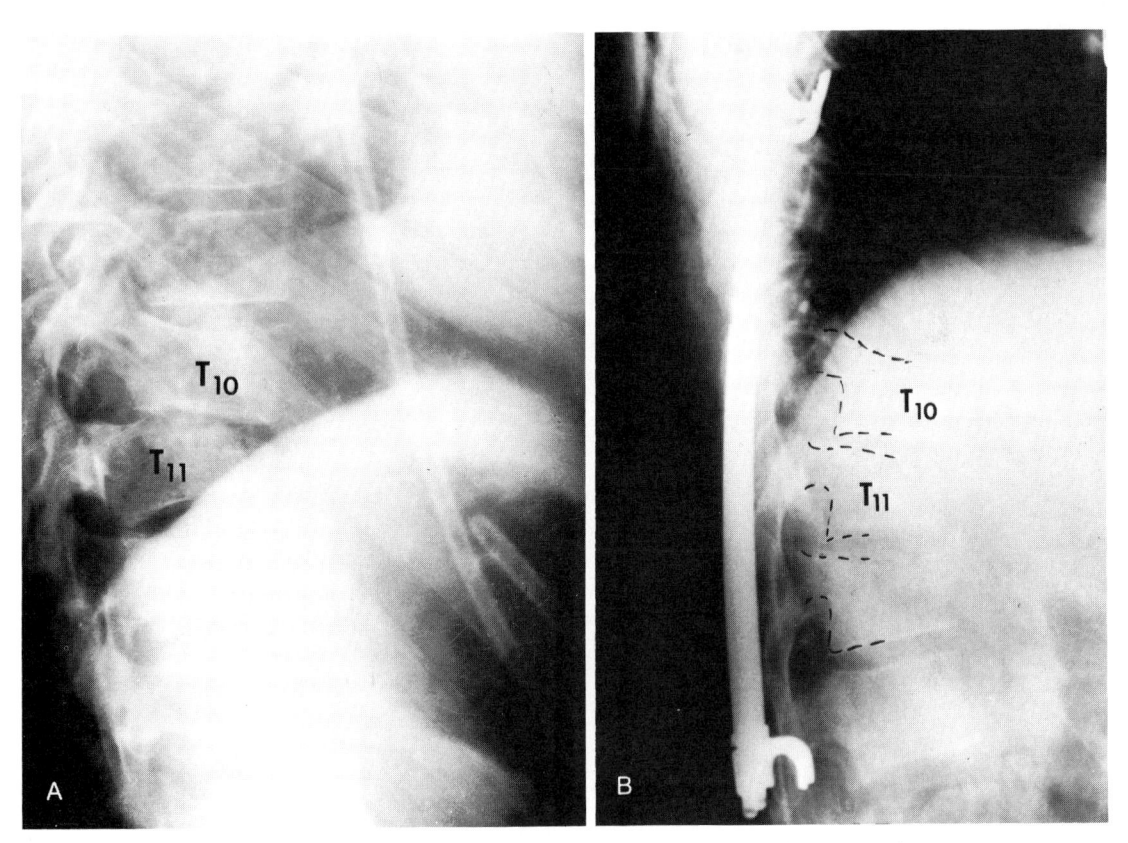

Figure 20–15. Open reduction and anatomic realignment of shear fracture dislocations is a useful procedure. A, In this case, the patient presented with an incomplete deficit. B, Anatomic realignment was obtained with a Harrington implant used as a three-point fixation device. Sublaminar wires will increase the stability but may be associated with a higher risk in the presence of an injured cord with epidural hematoma.

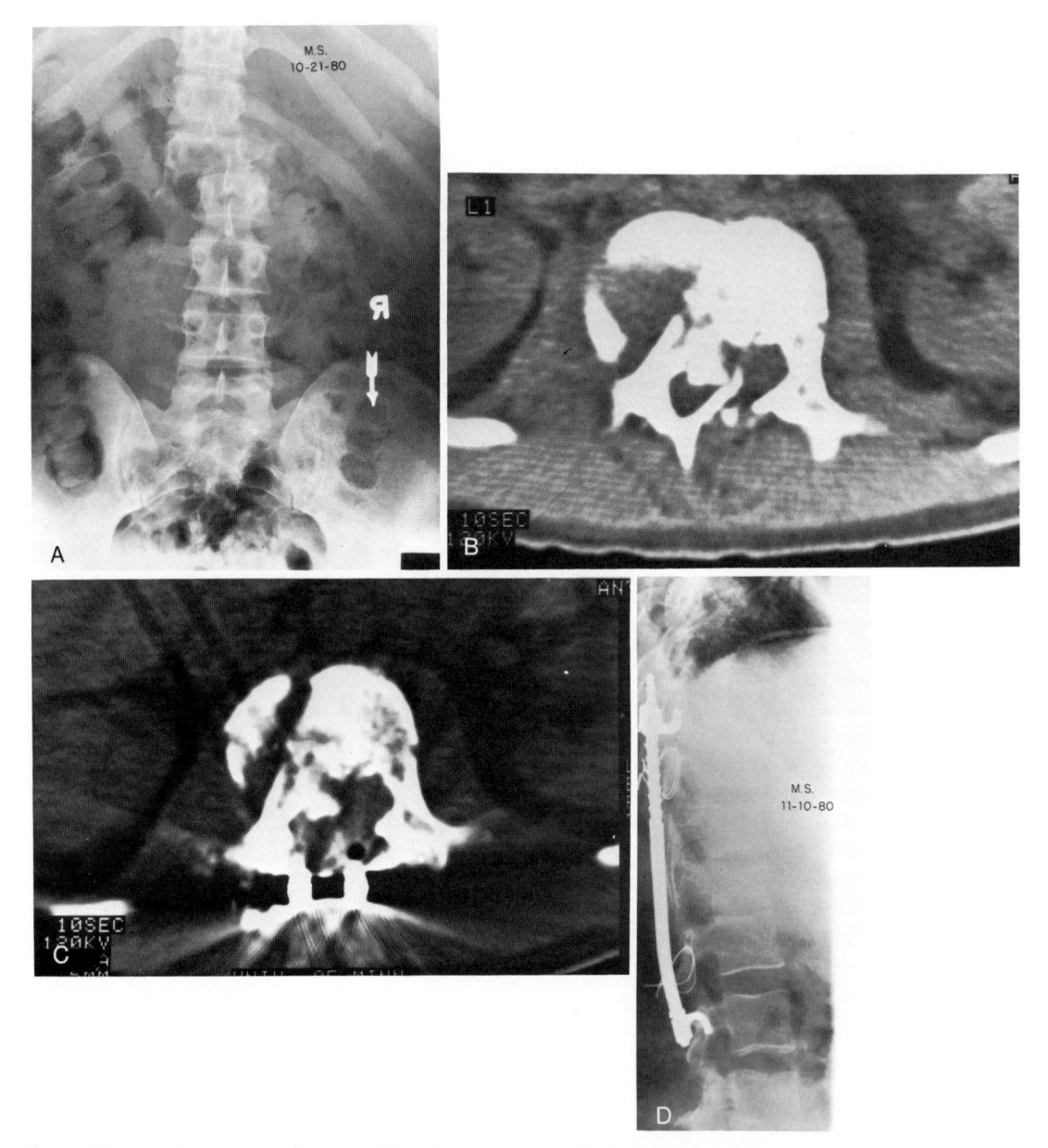

Figure 20–16. The preoperative x-ray (A) and CT scan (B) of a fracture dislocation of L1. The patient had an incomplete neurologic deficit. C and D, Stabilization posteriorly with posterolateral decompression was carried out. E, Because of residual bone in the canal a repeat posterolateral decompression was carried out. A third stage anterior spinal fusion was subsequently done because of deficient bone stock and a fear of late collapse. Although the patient had a complete neurologic recovery, the author would have favored a second stage anterior decompression and anterior fusion rather than a repeat posterolateral decompression.

Illustration continued on opposite page

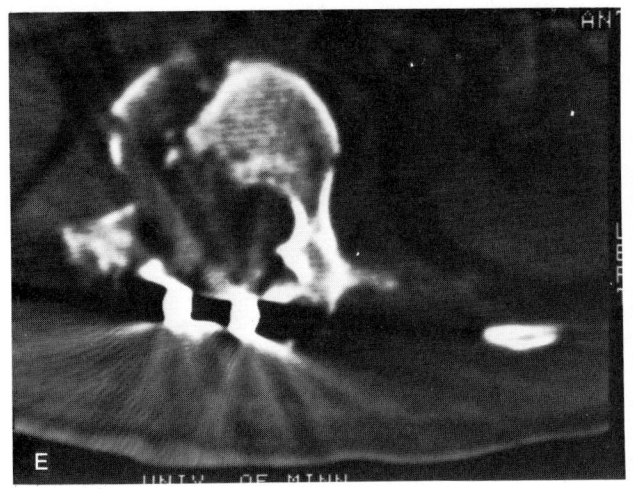

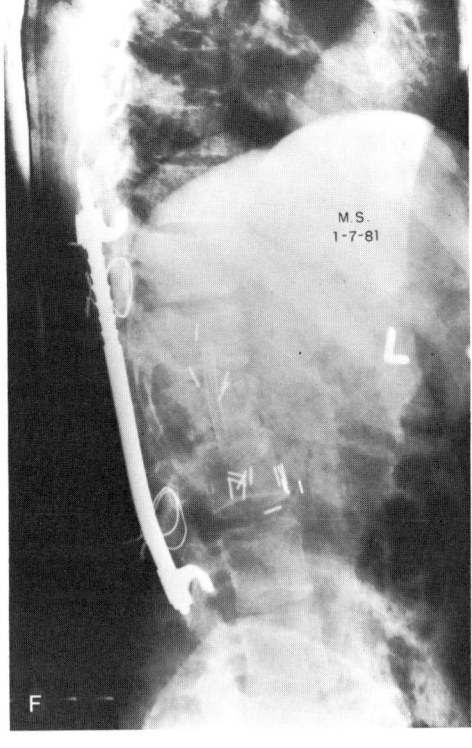

Figure 20–16 Continued.

most unlikely. In fact, according to Horal, there is no proof that the primary treatment in any way influences the later results. The association of spinal lesions in battered babies has been noted by Cullen[26] and this possible etiologic mechanism should always be kept in mind. Delayed onset paraplegia associated with spinal trauma without visualized radiographic abnormalities may also be the presenting symptom. Pang and Wilberger[99] noted that 52 per cent of children presenting with spinal cord injury without radiographic abnormalities showed delayed onset of paralysis up to four days after injury. Burke[23] has also noted a high incidence (80 per cent) of spinal cord lesions in children with no evidence or minimal evidence of vertebral injury.

Treatment of acute injuries in children is the same as that for adults. For those patients showing anterior wedge fractures over multiple segments in the absence of neurologic deficit, treatment should be minimal. The author has found patients to be benefited by hyperextension bracing or casting. Longer follow-ups by Horal, however, have suggested that treatment of any kind does not affect a favorable long-term prognosis. If neurologic deficit is present, careful and complete radiographic evaluation is necessary. Decompression at the site of the compression would be indicated for neurologically involved patients.

The development of spinal deformity in the paralyzed child is a common event.[52, 77, 87] Over 90 per cent of patients sustaining paraplegia prior to the adolescent growth spurt will develop spinal deformity. This may occur even in patients who are older than 15 years of age.[80, 107] If laminectomy has been done, the risk of kyphosis is substantially increased.[24] This information is discussed more fully in the chapter on neuromuscular deformity. Suffice it to say that any child sustaining paraplegia prior to the adolescent growth spurt should be carefully followed for the development of any evidence of spinal deformity. Once a structural curve has developed, often one as small as 15 to 20 degress, orthotic treatment is indicated. Surgical stabilization is indicated for those patients with progressive spinal deformity uncontrolled by bracing during the growth periods or in those patients presenting with significant spinal deformity greater than 40 degrees once growth is complete. Spinal fusion with segmental instrumentation, in our experience, has proven the procedure of choice. If the patient presents with a fixed pelvic obliquity, more significant curvatures (i.e., greater than 70 degrees), and is skeletally immature, a combined anterior discectomy and fusion followed by a second stage posterior instrumentation with L-rod instrumentation to the pelvis would appear the procedure of choice.

SUMMARY

The management of spinal injuries has undergone radical and profound changes in the past decade. No doubt the next decade will see even a greater change in our current concepts of management of these patients. It is becoming more apparent that these patients are best managed in centers that have a developed expertise and interest in the spinal cord injured patient. Prior to the undertaking of any operative procedure the risk/benefit ratio should be carefully weighed, and if the procedure merely shortens the patient's recumbency by several weeks, a non-operative approach should be entertained. If surgery is elected, a clear indication of the rationale and the result to be expected should be determined. Sustained ongoing care and regular follow-up examinations are an important and necessary part of any treatment program.

References

1. Angtuaco, E. J. C., and Binet, E. F.: Radiology of thoracic and lumbar fractures. Clin. Orthop. Rel. Res., 189:43–57, 1984.
2. Aufdermaur, M.: Spinal injuries in juveniles: Necropsy findings in twelve cases. J. Bone Joint Surg., 56B:13, 1974.
3. Bedbrook, G. M.: Fracture dislocations of the spine with and without paralysis: a case for conservatism and operative techniques. In Lynch, R., Hoaglund, F. T., and Riseborough, E. (eds.): Controversies and Orthopaedic Surgery. Philadelphia, W. B. Saunders, p. 423, 1982.
4. Bedbrook, G. M.: Pathological principles in the management of spinal cord trauma. Paraplegia, 4:43, 1966.
5. Bedbrook, G. M.: Spinal injuries with tetraplegia and paraplegia. J. Bone Joint Surg., 61B:267, 1979.
6. Bedbrook, G. M.: Stability of spinal fractures and fracture dislocation. Paraplegia, 9:27–43, 1975.
7. Bedbrook, G. M.: Treatment of thoracolumbar dislocation and fracture with paraplegia. Clin. Orthop., 112:27–43, 1975.
8. Bedbrook, G. M.: Use and disuse of surgery in lumbo-dorsal fractures. J. West Pacific Orthop. Assoc., 6:26, 1969.
9. Bernard, T. N., Jr., Whitecloud, T. S., Rodriguez, R. P., and Haddad, R. J., Jr.: Segmental spinal instrumentation in the management of fractures of the thoracic and lumbar spine. South. Med. J., 76:1232–1236, 1983.
10. Bohler, L.: The Treatment of Fracture. 5th Ed., New York, Grune & Stratton, p. 323, 1956.
11. Bohlman, H. H.: Late, progressive paralysis and pain following fractures of the thoracolumbar spine. In Proceedings of the American Academy of Orthopaedic Surgeons. J. Bone Joint Surg., 58A:728, 1976.
12. Bohlman, H. H., and Eismont, F. J.: Surgical techniques of anterior decompression and fusion for spinal cord injuries. Clin. Orthop. Rel. Res., 154:57, 1981.
13. Bohlman, H. H., and Freehafer, A.: Late anterior decompression of spinal cord injuries. J. Bone Joint Surg., 57A:1025, 1975.
14. Bradford, D. S.: Management of injuries to the thoracolumbar spine. In Evarts C. M. (ed.): Surgery of the Musculoskeletal System. New York, Churchill-Livingstone, p. 281, 1983.
15. Bradford, D. S.: The role of the anterior approach in the management of spinal deformities. In Dickson, R., and Bradford, D. S. (eds.): The Management of Spinal Deformities. London, Butterworths Intl. Medical Review, p. 275, 1984.
16. Bradford, D. S.: The role of internal fixation and spine fusion in thoracic and lumbar spine fractures. In Chou, C. N., and Seljeskog, E. L. (eds.): Spinal Deformity and Neurologic Dysfunction. New York, Raven Press, 1978.
17. Bradford, D. S.: Spinal instability: orthopaedic perspective and prevention. Clin. Neurosurg., 27:591–610, 1980.
18. Bradford, D. S., Akbarnia, B., Winter, R. B., and Seljeskog, E.: Surgical stabilization of fracture and fracture-dislocations of the thoracic spine. Spine, 2:185, 1977.
19. Bradford, D. S., and McBride, G. G.: Thoracic and lumbar spine fractures with incomplete neurologic deficit. A correlative study on the adequacy of decompression vs. neurologic return. Orthop. Trans., 8:159, 1984.
20. Bradford, D. S., Winter, R. B., Lonstein, J. E., and Moe, J. H.: Techniques of anterior spinal surgery in the management of kyphosis. Clin. Orthop. Rel. Res., 128:129, 1977.
21. Bryant, C. E., and Sullivan, J. A.: Management of thoracic and lumbar spine fractures with Harrington distraction rods supplemented with segmental wiring. Spine, 8:532–537, 1983.
22. Burke, D. C., and Murray, D. D.: The management of thoracic and thoraco-lumbar injuries of the spine with neurological involvement. J. Bone Joint Surg., 58B:72–78, 1976.
23. Burke, D. S.: Traumatic spinal paralysis in children. Paraplegia, 11:268, 1974.
24. Cattell, H. S., and Clark, G. H.: Cervical kyphosis and instability following multiple laminectomies in children. J. Bone Joint Surg., 49A:713, 1967.
25. Chance, G. Q.: Note on a type of flexion fracture of the spine. Br. J. Radiol., 21:452–453, 1948.
26. Cullen, J. C.: Spinal lesions in battered babies. J. Bone Joint Surg., 57B:364, 1975.
27. Cusick, J. F., Myklebust, J., Zyvoloski, M., et al.: Effects of vertebral column distraction in the monkey. J. Neurosurg., 57:651–659, 1982.
28. Davies, W. E., Morris, J. H., and Hill, V.: An analysis of conservative (non-surgical) management of thoracolumbar fractures and fracture-

dislocations with neural damage. J. Bone Joint Surg., 62A:1324–1327, 1980.
29. Denis, F.: The three column spine and its significance in the classification of acute thoracolumbar spinal injuries. Spine, 8:817, 1983.
30. Denis, F., Armstong, G. W. D., Searls, K., and Matta, L.: Acute thoracolumbar burst fractures in the absence of neurologic deficit. Clin. Orthop. Rel. Res., 189:142–149, 1984.
31. Denis. F., Ruiz, H., and Searls, K.: Comparison between square-ended distraction rods and standard round-ended distraction rods in the treatment of thoracolumbar spinal injuries. Clin. Orthop. Rel. Res., 189:162–167, 1984.
32. De Oliveira, J. C.: A new type of fracture dislocation of the thoracolumbar spine. J. Bone Joint Surg., 60A:481, 1978.
33. DeWald, R. L.: Burst fractures of the thoracic and lumbar spine. Clin. Orthop. Rel. Res., 189:150–161, 1984.
34. Dick, I. L.: The treatment of traumatic paraplegia in fractures of the lumbo-dorsal spine. Edinburgh Med. J., 60:249, 1953.
35. Dickson, J. H., Harrington, P. R., and Erwin, W. D.: Results of reduction and stabilization of the severely fractured thoracic and lumbar spine. J. Bone Joint Surg., 60A:799–805, 1978.
36. Dolan, E. J., Tator, C. H., and Endrenyi, L.: The value of decompression for acute experimental spinal cord compression injury. J. Neurosurg., 53:749–755, 1980.
37. Dolan, E. J., Transfeldt, E. E., Tator, C. H., et al.: The effect of spinal distraction on regional spinal cord blood flow in cats. J. Neurosurg., 53:756–764, 1980.
38. Donovan, W. H., and Dwyer, A. P.: An update on the early management of traumatic paraplegia (nonoperative and operative management). Clin. Orthop. Rel. Res., 189:12–21, 1984.
39. Dorr, L. D., Harvey, J. P., Jr., and Nickel, V. L.: Clinical review of the early stability of spine injuries. Spine, 7:545–550, 1982.
40. Dunn, H. K.: Anterior stabilization of thoracolumbar injuries. Clin. Orthop. Rel. Res., 189: 116–124, 1984.
41. Dunn, H. K.: Neurologic recovery following anterior spinal canal decompression in thoracic and lumbar injuries. Orthop. Trans., 8:160, 1984.
42. Dunn, H. K., and Daniels, A. U.: Anterior spine stabilization and implant system. Orthop. Trans., 5:18, 1981.
43. Erickson, D. L., Leider, L. L., Jr., and Brown, W. E.: One-stage decompression-stabilization for thoracolumbar fractures. Spine, 2:53–56, 1977.
44. Ferguson, R. L., and Allen, B. L., Jr.: A mechanistic classification of thoracolumbar spine fractures. Clin. Orthop. Rel. Res., 189:77–88, 1984.
45. Flesch, J. R., Leider, L. L., Erickson, D. L., et al.: Harrington instrumentation and spine fusion for thoracic and lumbar spine fractures. J. Bone Joint Surg., 59A:143, 1977.
46. Foo, D., and Rossier, A. B.: Post-traumatic spinal epidural hematoma. Neurosurgery, 11:25–32, 1982.
47. Fountain, S. S.: A single-stage combined surgical approach for vertebral resections. J. Bone Joint Surg., 61A:1011–1017, 1979.
48. Frankel, H. L., Hancock, D. O., Hyslop, G., et al.: The value of postural reduction in the initial management of closed injuries of the spine with paraplegia and tetraplegia. Paraplegia, 7:179, 1969.
49. Gaines, R. W., Breedlove, R. F., and Munson, G.: Stabilization of thoracic and thoracolumbar fracture-dislocations with Harrington rod and sublaminar wires. Clin. Orthop. Rel. Res., 189: 195–203, 1984.
50. Gaines, R. W., and Humphreys, W. G.: A plea for judgement in management of thoracolumbar fractures and fracture-dislocations. A reassessment of surgical indications. Clin. Orthop. Rel. Res., 189:36–42, 1984.
51. Gertzbein, S. D., McMichael, D., and Tile, M.: Harrington instrumentation as a method of fixation in fractures of the spine: a critical analysis of deficiencies. J. Bone Joint Surg., 64B:526, 1982.
52. Gillespie, R., and Wedge, J. H.: The problems of scoliosis in paraplegic children. J. Bone Joint Surg., 56A:1767, 1974.
53. Green, B. A., Callahan, R. A., Klose, K. J., and De La Torre, J.: Acute spinal cord injury: current concepts. Clin. Orthop. Rel. Res., 154:125–135, 1981.
54. Guttman, L.: Spinal Cord Injuries: Comprehensive Management and Research. Oxford, Blackwell Scientific Publications, p. 152, 1976.
55. Guttman, L.: Spinal deformities in traumatic paraplegics and tetraplegics following surgical procedures. Paraplegia, 7:38, 1969.
56. Guttman, L.: Surgical aspects of the treatment of traumatic paraplegia. J. Bone Joint Surg., 31B:339, 1949.
57. Hardy, A. G.: The treatment of paraplegia due to dislocations of the dorso-lumbar spine. Paraplegia, 3:112–119, 1965.
58. Harrington, P. R.: Instrumentation in spine instability other than scoliosis. S. Afr. J. Surg., 5:7, 1967.
59. Hasday, C. A., Passoff, T. L., and Perry, J.: Gait abnormalities arising from iatrogenic loss of lumbar lordosis secondary to Harrington instrumentation in lumbar fractures. Spine, 8:501, 1983.
60. Holdsworth, F. W.: Fractures, dislocations and fracture-dislocations of the spine. J. Bone Joint Surg., 45B:6, 1963.
61. Holdsworth, F. W.: Fractures, dislocations and fracture-dislocations of the spine. J. Bone Joint Surg., 52A:1534, 1970.
62. Holdsworth, F. W., and Hardy, A.: Early treatment of paraplegia from fractures of the thoracolumbar spine. J. Bone Joint Surg., 35B:540–550, 1953.
63. Hone, M., and Cornish, B.: Personal communication, 1968. Cited by Bedbrook, G. M.: Use and disuse of surgery in lumbo-dorsal fractures. J. Western Pacific Ortho. Assoc., 6:5–26, 1969.
64. Horal, H., Nachemson, A., and Scheller, S.: Clinical and radiological long term follow-up of vertebral fractures in children. Acta Orthop. Scand., 43:491, 1972.
65. Hubbard, D. D.: Injuries of the spine in children and adolescents. Clin. Orthop., 100:56, 1974.
66. Jacobs, R. R., Asher, M. A., and Snider, R. K.: Thoracolumbar spinal injuries. A comparative study of recumbent and operative treatment in 100 patients. Spine, 5:463–477, 1980.
67. Jacobs, R. R., and Casey, M. P.: Surgical man-

agement of thoracolumbar spinal injuries. Clin. Orthop. Rel. Res., 189:22–35, 1984.
68. Jelsma, R. K., Rice, J. F., Jelsma, L. F., and Kirsch, P. T.: The demonstration and significance of neural compression after spinal injury. Surg. Neurol., 18:79–92, 1982.
69. Kahanovitz, N., Bullough, P., and Jacobs, R. R.: The effect of internal fixation without arthrodesis on human facet joint cartilage. Clin. Orthop. Rel. Res., 189:204–208, 1984.
70. Kaneda, K., Abumi, K., and Fujaya, M.: Burst fractures of the thoracolumbar and lumbar spine with neurologic involvement, anterior decompression and fusion with instrumentation. Orthop. Trans., 7:16, 1983.
71. Katznelson, A. M.: Stabilization of the spine in traumatic paraplegia. Paraplegia, 7:33, 1969.
72. Kaufer, H.: The thoracolumbar spine. In Rockwood, A., Jr., and Green, D. P. (eds.): Fractures. Philadelphia, J. B. Lippincott, pp. 1036–1085, 1972.
73. Kaufer, H., and Hays, J. T.: Lumbar fracture dislocations. J. Bone Joint Surg., 48A:712, 1966.
74. Keene, J. S.: Radiographic evaluation of thoracolumbar fractures. Clin. Orthop. Rel. Res., 189:58–64, 1984.
75. Kelly, R. P., and Whitesides, T. E.: Treatment of lumbodorsal fracture dislocations. Ann. Surg., 167:705–717, 1968.
76. Kempf, I., Renault, D., LeMaguet, A., et al.: Biomechanical study of dorsolumbar spine osteosynthesis with reversed Harrington rods and hooks and Roy-Camille plates. Acta Orthop. Bel., 46:829–837, 1980.
77. Kilfoyle, R. M., Foley, J. J., and Norton, P. L.: Spine and pelvic deformity in childhood and adolescent paraplegia. J. Bone Joint Surg., 47A:659, 1965.
78. Kostuick, J. P.: Anterior fixation for fractures of the thoracic and lumbar spine with or without neurologic involvement. Clin. Orthop. Rel. Res., 189:103–115, 1984.
79. Kostuick, J. P.: Anterior spinal cord decompression for lesions of the thoracic and lumbar spine, techniques, new methods of internal fixation results. Spine, 8:512–531, 1983.
80. Lancourt, J. E., Dickson, J. H., and Carter, R. E.: Paralytic spinal deformity following traumatic spinal cord injury in children and adolescents. J. Bone Joint Surg., 63A:47–53, 1981.
81. Larson, S. J., Holst, R. A., Hemmy, D. C., and Sances, A., Jr.: Lateral extracavity approach to traumatic lesions of the thoracic and lumbar spine. J. Neurosurg., 45:628–637, 1976.
82. Lewis, J., and McKibben, B.: The treatment of unstable fracture-dislocations of the thoracolumbar spine accompanied by paraplegia. J. Bone Joint Surg., 56B:603, 1974.
83. Luque, E. R., Cassis, N., and Ramirez-Wiella, G.: Segmental spinal instrumentation in the treatment of fractures of the thoracolumbar spine. Spine, 7:312–317, 1982.
84. Maiman, D. J., Larson, S. J., and Benzel, E. C.: Neurological improvement associated with late decompression of the thoracolumbar spinal cord. Neurosurgery, 14:302–307, 1984.
85. Malcolm, B. W., Bradford, D. S., Winter, R. B., and Chou, S. N.: Post traumatic kyphosis: a review of 48 surgically treated patients. J. Bone Joint Surg., 63A:891, 1981.
86. Malgaine, J.: Traite des fractures et des luxations. Vol. 1, p. 410, Vol. 2, p. 318, Paris, 1847.
87. Mayfield, J. K., Erkkila, J. C., and Winter R. B.: Spine deformity subsequent to acquired childhood spinal cord injury. J. Bone Joint Surg., 63A:1401, 1981.
88. McAfee, P. C., and Bohlman, H. H.: Complications of Harrington instrumentation in thoracolumbar fractures—10 year experience. Presented at the 19th Annual Meeting of the Scoliosis Research Society, Orlando, Florida, September 19–22, 1984.
89. McAfee, P. C., Yuan, H. A., Fredrickson, B. E., and Lubicky, J. P.: The value of computed tomography in thoracolumbar fractures. An analysis of 100 consecutive cases and a new classification. J. Bone Joint Surg., 65A:461–473, 1983.
90. McAfee, P. C., Yuan, H. A., and Lasda, N. A.: The unstable burst fracture. Spine, 7:365–373, 1982.
91. McBride, G. G., and Bradford, D. S.: Vertebral body replacement with a femoral neck allograft and vascularized rib strut graft—a technique for treating post-traumatic kyphosis with neurologic deficit. Spine, 8:406–415, 1983.
92. McEvoy, R. D., and Bradford, D. S.: The management of burst fractures of the thoracic and lumbar spine: experience in 59 patients. Orthop. Trans., 7:480, 1983.
93. Mino, D. E., Yuan, H. A., Frederickson, B. E., and Stauffer, E. S.: Non-operative management of lumbar burst fractures. Presented at the 19th Annual Meeting of the Scoliosis Research Society, Orlando, Florida, September 19–22, 1984.
94. Morgan, R., Brown, J. C., and Bonnett, C.: The effect of laminectomy on the pediatric spinal cord injured patient. J. Bone Joint Surg., 56A:1767, 1974.
95. Morgan, T. H., Wharton, G. W., and Austin, G. N.: The results of laminectomy in patients with incomplete spinal cord injuries. Paraplegia, 9:14, 1971.
96. Nicoll, E. A.: Fractures of the dorso-lumbar spine. J. Bone Joint Surg., 31B:376, 1949.
97. Nykamp, P. W., Levy, J. M., Christensen, F., et al.: Computed tomography for a bursting fracture of the lumbar spine. J. Bone Joint Surg., 60A:1108–1109, 1978.
98. Osebold, W. R., Weinstein, S. L., and Sprague, B. L.: Thoracolumbar spine fractures; results of treatment. Spine. 6:13, 1981.
99. Pang, P., and Wilberger, J. E.: Spinal cord injury without radiographic abnormalities in children. J. Neurosurg., 57:114, 1982.
100. Park, W. M., McCall, I. W., McSweeney, T., and Jones, B. F.: Cervicodorsal injury presenting as sternal fracture. Clin. Rad., 31:49–53, 1980.
101. Paul, R. L., Michael, R. H., Dunn, J. E., and Williams, J. P.: Anterior transthoracic surgical decompression of acute spinal cord injuries. J. Neurosurg., 43:299–307, 1975.
102. Pennybacker, J. B.: The treatment of traumatic paraplegia. J. Bone Joint Surg., 35B:517, 1953.
103. Pierce, D. S.: Spinal cord injury with anterior

decompression, fusion, and stabilization and early rehabilitation. J. Bone Joint Surg., 51A:1675, 1969.
104. Posner, I., White, A. A., Edwards, W. T., and Nayaes, W. C.: A biomechanical analysis of clinical stability of the lumbar and lumbo-sacral spine. Spine, 7:374, 1982.
105. Post, M. J. D., Green, B. A., Quencer, R. M., et al.: The value of computed tomography in spinal trauma. Spine, 7:417–431, 1982.
106. Purcell, G. A., Markolf, K. L., and Dawson, E. G.: Twelfth thoracic-first lumbar vertebral mechanical stability of fractures after Harrington-rod instrumentation. J. Bone Joint Surg., 63A:71–78, 1981.
107. Renshaw, T. S.: Paralysis in the child; orthopaedic management. In Bradford, D. S., and Hensinger, R. (eds.): The Pediatric Spine. New York, Thieme-Stratton, pp. 118–130, 1985.
108. Riska, E. B.: Anterolateral decompression as a treatment of paraplegia following vertebral fracture in the thoracolumbar spine. Int. Orthop., 1:22, 1976.
109. Roaf, R.: A study of the mechanics of spinal injuries. J. Bone Joint Surg., 42B:810–823, 1960.
110. Roberts, J. B., and Curtis, P. H.: Stability of thoracic and lumbar spine in traumatic paraplegia following fracture or fracture dislocation. J. Bone Joint Surg., 52A:1115, 1970.
111. Rossier, A. B.: Rehabilitation of the spinal cord injury patient. West Caldwell, NJ, Ciba-Geigy Corporation, 1975.
112. Roy-Camille, R.: Chirurgie de L'arthrose rachidienne et du Disque Intervertebral. Grandes Deformations acquises Rachidiennes Infections Rachidiennes. Masson, Paris, 1984.
113. Smith, W. S., and Kauffer, H.: Patterns and mechanisms of lumbar injuries associated with lap seat belts. J. Bone Joint Surg., 51A:239, 1969.
114. Soreff, J.: Assessment of the late results of traumatic compression fractures of the thoracolumbar vertebral bodies. Stockholm, Karolinska Hospital, pp. 1–88, 1977.
115. Stauffer, E. S.: Current concepts review; internal fixation of fractures of the thoracolumbar spine. J. Bone Joint Surg., 66A:1136, 1984.
116. Stauffer, E. S.: Surgical management of trauma to the spine. In Evarts, C. M. (ed.): Surgery of the muscoskeletal system. New York, Churchill Livingstone, p. 211, 1983.
117. Sullivan, J. A.: Sublaminar wiring of Harrington distraction rods for unstable thoracolumbar spine fractures. Clin. Orthop. Rel. Res., 189:178–185, 1984.
118. Sutherland, C. J., Miller, F., and Wang, G. J.: Early progressive kyphosis following compression fractures. Two case reports from a series of "stable" thoracolumbar compression fractures. Clin. Orthop. Rel. Res., 173:216–220, 1983.
119. Wenger, D. R., and Carollo, J. J.: The mechanics of thoracolumbar fractures stabilized by segmental fixation. Clin. Orthop. Rel. Res., 189:89–96, 1984.
120. White, A. A., and Panjabi, M. M.: Clinical Biomechanics of the Spine. Philadelphia, J. B. Lippincott, 1978.
121. White, A. A., and Panjabi, M.: Clinical instability of the spine. In Evarts, C. M. (ed.): Surgery of the Musculoskeletal System. New York, Churchill Livingstone, p. 219, 1983.
122. White, R. R., Newberg, A., and Seligson, D.: Computerized tomographic assessment of the traumatized dorsolumbar spine before and after Harrington instrumentation. Clin. Orthop., 146:150–156, 1980.
123. Whitesides, T. E., Jr.: Traumatic kyphosis of the thoracolumbar spine. Clin. Orthop., 128:78–92, 1977.
124. Whitesides, T. E., Kelly, R. P., and Howland, S. C.: The treatment of lumbodorsal fracture-dislocations. J. Bone Joint Surg., 52A:1267, 1970.
125. Whitesides, T. E., Jr., and Shah, S. G. A.: On the management of unstable fractures of the thoracolumbar spine: rationale for use of anterior decompression and fusion and posterior stabilization. Spine, 1:99–107, 1976.
126. Willen, J.: Unstable Thoracolumbar Fractures; An Experimental Clinical Study. Sweden, Goteborg University, 1984.
127. Wyard, G., and Bradford, D.: Spinal injuries in a multiple trauma patient. Minn. Med., 58:536–539, 1976.
128. Yamada, K., and Ikata, T.: Early treatment of traumatic paraplegia and tetraplegia by a new method using a rolling plaster jacket or a rocking plaster shell. Paraplegia, 6:238, 1969.
129. Yosipovitch, Z., Robin, G. C., and Makin, M.: Open reduction of unstable thoracolumbar spinal injuries and fixation with Harrington rods. J. Bone Joint Surg., 59A:1003–1015, 1977.
130. Young, B., Brooks, W. H., and Tibbs, P. A.: Anterior decompression and fusion for thoracolumbar fractures with neurologic deficits. Acta Neurochir., 57:287–298, 1981.

21

COMPLICATIONS OF TREATMENT

John E. Lonstein, M.D.

Corrective spinal surgery is a major undertaking. A thorough knowledge of possible complications—their occurrence, recognition, and prevention—is essential for the care of the patient with a spinal deformity.[67, 88, 91-94] Complications may be classified as occurring as a result of either non-operative therapy or operative therapy. The latter group is subdivided into intraoperative and postoperative complications and immediate or delayed complications.

NON-OPERATIVE COMPLICATIONS

Traction

Complications from the use of traction for the treatment of deformities (see Chapter 8, pp. 113–116) may be caused by the traction device (halo, femoral pins, iliac pins) or may occur as a result of the actual traction.

HALO[107]

Infected Pins. Infected halo pins are the most common problem found with the use of the halo.[101, 105] The skin surrounding the pin becomes infected, with resultant edema, erythema, drainage, and tenderness. The localized infection may spread to the skull, leading to osteomyelitis.[144] With the bone resorption that occurs as a result of the infection, the pin becomes loose, and if it is excessively tightened, skull penetration can occur. The infection can extend intracranially either directly or by venous channels, resulting in a subdural or intracerebral abscess.[62, 64, 135, 142]

Daily pin care is important in the prevention of this problem. This procedure is performed twice daily. Education of the parent or the person who will be caring for the patient is essential to assure adequate home care following discharge. The hair in the immediate vicinity (1½ cm. diameter area) of the pin is cut short so that the pin/scalp junction can be visualized. Alcohol or peroxide solution is used to clean the area; all crusting or exudate should be removed. An iodine-containing solution such as Betadine is applied to the area. It is desirable that the entire scalp and hair be washed at least twice a week; more frequent washings are necessary in patients with oily scalps. With daily pin care, pin loosening is rare. Pin tightening after the first day of application may lead to bone resorption and pin penetration intracranially. A painful pin site indicates loosening or infection.

When the pin site becomes infected, the pin is removed and a new pin is inserted in an adjacent halo pin hole, using the technique described in Chapter 8. Local care of the infection is usually sufficient. With cellulitis and drainage, systemic antibiotics specific to the organism cultured from the drainage are given.

If osteomyelitis develops, debridement is essential. When there is an infection or continued drainage with symptoms of headache, visual changes, seizure, or drowsiness, the possibility of intracranial spread of the infection must be entertained. The halo is removed, a CT scan is useful in confirming the diagnosis, and the abscess is appropriately drained.[62]

Pin Loosening. Pin loosening can occur without pin infection. When there is a loose pin with associated pain, the pin is carefully tightened. If the loosening recurs, rather than continually tightening the pin and increasing the danger of skull penetration,[105] additional pins are added so that the forces can be distributed over six or eight pin sites.

Halo Slippage. When the halo is properly applied below the maximal diameter of the skull, slippage is rare. When slippage occurs reapplication of the halo is necessary. Slippage is also common in uncooperative patients or in cases in which large distractive forces are being used. In these cases increasing skull fixation with the use of six or eight halo pins will help prevent slippage.

FEMORAL PINS

Pin Tract Infection. Owing to the motion of the pin in the thigh, drainage is common and infection frequent. The use of Plaster of Paris to incorporate the pins eliminates the motion, and drainage and infection are unusual. When these problems occur, the pin is removed and the infection treated with local care. Because the infection is usually mild and localized, this treatment is generally successful. With more extensive infection with systemic manifestations, and even osteomyelitis, appropriate systemic antibiotics are added, with debridement where necessary.

Pin Loosening. With poor insertion technique or very osteoporotic bone, the femoral pin may cut out of the bone. If doubt exists, a radiograph will confirm that the pin is not in the femur. The pin is removed and reinserted, care being taken to place it in the distal femoral diaphysis, not the metaphysis.

HALOPELVIC TRACTION

The use of halopelvic traction using the halopelvic apparatus (halo loop) has been abandoned at this Center. Numerous complications have been described,[27, 45, 68, 104, 105, 114, 137, 138, 152] including laceration of the peritoneum and bowel,[104] infected pelvic pins,[104, 105] pin breakage, increased neurologic deficit,[104, 105] and osteoporosis. Cervical spine problems were found in a high percentage of patients undergoing halopelvic distraction.[104, 105, 137, 138] These included degenerative changes of the facet joints of the cervical spine,[138] avascular necrosis of the dens,[137] separation of the atlantoaxial joint, loss of cervical lordosis, and avulsion of the ring apophysis of C2.

NEUROLOGIC PROBLEMS

The most feared complication of distraction is paralysis, which may be paresis, paraplegia, quadriparesis, quadriplegia, or cranial or peripheral nerve deficit.

Paraplegia and Quadriplegia. Quadriplegia or paraplegia can occur as a result of traction or of surgery. It may be complete or partial, and is flaccid at first, then spastic later.

Spinal cord lesions have been reported with the use of both halofemoral and halopelvic traction, being more common with the latter.[89, 104, 108] The majority of reported cases occur preoperatively with distraction in the patient with kyphosis or postoperatively after fusion or a releasing procedure (osteotomy or wedge excision of rigid deformities). In a severe deformity, the spinal cord occupies the shortest route in the spinal canal; it is situated along the concavity of the deformity. In kyphosis, it is stretched anteriorly against the vertebral bodies, since the rigid apex does not change as the spine is elongated (Fig. 21–1).

The usual problem is kyphosis in the upper thoracic spine, which places the cord "at risk." The blood supply to the cord shows a critical vascular zone from the fourth to the ninth thoracic segment.[29] Dommisse has shown this area to have the fewest radicular branches and the fewest cord perforators.[30] In addition, the spinal canal is narrowest in this area, and the spinal cord has its least flexibility or elasticity between flexion and extension.[10]

With traction, the cord is pulled against the anterior bone with resultant circulatory changes and edema, which tip the normal balance of cord blood flow.[148] It is necessary to recognize "cords at risk" whenever possible. If vascular changes due to deformity, rigid kyphosis, or diastematomyelia exist, distraction would be contraindicated. Correction in these cases should be carried out with caution. Careful monitoring of neurologic function is necessary in all patients in traction. The earliest signs of cord dysfunction are urinary incontinence or retention, dysaesthesias or a heavy feeling in the legs. These signs occur a few hours prior to paraplegia. Immediate reduction or cessation of traction is necessary. After recovery has occurred, it is possible to carefully and slowly reinstitute the distraction with careful neurologic monitoring, even to levels beyond

COMPLICATIONS OF TREATMENT

Figure 21–1. The effects of traction on congenital kyphosis. A, Type I congenital kyphosis with two hemivertebrae at the apex of the deformity. Note that the spinal cord is tented over the apex of the kyphosis. B, Longitudinal traction is applied. The apical area is rigid, and no correction occurs. The spine adjacent to the apex lengths, and the kyphosis improves. As the apical area is unchanged, the spinal cord is pulled against the apical bone with paralysis resulting.

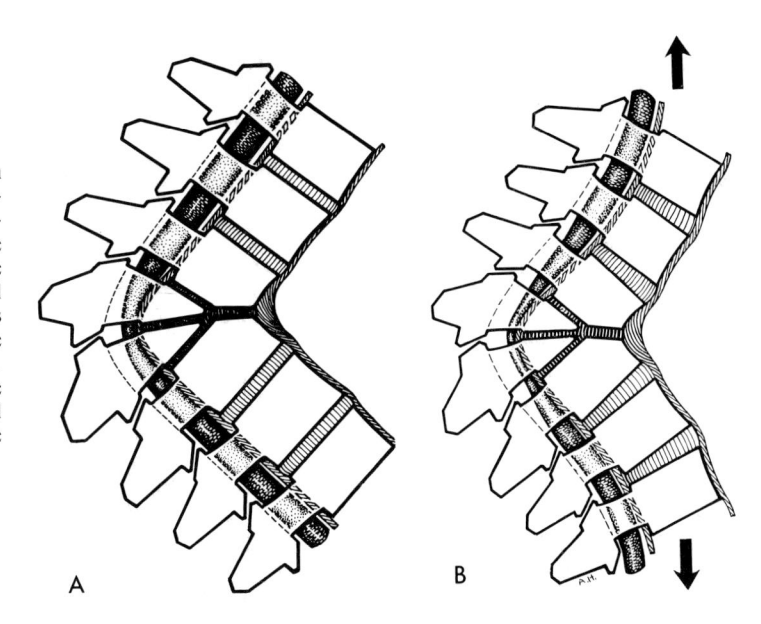

those which produced the original neurologic deficit.

Cranial Nerve Lesions. Cranial nerve palsies can occur during the use of distraction. The most common of these is at the sixth cranial nerve (abducens) with loss of lateral gaze. This paralysis is usually unilateral but may be bilateral.[89, 105, 131] Palsies of the lower cranial nerves, the ninth, tenth, eleventh, or twelfth, can occur with weakness of tongue motion and difficulty in speech or swallowing. Recurrent laryngeal nerve palsy, resulting in speech difficulty, can occur,[105] and we have also seen a case of a Horner's syndrome when traction was used in a rigid congenital cervical scoliosis with marked head tilt. Traction can also affect the medulla, causing respiratory palsy and respiratory arrest. We have a case in which distraction applied during cast application in a patient with congenital scoliosis resulted in respiratory arrest. Immediate release of traction resulted in return of spontaneous respiration.

Traction on the cranial nerves affects those with long intracranial courses that pass over bony prominences, the abducens over the petrous temporal bone and the lower cranial nerves at their site of exit from the skull. With elongation of the nerve fibers, the vessels are obliterated, the venules because of their low intraluminar pressure are the first affected.[79] This results in interruption of conduction with preservation of anatomical continuity—Seddon's neuropraxia.[122] Partial loss of conduction results in paresis, complete loss in paralysis. These cranial nerve palsies are prevented by careful daily neurologic monitoring with reduction or cessation of traction if problems occur. When recovery has occurred, traction may be slowly and carefully resumed. In general, cranial nerve palsies are temporary and resolve with prompt release of traction, but complete recovery may take up to a year, as in a case described by O'Brien.[105]

Brachial Plexus Lesions. Traction can also result in neuropraxia of the brachial plexus; the fifth and sixth cervical roots and the first thoracic root are more commonly affected. The upper roots are affected because of their nearly vertical course, the lower ones because of traction over the first rib. The pathogenesis is the same as that described for cranial nerves. Seddon[122] has shown that the nerve fibers are affected in order of their size; motor fibers are thus affected first. Clinically motor weakness is common and sensory loss minimal. With immediate release of traction, recovery is usually rapid and complete.

Prevention. Prevention of nerve or cord lesions is by recognition of high risk cases. Careful daily neurologic examinations are essential in evaluating cranial nerve, brachial plexus, and spinal cord function. These examinations should be done daily by the physician and at least once a shift by the nursing personnel. The early signs of cord dysfunction—urinary retention, incontinence, or a heavy or burning feeling in the legs—must be promptly recognized, reported to the physician, and acted upon in order to prevent irreversible cord damage.

PRESSURE SORES

As has been shown in large spinal cord injury units, this previously common problem can be prevented. A patient in bed or in traction has decreased mobility. In addition, a large number of these patients have decreased or absent skin sensibility. With prolonged, constant pressure on the skin over bony prominences (sacrum, scapulae) skin circulation is decreased and breakdown occurs. Constant attention to skin nutrition and pressure is necessary to prevent breakdown. The patient is placed on a foam mattress, and in patients with marked bony prominences (sacrum, ribs) an area is cut out in the foam and a pressure relieving pad is placed. The patient is turned every two hours day and night, being positioned sequentially supine and on both sides. The skin is inspected for areas of redness, which is the first sign of increased pressure. These areas are massaged to restore skin circulation and are carefully watched. If skin breakdown is imminent, the localized pressure is further decreased with the use of a foam donut that distributes the pressure around the bony prominence and not over it.

THROMBOPHLEBITIS

The incidence of thrombophlebitis in scoliosis surgery is low. Uden has reported an incidence of 0.7 per cent in 1229 scoliosis procedures in Scandinavia.[139] The presentation can be with the classic signs of fever, pain, and muscle tenderness or the first sign may be a pulmonary embolus, the venous thrombosis being asymptomatic and only demonstrable on phlebography.[102, 145]

The thrombophlebitis can occur either preoperatively in traction or postoperatively, and in rare cases may be due to compression of the axillary or femoral vein at the edge of the cast. Prevention is by maintaining venous flow in the lower extremities. Antiembolic stockings are worn by *all* patients, and regular leg exercises are encouraged. Aspirin or other antithrombotic agents are used in adults with a prior history of thrombophlebitis.[134] The best prevention is to minimize the time a patient spends in bed by careful selection of candidates for halo traction and by the use of early ambulation postoperatively.

Careful cast trimming around the axillae and groin is necessary to eliminate this possible cause of venous occlusion. In addition, the use of casts extending to the thighs should only be used when absolutely necessary.

Cast

PRESSURE SORES (Fig. 21–2)

With the use of cast immobilization postoperatively the most common complication seen is a pressure sore. Any constant excessive pressure by the cast in a localized area, especially over bony prominences, results initially in erythema and pain. With continued pressure the skin circulation is impaired, the pain decreases as the sensory nerve endings also become ischemic, and skin breakdown occurs. The pressure sore is initially a superficial skin defect, but with time it extends to the underlying subcutaneous tissue and then to the underlying muscle and bone. The area becomes superficially infected with a serous and a subsequent purulent discharge. Drainage and malodor are often the first signs of a pressure sore, especially in the patient with anaesthetic skin. The most common sites are over bony prominences—sacrum, iliac spines, scapulae, clavicles, rotational rib prominence—and under a sharp edge or irregular area in the cast.

With careful attention to detail in cast application these problems are reduced. All bony prominences need to be adequately padded. The padding should *not* be placed *over* the bony prominence, as this only increases the localized pressure. The central area of a piece of felt is cut out; the felt is cut radially to fit around the bony prominence. In this way the pressure is distributed over a wide area *around* the bony prominence and is not localized. In addition, during application of the plaster, direct pressure over the bony prominence is avoided.

In the first few days in the new cast, the skin under the cast must be frequently inspected for reddened or painful areas. These areas are immediately relieved, and if necessary felt padding is added, the pad being placed *around* and not over the bony prominence. In cases with a very bony prominence, rib prominence or sharp kyphosis, the cast is windowed in this area so that the skin can be inspected and padding added around the prominence. After discharge the patient's family continues this skin inspection.

Early detection is essential, as once a pressure area develops, it can rapidly increase in

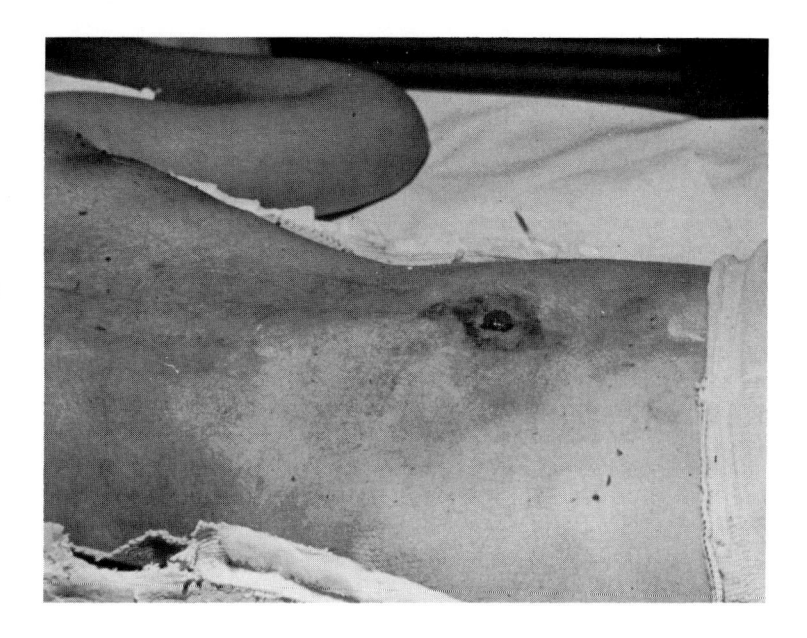

Figure 21–2. Pressure sore found under a cast.

size and depth. Once diagnosed, the cast must be windowed widely in the area of the skin breakdown. Local care with debridement as necessary is performed with frequent changes of the overlying sterile dressings. With the relief of pressure and local care, the pressure sore usually heals without difficulty.

FEMORAL CUTANEOUS NERVE IRRITATION

The edge of the cast or brace can compress the anterior femoral cutaneous nerve with resultant parasthesia in the anterior thigh. Compression is relieved by undercutting the cast's edge (or by relieving the brace) in the area of the anterior superior iliac spine to provide adequate room for the nerve.

VASCULAR COMPRESSION OF THE DUODENUM[4, 7, 16, 40, 48, 61, 87, 113, 123, 126]

Vascular compression or obstruction of the duodenum is an obstruction of the third part of the duodenum by the superior mesenteric artery. This syndrome is also known as cast syndrome or superior mesenteric artery syndrome. It has been reported in patients with scoliosis, multiple trauma, burns, or conditions requiring the application of body or spica casts. In scoliosis, the syndrome occurs in patients who are usually thin and asthenic following correction of the curve by a cast, instrumentation, a brace, or traction. As a result of correction of the curve, the angle between the superior mesenteric artery and the aorta is narrowed. The third part of the duodenum, which lies in this angle, is pinched and compressed, with resultant obstruction (Fig. 21–3A).

The syndrome presents as a high intestinal obstruction with nausea and vomiting. The vomiting decompresses the stomach giving asymptomatic intervals of many hours prior to the next episode. The vomitus usually contains bile. There is minimal bowel distension because the obstruction is high, but occasionally epigastric fullness may develop as the stomach distends. The abdomen is soft, with tenderness in the epigastrium to deep palpation. Bowel sounds are normally active or may be hypoactive with flatus and stool still being passed. The diagnosis is difficult postoperatively owing to nausea and vomiting associated with analgesic use and the distension due to ileus and aerophagia. Distension of the stomach accentuates the downward pressure on the duodenum. Prolonged vomiting will result in dehydration and hypovolemia with hypokalemic alkalaosis. If untreated, shock, oliguria, gastric rupture, and even death can occur.[40, 72]

A high level of suspicion is necessary for the early diagnosis. Radiographic studies confirm the diagnosis.[49] A plain film of the abdomen may show gastric and duodenal distension with very little gas in the remainder of the bowel. Contrast studies using Gastrografin (not barium) demonstrate obstruction of the third part of the duodenum. There is delayed gastric emptying, and the

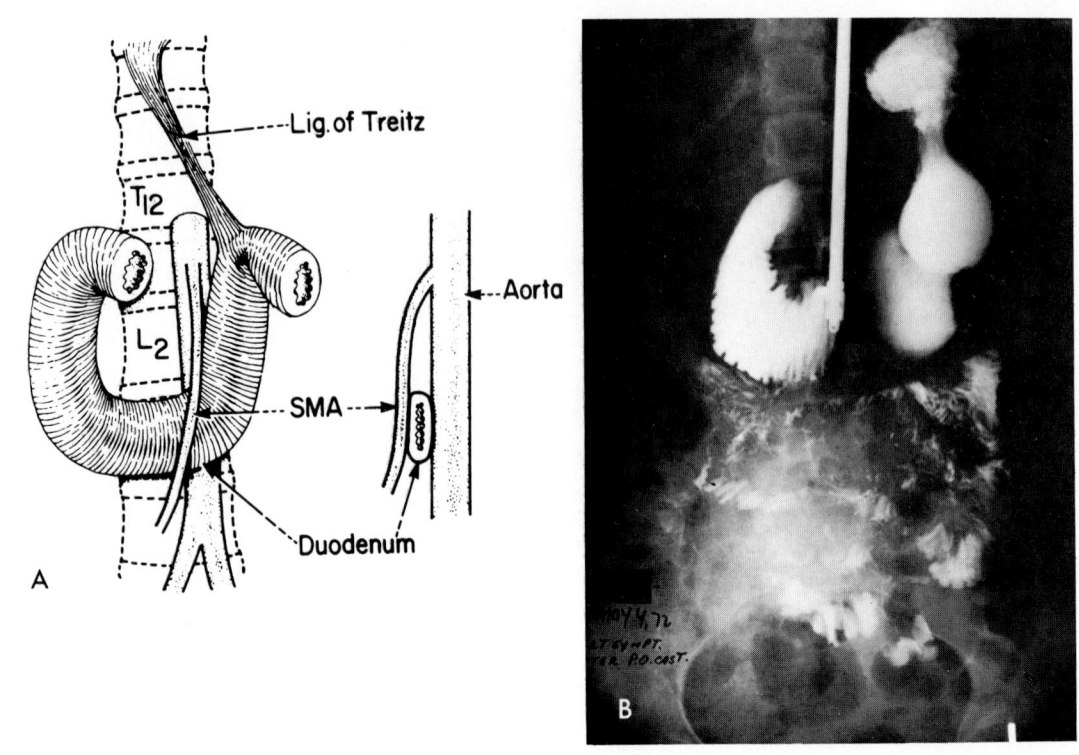

Figure 21–3. Vascular compression of the duodenum. *A*, Diagrammatic representation of the third part of the duodenum to show the site of the duodenal compression. The third part of the duodenum passes between the superior mesenteric artery (SMA) anteriorly and the aorta and vertebral column posteriorly. Any reduction of the angle between the SMA and aorta will compress the duodenum. (Reprinted with permission from Skandalakis, J. E., et al., Contemp. Surg., *10*:33, 1977.) *B*, C. W., a 16 year old girl with idiopathic scoliosis and a 60 degree right thoracic curve. In a preoperative cast this was corrected to 19 degrees, and on the day of surgery the correction was 20 degrees. One week later a postoperative cast was applied, and she was ambulated. A day later she presented with nausea and vomiting. A Gastrografin swallow showed obstruction of the third part of the duodenum. The cast was removed and the patient kept supine with nasogastric suction to decompress the stomach. The obstruction resolved with this therapy, and a second postoperative cast was applied without recurrence of the obstruction.

proximal duodenum is dilated with increased (or reverse) peristalsis (Fig. 12–3*B*). Delayed films are necessary to see if any contrast material passes the obstruction, thus differentiating a complete from a partial obstruction.

Initial treatment includes general treatment of a bowel obstruction—oral intake restriction, nasogastric suction, intravenous fluid administration, and fluid and electrolyte balance monitoring. Specific measures include positioning the patient in the left lateral decubitus position with elevation of the foot of the bed; this position encourages relief of the obstruction. This positioning is important, and if the syndrome occurs while the patient is in a cast, cast removal is usually not necessary. Generally with the above regimen the obstruction regresses after 48 to 72 hours. Oral intake is carefully restarted with soft solids followed by regular diet. If the obstruction persists beyond 48 to 72 hours, hyperalimentation is a useful adjunct to this treatment.[55] This helps maintain the patient's nutritional state.

In rare cases in which the non-operative treatment fails, surgical intervention is indicated. The procedure of choice is a side to side duodenojejunostomy. Other techniques to relieve the obstruction, release of the ligament of Treitz or a gastrojejunostomy, are less effective.

Braces[5, 6, 52, 63, 74]

Problems and complications specifically related to braces have been fully discussed in Chapter 7, page 106.

OPERATIVE COMPLICATIONS

Intraoperative Complications[8, 34, 106]

Intraoperative cardiac arrest may occur from anoxia, blood replacement problems, or air embolism. Anoxia is the most frequent cause of this rare complication. An adequate airway, maintained throughout the procedure, is the best way to prevent anoxia. Scoliosis surgery is often associated with substantial blood loss. In our experience, this problem occurs more frequently in paralytic deformities, adult scoliosis, or salvage two-stage procedures. In addition, intraoperative trauma to the intercostal artery during surgery (anterior or posterior), to the gluteal artery during bone graft removal, or to the iliac vessels during the anterior lumbar approach will result in rapid, excessive blood loss. The loss may be minimized by careful technique. The loss should be monitored by accurate measurement of drainage and weighing of all the sponges used, and the replacement is carefully calculated. Inadequate replacement leads to hypovolemia, shock, cardiac arrest, or cerebral ischemia. Excessive transfusion raises the central venous pressure, resulting in cardiac decompensation, acute pulmonary edema, and cardiac arrest. Volume replacement is particularly critical in children and in patients who are below average size for their age (e.g., those with paralytic diseases, multiple congenital anomalies).

The blood loss replacement and transfusion problems are discussed in Chapter 22.

A problem with stored blood is the possibility of transfusion of microemboli which occlude the pulmonary microcirculation, resulting in a "shock lung syndrome."[13, 22] To prevent these emboli from reaching the circulation, micropore filters are used to filter these microemboli of disintegrated cells from the blood.[22, 127] These filters should be changed when large volumes of blood replacement are necessary. In addition, the blood needs to be warmed, as the rapid administration of large volumes of cold blood can result in hypothermia, cardiac cooling, and cardiac arrest.

A rare cause of cardiac arrest is air embolism.[23, 83] Air can enter the circulation through the intravenous line, especially when blood is transfused under pressure. Air can also enter the circulation through the decorticated bone, especially if large venous channels are present. The air enters the circulation during expiration when the intraosseous intravascular pressure falls, and also during the "wake up test" if the patient becomes light. A positive pressure with expiration must be maintained.

Air embolism is diagnosed by a sudden drop in pressure associated with a "roaring train" cardiac murmur. With intracardiac shunts, blood and air enter the left heart with a possibility of cerebral air embolism. Careful monitoring of end tidal CO_2 is the earliest sign of this complication, with a rise in end tidal nitrogen. Treatment is by administration of pure oxygen with pressure on the abdomen, which increases the pressure in Batsen's plexus and thus the intraosseous venous plexus. If significant amounts of air enter the heart, the patient should be turned over, and cardiac aspiration is indicated.

When an intraoperative cardiac arrest occurs, the incision is rapidly packed with gauze sponges and closed with towel clips. The patient is then turned over, and resuscitative measures are carried out. When resuscitation is complete, the wound is irrigated and sutured with the patient on the side.

NEUROLOGIC INJURY[150]

Neurologic injury may occur from direct injury to the cord or nerves or from excessive traction during correction. Direct injury may occur during posterior procedures, anterior fusion, disc excision, cord decompression, or closure of a wedge osteotomy during a hemivertebra excision or corrective osteotomy. In cases in which there are large laminar defects—spina bifida deformities, neurofibromatosis with erosion of the lamina or bone graft, or in post-laminectomy deformities—the spinal cord can be injured during exposure. Careful surgical techniques can prevent these injuries. The possibility of laminar or graft defects must always be considered during exposure when the anatomy appears unusual.

Paraplegia was almost non-existent in the days of plaster cast correction. Since the advent of instrumentation, forceful corrective techniques, and the treatment of severe rigid deformities, paraplegia has been more commonly reported.[14, 73, 81, 108, 114, 128, 152, 153] The neurologic loss can be associated with instrumentation, anterior or posterior fusion, or osteotomies.

During Harrington instrumentation, the distractive force is exerted on *all* tissues, including the spinal cord. The interruption of the blood supply to the cord is thought to be the cause of the paralysis. These changes are similar to those described in relation to traction complications (page 466). The additive effects of traction and decreased spinal cord blood flow have been shown by Grundy and coworkers,[57] Dolan and coworkers,[28] and Cusick and coworkers,[24] indicating a danger of distraction with hypotensive anaesthesia.[11, 56] Paraplegia is more common in congenital spine deformities,[81] especially in patients with cord tethering by a tight filum terminale, diastematomyelia, or other types of spinal dysraphism. A high incidence of paraplegia also occurs in the treatment of severe rigid deformities[112, 129] or kyphosis.

The paraplegia can occur during surgery, and thus presents when the patient awakens from the anesthesia. The paraplegia can also be delayed, usually developing in the first 8 to 12 hours postoperatively, but it may be delayed for up to 72 hours.[77, 149] The evidence for a vascular etiology was shown by Ponte[111] who described two cases in which paraplegia associated with hypovolemia developed in the postoperative period after spinal fusion and Harrington instrumentation. While arrangements were made for emergency rod removal, the blood volume and thus blood pressure were restored with blood transfusions, and the paraplegia disappeared. In the delayed type of paralysis the first signs of altered cord function present as muscle weakness, bladder paralysis, or sensory changes, usually parasthesiae of a burning or tingling nature. The paraparesis can rapidly progress to complete paraplegia.

Patients who are at a high risk for developing neurologic problems should be recognized with adequate preoperative evaluation, including myelography.[103, 125] If instrumentation is planned in these cases, it is best used with extreme caution and intraoperative monitoring. If correction is necessary in severe rigid curves, anterior osteotomies are often indicated to mobilize the spine and allow safe correction. Operations that "shorten" the long side of the curve may be preferable to those that stretch the short side of the curve.

Intraoperative monitoring of cord function is an integral part of any procedure in which distraction or a marked corrective force is planned.[17, 38, 41, 60, 66, 98, 99, 130, 140, 141] It is discussed fully in Chapter 22. All but one case of a "positive" wake up test (i.e., inability to move the toes) in Stagnara's experience have been in curves greater than 120 degrees.[129] We have seen a positive test in a case of idiopathic scoliosis with only a 57 degree right thoracic curve. Intraoperative cord monitoring is of no value in delayed onset paraplegia. Cases have been presented in which the electronic monitoring was normal, and on awakening, paraplegia was present.[46, 77, 118] Postoperative monitoring is essential for a minimum of 24 hours. The early diagnosis of neurologic impairment is essential, as it has been shown that prompt removal of the instrumentation gives the greatest chance of return of normal function; there is a direct correlation between neurologic recovery and the interval between the onset of impairment and removal of Harrington instrumentation.[81] With a delay of under three hours after onset of paraplegia, the chance of recovery is excellent, but if the delay is over six hours, the chance of recovery is low. Laminectomy is *not* necessary in these cases unless there is specific reason to suspect the presence of a bone fragment of hematoma in the spinal canal.

In rare cases, paraplegia can follow a spine fusion in which instrumentation is not used; this is more common in congenital kyphosis or in cases in which a neurologic deficit existed preoperatively. In these cases a decreased blood supply to the spinal cord may be the cause of the neurologic deficit.

The advent and widespread use of Luque segmental spinal instrumentation[2, 80] has also resulted in a significant number of neurologic complications.[50, 65, 132] The rate in these cases as reported by Luque is 4.6 per cent transient and 0.6 per cent permanent neurologic sequelae;[80] King reported an incidence of 4 per cent neurologic complications.[73] Cord stretch or distraction by this powerful instrumentation, especially in rigid deformities, has a higher incidence of neurologic complications. The passage of the sublaminar wires also increases the neurologic risk because of cord contusion or nerve root impingement.[59, 73] Care in passage and handling of the wires is essential and is outlined Chapter 16. Neurologic impairment can present as nerve root hyperaesthesia or dysaesthesia or as cord damage with Brown Sequard Syndrome, paraparesis, or even paraplegia. With care in passage of wires and avoidance of excess force on correction, and anterior releases where indicated, these complications can be minimized.

During anterior instrumentation, it is possible to damage the spinal canal contents or nerve root by poor screw placement.

Dural Tear. Direct trauma to the dura during the surgical procedure results in a dural laceration with a leak of spinal fluid. This may be accompanied by trauma to the cord or cauda equina. This complication can occur during exposure, instrumentation, facet excision, osteotomy, or decortication; thus, care during surgery is necessary at all times. When the dura is lacerated, bone is removed to adequately visualize the tear. The dural opening is inspected and the dural sac contents examined for damage. Careful suture of the dura is performed, and when simple closure is not possible the defect is closed using a fascial or muscle graft. In rare cases a persistent spinal fluid leak occurs after surgery. The wound needs to be kept compressed, the patient is kept supine, and in addition antibiotic coverage is indicated. In persistent leaks, a cerebrospinal fluid bypass drainage via a C2 puncture should be considered.

PNEUMOTHORAX

A pneumothorax can occur during surgery for one of three reasons. The respirator can malfunction, forcing air into the lungs without allowing air to escape. The result is a tension pneumothorax (Fig. 21–4). A pulmonary bleb (congenital or emphysematous) can rupture spontaneously, also resulting in a tension pneumothorax. During the surgical procedure, the pleura can be damaged directly. This is more likely to occur when ribs are being resected as part of the surgical procedure either on the concavity to allow rod placement in severe deformities, or on the convexity in a thoracoplasty. The pneumothorax can either be diagnosed intraoperatively or present postoperatively with respiratory distress and anoxia. Intraoperative direct penetration is treated by insertion of a

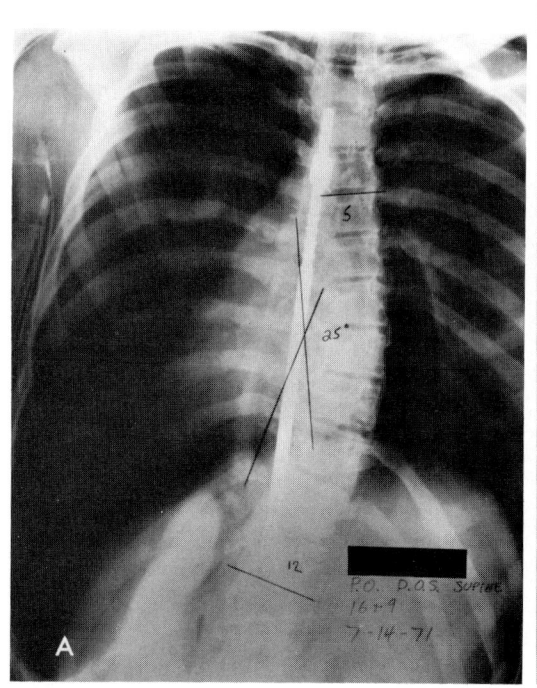

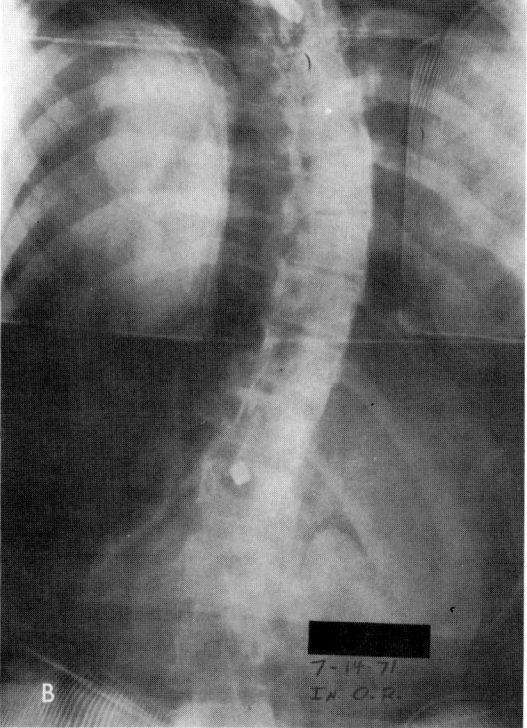

Figure 21–4. A, S.C., a 14 year old female who underwent a spinal fusion with Harrington instrumentation. In the recovery room she became cyanotic, and a chest x-ray revealed a large left pneumothorax. B, In reviewing the intraoperative marker x-ray, it is seen that the pneumothorax is present at this stage. On reviewing the case with the anesthesiologists, it was learned that for the early stages of the case there was respirator malfunction with a short expiratory phase and thus a build-up of positive pulmonary pressure. This pressure probably ruptured an area of congenital bulla formation. A chest catheter connected to underwater drainage was inserted.

chest tube. In the cases of tension pneumothorax a radiograph will confirm the diagnosis. Treatment consists of insertion of a chest tube and drainage to underwater suction.

HEMOTHORAX

Hemothorax can occur from rupture of a vessel, either an intercostal vessel along the rib or transverse process or a segmental vessel around the vertebral body. The vessels can be damaged because of penetration of an instrument following rib resection or during transverse process osteotomy. In addition, during anterior procedures the vessel can be damaged or the ligature around the vessel may become dislodged. Hemothorax should be suspected when chest tube output markedly increases and hypotension develops following anterior fusions, or when hypotension and respiratory distress follow posterior procedures. A chest radiograph will aid in the diagnosis. Treatment consists of thoracotomy and ligation of the lacerated vessel.

GLUTEAL ARTERY LACERATION

The superior gluteal artery can be lacerated by an osteotome or gouge at the greater sciatic notch while the iliac bone graft is being obtained. With subperiosteal exposure and a carefully placed Taylor retractor, the area of the sciatic notch is usually adequately protected. When the artery is lacerated, packing with gauze sponges rarely controls the hemorrhage. Usually enlarging the incision and removing bone from the area of the sciatic notch allows successful ligation of the artery. In cases in which this procedure is unsuccessful, the back wound is rapidly approximated, the patient is turned supine, and a laparotomy is performed to adequately visualize the vessel for ligation.

EXCESSIVE BLOOD LOSS

Excessive blood loss during surgery may occur from a variety of causes. It is more common in patients with osteoporotic bone, adults, patients with paralytic diseases, and patients who have been in a brace. The hemorrhage may be excessive throughout the whole procedure, or occur only with decortication. In our experience, coagulation studies have *not* been useful in demonstrating the cause. Careful meticulous technique will minimize this loss. Rarely, the hemorrhage is so extensive that the procedure must be terminated, the wound closed, and the fusion completed at a later time.

With anterior approaches, major vessels may be damaged leading to a sudden, large blood loss. Whenever the vertebral body is entered for an osteotomy, cord decompression, graft placement, or vertebrectomy, the vascular channels may bleed profusely. This must be controlled with the liberal use of bone wax, topical collagen, or thrombin-soaked Gelfoam, especially during the major resection of a vertebral body.

The role of hypotensive anesthesia and blood replacement with autotransfusion,[82] either predeposit of intraoperative, are discussed fully in Chapter 22.

BONE FRACTURE

During spinal fixation it is possible to fracture the bone at the site of the insertion of the instrumentation. This problem is more common in the patient with osteoporotic bone (neuromuscular disease, adults) or in the young patient. The occurrence may be lessened by careful technique in hook insertion and the avoidance of excess corrective forces. With the Harrington rod, the use of more than one rod or more than one hook at the ratchet end will help distribute the corrective forces.

Occasionally with anterior instrumentation the vertebral body is weak and will not hold the screw or the body will fracture. Methylmethacrylate has proven useful in augmenting the screw fixation in such cases (see Chapter 10).

PERITONEAL OR VISCERAL DAMAGE[31]

During anterior exposure of the thoracolumbar or lumbar spine, the peritoneum can be lacerated during the retroperitoneal dissection. All lacerations should be closed with catgut suture. Rarely, the abdominal viscera (bowel, spleen, liver, kidney, ureter) may be injured. The injury is usually recognized and appropriate treatment is performed. In some cases, especially with ureteric injury, the diagnosis is delayed and only made in the early postoperative period.

Early Postoperative Complications

PULMONARY PROBLEMS (Fig. 21–5)

Pulmonary problems with respiratory distress are a major postoperative complication

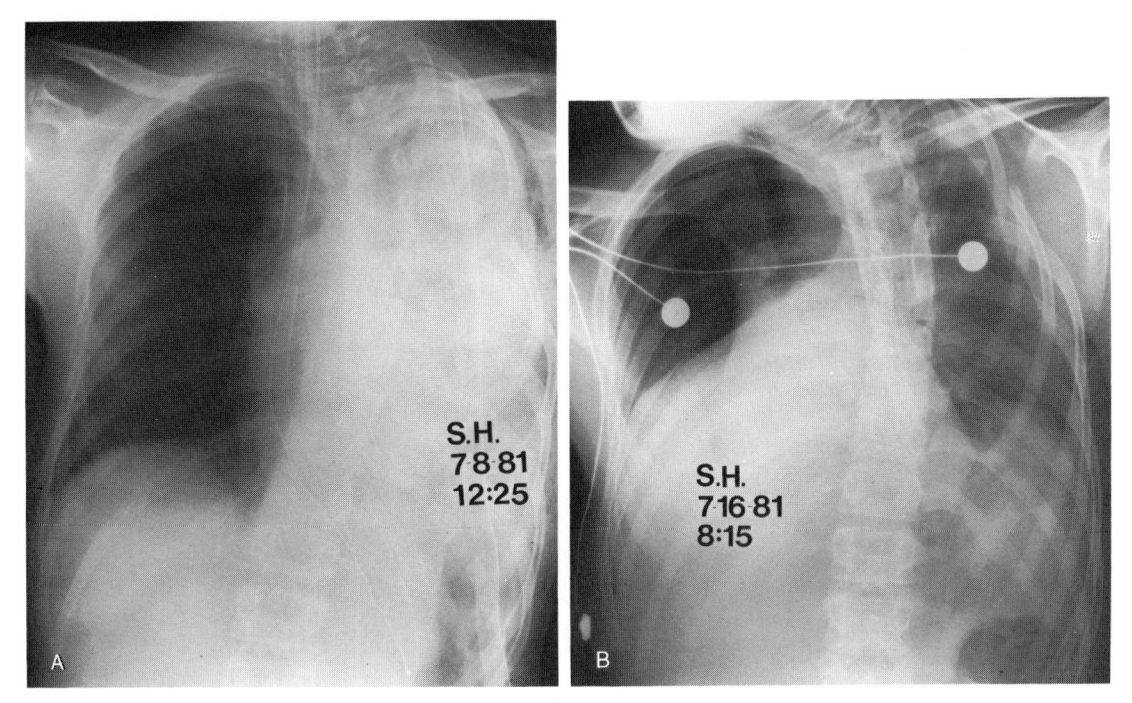

Figure 21–5. S.H., a 13+6 year old boy with post-laminectomy kyphosis underwent an anterior spinal fusion. A, The postoperative x-ray revealed a left hemothorax, which cleared after removing clots from the chest tube. B, A week later a chest x-ray revealed atelectasis of the right lower lobe. This was successfully treated with bronchoscopy and aspiration of the mucous plug.

in spinal surgery. These include atelectasis, pneumonia, pleural effusion, pneumothorax, shock lung, and respiratory failure. It has been shown that postoperative pulmonary functions in children undergoing scoliosis surgery are reduced when compared to peripheral surgery with decreased vital capacity, functional residual capacity, and total lung capacity.[120] A recent article stated that factors that related to an increased incidence of pulmonary problems in the postoperative period were: non-idiopathic scoliosis, mental retardation, anterior procedures, age 20 or more, and an obstructive component to the pulmonary function tests.[3] These pulmonary problems occur after both anterior and posterior approaches.[58] They are covered fully in the sub-chapter on Anesthesia.

Chylothorax is a rare complication that may occur after anterior approaches.[21, 36] It presents as an output of milky, odorless fluid which is sterile. It may also present following removal of the chest tube with progressive pleural effusion. Treatment consists of chest tube drainage and decreasing the patient's fat intake.

A rare cause of respiratory distress in spinal surgery is ARDS (acute respiratory distress syndrome).[13, 47] This has many causes, fluid overload, sepsis, microemboli, and usually presents two to five days postoperatively with fever, respiratory distress, reduced arterial oxygen, and marked radiographic changes. Prompt diagnosis and treatment as outlined in Chapter 22 is mandatory.

NEUROLOGIC PROBLEMS

Paralysis can present in the postoperative period and is discussed fully on page 471.

Acute hydrocephalus can occur after surgery in a child with myelodysplasia. The acute problem can follow excision of a non-functioning spinal cord during a posterior resection to correct a congenital kyphosis. Any surgical procedure on these children's spines can disturb the balance of cerebrospinal fluid formation and absorption, resulting in an acute increase in cerebrospinal fluid pressure. It is also possible for a ventriculoperitoneal shunt to be disturbed during an anterior approach to the spine. The child presents with restlessness, stupor, seizures, and papilloedema. Prompt diagnosis followed by neurosurgical consultation and an emergency shunting procedure is necessary.

WOUND INFECTION[33, 71, 78, 136]

An early review of wound infections in scoliosis surgery showed a high rate of infection with an overall incidence of 9.3 per cent, and the rate in adults being 20 per cent.[78] A recent review of 7,769 surgical procedures from 1950 to 1982 revealed an overall infection rate of 2.5 per cent, 2.6 per cent in posterior procedures and 0.9 per cent in anterior procedures.[136] The factors that were related to a higher infection rate were identified. The etiology of the deformity was related to the incidence; the infection rate in myelodysplasia was 7.9 per cent, in cerebral palsy was 2.5 per cent, and in idiopathic scoliosis was 1.4 per cent. In children under age 20, the infection rate was 1.5 per cent and it was 2.7 per cent for adults over age 20. The use of instrumentation was associated with an increased infection rate, the rate was 3.6 per cent with instrumentation and 1.5 per cent without instrumentation. The infection rate was greater in longer operations, which were associated with greater blood loss. The use of the preoperative traction was also associated with a higher infection rate (10.4 per cent) as was previous spine surgery (6.8 per cent), especially if this surgery had led to an infection (22 per cent). The use of allograft did *not* result in an increase in the infection rate.

Since 1972, the use of prophylactic antibiotics has resulted in a decrease in the infection rate from 4.4 per cent before antibiotics to 1.2 per cent with antibiotics. The effect of antibiotics is most marked in patients with idiopathic scoliosis in whom the infection rate without antibiotics was 2.3 per cent and with antibiotics 0.1 per cent. This importance of prophylactic antibiotics in spine surgery is well documented.[18, 35, 96, 97, 100, 109, 121]

Early diagnosis and prompt treatment are necessary to adequately treat wound infections.[37, 44] Any temperature elevation is viewed with suspicion, and the wound is inspected for erythema, edema, and tenderness. When an infection is suspected, a culture is obtained after adequate surgical preparation of the wound area. Aspiration is performed lateral to the incision, and the aspirate is cultured. The sedimentation rate and white cell count are *not* useful in diagnosis unless serial examination shows a rising level. If the wound is highly suspicious, one should *not* wait for culture results. When an infection is diagnosed or the possibility is high, the patient is taken to surgery. The entire wound is opened down to the bone graft and debrided and thoroughly irrigated. Additional cultures are taken, and after complete debridement, irrigation and suction tubes are inserted. The bone graft is removed, thoroughly washed, and replaced, and the instrumentation is left in situ. The wound is closed as if it were primary closure of a clean wound. The irrigation and suction system are continued for a total of three to five days. Antibiotics are started in large doses preoperatively, and if necessary are changed when the sensitivity results are available. The antibiotics are usually continued for ten days intravenously and six weeks orally.

At the end of five days, if the patient is afebrile, the wound benign, and the white cell count and sedimentation rate falling, the irrigation is discontinued and all tubes are connected to suction for 24 hours. The tubes are then removed. Culture of the suction drainage is of no benefit. The care of wound infections by suture removal and packing is condemned, as the infection is inadequately treated, the hospitalization prolonged, and the cosmetic result poor (Fig. 21–6).

In some cases the infection recurs after adequate treatment as outlined, *or* at the time of debridement the control of the infection is in doubt. In these cases the wound is packed open, redressed in the operating room, and when clean (usually three to five days later) a delayed primary closure is performed. In the rare cases in which this is not possible, the wound is allowed to granulate by secondary intention.

It must be emphasized that the bone graft and instrumentation should *not* be removed. The pseudarthrosis rate is higher after an infection. With this regimen the infection is controlled, and the outcome of the scoliosis and infection are satisfactory.

GENITOURINARY TRACT PROBLEMS

Urinary retention is common in the postoperative period in scoliosis patients. Catheterization is often necessary in these patients. There is a direct correlation between the number of straight catheterizations and onset of urinary infection in the adolescent female.[143] This is different from the case of paraplegia with clean, intermittent self-catheterization.[53, 76] In the postoperative patient, the use of an indwelling catheter is also

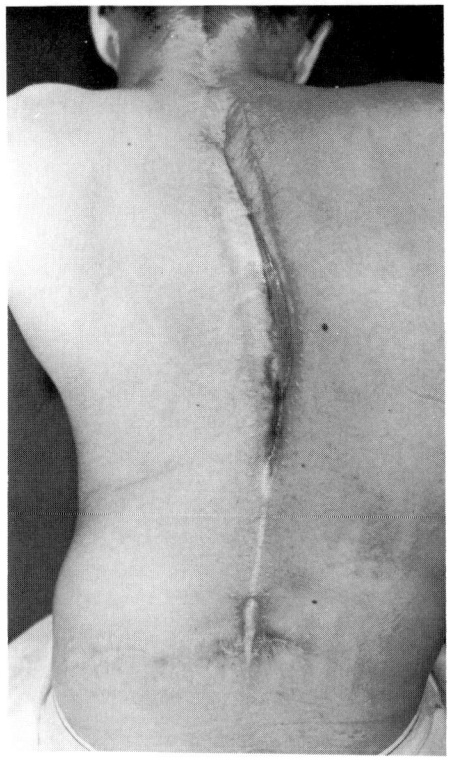

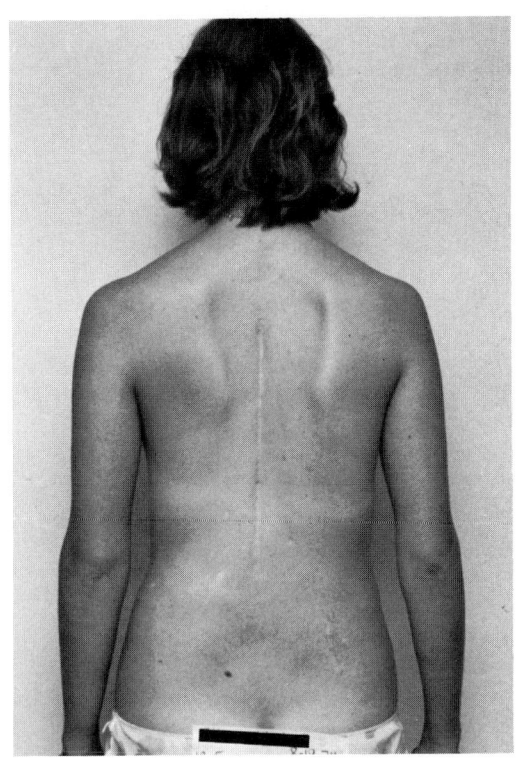

Figure 21–6. A, Cosmetic result of treatment of a wound infection in a 16 year old boy with myelodysplasia treated with wound debridement, open packing, and closure by granulation and epithelialization. Total hospitalization was four months. B, Cosmetic result of treatment of wound infection in a 13+8 year old girl with idiopathic scoliosis treated by debridement and wound closure over irrigation-suction tubes. Additional hospitalization for treatment of the infection was 10 days.

associated with a high urinary infection rate.[75, 110] Intermittent catheterization in the female also leads to damage to the short urethra; with resultant stricture formation. Thus an indwelling catheter is preferred as it monitors the urine output, prevents bladder overdistension; and prevents repeated urethral trauma in the female. After removal of the catheter, the urine is cultured 24 hours later and any infection appropriately treated.

Damage to the genitourinary system is possible during the course of dissection in an anterior approach. In addition, mechanical correction of severe curves has been reported to result in angulation of the ureter with resultant obstruction.[110] Angulation may be the result of positioning in the tuck position.[70] Rarely, the retroperitoneal dissection can cause retroperitoneal fibrosis and paraurethral scarring with resultant hydronephrosis.[20, 32, 85, 124] These require late re-exploration of the retroperitoneal space with release of the scarring.

GASTROINTESTINAL TRACT PROBLEMS

Ileus occurs rarely, unless morphine is used postoperatively. It is frequently seen in cases of anterior retroperitoneal approaches. In posterior fusions, bowel sounds usually return a day or two after surgery. In anxious patients and in cases of air swallowing (aerophagia) the ileus can be more marked. This was seen with the use of intermittent positive-pressure breathing (IPPB) postoperatively but is rare with the current routine use of incentive spirometry, which actually is more efficient for postoperative pulmonary care.[19]

In anterior fusions a nasogastric tube is routinely used until bowel sounds return, and then oral feeding is slowly instituted. Prolonged ileus occasionally occurs with extensive retroperitoneal bleeding and a retroperitoneal hematoma. In these cases it is imperative to wait for satisfactory bowel sounds before discontinuing the nasogastric suction and starting oral feeding.

Acute cholecystitis has been seen following spinal fusion. This presents as an acute abdomen in an adult in the early postoperative period.[15, 42] The factors in its etiology are thought to be dehydration, fever, fasting, anesthesia, and narcotics, all of which lead to contraction of the sphincter of Oddi and concentration of the bile. In addition, there is hemolysis and there may be an anatomic change in the celiac axis with interruption of the blood supply by way of the celiac artery. A high index of suspicion is necessary to make the diagnosis; a non-functioning cholecystogram confirms the diagnosis. Exploration and cholecystectomy may be necessary in these cases.

Postoperative nausea and vomiting may be indicative of vascular obstruction of the duodenum. This is discussed fully on page 469.

BLOOD REACTION AND HEPATITIS

With the extensive use of blood replacement for scoliosis surgery, problems with transfusions frequently occur.[12, 151] Mild transfusion reactions (fever, skin eruptions) are common, but anaphylaxas is rare in our experience. With skin eruptions, the transfusion is stopped, and Benadryl administered. Occasionally difficulty is encountered in crossmatching blood, especially when prior surgery has been performed and antibodies are present that make crossmatching difficult. This problem can be decreased with the use of predeposit autologous transfusions. Three units of blood are drawn from the patient at weekly intervals, starting three weeks preoperatively. This blood is stored and transfused at the time of surgery.[84] This volume of replacement is usually sufficient for the routine one stage procedure. When extreme difficulty is experienced in obtaining compatible blood, the autologous blood can be drawn and frozen, allowing storage over many months and thus the capability of getting a large volume of blood for the surgical procedure.

Disease in the donor, for example, hepatitis, syphilis, and acquired immune deficiency syndrome (AIDS), can be transmitted with blood transfusions. These problems in our experience are rare. Hepatitis is eliminated with the detection of hepatitis B surface antigen (HBsAg),[146] syphilis with a serologic test (VDRL) and rapid plasma reagin (RPR) test, and AIDS by the detection of antibodies against the HTLV-III virus.[119] A high standard of service by local blood transfusion services or the Red Cross helps to minimize these problems. A study to modify post-transfusion hepatitis by Gamma globulin administration has not been shown to change the hepatitis rate significantly.[95]

INSTRUMENTATION DISLODGEMENT[57]

In the postoperative period, the upper hook of the Harrington rod may dislodge from its fixation site. This occurs for one of a number of reasons—excessive force, weak bone, or faulty hook placement.

Upper hook dislodgement more commonly occurs when thoracic kyphosis is not recognized during instrumentation and thus the rod is not adequately contoured to conform to the sagittal contours of the spine. The lateral x-ray must be evaluated preoperatively so that the sagittal contours are appreciated and appropriate rod contouring performed.

In rare cases rod dislodgement may occur in a restless or uncooperative patient (e.g., cerebral palsy, mental retardation, children) Here additional internal stabilization (sublaminar wires, a compression rod) is used, and if necessary a cast is applied either immediately while the patient is under the same anesthetic for the fusion, or in the early postoperative period. In rare cases the compression hooks may dislodge, either at the ends in the treatment of kyphosis, or in the middle when the compression rod is used to increase spine stability in the treatment of severe curves.

Rod slippage through the upper distraction hook is possible when the ratchets are not stabilized with a wire hoop of C ring. A Luque rod can also slip if the "L" is not fixed either to the spinous process of by a sublaminar wire at the short end of the "L." Careful technique is necessary to prevent these complications from occurring.

Dislodgement is usually diagnosed when an upright radiograph is taken in the postoperative immobilization, and a loss of correction is seen. The hook is displaced laterally on the frontal view, with a posterior displacement on the lateral x-ray. These x-rays are compared with the immediate postoperative supine films for correction and hook position. The dislodgement sometimes occurs after discharge, and in these cases it is diagnosed by a prominence in the upper incision area or on the routine one month postoperative radiographs. Hook displacement accompanied by a loss of correction or a very prominent hook, is treated by re-operation and hook re-insertion (Fig. 21-7). Re-insertion is usually one or two vertebrae cephalad to the original insertion. The causal factor is addressed and treated (i.e., adequate hook insertion, rod contouring for kyphosis, double upper hooks, or the addition of stabilizing sublaminar wires). In some rare cases there is minimal loss of correction, and in these cases careful serial x-rays are used to check for loss of correction. With loss of correction re-insertion is performed, and if no loss occurs immobilization is continued until the fusion is solid.

In anterior instrumentation, screw pullout or tilting can occur, being more common at the ends of the instrumentation. These problems are usually due to excessive force being used during anterior instrumentation, especially when the vertebral bone is of poor quality. Care during screw insertion and instrumentation will minimize this problem (See Chapter 10).

Late Postoperative Complications

INFECTION

Late infections or wound problems can present after the patient has left the hospital. Infection may present months to years after surgery, usually as a draining sinus. The treatment is the same as an initial infection, with the addition of a sinogram preoperatively so that the whole sinus tract can be excised during the operative procedure.

In rare cases, superficial wound separation occurs after the patient is discharged. This wound must be inspected, and after adequate sterile preparation, probed to see if there is an accompanying deep infection. In the latter cases there are accompanying systemic signs and symptoms plus swelling, erythema, and tenderness of the wound. In the case of deep infection, the wound is opened in toto and treated as described on page 476. If there is a localized separation without a wound infection, in our experience it is best treated with local repeat debridements and packing, allowing the area to granulate, close, and epithelialize. This can even occur when there is exposed instrumentation in the depths of the wound.

PSEUDARTHROSIS

Failure to obtain a solid fusion at one or more levels is a serious problem in spinal surgery. The pseudarthrosis rate has been reduced by advances in scoliosis care especially use of facet fusions, autologous iliac cancellous bone, addition of banked bone, instrumentation, early mobilization, and adequate postoperative immobilization. Pseudarthroses can occur despite the best efforts of the surgeon. The ultimate test of any new instrumentation or technique can only be judged by the fusion rate using the new instrumentation or technique. The ability of a new technique to obtain dramatic correction will be negated by the failure to obtain spine stabilization with an adequate fusion.

Pseudarthroses are more common in the lumbar spine, particularly in the lumbosacral (L4 to S1) and thoracolumbar (T11 to L1) areas. Certain predisposing factors have been well documented. Pseudarthroses are more common in adults,[75] increasing with increasing age.[25] Certain diagnoses, paralytic curves, neurofibromatosis, kyphosis, are associated with an increased pseudarthrosis rate.[86] The treatment of kyphosis with a posterior fusion alone, with the fusion mass being placed in tension, is associated with a higher percentage of failure.

Diagnosis can occur early or late. Early recognition is important. Routine supine oblique radiographs taken at the time of the removal of the postoperative immobilization are carefully examined for adequacy of the fusion. The fusion mass is carefully inspected for any defects crossing it, all visible facets being evaluated. A facet joint that is easily visible and not obliterated indicates a possible area of weakness; the defects in the fusion mass usually pass through these unfused facets (Fig. 21-8). In an anterior fusion the defect is seen as an open intervertebral space. These areas are also very tender to palpation and percussion. There is usually no loss of correction yet, as the instrumentation and the immobilization have supported the spine and maintained correction. If a pseudarthrosis is diagnosed, the treatment depends on the quality of the fusion; if the fusion is still generally immature and non-trabeculated then continued immobilization is indicated. If, on the other hand, the fusion is well trabeculated with obvious defects present, the pseudarthroses are repaired unless they are absoutely painless with no loss of correction.

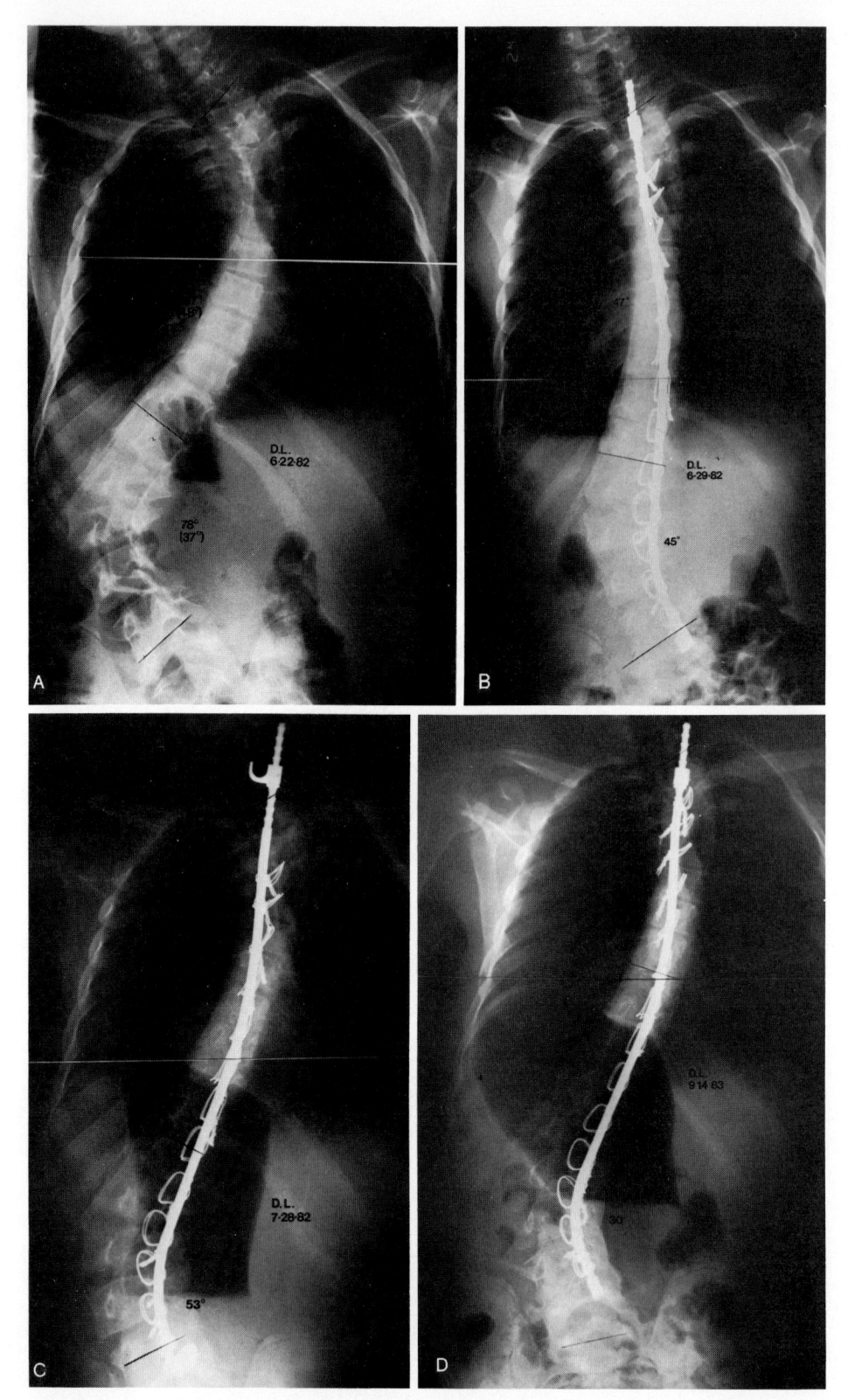

Figure 21–7. *A*, D.L., a 16 year old boy with cerebral palsy, had curve progression, and a sitting x-ray showed a right thoracic curve of 87 degrees and a left lumbar curve of 78 degrees. *B*, A posterior fusion with Harrington rod and sublaminar wires was performed; the postoperative x-ray showed correction to 47 degrees and 45 degrees. *C*, The one month postoperative x-ray showed dislodgement of both hooks with loss of correction to 58 degrees and 53 degrees. *D*, The hooks were re-inserted, and 14 months later the fusion was solid with recorrection obtained.

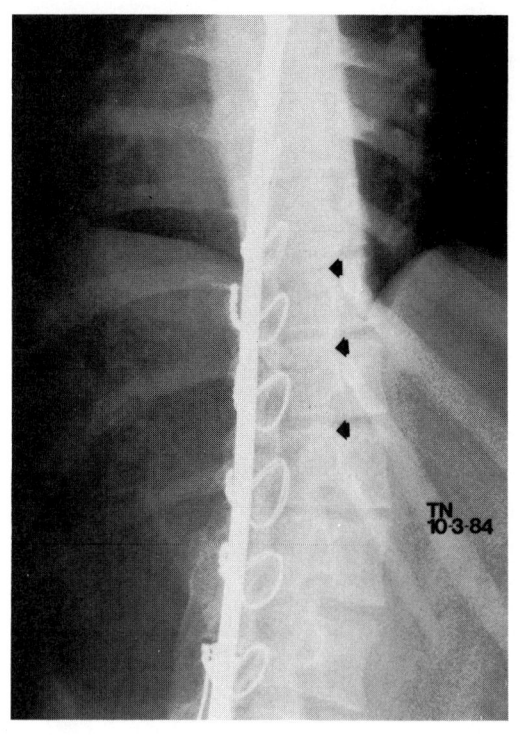

Figure 21–8. Oblique x-ray at 16 months postoperative of a 15 year old girl with idiopathic scoliosis shows defects of the fusion at the facet joints (*arrows*). A solid fusion in the lumbar area is well seen.

In patients fused while they are still growing, other clues to the presence of a pseudarthrosis may be present. The weak area in the graft allows the graft to elongate, and if the Harrington rods are present, the rod is "pulled" out of the lower hook. In addition, the disc space opposite the pseudarthrosis is wide as growth continues, but the other discs become narrowed as the vertebral body growth continues at the expense of the disc space.

A pseudarthrosis may not be diagnosed on the post-immobilization x-rays, but may present later as a loss of correction with height loss, back pain, increasing deformity, or instrumentation failure (Fig. 21–9). The increase in deformity can either be an increase in the scoliosis, or if the fusion is wide, increase in kyphosis. Localized pain and tenderness are often present at the area of pseudarthrosis. The pseudarthrosis can be seen on frontal or supine oblique views as a defect crossing the fusion mass in a serpentine manner. The defect is more visible now as the fusion mass is well trabeculated and of a uniform density. In anterior or combined anterior and posterior fusions a defect is seen anteriorly with a disc not fused while the other disc spaces are obliterated with trabeculae crossing the disc space. Instrumentation breakage is a sign of a weakness in the fusion until proven otherwise.[39] Stress x-rays are useful in difficult cases, especially in those with no instrumentation.[116, 117] The use of bone scans has not proven to be useful to diagnose pseudarthroses;[54] the best diagnostic aid is adequate supine oblique views of good quality.

Treatment of a pseudarthrosis presenting late depends on the manifestation. When it presents with pain, loss of correction, or increasing deformity, repair as outlined on page 394 is indicated. In rare cases in which an obvious pseudarthrosis is visible with or without instrumentation failure and there is *no* pain, increasing deformity, or loss of correction, observation is indicated. In some of these cases the fibrous tissue in the defect maintains spine stability and *no* repair is necessary.

Prevention of deformity involves the technique of meticulous exposure, facet excision, decortication, and the addition of sufficient fusion bone—autologous iliac bone augmented by banked bone when quantity is insufficient. In deformities associated with a high pseudarthrosis rate, the addition of an anterior fusion has markedly decreased the incidence (neurologic diseases, adults, kyphosis).

INSTRUMENTATION PROBLEMS

Late instrumentation problems include displacement or breakage (Fig. 21–10). Breakage of the instrumentation (rods or anterior fixation) is usually associated with a pseudarthrosis. The most common failure point of the Harrington distraction rod is at the junction of the solid portion of the rod and the ratchets (Fig. 21–11). It is axiomatic that broken instrumentation suggests a pseudarthrosis and is *not* the metal but the fusion that has failed. Rarely will the rod break if the fusion is solid.[39] This is because of rod breakage while the fusion is healing and thus no fusion weakness exists. When a rod breaks and there is loss of correction, the broken ends separate and the rod alignment is lost (Fig. 21–12). When a Dwyer cable breaks, a few strands break first, the area unravels and the whole cable breaks, this breakage being opposite a disc space that is not fused.

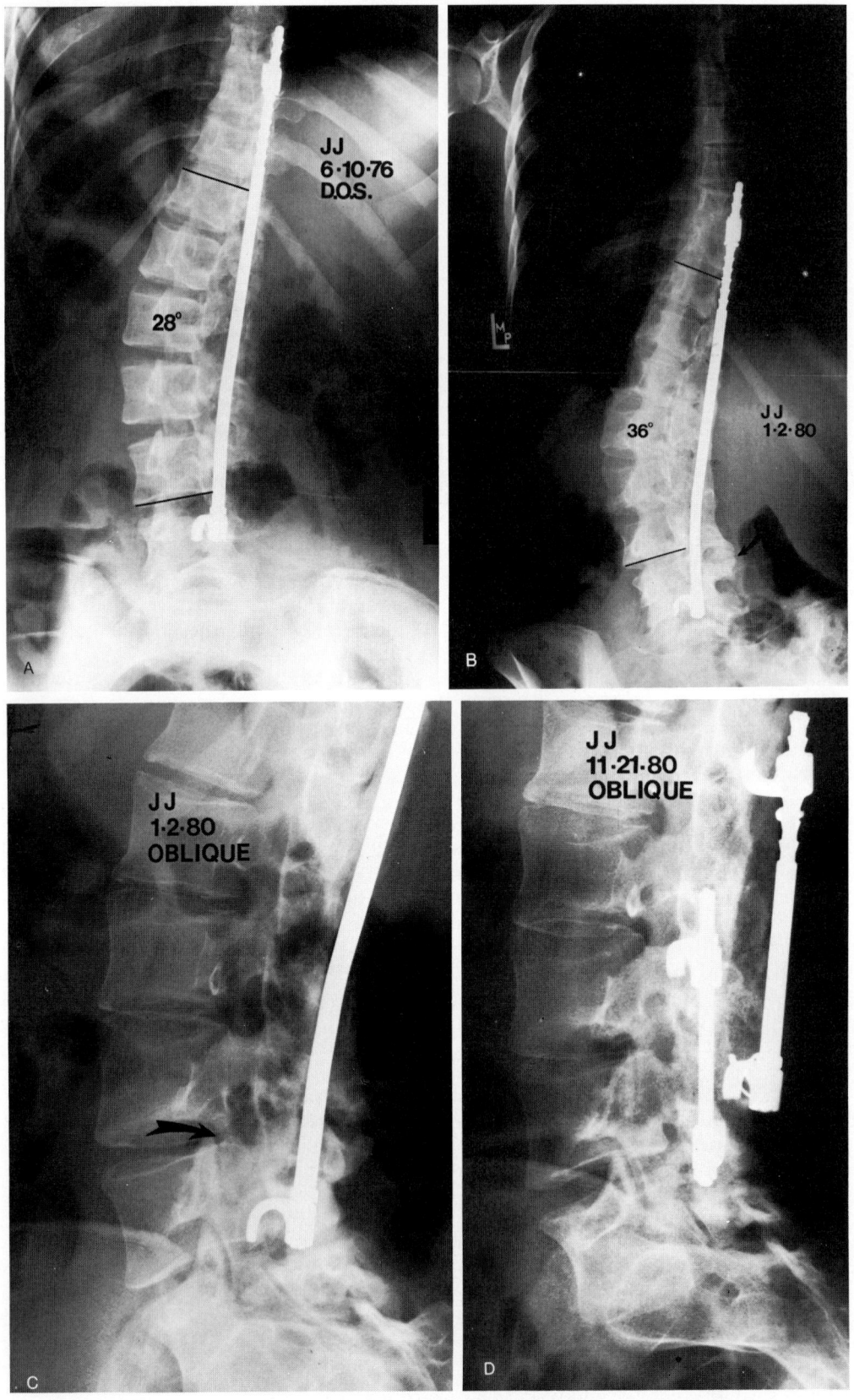

Figure 21–9. *See legend on opposite page.*

COMPLICATIONS OF TREATMENT

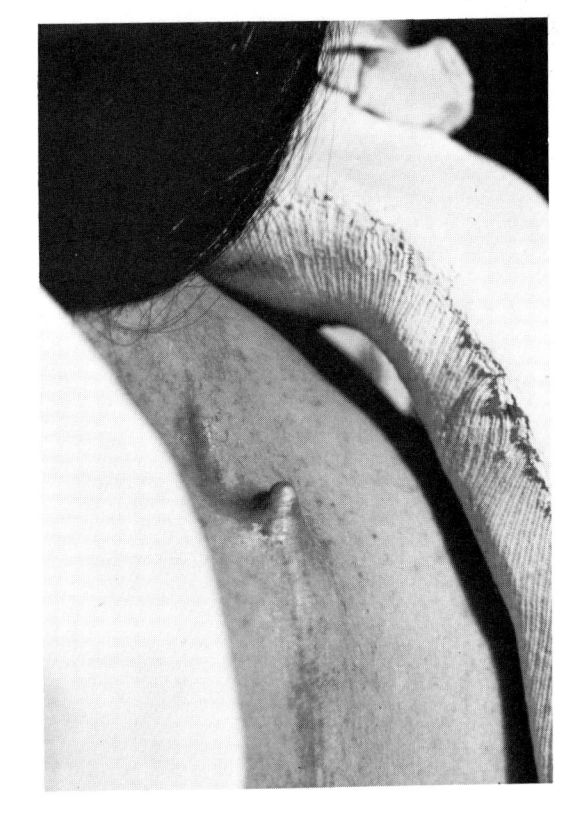

Figure 21–10. Clinical photograph of a patient in a halo cast showing the upper end of the Harrington distraction rod tenting the skin. The upper hook had cut out, and the rod became palpable. Operative reinsertion was necessary.

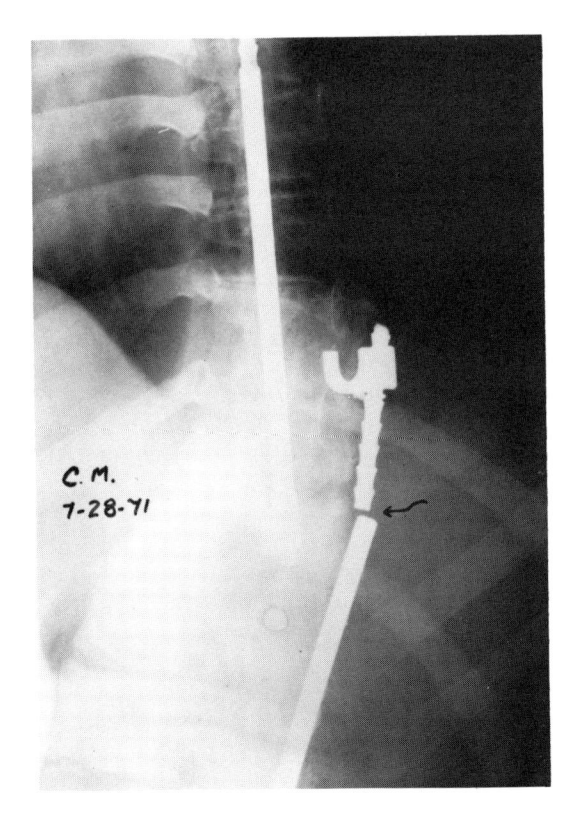

Figure 21–11. An oblique x-ray in a 15 year old girl, who had a posterior fusion for idiopathic scoliosis a year previously, shows breakage of the Harrington rod at the junction of the solid and ratchet area opposite the pseudarthrosis of the fusion.

Figure 21–9. A, This girl with idiopathic scoliosis had a posterior fusion with instrumentation on June 10, 1976, at the age of 15+3. B, She presented three and a half years later with lumbar pain; the anteroposterior x-ray showed loss of correction and a pseudarthrosis at L4–L5. C, An oblique view confirmed the defect through the lumbar facet. D, A pseudarthrosis repair and re-instrumentation was performed, and ten months later she was painfree with a solid fusion.

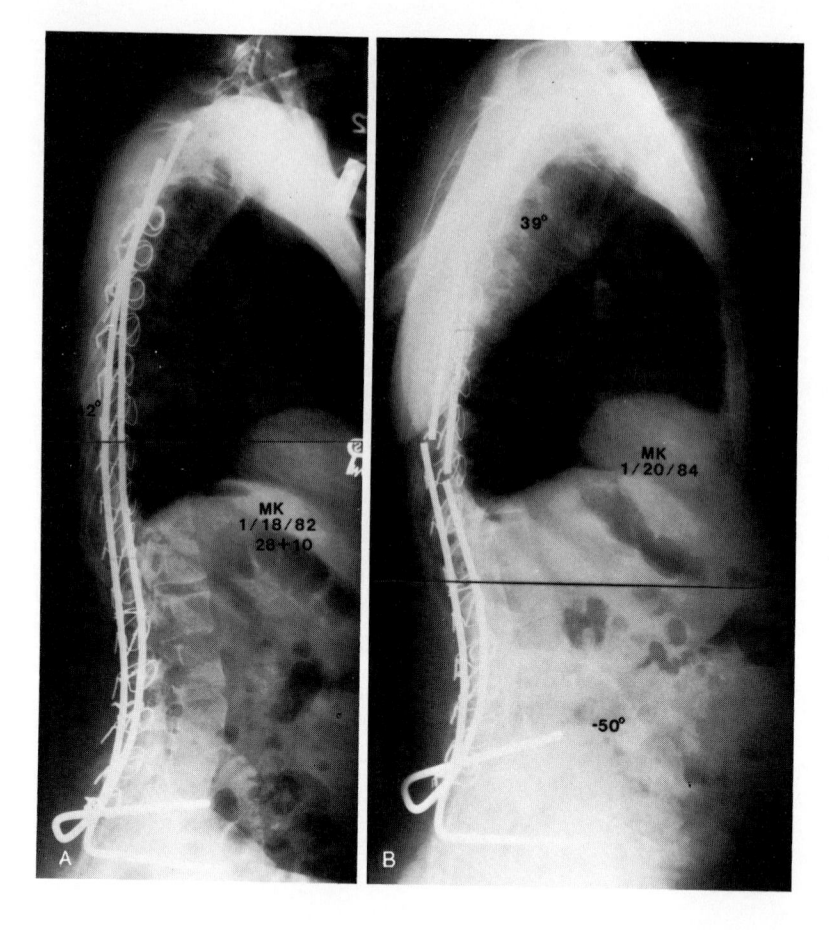

Figure 21–12. *A*, M.K., a 28+10 year old female with post polio scoliosis had a posterior fusion with Luque instrumentation utilizing 3/16-inch rods. *B*, Two years later there was loss of correction, pain, and rod breakage due to a pseudarthrosis of the fusion. Pseudarthrosis repair and re-instrumentation was performed.

With the use of sublaminar wires, wire breakage can occur. This is diagnosed radiographically and is due to excess force on the wire or overstressing and weakening of the wire during tightening.

Instrumentation displacement can occur late with hook displacement, or cut out; or screw tilting or displacement in the vertebral body (Fig. 21–13). Unless accompanied by other problems, for example, pseudarthrosis, prominence, these displacements do not need treatment. Anterior instrumentation displacement or breakage has been associated with erosion of the aorta with aortic aneurysm. This complication has also been described with anterior instrumentation alone owing to the bulk of metal (e.g., the Dunn device) next to the great vessels. These aneurysms are often fatal.

The end of the instrumentation may be prominent under the skin. This can be due to the prominent end of a rod, or due to prominent hooks or wires. A protective bursa develops around the prominent metal. This is often painful, and occasionally skin breakdown occurs. Trimming the rod, or removal of prominent hooks or wires is often necessary.

Lengthening of Curve. Lengthening of the curvature ("adding on") is an extension of the curvature to include vertebrae that originally were *not* a part of the curve. This may occur as a result of improper selection of the fusion area, by failure to include all rotated vertebrae into the fusion. The curve may stop at the twelfth thoracic vertebra, but the rotation continues into the lumbar spine. In this case the fusion must include all the rotated vertebrae and not follow the arbitrary rule to fuse one vertebra below and above the end vertebrae.

Adding on can occur even with proper selection of the fusion area. In some patients fused before the adolescent growth spurt, the original curve may extend, and adjacent unfused vertebrae subsequently become part of the curve. The use of prolonged immobilization in these young fusions may control curve lengthening.

Bending of the Fusion. A fusion performed before the adolescent growth spurt may bend. The fusion mass is living bone,

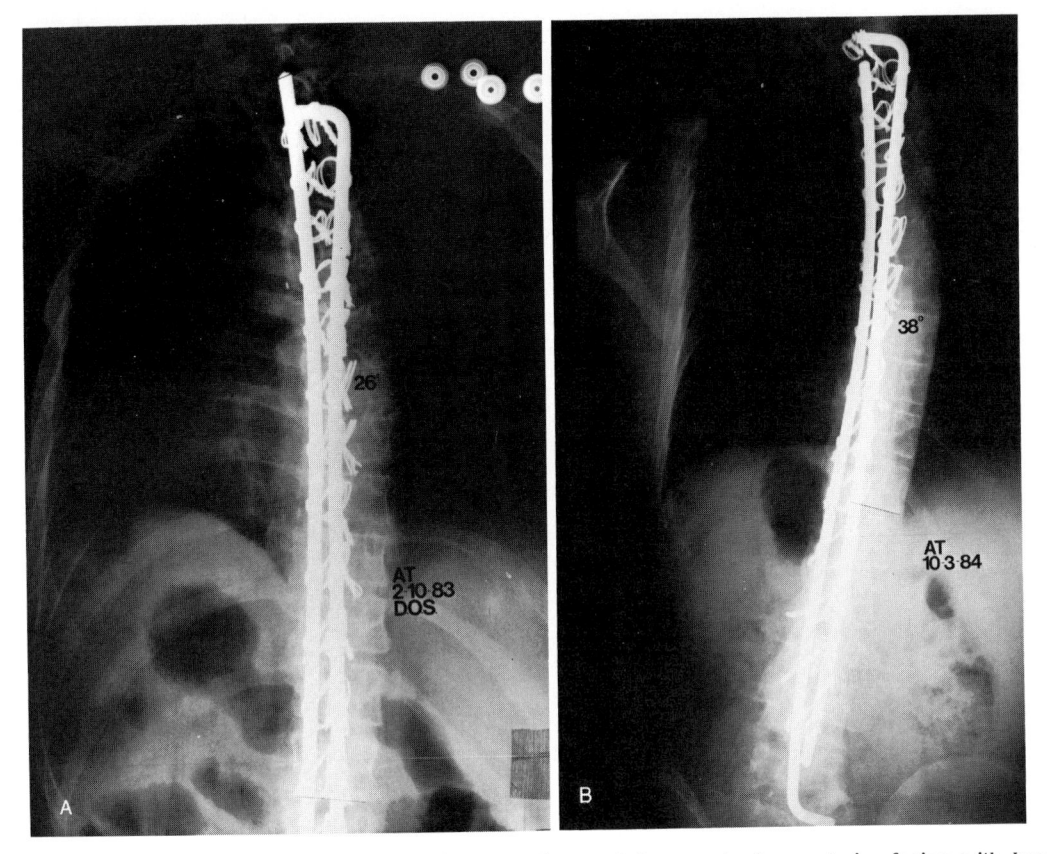

Figure 21-13. A, A.T., a 25 year old male with muscularum deformans had a posterior fusion with Luque instrumentation. Note the rod overlap superiorly. There was no pain postoperatively, but the rod was noted to slip. B, A year and ten months later the fusion was solid, there was no pain, and the rod slippage had not changed. A wire loop around the L of the Luque rod would have prevented rod slippage.

and does not increase in length if solid. The fusion may rather remodel and bend, with microfractures occurring on the convexity (the side of tension). The result is bending of the fusion and increase of the curvature. Bending is prevented by good surgical technique to provide a strong thick fusion mass that is protected until the bone is healed and mature. In some cases of thick strong fusions at a young age, the anterior growth causes the spine to rotate around the thick fusion. This results in loss of correction or more commonly increasing rotational prominence with no curve change. This can be prevented by performing an anterior fusion to control the anterior growth.

Stunting of Trunk Growth. Extensive fusion at a young age produces shortening of trunk height, since the fusion mass does not elongate. Long-term studies by Moe and Sundberg[90] and Winter[147] of patients undergoing fusion before the age of 10 showed an average lengthening of the fusion mass to be only 1 mm. in five years. It is understood that with a severe progressive deformity in a child a short, straight fused spine is better than an even shorter crooked spine, which would result if the fusion were not performed. Fusion in the young can be postponed with the use of an orthosis or the use of a rod without a fusion (see Chapter 11). In congenital scoliosis the area involved does *not* have normal growth potential, and a long fusion is necessary. The stunting of growth that is seen is due to the underlying deformity, the fusion only stabilizes the area, preventing progression.

When fusions are indicated in the young, the minimal fusion should be performed to control the curve. If necessary, prolonged bracing plus a rod without a fusion are used to control the remainder of the spine; the definitive fusion is performed in adolescence.

Lordosis. Lordosis in the area of fusion is caused by a posterior epiphysiodesis effect with continuance of anterior growth. It is caused by a long fusion in a young child, in whom the fusion mass is thin and easily bent by the anterior growth. In our experience this problem is rare.[90, 147] When this problem occurs, anterior epiphysiodesis and thickening of the fusion posteriorly are indicated. If this problem is severe, combined anterior-posterior osteotomy and reconstruction are indicated.

Loss of Lumbar Lordosis. Fusion of the lumbar spine with flattening of the spine eliminates the normal lumbar lordosis. This problem was rare before the use of Harrington instrumentation, but a straight distraction rod inserted from the thoracic area to the sacrum may cause the normal lordosis to be decreased or eliminated. This condition is commonly associated with a pseudarthrosis in the low lumbar area, usually at the lumbosacral junction. In polio patients this problem occurs in association with weak quadriceps and hip flexion contractures.

The forces on the spine can result in true kyphosis in the lumbar area, and is commonly associated with kyphosis above the fusion. The patient presents with a forward leaning gait and compensates by hyperextension of the thoracic spine or by knee flexion, which results in a fatiguing, awkward gait.

Prevention of this complication is by preservation of lumbar lordosis. A contoured distraction rod should be used. The rod has a tendency to rotate, but a square-ended Moe rod and Moe hook will prevent this. In addition, a compression rod can be added on the concavity to maintain the lordosis. An alternative is to use a Luque rod contoured to maintain the lumbar lordosis. This complication is treated by rod removal, pseudarthrosis repair, and a closing wedge lumbar osteotomy (see Chapter 18).[1, 26]

In the treatment of lumbar or thoracolumbar curves with anterior compression instrumentation (Dwyer or Zielke), placement of the screws anteriorly results in loss of lordosis and even true kyphosis. Care in screw insertion and placement of bone blocks anteriorly maintain the lumbar lordosis (see Chapter 10).

MISCELLANEOUS PROBLEMS

Other complications that are specific for spinal fusions have been described; only single cases have been reported.

Acquired spondylolysthesis has occurred after fusion to the lower lumbar spine (L4 or L5). The spondylolysthesis occurred postoperatively and required rod removal and fusion extension.[43, 133] A fusion to the upper thoracic area (T1) complicated by a bilateral facet subluxation at C6 and C7 was reported by Drennan; the subluxation was reduced with a halo and successfully held with a posterior fusion.

Other rare complications include thoracic outlet syndrome,[50] bronchial compression,[69] and spinal stenosis due to a Harrington hook.[9]

References

1. Adams, J. C.: Techniques, dangers and safeguards in osteotomy of the spine. J. Bone Joint Surg., 34B:226, 1952.
2. Allen, B. L., Jr.: Segmental spinal instrumentation with L-rods. American Academy of Orthopaedic Surgeons Instructional Course Lectures 32:202–208, 1983.
3. Anderson, P. R., Puno, M. R., Lovell, S. L., and Swayze, C. R.: Postoperative respiratory complications in non-idiopathic scoliosis. Acta Anaesthesiol. Scand., 29:186–192, 1985.
4. Barner, H. B., and Sherman, D. C.: Vascular compression of the duodenum. Surg. Gynecol. Obstet., 117:103, 1963.
5. Berg, U., and Aaro, S.: Long term effects of Boston brace treatment and renal function in patients with idiopathic scoliosis. Clin. Orthop., 180:169–172, 1983.
6. Bernstein, A. E., and Warner, G. M.: Onset of anorexia nervosa after prolonged use of the Milwaukee brace. Psychosomatics, 24:1033–1034, 1983.
7. Bisla, R. S., and Louis, H. J.: Acute vascular compression of the duodenum following cast application. Surg. Gynecol. Obstet., 140:563–566, 1975.
8. Boas, E. P.: The cardiovascular complications of kyphoscoliosis with report of a case of paroxysmal auricular fibrillation in a patient with severe scoliosis. Am. J. Med. Sci., 166:89–95, 1923.
9. Bowen, J. R., and Ferrer, J.: Spinal stenosis caused by a Harrington hook in neuromuscular disease. Clin. Orthop., 180:179–181, 1983.
10. Breig, A.: Biomechanics of the Central Nervous System. Stockholm, Almquist and Wiksell, 1966.
11. Brodkey, J. S., Richards, D. E., Blasingame, J. P., et al.: Reversible spinal cord trauma in cats: additive effects of direct pressure and ischemia. J. Neurosurg. 37:591–593, 1972.
12. Broude, A. I.: Transfusion reactions from contaminated blood: their recognition and treatment. New Engl. J. Med., 258:1289, 1958.
13. Brown, L. P., and Stelling, F. H.: Fat embolism as a complication of scoliosis fusion. J. Bone Joint Surg., 56A:1764, 1974.
14. Buchner, H., Pink, P., and Reinisch, H.: Funfjahrige erfahrungen mit dem Harrington-Stab bei der operativen Behandlung der Skoliose. Arch. Orthop. Unfallchir., 80:343, 1974.
15. Bunch, W. H.: Cholecystitis following spinal fu-

sion. Presented at the Annual Meeting of the Scoliosis Research Society, Lexington, KY., 1975.
16. Bunch, W., and Delaney, J.: Scoliosis and acute vascular compression of the duodenum. Surgery, 67:901, 1970.
17. Bunch, W. H., Scarff, T. B., and Trimble, J.: Current concepts review—spinal cord monitoring. J. Bone Joint Surg., 65A:707–709, 1983.
18. Byrd, H. J., Hughes, J. L., and Sauer, B.: An evaluation of cefoxitin in the prevention of postoperative infections following orthopedic surgical procedures. Orthopaedics, 8:69–71, 1985.
19. Celli, B. R., Rodriguez, K. S., and Snider, G. L.: Controlled trial of intermittent positive pressure breathing, incentive spirometry and deep breathing exercises in preventing pulmonary complications in abdominal surgery. Am. Rev. Resp. Dis., 130:12–15, 1984.
20. Cleveland, R. H., Gilsanz, V., Lebowitz, R. L., and Wilkinson, R. H.: Hydronephrosis from retroperitoneal fibrosis and anterior spinal fusion. J. Bone Joint Surg., 60A:996, 1978.
21. Colletta, A. J., and Mayer, P. J.: Chylothorax: an unusual complication of anterior thoracic interbody spinal fusion. Spine, 7:46–49, 1982.
22. Connell, R. S., and Swank, R. L.: Pulmonary microembolism after blood transfusions. Ann. Surg., 177:40, 1973.
23. Curtis, B. H.: Air embolism as a complication of spine fusion. J. Bone Joint Surg., 54A:201, 1972.
24. Cusick, J. F., Jyklebust, J., Syvoloski, M., et al.: Effects of vertebral column distraction in the monkey. J. Neurosurg., 57:651–659, 1982.
25. Dawson, E. G., Caran, A., and Moe, J. H.: Surgical management of scoliosis in the adult. J. Bone Joint Surg., 55A:437, 1973.
26. Denis, F., and Moe, J. H.: Iatrogenic loss of lumbar lordosis. Presented at Annual Meeting of Scoliosis Research Society, Ottawa, Canada. September, 1976.
27. Dewald, R. L., and Ray, R. D.: Skeletal traction for the treatment of severe scoliosis. J. Bone Joint Surg., 52A:233, 1970.
28. Dolan, E. H., Transfeldt, E. E., Tator, C. H., et al.: The effect of spinal distraction on regional spinal cord blood flow in cats. J. Neurosurg., 53:756–764, 1980.
29. Dommisse, G. F.: The blood supply of the spinal cord. J. Bone Joint Surg., 56B:225, 1974.
30. Dommisse, G. F.: The Arteries and Veins of the Human Spinal Cord from Birth. Edinburgh, Churchill Livingstone, 1975.
31. Dwyer, A. F., and Shafer, M. F.: Anterior approach to scoliosis. J. Bone Joint Surg., 56B:218, 1974.
32. Dwyer, A. P., et al: The late complications following Dwyer anterior spinal instrumentation in the management of scoliosis. Presented at the Annual Meeting of the Scoliosis Research Society, Lexington, Kentucky, 1975.
33. Dwyer, A. P.: Paravertebral infection following Dwyer anterior spinal instrumentation. Presented at the Annual Meeting of the Scoliosis Research Society, Lexington, Kentucky, 1975.
34. Dykes, M. H., Fuller, J. E., and Goldstein, L. A.: Sudden cessation of cardiac output during spinal fusion. Anaesth. Analg. Rev. 33:47–60, 1976.
35. Eftekhar, N. S.: Prevention is the best treatment for infection in implant surgery. Orthop. Rev., 8:25–28, 1979.
36. Eisenstein, S., and O'Brien, J. P.: Chylothorax—a complication of Dwyer anterior instrumentation. Br. J. Surg., 64:339–341, 1977.
37. Ellner, P. D.: Laboratory procedures to determine infections in orthopaedic surgery. Orthop. Rev., 8:37–45, 1979.
38. Engler, G. L., Spielholtz, N. I., Bernhard, W. N., et al.: Somatosensory evoked potentials during Harrington instrumentation for scoliosis. J. Bone Joint Surg., 60A:520–532, 1978.
39. Erwin, W. D., Dickson, J. H., and Harrington, P. R.: Clinical review of patients with broken Harrington rods. J. Bone Joint Surg., 62A:1302–1307, 1980.
40. Evarts, C. M., Winter, R. B., and Hall, J. E.: Vascular compression of the duodenum associated with the treatment of scoliosis. J. Bone Joint Surg., 53A:431, 1971.
41. Faust, D., and Happel, L. T.: Cortical evoked potentials in spinal surgery. Orthopedics, 7:44–48, 1984.
42. Floman, Y., Micheli, L. J., Barker, W. D., and Hall, J. E.: Acute cholecystitis following the surgical treatment of spinal deformities in the adult. Clin. Orthop., 151:205–209, 1980.
43. Friedman, R. J., and Micheli, L. J.: Acquired spondylolisthesis following scoliosis surgery. Clin. Orthop., 180:132–134, 1984.
44. Gaines, D. L., Moe, J. H., and Bocklage, J.: Management of wound infections following Harrington instruments and spine fusion. J. Bone Joint Surg., 52A:404, 1970.
45. Gardner, A. D., O'Brien, J. P., and Hodgson, A. R.: Accurate electronic measurement of the forces applied to the spine during halo-pelvic traction. Presented at the Annual Meeting of the Scoliosis Research Society, Louisville, Kentucky, September, 1975.
46. Ginsburg, H., Shetter, A., and Raudzens, P.: Postoperative paraplegia with preserved intraoperative somatosensory evoked potentials. Orthop. Trans. 8:161, 1984.
47. Gittman, J. E., Buchanan, T. A., Fisher, B. J., et al.: Fatal fat embolism after spinal fusion for scoliosis. JAMA, 249:779–781, 1983.
48. Gray, S. W., Akin, J. T., Milsap, J. H., and Skanalakis, J. E.: Vascular compression of the duodenum. Contemp. Surg., 9:37, 1976.
49. Griffiths, G. J., and Whitehouse, G. H.: Radiological features of vascular compression of the duodenum occurring as a complication of the diagnosis of scoliosis (cast syndrome). Clin. Radiol., 29:77, 1978.
50. Grimer, R. J., Milligan, P. J., and Thompson, A. G.: Thoracic outlet syndrome following correction of scoliosis in a patient with cervical ribs. J. Bone Joint Surg., 65A:1172–1173, 1983.
51. Grundy, B. L., Nash, C. L., and Brown, R. H.: Anterior pressure manipulation alters spinal cord function during correction of scoliosis. Anaesthesiology, 54:249–253, 1981.
52. Gryboski, J. D., Kocoshis, S. A., Seachore, J. H., et al.: "Body Brace" esophagitis, a complication of kyphoscoliosis therapy. Lancet, 2:449–451, 1978.
53. Guttmann, L, and Frankel, H.: The value of intermittent catheterization in the management

of traumatic paraplegia and tetraplegia. Paraplegia, 4:63, 1966.
54. Hannon, K. M., and Wetta, W. J.: Failure of Technetium bone scanning to detect pseudarthroses in spinal fusion for scoliosis. Clin. Orthop., 123:42–44, 1977.
55. Hardy, J. M., Cooke, R. W., and Einbund, M.: Hyperalimentation in the treatment of "cast syndrome." J. Bone Joint Surg., 54A:200, 1972.
56. Hardy, R. W., Nash, C. L., and Brodkey, J. S.: Follow-up report: Experimental and clinical studies in spinal cord monitoring. The effect of pressure anoxia and ischaemia on spinal cord function. J. Bone Joint Surg., 55A:435, 1973.
57. Harrington, P. R.: Technical details in relation to the successful use of instrumentation in scoliosis. Orthop. Clin. North Am., 3:49, 1972.
58. Hendrix, R. W., Matalon, T. S., Calenoff, L., et al.: Pulmonary complications following spinal instrumentation. Contemp. Orthop., 3: 423–430, 1981.
59. Herring, J. A., Fitch, R., Wenger, D., et al.: Segmental spinal instrumentation—a review of early results and complications. Orthop. Trans., 8:172, 1984.
60. Hoppenfeld, S., Gross, A., and Andrews, C.: The ankle clonus test—an alternative to the Stagnara wake up test and somatosensory evoked potentials in the assessment of spinal cord damage in the treatment of scoliosis with Harrington rod instrumentation. Orthop. Trans., 9:118, 1985.
61. Hughes, J. P., McEntire, J. D., and Setze, T. K.: Cast syndrome. Arch. Surg., 108:230, 1974.
62. Humbyrd, D. E., Latimer, R., Lonstein, J. E., and Samberg, L. C.: Brain abscess as a complication of halo traction. Spine, 6:365–368, 1981.
63. Jacobsen, S. T., and Crawford, A. H.: Brachial plexus injury following Risser hyperextension casting for Scheuermann's disease. Orthopaedics, 5:1183–1185, 1982.
64. Jamieson, K. G., and Yelland, J. D. N.: Cerebral abscess due to skull fracture. Aust. N.Z. J. Surg., 34:301, 1965.
65. Johnson, C. E., Norris, R., Burke, S. W., et al.: Delayed paraplegia following segmental spinal instrumentation. Presented at the Annual Meeting of the Scoliosis Research Society, Orlando, Florida, September, 1984.
66. Jones, E. T., Mathews, L. S., and Hensinger, R. N.: The wake-up technique as a dual protector of spinal cord function during spine fusion. Clin. Orthop., 168:113–118, 1982.
67. Kahanovitz, M., and Levine, D. B.: Iatrogenic complications of spinal surgery. Contemp. Orthop., 2:23–42, 1984.
68. Kalamchi, A., Yau, A. C. M. C., O'Brien, J. P., and Hodgson, A.: Halo pelvic distraction apparatus. J. Bone Joint Surg., 58A:1119, 1976.
69. Karroll, M., Hernandez, R. J., and Wessel, H. U.: Computed tomography diagnosis of bronchial compression by the spine after surgical correction of scoliosis. Pediatr. Radiol., 14:335–336, 1984.
70. Keim, H. A., and Weinstein, J. D.: Acute renal failure—a complication of spine fusion in the tuck position. J. Bone Joint Surg., 52A:1248, 1970.
71. Keller, R. B., and Pappas, A. M.: Infection after spinal fusion using internal fixation instrumentation. Orthop. Clin. North Am., 3:99, 1972.
72. Kennedy, R. H., and Cooper, M. J.: An unusually severe case of cast syndrome. Postgrad. Med. J., 59:539–540, 1983.
73. King, A. G.: Complications in segmental spinal instrumentation. In Luque, E. (ed.):Segmental Spinal Instrumentation. Thorofare, N. J., Slack, Inc., pp. 301–330, 1984.
74. Kling, T. F., Drennan, J. C., and Gryboski, J. D.: Esophyagitis complicating scoliosis management with the Boston Thoracolumbosacral Orthosis. Clin. Orthop., 159:208–210, 1981.
75. Kostuik, J. P., Israel, J., and Hall, J. E.: Scoliosis surgery in adults. Clin. Orthop., 93:225, 1973.
76. Lapides, J., Diokno, A. C., Silber, S. J., and Lowe, B. S.: Clean, intermittent self catheterization in the treatment of urinary tract disease. J. Urol., 107:458, 1972.
77. Letts, R. M., and Hollenberg, C.: Delayed paresis following spinal fusion with Harrington instrumentation. Clin. Orthop. Rel. Res., 125:45–48, 1977.
78. Lonstein, J., Winter, R., Moe, J., and Gaines, D.: Wound infection with Harrington instrumentation and spine fusion for scoliosis. Clin. Orthop., 96:22, 1973.
79. Lundborg, G., and Rydevik, B.: Effects of stretching the tibial nerve of the rabbit. A preliminary study of the intraneural circulation and the barrier function of the perineurium. J. Bone Joint Surg., 55B:390, 1973.
80. Luque, E. R.: The anatomic basis and development of segmental spinal instrumentation. Spine, 7:256–259, 1982.
81. MacEwen, D. G., Bunnell, W. P., and Sriram, K.: Acute neurological complications in the treatment of scoliosis. J. Bone Joint Surg., 57A:404, 1975.
82. MacEwen, D. G., and Cowell, H. R.: Autogenous transfusion for spinal surgery in children. J. Bone Joint Surg., 56A:440, 1974.
83. McCarthy, R. E., Mertz, J. D., Lonstein, J. E., and Kuslich, S. D.: Air embolism in spinal susrgery. Presented at the Annual Meeting of the Pediatric Orthopedic Society of North America, San Antonio, Texas, May, 1985.
84. McCollister, E. C.: Intraoperative autotransfusion in surgery for scoliosis—a preliminary report. J. Bone Joint Surg., 56A:1764, 1974.
85. McMaster, W. C., and Silber, I.: An urologic complication of Dwyer instrumentation. J. Bone Joint Surg., 57A:710, 1975.
86. May, V. R., and Mauck, W. R.: Exploration of the spine for pseudarthrosis following spinal fusion in the treatment of scoliosis. Clin. Orthop., 53:115–122, 1967.
87. Meznik, F., Pfluger, G., Zhuber, K., and Zekert, F.: Zur entstehung und behandlung des sogenannten "cast syndroms" nach skoliose operationen. Z. Orthop., 113:174–180, 1975.
88. Micheli, L. J., and Hall, J. E.: Complications in the management of adult spinal deformities. In Epps, C. H. (ed.): Complications in Orthopaedic Surgery. Philadelphia, J. B. Lippincott, pp. 1039–1072, 1978.
89. Moe, J. H.: Complications of scoliosis treatment. Clin. Orthop., 53:21, 1967.
90. Moe, J. H., and Sundberg, B.: A clinical study of spine fusion in the growing child. J. Bone Joint Surg., 46B:784, 1964.
91. Moe, J. H., Winter, R. B., Bradford, D. S., et al.:

Scoliosis and Other Spinal Deformities, Philadelphia, W. B. Saunders, 1978.
92. Morbidity Report. Scoliosis Research Society Meeting. Hartford, Connecticut, September, 1971.
93. Morbidity Report. Scoliosis Research Society Meeting. Wilmington, Delaware, September, 1972.
94. Morbidity Report. Scoliosis Research Society Meeting. Gothenburg, Sweden, September, 1973.
95. Morgenstern, J. M., Hassmann, G. C., and Keim, H. A.: Modifying post-transfusion hepatitis by gamma gobulin in spinal surgery. Orthop. Rev., 4:29, 1975.
96. Munster, A. M., Weidner, J., and Gibson, G.: Prophylactic antibiotics in surgery. JAMA, 241:717–718, 1979.
97. Nash, C. D., and Keim, H. A.: Prophylactic antibiotics in spinal surgery. Orthop. Rev., 11:27–30, 1973.
98. Nash, C., Lorig, R. A., Schatzinger, L. A., et al.: Spinal cord monitoring during operative treatment of the spine. Clin. Orthop. Rel. Res., 126:100–105, 1977.
99. Nash, C. L., Schatzinger, L., and Lorig, R.: Intraoperative monitoring of spinal cord function during scoliosis surgery. J. Bone Joint Surg., 56A:1765, 1974.
100. Nelson, C. L.: Preventive antibodies in orthopedic surgery. J. Surg. Pract., 7:16–25, 1978.
101. Nickel, V. L., Perry, J., Garret, A., and Heppenstall, M.: The halo. J. Bone Joint Surg., 52A:1400, 1968.
102. Nillius, A., Willner, S., Arborelius, M., and Nylander, G.: Combined radionucleotide phlebography and lung scanning in patients operated on for scoliosis with Harrington procedure. Clin. Orthop., 152:241–246, 1980.
103. Nordwall, A., and Wikkelso, C.: A late neurological complication of scoliosis surgery in connection with syringomyelia. Acta Orthop. Scand., 50:407–410, 1979.
104. O'Brien, J. P., Yau, A. C., Smith, T. K., and Hodgson, A. R.: Halo pelvic traction. J. Bone Joint Surg., 53B:217, 1971.
105. O'Brien, J. P.: The halo pelvic apparatus. Acta Orthop. Scand. (Suppl.), 163:79, 1975.
106. Pasteyer, J., Jean, N., Merckx, J., et al.: Accidents de l'anesthesie au cours de la chirurgie des scolioses. Anaesth. Anal. Rev., 33:47–60, 1976.
107. Perry, J.: The halo in spinal abnormalities. Orthop. Clin. North Am., 3:69–80, 1972.
108. Pinto, W. C.: Complications of surgical treatment of scoliosis. Israel J. Med. Sci., 9:837, 1973.
109. Polk, H. C., Trachtenberg, L. O., and Finn, M. P.: Antibiotic activity in surgical incisions. JAMA, 244:1353–1354, 1980.
110. Ponder, R. C., Dickson, J. H., Harrington, P. R., and Erwin, W. D.: Results of Harrington instrumentation and fusion in the adult idiopathic scoliotic patient. J. Bone Joint Surg., 57A:797, 1975.
111. Ponte, A.: Postoperative paraplegia due to hypercorrection of scoliosis and drop in blood pressure. J. Bone Joint Surg., 56A:444, 1974.
112. Pouliquen, J. C., Rigault, P., Canevet, M., and Buyonvarch, G.: Les complications medullaires de la chirurgie des deviations rachidiennes. Chir. Pediatr., 21:215–224, 1980.
113. Puranik, S. R., Keiser, R. P., and Gilbert, M. G.: Arteriomesenteric duodenal compression in children. Am. J. Surg., 124:334–339, 1972.
114. Ransford, A. O., and Manning, C. W. S. F.: Complications of halo-pelvic distraction for scoliosis. J. Bone Joint Surg., 57B:131, 1975.
115. Raphael, B. G., Lackner, H., and Engler, G. L.: Disseminated intravascular coagulation during surgery for scoliosis. Clin. Orthop., 162:41–46, 1982.
116. Risser, J. C., and Norquist, D. M.: A followup study of the treatment of scoliosis. J. Bone Joint Surg., 40A:555, 1958.
117. Risser, J. C., Iqbal, Q. M., Nagata, K., and Azevedo, G.: Early non-operative diagnosis of spinal pseudarthrosis. Int. Surg., 67:181–186, 1982.
118. Schmitt, E. W.: Post-instrumentation paraplegia and a negative Stagnara test—a case report. Presented at the Annual Meeting of the Scoliosis Research Society, Boston, Massachusetts, September, 1978.
119. Schmitt, V., and Sandler, S. G.: HTLV-III antibody testing. American Red Cross National Headquarters BSV, No. 85–2, January 15, 1985.
120. Schur, M. S., Brown, J. T., Kafer, E. R., et al.: Postoperative pulmonary function in children—comparison of scoliosis with peripheral surgery. Am. Rev. Respir. Dis., 130:46–51, 1984.
121. Schurman, D. J., and Woolson, S. T.: Prophylactic antibiotics in orthopaedic surgery. Orthopedics, 7:1603, 1984.
122. Seddon, H. J.: Peripheral nerve injuries. M.R.C. Special Report Series, No. 82. Her Majesty's Stationery Office, 1954.
123. Shalding, B.: The so-called superior mesenteric artery syndrome. Am. J. Dis. Child., 130:1371, 1976.
124. Silber, I., and McMaster, W.: Retroperitoneal fibrosis with hydronephrosis as a complication of the Dwyer procedure. J. Pediatr. Surg., 12:255, 1977.
125. Simurda, M. A.: Arteriovenous fistula and neurological sequelae of spinal fusion. J. Bone Joint Surg., 51B:193, 1969.
126. Skandalakis, J. E., Akin, J. T., Milsap, J. H., and Gray, S. W.: Vascular compression of the duodenum. Contemp. Surg., 10:33, 1977.
127. Solis, R. T., and Gibbs, M. B.: Filtration of microaggregates in stored blood. Transfusion, 12:245, 1972.
128. Stagnara, P.: Utilization of Harrington device in the treatment of scoliosis. In Chapchal, G. (ed.): Symposium in Jijmegen, Netherlands, Stuttgart, George Thieme, p. 61. 1973.
129. Stagnara, P.: Personal communication, 1975.
130. Sudhir, K. G., Smith, R. M., Hall, J. E., et al.: Intraoperative awakening for early recognition of possible neurologic sequelae during Harrington rod spinal fusion. Anesth. Analg. (Cleve), 55:526–528, 1976.
131. Telfer, R. B., Hoyt, W. F., and Schwartz, H. S.: Crossed eyes and halo-pelvic traction. (Letter to Editor.) Lancet, 2:922, 1971.
132. Thompson, G. H., Wilber, R. B., Shaffer, J. W., et al.: Complications of segmental spinal instrumentation in spinal deformities. Orthop. Trans., 9:123, 1985.

133. Tietjen, R., and Morgenstern, J. M.: Spondylolisthesis following surgical fusion for scoliosis. Clin. Orthop., *117*:176–178, 1976.
134. Tillberg, G.: Prophylaxis and postoperative venous thrombosis. Acta Orthop. Scand. (Suppl.), *158*:3, 1974.
135. Tindall, G. T., Flanagan, J. F., and Hashold, B. S.: Brain abscess and osteomyelitis following skull fracture. Arch. Surg., *79*:114, 1959.
136. Transfeldt, E. E., Lonstein, J. E., Winter, R. B., et al.: Wound infections in reconstructive spinal surgery. Orthop. Trans., *9*:128, 1985.
137. Tredwell, S. J., and O'Brien, J. P.: Avascular necrosis of the proximal end of the dens. J. Bone Joint Surg., *57A*:201, 1972.
138. Tredwell, S. J., and O'Brien, J. P.: Apophyseal joint degeneration in the cervical spine following halo-pelvic distraction. Presented at the Annual Meeting of the Scoliosis Research Society, Louisville, Kentucky, September, 1975.
139. Uden, A.: Thomboembolic complications following scoliosis surgery in Scandinavia. Acta Orthop. Scand., *50*:175–178, 1979.
140. Vauzelle, C., Stagnara, P., and Jouvinroix, P.: Functional monitoring of spinal cord during spinal surgery. J. Bone Joint Surg., *55A*:441, 1973.
141. Vauzelle, C., Stagnara, P., and Jouvinroix, P.: Functional monitoring of spinal cord during spinal surgery. Clin. Orthop., *93*:173, 1973.
142. Victor, D. E., Bresnan, M. J., and Keller, R. B.: Brain abscess complicating the use of halo traction. J. Bone Joint Surg., *55A*:635, 1973.
143. Wade, G. H.: The relationship between urinary retention, multiple straight catheterizations, and the incidence of urinary tract infection in the female adolescent following a posterior spinal fusion. Orthop. Nursing, *1*:23–27, 1982.
144. Weisl, H.: Unusual complications of skull caliper fracture. J. Bone Joint Surg., *54B*:143, 1972.
145. Whitehouse, G. H., and Griffiths, G. H.: The phlebographic demonstration of venous thrombosis occurring during the treatment of scoliosis. Clin. Radiol., *29*:579–583, 1978.
146. Widman, F. K. (ed.): Technical manual of the American Association of Blood Banks. 8th Ed., Washington, D.C., American Association of Blood Banks, 325–327, 1981.
147. Winter, R. B.: The effects of early fusion on spine growth. *In* Zorab, P. A. (ed.): Scoliosis and Growth. Edinburgh, Churchill Livingstone, 1971.
148. Winter, R. B., Moe, J. H., and Wang, J. F.: Congenital kyphosis. J. Bone Joint Surg., *55A*:223, 1973.
149. Winter, R. B.: Congenital kyphoscoliosis with paralysis following hemivertebra excision. Clin. Orthop., *119*:116–125, 1976.
150. Winter, R. B.: Treatment of scoliosis and possible neurologic complications. *In* Chou, S. H., and Seljeskog, E. L. (eds.): Spine Deformities and Neurologic Dysfunction. New York, Raven Press, pp. 209–230, 1978.
151. Young, L. E.: Complications of blood transfusions. Ann. Int. Med., *61*:136, 1964.
152. Zielke, K., and Pellin, B.: Halo-pelvic traktion-Minderung ihrer Gefharen durch Vereinfachung der Anwendung. Z. Orthop., *112*:351, 1974.
153. Zielke, K., and Pellin, B.: Das neurologische risiko der Harrington operation. Arch. Orthop. Unfallchir., *83*:311–322, 1975.

22

MISCELLANEOUS PROBLEMS

Benign and Malignant Tumors of the Spine

David S. Bradford, M.D.

Tumors of the spine often have an insidious onset, resulting in variable complaints on the part of the patient. Furthermore, they often pose a diagnostic dilemma because the management is, for the most part, dependent on the nature of the tumor, the presence or absence of associated spinal deformity, and the presence or absence of a neurologic deficit. A thorough and detailed radiographic evaluation associated with adequate biopsy material for examination is usually necessary for proper and expeditious care.

Roentgenograms should be of excellent quality, and the routine x-rays should be supplemented with oblique projections as well as tomography. A bone scan is particularly helpful in certain lesions (e.g., osteoid osteoma) to facilitate location of the lesion and visualization of detail not well seen on routine radiographs. Arteriography is also helpful in evaluating the extent of the tumor, the location of major feeder vessels, and in providing a vehicle for embolization as a primary treatment or in association with resection. CT scanning has proven of immense benefit particularly in association with metrizamide myelography in demonstrating the extent of the lesion and the presence or absence of dural compression.[9, 12, 31, 33, 37, 47, 57, 66] Finally, the use of magnetic resonance imaging may be particularly helpful in defining the extent of soft tissue involvement.[47]

BIOPSY

Open or closed vertebral biopsy is often indicated in order to establish a diagnosis of a primary or a metastatic tumor to the spine. An excisional biopsy for benign-appearing and symptomatic lesions such as osteoid osteoma is usually possible. On the other hand, the needle biopsy or an incisional biopsy is usually necessary for more malignant-appearing metastatic tumors to the vertebral column. In general, we agree with the recommendation recently made by Dunn[17] that closed biopsy techniques are most useful for lesions involving the lumbar spine, whereas open biopsy techniques are more useful for lesions involving the thoracic spine. Biopsy technique using a Craig needle as described by Ottolenghi has proved most useful in our experience.[49] In the thoracic spine we have preferred to do an open biopsy because of the risk of neurologic damage, pneumothorax, or hemothorax from a closed biopsy. An open biopsy may be performed through a costotransversectomy approach, or through a transpedicular approach as described first by Michele and Krudger.[46] With the transpedicular approach, the skin and subcutaneous tissue are reflected 1 to 2 cm. lateral to the midline and the approach is through the paravertebral muscles. The superior facet is identified and a hole is made just over the pedicle with a small osteotome and drill. This hole then overlies the involved pedicle and a small curette may be passed safely within the pedicle into the centrum of the vertebral body, obtaining ample material for histologic evaluation.

BENIGN TUMORS OF THE SPINE

Benign tumors of the spine include osteoid osteoma, osteoblastoma, aneurysmal bone cyst, hemangioma, histiocytosis-x, and osteochondromas.

Osteoid Osteoma

The name osteoid osteoma was first proposed by Jaffe in 1935 to designate a benign, neoplastic lesion of bone characterized by a core of nidus-like focus and reactive parafocal bone thickenings.[33] These lesions may cause a painful scoliosis and indeed pose a diagnostic dilemma, since routine radiographs may not initially visualize the lesion.

The clinical features have been well described.[1, 21, 22, 25, 30, 41, 52, 58] Osteoid osteoma of the spine affects males more frequently than females. The onset of symptoms is usually during the second decade of life, although cases have been reported in patients under five and over 40 years of age. The lesions are almost invariably located in the posterior elements of the vertebra; however, four cases have been reported in which the lesion involved the vertebral body.[30, 60] The lumbar spine is the area most commonly involved, followed by the cervical and then the thoracic area.[71]

Pain is by far the most common symptom and is usually described as a localized ache that increases with time. The pain may be aggravated by motion, and it is not always relieved by aspirin. Sometimes it is more severe at night, or may be increased by coughing, sneezing, or defecation. Radicular pain is common, particularly when the lesion involves the lumbar spine. We have had one patient who had no pain and was treated for scoliosis with a Milwaukee brace for two years until the correct diagnosis was made.

Physical findings reveal tenderness and marked muscle spasm at the site of the lesion. Neurologic involvement may be present. This may present as weakness of the limb, cutaneous hypesthesia, positive straight leg raising, and deep tendon reflex changes. Atrophy has been reported, but it is not clear whether this is from disuse secondary to radicular pain or whether it is caused by neurologic involvement.

Scoliosis is common but may not be present if a lesion involves the spinous processes, sacrum, or vertebral body. The scoliosis is usually associated with torticollis of the cervical spine and pelvic obliquity in the lumbar spine. The magnitude of the scoliosis is variable. The curvature may present as a typical C-shaped curve but the so-called typical idiopathic curvature is also seen in association with osteoid osteoma. The lesion is almost invariably located on the concave side of the curvature and often in the apical posterior elements. The scoliosis usually demonstrates minimal correctability on side bending.

The radiographic appearance is usually characteristic[8, 20, 36, 64] and consists of a central radiolucency with a surrounding sclerotic reaction (Fig. 22–1). This x-ray appearance may not always be present. The initial x-rays may, in fact, be negative since the lesion may

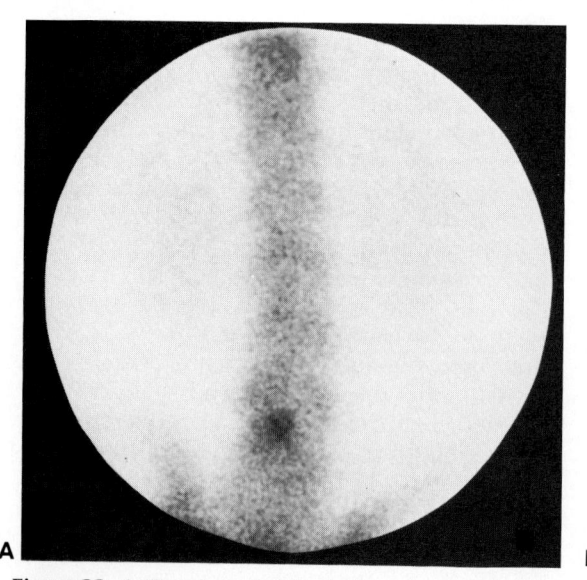

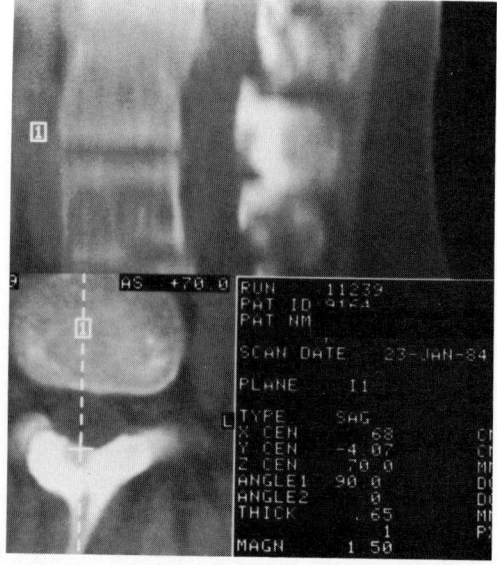

Figure 22–1. The characteristic findings on radioactive bone scan (A) and CT scan (B) in a patient with an osteoid osteoma.

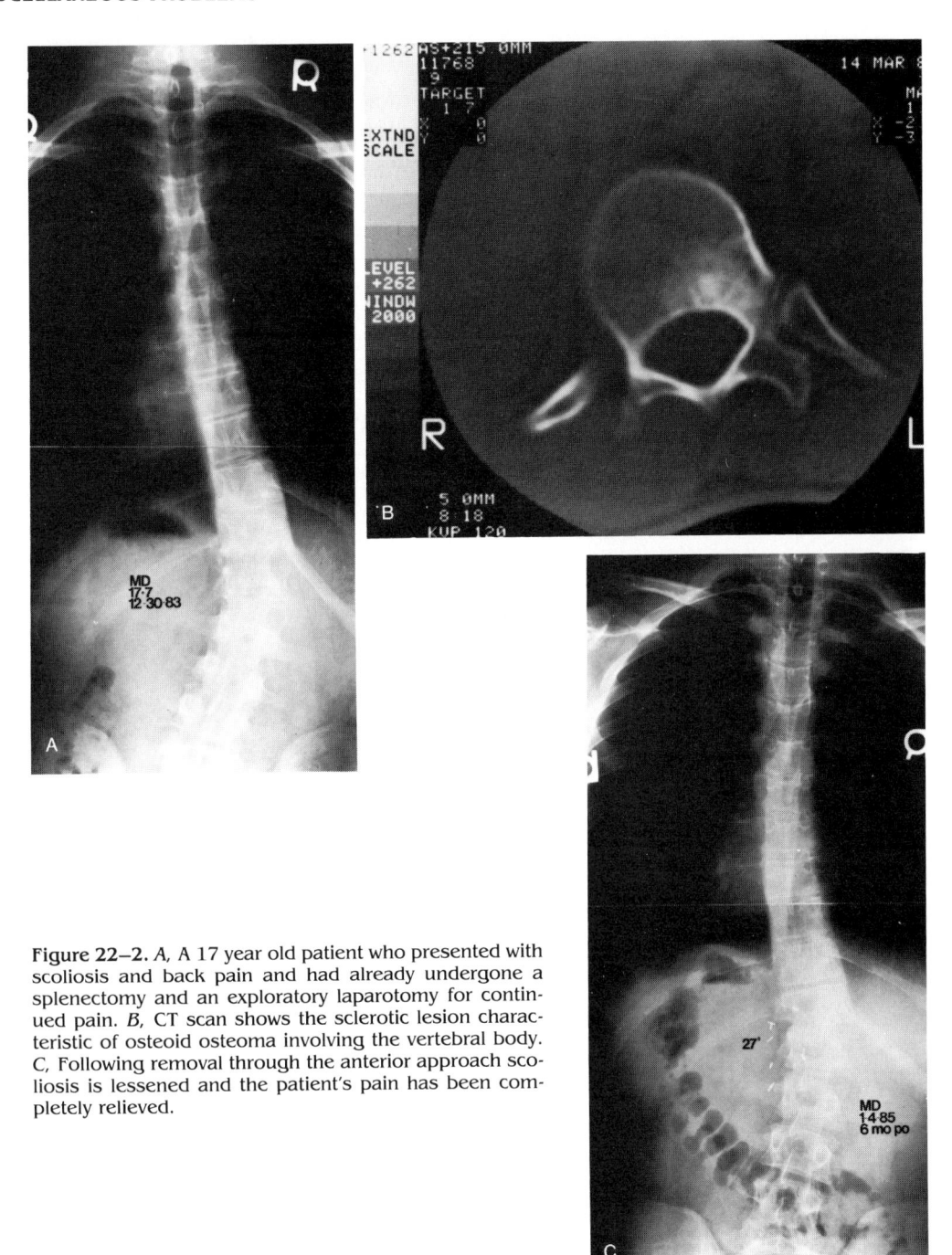

Figure 22–2. *A*, A 17 year old patient who presented with scoliosis and back pain and had already undergone a splenectomy and an exploratory laparotomy for continued pain. *B*, CT scan shows the sclerotic lesion characteristic of osteoid osteoma involving the vertebral body. *C*, Following removal through the anterior approach scoliosis is lessened and the patient's pain has been completely relieved.

produce pain, before it is radiographically detectable. Tomography of the spine is helpful, as is a bone scan, in identifying a suspected osteoid osteoma.[32, 48, 55] In fact, the intraoperative localization of the lesion as reported by Rinsky and Israeli[55] might be considered. Computerized tomography has likewise been beneficial in our experience and that reported by others.[70] Sclerosis has been identified as crossing the intervertebral space from lesions in the vertebral body[30] as well as lesions involving the posterior element.[40]

Most authors have commented on the length of time between the onset of symptoms and the diagnosis. Indeed, it is most common to have one or more other diagnoses entertained before the correct one is made.[10, 62]

The diagnoses most frequently considered are lumbosacral strain, herniated nucleus pulposus, idiopathic scoliosis, arthritis, osteochondritis, hysteria, infection, and cord tumor.

Treatment consists of thorough removal of the lesion (Fig. 22–2).[36] The natural history of spinal lesions has not been well described but incomplete removal is likely to be associated with recurrence of the tumor.[16] Spontaneous healing after the appearance of symptoms has also been reported.[59] Persistent pain and deformity after removal of the lesion should lead one to suspect incomplete removal or recurrence or a multifocal lesion.[62]

There appears to be little reason or advantage to proceed with spinal fusion at the time of surgical excision. Although the curvatures are relatively inflexible preoperatively, with removal of the nidus the scoliosis will usually improve. It may take six months to a year until the patient's flexibility returns. If the curvature is moderately severe (> 40 degrees) and the spine has been rendered unstable by removal of the articular facets and pedicle, consideration should be given to spine fusion at the time of tumor removal.

Osteoblastoma

Benign osteoblastoma is an uncommon tumor that accounts for fewer than 1 per cent of all bone tumors.[37] More than 40 per cent of reported cases have been located in the spine and more than half of these had an associated scoliosis.[43] Although there are a large number of reports describing this lesion of the spine,[2, 13, 17, 42] the larger series is that reported by Marsh and coworkers.[43] In a study of 197 cases, they found that 41 per cent of the lesions involved the spine, the male to female ratio was 2:1, and 80 per cent of the patients were under 30 years of age.

In lesions involving the spine, pain is the characteristic presenting complaint, and scoliosis has been reported in more than half of the patients whose tumor arose in the thoracolumbar spine or ribs.[2, 43, 44]

Although there may be no distinguishing radiographic picture in many cases, some authors[38, 43] have felt that the lesion usually shows an expanded cortex, virtually always separated from the surrounding soft tissue by a thin rim of reactive bone. Some osteoblastomas may demonstrate sclerosis of surrounding bone.[6] Rarely, if ever, does a lobulated or soap bubble appearance develop. Tomograms and computerized tomography may be of help, particularly in preoperative planning.

The treatment of choice is complete excision of the tumor. Incomplete curettage may result in tumor recurrence.[18] Radiotherapy does not alter the course of the disease and appears to be contraindicated.[43, 44] Although the lesion is considered benign by most authors, there are three case reports of pulmonary metastasis in the absence of radiotherapy.[45]

If the diagnosis is made early, usually within six months, the scoliosis is reversible after excision of the tumor. In the event of a late diagnosis, in the presence of structural changes[2, 54] or when the spine is destabilized through a more radical excision, correction and stabilization of the curvature would be desirable.

Aneurysmal Bone Cyst

Aneurysmal bone cyst is a tumor-like bone condition characterized by a rapidly expansile hyperemic osteolytic process. Although it was first reported as an ossified hamartoma,[34, 69] Jaffe and Lichenstein determined the true nature of the lesion and coined the name aneurysmal bone cyst. The etiology is unknown.

Clinical symptoms consist of a rapid evolution of pain in the spine, often accompanied by radicular symptoms in the legs and the trunk secondary to cord compression.[11, 26, 53, 61] The differential diagnosis consists of a giant cell tumor or a cavernous hemangioma. Giant cell tumors usually tend to occur in older patients, being rare below age 20, and are usually found in the sacrum. A cavernous hemangioma usually affects the vertebral body, whereas an aneurysmal bone cyst affects the neural arch or both the posterior elements and the body.

Radiographically the appearance is characterized by osteolysis of the vertebra, progressive destruction of bone with poor demarcation that may resemble a malignancy, and ballooning out of the bone with a thin shell and osseous septa. In fact, the bone cortex may be so thin that it is invisible on x-ray. The later radiographic features include progressive ossification of the tumor mass. The tumor has the ability to cross the intervertebral space and involve adjacent vertebrae, which is most uncommon in other forms of benign or even malignant tumors of the spine, except cordoma.[6] In the presence of a neurologic deficit, myelography invariably shows a block. Scoliosis or kyphosis with osteolysis in the concavity of the curvature may be noted.[60]

Because of the inaccessible location and the large size of the lesion, complete surgical removal may not be possible.[6] Furthermore, extensive and profuse hemorrhage may develop with the primary surgical approach. It is known that the lesion is sensitive to irradiation, and complications from radiation myelopathy and post-radiation sarcoma are well appreciated.[50, 59, 68] Occasionally, low dose radiation may be preferred over surgery (Fig. 22–3).

At our center, we would recommend en bloc excision. Embolization of the tumor before surgery may prove a useful adjunct.[3, 14, 19] It should be recognized that incomplete curettage often leads to resolution of the tumor.[68] Following curettage of the tumor, bone grafting is carried out and the patient is carefully followed with repeated radiographic evaluation to determine the healing of the lesion and the possible development of spinal deformity. In the presence of spinal deformity and more extensive lesions, a combined approach may be necessary followed by internal fixation and spine fusion (Fig. 22–4).

Hemangioma

Hemangioma of the vertebral column is a vascular hamartoma orginating from an excluded area of embryonal angioblastic tissue.[60] The lesion is rare.[6] Often these lesions are seen parenthetically on review of routine spine x-rays. They are characterized by thickened vertical trabecular patterns of bone and, according to Jaffe in 1958, at autopsy these lesions show only telangiectasia or varicosity of the osseous veins and should not be called true hemangiomas. True hemangiomas present as an expansile or lucent lesion in the vertebral body, often associated with compression fracture, producing pain and neurologic symptoms. The radiographic findings are suggestive of a benign process that may show radiolucency in the vertebral body as well as the posterior arch. An associated compression fracture of the vertebra is not uncommon. In patients with neurologic findings or symptoms, myelographic obstruction may be demonstrated secondary to an extradural mass. The mass consists of an extension of the hemangioma into the extraosseous tissue.[6, 60]

When pain only is the symptom, low dose radiation may prove useful.[60] When there is neurologic dysfunction, anterior decompression and excision plus anterior spinal fusion is the treatment of choice. Embolization of the feeding artery may facilitate excision.[29]

Histiocytosis-X

Of the lesions most likely to be seen by the orthopaedic surgeon involving the reticuloendotheliosis triad, eosinophilic granuloma would be the more common one. Eosinophilic granuloma usually presents as a solitary lesion during childhood, although at times the site may be multiple.[56, 63] Patients with this lesion often present with pain and on x-ray showing collapse of the vertebra diagnosed as vertebra plana. Biopsy has been recommended when the typical characteristic radiographic appearance is not present.[60] For the most part, this lesion is benign and will usually heal spontaneously, although chemotherapy and moderate dose radiation therapy have been used with some success. If the patient develops kyphosis as a result of vertebral collapse, bracing is indicated. If neurologic symptoms develop, anterior decompression with anterior spinal fusion is the treatment of choice (Fig. 22–5).

Giant Cell Tumor

Giant cell tumor is an uncommon lesion of the spinal column. In the Mayo Clinic series, only 12 per cent of 264 giant cell tumors in their files involved the spine.[12] Radiographically the tumor presents as a radiolucent lesion, involving the vertebral body in 50 per cent of the cases, and it may involve the posterior element as well.[6] The scoliosis or kyphosis may be associated with the collapse of the vertebra secondary to the tumor. The treatment is curettage and bone grafting.

PRIMARY AND METASTATIC MALIGNANT SPINAL TUMORS

Primary malignant bone tumors of the spine are uncommon. These would include malignant giant cell tumors, chondrosar-

Text continued on page 500

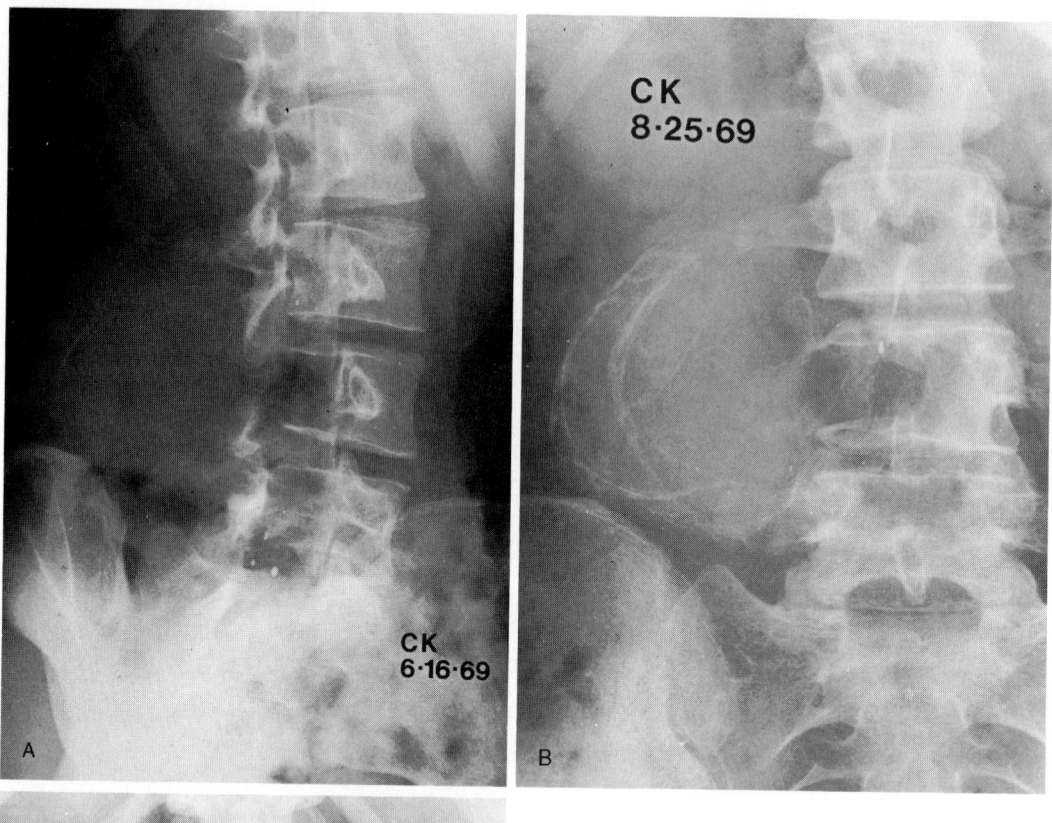

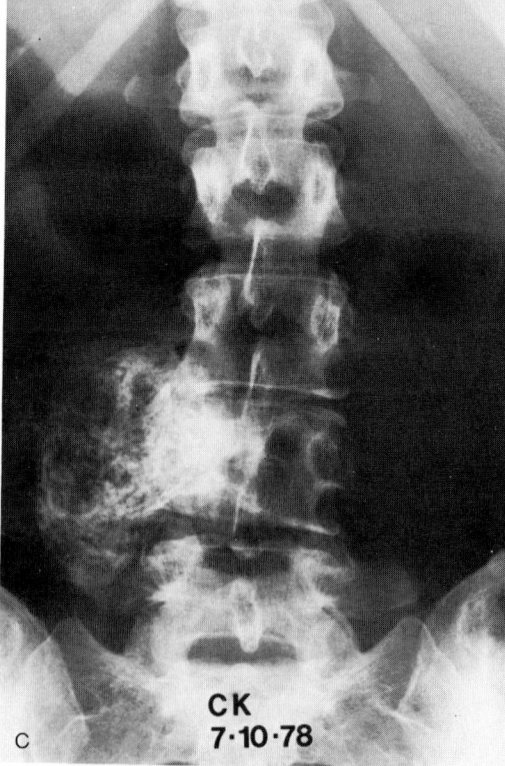

Figure 22–3. A, A very large extremely vascular aneurysmal bone cyst was diagnosed by needle biopsy on this patient. Surgery was deemed ill advised. Low dose radiation was carried out (Cobalt 2400 rads) in June of 1969. B, Early healing was apparent two months later. C, At follow-up seven years later complete sclerosis of the lesion was well demonstrated.

MISCELLANEOUS PROBLEMS

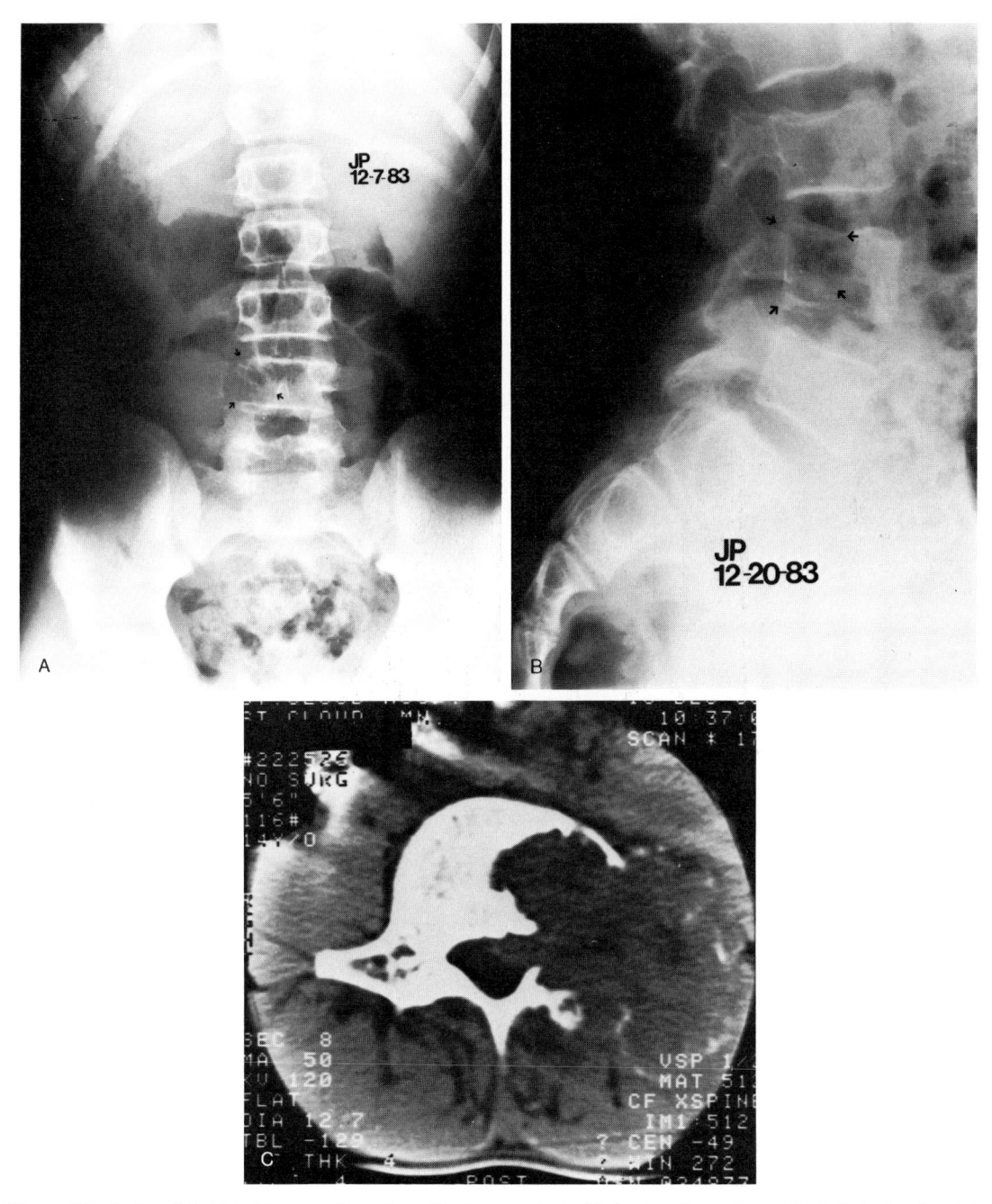

Figure 22–4. *A* and *B,* This 14 year old male patient presented with back pain and an osteolytic lesion involving the fourth vertebral body. *C,* CT scan revealed a large lytic defect confirmed on biopsy as an aneurysmal bone cyst.

Illustration continued on following page

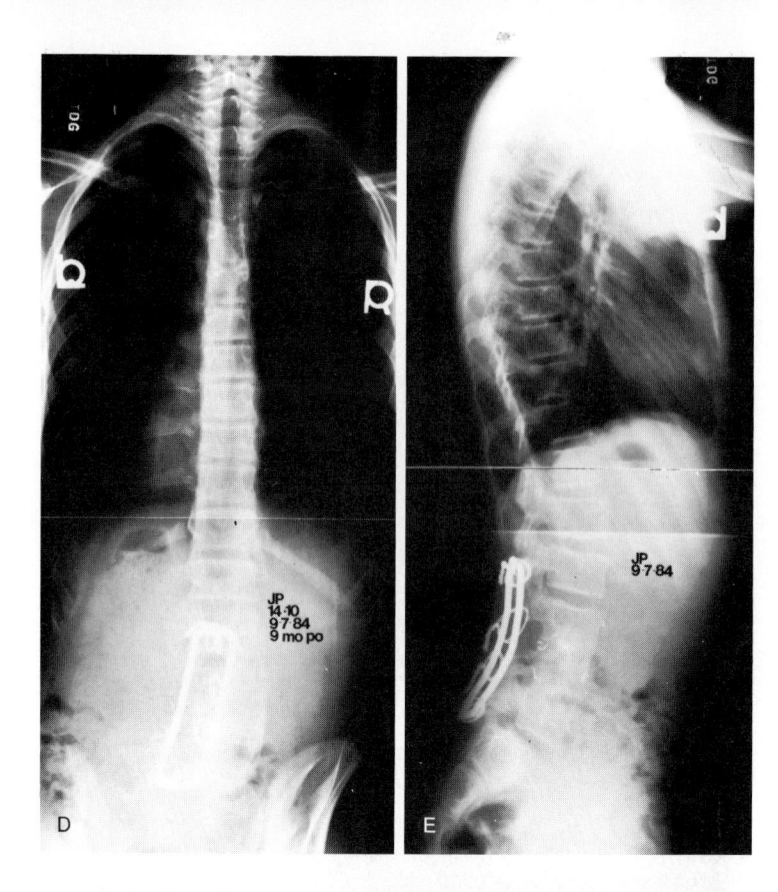

Figure 22–4 *Continued.* D and E, Following combined anterior/posterior resection with O ring stabilization, a solid arthrodesis was achieved and the patient's symptoms were relieved. Prior to resection the lesion was embolized.

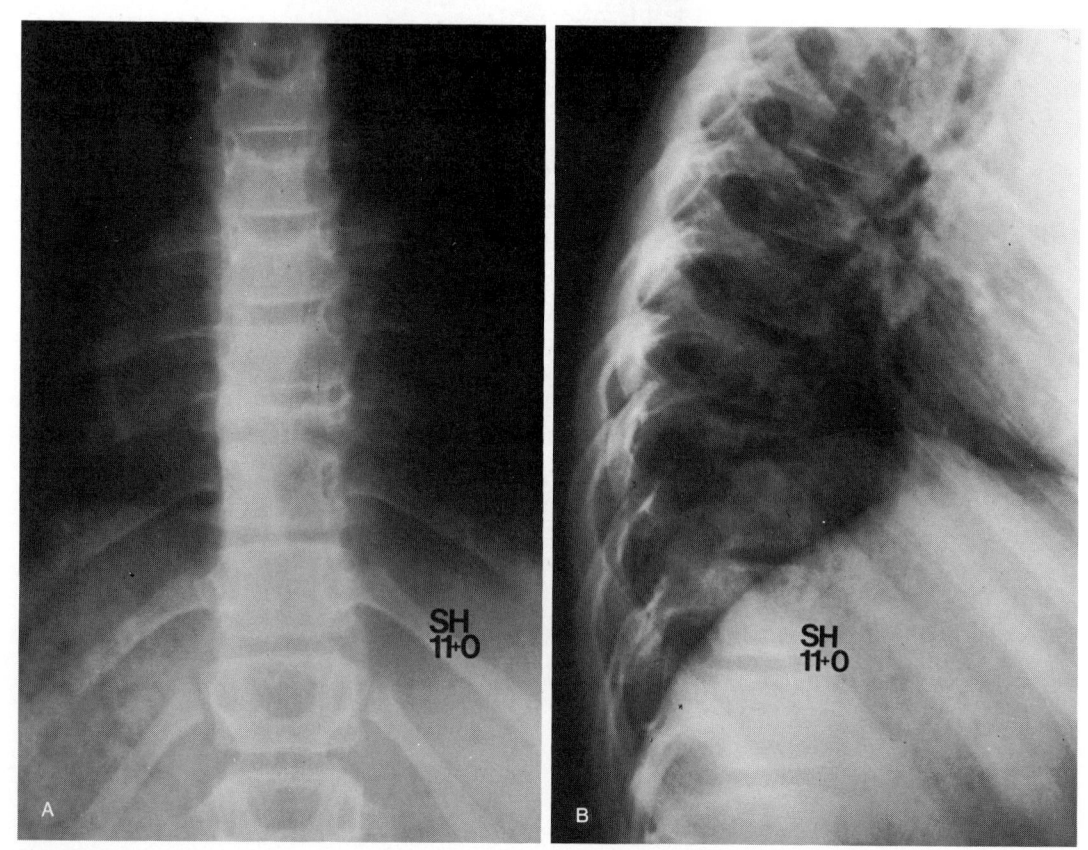

Figure 22–5. A and B, The radiographic appearance of an eosinophilic granuloma. Anterior decompression and anterior fusion may be necessary in the presence of bone collapse and neurologic deficit.

MISCELLANEOUS PROBLEMS 499

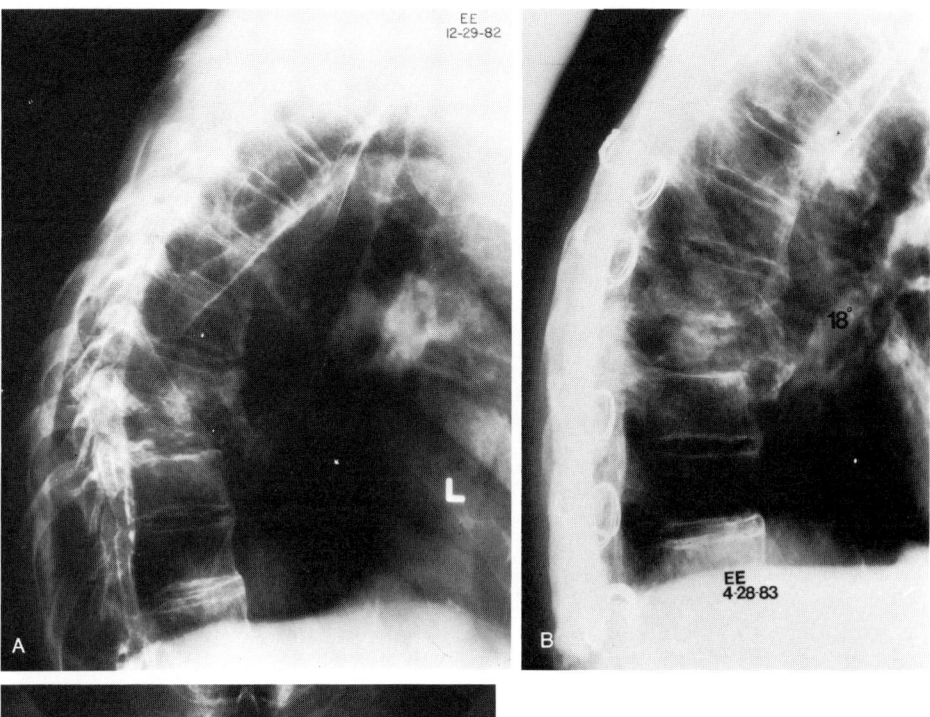

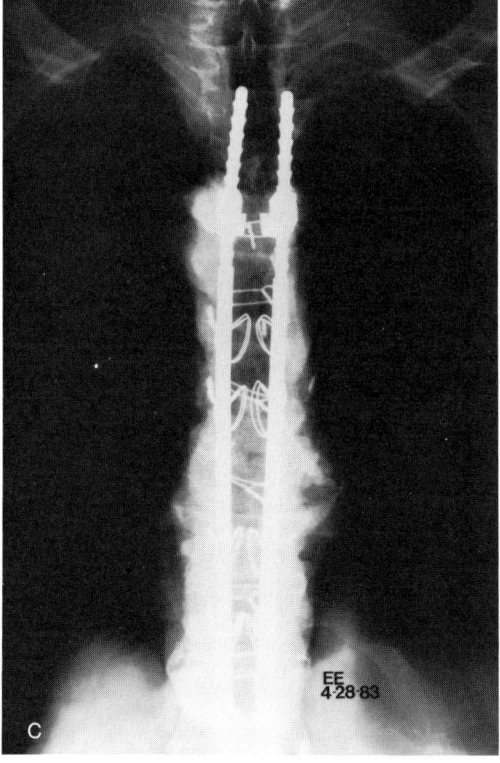

Figure 22–6. *A*, *B*, and *C*, This patient presented with metastatic tumor, back pain, and progressive kyphosis. He was neurologically intact. Posterior stabilization alone with Harrington rods, sublaminar wires, and methylmethacrylate provided him with pain relief and immediate mobility.

coma, osteogenic sarcoma, fibrosarcoma, and cordoma.[5, 12, 44, 65] Our experience with these lesions is limited. Prognosis for the most part is poor. Good longterm results following radical resections for sacral cordomas have been reported by Stener.[67]

METASTATIC DISEASE OF THE SPINE

The skeleton is the third most frequent site for metastatic disease, and within the skeletal system the vertebral column is the most commonly affected.[33] Although x-ray evidence of metastasis does not become apparent until 30 to 50 per cent of a bone is destroyed, Jaffe has estimated that 70 per cent of people who die from cancer show evidence of skeletal metastasis, with the thoracic spine being the most common area of involvement. Gilbert and coworkers[24] have noted that lung and breast tumors are the most common metastatic lesions in the thoracic spine.

Metastatic disease to the spine poses two problems for the spinal surgeon: (1) spinal instability secondary to fracture from osteolysis of the bone, and (2) spinal cord compression secondary to extradural compression, pressure from intradural metastasis (rare), or pressure secondary to angulation following vertebral body collapse or fracture dislocation. Cord compression may occur over several levels in the same patient, and this should be appreciated before treatment is begun.[7]

The primary complaint of patients with spinal metastasis is back pain of a severe, almost unremitting nature. It is aggravated by activity and not particularly relieved by rest. Radicular pain may be present along with a progressive neurologic deficit. With a rapid progressive paraplegia chances of neurologic recovery are poor, even with prompt treatment.[7, 17]

Surgery is indicated in these patients for continued progressive pain uncontrolled by conservative management or the occurrence of neurologic dysfunction. Following radiographic evaluation and biopsy as previously discussed, surgical stabilization alone is carried out in cases in which neurologic dysfunction is not present.

For stabilization, several options are available. Treatment may consist either of bone, metal, or methylmethacrylate constructs alone or in combination. Surgical implants may be used either posteriorly or anteriorly. Where neurologic dysfunction is not a problem, we have generally favored posterior stabilization in situ using Harrington implants or L-rods supplemented with methacrylate as necessary (Fig. 22–6). Radiation and chemotherapy then proceed as recommended by the oncologist. We have generally

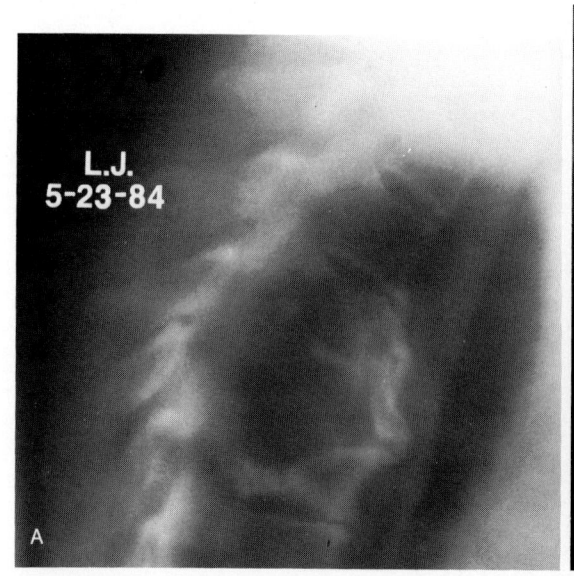

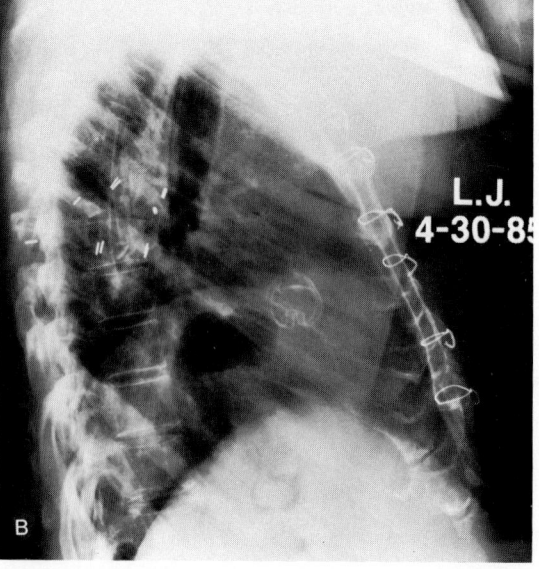

Figure 22–7. In the presence of a neurologic deficit secondary to metastatic tumor, decompression with stabilization is indicated. A, L.J. presented with a solitary myeloma. B, He was managed successfully with anterior decompression, vascularized rib grafting, and postoperative radiation. He has continued to do well one year after surgery and remains neurologically normal, without evidence of recurrence.

MISCELLANEOUS PROBLEMS

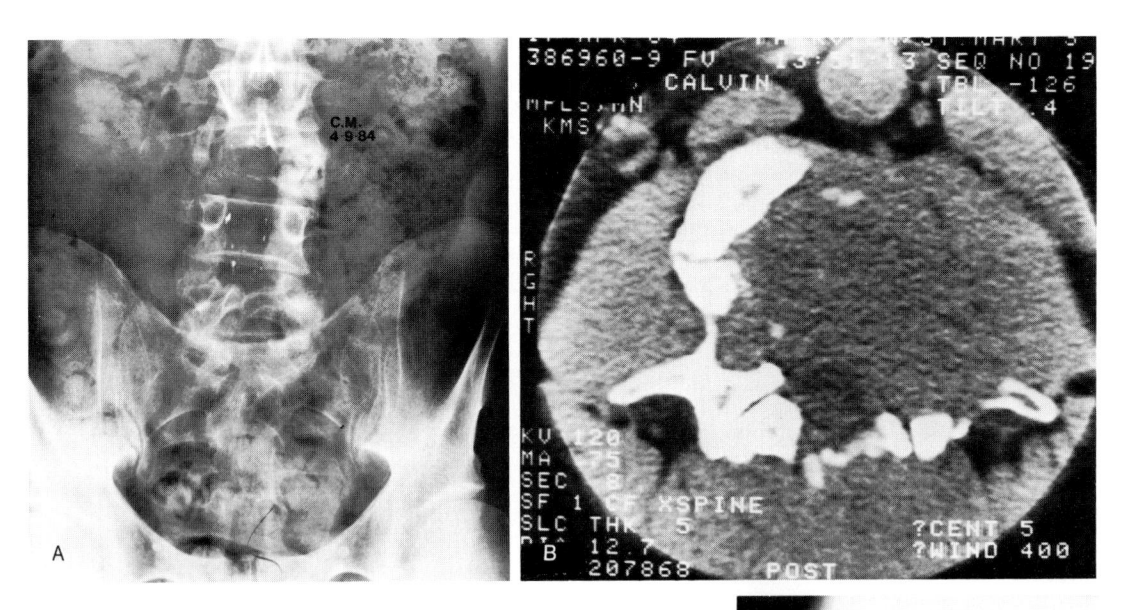

Figure 22–8. A, B, and C, Severe destructive lesions with loss of bone stock may require more extensive resection and fixation. C.M. presented with a solitary plasma cytoma following anterior resection, fusion, and stabilization. A second stage posterior approach was carried out consisting of Steffe plate fixation and fusion. His postoperative course has remained satisfactory.

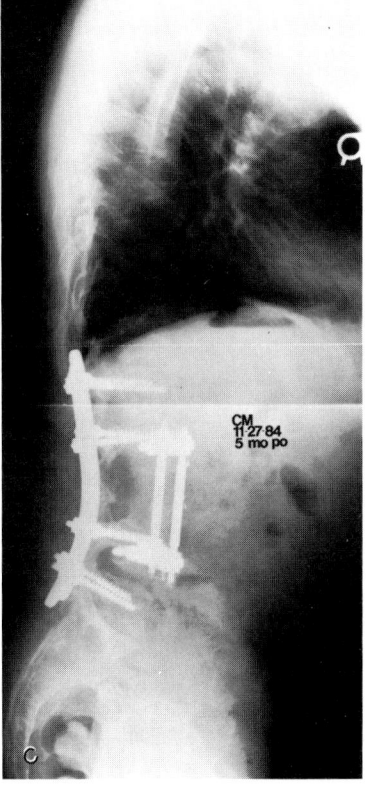

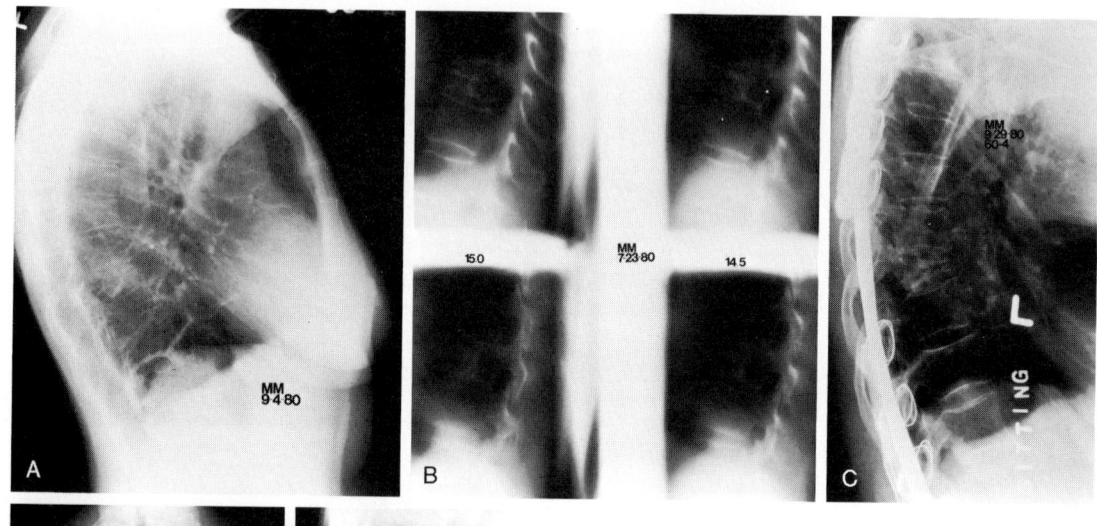

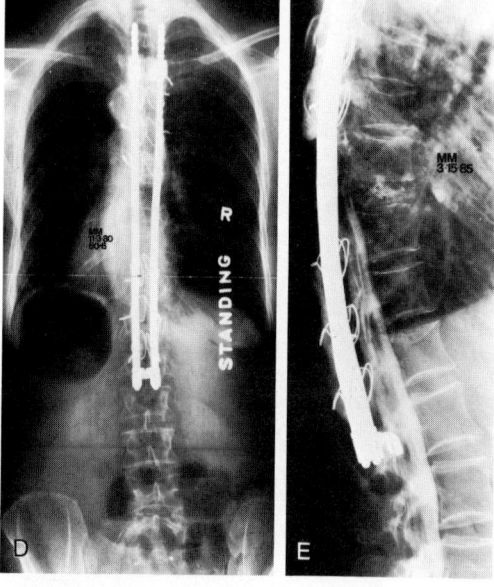

Figure 22–9. *A* and *B*, M.M. presented with metastatic breast carcinoma and progressive neurologic deterioration. It was felt her clinical condition did not allow an anterior transthoracic approach. *C* and *D*, Following a posterior decompression, stabilization was carried out with Harrington rods, sublaminar wires, and methylmethacrylate. Five years later (*E*) she had a recurrence of her symptoms and progressive neurologic deficit. Reexploration was undertaken but the results were unsatisfactory because of severe hemorrhage. Patient's course has deteriorated but she had significant relief over the five year interval.

added a posterior spinal fusion with instrumentation unless the life expectancy is so short that arthrodesis would appear to offer little benefit.

In the presence of spinal cord compression, two options are available: (1) a posterior laminectomy with decompression and surgical stabilization with Harrington or other metallic implants[35, 51] or anterior decompression and anterior spinal fusion. In a series of patients treated by posterior decompression without stabilization, Hall and McKay in 1973[27] noted that only 9 per cent of their patients with anteriorly located tumors improved neurologically, whereas 39 per cent of patients with tumors located posteriorly received benefit. Harrington[28] in a series of 14 patients treated by anterior decompression and stabilization with methylmethacrylate and metal showed neurologic improvement in all but one patient, with pain relief in all 14 patients. Dunn has likewise recommended a primary anterior approach with decompression, instrumentation, and fusion.[17]

When presented with a patient with metastatic tumor to the spine and progressive neurologic deterioration secondary to compression anteriorly, we have generally favored an initial anterior approach with anterior cord decompression and anterior fusion with strut bone grafts. Steroids are administered preoperatively, and radiation is begun postoperatively as recommended by the oncologist. In general, we have not favored anterior implants unless the bone stock of the vertebral body proximally and distal to the tumor is intact and strong without evidence of tumor invasion. If implants are used, fixation may be increased with the use of methylmethacrylate. Vascularized rib grafts may be helpful if the tumor is located at a single or double level and the area can be spanned comfortably to normal bone (Fig. 22–7). If stability is not optimal following anterior decompression and anterior fusion with rib or fibula strut grafts, a second stage posterior spinal fusion with instrumentation is carried out one to two weeks later (Fig. 22–8). If the patient's clinical condition is poor and a thoracotomy appears ill advised, a posterior decompression laminectomy with implant stabilization and fusion is carried out (Fig. 22–9). Patients are ambulated or mobilized shortly after surgery, and an underarm body brace may be prescribed if fixation is less than satisfactory.

References

1. Akbarnia, B. A., Bradford, D. S., and Winter, R. B.: Osteoid osteoma of the spine—an analysis of 14 patients. Orthop. Trans., 6(1):4, 1982.
2. Akbarnia, B. A., and Rooholamini, S. A.: Scoliosis caused by benign osteoblastoma of the thoracic or lumbar spine. J. Bone Joint Surg., 63A:1146–1155, 1981.
3. Allison, D. J.: Therapeutic embolization. J. Bone Joint Surg., 64B:151–152, 1982.
4. Barron, K. D., Hirano, A., Araki, S., and Ferry, R. D.: Experiences with metastatic neoplasms involving the spinal cord. Neurology, 9:91, 1959.
5. Barwick, K. W., Huvos, A. G., and Smith, J.: Primary osteogenic sarcoma of the vertebral column. Cancer, 46:595, 1980.
6. Beabout, J. W., McLeod, R. A., and Dahlin, D. C.: Benign tumors. Semin. Roentgenol., 14:33–43, 1979.
7. Bolland, P. J., Lane, J. N., and Sundaresan, N.: Metastatic diseases of the spine. Clin. Orthop., 169:95, 1982.
8. Caldicott, W. J. H.: Diagnosis of spinal osteoid osteoma. Radiology, 92:1192–1195, 1969.
9. Campanacci, M.: Tumori delle ossa e delle parti molli. Bologna, A. Gaggi, 1981.
10. Coley, B. L., and Lenson, N.: Osteoid osteoma. Am. J. Surg., 77:3–9, 1949.
11. Dabska, M., and Buraczewsky, J.: Aneurysmal bone cyst. Cancer, 23:371–389, 1969.
12. Dahlin, D. C.: Bone Tumors. Springfield, Charles C Thomas, 1978.
13. Davis, N. A., Dooley, B. J., and Bardsley, A.: Benign osteoblastoma. Aust. N.Z. J. Surg., 46:37–43, 1976.
14. Dick, H. M., Bigliani, L. U., Michelsen, W. J., et al.: Adjuvant arterial embolization in the treatment of benign primary bone tumors in children. Clin. Orthop., 139:133–141, 1979.
15. Doron, Y., Gruszkiewicz, J., Gelli, B., and Peyser, E.: Benign osteoblastoma of vertebral column and skull. Surg. Neurol., 7:86–90, 1977.
16. Dunlop, J. A. Y., Morton, K. S., and Elliott, G. B.: Recurrent osteoid osteoma. Report of a case with a review of the literature. J. Bone Joint Surg., 52B:128–133, 1970.
17. Dunn, H. K.: Tumors of the thoracic and lumbar spine. In Evarts, C. M. (eds.): Surgery of the Musculoskeletal System, Vol. 2, New York, Churchill Livingstone, p. 191, 1983.
18. Eisenbrey, A. B., Huber, P. J., and Rachmaninoff, N.: Benign osteoblastoma of the spine with multiple recurrences. Case report. J. Neurosurg., 31:468–473, 1969.
19. Feldman, F., Casarella, W. J., Dick, H. M., and Hollander, B. A.: Selective intraarterial embolization of bone tumors. A useful adjunct in the management of selected lesions. J. Roentgenol., 123:130–135, 1975.
20. Flaherty, R. A., Pugh, D. G., and Dockerty, M. B.: Osteoid osteoma. Am. J. Roentgenol., 76:1041–1051, 1956.
21. Freiberger, R. H., Loitman, B. S., Helpern, M., and Thompson, T. C.: Osteoid osteoma. A report on 80 cases. Am. J. Roengtenol., 82:194, 1959.
22. Freiberger, R. H.: Osteoid osteoma of the spine.

A cause of backache and scoliosis in children and young adults. Radiology, 75:232, 1960.
23. Gertzbein, S. D., Cruickshank, B., Hoffman, H., et al.: Recurrent benign osteoblastoma of the second thoracic vertebra. A case report. J. Bone Joint Surg., 55B:841–847, 1973.
24. Gilbert, R. N., Kim, J. M., and Posner, J. B.: Epidural spinal cord compression from metastatic tumor: diagnosis and treatment. Ann. Neurol., 3:40, 1978.
25. Golding, J. S. R.: The natural history of osteoid osteoma. With a report of 20 cases. J. Bone Joint Surg., 36B:218, 1954.
26. Gruszkiewicz, J., Doron, Y., Peyser, E., et al.: Aneurysmal bone cyst of spine. Acta Neurochir., 66:109–121, 1982.
27. Hall, A. J., and Mackay, N. N.: The results of laminectomy for compression of the cord or cauda equina by extradural malignant tumor. J. Bone Joint Surg., 55B:497, 1973.
28. Harrington, K. D.: The use of methylmethacrylate for vertebral body replacement and anterior stabilization of pathological fracture dislocations of the spine, due to metastatic disease. J. Bone Joint Surg., 63A:36, 1981.
29. Hekster, R. E. M., Luyendijk, W., and Tan, T. I.: Spinal-cord compression caused by vertebral haemangioma relieved by percutaneous catheter embolisation. Neuroradiology, 3:160–164, 1972.
30. Heiman, M. L., Cooley, C. J., and Bradford, D. S.: Osteoid osteoma of a vertebral body. Clin. Orthop., 118:159, 1976.
31. Huvos, A. G.: Bone Tumors: Diagnosis, Treatment, and Prognosis. Philadelphia, W. B. Saunders, 1979.
32. Israeli, A., Zwas, S. T., Horoszowski, H., and Farine, I.: Use of radionuclide method in preoperative and intraoperative diagnosis of osteoid osteoma of the spine. Case report. Clin. Orthop. Rel. Res., 175:194–196, 1983.
33. Jaffe, H. L.: Tumors and Tumorous Conditions of the Bones and Joints. Philadelphia, Lea & Febiger, 1958.
34. Jaffe, H. L., and Lichtenstein, L.: Solitary inicameral bone cysts with emphasis of the roentgen picture, the pathologic appearance and the pathogenesis. Arch. Surg., 44:1004–1024, 1942.
35. Jelsma, R. K., and Kirsch, P. T.: The treatment of malignancy of a vertebral body. Surg. Neurol., 13:189, 1980.
36. Keim, H. A., Reina, E. G.: Osteoid osteoma as a cause of scoliosis. J. Bone Joint Surg., 57A:159, 1975.
37. Lichtenstein, L.: Bone Tumors. St. Louis, C. V. Mosby, 1965.
38. Lichtenstein, L., and Sawyer, W. R.: Benign osteoblastoma. Further observations and report of 20 additional cases. J. Bone Joint Surg., 46A:755–765, 1964.
39. Livingston, K. E., and Perrin, R. G.: The neurosurgical management of spinal metastasis causing compression. J. Neurol., 49:889, 1978.
40. Lundeen, M. A., and Herring, J. A.: Osteoid osteoma of the spine: sclerosis in two levels. A case report. J. Bone Joint Surg., 62A:476–478, 1980.
41. Maclellan, D. I., and Wilson, F. C., Jr.: Osteoid osteoma of the spine. A review of the literature and report of six new cases. J. Bone Joint Surg., 49A:111, 1967.
42. McLeod, R. A., Dahlin, D. C., and Beabout, J. W.: The spectrum of osteoblastoma. Am. J. Roentgenol., 126:321–335, 1976.
43. Marsh, B. W., Bonfiglio, M., Brady, L. P., and Enneking, W. F.: Benign osteoblastoma: range of manifestations. J. Bone Joint Surg., 57A:1–9, 1975.
44. Marsh, H. O., and Choi, C. B.: Primary osteogenic sarcoma of the cervical spine originally mistaken for benign osteoblastoma. J. Bone Joint Surg., 52A:1467, 1970.
45. Merryweather, R., Middlemiss, J. H., and Sanerkin, N. G.: Malignant transformation of osteoblastoma. J. Bone Joint Surg., 62B:381–384, 1980.
46. Michele, A., and Krudger, F. J.: A surgical approach to the vertebral body. J. Bone Joint Surg., 31A:873, 1949.
47. Moon, K. L., Genant, H. K., and Holmes, C. A.: Muscular skeletal applications of nuclear magnetic resonance imaging. Radiology, 147:161, 1983.
48. Nelson, O. A., and Greer, R. B. III.: Localization of osteoid osteoma of the spine using computerized tomography. J. Bone Joint Surg., 65A:263–265, 1983.
49. Ottolenghi, C. E.: Aspiration biopsy in the diagnosis of lesions of the vertebral bodies. J. Bone Joint Surg., 37A:443, 1955.
50. Palmer, J.: Radiation myelopathy. Brain, 95:109–122, 1972.
51. Perrin, R. G., and Livingston, K. E.: Neurosurgical treatment of pathological fracture-dislocation of the spine. J. Neurosurg., 52:330–334, 1980.
52. Ponseti, I., and Barta, C. K.: Osteoid osteoma. J. Bone Joint Surg., 29:767, 1947.
53. Pou-Serradell, A., and Amat-Ballarin, L.: Aneurysmal bone cyst (Observation on two cases with neurological findings). Rev. Neurol. (Paris), 135:633–638, 1979.
54. Ransford, A. O., Pozo, J. L., Hutton, P. A. N., and Kirwan, O. G.: The behaviour pattern of the scoliosis associated with osteoid osteoma or osteoblastoma of the spine. J. Bone Joint Surg., 66B:16–20, 1984.
55. Rinsky, L. A., Goris, M., Bleck, E. E., et al.: Intraoperative skeletal scintigraphy for localization of osteoid-osteoma in the spine. J. Bone Joint Surg., 62A:143–144, 1980.
56. Rodrigues, R. J., and Lewis, H. H.: Eosinophilic granuloma of bone. Clin. Orthop., 77:183–187, 1971.
57. Ruge, D., and Wiltse, L. L.: Spinal Disorders: Diagnosis and Treatment. Philadelphia, Lea & Febiger, 1977.
58. Rushton, J. G., Mulder, D. W., and Lipscomb, P. R.: Neurologic symptoms with ostoid osteoma. Neurology, 5:794, 1955.
59. Sabanes, A. O., Dahlin, D. C., Childs, D. S., and Ivins, J. C.: Postradiation sarcoma of bone. Cancer, 9:528–542, 1956.
60. Savini, R., Giunti, A., Boriani, S.: Malignant spinal tumors. In Bradford, D. S., and Hensinger, R. (eds.): The Pediatric Spine. New York, Thieme and Stratton, pp. 131–154, 1985.
61. Schacked, I., Tarudor, R., Wolpin, G., and Orny, A.: Aneurysmal bone cyst of a vertebral body with acute paraplegia. Paraplegia, 19:294–298, 1981.
62. Schajowicz, F., and Lemos, C.: Osteoid osteoma and osteoblastoma. Closely related entities of

63. Seiman, L. P.: Eosinophilic granuloma of the spine. J. Pediatr. Orthop., 1:371–376, 1981.
64. Sherman, M. S.: Osteoid osteoma. Review of the literature and report of 30 cases. J. Bone Joint Surg., 29:918–930, 1947.
65. Solisio, E. O., Akbiyik, N., and Alexander, L. L.: Spinal cord compression from metastatic breast carcinoma: treatment by radiation therapy alone. J. Natl. Med. Assoc., 71:229, 1979.
66. Spjut, H. J., Dorfman, H. D., Fechner, R. E., and Ackerman, L. V.: Tumors of Bone and Cartilage: Atlas of Tumor Pathology. 2nd Series, Fascicle 5. The Armed Forces Institute of Pathology. Washington, D.C., 1971.
67. Stener, B.: Clinical Orthopaedics and Related Research Symposium on Neoplasms of the Spine. In Press.
68. Tillman, B. P., Dahlin, D. C., and Lipscomb, P. R.: Aneurysmal bone cyst. An analysis of 95 cases. Mayo Clinic Proc., 43:478–495, 1968.
69. Van Arsdale, W. W.: Ossifying haematoma. Ann. Surg., 18:8–17, 1893.
70. Wedge, J. H., Tchang, S., and MacFadyen, D. J.: Computed tomography in localization of spinal osteoid osteoma. Spine, 6:423–427, 1981.
71. Zwimpfer, T. J., Tucker, W. S., and Faulkner, J. F.: Osteoid osteoma of the cervical spine: case reports and literature review. Can. J. Surg., 25:637–641, 1982.

Spinal Cord Tumors

Robert B. Winter, M.D.

INTRODUCTION

Although spinal cord tumors are rare, they often manifest themselves by producing a scoliosis in the growing child. Therefore, a tumor must always be considered in the differential diagnosis of scoliosis.

CLASSIFICATION

Spinal cord tumors may be divided into extradural and intradural types. Extradural tumors are usually malignant; they are metastases from primary tumors as well as reticuloendothelial malignancies. A major exception to this is the benign neurofibroma, which customarily extends into the spinal canal through a foramen from its primary paraspinal origin. Intradural tumors are further subdivided into intramedullary and extramedullary types.

The intramedullary tumors more commonly cause scoliosis. The intramedullary tumors are the gliomas and ependymomas; the most common scoliosis-producing tumor that we see in our clinics is an astrocytoma. All series reporting spinal cord tumors in children note the long delay in diagnosis.[3, 20] Syringomyelia is also an intramedullary space-occupying lesion, but it is not a neoplasm.

There are also intradural, extramedullary tumors such as neurofibromas, meningiomas, lipomas, and dermoids. These often produce neurologic symptoms and findings, but seldom cause scoliosis. Neurofibromas are often seen in patients with spine deformity due to neurofibromatosis. The curvature in these cases is due to the primary disease, not the neurofibroma. If a patient presents with a neurofibromatosis scoliosis (no kyphosis) and a neurologic deficit, that deficit will usually be due to either an intradural or extradual neurofibroma. If, however, the patient has kyphoscoliosis, the neurologic deficit may be caused by either the kyphosis or a tumor. Careful myelography with CT scanning or MRI scanning is necessary to distinguish between these two problems.

DIAGNOSIS

Clinical

Spinal cord tumors may occur at any age, but are most common in children and more common in young children than adolescents. The inability of a young child to articulate a complaint is one of the causes for late diagnosis. The presenting complaint may be scoliosis, pain, irritability, a "stiff" spine, bed-wetting, a limp, an abnormal gait, itching, or change of bowel habits. Back pain is the most common complaint.

Extremely careful examination is the key to diagnosis. The child will either stand erect or slightly deviated to one side. On bending forward, there may be restriction of the bending, and/or deviation to one side.[1, 2, 5, 9, 16] This persistent deviation to one side on forward bending is an extremely valuable sign, and if present the situation should be viewed with concern (Fig. 22–10). Other irritative lesions

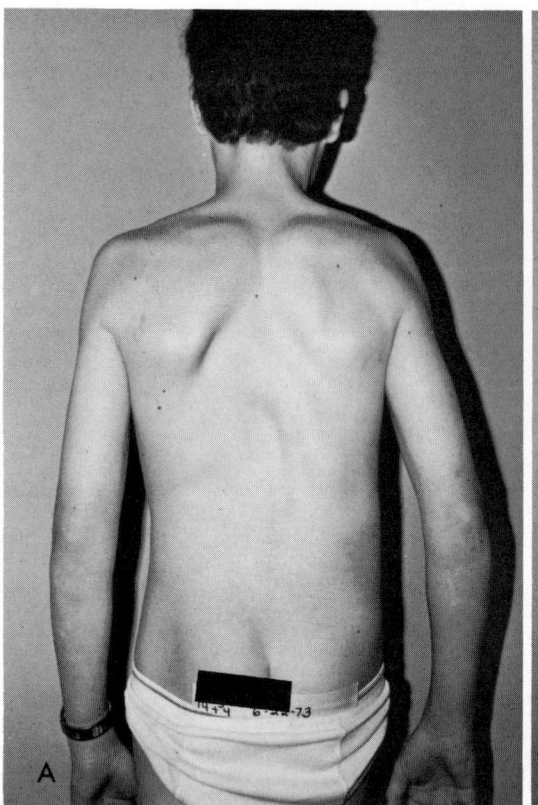

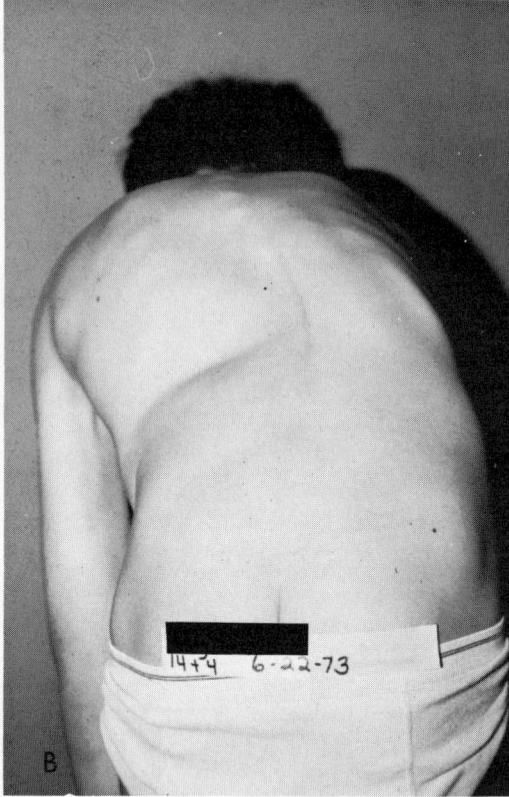

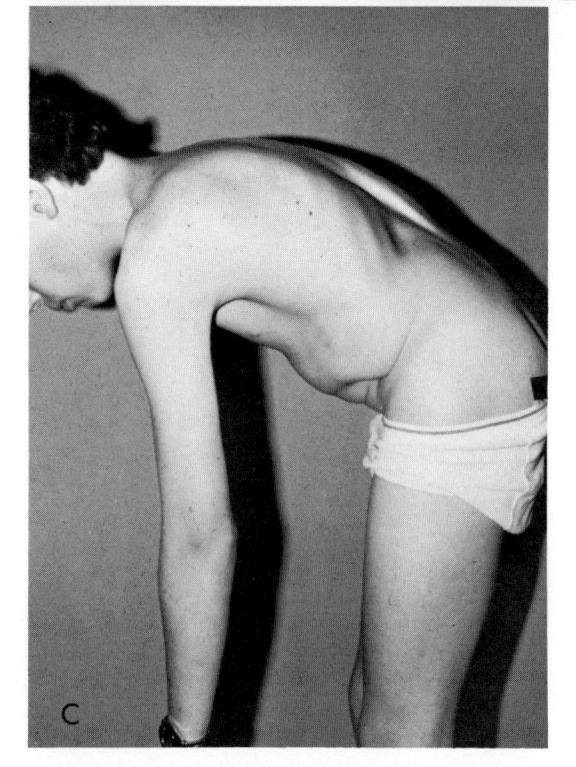

Figure 22–10. *A*, D.W. This 14+4 year old boy presented with a spine deformity that had been diagnosed two years earlier and treated with exercises. This posterior view of his back showed decompensation to the left and a rigid lumbar scoliosis with lumbar muscle spasm. *B*, Forward bending showed the marked lumbar muscle spasm with deviation of the trunk to the left. *C*, Side view of forward bending shows the spinal rigidity with restriction of forward bending. Neurologic examination showed minor sensory and proprioceptive loss in one leg.

Illustration continued on opposite page

MISCELLANEOUS PROBLEMS

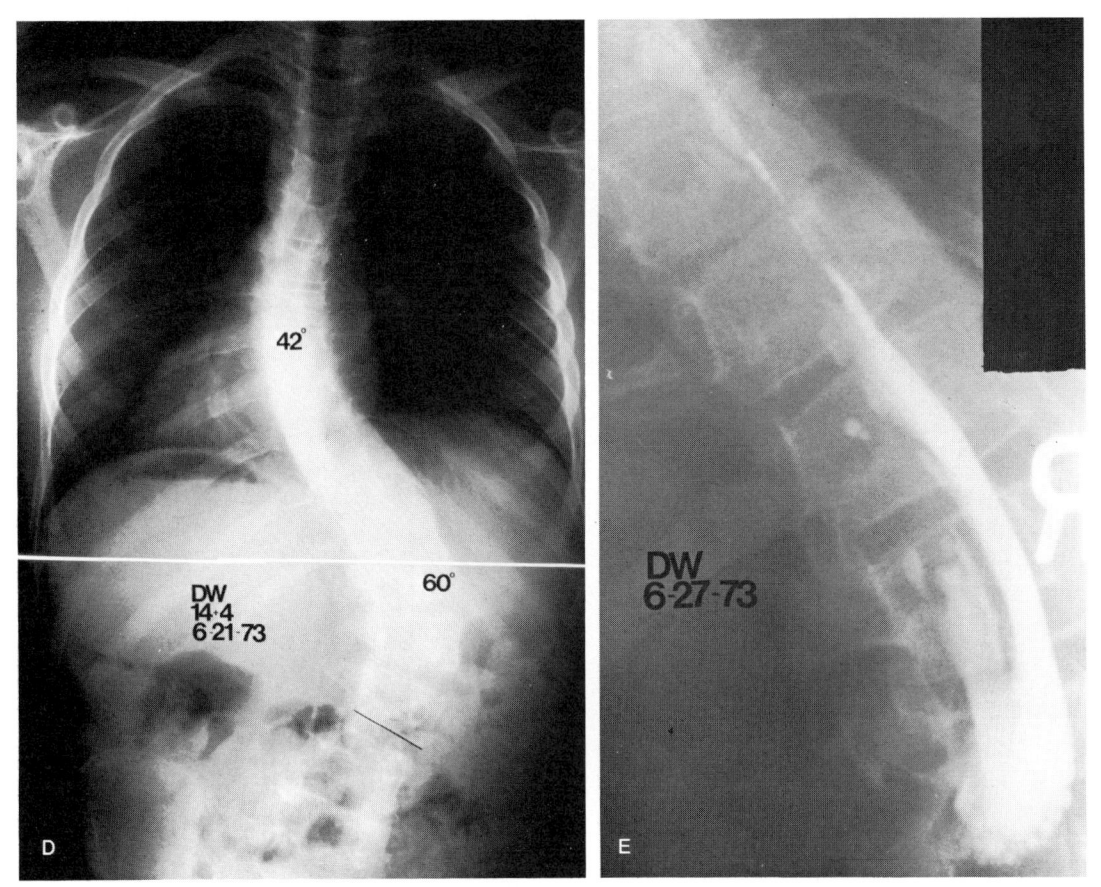

Figure 22–10 *Continued.* D, Anteroposterior standing x-ray shows a left thoracic curve of 42 degrees and a right lumbar curve of 60 degrees. The marked decompensation to the left is noted. The presence of a left thoracic curve is very suspicious, as it is rare in "idiopathic" scoliosis. E, Myelogram shows widening of the whole spinal cord with only a trickle of dye alongside the cord. At surgery an ependymoma of the whole cord was found, which was partially resected in a two-stage procedure.

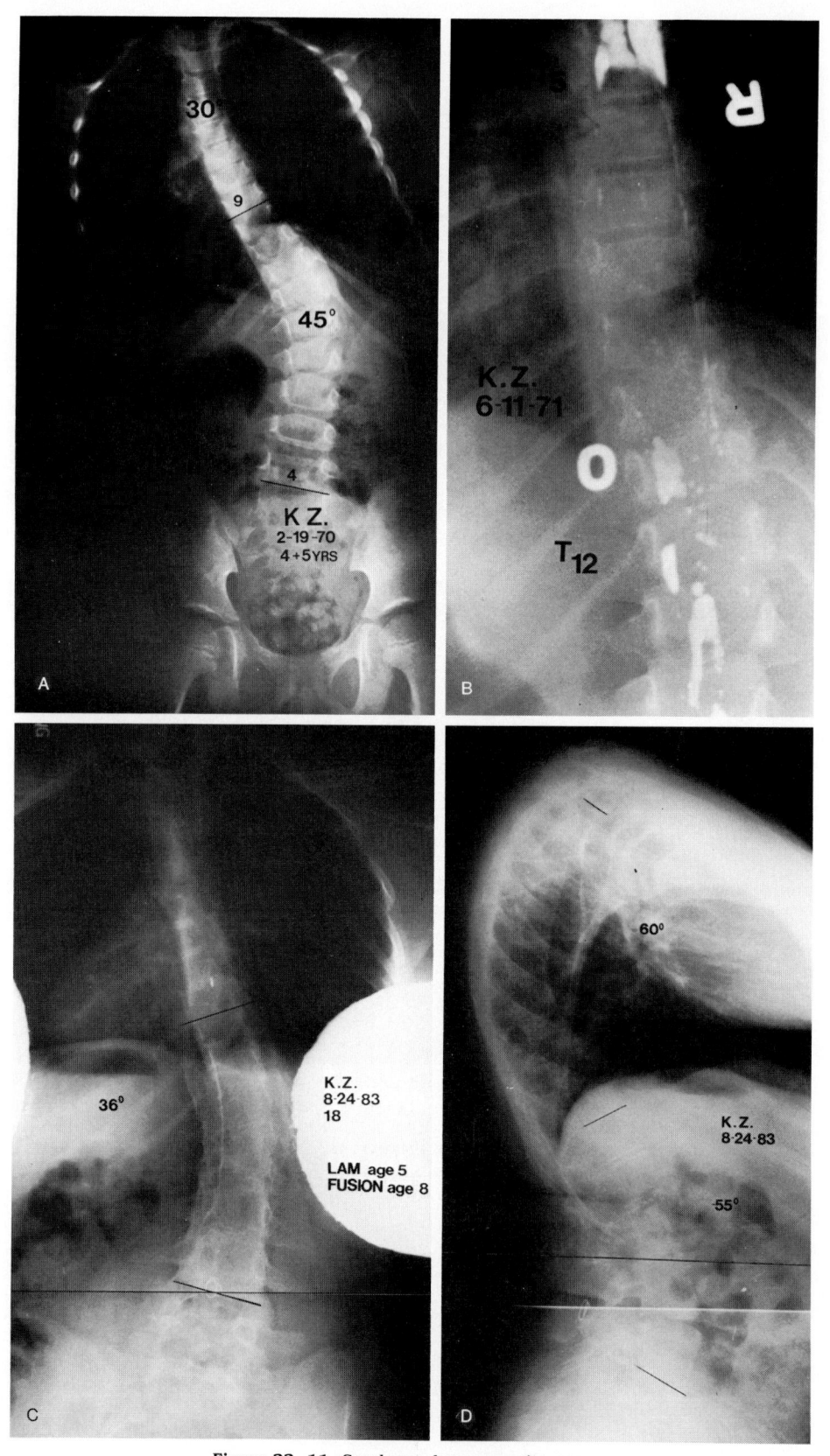

Figure 22–11. *See legend on opposite page.*

such as spondylolisthesis, herniated discs, vertebral tumors, and infections may also produce this finding.

Weakness is one of the most common early presentations of spinal neoplasms in children.[20] When the onset is major, (i.e., paraparesis or paraplegia) the diagnosis is quickly made. More often the onset is very gradual and the weakness is difficult to detect. The child may have only a slight gait change, a limp, a "dragging" of one foot, or merely a slowing down of play activities.

Sensory changes are very difficult to detect and are seldom verbalized by the child. One of our patients with an astrocytoma had unilateral abdominal itching as her major complaint (Fig. 22–11). That and her scoliosis were the only findings.

Sphincter disturbance is virtually impossible to detect in the infant or toddler, but in the child who has been toilet trained, a regression of function is cause for concern. Constipation, fecal soiling, bedwetting, and stress incontinence should be investigated.

Musculoskeletal findings can be scoliosis, a limp, back pain or spasm, or a foot deformity. Back pain in children, as stated previously, is usually caused by some specific organic defect, and a diligent search for that defect is mandatory.[4, 7] A child with a foot deformity or weakness must always have a back examination both clinically and radiologically. Scolioses not fitting the usual and customary patterns should always be suspect (Fig. 22–12).[7]

Radiologic

The plain anteroposterior and lateral films often reveal signs of intraspinal pathology. Enlarged foramina are either caused by dural ectasia or a dumbbell tumor of neurofibromatosis. An increase of interpedicular distance is a sign of spinal dysraphism (see Chapter 12) or a slowly growing intraspinal tumor or syringomyelia.[18] Are the pedicles of normal shape or thinned?[8]

Myelography, preferably with water-soluble media, is the key to accurate diagnosis. The spinal tap will usually reveal an elevated protein content and the tumor may block the passage of the contrast material. A "negative" myelogram in a few children is far better than missing the diagnosis because of reluctance to perform a myelogram on a child. Unexplained back pain, deviation on forward bending, and an unusual curve pattern are adequate reasons for performing a myelogram, *even if the routine neurologic examination is normal!*[8]

Magnetic Resonance Imaging (MRI) has proven highly beneficial for the diagnosis of spinal cord tumors and syringomyelia. It is rapidly replacing myelography in our clinics.

TREATMENT

The treatment of all spinal cord tumors is laminectomy, inspection of the lesion, excision if possible,[12] or biopsy if not.[15] Radiation may be used for certain tumors, especially the more severe grades of astrocytoma. At our institution, a Grade I astrocytoma is no longer irradiated as the chance for death from post-radiation sarcoma is higher than that from the tumor. These tumors, both low grade astrocytomas and ependymomas, characteristically do not metastasize.[17] They may cause paraplegia but not death, unless they involve the centers of respiration.

All too often we have seen patients with severe spinal deformity resulting from the tumor, the paralysis, or the laminectomy in whom treatment of the deformity has been withheld in the false expectation that the child would die. These deformities are discussed in more detail in the section on postlaminectomy deformities (pp. 513–522). In most circumstances, it is best to be optimistic and to expect the child to survive and func-

---

Figure 22–11. *A*, A four year old girl with an unusual pattern, 45 degree scoliosis. Her chief complaint was itching on the abdominal wall. A Milwaukee brace was prescribed on the mistaken diagnosis of "infantile idiopathic scoliosis." *B*, About a year later, she was noted to drag her left leg and she was found to have left leg weakness and hyperactive reflexes. This myelogram was obtained; it shows a large intramedullary tumor extending from T5 to T11. A biopsy revealed an astrocytoma, Grade II, and she received 4000 rads of radiation to the tumor. *C*, She subsequently developed increasing spinal deformity owing to both the tumor and the laminectomy. She had both anterior (T4 to T12) and posterior (T3 to L4) fusion at age 8 years. She was last seen in 1983 at the age of 18. One centimeter atrophy of the left calf and a positive left Babinski reflex were the *only* residual neurologic deficits. *D*, A lateral radiograph at age 18. She had had a 72 degree thoracic kyphosis prior to the fusion. No instrumentation was used because of the extensive (T4 to T12) laminectomy and the intramedullary tumor. The anterior fusion was from T4 to T12 and the posterior one from T3 to L4.

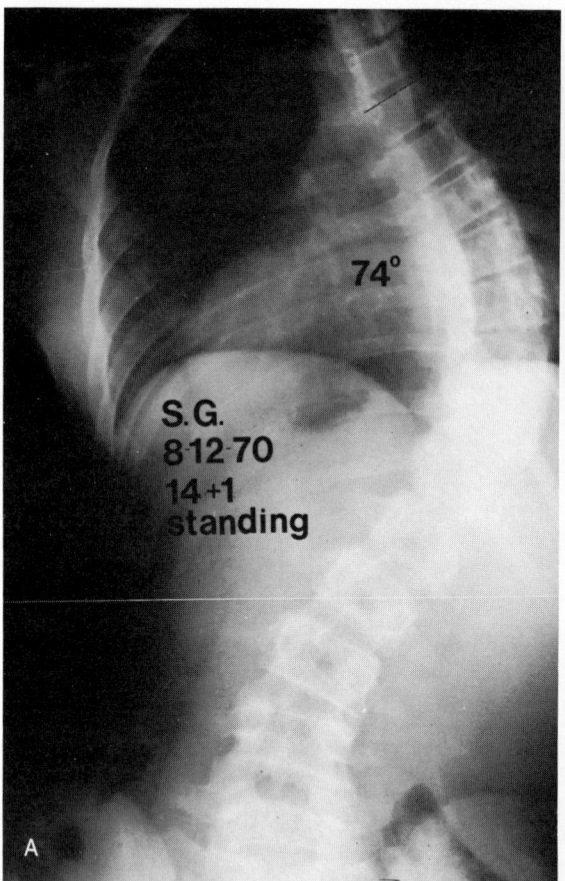

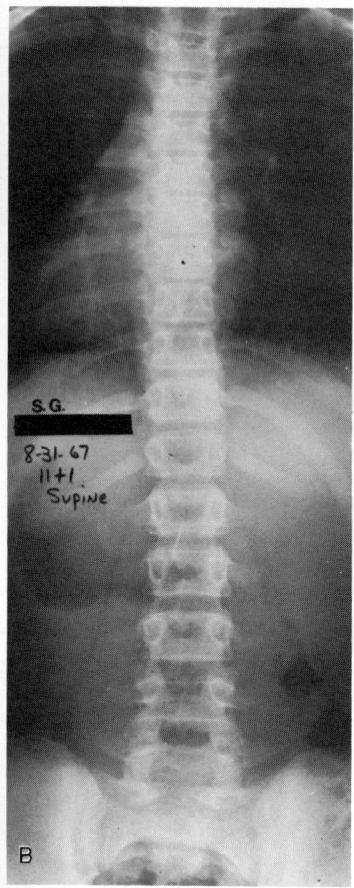

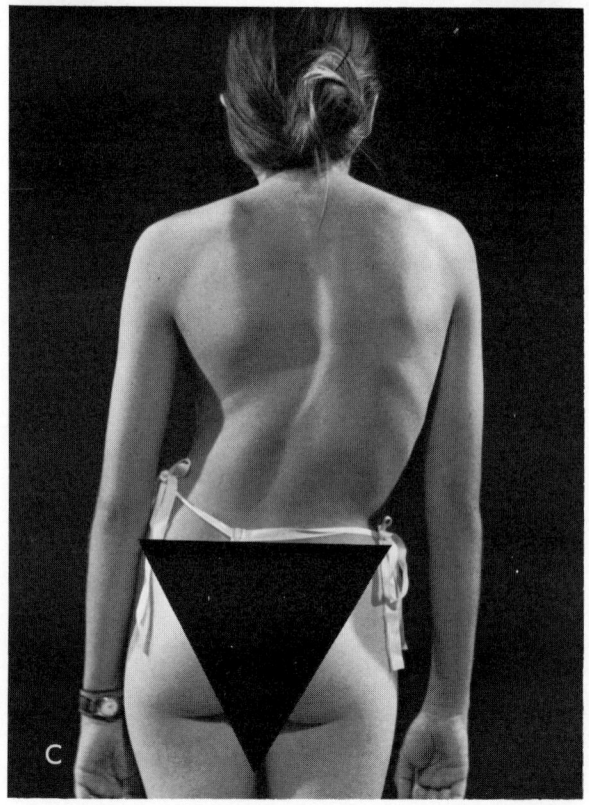

Figure 22–12. *A*, This 14+1 year old girl presented with a 74 degree curve. Neurologic examination was normal. She had no back pain, no limitation of forward bending, and no deviation on forward bending. *B*, This supine x-ray was taken three years previously and showed a minimal curve. *C*, This clinical photograph showed deformity and decompensation. No spinal rigidity was present on forward bending.

A spinal fusion and Harrington instrumentation was carried out with no complication and an excellent result. Six years later, following the birth of her first child, there was a sudden onset of leg weakness. A myelogram showed a spinal cord tumor, which on exploration was diagnosed as a very low grade astrocytoma. In retrospect this tumor was probably present on initial presentation, but there were no clues to its presence other than the rapid progression of the scoliosis.

tion well in life. With this attitude, the child will be carefully followed, any deformity detected early, and appropriate treatment promptly instituted.

It is very helpful if the responsible orthopaedic surgeon "scrubs in" with the neurosurgeon at the time of the laminectomy so that the length and width of the laminectomy is precisely known. The relationship with the family is also strongly maintained with this procedure.

Bracing is usually started immediately if there was a scoliosis existing prior to the laminectomy, or if the laminectomy involved the thoracic or thoracolumbar spine. Curvatures, either scolioses, kyphoses, or lordoses, which are progressive despite the laminectomy and brace treatment, should be surgically stabilized. A kyphosis in the area of laminectomy requires an anterior fusion to become solid. Posterior fusion of the curve area without laminectomy, and transverse process fusion in the area of laminectomy are also needed (see Fig. 22–11).

References

1. Bennett, G. D.: Tumors of cauda equina and spinal cord. Report of four cases in which marked spasm of erector spinal and hamstring muscles was an outstanding sign. JAMA, 89:1480–1483, 1927.
2. Boldrey, E., Adams, J. E., and Brown, H. A.: Scoliosis as a manifestation of disease of the spinal cord. Arch. Neurol. Psychiatry, 61:528, 1949.
3. Citron, N., Edgar, M. A., Sheehy, J., and Thomas, D. G. T.: Intramedullary spinal cord tumors presenting as scoliosis. J. Bone Joint Surg., 66A:513–517, 1984.
4. Craig, W. McK.: Need for consideration of intraspinal tumors as a cause of pain and disability. JAMA, 164:436–437, 1957.
6. Colloz, J. E., Queneau, P., Canlorbe, R., and Rubin, S.: Modifications de la Statique Rachidienne au Cours des Compressions Medullaires Pour Tumeur Chez. l'Enfant. Arch. Franc. Pediatr., 20:309, 1963.
7. Dubousset, J., Queneau, P., and Lacheretz, C.: Stiff and painful scoliosis in children. Rev. Chir. Orthop., 57:215–225, 1971.
8. Ekelund, L., and Cronquist, S.: Roentgenological changes in spinal malformations and spinal tumors in children. Radiology, 13:541, 1973.
9. Fraser, R. D., Paterson, D. C., and Simpson, D. A.: Orthopedic aspects of spinal tumors in children. J. Bone Joint Surg., 59B:143, 1977.
10. Grant, F. C., and Austin, G. M.: The diagnosis, treatment, and prognosis of tumors affecting the spinal cord in children. J. Neurosurg., 13:535, 1956.
11. Hoft, H., Ransohoff, J., and Carter, S.: Spinal cord tumors in children. Pediatrics, 23:1152, 1959.
12. Horrax, G., and Henderson, D. G.: Encapsulated intramedullary tumor involving the whole spinal cord from medulla to conus: complete enucleation with recovery. Surg. Gynecol. Obstet., 68:814–819, 1939.
13. Jorgensen, J., Oresen, N., and Poulsen, J. O.: Intraspinal tumors in the first two decades of life. Acta Orthop. Scand., 47:391–396, 1976.
14. Paillas, J. E., Vogouroux, R., Serratrice, G., and Courson, B.: Compressions medullaires D'origine Tumorale Chez l'Enfant. Sem. Hop., 39:2663, 1963.
15. Pool, J. L.: The surgery of spinal cord tumors. Proc. Congress Neurosurg., 17:310, 1970.
16. Richardson, F. L.: A report of 16 tumors of the spinal cord in children; the importance of spinal rigidity as an early sign of disease. J. Pediatr., 57:42, 1960.
17. Shuman, R. M., Ellsworth, C. A., and Leech, R. W.: The biology of childhood ependymomas. Arch. Neurol., 32:731, 1975.
18. Simril, W. A., and Thurston, D.: The normal interpedicular space in the spine of infants and children. Radiology, 64:340–347, 1955.
19. Srien, H. J., Thelen, E. P., and Keith, H. M.: Intraspinal tumors in children. JAMA, 155:959–961, 1954.
20. Tachdjian, M. O., and Matson, D. D.: Orthopaedic aspects of intraspinal tumors in infants and children. J. Bone Joint Surg., 47A:223, 1965.
21. Till, K.: Observations on spinal tumors in childhood. Proc. R. Soc. Med., 52:333–336, 1959.
22. Toumey, J. W., Poppen, J. L., and Hurley, M. T.: Cauda equina tumors as cause of the low back syndrome. J. Bone Joint Surg., 32A:246–256, 1950.

Hysterical (Conversion) Scoliosis

Robert B. Winter, M.D.

Although unusual, scoliosis as a psychosomatic manifestation can occur, and the astute physician should be aware of this possibility (Fig. 22–13).

Three cases were reported by Gillette,[2] one a boy age 7, one a girl age 6, and the third a female age 20 with both a hysterical lateral curve and a hysterical club foot. Schulthess[4] shows an example of an adolescent female also with a hysterical lateral curve and hysterical club foot.

Blount and coworkers reported eight cases in 1974.[1] The curve patterns were not characteristic of any structural or other functional

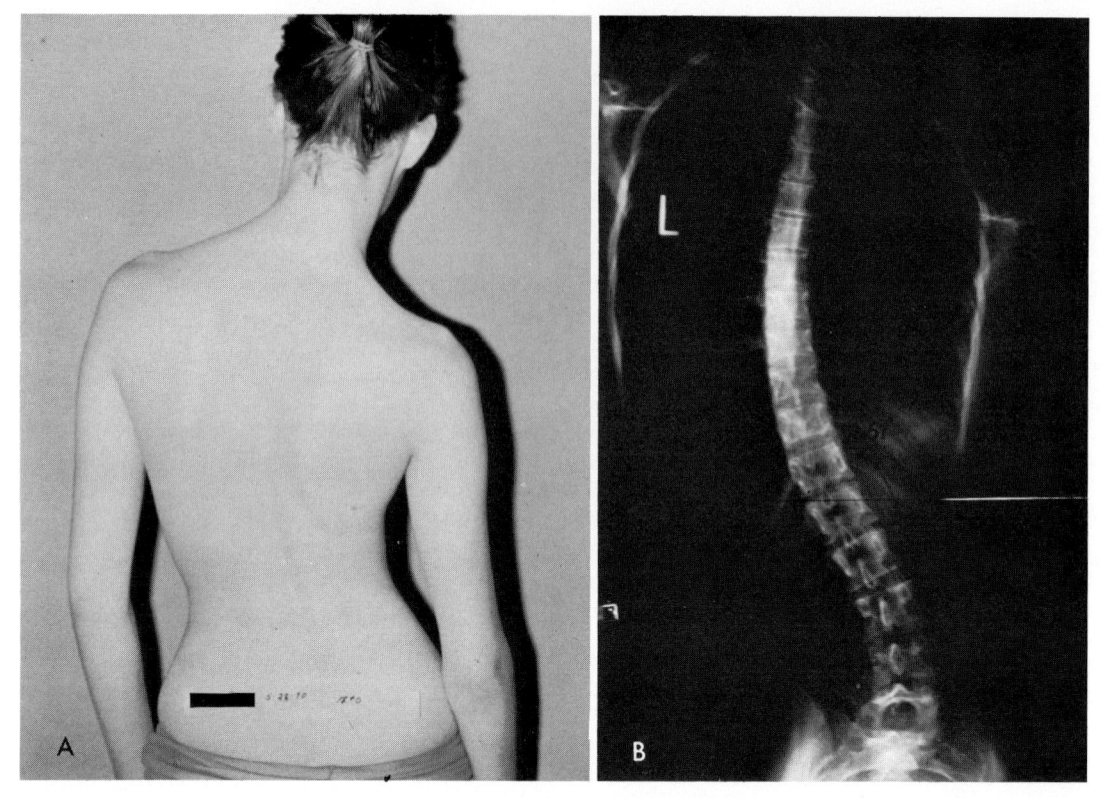

Figure 22–13. *A,* An 18 year old female with a long left curvature. There was no true rotation on forward bending. The curve persisted in the prone position but disappeared when supine. The curve also disappeared during sleep or anesthesia. *B,* The x-ray, which shows a long, sweeping curve extending into the cervical spine but without rotation, is highly suspicious for hysteria just by its pattern. This girl required extensive psychiatric treatment.

curves. They looked like children bending voluntarily in unusual positions.

Perves[3] reported five cases in 1976. All were female, with the ages ranging from 9 to 25. He felt all the patients had a "disturbed or unfavorable social milieu."

The peculiar position may be held throughout the examination. It may be present standing and disappear while prone or supine. It may persist while prone but with distraction may then vanish. A few may disappear only while asleep or under an anesthetic.

There is no true structural rotation. Shoulder elevation is usually quite pronounced but out of proportion for the curve. The patient may have other psychosomatic manifestations that give clues to the diagnosis. For example, one of Blount's patients, a male aged 16, had a collection of 23 lawn sprinklers.

A high index of suspicion and astute clinical diagnosis are the keys to this problem. A thorough neurologic exam is essential. Treatment is psychiatric. Orthopedic treatment by exercises, braces, or surgery is contraindicated.

References

1. Blount, W. P., Waldram, D. W., and Dicus, W. T.: The diagnosis of "hysterical" (conversion) scoliosis. Presented to Scoliosis Research Society, 1974. J. Bone Joint Surg., 56A:1766, 1974.
2. Gillette, A. J.: Quotation from Am. Orthop. Assoc. News, VI:11, Jan., 1914.
3. Perves, A.: Scolioses psychogeniques. Paper presented at the French Scoliosis Society, 1976.
4. Schulthess, W., *In* Jaochimstal: Handbuch der Orthop. Chirurgie, vol. II, p. 1012, Jena, Verlag Von Gustav Fisher, 1905–1907.

Post-Laminectomy Spine Deformity

John E. Lonstein, M.D.

A large number of laminectomies are performed every year for the excision of ruptured lumbar intervertebral discs and the treatment of lumbar spinal stenosis. Deformities following these laminectomies are rare; the most common problem is subluxation if the facets are removed. Increase in an existing kyphosis occurs with the treatment of cord compression by laminectomy (see page 540).

Multilevel laminectomies are performed less frequently. The most common occurrence of deformity following these laminectomies is in children.[5, 9, 10, 18, 20, 23] These laminectomies are performed for intraspinal pathology, mainly malignant spinal cord tumors.[11, 13] With the aggressive treatment of these malignant tumors by laminectomy and excision, radiotherapy, and chemotherapy, a large number of children are surviving and presenting to the orthopaedic surgeon with a severe post-laminectomy spine deformity.

INCIDENCE

The occurrence of post-laminectomy spine deformity is rare in adults but occurs in children treated for spinal cord tumors. The first report of this problem is that of Bette and Englehardt,[1] who in 1955 reported three cases of post-laminectomy deformities. Haft, in 1959, reported 30 children who had laminectomy for spinal cord tumors, and of the 17 with adequate follow-up, 10 developed spine deformity (33 per cent).[8] In Tachdjian and Matson's series of 115 children with spinal cord tumors, 46 developed spine deformity (40 per cent).[19] Boersma reported that half of the 51 children in his series developed spine deformity after laminectomy for spinal cord tumors.[2] Dubousset and associates, in 1970, reported on 55 children, 78 per cent of whom developed late post-laminectomy spine deformity.[6] Fraser, in 1977, reported that 35 per cent of the 29 children in his series developed post-laminectomy spine deformity.[7] A recent report of Yasuoka and co-workers reported that 46 per cent of patients under age 25 with a laminectomy developed post-laminectomy deformity.[23] Taking all these series together, the incidence of deformity is 50 per cent.

TYPES OF DEFORMITIES

Kyphosis is the most common deformity found following multiple level laminectomies, often with an associated mild scoliosis.[12, 19, 21] When other conditions that can cause a spine deformity are eliminated, Yasuoka and co-workers found that the age at which the laminectomy was performed was related to the incidence of deformity. In the 26 patients under age 15, 12 (46 per cent) developed a deformity, whereas only 2 of the 32 patients (6 per cent) aged 15 to 24 developed a deformity, and both of these were mild and non-progressive. In addition, the level of the laminectomy correlated with the incidence of deformity. All the cervical or cervicothoracic laminectomies were followed by deformity, as were 36 per cent of those at the thoracic level and none at the lumbar level; however, follow-up was incomplete in these latter two groups.[22]

The kyphosis may be either short and angular or a gradual rounded deformity. The configuration depends on the character of the laminectomy, as discussed subsequently. The kyphoses are progressive, and in the author's series led to cord compression in five cases.[12]

Scoliosis occurs less frequently, but usually occurs in the area of laminectomy and is associated with kyphosis. Less commonly scoliosis occurs below the area of laminectomy and is related to paralysis resulting from the cord tumor or its treatment. In rare cases the scoliosis is the first sign of a cord tumor, with progression occurring after laminectomy.

Lordosis is common after cervical laminectomies, giving the so-called swan neck deformity. If the laminectomy extends to the upper thoracic area, a severe cervicothoracic or high thoracic kyphosis is also present. Lordosis also occurs as a compensatory curve above a thoracic kyphosis. In the lumbar area, an extensive laminectomy will result in lumbar hyperlordosis (Fig. 22–14).

PATHOGENESIS

The most important factor in the development of the deformity is mechanical. The posterior ligament complex plays an important stabilizing role, which is complemented by normal muscle tone. Gravity normally exerts a flexion bending movement on the thoracic spine, which is resisted by the posterior ligament complex and spine extensors. After laminectomy there is disruption of the posterior ligament complex with removal of the interspinous ligaments, spinous processes, and laminae with complete or partial removal of the facet joints. With this loss of posterior stability and loss of extensor muscle function, the normal flexion forces produce kyphosis.[16]

Many of the conditions for which laminectomies are performed can of themselves produce a spinal deformity (e.g., trauma, neurofibromatosis, and syringomyelia). If these conditions are excluded from a series of post-laminectomy deformities, the effect of the *laminectomy alone* on the production of the deformity can be evaluated. This was done by Yasuoka and coworkers,[22] giving the differences with age and level of laminectomy as mentioned above. They found no correlation between the deformity and the number of laminae removed, but their number of patients was small.

Yasuoka and coworkers, in reviewing 12 patients (9 children and 3 adults) who underwent surgery for the post-laminectomy deformity or instability, shed light on the pathogenesis.[22] The children had increased wedging or excessive motion, whereas subluxation occurred in the adults. In children there is a large cartilaginous growth plate. With the laminectomy and loss of the posterior stability, kyphosis develops. This exerts increased stress on the anterior part of the vertebral body and growth plate, which results in decreased growth and subsequent wedging. With time, the kyphosis and vertebral wedging increase (Fig. 22–15). This results in a long, gradual rounded deformity.

Another important factor in the development of the deformity is the integrity of the

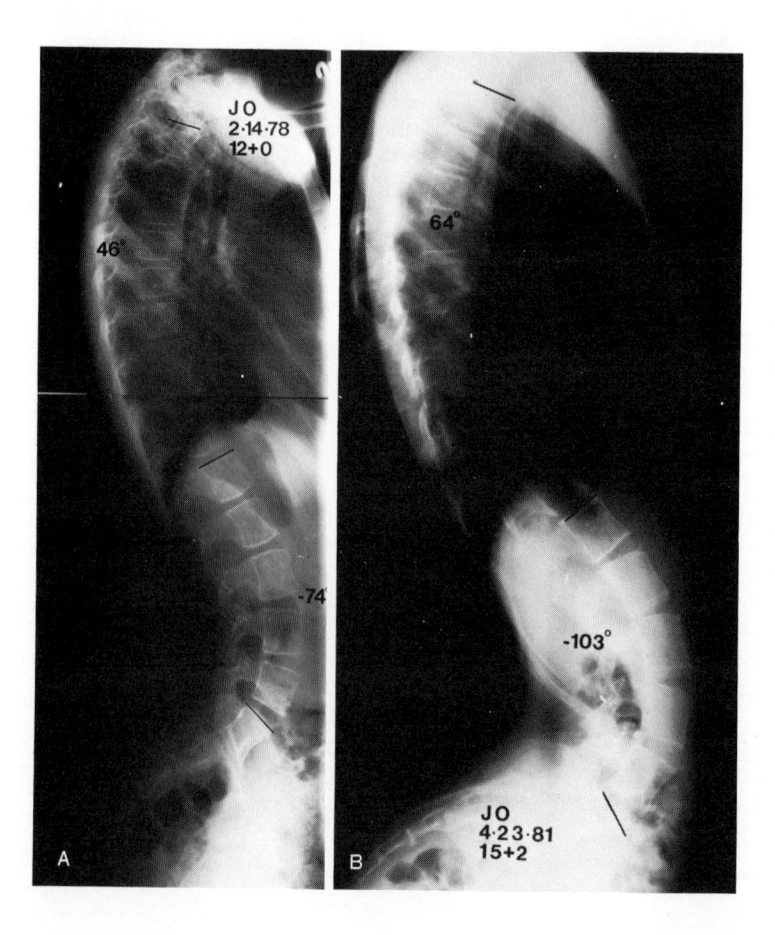

Figure 22–14. *A*, J.O. presented at age 12 with lumbar back pain and a stiff lumbar spine. The lateral radiograph shows a lumbar lordosis of −74 degrees. A spinal cord tumor was diagnosed two years later, and the patient underwent partial excision of a lumbar ependymoma of the filum terminale and postoperative irradiation. *B*, This radiograph one year after laminectomy shows increase of the lumbar lordosis to −103 degrees.

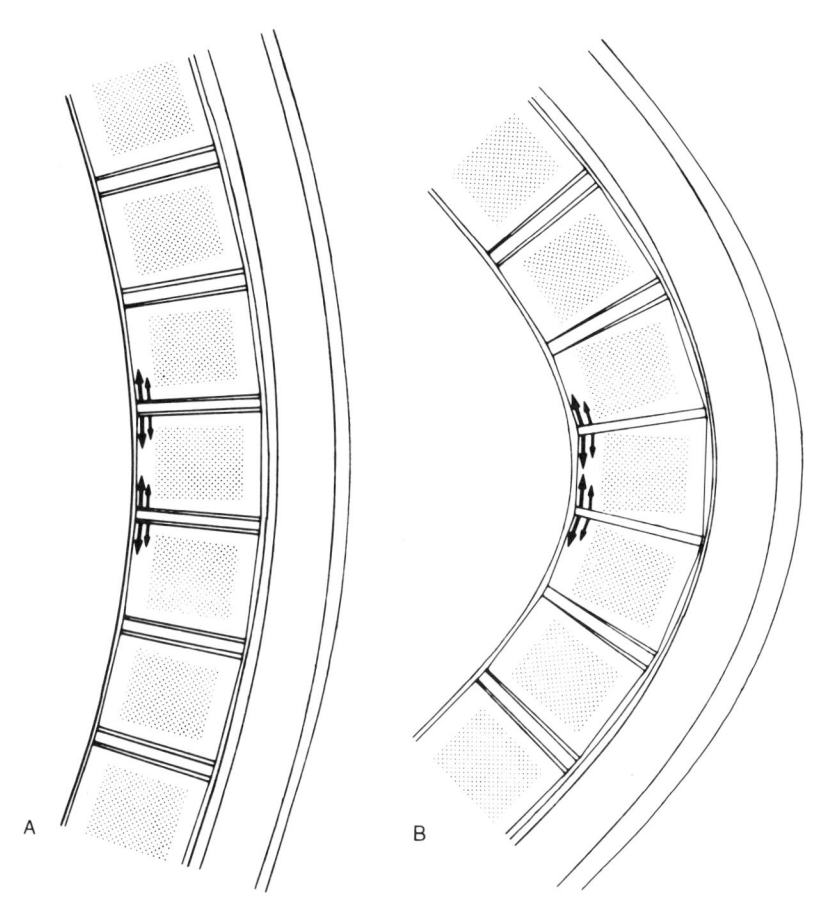

Figure 22–15. A, Child's spine after laminectomy, showing increased pressure on the cartilaginous portion of the vertebra anteriorly. B, With time, there is decreased cartilage growth with wedging of the vertebra. (Reprinted with permission from Yosouka, S., et al.: Pathogenesis and prophylaxis of post-laminectomy deformity of the spine after multiple level laminectomy: difference between children and adults. Neurosurgery, 9:145–152, 1981.)

facet joints. The role of the facets in stability has been shown in animal[15] and cadaver[16] experiments as well as clinically.[6] No adult with a simple laminectomy develops a deformity unless a facetectomy has been performed. In post-laminectomy deformities, a correlation between the facet integrity and deformity is found when the laminectomy is diagrammatically represented using the technique of Dubousset and associates (Fig. 22–16).[6] If the facets are completely removed at one level, a sharp angular kyphus develops, with the apex at this level. The intervertebral foramen is enlarged in this area, and the disc space opens posteriorly (Fig. 22–17). In addition, if the facet is partially removed on one side, a sharp angular scoliosis develops in addition to the kyphosis (Fig. 22–17). If the facets are preserved in part, or completely, a gradual rounding kyphosis develops as described before (Fig. 22–18). By careful evaluation of the post-laminectomy x-rays and with examination of the facet joints, an accurate prediction of the potential deformity can be made.

In the pathogenesis of the spine deformity, factors other than the mechanical ones mentioned are important. Radiotherapy damages the growth plates, adding to the deformity (see page 547). The tumor can destroy local tissue, for example, bone destruction by an eosinophilic granuloma. A spinal cord tumor can cause extensive paralysis of the paraspinal muscles; this may be undetected clinically, but it adds to the increasing deformity. If the paralysis due to the tumor is complete and if the paralysis occurs in a patient under the age of ten and is a high paralysis, 100 per cent of these patients develop a collapsing paralytic deformity.[3, 4]

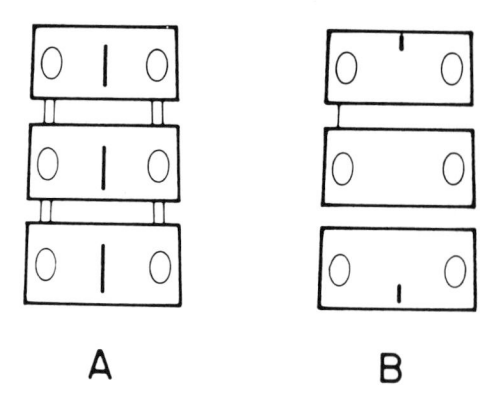

Figure 22–16. *A*, Normal spine. Vertebral bodies with intact spinous processes and pedicles. The facet joints are represented by two parallel lines joining the vertebral bodies on each side. *B*, Laminectomy. The spinous processes are removed. On the left, the facet is partially removed and a single line is drawn; on the right, the facet removal is complete and no line is drawn. (Reprinted with permission from Lonstein, J. E.: Post-laminectomy kyphosis. *In* Chou, S. N., Seljeskog, E. L. (eds.): Spinal Deformity and Neurological Dysfunction. New York, Raven Press, p. 53–63, 1978.)

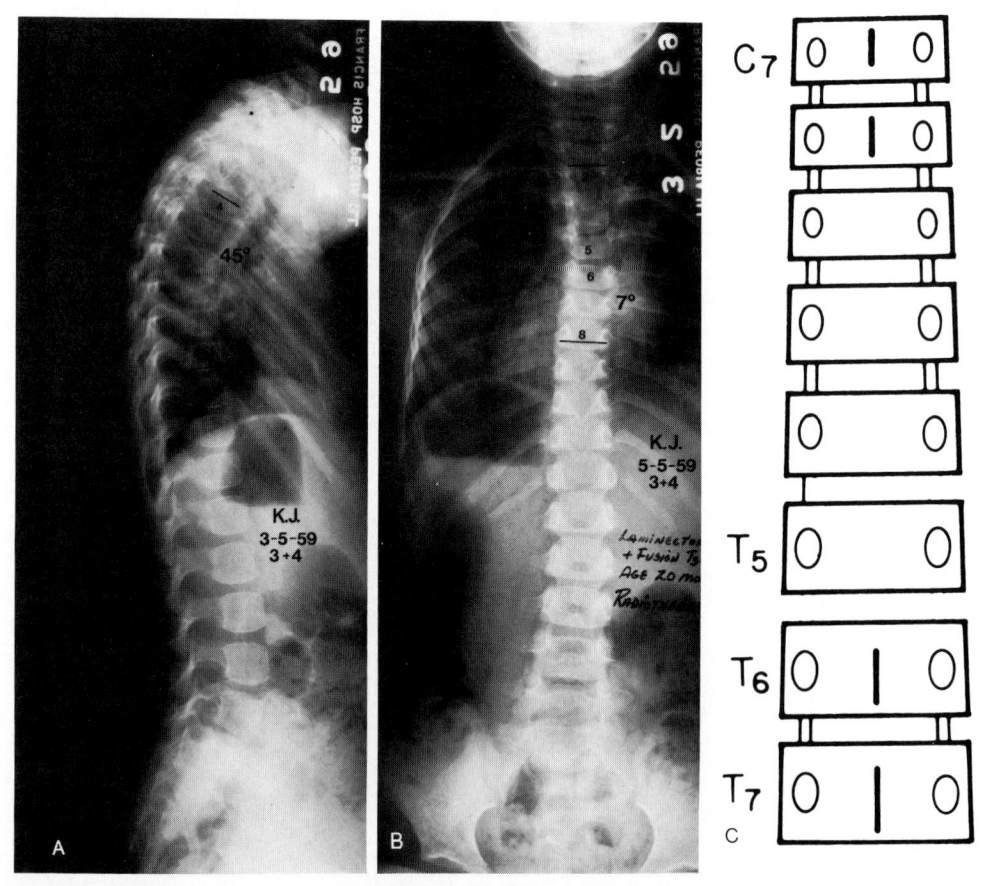

Figure 22–17. *A*, K.J. This female had a laminectomy from T3 to T6 at 20 months for excision of a neuroblastoma of the spinal cord with postoperative irradiation. A lateral x-ray at age 3 + 4 years showed a 45 degree kyphosis. *B*, Anteroposterior x-ray at age 3 + 4 showed a minimal 7 degree right thoracic kyphosis. The absent facet joints bilaterally at the T5-T6 junction are well seen. In addition, there is no facet on the right at T4-T5. This x-ray was used for the diagram in *C*. *C*, Laminectomy. There is a T2 to T6 laminectomy with no facets between T4 and T5 on the right and bilaterally between T5 and T6. In addition, partial facet removal occurred between T4 and T5 on the left.

Illustration continued on opposite page

MISCELLANEOUS PROBLEMS 517

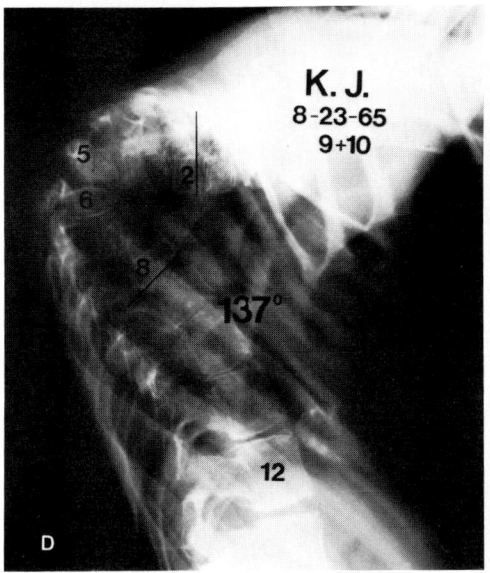

Figure 22–17 *Continued.* D, Standing lateral x-ray at age 9+10 years shows a sharp angular kyphosis measuring 137 degrees. Note that the maximal deformity is between T5 and T6, the site of complete facet removal. The disc space is open posteriorly, and there is an enlarged foramen at this level. E, Standing anteroposterior x-ray at age 9+10 years shows a 78 degree right thoracic scoliosis. Note in C that less stability exists on the right side as the facets are removed at two levels on this side.

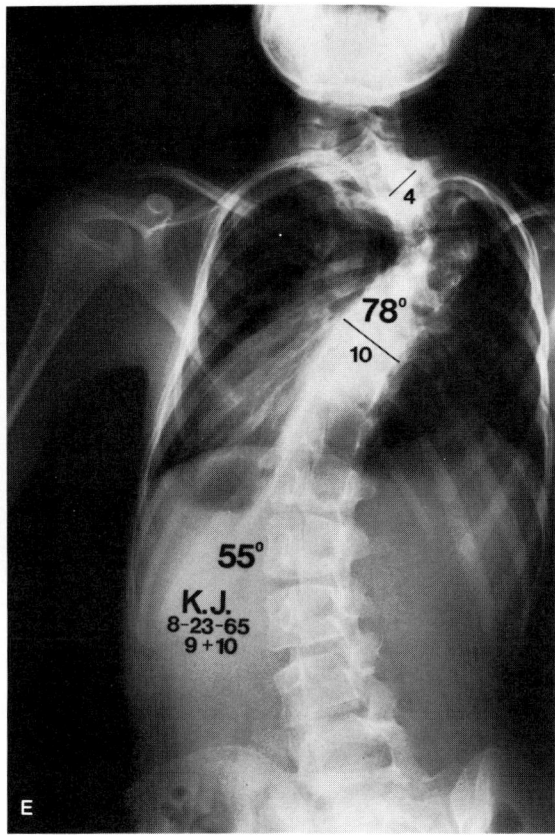

TREATMENT

The first rule is prevention of the deformities. Osteoplastic laminectomies are being performed with reconstruction of the lamina, and this may, we hope, prevent some deformities.[17] The facet joints should be preserved whenever possible. Consultation between the neurosurgeon and the orthopaedic surgeon is desirable at the time the tumor is treated. The ideal is for the orthopaedic surgeon to view the extent of the laminectomy at the time of surgery.

Postoperatively the child is carefully followed, and at the first sign of progressive kyphosis, a cast or brace is fitted to control the deformity. In the author's experience, this non-operative control is usually only temporary, giving lasting control in only few cases (2 of 17).[14]

If the deformity progresses in the brace or if the child presents with a marked deformity, a spinal fusion should be performed. There are two exceptions to this. One is the patient with an extremely poor prognosis related to a very malignant tumor. This is rare today, as with more aggressive care of these tumors, more children are surviving. The other exception is an extensive laminectomy and facet excision performed for a tumor of low malignancy. In these cases a more aggressive surgical approach is warranted with early spine fusion, even before the inevitable deformity develops.

The surgical approaches available are posterior, anterior, or the combined approach. A small amount of bone surface is available posteriorly after a wide laminectomy. This makes fusion difficult. A recent review of our experience in 45 patients showed the pseudarthrosis rate was 33 per cent with posterior fusion alone, 22 per cent with anterior fusion alone, and 9.5 per cent in combined anterior and posterior fusions.[14] The combined approaches are thus the treatment of choice. In the anterior fusion the whole disc must be excised *back* to the posterior longitudinal ligament. If any posterior anulus and cartilage are not removed, posterior growth is still possible, as the posterior fusion tends to be thin. This growth will result in a pseudarthrosis or in an increasing deformity, with

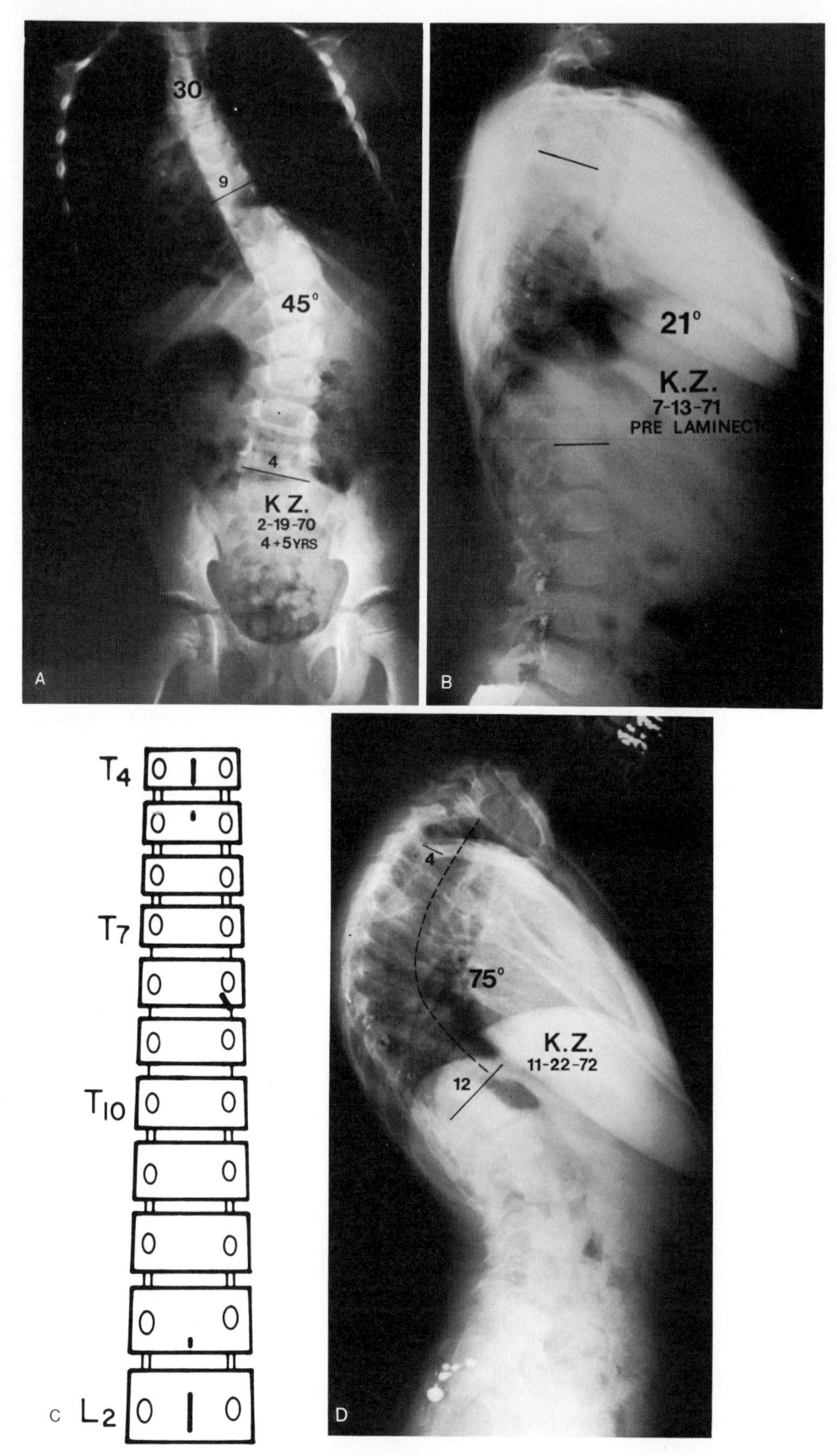

Figure 22–18. *See legend on opposite page.*

MISCELLANEOUS PROBLEMS 519

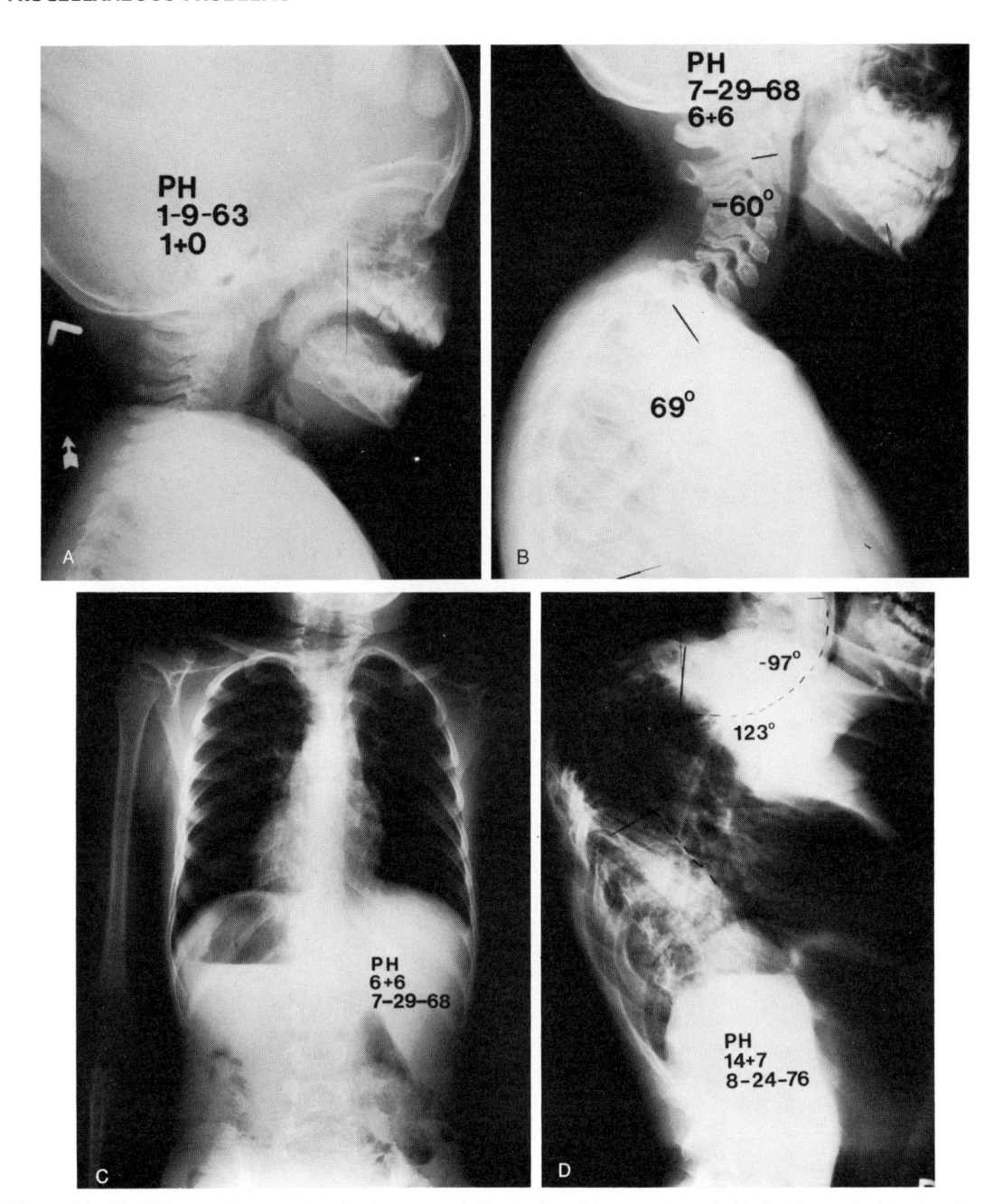

Figure 22–19. P.H. was diagnosed as having a cervical spinal cord tumor at age 1. He had a cervical laminectomy and postoperative irradiation for the astrocytoma. A, This radiograph prior to the laminectomy shows no deformity. B, Five years and six months later there was a −60 degree lordosis, and a 69 degree high thoracic kyphosis, and no scoliosis (C). There was residual paralysis of the right upper extremity. D, At age 14+7 he presented with a progressing deformity with 123 degrees of high thoracic kyphosis and −97 degrees of cervical lordosis.

Illustration continued on following page

Figure 22–18. A, K.Z. This female presented at the age of 4+5 with a 49 degree right thoracolumbar scoliosis. This was diagnosed as infantile idiopathic scoliosis and a Milwaukee brace was fitted. B, Lateral x-ray at the age of 5+10 years shows a 21 degree thoracic kyphosis. The child had a complaint of back pain on initial presentation as well as itching around the chest cage. A spinal cord tumor was diagnosed and laminectomy performed. A spinal cord astrocytoma was found, and postoperative irradiation was given. C, Diagram of laminectomy from T6 to T12, showing partial facet removal bilaterally from T7 to T10. D, Lateral x-ray at 14 months postlaminectomy shows a gradual, rounding kyphosis of 75 degrees.

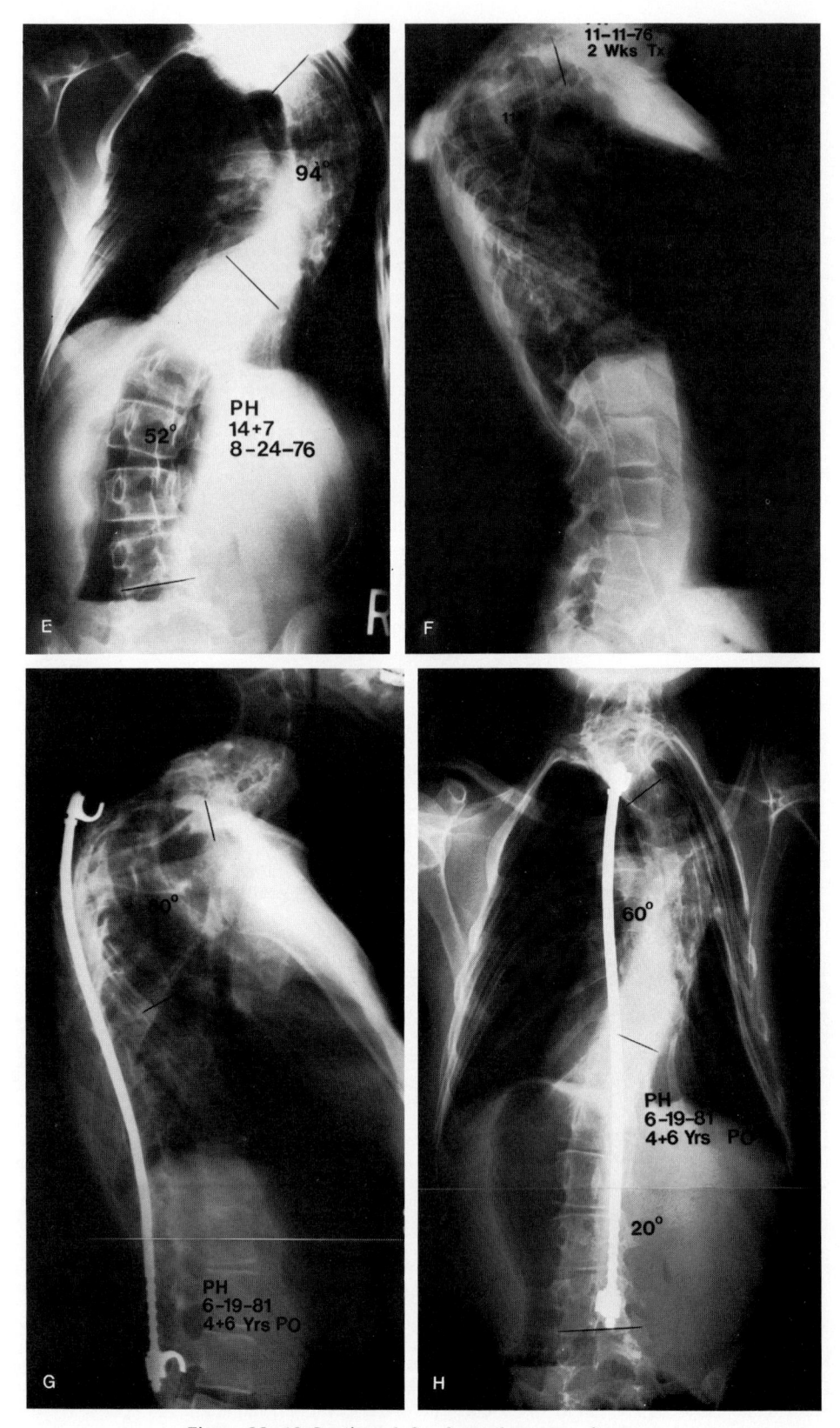

Figure 22–19 Continued. See legend on opposite page.

the anterior fusion acting as a type II congenital kyphosis. The disc and cartilage are thus completely removed, and the fusion is performed using the rib as an inlay strut graft. The vertebral bone and any additional chips of rib bone are placed in the disc spaces. One to two weeks later a posterior fusion is performed, which extends into the compensatory lordotic curves. Instrumentation is usually impossible posteriorly either because the bone is too soft in a young child or because the kyphus is too angular. Postoperatively a halo cast is often used because the deformity is in the high thoracic area and this is the most effective way to immobilize this area.

Cases presenting late with angular kyphosis and scoliosis may benefit from preoperative correction using halo wheelchair traction. A two-stage anterior and posterior fusion is performed, usually using bypass strut grafts with an anterior fibular graft. If there is marked scoliosis, the approach is easier on the side of the convexity of the scoliosis. In these cases, every attempt must be made to place the graft in the weight-bearing line of the spine.

A posterior fusion is performed one to two weeks later. In the area of the laminectomy, strips of bone are placed laterally. If possible, instrumentation, using large compression rods (3/16 inch or .48 cm.) or large Luque rods (1/4 inch or .64 cm.) with sublaminar wires passed around the transverse processes or through the foramina, is placed. If there is an associated paralytic scoliosis, this is appropriately treated with fusion and instrumentation at the same time (Fig. 22–19). If no instrumentation is used or the kyphosis is unstable, the patient needs to be kept supine in a halo cast for appropriately four months, with continued immobilization when ambulatory.

References

1. Bette, H., and Englehardt, H.: Folgezustande von Laminektomie an der Halswirbelsaule. Z Orthop., 85:564–573, 1955.
2. Boersma, G.: Curvatures of the Spine Following Laminectomies in Children. Amsterdam, Born, p. 257, 1969.
3. Brown, H. P.: Spine deformity subsequent to spinal cord injury. Orthop. Sem. Rancho Los Amigos Hosp., 5:41, 1972.
4. Brown, H. P., and Bonnett, C. C.: Spine deformity subsequent to spinal cord injury. J. Bone Joint Surg., 55A:441, 1973.
5. Cattell, H. E., and Clark, L. G.: Cervical kyphosis and instability following multiple laminectomies in children. J. Bone Joint Surg., 49A:713, 1967.
6. Dubousset, J., Guillaumat, M., and Mechin, J. F.: Paper presented to Neurosurgical Congress on Infants, Versailles, 1970. In Rougerie, J. (ed.): Les Compressions Medullaires non Traumatiques de l'Enfant. Paris, Masson et Cie, p. 185, 1973.
7. Fraser, R. D., Patterson, D. C., and Simpson, D. A.: Orthopaedic aspects of spinal tumors in children. J. Bone Joint Surg., 59B:143–151, 1977.
8. Haft, H., Ransohoff, J., and Carter, S.: Spinal cord tumors in children. Pediatrics, 23:1152, 1959.
9. Haritonova, K. I., Tziuian, J. L., and Ekshtadt, N. K.: Orthopaedic sequelae of laminectomy. Orthop. Traumatol. Protez., 11:32, 1974.
10. Jenkins, D. H. R.: Extensive cervical laminectomy—long term results. Br. J. Surg., 60:852–854, 1973.
11. Lonstein, J. E., Winter, R. B., Bradford, D. S., et al.: Post-laminectomy spine deformity. J. Bone Joint Surg., 58A:727, 1976.
12. Lonstein, J. E.: Post-laminectomy kyphosis. Clin. Orthop., 128:93–100, 1977.
13. Lonstein, J. E.: Post-laminectomy kyphosis. In Chou, S. N., and Seljeskog, E. L. (eds.): Spinal Deformity and Neurological Dysfunction. New York, Raven Press, pp. 53–63, 1978.
14. Lonstein, J. E., and Cho, J. L.: The treatment of post-laminectomy spinal deformity. In preparation.
15. Munechika, Y.: Influence of laminectomy on the stability of the spine: an experimental study with special reference to the extent of the laminectomy and resection of the intervertebral joint. J. Jpn. Orthop. Assoc., 47:111–126, 1973.
16. Panjabi, M. M., White, A. A., and Johnson, R. M.: Cervical spine mechanics as a function of transection on components. J. Biomech., 8:327–336, 1975.
17. Raimondi, A.: Personal communication to Fraser, 1974. Quoted in Fraser et al: Orthopaedic aspects of spinal tumors in children. J. Bone Joint Surg., 59B:143–151, 1977.
18. Rogers, L.: The surgical treatment of cervical spondylotic myelopathy. Mobilization of the complete cervical cord into an enlarged canal. J. Bone Joint Surg., 43B:3–6, 1961.
19. Tachdjian, M. O., and Matson, D. D.: Orthopaedic aspects of intraspinal tumors in infants and children. J. Bone Joint Surg., 47A:223, 1965.

Figure 22–19 Continued. E, He also had 94 degrees of right thoracic scoliosis. F, After two weeks of halo wheelchair traction the kyphosis was reduced to 114 degrees, and the patient underwent an anterior fusion with strut grafting of the kyphosis, with a second stage posterior fusion from C2 to L4 for both the cervical lordosis and paralytic scoliosis; a Harrington distraction rod was used for the scoliosis. G, He was immobilized in a halo cast for 6 months followed by a Milwaukee brace for 4 months, the fusion being solid at this time. Four and a half years later there was no loss of correction, with the kyphosis stable at 80 degrees. H, The scoliosis was reduced to 60 degrees with good thoracopelvic balance.

20. Teng, P.: Spondylosis of the cervical spine with compression of spinal cord and nerve roots. J. Bone Joint Surg., 42A:392–407, 1960.
21. Vlach, O., Muller, I., and Slechta, J.: On the kyphotization of the spine after laminectomy. Acta Chir. Orthop. Traumatol. Cech., 48:112–116, 1981.
22. Yasuoka, S., Peterson, H., Laws, E. R., Jr., et al.: Pathogenesis and prophylaxis of post-laminectomy deformity of the spine after multiple level laminectomy; difference between children and adults. Neurosurgery, 9:145–152, 1981.
23. Yasuoka, S., Peterson, H. A., and MacCarty, C. S.: Incidence of spinal column deformity after multilevel laminectomy in children and adults. J. Neurosurg., 57:441–445, 1982.

Dwarfs
Robert B. Winter, M.D.

INTRODUCTION

By defintion, dwarfs have a disproportionate short stature, as compared to midgets, whose body proportions are normal.[55] In dwarfs, the disorder of bone growth and maturation often affects some part of the skeleton with greater intensity, creating disproportionate growth between the axial and the appendicular skeleton and between different parts of the extremities.

Dwarfs have been described from earliest times. In Egypt they were esteemed as gods or art figures. In the middle ages they lived with royalty and served as counselors and were the subjects of painters (Fig. 22–20). By the 1800's dwarfs had been relegated to circuses and "freak" shows. It is only recently that they have been recognized for what they really are—intelligent, contributing members of society.

The most significant problem of dwarfs is not their short stature, but the associated medical problems. Most of these affect the musculoskeletal system, with the spine usually being involved. Disorders of the spine can lead to deformity, even greater shortness, pain, respiratory compromise, minor or major neural defects, and even death.

There are a large number of dwarfing conditions. The more common types, and the types with more significant spinal involvement, will be discussed in this section. The reader is referred to the review by Bethem and associates[10] in which the spinal problems of the various disorders are discussed in detail. Other good general reviews are those by Bailey,[4] Beighton,[6] Eulert,[17] Jones and Hensinger,[25] Kopits,[29] Nelson,[50] Spranger and coworkers,[61] and Stanescu and coworkers.[62]

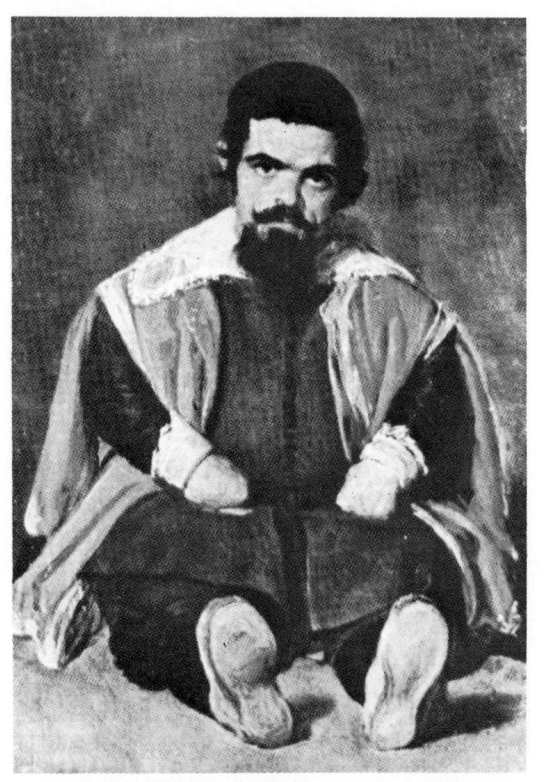

Figure 22–20. Portrait of Sebastian de Morra, a dwarf in the court of Prince Baltasar Carlos of Spain, painted by Diego Velázquez in 1643.

ACHONDROPLASIA[46, 52, 58]

Achondroplasia is the most common form of dwarfism. It is transmitted as an autosomal dominant. The condition is obvious at birth. About 90 per cent of cases are due to a new mutation, the parents being unaffected.[3, 38]

The classic appearance of these patients is a short-limbed rhizomelic (proximal segments shorter than distal segments) dwarf with a slightly enlarged head and depressed base of the nose.

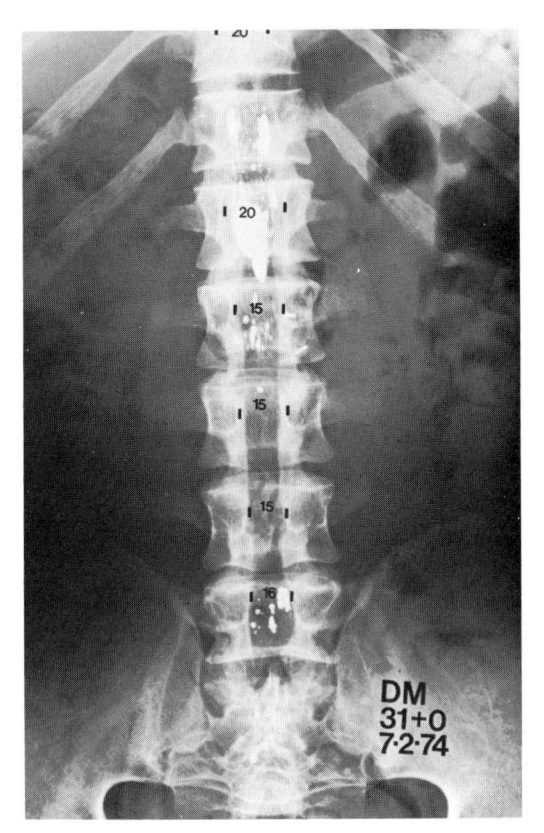

Figure 22–21. The decreasing interpediculate distance of the lumbar spine is well seen in this 31 year old male with achondroplasia. He had had a laminectomy for spinal stenosis three years earlier.

The spine is of normal length; all of the shortening occurs in the extremities. The most diagnostic finding in the spine is the narrow interpediculate distance in the lumbar spine, which gradually decreases from the upper to the lower lumbar spine.[13, 51] This narrow interpediculate distance is coupled with a shortness of the pedicles to create a spinal canal with a decreased cross sectional area (spinal stenosis) (Fig. 22–21).

Although the canal is narrow from birth, symptoms of spinal stenosis are not found in children, are rare in adolescents, and have an average onset at age 38.[1, 8, 16, 19, 59, 66] This suggests that other factors, such as disc degeneration, disc herniation,[56] increasing lumbar lordosis, and facet joint degeneration with hypertrophic spurring, are important in the development of neural symptoms.

The non-operative treatment of the patient with symptomatic spinal stenosis is a brace that reduces the lumbar lordosis. This will often "open up" the spinal canal sufficiently to relieve the claudication symptoms. Patients with more advanced neurologic deficits and patients who do not respond to the brace should have a laminectomy. The laminectomy usually extends from about L2 to S2, and should *not* extend proximally into the thoracolumbar junction (which will result in a kyphos). Most importantly, the laminectomy should extend laterally to the pedicles but, at the same time, the integrity of the facet joints should not be violated. This requires "undercutting" to enlarge the canal, usually removing some of the ventral part of the superior articular facets. The foramina, as well as the canal, are small, making both lateral recess release and foraminal release important (Figs. 22–22 and 22–23).[41, 42]

Kyphosis

The second problem common in achondroplasts is a thoracolumbar kyphosis. All newborns with achondroplasia have a mild thoracolumbar kyphosis, and this may be associated with anterior wedging of the apical vertebra. As the extensor muscles develop, the kyphosis usually resolves to the normal configuration. In about 30 per cent of patients a persistent kyphosis remains, and about one third of these develop a major progressive thoracolumbar kyphosis. The wedging of the apical vertebra may become so severe as to mimic a congenital anterior hemivertebra. Left untreated, this kyphosis can result in loss of height, severe cosmetic deformity, and paraplegia (Fig. 22–24).

The best treatment for this kyphosis problem is its prevention. Achondroplastic children with thoracolumbar kyphosis that does not spontaneously resolve, or is progressive, should be treated in a brace that provides a hyperextension moment at the thoracolumbar junction. This can be accomplished by a Milwaukee brace or a TLSO with appropriate design for the problem.[22]

Major kyphoses are beyond the ability of a brace to control or correct them and require surgical stabilization. As with other major kyphosis problems, posterior fusion alone is insufficient. Anterior surgery is essential, first resecting the contracted anterior longitudinal ligament and the anulus throughout the kyphotic area, then correcting the kyphosis with an anterior distractor (Santa Casa, Slot), and stabilizing the kyphosis in the corrected position with a strut graft, using rib, fibula, or both as necessary. A posterior fusion is done at a second stage; any instru-

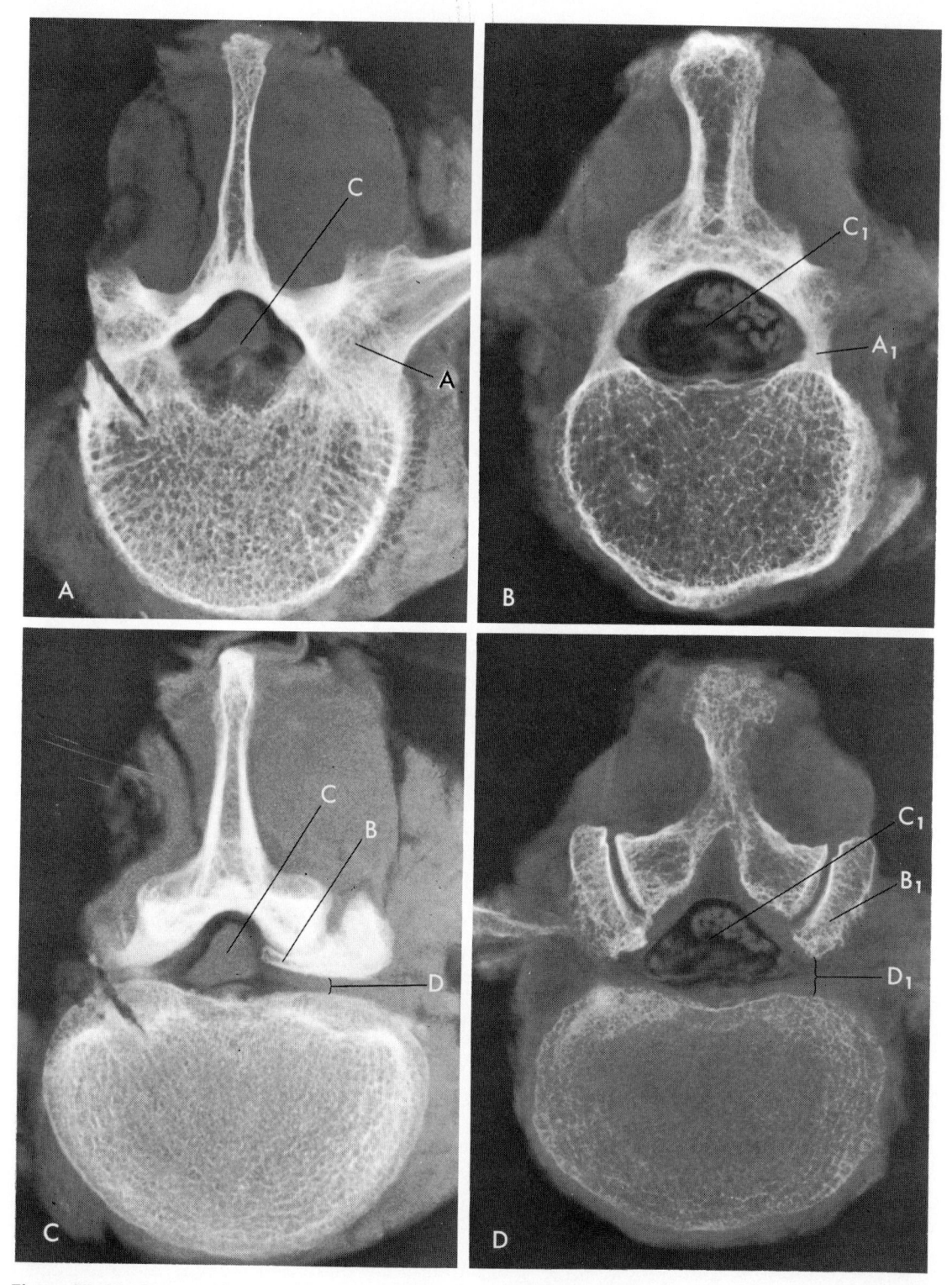

Figure 22–22. Cross-sections of the lumbar spine of an achondroplast (*A* and *C*) are compared to a matched nonachondroplast (*B* and *D*). In the achondroplast the pedicles are broader and shorter (A) when compared to the normal (A_1). The facet joints are hypertrophied encroaching on the spinal canal (B), no encroachment being present in the nonachondroplast (B_1). The total cross sectional area of the spinal canal in the achondroplast is decreased (C) when compared to the nonachondroplast (C_1), leaving just enough space for the spinal cord. The nerve root foramen in the achondroplast is markedly narrowed (D) when compared to the nonachondroplast (D_1).

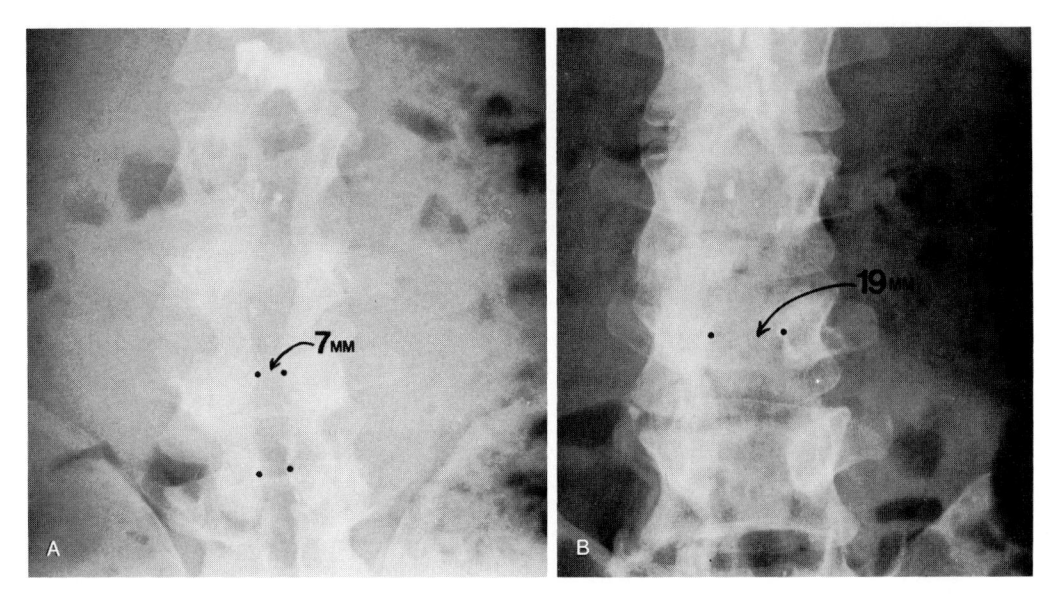

Figure 22–23. A, An achrondroplasia patient who presented with spinal stenosis symptoms despite a previous laminectomy. The x-ray shows an inadequate laminectomy, only 7 mm. of space between the residual bone impingement. B, The same patient after repeat laminectomy with removal of bone back to the medial border of the pedicles. This provides 19 mm. of space without bony impingement. Because of the radical facet removal on the right side, an interbody fusion was done at a second stage.

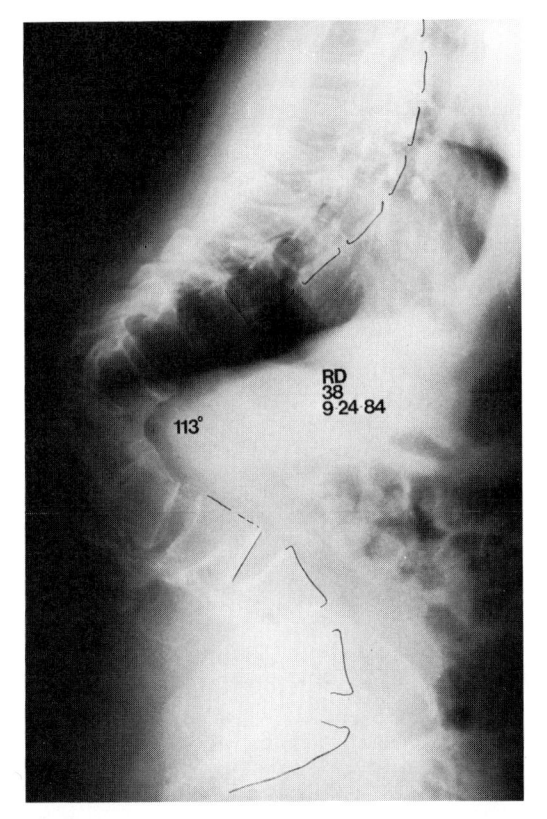

Figure 22–24. A 38 year old man seen for progressive paraparesis due to a thoracolumbar kyphosis.

mentation that penetrates the narrow spinal canal, either Harrington hooks or Luque wires, must be avoided. Casting in hyperextension is maintained until the fusion is solid (Fig. 22–25).

Finally, the patient with severe kyphosis presenting with paraparesis should be treated by anterior spinal cord decompression, anterior strut graft fusion, and posterior fusion. Laminectomy is contraindicated for this problem.

Scoliosis

Scoliosis can occur in the achondroplast and is more common than has been previously appreciated. Of Langer's series, 75 per cent had at least a mild degree of scoliosis.[37] Progression can occur and should be treated with a brace. If necessary, fusion can be done, but posterior instrumentation should be avoided because of the small canal. Paraplegia has been reported due to instrumentation (Fig. 22–26).

Low Back Pain

Low pack pain is common in almost all achondroplasts and may even begin in child-

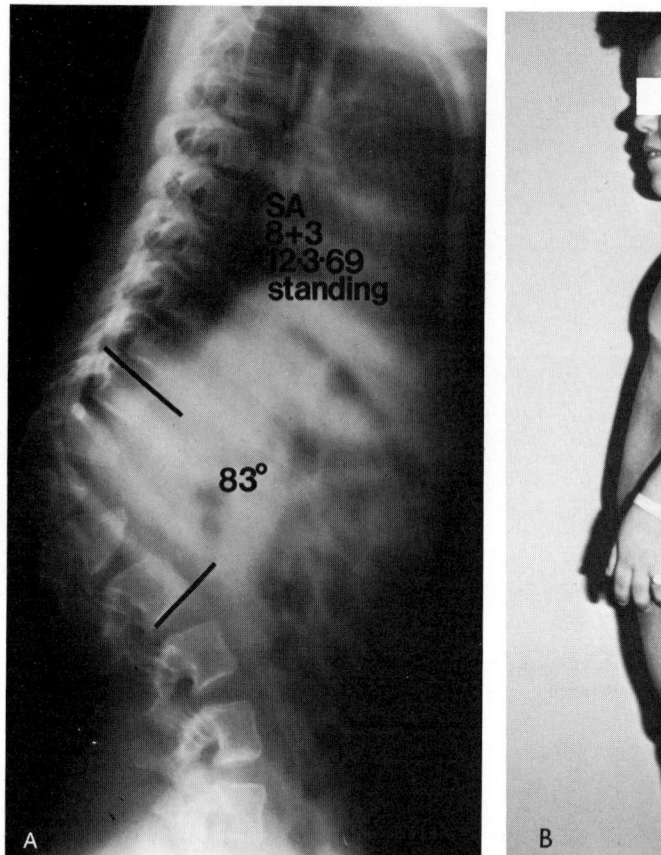

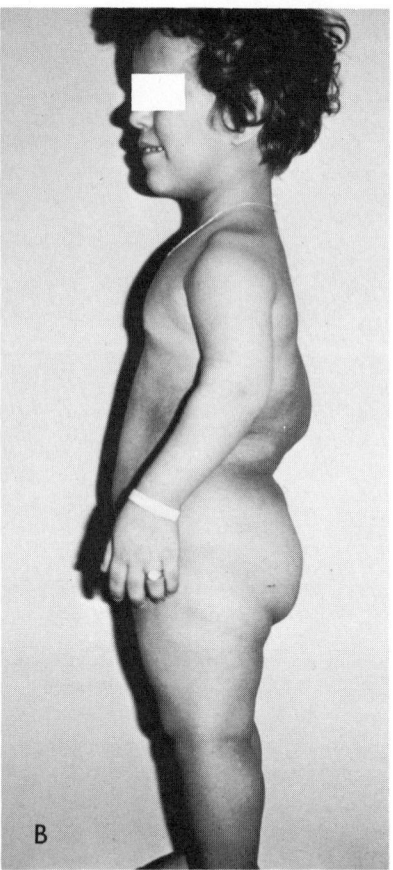

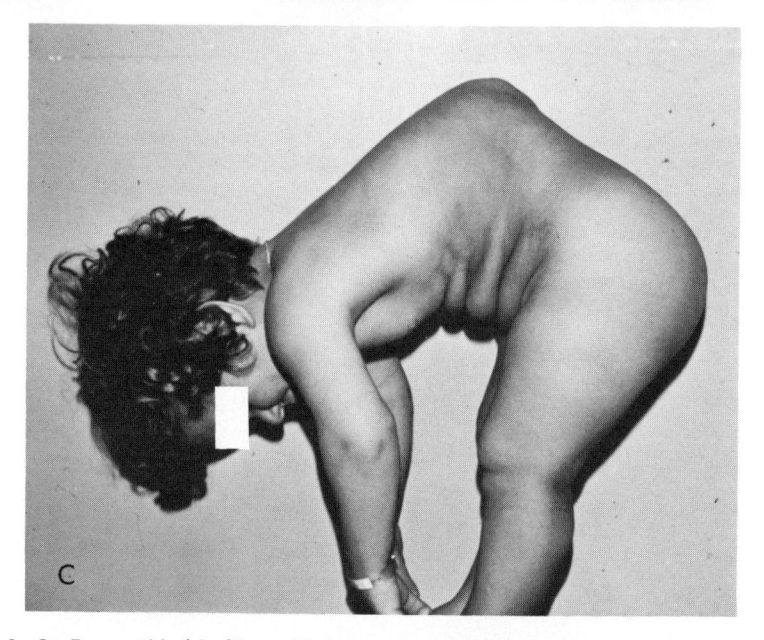

Figure 22–25. *A*, An 8+3 year old girl with an 83 degree thoracolumbar kyphosis due to achondroplasia. Brace treatment should have been done at this time, but she was only observed. (Reprinted with permission from Bethem, et al.: Spinal disorders of dwarfism. J. Bone Joint Surg., 63A:1412–1425, 1981.) *B*, Initial clinical photographs show the short limbs with marked proximal shortening, enlarged head, and depressed base of nose. The thoracolumbar kyphosis is well seen on forward bending (*C*).

Illustration continued on opposite page

MISCELLANEOUS PROBLEMS

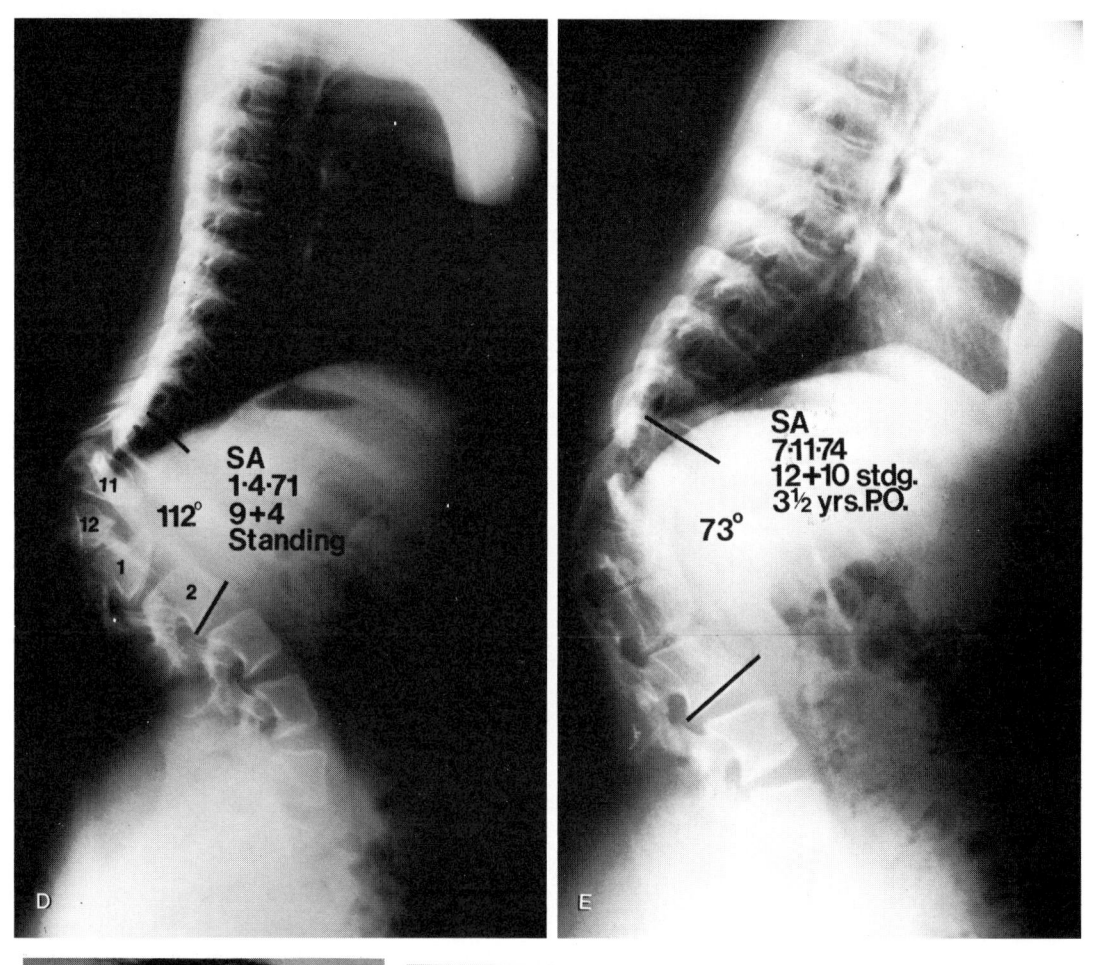

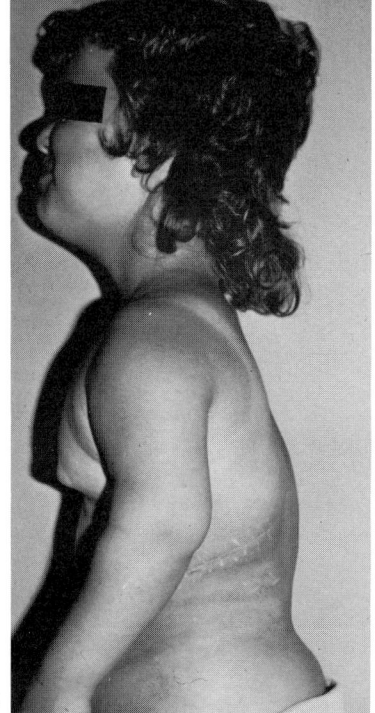

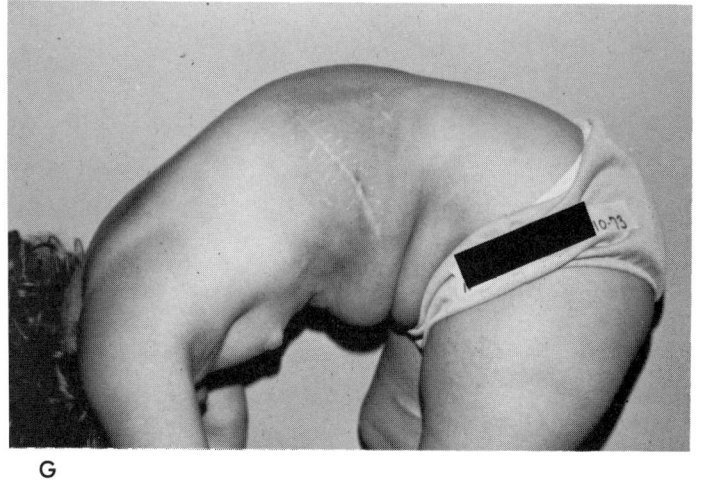

Figure 22–25 *Continued. D,* When she presented at our clinics in 1971 at the age of 9+4, her kyphosis had increased to 112 degrees and was now beyond bracing. She was neurologically normal. *E,* At age 12+10, 3½ years after combined anterior and posterior fusion, her kyphosis measures 73 degrees. The posterior fusion was too short and should have extended proximally another three vertebrae. *F,* Lateral clinical photograph 2½ years postoperatively shows the markedly improved kyphosis. *G,* The improvement is well seen on forward bending.

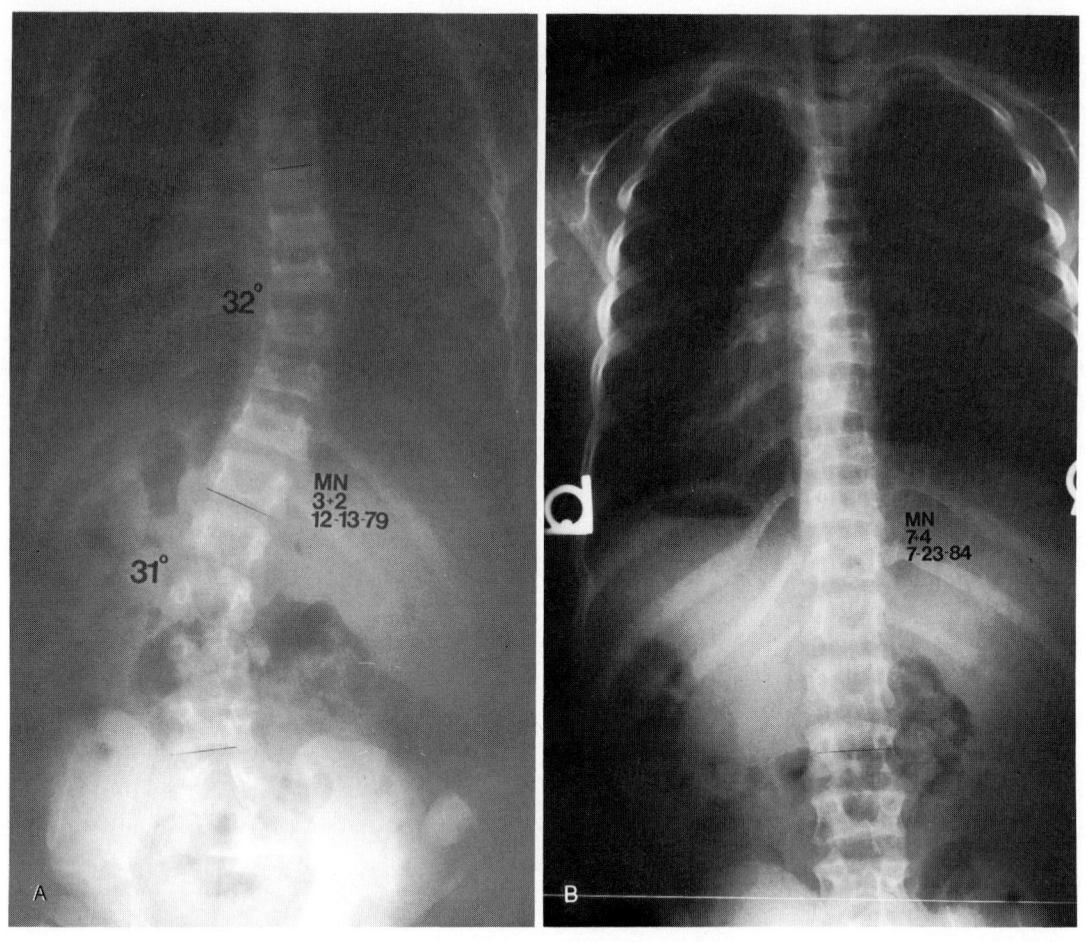

Figure 22–26. A, A 3 year old male with achondroplasia presented with these 32 and 31 degree progressive curves. A TLSO was prescribed and worn for 3 years. B, The same patient at age 7, one year after brace removal.

hood. It appears to be associated with the mechanical disadvantage of the increased lumbar lordosis. It is worse in the standing position and is relieved by "hunkering," or sitting in a squatting position, decreasing the lumbar lordosis and increasing the volume of the lumbar spinal canal. Lumbar back pain can be helped by an orthosis that decreases the lumbar lordosis.

HYPOCHONDROPLASIA

Hypochondroplasia is a form of short-limbed rhizomelic dwarfism with an autosomal dominant mode of inheritance.[5] It closely resembles achondroplasia, but the difference is important, as these patients seldom have spine problems and do not develop paraplegia; scoliosis has not been reported.

Radiologically, there is minimal interpediculate narrowing, the pelvis is normal, and there is only a slight flaring of the long bones at the metaphyseal-epiphyseal junction.

DIASTROPHIC DWARFISM[2, 9, 21, 23, 35, 63, 65, 67, 68]

The word diastrophic is based on a Greek word meaning twisted, tortuous, or crooked and was used by Lamy and Maroteaux to describe this severe type of dwarfism.[33] It is inherited as an autosomal recessive.

The dwarfing is severe. There are contractures of many joints, especially the elbows, hips, and knees. There is severe and rigid talipes equinovarus, and the hands show a short and radially directed thumb ("hitchhiker's thumb"). The ears are also deformed, with cystic swelling early in life. Spinal problems are frequent and may be severe.

The most common spinal problem is scoliosis, which occurs in about 80 per cent of patients.[53] These curvatures tend to occur early and may progress severely. A progressive curve must be treated aggressively since catastrophic deformity can result, making an already short person even shorter, and significantly affecting pulmonary function.

The treatment of choice is the Milwaukee brace. A skilled orthotist is required in order to adequately fit a dwarfed child. The brace should be applied before the scoliosis reaches 40 degrees.

If bracing is unsuccessful, fusion should be done to arrest progression. There is often reluctance to fuse the spine in a dwarf, but failure to fuse will result in an even shorter person (Fig. 22–27).

Cervical kyphosis can occur in this condition and may result in quadriplegia.[26] The cervical spine should always be radiologically examined. Odontoid hypoplasia and upper cervical instability, so common in other dwarfing problems, are not seen in diastrophic dwarfism. If cervical kyphosis is noted early in life, it should be treated with a Milwaukee brace, as successful results have been seen. Progressive kyphosis despite bracing should be treated by anterior fusion before quadriplegia develops. A halo cast should be used postoperatively (Figs. 22–28 and 22–29).

SPONDYLOEPIPHYSEAL DYSPLASIA[15, 44, 60, 64]

Spondyloepiphyseal dysplasia (SED) encompasses a large group of conditions in which there are changes both in the spine and in the epiphyses of the long bones. There are several different subclassifications, but the one most commonly used is that of Bailey.[4] He described four major groups: (1) spondyloepiphyseal dysplasia congenita, (2) pseudoachrondroplasia, (3) pseudo-Morquio's disease, and (4) spondyloepiphyseal dysplasia tarda.

Involvement of the spine varies according to the specific type. The first three types have marked platyspondyly, biconvexity of the vertebral bodies, and anterior vertebral wedging (especially at the thoracolumbar junction). The tarda form has only mild changes of vertebral shortening, pedicle shortening, and narrowed intervertebral discs.[34, 43]

Spinal problems are most common with SED congenita and consist of scoliosis, kyphoscoliosis, and odontoid hypoplasia with upper cervical instability.

Scoliosis and kyphoscoliosis are most common in the thoracic or thoracolumbar area. If the curve is progressive and less than 40 degrees, a Milwaukee brace should be used. If the curve is more severe or the brace has failed, then fusion should be done.

Upper cervical instability is common in SED congenita; therefore, cervical flexion and extension radiographs should be done in all patients and should be repeated as they grow.[28] Progressive instability should be treated by fusion before quadriparesis or sudden death occurs. A progressive slowing of play activities is usually the first sign of neurologic involvement. There may be no "hard" neurologic findings at that time.

A C1-C2 fusion is necessary if there is instability. This is done posteriorly using delicate air drill decortication and cancellous autogenous bone graft. Internal fixation with wires is not recommended, and a halo cast should be used following the fusion (Fig. 22–30).[27]

MULTIPLE EPIPHYSEAL DYSPLASIA

This is a group of disorders defined by Maroteaux as having changes in the long bones limited to the epiphyses. The spinal lesions are confined to the growth plates without severe distortion of the vertebral shape. The spinal problems are back pain and kyphosis; the back pain starts in the adolescent years and increases with age. The kyphosis resembles Scheuermann's disease and if progressive can be treated with a Milwaukee brace if it is in the thoracic area or a TLSO if it is in the thoracolumbar area.

THE MUCOPOLYSACCHARIDOSES[45, 49]

This group of disorders is different from all the rest because of the known disturbances of mucopolysaccharide metabolism. To the orthopaedist the most important is Morquio's disease, in which there is a disturbance of keratan sulfate metabolism.[36]

Kyphosis, occurring at the thoracolumbar junction, is also common to all these conditions and should be treated if significant or progressive.[20] Atlanto-axial instability secondary to odontoid hypoplasia and lax ligaments is common and may result in spinal cord compression with quadriparesis and even death.[12, 40] Flexion-extension radiography of the cervical spine is mandatory in

Text continued on page 535

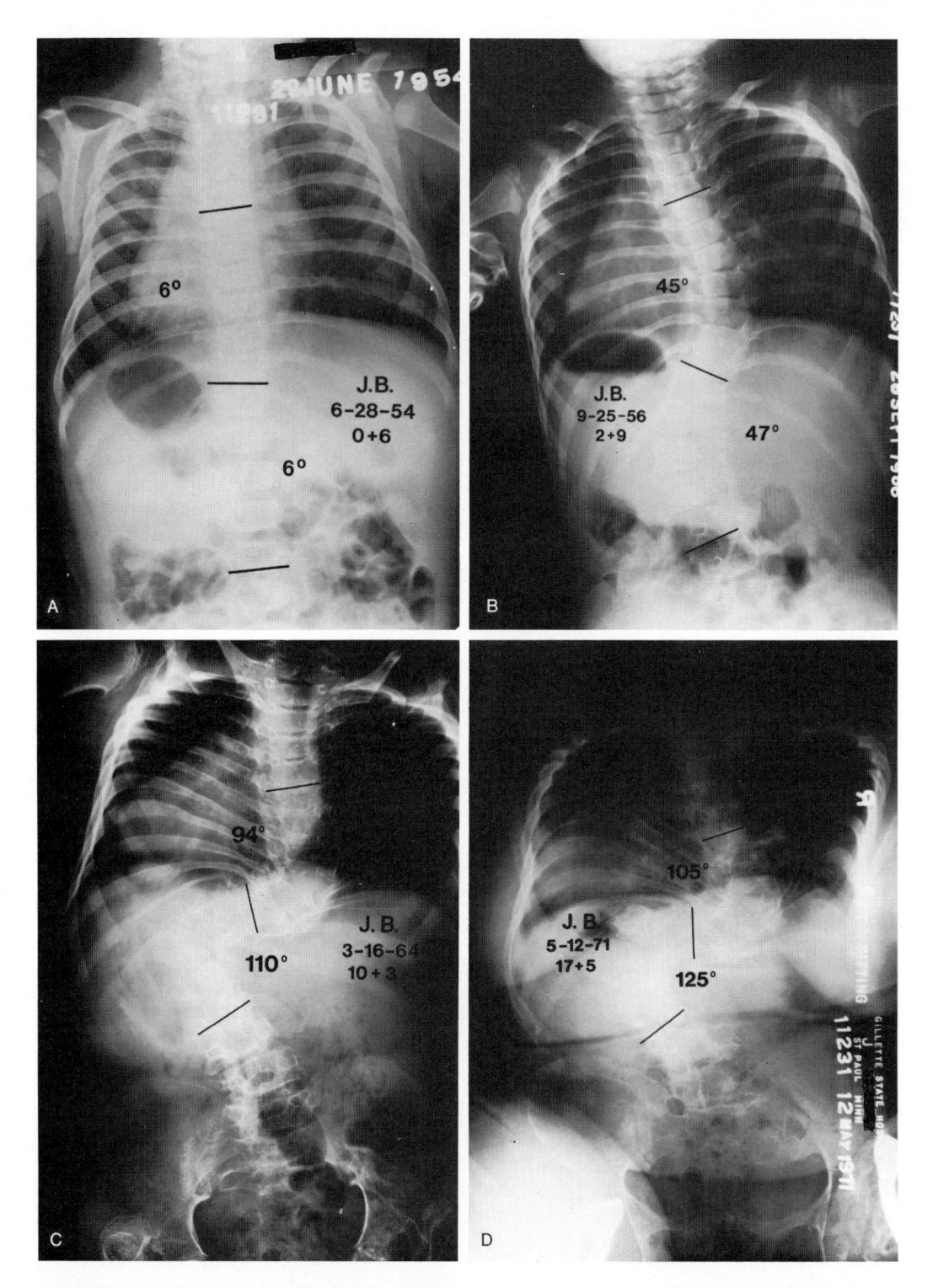

Figure 22–27. *A*, A 6 month old girl with diastrophic dwarfism. There are two 6 degree scolioses. *B*, By age 2+9 years, the curves had increased to 45 and 47 degrees. No treatment was given. *C*, At age 10+3, the curves were 94 and 110 degrees. Still no treatment was given. *D*, When last seen at age 17, the curves were 105 and 125 degrees. There was also a severe kyphosis (102 degrees) at the thoracolumbar area. (Reprinted with permission from Bethem, et al.: Disorders of the spine in diastrophic dwarfism. J. Bone Joint Surg., 62A:529–536, 1980.)

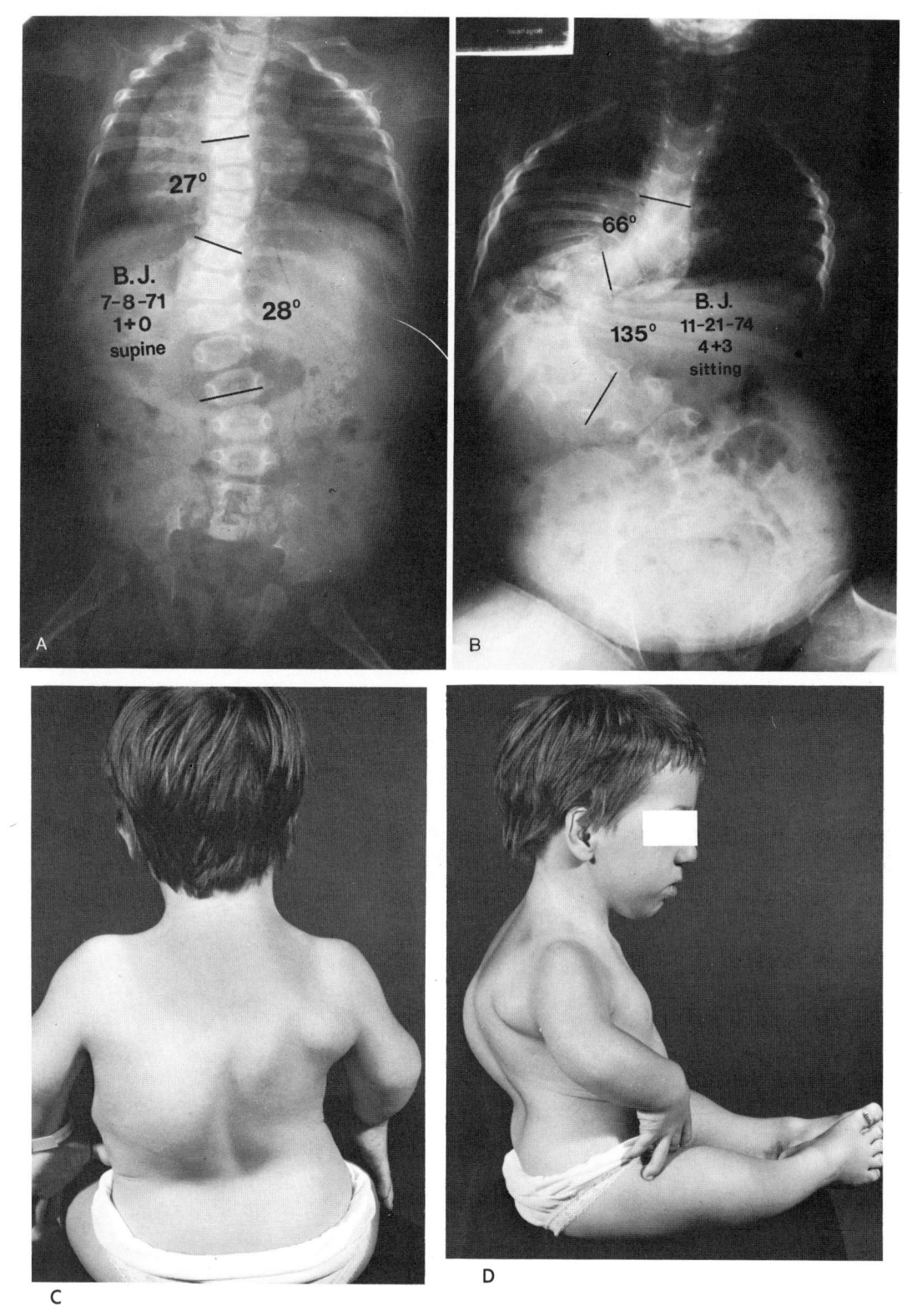

Figure 22–28. A, A one year old girl with scolioses of 27 and 28 degrees secondary to diastrophic dwarfism. No treatment was given. B, When first seen at Gillette Children's Hospital, her curves were 66 degrees and 135 degrees. C and D, Clinical back and side views show typical short-limbed dwarfism with marked spinal deformity.

Illustration continued on following page

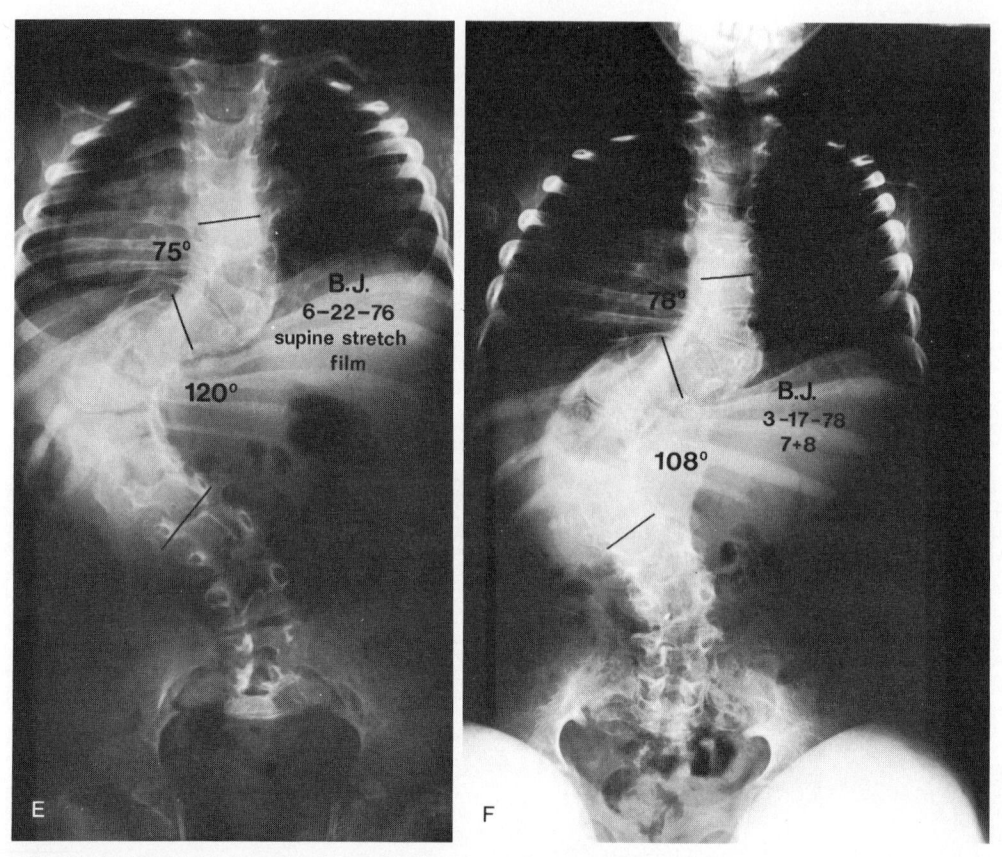

Figure 22–28 *Continued. E*, A supine "stretch" film showed correction to 75 degrees and 120 degrees. She was treated by posterior fusion, correction in a halo cast, bedrest for 6 months, augmentation of the posterior fusion, and then 12 months of ambulatory support in a Milwaukee brace. *F*, A 2 year follow-up (3 months after removal of all support) shows a solid fusion and curves of 78 degrees and 108 degrees. She has remained solid without change since that time.

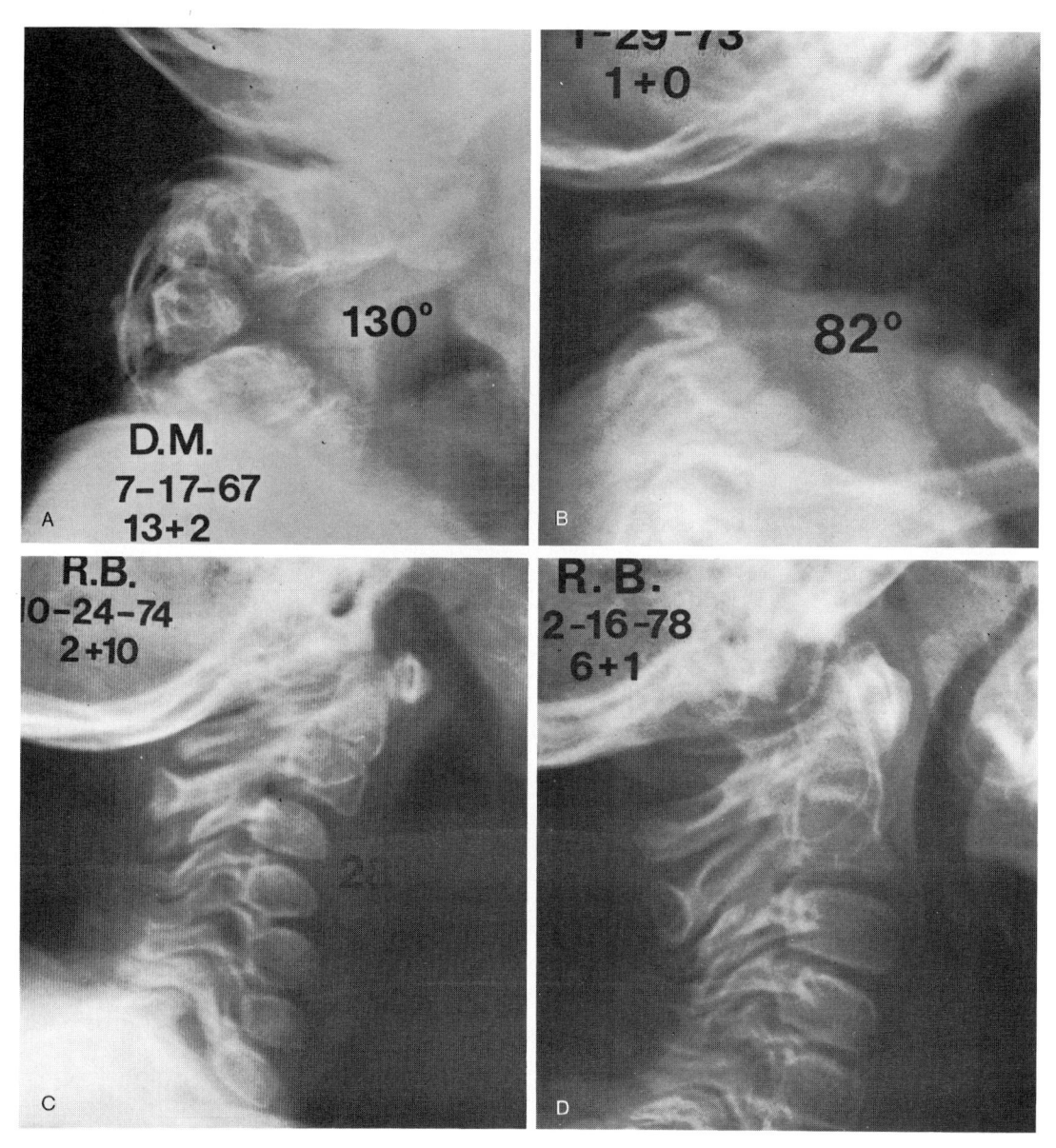

Figure 22–29. A, A 13 year old boy with diastrophic dwarfism and a severe, 130 degree cervical kyphosis. Neurologic symptoms first began at age 7 and became severe at this time; he died of complications of his quadriplegia at age 18. B, This one year old girl had a severe cervical kyphosis of 82 degrees. No treatment was given. C, By age 2 + 10 years, the kyphosis had spontaneously reduced to 28 degrees. D, By age 6, the kyphosis was gone. (B, C, and D reprinted with permission from Bethem, et al.: Disorders of the spine in diastrophic dwarfism. J. Bone Joint Surg., 62A:529–536, 1980.)

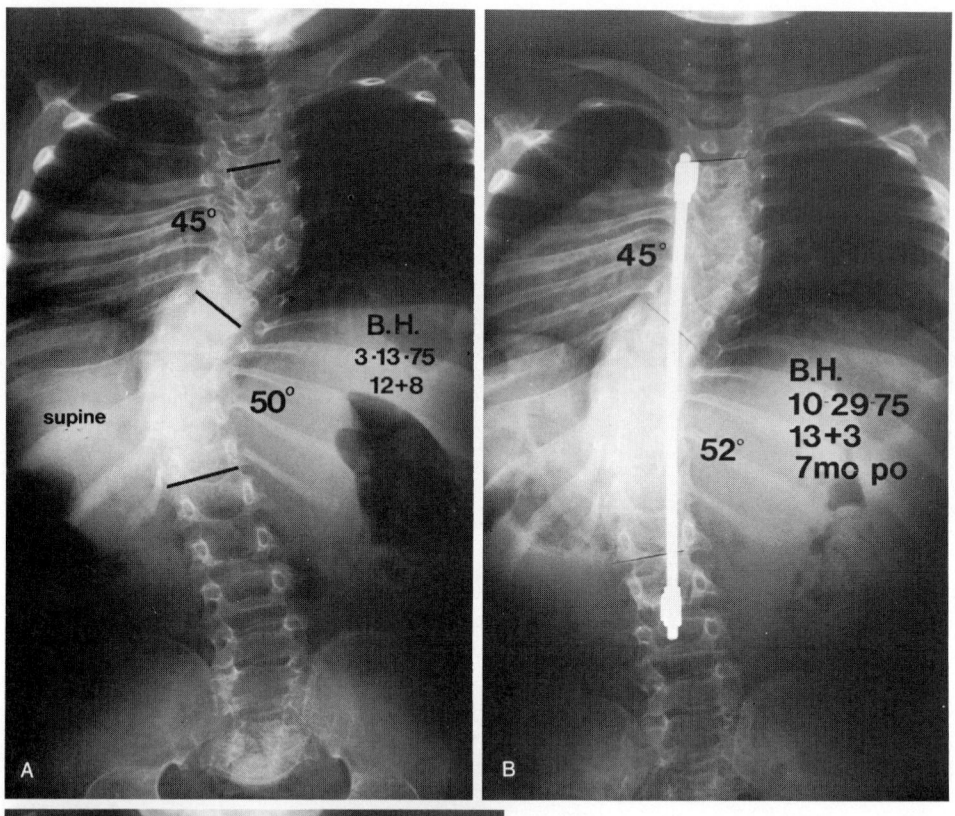

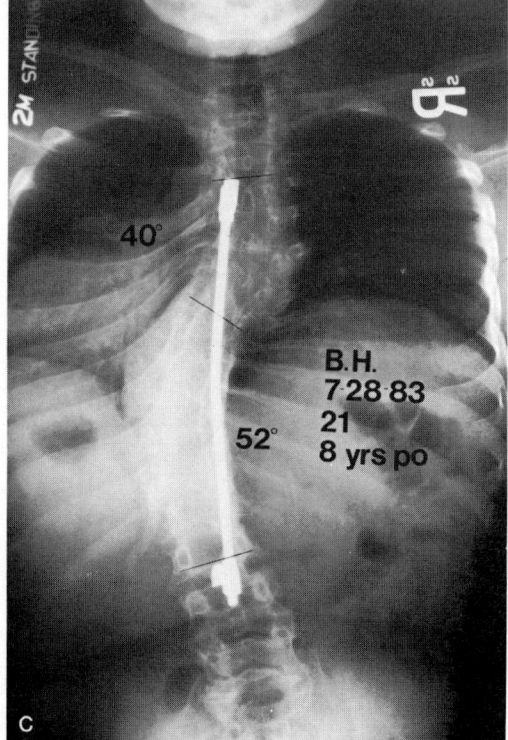

Figure 22–30. *A*, A 12 year old male with SED congenita. There were double structural thoracic curves refractory to brace treatment. Fusion was scheduled. *B*, Seven months after surgery the cast was removed. His curves measured 45 degrees and 52 degrees, showing the severe rigidity of his curves. *C*, Eight years after surgery, the curves were the same.

patient evaluation. If kyphosis is present, it should be treated by arthrodesis (Figs. 22–31 and 22–32).

CHONDRODYSTROPHIA CALCIFICANS CONGENITA

This condition, first described by Conradi in 1914,[14] has a wide spectrum of presentation; the more severe forms result in death during the first year of life.[18, 57] Those who survive may develop scoliosis or atlanto-axial instability. This is the only form of dwarfism in which the scoliosis is congenital, that is, due to hemivertebrae or other anomalies. Only four patients have been seen at our center and all four were congenital. Bracing has not been successful and early fusion was necessary in all. Atlanto-axial instability has been reported (Fig. 22–33).[11]

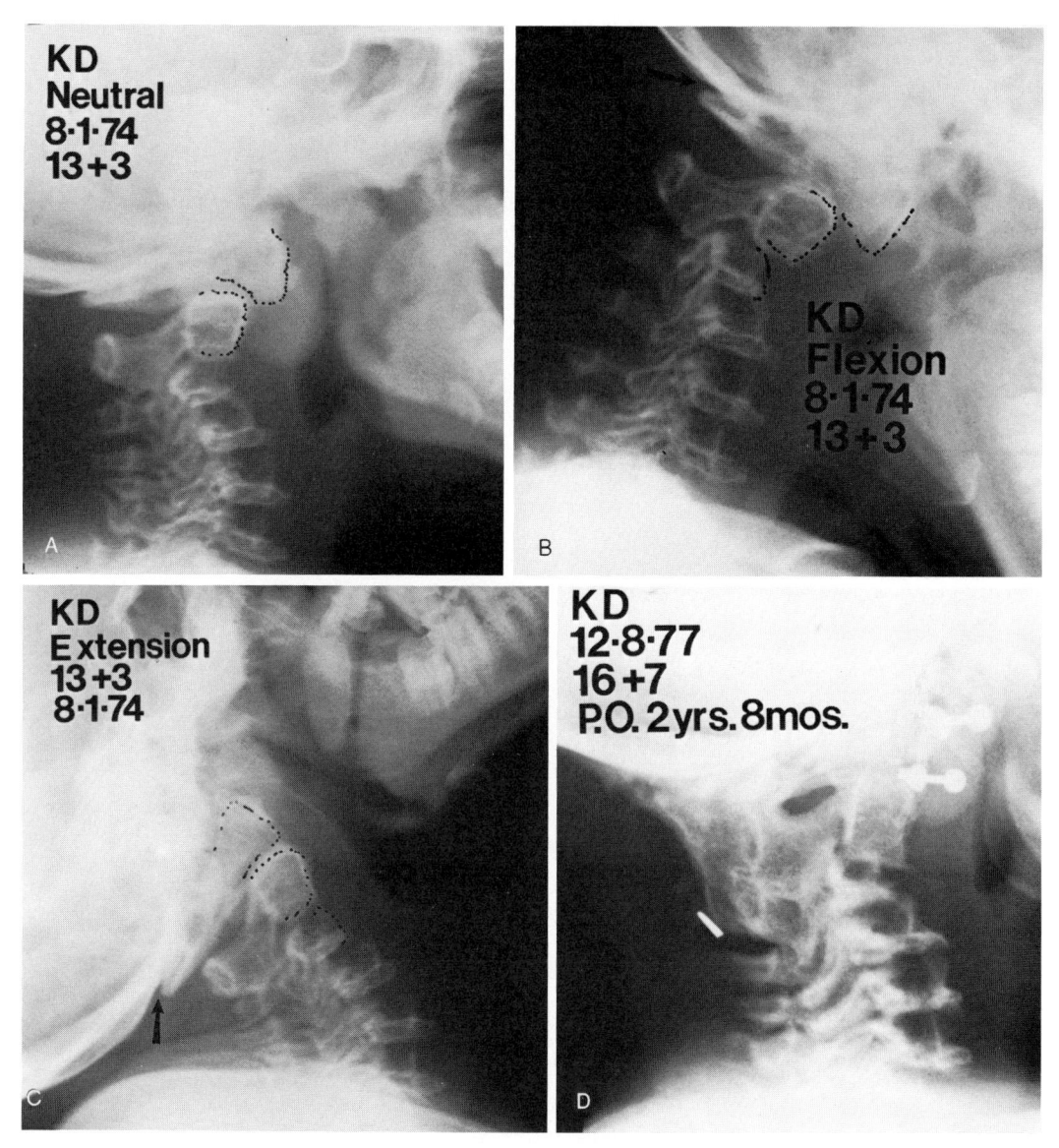

Figure 22–31. A, A 13 year old girl with Morquio's disease and foreward subluxation of C1 on C2. There were no objective neurologic findings but her play activities had slowed down considerably. B, In flexion, there is marked displacement forward of C1 on C2, and the posterior ring of C1 remains fixed to the occiput, suggesting occipitalization of the ring of C1. Note also the kyphosis of the bodies of C2, C3, and C4. C, In extension, the relationship of C1 and C2 returns to normal and the C2 to C4 kyphosis is markedly improved. D, Two years, eight months following occiput to C2 arthrodesis, the fusion is solid, and the patient's activity level has returned to normal. (Reprinted with permission from Bethem, et al.: Disorders of the spine in diastrophic dwarfism. J. Bone Joint Surg., 62A:529–536, 1980.)

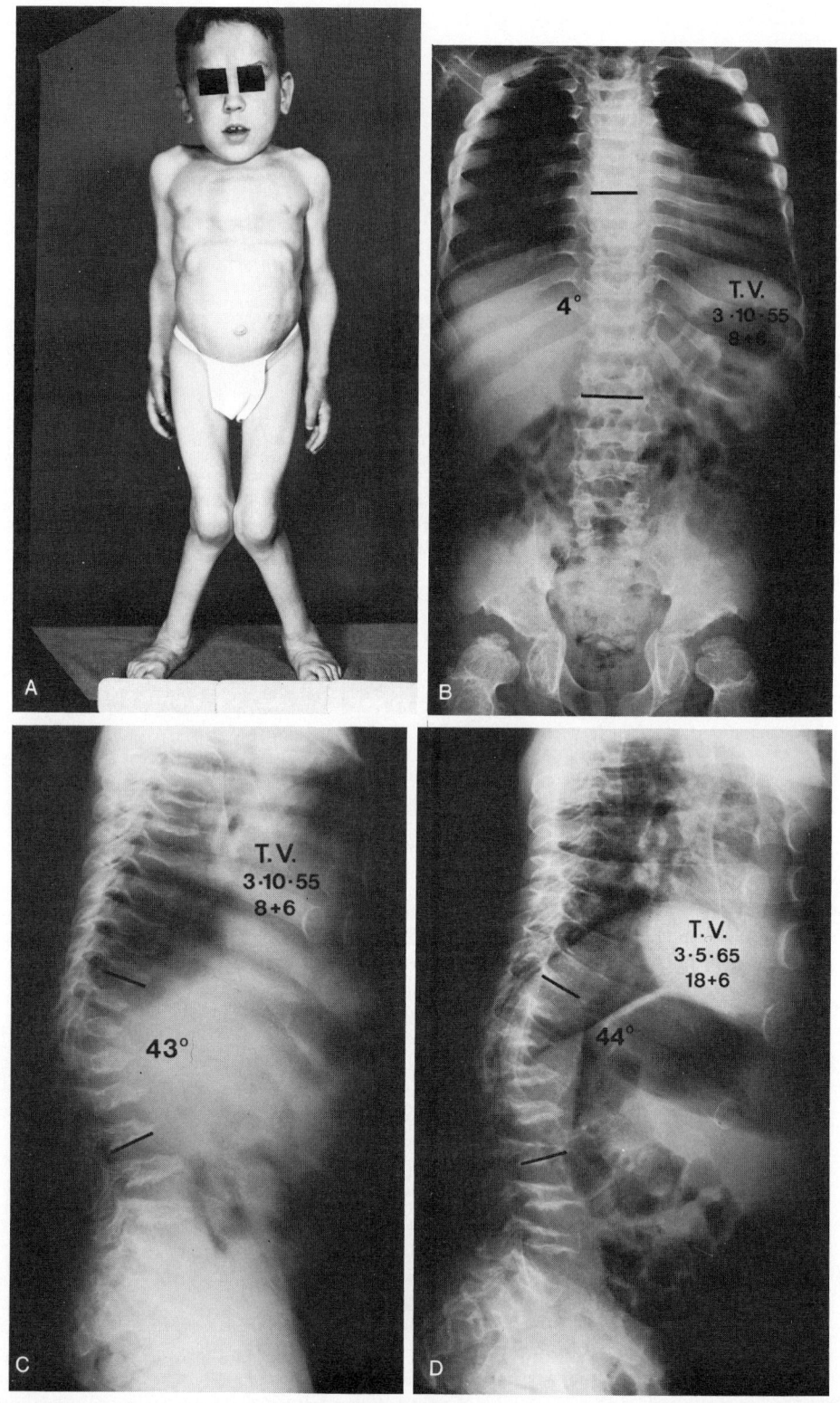

Figure 22–32. *A*, An 8 year old boy with Morquio's disease. The chest deformity, genu valgum, and flat feet are typical. *B*, An anteroposterior radiograph of his spine shows the platyspondylisis, the lack of any scoliosis, and the abnormal hip development. *C*, A lateral radiograph at age 8+6, demonstrating the classic bullet-shaped vertebrae and a 43 degree thoracolumbar kyphosis. *D*, The same patient at age 18. There was no increase in the kyphosis. The vertebrae remain short in height and deformed. (Reprinted with permission from Bethem, et al.: Spinal disorders of dwarfism. J. Bone Joint Surg., 63A:1412–1425, 1981.)

MISCELLANEOUS PROBLEMS

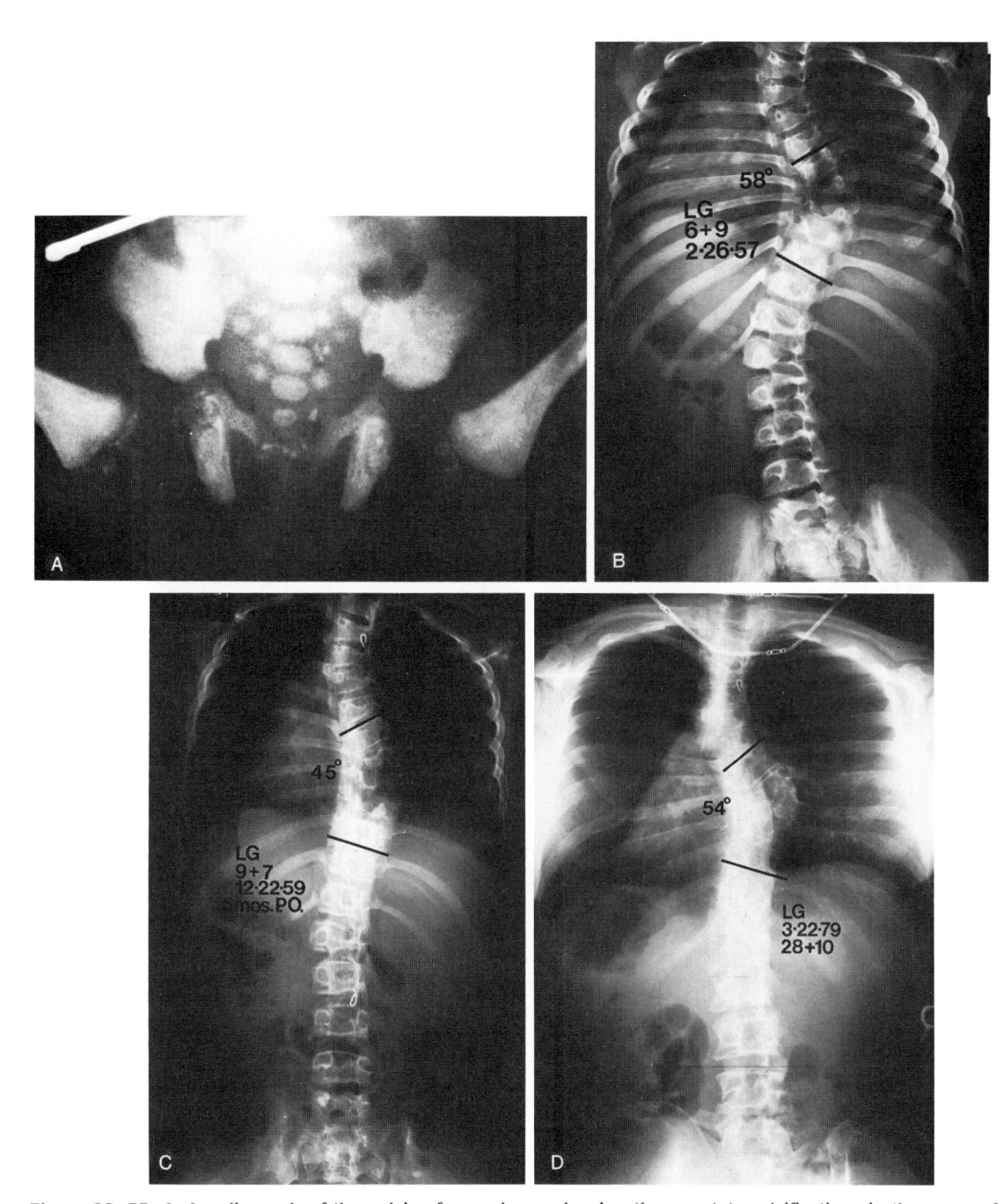

Figure 22–33. *A*, A radiograph of the pelvis of a newborn, showing the punctate calcifications in the areas of developing cartilage ("stippled" epiphyses). *B*, The same patient, at age 6+9, with a 58 degree scoliosis from T5 to T10. She was placed in a Milwaukee brace at this time, which was not successful in curve control. *C*, In July of 1959, she had a posterior spine fusion from T2 to L2, with Risser cast correction. This radiograph was taken five months later at the time of a cast change. *D*, A follow-up 19 years later at age 28. The curve was 54 degrees, the fusion solid, and she had no complaints. Despite her short stature, she was fully employed as an occupational therapist. (*B* and *D* reprinted with permission from Bethem, et al.: Disorders of the spine in diastrophic dwarfism. J. Bone Joint Surg., 62A:529–536, 1980.)

METATROPIC DWARFISM[24, 39, 47, 54]

Patients with metatropic dwarfism resemble achondroplastic dwarfs during infancy and Morquio's disease patients later in life. This type of dwarfism appears to be autosomal recessive. In the newborn, the spine shows a delay in ossification of the vertebral bodies, but well-ossified posterior elements. Platyspondyly persists during growth.

Scoliosis usually presents at an early age, with marked progression being common. There is also a significant degree of kyphosis. Odontoid hypoplasia with atlanto-axial instability is common and usually requires arthrodesis.

KNIEST SYNDROME[32]

Kniest syndrome is a rare form of dwarfism, and is difficult to separate from metatrophic dwarfism and spondyloepiphyseal dysplasia congenita. There is marked platyspondyly and kyphosis has been noted. Peripheral joint contractures can be severe.

SPONDYLOEPIMETAPHYSEAL DYSPLASIA[7, 31]

This rare lesion, spondyloepimetaphyseal dysplasia, produces severe kyphoscoliosis, often being lethal during growth. Lax ligaments and blue sclerae are typical. The two patients seen at our center have both had severe deformity, and both required fusion. One had progressive kyphosis and died of respiratory insufficiency at age 20 years.

SUMMARY

Spinal problems are common in all of the dwarfing conditions, and depending upon which condition is present various problems may exist. An accurate diagnosis is thus important and adequate consultation should be sought.

Spinal stenosis, with or without cauda equina compression, is unique to achondroplasia. Mid-cervical kyphosis is seen only in diastrophic dwarfism.

Odontoid hypoplasia with atlanto-axial instability is not seen in achondroplasia or diastrophic dwarfism, but is notable in Morquio's disease, SED congenita, chondrodystrophia calcificans congenita, and metatrophic dwarfism. This instability can lead to quadriparesis and even death. Upper cervical arthrodesis is often necessary.[30]

Scoliosis and kyphoscoliosis are especially troublesome in diastrophic dwarfism, SED congenita, frontometaphyseal dysplasia,[48] and spondyloepimetaphyseal dysplasia. Thoracolumbar kyphosis can be a major problem in achondroplasia, Morquio's disease, metatropic dwarfism, and Kniest syndrome.

References

1. Alexander, E.: Significance of the small lumbar spinal canal: cauda equina compression syndromes due to spondylosis. Part 5: Achondroplasia. J. Neurosurg., 31:513–519, 1969.
2. Amuso, S. T.: Diastrophic Dwarfism. J. Bone Joint Surg., 50A:113, 1963.
3. Bailey, J. A.: Orthopaedic aspects of achondroplasia. J. Bone Joint Surg., 52A:1285–1301, 1970.
4. Bailey, J. A.: Disproportionate Short Stature. Philadelphia, W. B. Saunders, 1973.
5. Beals, R. K.: Hypochondroplasia. J. Bone Joint Surg., 51A:728–736, 1969.
6. Beighton, P.: Orthopaedic problems in dwarfism. J. Bone Joint Surg., 62B:116, 1980.
7. Beighton, P. H., and Koslowski, K.: Spondylo-epimetaphyseal dysplasia with joint laxity and severe progressive kyphoscoliosis. Skeletal Radiol., 5:205–212, 1980.
8. Bergstrom, K., Laurent, U., and Lundberg, P. O.: Neurological symptoms in achondroplasia. Acta Neurol. Scand., 47:59–70, 1971.
9. Bethem, D., Winter, R. B., and Lutter, L.: Disorders of the spine in diastrophic dwarfism. A discussion of nine patients and review of the literature. J. Bone Joint Surg., 62A:529–536, 1980.
10. Bethem, D., Winter, R. B., Lutter, L., et al.: Spinal disorders of dwarfism: review of the literature and report of 80 cases. J. Bone Joint Surg., 63A:1412–1425, 1981.
11. Bethem, D.: Os odontoideum in chondrodystrophia calcificans congenita, a case report. J. Bone Joint Surg., 64A:1385–1386, 1982.
12. Blaw, M. D., and Langer, L. O.: Spinal cord compression in Morquio-Brailsford disease. J. Pediatr., 74:593–600, 1969.
13. Caffey, J.: Achondroplasia of pelvis and lumbosacral spine. Am. J. Roentgenol., 80:449–457, 1958.
14. Conradi, E.: Vorzeitges Auftreten von Kochen und eigenartigen Verkalkungskernen bei Chondrodystrophia fetalis Hypoplastica: Histologische und Rontgenuntersuchungen. J. Kinderheilkd., 80:86, 1914.
15. Diamond, L. S.: A family study of spondyloepiphyseal dysplasia. J. Bone Joint Surg., 52A:1587–1594, 1970.
16. Duvisin, R. C., and Yahr, M. D.: Compression spinal cord and root syndromes in achondroplastic dwarfs. Neurology, 12:202–207, 1962.

17. Eulert, J.: Scoliosis and kyphosis in dwarfing conditions. Arch. Orthop. Traum. Surg., *102*:45–47, 1983.
18. Fairbank, H. A. T.: Dysplasia epiphysealis punctata. Synonyms: stippled epiphyses, chondrodystrophia calcificans congenita (Hunermann). J. Bone Joint Surg., *31B*:114–122, 1949.
19. Hancock, D. W., and Phillips, D. G.: Spinal compression in achondroplasia. Paraplegia, *3*:23–33, 1965.
20. Hensinger, R. N.: Kyphosis secondary to skeletal dysplasias and metabolic disease. Clin. Orthop., *128*:113–128, 1977.
21. Herring, J. A.: The spinal disorders in diastrophic dwarfism. J. Bone Joint Surg., *60A*:177, 1978.
22. Herring, J. A., and Winter, R. B.: Kyphosis in an achondroplastic dwarf. J. Pediatr. Orthop., *3*:250–252, 1983.
23. Hollister, D. W., and Lachman, R. S.: Diastrophic dwarfism. Clin. Orthop., *114*:61–69, 1976.
24. Johnston, C. E., II: Scoliosis in metatropic dwarfism. Orthopedics, *6*:491–498, 1983.
25. Jones, E., and Hensinger, R. N.: Spinal deformity in individuals with short stature. Orthop. Clin. North Am., *10*:877–890, 1979.
26. Kash, I. J., Sane, S. M., Samaha, F. J., and Briner, J.: Cervical cord compression in diastrophic dwarfism. J. Pediatr., *84*:862, 1974.
27. Koop, S., Winter, R., and Lonstein, J.: The surgical treatment of instability of the upper part of the cervical spine in children and adolescents. J. Bone Joint Surg., *66A*:403–411, 1984.
28. Kopits, S. E., Perovic, M. N., McKusick, V., et al.: Congenital atlantoaxial dislocations in various forms of dwarfism. *In* Proceedings of the American Academy of Orthopaedic Surgeons. J. Bone Joint Surg., *54A*:1349–1350, 1972.
29. Kopits, S. E.: Orthopaedic complications of dwarfism. Clin. Orthop., *114*:153–179, 1976.
30. Kopits, S. E.: Cervical myelopathy in dwarfism. Orthop. Trans., *3*:119, 1979.
31. Kozlowski, K., and Beighton, P.: Radiographic features of spondylo-epimetaphyseal dysplasia with joint laxity and progressive kyphoscoliosis. Fortschr. Roentgenstr., *141*:337–341, 1984.
32. Lachman, R. S., Rimoin, D. L., Hollister, D. W., et al.: The Kneist syndrome. Am. J. Roentgenol., *123*:805–814, 1975.
33. Lamy, M., and Maroteaux, P.: Le nanisme diastrophique. Presse Med., *68*:1977–1980, 1960.
34. Langer, L. O.: Spondyloepiphyseal dysplasia tarda. Hereditary chondrodysplasia with characteristic vertebral configuration in the adult. Radiology, *82*:833–839, 1964.
35. Langer, L. O.: Diastrophic dwarfism in early infancy. Am. J. Roentgenol., *93*:399–404, 1965.
36. Langer, L. O., and Carey, L. S.: The roentgenographic features of the KS mucopolysaccharidosis of Morquio (Morqui-Brailsford's Disease). Am. J. Roentgenol., *97*:1–20, 1966.
37. Langer, L. O., Bauman, P. A., and Gorlin, R. J.: Achondroplasia. Am. J. Roentgenol., *100*:12–26, 1967.
38. Langer, L. O., Bauman, P. A., and Gorlin, R. J.: Achondroplasia: clinical radiologic features with comment on genetic implications. Clin. Pediatr., *7*:474–485, 1968.
39. Larose, J. H., and Gay, B. B.: Metatropic dwarfism. Am. J. Roentgenol., *106*:156–161, 1969.
40. Lipson, S. J.: Dysplasia of the odontoid process in Morquio's syndrome causing quadriparesis. J. Bone Joint Surg., *59A*:340–344, 1977.
41. Lutter, L. D., and Langer, L. O.: Neurological symptoms in achondroplastic dwarfs—surgical treatment. J. Bone Joint Surg., *59A*:87–92, 1977.
42. Lutter, L. D., Lonstein, J. E., Winter, R. B., and Langer, L. O.: Anatomy of the achondroplastic lumbar canal. Clin. Orthop., *126*:139–142, 1977.
43. Maroteaux, P., Lamy, M., and Bernard, J.: La Dysplasie Spondylo-epiphysaire Tardire. Description Clinique et Radiologique. Presse Med., *65*:1205–1208, 1957.
44. Maroteaux, P., and Lamy, M.: Les Formes Pseudoachondroplasiques des Dysplasies spondylo-epiphysaires. Presse Med., *67*:383–386, 1959.
45. Maroteaux, P., Lamy, M., and Foucher, M.: La Maladie de Morquio: Etude Clinique, Radiologique et Biologique. Presse Med., *71*:2091–2094, 1963.
46. Maroteaux, P., and Lamy, M.: Achondroplasia in man and animals. Clin. Orthop., *33*:91–103, 1964.
47. Maroteaux, P.: Spondyloepiphyseal dysplasias and metatropic dwarfism. Birth Defects, *5*:35–41, 1969.
48. Medlar, R. C., and Crawford, A. H.: Frontometaphyseal dysplasia presenting as scoliosis. J. Bone Joint Surg., *60A*:392–394, 1978.
49. Morquio, L.: Sur une forme de dystrophie osseuse familiale. Arch. Med. Enf., *32*:129–140, 1929.
50. Nelson, M. A.: Orthopaedic aspects of the chondrodystrophies. The dwarf and his orthopaedic problems. Ann. R. Coll. Surg., *47*:185–210, 1970.
51. Nelson, M. A.: Spinal stenosis in achondroplasia. Proc. R. Soc. Med., *65*:1028–1029, 1972.
52. Ponseti, I. V.: Skeletal growth in achondroplasia. J. Bone Joint Surg., *52A*:701–716, 1970.
53. Poussa, M., Ryöppy, S., Ritsila, V., and Kaitila, I.: Spine in diastrophic dysplasia, report of 60 cases. Presented to the European Congress of Scoliosis and Kyphosis, Dubrovnik, Yugoslavia, October, 1983.
54. Rimoin, D. S., Siggers, D. C., Lachman, R. S., and Silberger, R.: Metatropic dwarfism, the Kneist syndrome, and the pseudoachondroplastic dysplasias. Clin. Orthop., *114*:70–82, 1976.
55. Rubin, P.: Dynamic Classification of Bone Dysplasias. Chicago, Year Book Medical Publishers, Inc., 1964.
56. Schreiber, F., and Rosenthal, H.: Paraplegia from ruptured disks in achondroplastic dwarfs. J. Neurosurg., *9*:648–651, 1952.
57. Selakovich, W. G., and White, J. W.: Chondrodystropia calcificans congenita. J. Bone Joint Surg., *37A*:1271–1277, 1955.
58. Silberman, F. N.: A differential diagnosis of achondroplasia. Radiol. Clin. North Am., *6*:223–237, 1968.
59. Spillane, J. D.: Three cases of achondroplasia with neurological compressions. J. Neurol. Neurosurg. Psychiatr., *15*:246–252, 1952.
60. Spranger, J. W., and Langer, L. O.: Spondyloepiphyseal dysplasia congenita. Radiology, *94*:313–323, 1970.
61. Spranger, J. W., Langer, L. O., and Wiedemann, H. R.: Bone dysplasias: an Atlas of Constitutional Disorders of Skeletal Development. Philadelphia, W. B. Saunders, 1974.
62. Stanescu, V., Stanescu, R., and Maroteaux, P.: Pathogenic mechanisms in osteochondrodysplasias. J. Bone Joint Surg., *66A*:817–836, 1984.

63. Stover, C., Hayes, J. Y., and Holt, J. F.: Diastrophic dwarfism. Am. J. Roentgenol., 89:914, 1963.
64. Suyiura, Y., Terashima, Y., Furukawa, T., and Yoneda, M.: Spondyloepiphyseal dysplasia congenita. Interm. Orthop., 2:47–51, 1978.
65. Taybi, H.: Diastrophic dwarfism. Radiology, 80:1–10, 1963.
66. Vogel, A., and Osborne, R. L.: Lesions of the spinal cord (transverse myelopathy) in achondroplasia. Arch. Neurol. Psychiatr., 61:644–662, 1949.
67. Walker, B. A., Scott, C. I., Hall, J. C., et al.: Diastrophic dwarfism. Medicine, 51:41–59, 1972.
68. Wilson, D. W., Chrispin, A. R., and Carter, C. O.: Diastrophic dwarfism. Arch. Dis. Child., 44:48–58, 1969.

Cord Compresssion
John E. Lonstein, M.D.

Neurologic deficits can be associated with scoliosis and kyphosis. They can be the cause of the spinal deformity (see Chapter 13) or may result from the deformity. There may be lesions that cause both the neurologic deficit *and* the deformity. Examples are spinal cord tumors, extramedullary tumors, trauma, bone tumors, or bone infections. Compression of the spinal cord by the deformity is discussed in this section.

INCIDENCE

There are numerous reports of this rare complication in the world literature;[10, 11, 12, 14, 15, 18] the majority are single case reports. The first report is that of McEwen in 1888, who reported a case successfuly treated by laminectomy.[12] The larger series reported are those of Marchetti and coworkers in 1968,[13] Roaf in 1964,[14] and Lonstein and associates in 1980.[11] This latter paper discusses forty-three patients with this complication from the Twin Cities Scoliosis Center. As with the other reported cases, the commonest cause of the spine deformity is congenital kyphosis; other causes of deformity are neurofibromatosis, inactive tuberculosis with kyphosis, post-laminectomy kyphosis, and numerous miscellaneous diagnoses. In all cases seen, kyphosis was the main spine deformity, either occurring alone or in combination with scoliosis. The kyphosis was severe, averaging 95 degrees, with 19 of the 43 patients having kyphosis over 100 degrees.[11]

In all the congenital kyphoses, the kyphosis was due to a failure of vertebral body formation—a posterior hemivertebra, classified as a Type I kyphosis by Winter and coworkers.[18] Scoliosis occurred in just under one third of cases, usually being minor except in neurofibromatosis when it was a major component of the deformity. Although the literature reports this complication as occurring with scoliosis alone, even idiopathic scoliosis, this has not been the author's experience. They have seen only one case of congenital scoliosis due to failure of vertebral body segmentation in which a fibrocartilaginous mass compressed the spinal cord at the level of the congenital vertebral anomalies.

The majority of the patients with this complication are males, with over two thirds of patients presenting under age 20. The kyphosis is most commonly in the thoracic spine; many are in the upper thoracic area. The neurologic deficit on presentation may be divided into minor, paraparesis, or paraplegia. A minor deficit is present if there is no alteration of daily life and activity, and if the deficit is only clonus, an abnormal reflex or minimal muscle weakness. All deficits short of complete paraplegia, resulting in an alteration in the functional level are classed as paraparesis. The majority of patients with cord compression due to the deformity present as paraparesis.

The exact incidence of this complication is unknown, but it is preventable. A common feature of reported cases is a kyphosis that was detected early, but *not* treated. With progression of the deformity, neurologic loss occurred, and the patients presented, on an average, over 10 years from the diagnosis of the deformity. Early and adequate treatment of the kyphosis would have prevented progression and subsequent spinal cord compression.

PATHOGENESIS

In analyzing the literature, certain common features are found, as mentioned previously.

In summary, this complication is commonest in severe kyphotic deformities (most often congenital), in the second decade of life, in males, and in the upper thoracic spine.

In severe kyphosis the spinal cord is stretched over the anterior bone, taking the shortest route across the deformity—the concavity of the curve. The dura is tethered to the skull at the foramen magnum and to the sacrum, and it has little elasticity. With increased flexion and increasing kyphosis, there is greater tension on the posterior dura, which compresses the spinal cord against the vertebral bodies anteriorly (Fig. 22–34). During the second decade and with the rapid growth spurt, there is slight differential growth between the bony spine and the spinal cord. An even more important factor is the rapid increase of the kyphosis during this growth spurt with increased angulation and increased cord compression.

A similar effect is seen in placing this deformity in longitudinal traction. If the kyphosis is rigid, traction lengthens the spine by correction of the compensatory lordotic areas above and below the rigid curve apex, which does not change at all. This results in increased tension on the spinal cord and increased neurologic loss (Fig. 22–35A). If the apex is flexible, on the other hand, traction will improve the apical area, reduce the pressure of the anterior compression, and improve the neurologic status (Fig. 22–35B).

There is a degree of normal elasticity in the spinal cord, allowing flexion and extension. With kyphosis, after maximal stretching, the spinal cord is under tension forces. Breig has shown that the spinal cord in the upper thoracic spine has the least elasticity.[1,2]

The combined anterior compression and traction reduce the blood supply of the spinal cord. The role of the blood supply has been emphasized by Stagnara in his discussions of cord compression.[17] Dommisse has described the segmental supply of the spinal cord as well as the anastomoses at the intervertebral foramina.[6,7] With compression and stretching of the spinal cord, the vessels will be compressed with resultant venous obstruction and reduced blood flow. With increased obstruction the arterial flow will decrease. This anoxia will result in decreased cord function and resultant neurologic loss.

An interesting finding is the high incidence of lesions of the high thoracic area. Three factors are important. The blood supply in this area is poorest because it has the fewest medullary feeders.[6,7] In addition, there are fewer perforating arteries arising from the anterior longitudinal arterial trunk (anterior spinal artery) in this area. The spinal cord in this area has the least elasticity;[1,2] the spinal canal is narrowest in this upper thoracic area. This combination of poor blood supply, decreased elasticity, and less space make the spinal cord in this area more sensitive to compression.

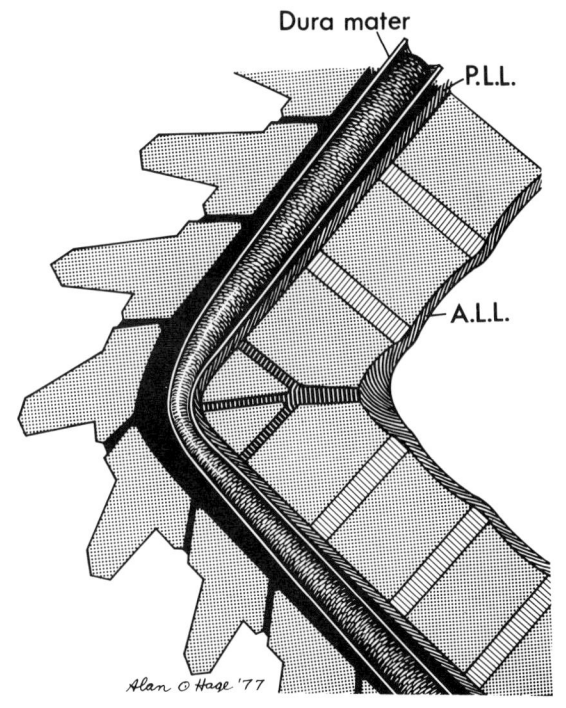

Figure 22–34. Diagrammatic representation of a congenital kyphosis, showing the compressed spinal cord at the apex of the deformity. The posterior dura is tight and compresses the spinal cord against the anterior bone at the apex of the deformity. A.L.L. = anterior longitudinal ligament; P.L.L. = posterior longitudinal ligament. (Reprinted with permission from Lonstein, et al.: Neurological deficits secondary to spinal deformity—a review of the literature and a report on 43 cases. Spine, 5:331–355, 1980.)

PRESENTATION

The neurologic loss may be of gradual onset or sudden onset with rapid deterioration, the latter presentation being more common. Rarely the onset follows some trauma, usually minor, (e.g., a fall, or direct trauma to the back in playing). The neurologic loss is classified as minor, paraparesis, or paraplegia.

With presentation of a spine deformity and

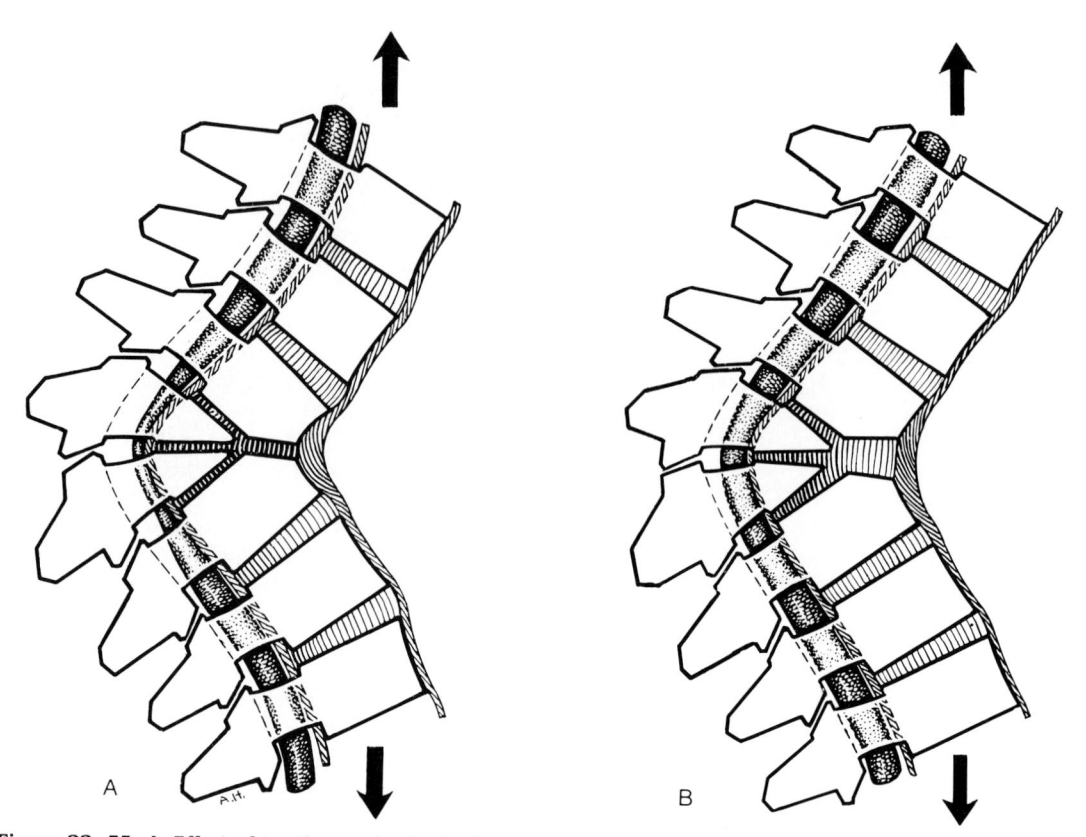

Figure 22–35. *A,* Effect of traction on kyphosis. In the case of a rigid kyphosis, the apical area will not change but the adjacent spine will be lengthened. This increases the tension on the spinal cord, with aggravation of neurological loss. *B,* When the kyphosis is flexible, traction will improve the apical area and reduce the pressure of the bone anteriorly on the spinal cord. (Reprinted with permission from Lonstein, et al.: Neurological deficits secondary to spinal deformity—a review of the literature and a report on 43 cases. Spine, 5:331–355, 1980.)

neurologic deficit, an accurate evaluation is essential to establish the diagnosis. A full history of the deformity is necessary. In addition, a history of the onset and progression of the neurologic loss is included. The physical examination should be complete, with emphasis on the spine deformity and neurologic examination.

After full radiologic evaluation of the spine deformity, the etiology of the deformity is diagnosed. Three possible correlations exist and must be differentiated. The neurologic deficit may be causing the deformity, may be a result of the deformity, or the two may be unrelated and a co-existing pathology is the cause of the neurologic loss. This is commonly an intraspinal tumor that is present in, for example, neurofibromatosis.

When kyphosis is absent, the occurrence of cord compression plus scoliosis should be viewed with suspicion. Patients with this combination have almost always shown a separate cause for the neurologic loss, for example, an arteriovenous malformation, a demyelinating disease of the spinal cord, or aorto-iliac occlusive disease with leg weakness due to ischemia. The authors have two cases of scoliosis causing cord compression; both patients have congenital scoliosis with a mass of fibrocartilage or bone associated with the congenital anomaly causing the cord compression, not the curve itself.

A myelogram is essential. It will reveal either an intrinsic lesion—spinal cord tumors, neurofibromas, meningiomas—or the presence of spinal cord compression at the apex of the kyphosis. In the latter situation there is narrowing of the dye column with complete or partial obstruction at the apex of the deformity. The myelographic technique of Gold and Leach,[8] which uses a large volume of pantopaque, has been replaced by the use of water-soluble dyes (metrizamide, amapaque) augmented by CT scanning and sagittal reconstruction, or by MRI when available. With this technique it is confirmed that

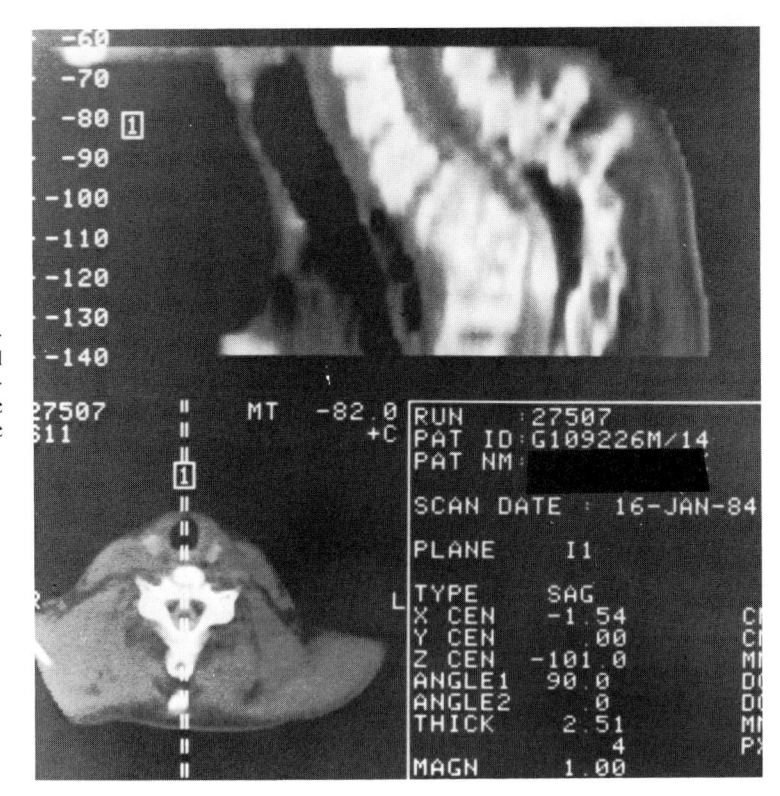

Figure 22–36. Sagittal reconstruction of CT scan in a case of cord compression due to healed tuberculosis. Note the anterior bone compressing the spinal cord at the apex of the deformity.

the compression is at the apex of the kyphosis and due to the anterior bone compressing the spinal cord. In addition, no intraspinal lesions are present (Fig. 22–36).

An additional evaluation of the deformity is necessary to evaluate the flexibility of the kyphosis. A hyperextension radiograph will show whether the apex of the kyphosis is rigid or flexible; this information is important in the treatment plan, especially with minor deficits or mild paraparesis.

TREATMENT PRINCIPLES

The treatment of cord compression due to untreated spine deformity can be non-operative or operative. Prolonged supine casting (5 to 12 months) is favored by the Europeans even in cases of a rigid kyphosis.[17] They report good results, probably because of reduction of the kyphosis in the horizontal position with rest, resulting in decreased compression and improved blood flow. It is our position that with a *rigid* kyphosis traction is dangerous, as it does *not* correct the apex of the deformity but puts increased tension on the spinal cord and increases the cord compression (see Fig. 22–35A). If, on the other hand, the kyphosis is flexible, correcting the kyphosis will improve the cord compression and perhaps the neurologic signs. In these cases, traction plays a role in treatment, as will be discussed.

The operative procedures for the treatment of cord compression include laminectomy, posterior decompression using the Hyndman Schneider technique, posterolateral decompression using the Capener approach, or an anterior transthoracic decompression. A laminectomy does *not* decompress the spinal cord, because the compressing bone is anterior.[4, 11] All the laminectomy achieves is loss of posterior stability, increase in the kyphosis, and deterioration of the neurologic deficit. Occasionally, with a laminectomy and incision of the dura posteriorly, the tight dura compressing the cord against the anterior bone is relieved, and improvement of the neurologic picture results. This tends to be only temporary as the kyphosis can increase owing to the posterior instability, and the neurologic picture usually deteriorates. An extension of the laminectomy was described by Hyndman and Schneider for removal of anterior bone.[10, 15] This technique is most applicable in patients with significant scoliosis and involves the removal of a large amount of bone—laminae, pedicle, transverse process, and ribs—to adequately visualize and remove the anterior bone. This leaves a very unstable spine, which requires stabilization anteriorly and posteriorly. This approach is sometimes applicable on a limited basis and combined with an anterior transthoracic decompression. Often with significant scoliosis combined with the kyphosis, it is the vertebral body plus the concave apical pedicle that are compressing the spinal cord. In this case, decompression using the anterior approach may be unsuccessful in completely removing the compressing bone, and a second stage posterolateral decompression is necessary.

The most successful approach for decompression is the anterior transthoracic approach, pioneered by Hodgson and Stock[9] for the treatment of spinal tuberculosis. This technique enables an approach to the apex of the deformity, allowing the surgeon to effectively remove the apical bone that is compressing the spinal cord (see Chapter 10).[4, 11] At the same time, the deformity is stabilized with an anterior strut graft fusion. In cases in which there is a very angular kyphosis, poor respiratory function, or the kyphosis is in an inaccessible area (high thoracic area), a Capener posterolateral decompression is used.[3] This technique, first described for the decompression of tuberculous spinal abscesses, approaches the spine laterally, and after removal of ribs, enables removal of anterior bone using an extrapleural approach. Stabilization of the deformity is still necessary at a second stage.

The treatment of cord compression due to the spinal deformity involves two principles, removal of the offending anterior compression and stabilization of deformity to prevent further progression (Figs. 22–37 and 22–38).

TREATMENT PLAN

After a myelogram confirms the diagnosis of compression due to the spine deformity, kyphosis or kyphoscoliosis, the treatment path depends on the neurologic picture. In a minor deficit, removal of the bone from anterior to the cord is not necessary. In these cases the deformity can be corrected and stabilized, and the minor signs will usually resolve. Correction can be by traction with flexible deformity, serial hyperextension casts, or at the time of stabilization. The correction is maintained by an anterior strut graft fusion and posterior spinal fusion. Depending on the stability and site of the deformity, the patient is placed either in a halo or a Risser-Cotrel cast and usually kept supine for three to four months, after which the cast is changed and the patient allowed to ambulate.

All patients with paraparesis or paraplegia should have a hyperextension x-ray to differentiate a flexible from a rigid kyphosis. If the kyphosis is flexible, the patient may be placed in cautious hyperextension halo-femoral traction with careful neurologic monitoring; this type of kyphosis occurs frequently in neurofibromatosis. The traction is gradually increased with careful monitoring over a period of weeks. When the impairment has improved to a minor deficit or to normal, the correction is held with an anterior fusion, which is reinforced one to two weeks later by a posterior fusion. When both scoliosis and kyphosis are present, it is usual to approach the spine on the concavity of the scoliosis. The discs are excised, and the strut grafts placed to stabilize both the kyphosis and scoliosis.

When the kyphosis is rigid on hyperextension or when there is no improvement in a flexible deformity after two to three weeks of traction, decompression is necessary. The best approach is anteriorly; both an anterior spinal cord decompression and an anterior spinal fusion should be performed while the patient is under the same anesthetic. The spine is approached via a thoracotomy for the thoracic spine or a thoracoabdominal approach for the thoracolumbar area. A wedge of bone is removed from in front of the spinal cord at the apex of the kyphosis, allowing the cord to move forward into the space created (see Chapter 10). Following the decompression, an anterior strut graft fusion is performed, and one to two weeks later a posterior fusion is usually necessary to increase the stabilization. In patients with severe scoliosis and rotation and in whom the concave apical pedicle is also compressing the cord, the decompression is completed during the posterior approach using a modified Hyndman Schneider decompression. This combined anterior and posterior approach has been shown to be the most effective method of cord decompression and spine stabilization.[11] Postoperatively patients are usually placed in halo traction or a Risser-Cotrel cast, and kept supine for three to four

MISCELLANEOUS PROBLEMS

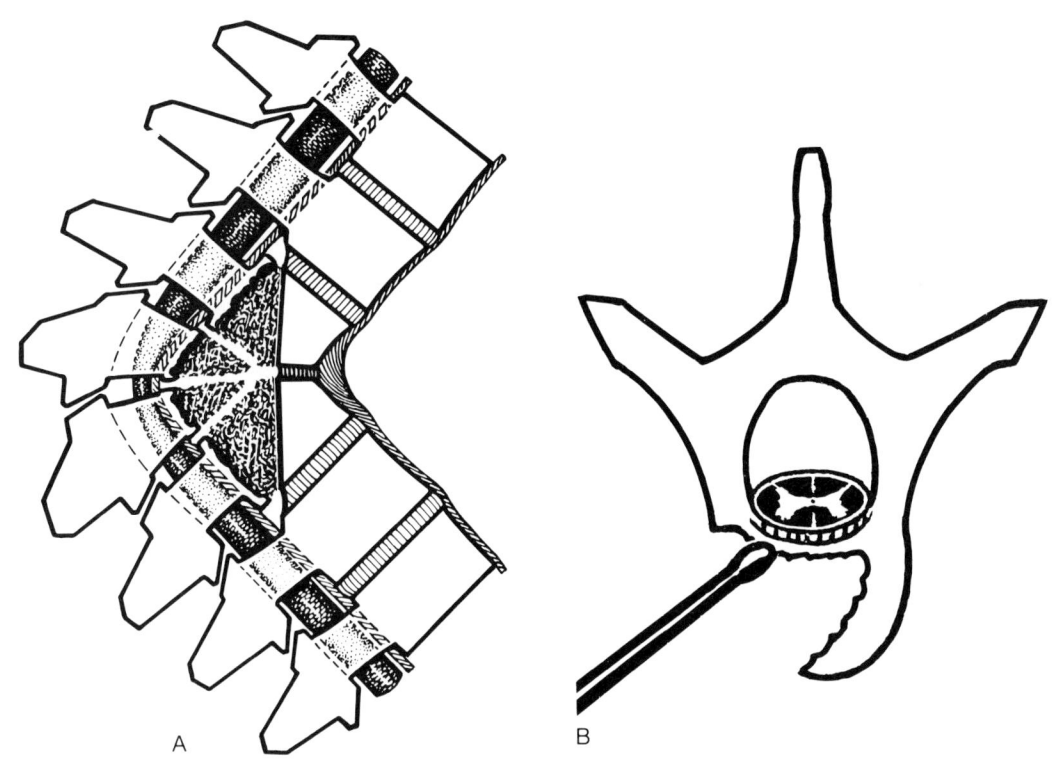

Figure 22–37. *A*, Diagrammatic representation of anterior spinal cord decompression. The spine at the apex of the kyphosis is visualized via a transthoracic approach. The bone at the apex of the kyphosis is removed, leaving the posterior cortex and far cortex intact. The posterior cortex is carefully removed, starting away from the apex and working towards the apex and towards the surgeon. *B*, Cross-section showing removal of remaining anterior bone, using a curette. (Reprinted with permission from Lonstein, et al.: Neurological deficits secondary to spinal deformity—a review of the literature and a report on 43 cases. Spine, 5:331–355, 1980.)

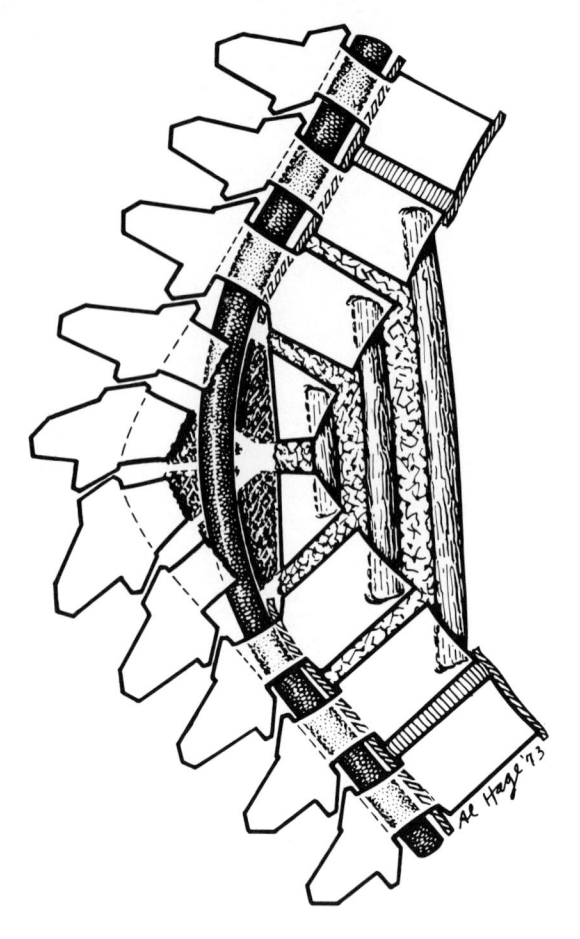

Figure 22–38. Decompression has been completed, and the spinal cord has moved forward into the area of excised bone. No bone remains compressing the cord, and spinal cord pulsations return. The intervertebral discs are excised, and an anterior strut graft fusion is performed. This is reinforced with a posterior fusion with Harrington instrumentation when possible. (Reprinted with permission from Lonstein, et al.: Neurological deficits secondary to spinal deformity—a review of the literature and a report on 43 cases. Spine, 5:331–355, 1980.)

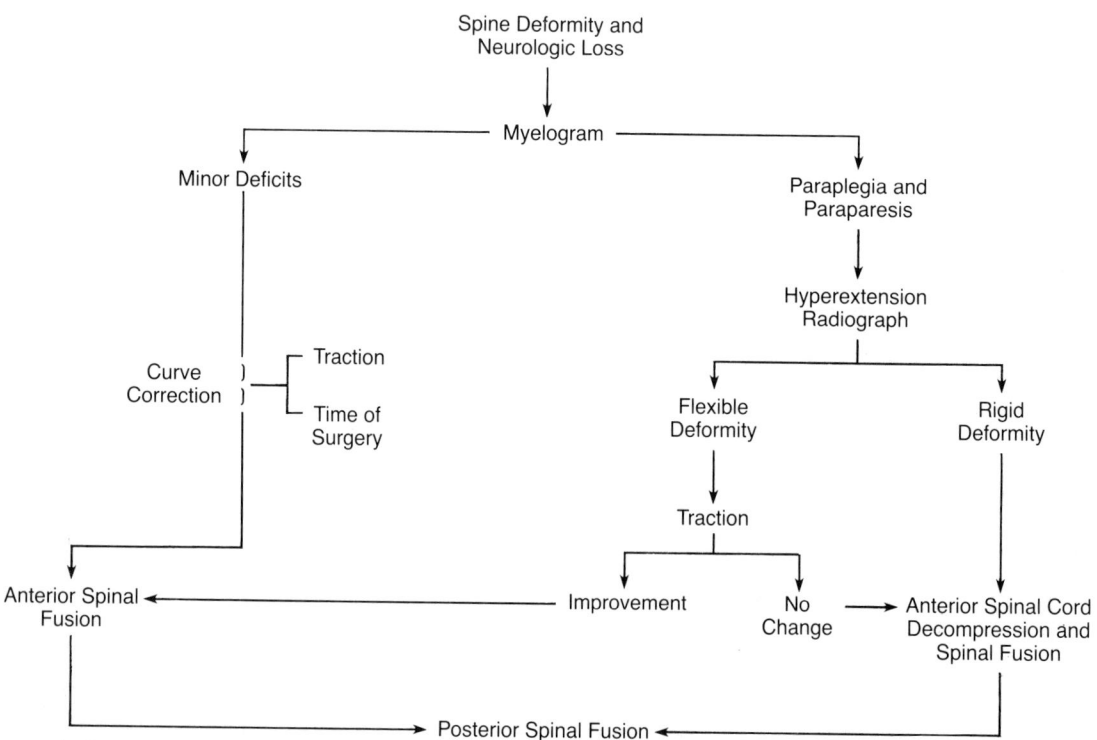

Figure 22–39. Outline of the treatment program for cord decompression and spinal deformity. (Reprinted with permission from Lonstein, et al.: Neurological deficits secondary to spinal deformity—a review of the literature and a report on 43 cases. Spine, 5:331–355, 1980.)

months. After this the cast is usually changed, the patient is allowed to ambulate, and immobilization is continued until the fusion is solid.

In very rare cases with severe angular kyphosis or a high thoracic deformity, the anterior approach is not practical and decompression is achieved via the Capener approach. An anterior fusion is still necessary to stabilize the kyphosis and prevent it's progressing. The Capener approach alone is an effective decompressive technique, but stabilization of the deformity must be performed with an anterior and posterior fusion.

The outline (Fig. 22-39) gives a logical approach to the treatment of cord compression resulting from a spine deformity. Early adequate treatment of kyphosis will stabilize the kyphosis, prevent progression, and make the aforementioned procedures of historical interest only. The best, most effective, and ideal treatment of this devastating complication of severe kyphosis is prevention.

References

1. Breig, A.: Biomechanics of the spinal cord in kyphosis and kyphoscoliosis. Acta Neurol. Scand., 40:196, 1964.
2. Breig, A.: Biomechanics of the Central Nervous System. Stockholm, Almquist and Wiksell, 1966.
3. Capener, N.: The evolution of lateral rachotomy. J. Bone Joint Surg., 36:173, 1954.
4. Chou, S. N.: The treatment of paralysis associated with kyphosis: role of anterior decompression. Clin. Orthop., 128:149-154, 1977.
5. Curtis, B. H., Fisher, R. L., and Butterfield, W. L.: Neurofibromatosis with paraplegia. J. Bone Joint Surg., 51A:843-861, 1969.
6. Dommisse, G. G.: The blood supply of the spinal cord. J. Bone Joint Surg., 56B:225, 1974.
7. Dommisse, G. G.: The Arteries and Veins of the Human Spinal Cord from Birth. New York, Longman, Inc., 1975.
8. Gold, L., Leach, D., Kieffer, S. A., et al.: Large volume myelography. Radiology, 97:531, 1970.
9. Hodgson, A. R., and Stock, F. E.: Anterior spine fusion. Br. J. Surg., 44:266, 1956.
10. Hyndman, D. R.: Transplantation of the Spinal Cord. Surg. Gynecol. Obstet., 84:460, 1947.
11. Lonstein, J. E., Winter, R. B., Moe, J. H., et al.: Neurological Deficits Secondary to Spinal Deformity—a review of the literature and report on 43 cases. Spine, 5:331-355, 1980.
12. MacEwen, W.: Case report in surgery of the brain and spinal cord. Br. Med. J., 2:302, 1888.
13. Marchetti, P. G., Faldini, A., and Ponte, A.: Il Trattamento Chirurgico delle Scoliosi. Report of 53rd Congress of the Italian Society for Orthopedics and Traumatology. Pisa, p.265, October, 1968.
14. Roaf, R.: Spinal deformity and paraplegia. Paraplegia, 2:112, 1964.
15. Schneider, R. S.: Transposition of the compressed spinal cord in kyphoscoliotic patients with neurologic deficits. J. Bone Joint Surg., 42A:1027, 1960.
16. Stagnara, P., and Pedriolle, R.: Elanjation vertebrale continue par platse a tendeurs. Rev. Orthop., 44:57-74, 1958.
17. Stagnara, P., Boulliat, G., Fauchet, R., and DuPeloux, J.: Considerations sur le traitement orthopedique des paraplegies cypho-scoliotiques. Rev. Neurol., 112:122-127, 1965.
18. Winter, R. B., Moe, J. H., and Wang, J. F.: Congenital kyphosis. J. Bone Joint Surg., 55A:223, 1973.

Spine Deformity Following Radiation

James W. Ogilvie, M.D.

INTRODUCTION

Radiation treatment plays an important role in the therapeutic approach to numerous malignancies, including the childhood tumors of neuroblastoma and Wilms' tumor.[21] These tumors occur in close proximity to the vertebral column, and thus may involve it by direct extension of the tumor, or the spinal column may be included in the treatment beam of postoperative radiation therapy. Low linear-energy-transfer radiation, such as gamma and roentgen rays, can be associated with serious disturbance of skeletal growth. Alterations of vertebral growth patterns can be noted as early as six months following therapeutic radiation, and spinal deformities in the coronal and sagittal planes can be experienced with ensuing growth.

As patients who have received life-saving therapeutic radiation grow into adulthood, the possibility of radiation carcinogenesis becomes important. This may require a 30 year follow-up or more,[18] and the effects of recurrent tumor, reparative process, radiation-induced tumor, and radiation-induced growth abnormalities or osteonecrosis must be differentiated.

With a knowledge of the natural history anticipated in a patient receiving a known amount of therapeutic radiation to the spinal column in childhood, it is possible to formulate a reasonable prognosis. The treatment plan may include the use of a spinal orthosis to minimize deformity, and in certain cases it may require surgical treatment to manage a progressive spine deformity.

HISTORY

Radiation biology as related to the skeletal system was first demonstrated by Perthes in 1903.[25] He noted a retarded development of osseous structures following exposure to roentgen rays. Morphologic changes in bone following roentgen radiation were studied by Racamier and Tribondeau, Salvetti, and in 1920, Segale documented definitive microscopic changes in the radiated long bones of skeletally immature rats.[27, 33, 34] Phemister documented radiation necrosis of bone and soft tissue in laboratory animals and also in tumor patients treated with radium needle implants.[26] Barr and others noted that roentgen exposure of 1,100 to 1,300 r was sufficient to interrupt epiphyseal growth in rats, although synovium and other periarticular soft tissues showed very little effect to radiation at this dosage.[3] The epiphyseal plate was found to be particularly sensitive to radiation. Engel, in 1935, was the first to produce experimental scoliosis in goats, dogs, and rabbits by exposing one side of the vertebral column to radium implants.[12] He felt that the resultant scoliosis was due to a direct effect on the cartilage growth plate, and not to soft tissue contractures. He noted that while there was no evidence of cartilage cell necrosis, there was no new bone formation in the radiation field.

These data plus that collected from other investigators confirm the fact that radiation can severely affect the longitudinal growth of the epiphyseal plate and cause a disturbance in metaphyseal remodeling.[28, 35] This results in diminished longitudinal growth of the bone and may produce characteristic changes both in metaphyses of long bones and in the vertebrae.

Schmorl was the first to assert that longitudinal growth of the vertebral body took place by enchondral ossification. This was demonstrated by Bick and Copel, confirming the concept that longitudinal growth of the vertebrae takes place at the cartilagenous endplate in a manner similar to the epiphysis in long bones.[5] Arkin and Simon expanded the work of Engel and produced scoliosis in rabbits, ascribing the scoliosis to a failure of longitudinal growth in the vertebrae rather than a soft tissue scarring.[2] Although the vertebrae were wedged into the concavity of the scoliosis, the epiphyseal plate was wider on the concavity, indicating failure of growth and ossification rather than external pressure as the pathogenesis of the scoliosis (Fig. 22–40). Arkin and co-workers in 1950 were the first to report a case of radiation-induced scoliosis in a human.[1] Their patient, a 19 month old female, was treated by nephrectomy for a Wilms' tumor. She received a total of 3,200 r during the pre- and postoperative periods. At the age of 13 years she was noted

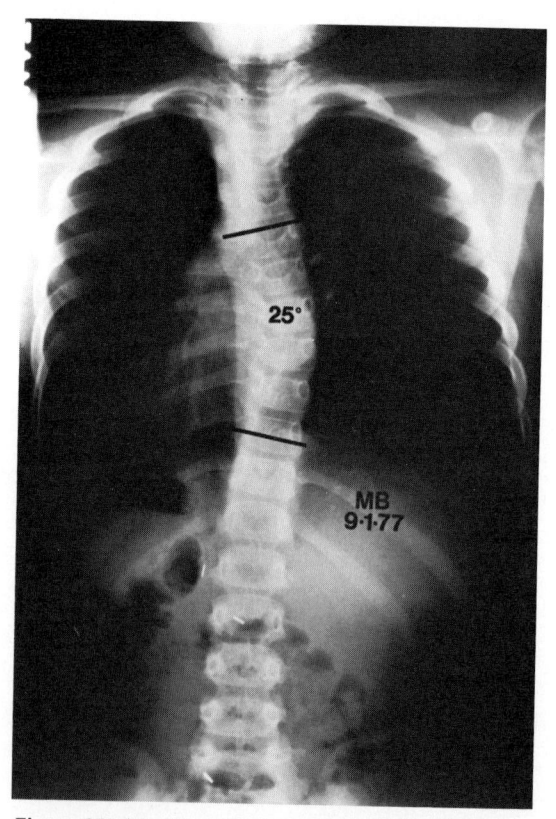

Figure 22–40. Therapeutic radiation and nephrectomy were used on this patient with Wilms' tumor. He subsequently developed a right thoracic 25 degree curve outside of the radiation field but no scoliosis in the lumbar spine. The pathogenesis of idiopathic and post-radiation scoliosis do not overlap.

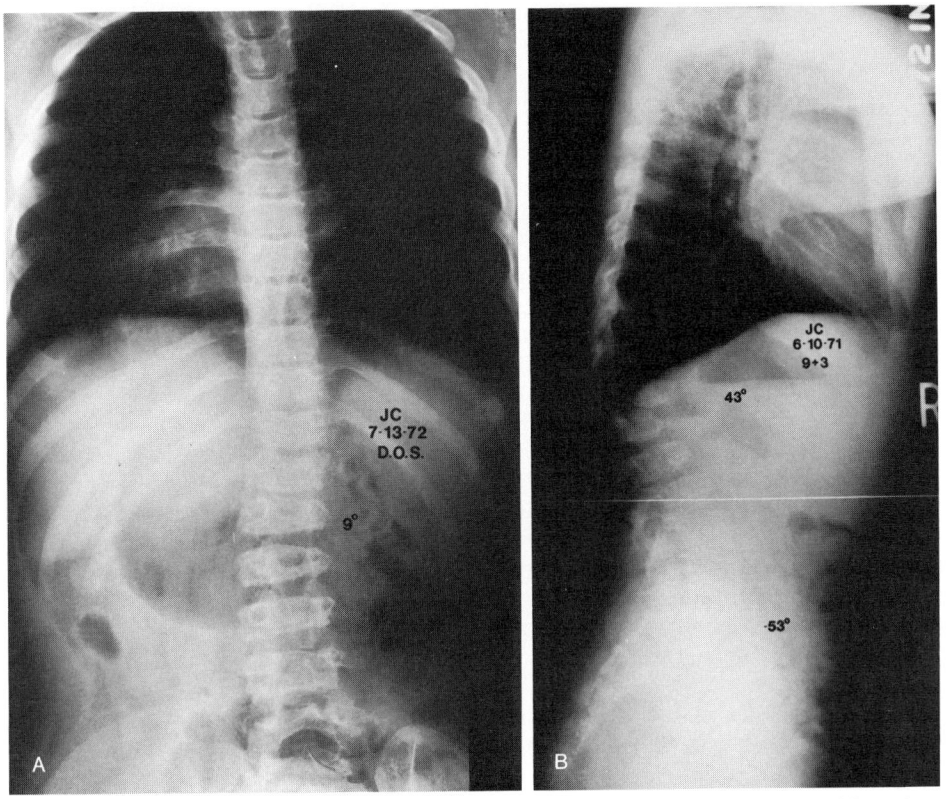

Figure 22–41. A and B, Irradiation effects on the growing spine. Vertebral endplate irregularities, "bone-within-a-bone" appearance, scoliosis, and kyphosis are noted in addition to hypoplasia of the right ilium and lower ribs.

to have scoliosis, which was correctly differentiated from an idiopathic adolescent curvature. Since then, numerous clinical reports have emerged, documenting the appearance of spine deformity following radiation therapy in children.[11, 13, 24, 31, 37]

Frantz reported an osteochondroma found in the distal femoral metaphysis of a child who had been treated with radiation for a hemangioma of the lower limb.[13] Subsequent reports have confirmed the occurrence of benign osteocartilaginous exostoses within the fields of treatment in 15 to 20 per cent of patients.[8, 23, 30] Katzman reported hypoplasia of the ilium and ribs on the side containing the radiation port in 15 of 20 patients.[16] The radiographic findings of involved vertebrae are similar to those of Morquio's disease, with a bone-in-bone appearance (Fig. 22–41). Anterior beaking is present along with vertebral endplate irregularities and smaller overall vertebral size.[23] Hyperluscent lung fields and associated soft tissue scarring, cutaneous hyperpigmentation, contractures, and underdevelopment of paraspinous muscles can also occur in the radiation field.[30]

Careful planning and documentation of the radiation field should allow exclusion of the iliac crests, gonads, and femoral heads. Vaeth reported that three of four women who received radiation for Wilms' tumor in childhood subsequently gave birth to normal children.[36].

Because of the difference of soft tissue and bone density, it is known that bone absorbs approximately four times as much low and medium energy radiation as does soft tissue.[20] In megavoltage radiation, such as that produced by Colbalt-60, there is proportionally less radiation absorbed by high density bone, and therefore higher voltage radiation is more efficient in delivering radiation to soft tissue when no primary effect is desired on osseous tissue.

Radiation-induced malignancy has also been reported following bone exposure of at least 3,000 r. The most frequent malignancy following bone irradiation is osteosarcoma; however, chondrosarcomas, giant cell sarcomas, and unclassified sarcomas have also been noted.[4] Cahan reported on 11 patients with osteosarcoma arising in the radiated bone at 6 to 22 years after radiation treatment.[7]

INCIDENCE

Any skeletally immature patient receiving more than 1,000 r exposure to the vertebral column is at risk for spine deformity. Fewer than 1,000 r usually produces no detectable changes in the vertebral body.[23] Controversy exists regarding the premise that megavoltage radiation causes fewer spine deformities than orthovoltage radiation. While the use of supervoltage radiation should theoretically result in a lower absorbed dose by the bony elements of the spine, there are no studies that conclusively resolve the question. Rutherford and Dodd reported a similar number of patients with radiation-induced scoliosis and rib and iliac hypoplasia in those who had received supravoltage and orthovoltage radiation treatment.[32] Since the periosteum and cartilage endplate are considered soft tissue, their exposure results in subsequent growth abnormalities.

Early assessment suggested that the symmetrical nature of the radiation fields had little effect on the severity of subsequent radiation scoliosis; however, this study involved a small number of patients with a relatively short follow-up.[31] Other studies, including those reported by Mayfield and others, have show that asymmetrical radiation fields have been associated with an increased number and severity of spine deformities.[19, 24, 30] Symmetrical portals for spinal irradiation more commonly result in kyphosis.

Donaldson and Wissinger studied 37 children following irradiation treatment for Wilms' tumor or neuroblastoma and found that 70 per cent had developed scoliosis, two of which required surgery.[10] In 81 patients who had been irradiated for Wilms' tumor, Riseborough noted 59 with scoliosis, 19 with kyphoscoliosis, and two with pure kyphosis.[29] Fourteen of those 59 patients had curves greater than 25 degrees. He also found that no child under the age of ten had a scoliosis curvature of more than 20 degrees. It has been noted in neuroblastoma patients treated with radiation, that 20 per cent developed spinal deformity significant enough to require treatment and that 7 per cent required subsequent surgical treatment.[18] In 59 consecutive Wilms' tumor patients receiving radiation treatment who were followed to the end of growth, Dubousset noted 40 per cent with scoliosis and 65 per cent with kyphotic deformities.[10]

Several principles seem well established when evaluating a pediatric patient who has undergone spinal column exposure to therapeutic radiation. There is little correlation between the individual changes of the vertebral body and the severity of curvature. A direct relationship exists between absorbed radiation and subsequent spine deformity. Absorbed radiation less than 1,000 r carries with it a minimal risk for subsequent orthopaedic difficulties. Mild curves are frequently seen in the 2,000 r group, and the most severe spine deformities have been associated with 3,000 r exposure. Radiation-induced malignancy is also increased in those patients receiving 3,000 r or more. It is also well established that the younger the patient at exposure, the greater the probability of spine deformity. The most serious disturbances occur in patients irradiated at less than two years of age. Radiation treatment given to those greater than four years of age is rarely associated with significant spinal deformity unless there has been surgical destabilization of the spine with laminectomy, or unless there has been bony erosion by the primary tumor. Any pediatric patient undergoing therapeutic radiation to the spine should have orthopaedic consultation and follow-up until skeletal maturity is reached.

Although surgery is the treatment of choice for Wilms' tumor and neuroblastoma, 3,000 r is the recommended dosage of therapeutic radiation in Group II and Group III Wilms' tumor patients, namely those patients in whom the tumor has extended beyond the kidney but has been completely excised, or those with residual non-hematogenous tumor confined to the abdomen.[21, 22] In these two groups, radiation plus actinomycin D and vincristine is recommended and has resulted in a four year relapse-free survival rate of 79 per cent. Since the incidence rate of Wilms' tumor is 7.8 per one million and neuroblastoma 16.6 per one million, significant numbers of children who have received radiation therapy to the vertebral column and chemotherapy are likely to survive into adulthood.[38] The problem of radiation-induced spine deformity will require continued vigilance.

PRINCIPLES OF TREATMENT

Our experience parallels that of other centers in that significant scoliosis is rarely present before the age of ten. As a patient experiences the adolescent growth acceleration, curves which have been relatively static over previous years may show a dramatic increase. When the curve has reached 20 degrees, as measured by the Cobb method, orthotic treatment has been used (Fig. 22–42). Whether this prevents progression in certain curves or merely delays progression is unclear, but orthoses are not generally effective in reducing these curvatures. Prolonged observation of a progressive radiation-induced spine deformity is not indicated. We have no experience with the use of surface electrode muscle stimulation in radiation-induced spine deformities, but the rigid nature of the curve and the primary defect in growth potential make these curves unlikely candidates for electrical stimulation. The use of a Milwaukee brace is traditional, however, since the apex of the scoliosis is usually below T9, a low profile orthosis can be employed until skeletal maturity. Careful assessment of the soft tissue is necessary in each patient. Extensive scarring or contracture may obviate the use of an orthosis. The age at which skeletal maturity occurs does not differ from non-radiated spines. If the coronal plane deformity reaches more than 40 degrees, surgical intervention should be considered, especially if kyphosis greater than 20 degrees accompanies the curvature. Pseudarthrosis and infection are both increased when surgery is performed on a previously radiated spine.[17, 29] The choice of fusion limits does not differ from idiopathic scoliosis curves. This should include the caudal-most vertebra that rests within the stable zone and one level cephalad to the upper neutral vertebra.

Healing is prolonged, and it may be desirable to supplement Harrington distraction rod posterior fusion with a repeat bone graft at six months following the initial surgery. The use of an autogenous cancellous bone graft from a non-radiated donor site is desirable.

Circumferential anterior-posterior fusion is required when the kyphotic component of the deformity is greater than 35 degrees in

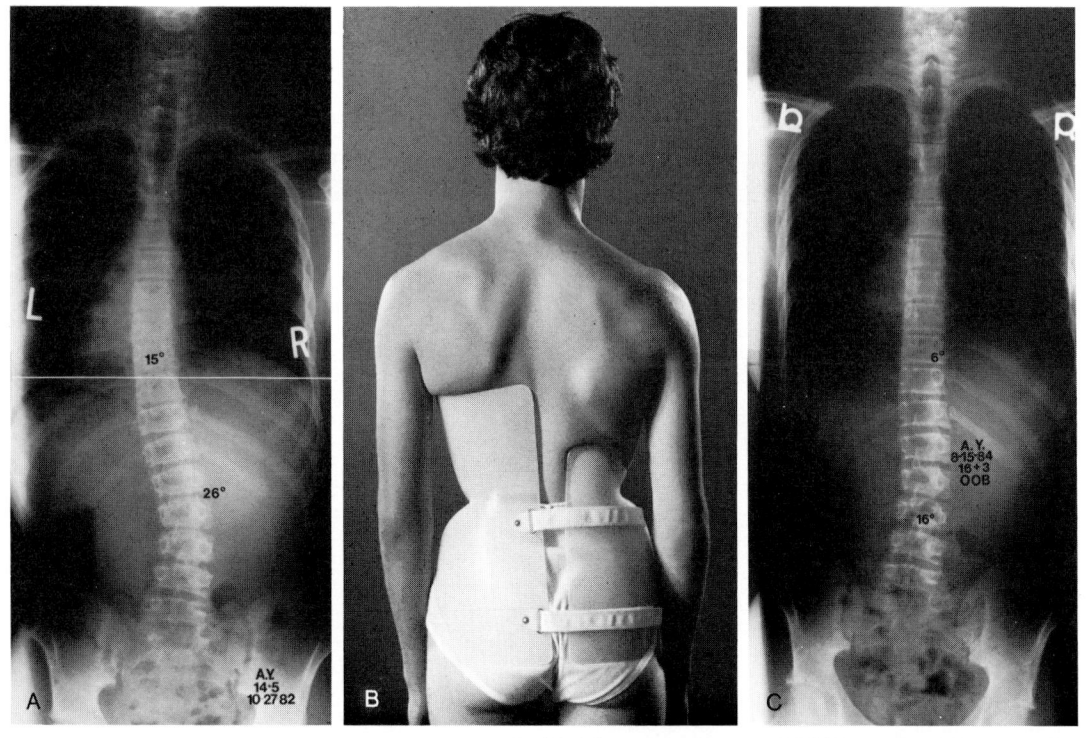

Figure 22–42. This 14+5 year old male was treated with left nephrectomy and 3000 r at age 16 months for a Wilms' tumor. His right lumbar scoliosis (A) was treated with a modified TLSO (B). At skeletal maturity his curve measured 16 degrees (C).

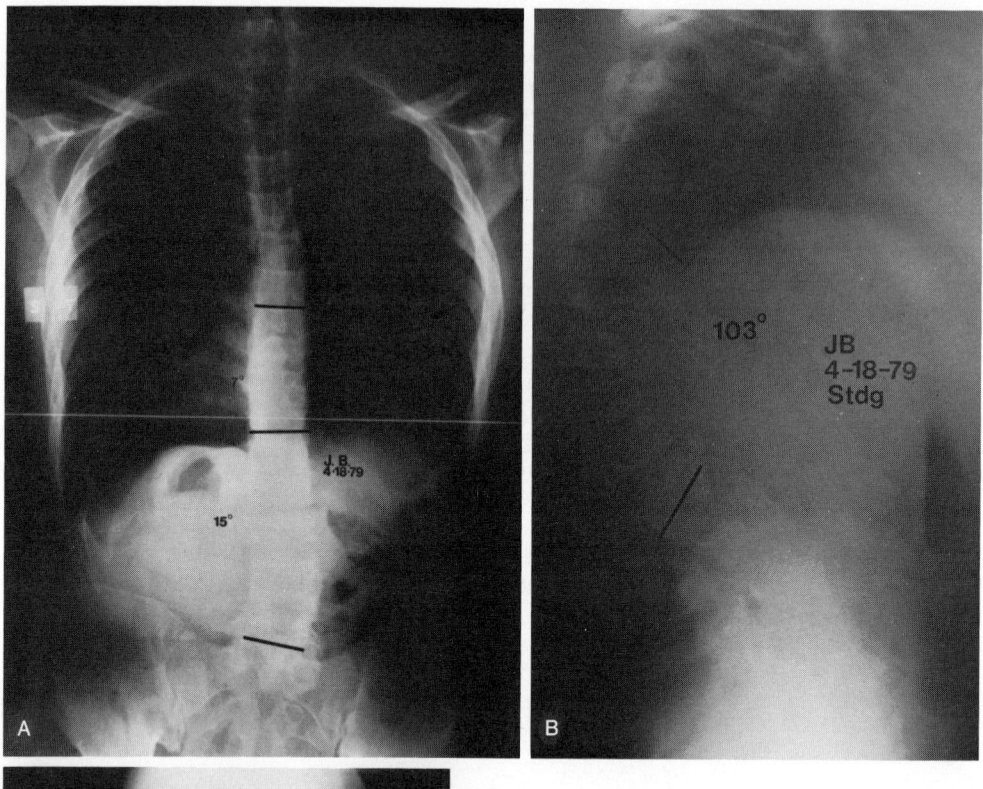

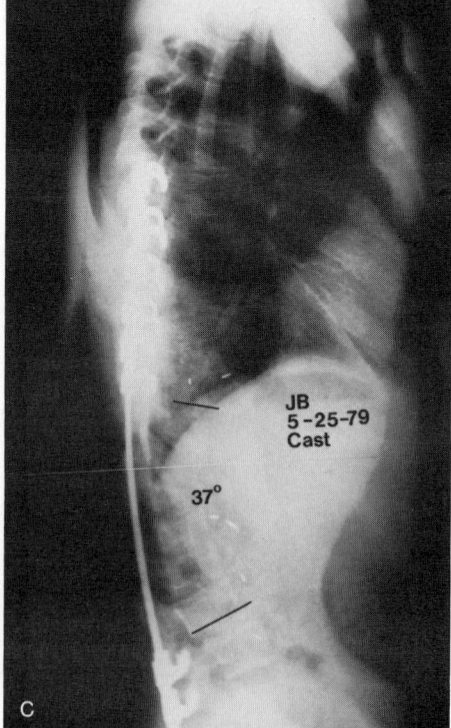

Figure 22–43. This 14+1 year old male was treated for Wilms' tumor with right nephrectomy and symmetrical portals of radiation. His 18 degree scoliosis (A) and 103 degree thoracolumbar kyphosis (B) were treated with anterior discectomy and rib strut grafting followed by posterior Harrington compression rods (C).

the lumbar area (Fig. 22–43). A greater degree of kyphus may be accepted in the thoracic spine. If a vascularized rib strut can be transferred from a non-radiated area, this too is ideal in utilizing an autogenous, rapidly healing anterior bone strut.[6] The use of segmental spinal instrumentation provides good fixation, however, we cannot confirm that the fusion rate is improved.

A total contact, low profile orthosis is routinely used for the six months following surgery. The decision whether to continue the orthosis, or proceed with supplemental bone graft at six months post-surgery should be individualized. Supplemental graft is seldom required in circumferential fusions. If fixation is questionable, or if bone healing has not advanced satisfactorily, one may elect to continue postoperative immobilization for an additional six months.

References

1. Arkin, A. M., Pack, G. T., Ransohoff, N. S., and Simon, N.: Radiation-induced scoliosis: a case report. J. Bone Joint Surg., 32A:401, 1950.
2. Arkin, A. M., and Simon, N.: Radiation scoliosis: an experimental study. J. Bone Joint Surg., 32A:396, 1950.
3. Barr, J. S., Lingley, J. R., and Gall, E. A.: The effect of roentgen irradiation on epiphyseal growth. Am. J. Roentgenol., 49:104, 1943.
4. Berdon, W. E., Baker, D. H., and Boyer, J.: Unusual benign and malignant sequelae to childhood radiation therapy. Am. J. Roentgenol., 93:545, 1965.
5. Bick, E. M., and Copel, J. W.: Longitudinal growth of the human vertebra. A contribution to human osteogeny. J. Bone Joint Surg., 32A:803, 1950.
6. Bradford, D. S.: Anterior vascular pedical bone grafting for the treatment of kyphosis. Spine. 5:318, 1979.
7. Cahan, W. G., Woodard, H. G., Higinbotham, H. L., et al.: Sarcoma arising in irradiated bone. Cancer, 1:3, 1948.
8. Cohen, J., and D'Angio, G. J.: Unusual bone tumors after roentgen therapy of children. Am. J. Roentgenol., 86:502, 1961.
9. D'Angio, G. J., Beckwith, J. B., Breslow, N. E., et al.: Wilms' tumor: an update. Cancer, 45:1791, 1980.
10. Donaldson, W. F., and Wissinger, H. A.: Axial skeletal changes following tumor dose radiation therapy. In proceedings of the American Orthopaedic Association. J. Bone Joint Surg., 49A:1469, 1967.
11. Dubousset, J.: Deformations rachidiennes post radiotherapique apres traitement du nephroblastome. Rev. Chil. Orthop., 66:441, 1980.
12. Engel, D.: Experiments on the production of spinal deformities by radium. Am. J. Roentgenol., 42:217, 1939.
13. Frantz, C. H.: Extreme retardation of epiphyseal growth from roentgen irradiation. Radiology, 55:720, 1950.
14. Heaston, D. K., Libshitz, H. J., and Chan, R. C.: Skeletal effects of megavoltage irradiation in survivors of Wilms' tumors. Am. J. Roentgenol., 133:389, 1979.
15. Hinkel, C. L.: The effect of roentgen rays upon the growing long bones of albino rats: II. Histopathological changes involving endochondral growth centers. Am. J. Roentgenol., 49:321, 1943.
16. Katzman, H., Waugh, T., and Berdon, W.: Skeletal changes following irradiation of childhood tumors. J. Bone Joint Surg., 51A:825, 1969.
17. King, J., and Stowe, S.: Results of spinal fusion for radiation scoliosis. Spine, 7:574, 1982.
18. Kohn, H. I., and Fry, R. J. M.: Radiation carcinogenesis. New Engl. J. Med., 310:504, 1984.
19. Mayfield, J. K., Riseborough, E. J., Jaffe, N., and Nehme, M. E.: Spinal deformity in children treated for neuroblastoma. J. Bone Joint Surg., 63A:183, 1981.
20. Moss, W. T., Brand, W. N., and Battifora, H.: The bone: response of normal bone to irradiation. In: Radiation Oncology: Rationale, Techniques, Results. 5th Ed. St. Louis, C. V. Mosby, 1979.
21. Moss, W. T., Brand, W. N., and Battifora, H.: Introduction to radiation oncology. In: Radiation Oncology: Rationale, Technique, Results, 5th Ed. St Louis, C. V. Mosby, 1979.
22. Moss, W. T., Brand, W. N., and Battifora, H.: The kidney. In: Radiation Oncology: Rationale, Technique, Results. 5th Ed. St. Louis, C. V. Mosby, 1979.
23. Murphy, F. D., and Blount, W. P.: Cartilaginous exostoses following irradiation. J. Bone Joint Surg., 44A:662, 1962.
24. Neuhauser, E. B. D., Wittenborg, M. H., Berman, C. Z., and Cohen, J.: Irradiation effects of roentgen therapy on the growing spine. Radiology, 59:637, 1952.
25. Perthes, G.: Ueber den einfluss der rontgenstrahlen auf epitheliol gewebe insbesondere auf das carcinom. Verh. Dsch. Ges. Chir., 32:525, 1903.
26. Phemister, D. B.: Radium necrosis of bone. Am. J. Roentgenol., 16:340, 1926.
27. Racamier, D., and Tribondeau, L.: A propos de l'action des rayons X sur l'osteogenese. Comp. Rend. Soc. Biol., 59:621, 1905.
28. Reidy, J. A., Lingley, J. R., Gall, E. A., and Barr, J. S.: The effect of roentgen irradiation on epiphyseal growth. J. Bone Joint Surg., 29:853, 1947.
29. Riseborough, E. J., Grabias, S. L., Burton, R. I., and Jaffe, N.: Skeletal alterations following irradiation for Wilms' tumor. J. Bone Joint Surg., 58A:526, 1976.
30. Rubin, P., Andrews, J. R., Swarm, R., and Gump, H.: Radiation induced dysplasias of bone. Am. J. Roentgenol., 82:206, 1959.
31. Rubin, P., Duthie, R. B., and Young, L. W.: The significance of scoliosis in postirradiated Wilms' tumor and neuroblastoma. Radiology, Vol. 79, No. 4, October 1962.
32. Rutherford, H., and Dodd, G. D.: Complications of radiation therapy: Growing bone. Semin. Roentgenol., Vol. IX, No. 1, Januray 1974.
33. Salvetti, E.: Einfluss der rontgenstrahlen auf die

bildung der knochennarbe. Dsche. Z. Chir., 28:130, 1914.
34. Segale, G. C.: Sull'azione biologica dei raggi rontgene del radium sulle cartilagini epifisarie. Radiol. Med., 7:234, 1920.
35. Tefft, M.: Radiation effect of growing bone and cartilage. Front. Radia. Ther. Oncol., 6:289, 1972.
36. Vaeth, J. M., Levitt, S. H., Jones, M. D., and Holtfreter, C.: Effects of radiation therapy in survivors of Wilms' tumor. Radiology, 79:560, 1962.
37. Whitehouse, W. M., and Lampe, I.: Osseous damage in irradiation of renal tumors in infancy and childhood. Am. J. Roentgenol., 70:721, 1953.
38. Young, J. L., Jr., and Miller, R. W.: Incidence of malignant tumors in U.S. children. J. Pediatr., 8:254, 1975.

Marfan's Syndrome

Robert B. Winter, M.D.

INTRODUCTION

Scoliosis occurs in 40 to 70 per cent of individuals with Marfan's syndrome.[3, 7, 10, 12, 16, 19] The scoliosis can be severe and can result in pain, marked cosmetic deformity, significant loss of pulmonary function, and even death from cor pulmonale. Because of the unique soft tissue features of this disease, treatment of the scoliosis and other spinal deformities of Marfan's syndrome can be quite different from those of other etiologies.

CLINICAL MANIFESTATIONS

Marfan's syndrome is a hereditary connective tissue disorder of unknown etiology that includes ocular, cardiovascular, and skeletal manifestations. It is inherited as an autosomal dominant trait.[9] It was first described by Marfan in 1896.[8] Recent studies have implicated a defect in collagen cross-linking.[4]

The ocular manifestations include subluxation or dislocation of the lens of the eye (ectopia lentis). This may be a subtle finding, and slit-lamp examination by an ophthalmologist may be necessary to confirm this defect.

The cardiovascular manifestations include aortic or mitral valve insufficiency, aortic arch dilitation, or dissecting aneurysm. The latter is frequently the cause of sudden death.

The skeletal manifestations include arachnodactyly, dolichomorphism, dolichocephaly, pectus excavatum, pectus carinatum, high-arched palate, ligamentous laxity, pes planus, scoliosis, thoracic lordosis, thoracolumbar kyphosis, and occasionally spondylolisthesis.

The differential diagnosis includes congenital contractural arachnodactyly, homocystinuria, Ehlers-Danlos syndrome, and mitral valve prolapse syndrome.[2, 5, 13, 14]

Since there is no specific biochemical test for Marfan's syndrome, the diagnosis is purely clinical. The diagnosis is not always easy, since not all patients have the classic triad of ectopia lentis, arachnodactyly, and cardiac valvular insufficiency. Patients with only questionable criteria for diagnosis have commonly been called "formes fruste" examples of the disease. It is not unusual to see a tall, thin adolescent with a scoliosis who also has a cardiac murmur. Echocardiographic evaluation may reveal a "floppy" mitral valve. In the absence of other objective criteria of Marfan's syndrome, this patient should *not* be labelled as having Marfan's syndrome. This is preferably called the "mitral valve prolapse syndrome."

The curve patterns in Marfan's syndrome closely resemble those of idiopathic scoliosis. Thoracic curves are usually to the right and lumbar to the left. Double major curves are frequent. Thoracic lordosis is very common and may be associated with a lumbar or thoracolumbar kyphosis. This reversal of the normal sagittal plane spinal alignment appears to be especially common in Marfan's syndrome and is important in the consideration of treatment.

REVIEW OF THE LITERATURE

There are several major reviews of scoliosis in Marfan's syndrome, including those by Orcutt and DeWald;[12] Robins, Moe, and Winter;[16] Savini, Cervellati, and Beroaldo;[17] Beneux and coworkers;[3] and Le Delliou.[7] Robins and associates reported on scoliosis in 35 patients, 27 with true Marfan's syndrome, and 8 with "forme fruste" disease. The scoliosis in the true Marfan's group averaged 64 degrees, and in the forme fruste group 79 degrees. Seventy-two per cent of the curves were painful. Fourteen patients were treated with a Milwaukee brace, and only five of these had a good result. Two had curves of such severity that brace treatment was inappropriate, and the other seven failed to respond to the brace and required surgery. The only brace successes were in the forme fruste type.

In this series 14 patients had spinal fusion, all posterior fusion with Harrington rods in eleven. The average correction was 41 per cent. Five patients had pseudarthrosis, four were successfully repaired, and one patient died of cardiac failure at age 11. There were no deaths or neurologic deficits caused by the surgery.

Orcutt and DeWald reported 35 patients with scoliosis out of 53 patients with known Marfan's syndrome. Six had brace treatment and seven surgery. Two had spondylolisthesis, one a Grade II, the other Grade IV. Careful cardiovascular evaluation was emphasized.

Beneux and coworkers reported 20 cases, 14 of which required surgical correction and stabilization. Three of these cases also required additional anterior fusion.

Savini and coworkers reported on 26 patients, 14 male and 12 female. In 23 scoliosis predominated, and in three kyphosis predominated. Many of the curves were severe, including one patient with two 180 degree curves. Only four patients had curves of less than 50 degrees. Patients with thoracic lordosis were noted to have decreased pulmonary function; one adult had a vital capacity of only 550 cc. Eight patients were treated non-operatively with braces or casts, and none of these treatments was successful. Seventeen patients had surgical treatment, the smallest scoliosis being 57 degrees, and the largest 180 degrees. The average correction was 43 per cent. Preliminary correction with halofemoral or halo suspension traction was found useful for the more major deformities. The patient with the two 180 degree curves was corrected to 90 degrees and 80 degrees, gained 400 cc. of vital capacity and 27 cm. in height! One patient in this series had severe spondylolisthesis. Two patients with severe spondylolisthesis (100 per cent slips) were reported by Winter.[20]

The most recent major report on spinal problems and their treatment is the thesis by LeDelliou from Lyon, France.[7] He reported on 59 patients, 43 with true Marfan's syndrome and 16 with forme fruste. Of the 59, 35 were female and 24 male. Double major curves were the most common in both groups, and the tendency for sagittal curve reversal was also noted, especially in the group with true Marfan's syndrome.

In the group with true Marfan's syndrome, the curves ranged from 11 degrees to 196 degrees, and in the forme fruste group from 23 degrees to 140 degrees. Only 19 of the 59 patients had scoliosis of less than 50 degrees, and only eight had scoliosis of less than 30 degrees. Eleven patients of the 59 had scolioses greater than 100 degrees. Flexibility (tested in suspension) ranged from 0 per cent to 60 per cent, and was most limited in the more severe and long-standing curves. An element of dystrophic dysplasia similar to neurofibromatosis was noted in one patient.

Non-operative treatment with braces or casts was attempted in 14 patients, four in Milwaukee braces, seven in the corset Lyonnaise, and three with both braces. Progression of the curve was halted in seven patients. Lumbar kyphosis was resistant to brace treatment. Surgery was done for 40 patients, 28 with true Marfan's syndrome and 12 with forme fruste disease. Thirty-four had Harrington instrumentation. Surgery was felt to be the treatment of choice for most patients with scoliosis due to Marfan's syndrome.

Fishman and coworkers[6] reported on five patients with dural ectasia (similar to that seen in neurofibromatosis) of the sacral area. This enlargement of the spinal canal occurs at the expense of the bony integrity of the lumbosacral area and can lead to lumbosacral pain and instability. The deficit in bony tissue can cause major problems in the surgical attempts to achieve fusion at the lumbosacral level.

PATIENT EVALUATION

The history should include specific questions concerning family history, not only of spine deformity, but also of lens abnormalities, cardiovascular problems, and sudden death. Is the curve painful? Is there shortness of breath?

The physical examination should include the eyes for lens dislocation, the palate for high arch, the chest for pectus excavatum or carinatum, the extremities for arachnodactyly, the fingers for hyperextensibility, and the foot for pes planus. The finger-wrist test and the thumb-in-fist test should be done.

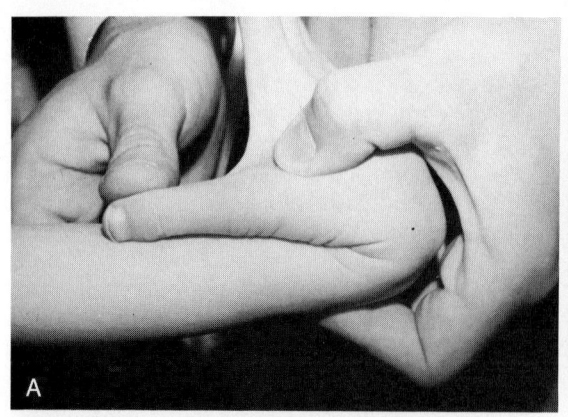

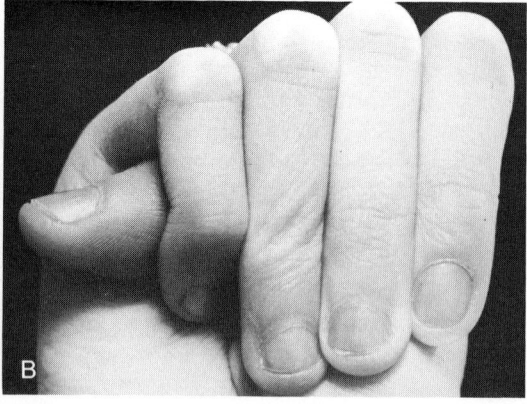

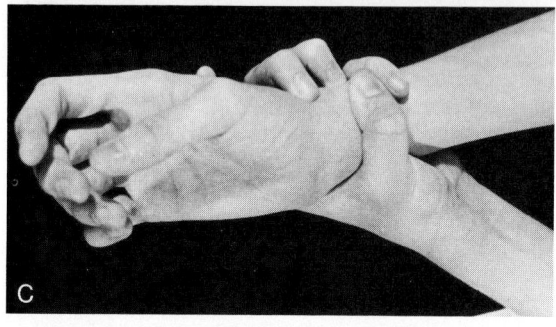

Figure 22–44. *A*, Ligamentous laxity in a young patient with Marfan's syndrome. *B*, Extension of the thumb beyond the ulnar border in a Marfan's patient. *C*, The ability to overlap the thumb and little finger around the opposite wrist, a sign of arachnodactyly.

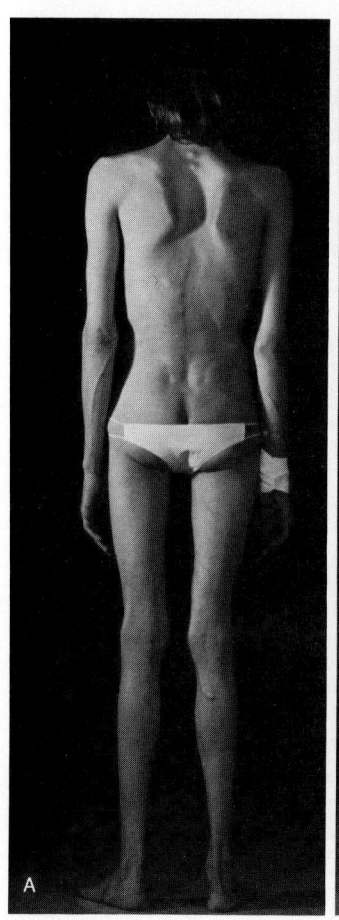

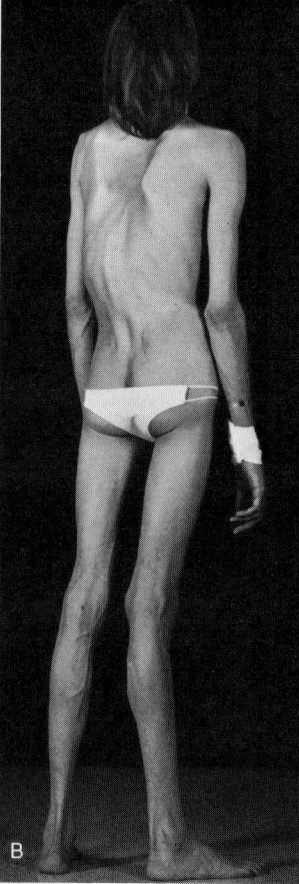

Figure 22–45. *A*, The posterior view of a tall (203 cm.) 17 year old male with Marfan's syndrome. He has a double major scoliosis pattern with 30 degree right thoracic and left lumbar curves. Thoracic lordosis can be seen. *B*, The same patient, in an oblique position, shows the marked reversal of sagittal plane alignment, with severe thoracic lordosis and lumbar kyphosis.

MISCELLANEOUS PROBLEMS

The heart should be examined for murmurs, especially those of mitral or aortic insufficiency. The spine should be reviewed for scoliosis, thoracic lordosis, lumbar or thoracolumbar kyphosis, and spondylolisthesis.

Ancillary studies include slit-lamp examination of the eyes, echocardiogram and electrocardiogram of the heart, and pulmonary function tests if there is major thoracic deformity, especially thoracic lordosis.[18]

Radiologic examination consists of standard spinal films, including both posteroanterior and lateral views. Presurgical films should include either bending or traction views to determine the curve flexibility. A spot lateral view of the lumbosacral area should be done if the full length lateral or clinical examination suggests spondylolisthesis. Myelography is not necessary except for the rare case showing dystrophic changes (Figs. 22–44 and 22–45).[9]

TREATMENT

Periodic Observation

Patients who are still in their growth years but have curves of less than 25 degrees are placed on serial observation, usually being seen at four month intervals. Patients who have completed growth, but who have unfused curves of 35 to 50 degrees should also be followed because of the risk of progression as adults. Observation at one year intervals is adequate for this group (Fig. 22–46).

Orthotic Treatment

Despite the relatively poor results of brace treatment, the occasional patient may benefit from bracing. Ideally this would be forme fruste type, or a documented progressive curve, still less than 45 degrees, with absence of thoracic lordosis and lumbar kyphosis. A Milwaukee brace is the orthosis of choice, since the increased flexibility of the soft tissues makes the patient susceptible to thoracic constriction if a circumferential orthosis is used. Curves progressing despite brace treatment should be fused. The only exception would be in the young patient (below age 10) who could benefit from instrumentation without fusion until a better age for fusion.

Surgical Treatment

The indication for surgery is a scoliosis of 45 degrees or more in the adolescent, or a painful curve, a progressive curve, or a curve

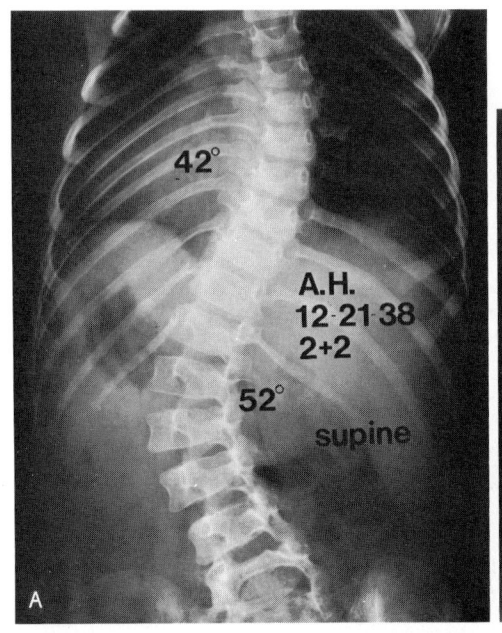

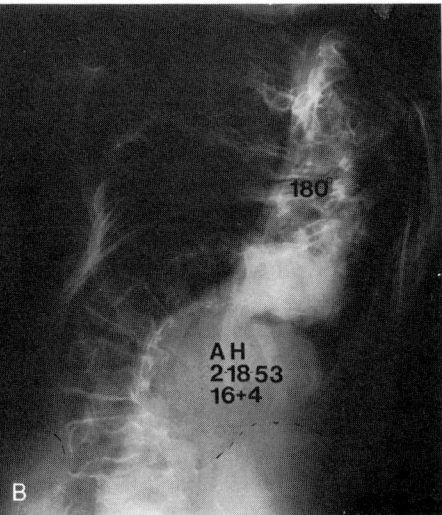

Figure 22–46. *A*, This two year old male was first seen at age two, already demonstrating curves of 42 degrees and 52 degrees. No treatment was given. *B*, When seen at age 16, his thoracic curve was 180 degrees and he had significant respiratory compromise.

over 50 degrees in the adult. The only contraindications to surgery are the presence of severe cardiac valvular insufficiency or dissecting aortic aneurysm. Valvular insufficiency can often be treated by cardiac surgery, and scoliosis surgery can be done subsequently.

The procedure of choice is posterior spine fusion with internal fixation by Harrington or Luque rods. The general techniques and choice of fusion are identical with those used in idiopathic scoliosis. Fusion to the sacrum is generally not necessary. Because of the frequency of thoracic lordosis, it is often advantageous to use sublaminar wiring in order to reconstitute thoracic kyphosis (Fig. 22–47). This can be done by posterior surgery alone in the teenager with a flexible curve, but may require preliminary discectomy in the more rigid adult lordosis.

A thoracolumbar or lumbar kyphosis should be tested preoperatively for correctibility by a supine hyperextension radiograph. If flexible, correction can be achieved by posterior surgery alone. If there is lack of correctibility, then anterior release, discectomy, and fusion should precede the posterior surgery. As much effort should be made to reconstitute normal sagittal plane alignment as is made to correct the scoliosis.

Preoperative skeletal traction, very popular 10 to 15 years ago, is used far less frequently now. Patients are being seen earlier now owing to better recognition and better awareness of the need for prompt surgical attention to the spine. Large and stiff single curves are

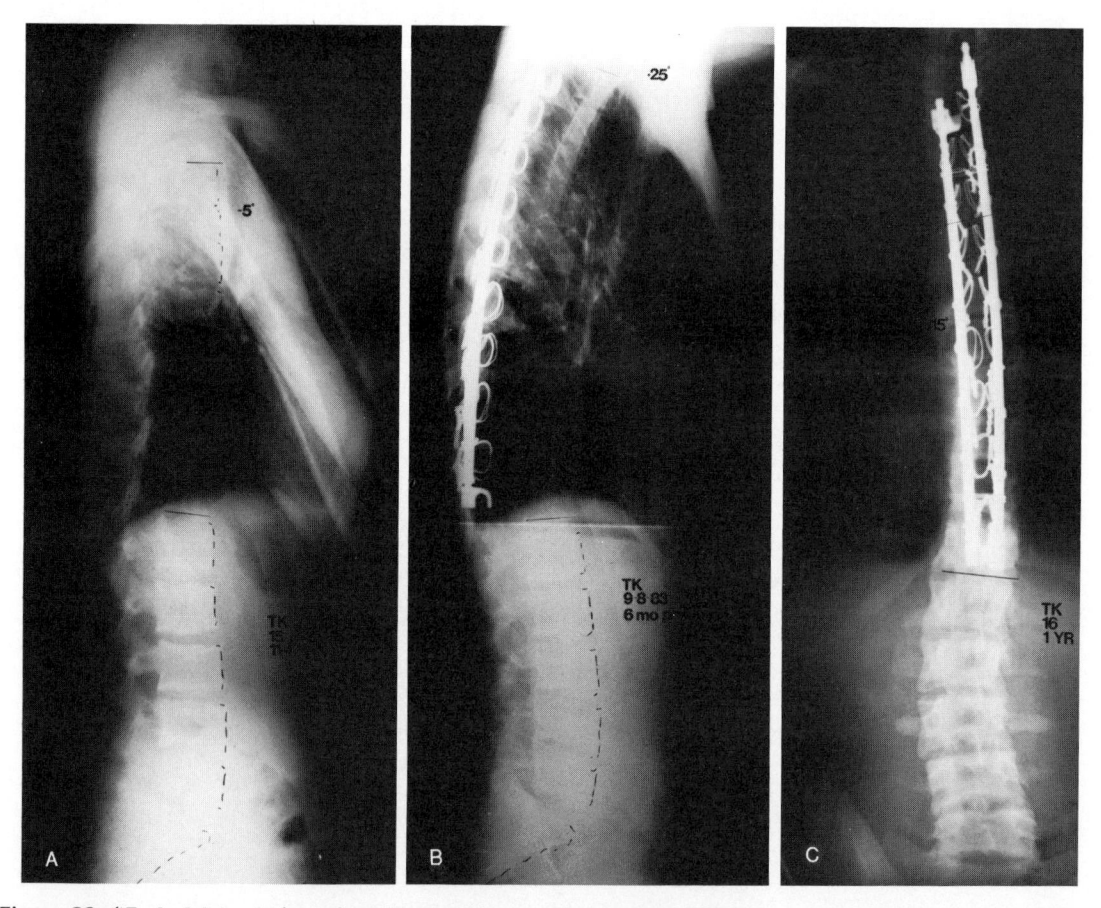

Figure 22–47. A, A lateral view of a 15 year old male with Marfan's syndrome. He had a 45 degree thoracic scoliosis, but his more major deformity was his thoracic hyperlordosis measuring −5 degrees (T2-T12). His vital capacity was 4.2 liters, a large volume for most people, but because of his height (202 cm.), it was a full liter below the expected normal. B, A lateral view six months after surgery shows reconstitution of a normal thoracic kyphosis (+25 degrees). This resulted in a measured gain of 1000 cc. of vital capacity and the ability to run for extended durations, a feat not possible before surgery. C, A posteroanterior view following surgery, showing the dural ¼ inch Harrington distraction rods and multiple sublaminar wires. Square-ended rods and square-holed lower hooks were used. The same result could have been achieved with dual heavy Luque rods.

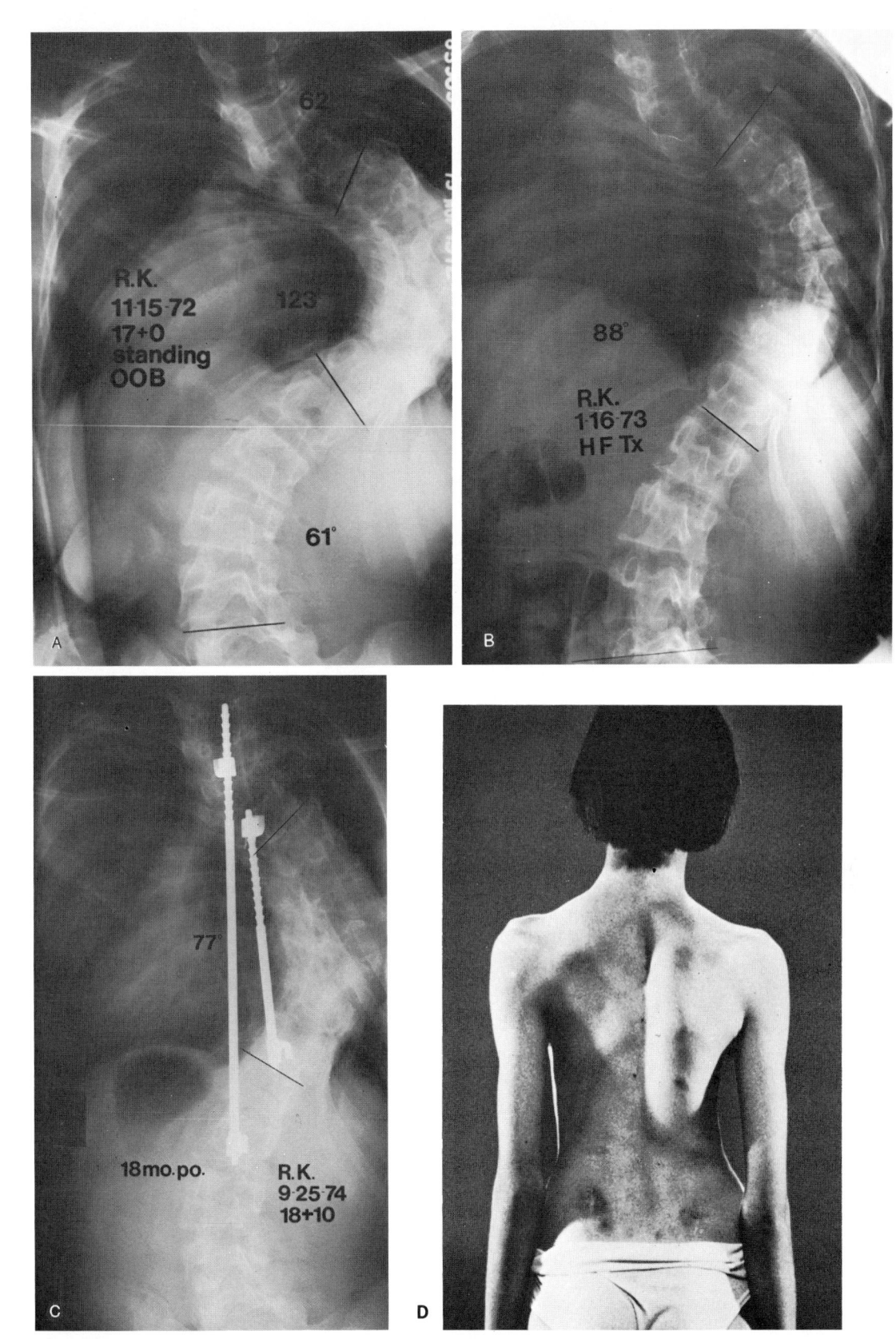

Figure 22–48. *A*, A 17 year old with a severe 123 degree curve associated with Marfan's syndrome. His vital capacity was markedly reduced. *B*, In halofemoral traction, his curve was reduced to 88 degrees. His vital capacity was improved by 500 cc., making his surgery safer. *C*, Eighteen months later, his curve was 77 degrees (it was 75 degrees at surgery). One single posterior operation was done. Anterior discectomy and fusion would have provided more correction, but at a higher risk because of his diminished vital capacity. *D*, His postoperative photograph.

better managed by preliminary discectomy than by traction. The best indications for traction are in the patient with large double major curves (e.g., 100 degrees/100 degrees or more) and the patient with significant cardiorespiratory compromise in whom traction could improve the pulmonary function so as to create a healthier patient at the time of surgery.

Attention to the sagittal plane deformity is quite important, as mentioned previously. Care must be taken when operating on a thoracic scoliosis not to have the lower limit of the fusion lie at the apex of a thoracolumbar or lumbar kyphosis.[1] In such a circumstance, the fusion should extend distally enough to control the kyphosis as well.

Some patients with Marfan's syndrome have been denied treatment based on a philosophy that they will die early from their cardiovascular disease. We do not agree with this, since the average life expectancy is 45, and it is improving with advances in cardiovascular surgery (Fig. 22–48).[11]

SUMMARY

Scoliosis is common in Marfan's syndrome, and has a strong tendency to progress to severe deformity. Pain is frequent in these curves. Non-operative treatment with orthoses has been successful in only a small percentage of patients. Surgical correction and stabilization has thus been the treatment of choice for most patients. Careful attention to sagittal plane alignment is critical, since reversal of normal patterns is frequent. Surgery should be directed just as much toward correction of sagittal plane deformity as toward the frontal plane (scoliosis) deformity.

References

1. Amis, J., and Herring, J.: Iatrogenic kyphosis: Complication of Harrington instrumentation in Marfan's syndrome. J. Bone Joint Surg., 66A:460–464, 1984.
2. Beals, R. K., and Heckt, F.: Congenital contractural arachnodactyly. J. Bone Joint Surg., 53A:987–993, 1971.
3. Beneux, J., Rigault, P., Poliquen, J. C., et al.: Les deviations rachidiennes de la maladie de Marfan chez l'enfant. Etude de 20 cas. Revue Chir. Orthop., 64:471–485, 1978.
4. Boucek, R. J., Noble, N. L., Gunta-Smith, A., and Butler, W. T.: The Marfan's syndrome, a deficiency in chemically stable collagen cross-links. New Engl. J. Med., 305:988–989, 1981.
5. Brenton, D. P., and Dow, D. J.: Homocystinuria and Marfan's syndrome. A comparison. J. Bone Joint Surg., 54B:277–298, 1972.
6. Fishman, E. K., Zinreich, S. J., Kumar, A. J., et al.: Sacral abnormalities in Marfan syndrome. J. Comput. Assist. Tomogr., 7:851–856, 1983.
7. LeDelliou, M.: Contribution a l'etude du syndrome de Marfan. Thesis, Universite Clande Bernard, Lyon, France, 1983.
8. Marfan, A. G.: Un cas de deformation congenitale des 4 membres plus prononcee aux extremities, caracterisee par l'allongement des os avec un certain degre d'amincissement. Bull. Soc. Med. Paris, 13:220–226, 1896.
9. McKusick, V. A.: Heritable Disorders of Connective Tissue. 4th ed. St. Louis, C. V. Mosby Co., 1972.
10. Morden, M. L., and Helfet, D.: Character of Spinal Deformities in Marfan's Syndrome. Am. Acad. Orthop. Surg., Anaheim, California, 1983.
11. Murdoch, J. L., Walter, B. A., Halpern, B. L., et al.: Life expectancy and causes of death in Marfan's syndrome. New Engl. J. Med., 286:804–808, 1972.
12. Orcutt, F. V., and DeWald, R. L.: The special problems which the Marfan syndrome introduces to scoliosis. J. Bone Joint Surg., 56A:1763, 1974.
13. Pyertiz, R. E.: Marfan syndrome. In Emergy, A., and Rimoin, D. (eds.): Principles and Practice of Medical Genetics. New York, Churchill Livingstone, pp. 820–835, 1983.
14. Pyeritz, R. E., and McKusick, V. A.: The Marfan syndrome: Diagnosis and management. New Engl. J. Med., 300:772–777, 1979.
15. Pyeritz, R. E., and McKusick, V. A.: Basic defects in the Marfan syndrome. New Engl. J. Med., 305:1011–1012, 1981.
16. Robins, P. R., Moe, J. H., and Winter, R. B.: Scoliosis in Marfan's syndrome, its characteristics and results of treatment of 35 patients. J. Bone Joint Surg., 57A:358–368, 1975.
17. Savini, R., Cervellati, S., and Beroaldo, E.: Le deformita vertebrali nella sindrome di Marfan. J. Ital. Orthop. Traumatol., 6:19–40, 1980.
18. Wanderman, K. L., Goldstein, M. S., and Faver, J.: Cor pulmonale secondary to severe kyphoscoliosis in Marfan's syndrome. Chest, 67:250–251, 1971.
19. Wilner, H. I., and Finby, J.: Skeletal manifestations in the Marfan syndrome. JAMA, 197:490–495, 1975.
20. Winter, R. B.: Severe spondylolisthesis in Marfan's syndrome. Report of two cases. J. Pediatr. Orthop., 2:51–55, 1982.

Arthrogryposis
Robert B. Winter, M.D.

Arthrogryposis was first described in 1841 by Otto. Stern, in 1923, is generally credited with originating the name arthrogryposis multiplex congenita. Scoliosis has been mentioned in numerous articles concerning the problem, but the incidence has varied from 0 per cent to 42 per cent. The cause of arthrogryposis is as yet unknown. The diagnosis may be quite difficult since there are no histologic, laboratory, or clinical tests specific for the condition. Many similar conditions are, thus, often included within this diagnosis.

The widely accepted diagnostic criteria include: (1) multiple flexion or extension contractures present at birth, (2) marked limitation of active and passive motion of the involved joints but relatively free motion over the small range of motion remaining, (3) cylindrical and fusiform joints, (4) intact sensation, (5) diminished or absent deep tendon reflexes, and (6) muscular atrophy (non-progressive). Skin creases over the joints are generally absent. Flexion contractures are usually associated with skin webbing across the joint.

Drummond and McKenzie[2] reported 50 patients with arthrogryposis. All had rigid contractures present at birth involving at least two extremities. Scoliosis occurred in 14 of the 50 patients reviewed, an incidence of 28 per cent. There were eight girls and six boys. Eight of the 14 patients had curves of at least 40 degrees by age 10. Only two of the 50 children died in childhood; both of these had severe scoliosis. Seven of the patients had congenital scoliosis associated with their arthrogryposis. Four children had long curves typical of paralytic scoliosis, and these occurred either in infancy or in early child-

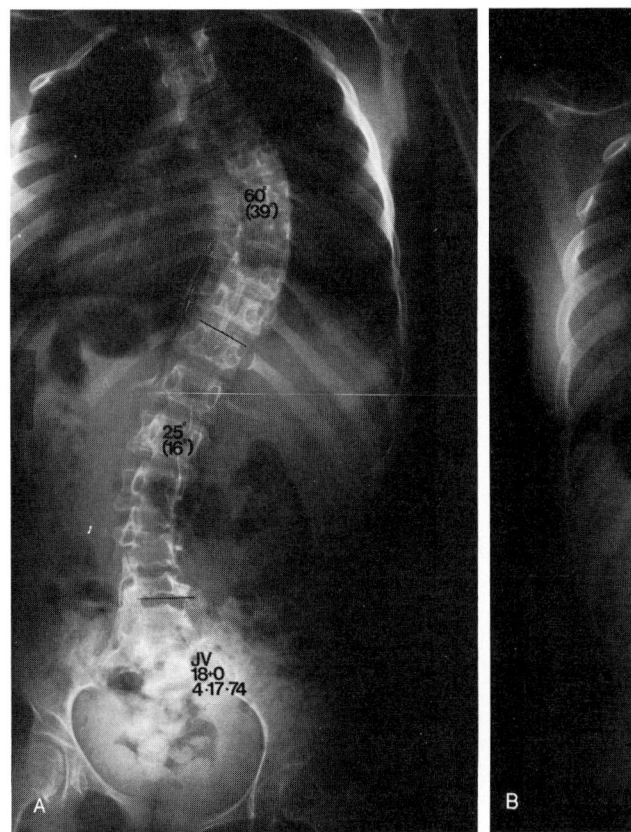

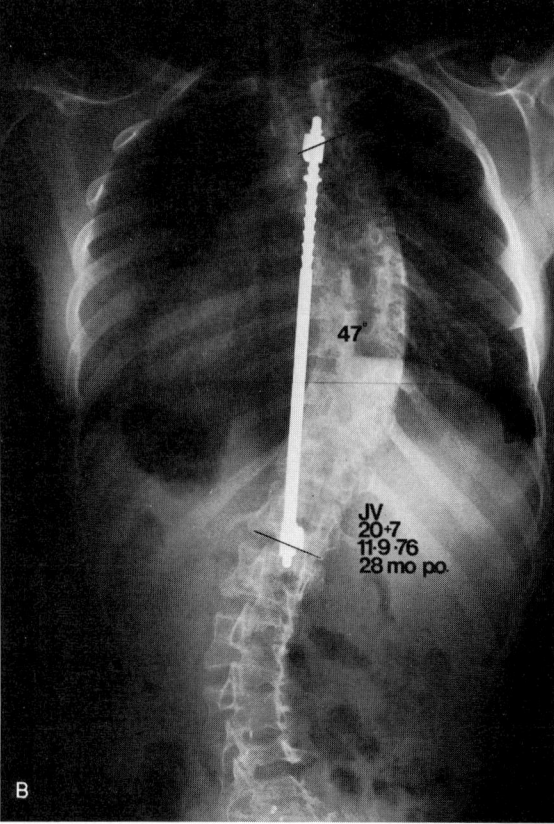

Figure 22–49. *A*, This 18 year old girl with arthrogryposis had a 60 degree right thoracic scoliosis and no pelvic obliquity. *B*, She was stabilized by a standard posterior fusion (T3-L1) with Harrington distraction rodding. A Risser cast was used postoperatively (surgery in 1974).

hood. These progressed to become long, rigid, decompensated curves. The authors recommended prompt treatment of the curve before it became severe.

Spencer, Millar, and Brown[5] reported on 112 patients with arthrogryposis of whom 35 had spinal deformity. Eight of these had congenital anomalies, usually defects of segmentation. Seventeen had collapsing paralytic type curves. Twenty-four had curves less than 20 degrees. The collapsing type of scoliosis appeared to be common to the patient who was severely involved and was non- or minimally ambulatory.

Herron, Westin, and Dawson[3] reviewed 88 patients with arthrogryposis and found scoliosis in 18. In most of the patients, the curvatures were progressive and became very structural quite early in the disease. They did not have good experience with bracing and found that when fusion was necessary, it usually had to be extended to the sacrum. Pelvic obliquity was a very significant problem.

The most recent report is by Bernstein[1] who reviewed 59 patient records, and found scoliosis to be present in 30 per cent. Two of these were congenital, one measuring 60 degrees and the other 70 degrees.

These curvatures are not easy to treat. Brace treatment appears to be satisfactory only for relatively flexible curves of 50 degrees or less, particularly in growing children. Exercises, stretching, and manipulation appear to have no benefit.

Often the patient has so many other significant handicapping problems that the scoliosis is ignored. This is not an appropriate form of management, since of all the problems the patient has, it is only the scoliosis that can be life-threatening.

Many patients thus come to surgery. The connective tissue is noted to be tough and tight, and the bones are osteoporotic. The percentage of correction is usually relatively small. In our personal experience, blood loss has been larger than in similar curves of idiopathic etiology. Fusion to the sacrum is often, but not always, necessary. It should be done if there is pelvic obliquity due to the scoliosis. Patients with congenital scoliosis should have treatment according to the rules for congenital scoliosis (see Chapter 12). The bones heal well, and pseudarthrosis has been minimal.

Segmental fixation with Luque instrumentation would appear to have significant advantage for these patients, although no such series has been reported. (Fig. 22–49).

References

1. Bernstein, S.: Arthrogryposis: long-term followup. Presented to the Pediatric Orthopaedic Study Group, Nashville, Tennessee, 1981.
2. Drummond, D., and McKenzie, D. A.: Scoliosis in arthrogryposis multiplex congenita. Spine, 3:146–151, 1978.
3. Herron, L. D., Westin, G. W., and Dawson, E. G.: Scoliosis in arthrogryposis multiplex congenita. J. Bone Joint Surg., 60A:293–299, 1978.
4. Siebold, R. M., Winter, R. B., and Moe, J. H.: The treatment of scoliosis in arthrogryposis multiplex congenita. Clin. Orthop., 0(103):191–198, 1974.
5. Spencer, D., Millar, E., and Brown, J. C.: Spinal deformity in arthrogryposis multiplex congenita. Presented to the Scoliosis Research Society, Hong Kong, 1977.

Osteogenesis Imperfecta
David S. Bradford, M.D.

Osteogenesis imperfecta is one of the most common hereditary disorders of connective tissue.[14] It is only in more recent times that the management of spinal deformities in this group of patients has been given the attention it rightfully deserves.[1–7, 10, 12, 18, 20, 25]

INCIDENCE AND NATURAL HISTORY

The classification of osteogenesis imperfecta has varied considerably from one reported series to the other. Looser, in 1906, classified the condition as either "congenita" or "tarda" and stated that both types were expressions of the same disease.[13] In the "congenita" form, the child had multiple fractures that occurred sometime before birth, micromelia, and caput membranacum. He felt this type was caused by an autosomal dominant mutation or could develop secondary to autosomal recessive inheritance. In the "tarda" form, fractures occurred at the time of birth or later. This type is inherited as an autosomal dominant trait with incomplete penetrance and variable expressivity. Seedorff[21] further divided this classification scheme based on the age of the first fracture into a "gravis" or a "levis" variety. Falvo[9] divided the tarda group into Type I and Type II, depending upon whether bowing of the long bones was present or not (Type I patients demonstrate bowing of the long bones, whereas type II patients do not). Sillence[22] more recently (1979) divided osteogenesis imperfecta patients into four groups, depending upon the mode of inheritance, the severity of the disease, and the presenting findings.

Since the classification of disease types has varied so much between different authors, an accurate portrayal of the incidence of scoliosis is difficult to establish. King and Bobechko,[12] using Seedorff's classification, found 43 per cent of patients with osteogenesis imperfecta "congenita" had scoliosis, whereas 70 per cent of the "tarda gravis" patients and 28 per cent of the tarda levis patients demonstrated scoliosis. Thoracic curves were most common. Falvo and co-workers, using their classification, found scoliosis in 92 per cent of patients with osteogenesis imperfecta. The incidence of scoliosis from other reported series has ranged from 50 to 80 per cent.[4-6, 18, 20]

Benson and associates[5] noted that, in 103 patients in whom x-rays were available for evaluation, 62 per cent of the patients had some degree of curvature. The percentage of patients with spinal deformity increased significantly after age five; before age five, 26 per cent of patients had curvatures, whereas in older children the figure rose to 82 per cent. When a curvature was noted, early progression could be expected. That progression may continue in the adult period, as supported by the recent work of Moorefield and Miller.[16] In fact, these authors noted that 50 per cent of their original 31 patients in the adult period had scoliosis, whereas in the childhood and adolescent periods, only 25 per cent had been noted to have scoliosis.

The etiology of spinal deformity is unknown. It may well be caused by a combination of several factors related to the softness or brittleness of the bone, which leads to compression fractures and vertebral collapse.[15, 16] Multiple fractures with alterations of vertebral growth plates,[14] laxity of ligaments with loss of intrinsic support to the spine, and abnormalities of the biochemistry and physiology of the intervertebral disc and soft tissues could all be associated with the pathogenesis of scoliosis and kyphotic curvatures. Paraplegia has been reported following manipulation of the spine.[26]

TREATMENT

The treatment of spinal deformities in isolated cases has been described.[2, 10, 12, 20] More recent and larger series have shown rather conclusively that non-operative treatment by orthotic devices has rarely if ever been successful, and may result in further chest wall deformity (Fig. 22-50).[5-7] In the largest series reported to date by Yong-Hing and MacEwen,[25] the authors have reviewed results of treatment in 121 patients from 51 orthopaedic surgeons in 14 countries. Of the 73 patients treated by bracing, the curvatures increased in all but 15 cases. It should be noted, however, that in only two of their cases had brace wear been discontinued and, in seven of the patients, brace treatment had been for less than 12 months. Sixty patients had undergone a spinal fusion, and complications had occurred in 33.

Our own experience would support the findings from these previous studies. Spinal bracing to control progressive scoliosis would appear ill advised and without benefit. Bracing has been of some help in controlling symptoms relating to kyphosis with compression fractures, however. It is also noted that patients with osteogenesis imperfecta may also have a decreased pulmonary function but this correlates more with the presence of scoliosis than the disease process itself.[8] Constructing braces and plaster casts that further compromise the chest cage can only aggravate this problem.

For progressive spinal curvatures, spinal fusion with instrumentation posteriorly is the procedure of choice. Although the bone stock appears deficient anteriorly and porotic based on x-ray evaluation, this is not necessarily true and in fact the posterior neural arch appears quite adequate to maintain fixation with a Harrington device or other metal construct. If the fixation appears in jeopardy and the bone is soft and osteoporotic, we would agree with Waugh[23] that the fixation may be more secure with the use of methylmethacrylate around the upper hook (Fig. 22-51). We have done segmental instrumentation with Luque rods and sublaminar wires

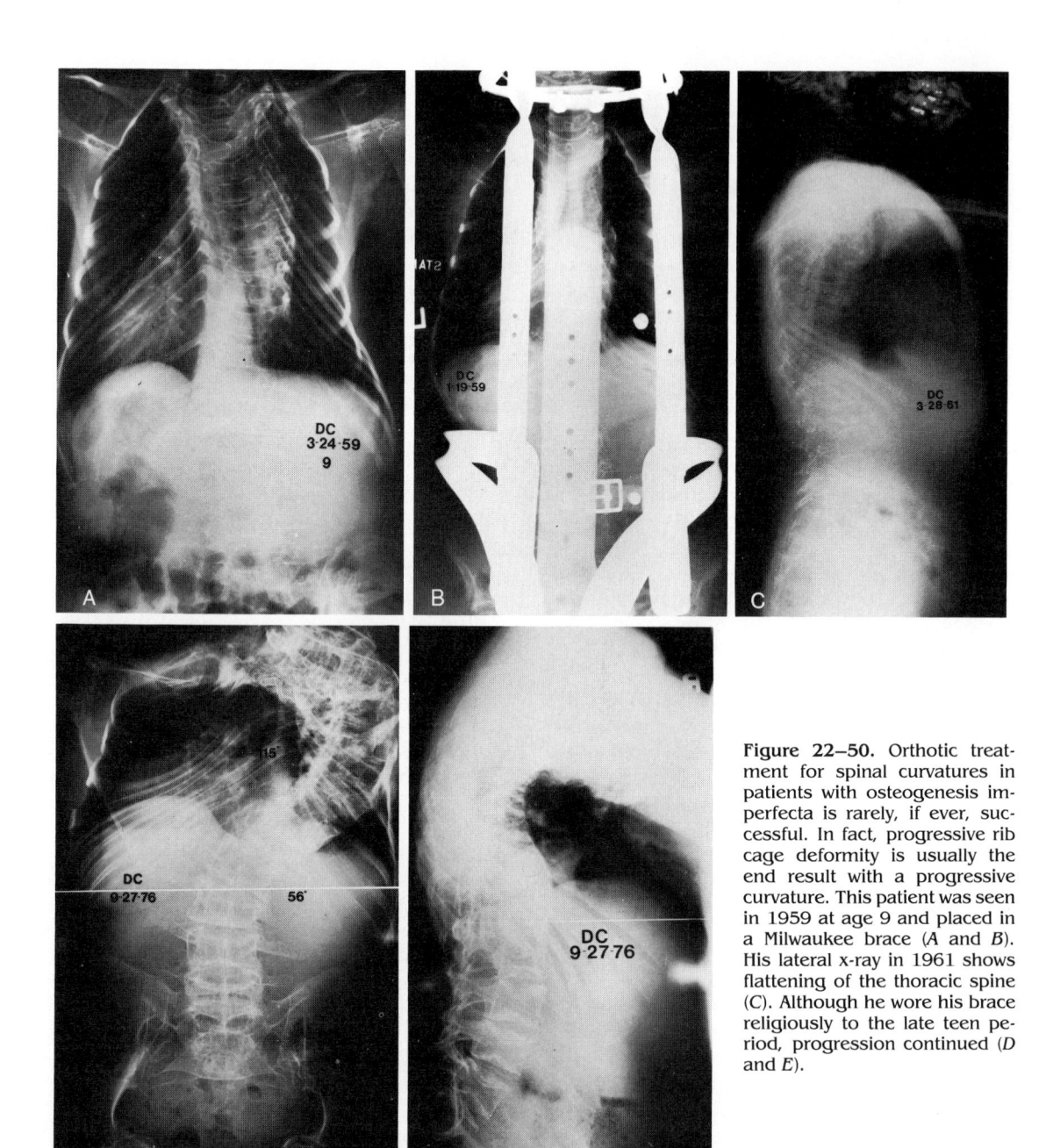

Figure 22–50. Orthotic treatment for spinal curvatures in patients with osteogenesis imperfecta is rarely, if ever, successful. In fact, progressive rib cage deformity is usually the end result with a progressive curvature. This patient was seen in 1959 at age 9 and placed in a Milwaukee brace (*A* and *B*). His lateral x-ray in 1961 shows flattening of the thoracic spine (*C*). Although he wore his brace religiously to the late teen period, progression continued (*D* and *E*).

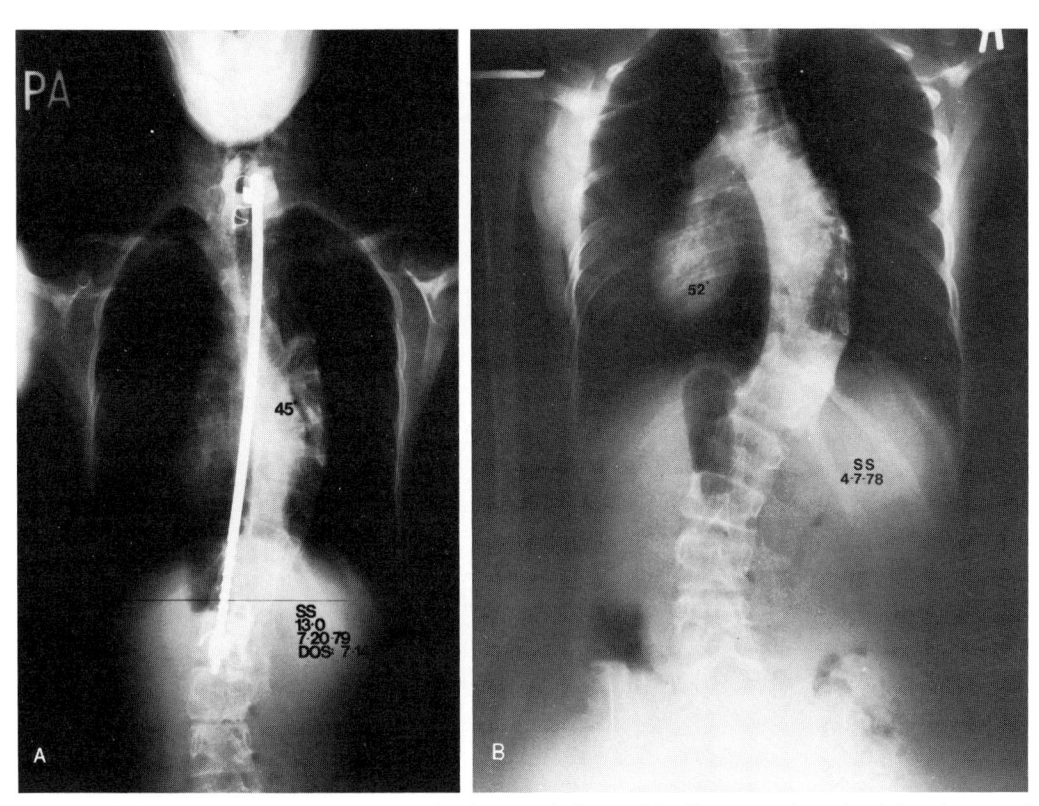

Figure 22–51. *A* and *B*, If a Harrington distraction implant is favored for the correction of a deformity associated with instrumentation, methacrylate fixation at the end hook sites has proved useful.

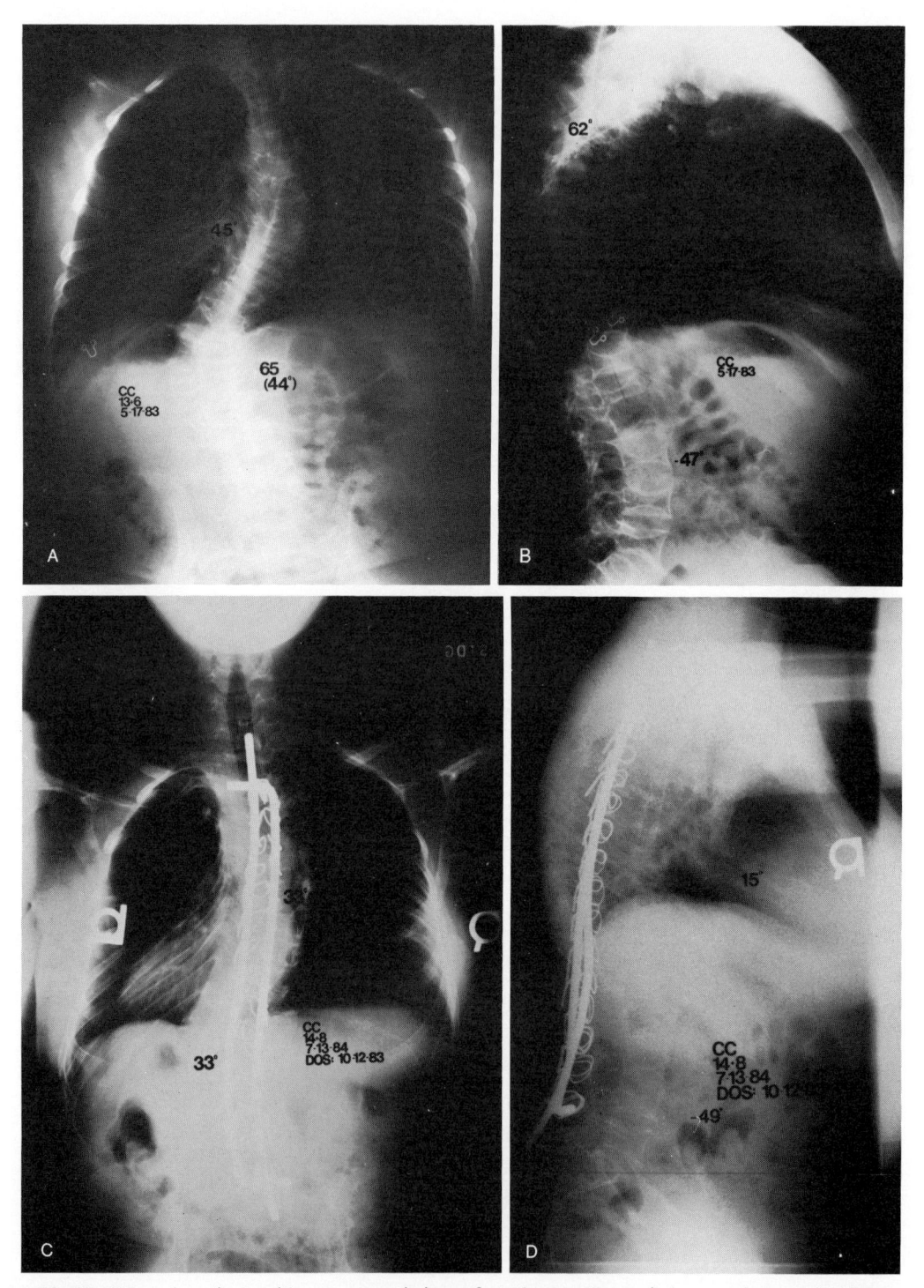

Figure 22–52. Although patients with osteogenesis imperfecta have osteopenic bone, adequate fixation usually may be obtained with segmental fixation. This patient with severe osteogenesis imperfecta obtained a satisfactory correction with a solid arthrodesis following spinal fusion with segmental instrumentation using the L-rod system. (*A* and *B*, Preoperative AP and lateral radiographs; *C* and *D*, follow-up AP and lateral radiographs.)

on several patients. Although again the bone is somewhat osteoporotic and it appears to bleed more than that in idiopathic cases, the security of fixation, the degree of correction, and the solidification of fusion have been most satisfactory. We would recommend the use of autogenous bone if possible, supplemented with bank bone if necessary.

It is our recommendation that if treatment is indicated for progressive curvatures, the treatment of choice is spinal fusion with instrumentation, preferably segmental instrumentation supplemented by external orthosis until fusion is solid (Fig. 22–52).

Spondylolisthesis may occur in association with osteogenesis imperfecta,[19] and this may either be of the pathologic variety with elongation of the pedicle, or lysis of the pars interarticularis.[17, 24] The management of this problem would be no different than the management of spondylolisthesis without osteogenesis imperfecta.

References

1. Albright, J. A.: Management overview of osteogenesis imperfecta. Clin. Orthop. Rel. Res., 159:80–87, 1981.
2. Albright, J. A., and Grunt, J. A.: Studies of patients with osteogenesis imperfecta. J. Bone Joint Surg., 53A:1415–1425, 1971.
3. Bauze, R. J., Smith, R., and Francis, M. J. O.: A new look at osteogenesis imperfecta. A clinical, radiological and biochemical study of 42 patients. J. Bone Joint Surg., 57B:1–12, 1975.
4. Beighton, P., Spranger, J., and Versveld, G.: Skeletal complications in osteogenesis imperfecta. A review of 153 South African patients. S. Afr. Med. J., 64:565–568, 1983.
5. Benson, D. R., and Donaldson, D. H.: The spine in osteogenesis imperfecta. J. Bone Joint Surg., 60A:925–929, 1978.
6. Benson, D. R., and Newman, D. C.: The spine and surgical treatment in osteogenesis imperfecta. Clin. Orthop. Rel. Res., 159:147–153, 1981.
7. Cristofaro, R. L., Hoek, K. J., Bonnett, C. A., and Brown, J. C.: Operative treatment of spine deformity in osteogenesis imperfecta. Clin. Orthop. Rel. Res., 139:40–48, 1979.
8. Falvo, K. A., Klain, D. B., and Krauss, A. N.: Pulmonary function studies in osteogenesis imperfecta. Am. Rev. Respir. Dis., 108:258, 1973.
9. Falvo, K. A., Root, L., and Bullough, P. G.: Osteogenesis imperfecta. Clinical evaluation and management. J. Bone Joint Surg., 56A:783, 1974.
10. Gitelis, S., Whiffen, J., and DeWald, R. L.: The treatment of severe scoliosis in osteogenesis imperfecta. Clin. Orthop. Rel. Res., 175:56–59, 1983.
11. Herndon, C. N.: Osteogenesis imperfecta: some clinical and genetic considerations. Clin. Orthop., 8:132, 1956.
12. King, J. D., and Bobechko, W. P.: Osteogenesis imperfecta. J. Bone Joint Surg., 53B:72–89, 1971.
13. Looser, E.: Zur Kenntnis der osteogenesis imperfecta und tarda (sogenannte idiopatische Osteopsathyrosis). Mitt. Grenzgeb. Med. Chir., 15:161–207, 1906.
14. McKusick, V. A.: Heritable Disorders of Connective Tissues, 4th ed. St. Louis, C. V. Mosby Co., 1972.
15. Milgram, J. W., Flick, M. R., and Engh, C. A.: Osteogenesis imperfecta: a histopathological case report. J. Bone Joint Surg., 55A:506–515, 1973.
16. Moorefield, W. G., and Miller, G. R.: Aftermath of osteogenesis imperfecta: the disease of adulthood. J. Bone Joint Surg., 62A:113–119, 1980.
17. Newman, P. H.: The etiology of spondylolisthesis. J. Bone Joint Surg., 45B:39, 1963.
18. Norimatsu, H., Mayuzumi, T., and Takahashi, T.: The development of the spinal deformities in osteogenesis imperfecta. Clin. Orthop. Rel. Res., 162:20–25, 1982.
19. Rask, M. R.: Spondylolisthesis resulting from osteogenesis imperfecta; report of a case. Clin. Orthop. Rel. Res., 139:164–166, 1979.
20. Renshaw, T. S., Cook, R. S., and Albright, J. A.: Scoliosis in osteogenesis imperfecta. Clin. Orthop. Rel. Res., 145:163–167, 1979.
21. Seedorff, K.: Osteogenesis imperfecta: a study of the clinical features and heredity based on 55 Danish families comprising 180 affected members. Opera ex Domo Biologiae Hereditariae Humanae Universitatis Hafniensis. Arhus: Universitetsforlaget, p. 20, 1949.
22. Sillence, D. O., Senn, A., and Danks, D. M.: Genetic heterogeneity in osteogenesis imperfecta. J. Med. Genet., 16:101–116, 1979.
23. Waugh, T. R.: The biomechanical basis for the utilization of methyl methacrylate in the treatment of scoliosis. J. Bone Joint Surg., 53A:194–195, 1971.
24. Wiltse, L.: Spinal Disorders, Diagnosis and Treatment. Philadelphia, Lea and Febiger, p. 199, 1977.
25. Yong-Hing, K., and MacEwen, G. D.: Scoliosis associated with osteogenesis imperfecta, results of treatment. J. Bone Joint Surg., 64B:36–43, 1982.
26. Ziv, I., Rang, M., and Hoffman, H. J.: Paraplegia in osteogenesis imperfecta. A case report. J. Bone Joint Surg., 65B:184–185, 1983.

Osteomyelitis
Robert B. Winter, M.D.

INTRODUCTION

Infection of the spine can lead to destruction of bone and result in spinal deformity. There are many different organisms that can infect the spine, but the most important by far is tuberculosis. The majority of this chapter will therefore deal with tuberculosis, with a smaller section on non-tuberculous infections.

TUBERCULOSIS

History

Tuberculosis is an ancient orthopaedic disease, having been noted in Egyptian mummies dating from 3000 B.C.[6] The first written description was given by Hippocrates (450 B.C.).[15] It was Sir Percival Pott who first accurately described the disease that bears his name, and his description included autopsy findings.[20]

Incidence

Tuberculosis is still prevalent in many parts of the world, especially Asia, Africa, Mexico, and parts of South America. In countries with adequate housing, good nutrition, and good public health preventive measures, the disease is almost extinct. However, an increasingly mobile world population has brought large numbers of infected individuals from underdeveloped countries into the more developed countries, thus making necessary a constant awareness for tuberculosis.

Site

The spine is frequently involved in tuberculosis. Hodgson reported that of 1000 consecutive cases of bone and joint tuberculosis, the spine was involved in 58.7 per cent.[18] This contrasts to non-tuberculous bone infections in which the spine is involved in only 2 to 5 per cent of cases.[22]

There is a marked predilection for involvement at the thoracolumbar junction, with a rapid fall-off above and below this level. However, any level from C1 to the sacrum can be involved. The high incidence at L1 is thought to be related to its close proximity to the kidneys. Seeding to the spine is thought to occur by way of Batson's venous plexus.[18] The sexes are equally susceptible as are all age groups. Children are most commonly affected in the underdeveloped countries and adults in the more developed countries.

Pathogenesis

Once the tubercle bacilli reach the vertebral body, infection is established and follows a definite pattern. The first stage is a prepurulent inflammatory reaction with Langhan's giant cells, epitheloid cells, and small inflammatory cells. Initially, the inflammation is closely related to the blood vessels but spreads rapidly, with thrombosis of vessels, cellular edema, and death. There is also a hypersensitivity immune reaction, adding to the inflammatory process. With the spread of the infection and tissue necrosis, a paraspinal abscess is formed.

The paraspinal abscess is the hallmark of active spinal tuberculosis and is the first visible radiologic sign. It is small at first and surrounded by edema of the paraspinal soft tissues. The abscess gradually enlarges as more tissues die. Initially the pus is fluid and greenish-yellow, but later in the disease process it becomes thicker and whiter with the consistency of toothpaste. After many years it becomes still thicker and even solid as calcification occurs. In the pus are small necrotic fragments of bone (sequestrae), cartilage, and granulation tissue.

As the abscess spreads, it strips the periosteum off the vertebrae, rendering them avascular. This avascular bone then has no resistance to the spreading infection. These avascular fragments of bone may be destroyed or become sequestrae. Bony sequestrae can displace posteriorly into the spinal canal and press against the spinal cord. The outer layers of the anulus fibrosus of the disc are continuous with the periosteum of the vertebrae and are elevated away from the

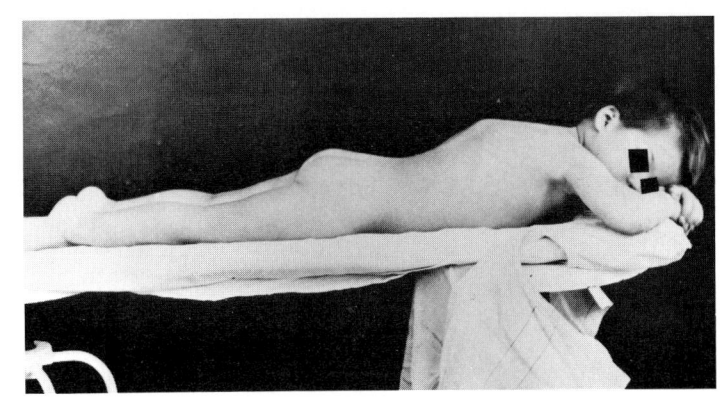

Figure 22–53. A 6 year old child with a thoracolumbar gibbus due to tuberculosis.

disc. The disc remains as an avascular and intact structure, and is not involved in the disease. If the bone above and below the disc becomes involved, the disc itself may become detached and float free in the pus.

The abscess cavity is surrounded by a wall of granulation tissue, with edema of the surrounding tissue. When the abscess is in contact with the dura, an inflammatory reaction that can result in pachymeningitis occurs. With healing of the infection, the granulation tissue becomes fibrous and may "strangulate" the cord, producing a late-onset and irreversible paraplegia.

With increasing pressure in the abscess, the body attempts to discharge the pus to the exterior, producing the classic paravertebral or psoas abscesses. These may spontaneously drain or require surgical drainage.

As the vertebral bodies are destroyed, the mechanical stability of the spine is lost and the combined effects of muscle tension and gravity result in spinal collapse. Since it is only the vertebral bodies and not the posterior elements that are destroyed, a kyphosis develops. The more vertebral bodies destroyed, the worse the kyphosis.

With control of the disease by the body's own defenses as well as medical treatment, the inflammation and the progressive bony destruction cease and gradual revascularization of the dead tissues take place. Spontaneous fibrous or even bony ankylosis of the vertebrae occurs. Despite apparent healing, tiny pockets of live bacteria may remain dormant for years. Later on, with decreased resistance owing to age, other disease, or steroid medication, the infection may reactivate and produce clinical disease once again.

In growing children, a progressive kyphosis can occur even though there is no progression of bony destruction. This is because of the destruction of the anterior vertebral growth plates. It is quite similar to the progressive congenital kyphosis due to congenital absence of these growth plates. Compensatory lordoses develop proximal and distal to the area of kyphosis. The lumbar vertebrae become tall and narrow rather than retaining the normal shorter and thicker structure (Figure 22–53).

Differential Diagnosis

In the advanced case, the findings are usually so classic as to leave little doubt as to the diagnosis. Vertebral destruction, kyphosis, disc sparing, and localized calcification are pathognomonic. In the early stages, the diagnosis may be much more difficult. Non-tuberculous infection and neoplasm are the two likely alternative diagnoses. Old, healed lesions may resemble congenital kyphosis.

Evaluation should include examination for other evidence of tuberculosis with Mantoux testing, sputum and gastric washings for tuberculosis, urine culture for tuberculosis, and chest roentgenogram for evidence of pulmonary tuberculosis.

Spinal radiographs should include supine anteroposterior and lateral views for bone detail, and laminograms (tomograms) or a CT scan for more precise detail. A CT scan is particularly valuable for detection of early disease and soft tissue spread.[2] It should be remembered that more than one area of the spine can be involved.

Needle biopsy to obtain samples for histology and culture is *not* recommended. Areas of necrosis, which are non-diagnostic and sterile, may be biopsied. In addition, there is considerable risk of hemorrhage. Open bi-

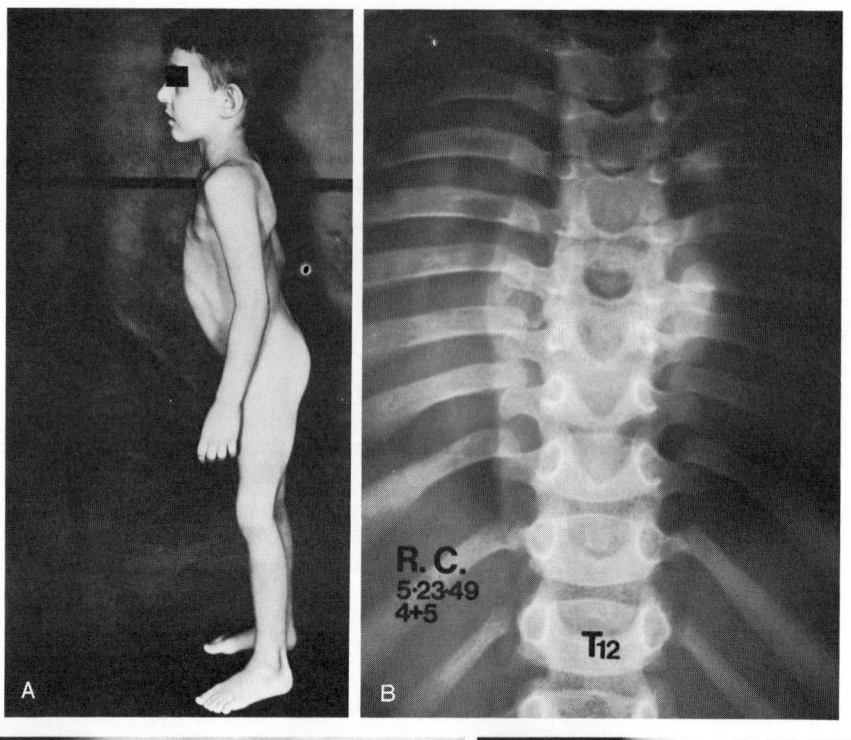

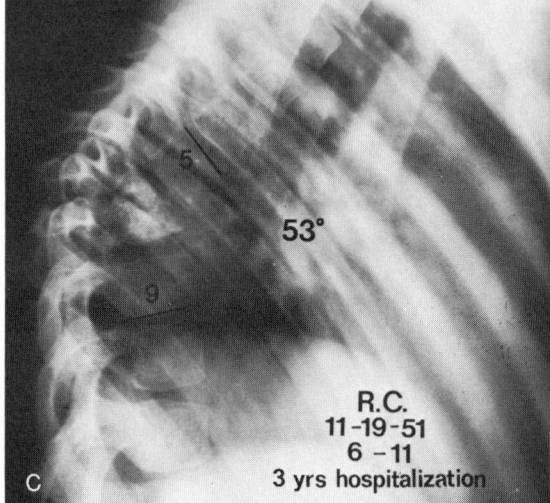

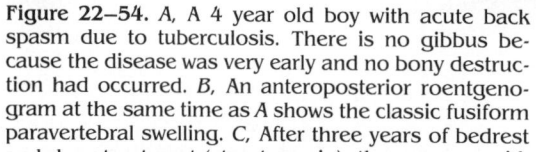

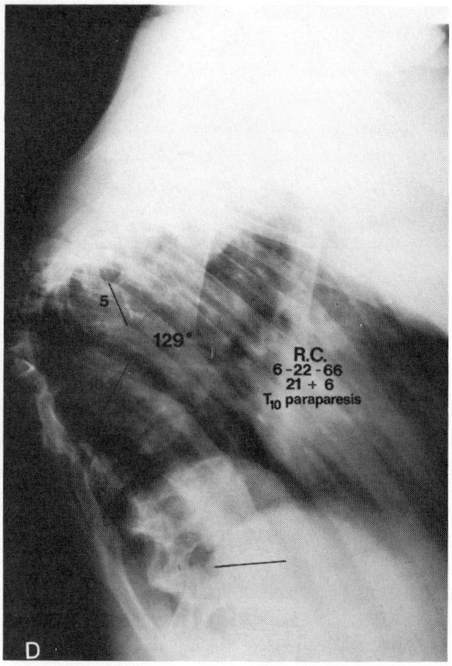

Figure 22–54. *A*, A 4 year old boy with acute back spasm due to tuberculosis. There is no gibbus because the disease was very early and no bony destruction had occurred. *B*, An anteroposterior roentgenogram at the same time as *A* shows the classic fusiform paravertebral swelling. *C*, After three years of bedrest and drug treatment (streptomycin), there was considerable collapse and a kyphosis of 53 degrees. At age 10 he developed sudden paraplegia, which was relieved by costotransversectomy and drainage of pus. A posterior fusion was done. *D*, At age 21 he again presented with slow onset paraplegia, but no sign of active disease. His posterior fusion had not prevented late collapse. His paraplegia was due to angulation and not to active disease. Anterior cord decompression and anterior fusion gave relief of his paralysis, and he had no further problems.

opsy via a transthoracic or retroperitoneal approach is preferable. Adequate sampling can be performed, drainage can be established, and thorough debridement done. Sensitivity testing should be done on the sample, since there is an increasing number of resistant strains (Fig. 22–54).

Treatment

HISTORICAL

In his 1779 monograph, Pott wrote, "The remedy for this dreadful disease consists merely in procuring a large discharge of matter."[3] Often a red-hot iron was applied to the bulging abscess in order to establish drainage.

With the introduction of aseptic surgery at the end of the nineteenth century, direct operative drainage became the procedure of choice. In 1891, Hadra, a German doctor practicing in Galveston, Texas, performed the first internal fixation of the spine; he used silver wire around the spinous processes in a case of tuberculosis.[13] Successful arthrodesis was first reported by Hibbs in 1911.[14]

The public health measures of sequestering active disease patients in sanitoria so they could receive "fresh air and sunshine" probably helped many of them to recover. However, equally important was the removal of infected patients so they could not infect others. The routine vaccination of cows and the killing of all infected cattle also removed the source of bovine tuberculosis. These measures markedly reduced the incidence and prevalence of tuberculosis in developed countries long before the advent of chemotherapy.

In 1945, streptomycin was introduced, the first drug to be effective against *Mycobacterium tuberculosis*. Para-aminosalicylic acid was developed in 1946 and isoniazid in 1951. Many other drugs have been more recently introduced.

Capener,[3] Cott and Alexander, and Griffiths are names important in the development of approaches to the abscesses and to the spine itself by the costrotransversectomy or "lateral rachotomy" route.[8] These techniques remained important until the development of the direct transthoracic approach by Hodgson and Stock in 1955.[16] This latter technique had actually been well described previously in Japan by Ito, Tsuchiya, and Asami[21] in 1934, but had not been widely accepted because antibiotics were not available.

There is no single best treatment for spinal tuberculosis; the proper treatment varies according to several factors. It is just as wrong to say that surgery is never indicated, as it is to say that surgery is always indicated. Antimicrobial therapy is fundamental to all treatment programs, usually 18 months of at least two and sometimes three different drugs. Streptomycin, isoniazid, and rifampin are the current drugs of choice.[20] Details of drug treatment are beyond the scope of this chapter and should be sought elsewhere.[20]

One treatment method is the use of drugs with no other form of therapy. The drugs are given on an outpatient basis with no bedrest, no brace, no cast, and no surgery. A second treatment method is drugs plus ambulatory support with a cast or brace. The third treatment method is surgical debridement of the lesion with bone grafting, casting, and drugs.

Considerable controversy existed as to the merits of these different treatment programs, and many scientific reports were written supporting one technique or another. Seldom were there any controls or matched groups, and it became impossible to know the relative value of any one technique. Finally, in the 1960's, the Medical Research Council of Great Britain formed a Working Party on Tuberculosis of the Spine, which set out to design and execute controlled studies of different treatment programs in various parts of the world. The study was restricted to thoracic and lumbar involvement in non-paralyzed patients (mostly children).

In Masan, Korea, ambulatory outpatient drug treatment was compared with the same drug treatment with an initial six month period of in-hospital bedrest.[24] In Pusan, Korea, ambulatory outpatient drug treatment was used in all, but one half of the patients were supported in a plaster cast.[25, 28] In Bulawayo, Rhodesia (Zimbabwe), ambulatory outpatient therapy was compared with simple surgical debridement.[26] In Hong Kong, debridement alone was compared with debridement and grafting.[27]

A favorable result in the study was defined as radiologically healed disease with all sinuses and abscesses healed, full physical activity, and no central nervous system involvement. In Masan, Pusan, and Bulawayo, the ambulant outpatient groups showed 88 per cent, 82 per cent, and 86 per cent favorable results. The use of six months of bedrest, nine months of casting, or open surgical debridement did not significantly alter the results.

In Hong Kong, debridement *and grafting* were compared with debridement alone. Results were analyzed at both five year[28] and ten year[29] intervals. At three years, both groups had the same percentage of healed lesions (87 per cent). At five years, the grafted group had 93 per cent solid bony fusion, whereas the debridement only group had 69 per cent solid bony fusion. At ten years, the incidence of bony fusion was the same, the grafted group having achieved bony union sooner. No patient in either group had developed a sinus, abscess, or neurologic deficit in the interval between five and ten years. The chief difference between the two groups was in the development of kyphosis. There was less loss of vertical height and less kyphosis in the grafted group, both differences being highly statistically significant.

In the Korean groups with no surgical debridement, only 46 per cent had bony fusion at five years compared with the 69 per cent with debridement and 93 per cent with grafting in Hong Kong. In addition, only one patient in Hong Kong developed subsequent paraparesis, whereas 43 developed paralysis while under treatment in the other centers.

In summary, ambulatory outpatient drug treatment will provide approximately 85 per cent of patients with healing of the active disease, a stable spine, and no paralysis. The other 15 per cent may have failure of tuberculous eradication, failure to prevent spinal collapse, or failure to prevent subsequent paraplegia. The addition of radical debridement, bone grafting, and cast protection can raise the true success rate to 95 per cent or better.

CURRENT TREATMENT, ACUTE DISEASE

Early Involvement, One Vertebra Only. In the early stages of the disease, the patient may present with malaise, night sweats, low grade fever, back pain, and back spasm. There will be the radiologic findings of destruction of one vertebra and paravertebral swelling. If the result of the Mantoux test is positive and the findings classic, then a presumptive diagnosis can be made and drug treatment started, usually with two drugs. The use of a cast or brace will make the patient more comfortable until the acute inflammatory process has subsided. In such an early situation with only one vertebra involved, surgical treatment is not necessary unless there is a failure of this non-operative approach. Drug treatment is usually for 18 months.

Early Involvement, Two or More Vertebrae. When there is destruction of two or more vertebral bodies, the above management is not adequate unless there are no facilities for operative treatment. We feel that the Hodgson approach of direct anterior exposure, debridement of the abscess and its contents back to raw bleeding bone, and the insertion of autogenous bone grafts is the procedure of choice.[1, 17] This surgery is done after a short period of drug treatment, bedrest, and nutritional build-up. Posterior fusion is also done in order to provide more stability and prevent progressive kyphosis.[12]

Pinto and Avanzi[31] have advocated the use of an anterior distracting device (see discussion of the Santa Casa distractor) and rib strut grafts, the distracting device being only temporary in order to achieve correction of the kyphosis; the correction is held by the strut grafts. Posterior fusion is also done. A cast is used postoperatively for nine months.

More recently, Cardosa and coworkers[4] reported on the use of bone chips anteriorly rather than strut grafts. One to two weeks later a posterior spinal fusion with Luque instrumentation was performed. No cast or brace was used. Their average kyphosis in 22 cases was 69 degrees preoperatively and 39 degrees postoperatively.

Active tuberculosis of the cervical spine often results in paralysis, and it requires aggressive treatment with anterior debridement, anterior fusion, and halo cast support. Posterior fusion is not necessary.[19] Transoral decompression may be necessary for C1 involvement.[11]

Acute Disease with Spinal Cord Involvement. Although bedrest, casting, and drug treatment can result in reversal of paralysis in some cases, the results are both better and much more rapid with a surgical approach. After a brief period of a few days with bedrest, drug treatment, nutritional support, and general evaluation, an anterior approach should be done. The abscess and its contents are removed, and the dura is thoroughly exposed throughout the diseased area. Bone grafts are added, either struts or chips, depending on the technique being utilized. The

MISCELLANEOUS PROBLEMS 573

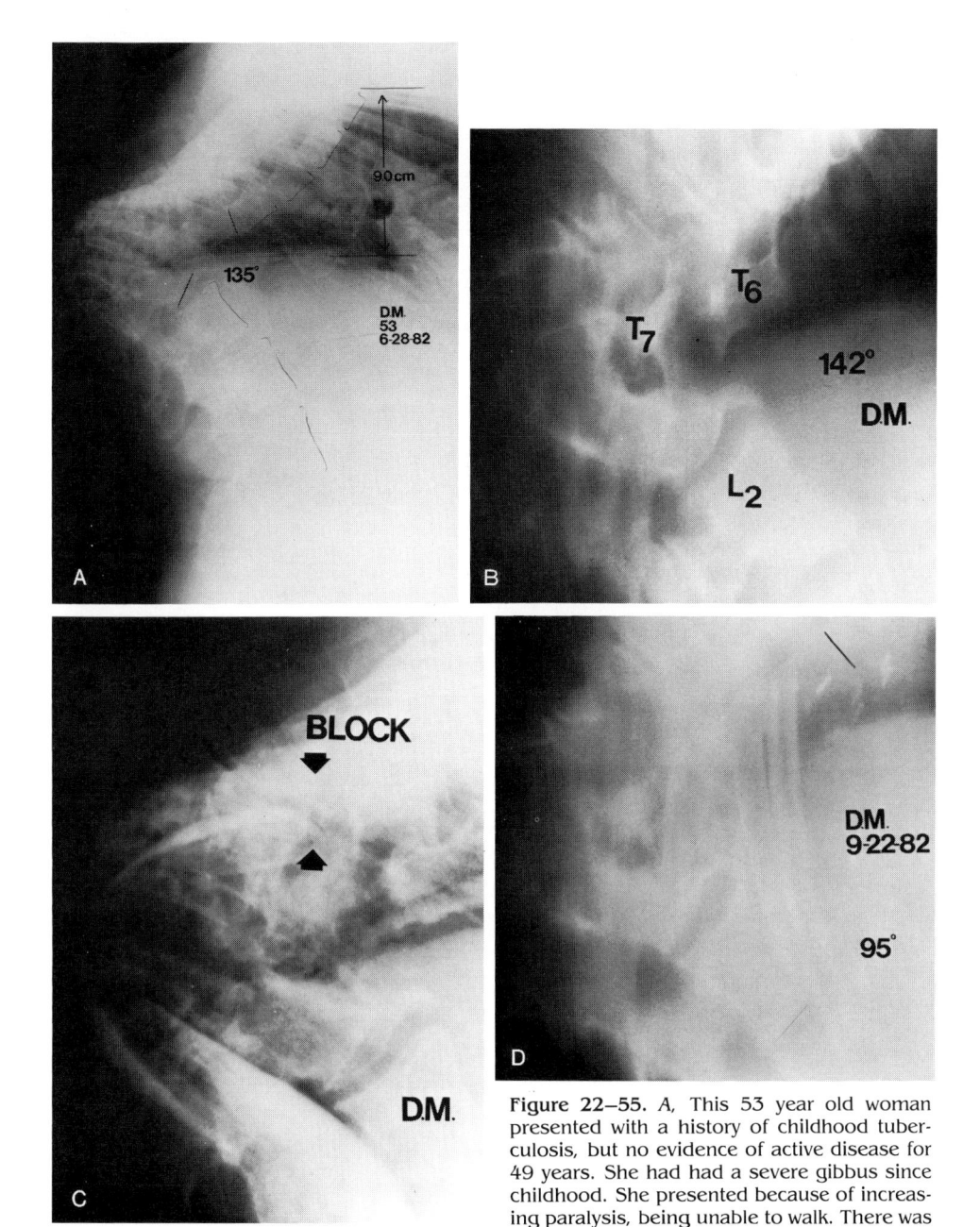

Figure 22–55. *A*, This 53 year old woman presented with a history of childhood tuberculosis, but no evidence of active disease for 49 years. She had had a severe gibbus since childhood. She presented because of increasing paralysis, being unable to walk. There was only 9.0 cm. from her diaphragm to the lung apex. *B*, A lateral tomogram showed the 142 degree gibbus, a solid bony ankylosis at the apex, and a destructive lesion at T6-T7. *C*, A myelogram (high volume) showed the contrast material flowed easily around the apex of the gibbus, but was blocked at T6-T7. This area was explored by a costotransversectomy, and granulation tissue was found. The dural sac was decompressed. Tuberculosis organisms were identified and antibiotics started. *D*, After securing good antibiotic control, the area was approached through a transthoracic, retroperitoneal exposure. Further debridement was done back to raw, bleeding bone, and area was grafted with autogenous rib and iliac crest bone, using a Santa-Casa distractor to gain some correction (95 degrees). Within three months she was neurologically normal and has remained so for four years.

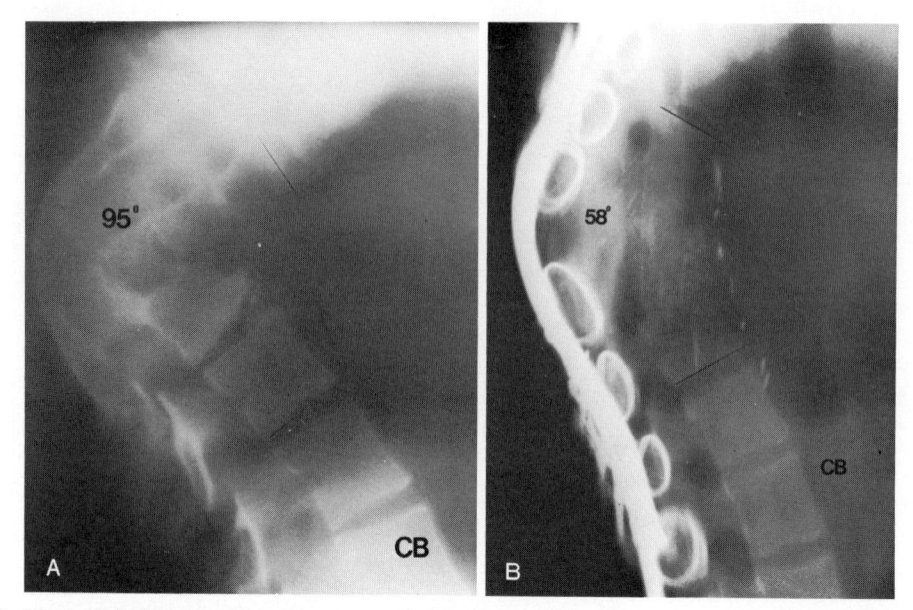

Figure 22–56. *A*, This 35 year old woman presented to our center with a sharp, angular 95 degree kyphosis. She had had a short posture fusion at the age of 5. After that posterior fusion, she had awakened with paraplegia and has remained paraplegic ever since, except that she had preservation of bowel and bladder function. About four months prior to being seen at our center, her bladder and bowels began to lose function in addition to which she noticed decreasing height and increasing respiratory difficulties. The goals of treatment in her case were (1) to remove bone in front of the spinal cord and (2) to reconstitute better thoracic height and shape to give her better lung volume. *B*, Her surgical procedure consisted of the approach described by Luque; first anterior vertebrectomy of the entire area of gibbus back to the dura, allowing the dura to move forward. All of the bone removed from the bodies was replaced anterior to the dura as well as rib chips. No strut graft was used.

Two weeks later a large posterior wedge was removed from her previous fusion mass, and Luque rodding was instituted to diminish the kyphosis and stabilize the spine. Her 95 degree kyphosis was reduced to 58 degrees.

posterior surgery is done one to two weeks later. Postoperative support is maintained until the fusion is absolutely solid. Bedrest is usually continued until the paralysis has recovered. Even complete paraplegia of several months' duration can be partially or totally reversed. Because the onset of the paralysis is usually slow and gradual, the lesion does not have the same bad prognosis as does an acute traumatic paraplegia. Chahal and Jyoti[5] reported on 29 patients with paralysis of whom, at followup, only three had any paralysis, and two of these were very mild.

CURRENT TREATMENT, LATE KYPHOTIC DEFORMITY

Often patients present to spinal centers with severe kyphosis secondary to old, healed tuberculosis. There is no longer any active infection, but the patient may have kyphotic progression due to mechanical factors. Pain in the gibbus, pain in the compensatory lumbar or cervical lordoses, decreased pulmonary function, or paralysis may be present because of the deformity and not the abscess formation.

Treatment often depends on the presenting problem. Progressive kyphosis needs stabilization. Loss of pulmonary function needs spinal realignment in order to increase lung volume. Paralysis needs anterior decompression and sometimes stabilization.

Treatment of the kyphosis is difficult owing to the rigidity of the deformity. Both anterior and posterior surgery are always necessary. Yau and associates[33] have recommended a posterior wedge osteotomy of the ankylosed posterior elements first, an anterior osteotomy second, correction with a halopelvic device third, and posterior instrumentation and fusion last. The many complications associated with the halopelvic device have made this program both arduous and risky.

More recently, we have favored a two-stage approach in which the anterior osteotomy is done first with abundant chip grafting and at the second stage a posterior closing wedge osteotomy is done with instrumentation and fusion. This obviates the need for four stages and the halopelvic device.

For the patient with late deformity and paralysis, anterior decompression is critical. Laminectomy is totally useless. If the kyphosis is acceptable and the spine stable, no fusion is necessary. If correction is desired, then anterior fusion is done at the time of the anterior decompression and, two weeks later, a posterior osteotomy, fusion, and instrumentation are done in order to achieve both correction and stabilization. As pointed out by both DuToit[9] and Otani and coworkers,[30] the aorta may be kinked at the angle of the kyphosis. A preoperative aortogram or MRI scan may be useful in a patient with late tuberculous kyphosis. The surgeon can thereby better choose the side of approach. Preoperative myelography, CT scan, or MRI scan should also be done to be sure of the level of cord compression (Figs. 22–55 and 22–56).

NON-TUBERCULOUS INFECTION[7, 10, 23, 32]

A long list of other organisms may cause vertebral osteomyelitis. These include *Staphylococcus*, *Brucella*, *Escherichia coli*, *Aerobacter*, *Proteus*, *Pseudomonas*, and even fungi and parasites. Patients with osteomyelitis of these causes more often have disc space loss early and bone loss later. Acute diagnosis is of the utmost importance and needle biopsies are useful. Open biopsies should be done if needle biopsies are non-diagnostic or in an area best not approached with a needle. Appropriate antibiotics should be used in large doses. Debridement should be reserved for those cases that fail to respond to antibiotic therapy, large abscesses, or paraplegia. The rare cases with severe bone loss may require bone grafting anteriorly with fusion and instrumentation posteriorly. As shown by Eismont and coworkers[10] in a review of 61 patients with pyogenic and fungal osteomyelitis, laminectomy is useless for paralysis; anterior decompression is essential.

References

1. Bailey, H. L., Gabriel, M., Hodgson, A. R., and Shin, J. S.: Tuberculosis of the spine in children. Operative findings and results in 100 consecutive patients treated by removal of the lesion and anterior grafting. J. Bone Joint Surg., 54A:1633–1657, 1972.
2. Brant-Zawadski, M., Burke, V. D., and Jeffrey, R. B.: CT in the evaluation of spine infection. Spine, 8:358–364, 1983.
3. Capner, N.: The evolution of lateral rachotomy. J. Bone Joint Surg., 36B:173, 1954.
4. Cardoso, A., Flores, A., and Galvan, R.: Segmental Instrumentation in Pott's Disease. Scoliosis Research Society, 1984; Orthop. Trans. 9:125, 1985.
5. Chahal, A. S., and Jyoti, S. P.: The radical treatment of tuberculosis of the spine. Intern. Orthop. (SICOT), 4:93–99, 1980.
6. Derry, O. G.: Pott's disease in ancient Egypt. Med. Press. Circ., pp. 196–200, July, 1938.
7. Digby, J. M., and Kersley, J. B.: Pyogenic non-tuberculous spinal infections, an analysis of 30 cases. J. Bone Joint Sug., 61B:47–55, 1979.
8. Dott, N. M.: Skeletal traction and anterior decompression in the management of Pott's paraplegia. Edinb. Med. J., 54:62, 1947.
9. DuToit, G.: Anterior spinal cord decompression in kyphosis with particular reference to healed tuberculosis. J. Bone Joint Surg., 66B:455, 1984.
10. Eismont, F. J., Bohlman, H. H., Soni, P., et al.: Pyogenic and fungal vertebral osteomyelitis with paralysis. J. Bone Joint Surg., 65A:19–29, 1985.
11. Fang, D., Leong, J. C. Y., and Fang, H. S. Y.: Tuberculosis of the upper cervical spine. J. Bone Joint Surg., 65B:47–50, 1983.
12. Fountain, S. S., Hsu, L. C. S., Yau, A. C. M. D., and Hodgson, A. R.: Progressive kyphosis following solid anterior spine fusion in children with tuberculosis of the spine. J. Bone Joint Surg., 57A:1103, 1975.
13. Hadra, B. E.: Wiring the vertebrae as a means of immobilization in fractures and Pott's disease. Med. Times Register 22:423, 1891, reprinted in Clin. Orthop., 112:4, 1975.
14. Hibbs, R. A.: An operation for progressive spinal deformities. N.Y. Med. J., 93:1013, 1911.
15. Hippocrates: The Genuine Works of Hippocrates. Translated by F. Adams. London, The Sydenham Society, 1849.
16. Hodgson, A. R., and Stock, F. E.: Anterior spinal fusion. A preliminary communication on the radical treatment of Pott's disease and Pott's paraplegia. Brit. J. Surg., 44:266–275, 1956.
17. Hodgson, A. R., Stock, F. E., Fang, H. S. Y., and Ong, G. B.: Anterior spinal fusion. The operative approach and pathological findings in 412 patients with Pott's disease of the spine. Brit. J. Surg., 48:172–178, 1960.
18. Hodgson, A. R., Skinsnes, O. K., and Leong, C. Y.: The pathogenesis of Pott's paraplegia. J. Bone Joint Surg., 49A:1147–1156, 1967.
19. Hsu, L. C. S., and Leong, J. C. Y.: Tuberculosis of the lower cervical spine (C2-C7), a report on 40 cases. J. Bone Joint Surg., 66B:1–5, 1984.
20. Hsu, L. C. S., and Yau, A. C. M. C.: Tuberculosis of the spine. In Bradford, D. S., and Hensinger, R. (eds.): The Pediatric Spine. New York, Thieme-Stratton, pp. 68–79, 1985.
21. Ito, H., Tsuchiya, J., and Asami, G.: A new radical operation for Pott's disease. J. Bone Joint Surg., 16:499, 1934.
22. Kulowski, J.: Pyogenic osteomyelitis of the spine. An analysis and discussion of 102 cases. J. Bone Joint Surg., 18:343–364, 1936.
23. Malawski, S. K.: Pyogenic infection of the spine. Intern. Orthop. (SICOT), 1:125–131, 1977.

24. Medical Research Council Working Party on Tuberculosis of the Spine: A controlled trial of ambulant out-patient treatment and in-patient rest in bed in the management of tuberculosis of the spine in young Korean patients on standard chemotherapy. A study in Masan, Korea. J. Bone Joint Surg., 55B:678–697, 1973.
25. Medical Research Council Working Party on Tuberculosis of the Spine: A controlled trial of plaster-of-Paris jackets in the management of ambulant out-patient treatment of tuberculosis of the spine in children on standard chemotherapy. A study in Pusan, Korea. Tubercle, 54:261–282, 1973.
26. Medical Research Council Working Party on Tuberculosis of the Spine: A controlled trial of debridement and ambulatory treatment in the management of tuberculosis of the spine in patients on standard chemotherapy. A Study in Bulawayo, Rhodesia. J. Trop. Med. Hyg., 77:72–92, 1974.
27. Medical Research Council Working Party on Tuberculosis of the Spine: A controlled trial of anterior spinal fusion and debridement in the surgical management of tuberculosis of the spine in patients on standard chemotherapy. A study in Hong Kong. Br. J. Surg., 61:853–866, 1974.
28. Medical Reserach Council Working Party on Tuberculosis of the Spine: A five year assessment of controlled trials of in-patient and out-patient treatment in plaster-of-Paris jackets for tuberculosis of the spine in children on standard chemotherapy. J. Bone Joint Surg., 58B:399, 1976.
29. Medical Research Council Working Party on Tuberculosis of the Spine: A 10 year assessment of a controlled trial comparing debridement and anterior spinal fusion in the management of tuberculosis of the spine in patients on standard chemotherapy in Hong Kong. J. Bone Joint Surg., 64B:393–398, 1982.
30. Otani, K., Satomi, K., Fujimura, Y., et al.: Spinal osteotomy to correct kyphosis in spinal tuberculosis. Intern. Orthop. (SICOT), 3:299–235, 1979.
31. Pinto, W. C., and Avanzi, O.: Surgical treatment of Pott's disease. Presented to the Spinal Symposium, Jerusalem, Israel, April, 1983.
32. Samra, Y., Hertz, M., Shakad, Y., et al.: Brucellosis of the spine, report of 3 cases. J. Bone Joint Surg., 64B:429–431, 1982.
33. Yau, A. C. M. C., Hsu, L. C. S., O'Brien, J. P., and Hodson, A. R.: Tuberculous kyphosis treatment with spinal osteotomy, halo pelvic distraction and anterior and posterior fusion. J. Bone Joint Surg., 56A:1419, 1974.

Congenital Heart Disease And Scoliosis

Robert B. Winter, M.D.

INTRODUCTION

There is a strong relationship between scoliosis and congenital heart disease. The incidence of "idiopathic-like" scoliosis in patients with congenital heart disease is 10 times that of idiopathic scoliosis in the population as a whole. In addition, patients with congenital scoliosis may have a co-existent congenital heart defect. The significant problems of patient management make this a relevant subject.

LITERATURE REVIEW

Several authors have commented upon the increased incidence of scoliosis in patients with congenital heart disease.[1, 3, 4, 5, 7, 9, 10, 11] If these were all congenital scoliotics, we would not be very surprised. However, most of these scoliotics have an idiopathic type curvature. By this it is meant that there are no visible vertebral anomalies and no curve at birth, and the patterns of curvature as well as the behavior of the curve are quite similar to idiopathic scoliosis.

The reader is referred to the excellent paper by Reckles and coworkers from the Mayo Clinic,[8] who have analyzed this problem in detail. They found the incidence of congenital heart defects among the adolescent scoliosis population was 5 per cent, a figure 10 times greater than the incidence of congenital heart disease in the population at large. The incidence of idiopathic-like scoliosis with curves greater than 20 degrees among patients with congenital heart defects (followed for at least 10 years after cardiac surgery) was 8.5 per cent. This is 10 times greater than the population at large. These same authors found no significant correlation between scoliosis and sex, type of cardiac anomaly, size of heart, side of heart, side of aortic arch, cyanosis, age at surgery, number and type of surgical incisions, number and side of ribs removed, or number and type of surgical procedures.

Luke and McDonnell[4] reviewed 3540 patients with congenital heart disease. There were 850 with cyanotic heart disease. Of these, 51 (6 per cent) had scoliosis. There were 2690 with non-cyanotic heart disease. Of these, 22 (0.8 per cent) had scoliosis. They felt that there was definitely a strong correlation with cyanotic heart disese. They found no correlation with the side of the aortic arch or the side of the thoracotomy and the side of the scoliosis. There was no relationship between the severity of cyanosis and the severity of the curve.

Roth and associates[9] reviewed 500 consecutive patients in the heart clinic at Boston Children's Hospital. Scoliosis of greater than 10 degrees was noted in 12 per cent, and scoliosis greater than 20 degrees in 4.6 per cent. There was a 28.4 per cent incidence in those with cyanotic heart disease versus 8.7 per cent in those with non-cyanotic heart disease. The lower the arterial oxygen saturation, the greater was the incidence of scoliosis. The highest incidence, however, was in patients with simple coarctation, 30 per cent of whom had curves of 10 degrees or more[7] (35 out of 115). Forty per cent of the males and 26 per cent of the females with coarctation had scoliosis. Twenty-eight curves were between 10 and 19 degrees. Six curves were between 20 and 29 degrees, and only one curve was severe.

Zorab[12] has noted that electrocardiographic abnormalities indicate true heart conditions and cannot be attributed to alterations of the thorax by the curve.

Thus, in summary, there is a high incidence of idiopathic type scoliosis in patients with congenital heart disease. There is probably a strong correlation with cyanotic heart disease.

TREATMENT

Because the patient with congenital heart disease is usually under treatment by the medical profession, there should be no difficulty in early detection of scoliosis. Scoliosis should be sought in all chest x-rays in these patients. If a curve of 10 degrees or more is noted, consultation with an orthopedist knowledgeable about scoliosis should be obtained. Progressive curves of 15 degrees or more and established curves of 20 degrees or more should be treated aggressively by bracing in the growing child. One should be even more aggressive about starting brace treatment early in these children because (1) we have the feeling that the larger curves do less well in braces than do the usual idiopathic, and (2) the surgical risks may be much higher.

Children with congenital heart disease, especially those with cyanotic heart disease, are slow to reach the end of growth. Treatment must continue until skeletal growth is complete, no matter what the chronologic age. The techniques of bracing are no different from those used with idiopathic scoliosis (see Chapter 11).

A patient with congenital heart disease should not be denied adequate scoliosis surgery. However, surgical treatment presents special hazards and problems. Bunch[2] pointed out that patients with cyanotic congenital heart disease may have "functional thrombocytopenia" with low normal platelet counts, normal Factor VIII, and decreased Factor V. Congenital heart patients tolerate variations in fluid replacement poorly during surgery, so the volumes must be precisely measured. A central venous pressure catheter is strongly recommended along with controlled monitoring of blood gases. For patients with heart block or other arrhythmias, a transvenous pacemaker can be extremely valuable.

Surgery of congenital heart patients should always be undertaken in an institution capable of performing such monitoring activity, in terms of both equipment and personnel. The principles of surgery are the same as for the patient with idiopathic scoliosis.

References

1. Beals, R. V., Kenney, K. H., and Lees, M. H.: Congenital heart disease and idiopathic scoliosis. Clin. Orthop., 89:112–116, 1972.
2. Bunch, W. H., and Komp, D. M.: Surgical correction of scoliosis in a child with hemostatic abnormalities secondary to congenital heart disease. Clin. Orthop., 89:139–142, 1972.
3. Jordan, C. E., White, R. I., Fisher, K. C., et al.: The scoliosis of congenital heart disease. Am. Heart. J., 84:463–469, 1972.
4. Luke, M. J., and McDonnell, E. J.: Congenital heart disease and scoliosis. J. Pediatr., 73:725–733, 1968.
5. Marisaki, N.: Spinal scoliosis associated with congenital heart disease. J. Japn. Orthop. Assoc., 38:699–700, 1964.
6. Nilsen, N. Ö.: Anomalies in derivatives from the visceral arches combined with congenital heart defects. Scand. J. Thorac. Cardiovasc. Surg., 3:211–214, 1969.
7. Poitras, B., Rosenthal. J., and Hall, J.: Scoliosis

and coarctation of the aorta. J. Pediatr., 86:476–477, 1975.
8. Reckles, L. N., Peterson, H. A., Bianco, A. J., and Weidman, W. H.: The association of scoliosis and congenital heart disease. J. Bone Joint Surg., 57A:449–455, 1975.
9. Roth, A., Rosenthal, A., Hall, J. E., and Mizel, M.: Scoliosis and congenital heart disease. Clin. Orthop., 93:95–102, 1973.
10. White R. I., Jordan, C. E., Fisher, K. C., et al.: Skeletal changes associated with adolescent congenital heart disease. Am. J. Roentgenol., 116:531–538, 1972.
11. Wright, W. D., and Niebauer, J. J.: Congenital heart disease and scoliosis. J. Bone Joint Surg., 38A:1131–1136, 1956.
12. Zorab, P.: The cardiac aspects of scoliosis. Scoliosis Research Society, 1973.

Scoliosis And Congenital Limb Deficiency

Robert B. Winter, M.D.

INTRODUCTION

Although isolated case reports appeared earlier, such as that by Epps,[1] scoliosis in association with congenital upper limb deficiency was not recognized as an entity until the report by Makley and Heiple in 1970.[3] The authors of this book have also noted the strong relationship between congenital upper limb deficiency (complete or partial) and an idiopathic appearing scoliosis.

INCIDENCE

In the review by Makley and Heiple there were 27 patients with major limb deficiencies. There were 18 patients with radial hemimelia. Of these, nine had scoliosis and seven of the nine had an idiopathic type scoliosis. There were six patients with ulnar hemimelia, four of whom had scoliosis, and all four were idiopathic type. Three patients had amelia or phocomelia, and two of these had scoliosis, both idiopathic type. Thus, the incidence of significant scoliosis was 48 per cent. Five patients underwent spine fusion. Congenital anomalies were not noted at surgery.

Makley and Heiple found no increased incidence of scoliosis in minor limb anomalies, such as syndactylism or hypoplasia. Congenital anomalies of the upper extremities, especially Sprengel's deformity (congenital elevation of the scapula), are frequently associated with congenital scoliosis. Such congenital scolioses may or may not be a problem. For information on this, the reader is referred to Chapter 12, Congenital Spine Deformity.

In 1983, Powers and coworkers reported a review of all patients seen at the Chicago Shrine Amputee Clinic between 1927 and 1980.[5] One hundred and thirty patients had limb deficiency. Of these, 24 or 18 per cent had spine problems. Twenty-one (16 per cent) had scoliosis of 10 to 88 degrees. Two thirds of these had a diagnosis of scoliosis prior to age six. Of the bilateral amelia patients 100 per cent had scoliosis, and 50 per cent of the unilateral amelia patients had scoliosis. Thirteen per cent of the radial hemimelia patients and 20 percent of the ulnar hemimelia patients had scoliosis. There was no relationship between the side of the amelia and the side of the scoliosis.

Six patients were placed in a Milwaukee brace; five of the six did not tolerate the brace well. Four patients, all of whom had been unsuccessfully tried in braces, underwent surgical treatment.

Nel and DuToit published a report in 1983, reviewing 104 patients from South Africa with congenital upper limb anomalies of whom seven had an idiopathic type scoliosis.[4] This is 6.7 per cent of the population, much higher than the general population of South Africa. All of these patients had a structural scoliosis of at least 10 degrees. In the amelia, hemimelia, and phocomelia groups, there was a 40 per cent incidence of idiopathic type scoliosis. Of the seven patients with scoliosis, the range was from 30 to 140 degrees.

The most recent report is that by Lester and associates, who reviewed the experience at the Elizabethtown, New Jersey, Crippled Children's Hospital.[2] There were 15 patients with a scoliosis of 10 degrees or more. Of these 15, 13 had an idiopathic type curve and

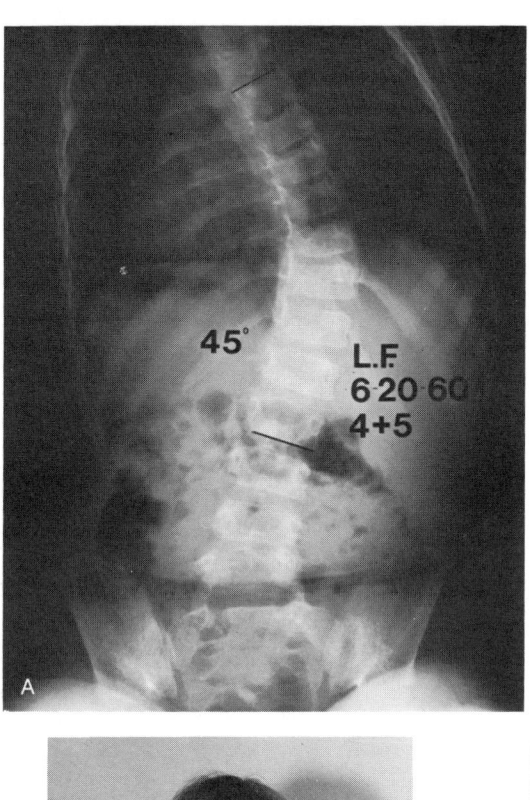

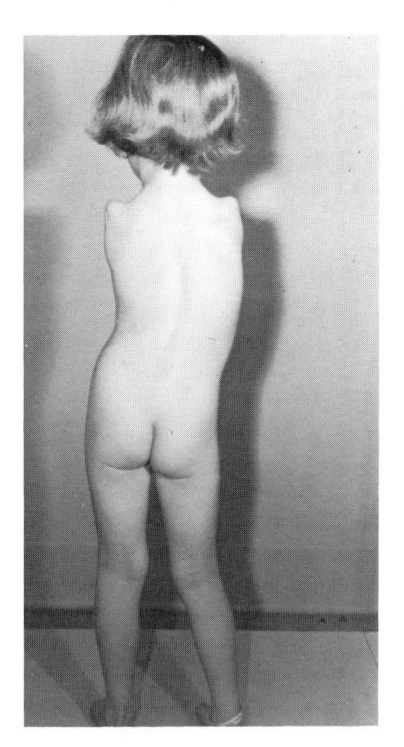

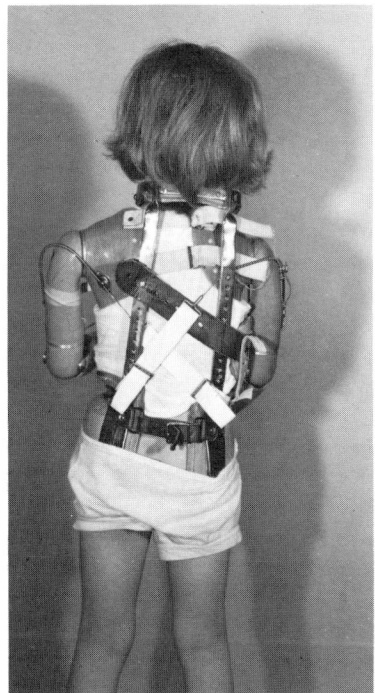

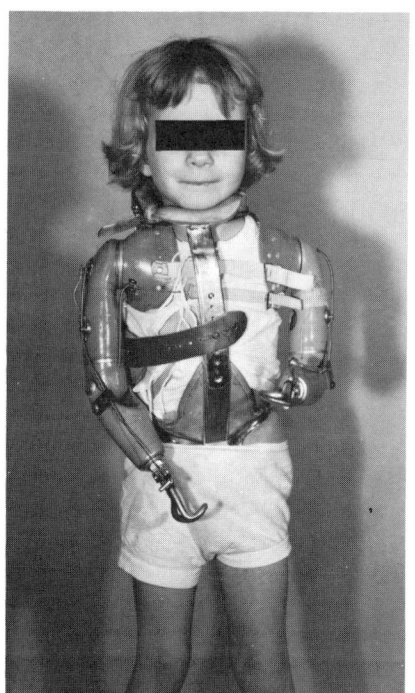

Figure 22–57. A, A 4+5 year old girl presented with a 45 degree T6 to L2 idiopathic-type curve. A radiograph at age 3+10 years, just seven months previously, had shown a 30 degree curve. Treatment with a Milwaukee brace was begun immediately. B, A photograph at age 4+5 years. C, A photograph at age 6 showing the Milwaukee brace plus bilateral upper extremity prostheses. D, An anterior view showing the Milwaukee brace and the prostheses. She had voluntary control over both elbow joints and both terminal devices.

Illustration continued on following page

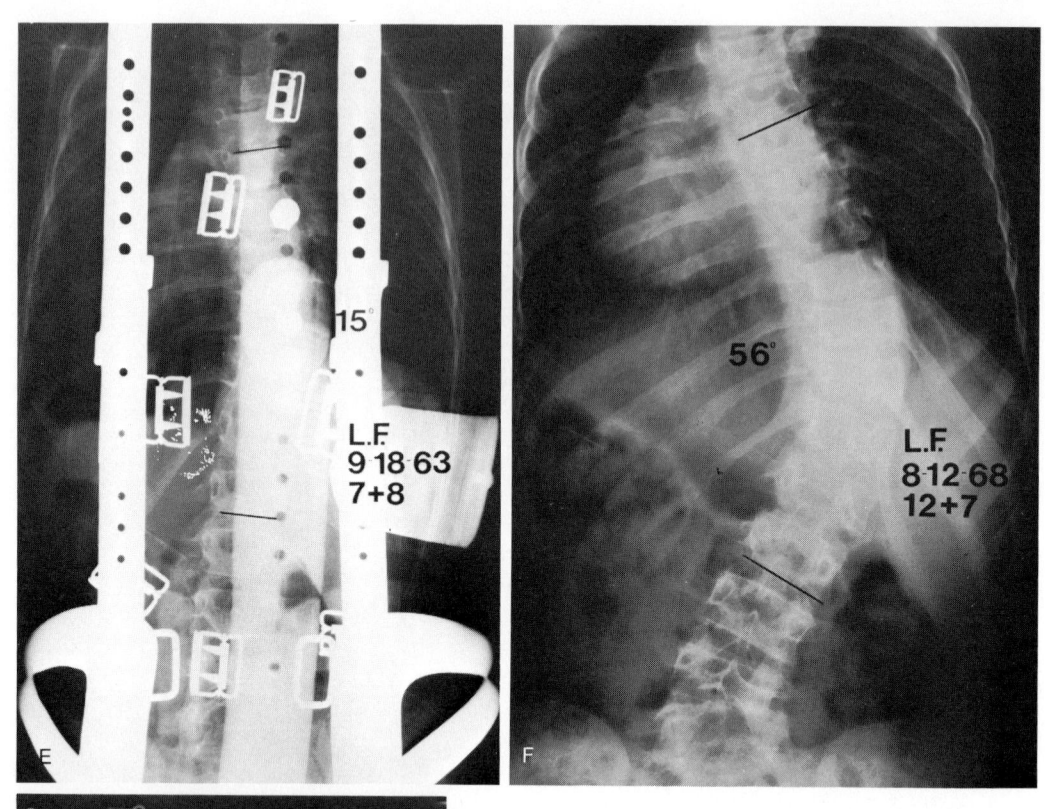

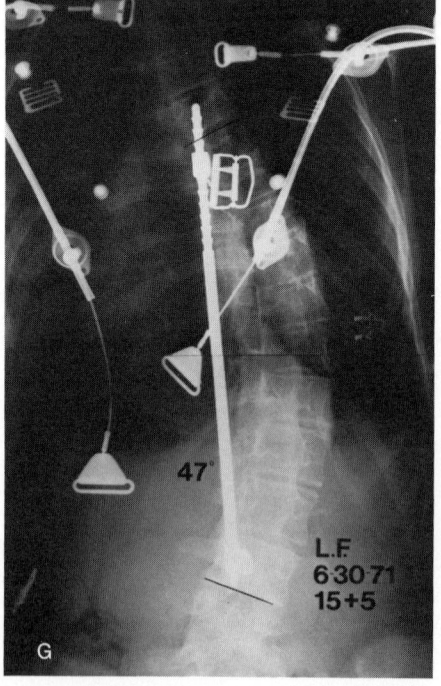

Figure 2–57 *Continued.* E, A radiograph in the brace at age 7 + 8 years. The curve is well controlled at 15 degrees. F, A radiograph at age 12 + 7 years, showing an increase of the curve to 56 degrees. This is typical of such a curve at the adolescent growth spurt. Fusion was done at this time. G, A radiograph three years after surgery. The fusion was solid, but had some bending after becoming solid. The patient subsequently became employed in a bank and requires assistance only in donning her prostheses each morning.

two a congenital type of curve. Scoliosis was noted in 25 per cent of amelia patients. Of the 13 patients with idiopathic type scoliosis of 10 degrees or more, two had bilateral amelia and 11 had unilateral amelia. This series had a lesser degree of curvature than most other series, the largest curve being 32 degrees.

In summary, the incidence of scoliosis in patients with major congenital limb deficiencies is extremely high, and most of these curvatures are of an idiopathic type rather than congenital.

TREATMENT

These curves may appear at any time during growth, but they have a strong tendency to develop in the infantile (0 to 3) and juvenile (3 to 10) years. Because of the many years of growth remaining, very severe curves are possible if treatment is not instituted.

There has been a disturbing tendency to avoid treating these curves because of the limb deficiency problem. All too often the statement is made: "The child cannot tolerate a brace because of the need to use the feet." Such a philosophy has frequently resulted in a short, severely deformed child with poor pulmonary function and reduced self-image far beyond that due to the limb deficiency.

Bracing is feasible if applied early and maintained consistently so that the child learns to adapt to both the brace and limb deficiency. Braces that constrict the thorax are not recommended because of their tendency to diminish rather than to improve pulmonary function. Thus, the Milwaukee brace is the brace of choice for such curvatures (Fig. 22–57).

The use of electrical stimulation would be highly advantageous to these children; as of this writing (1986), no reports are available of such treatment.

Significant curvatures developing in small children can be treated by subcutaneous Har-

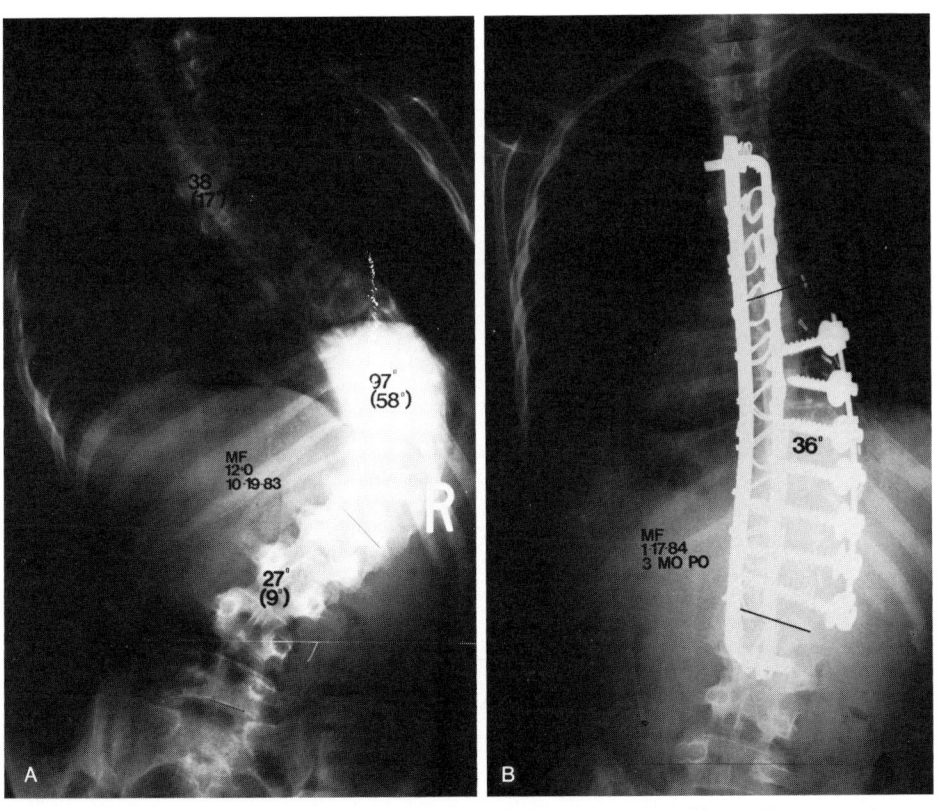

Figure 22–58. *A,* This 12 year old girl had total amelia of both upper extremities and presented to our Center with a 97 degree T6 to L2 idiopathic-type scoliosis. On bending films, the curve corrected to 58 degrees. Because of the rigidity of the curve, and the desire to avoid fusing down to L4, an anterior fusion with a Zielke device was done first, followed one week later by a Luque procedure posteriorly. *B,* A radiograph three months after her surgery shows correction to 36 degrees. No cast or brace was used.

rington instrumentation without fusion, periodic lengthening of the rod, and then fusion when more adequate spine length has been achieved. This approach is no different than in other children with recalcitrant juvenile or infantile idiopathic scoliosis. We have in our clinics one patient who was successfully managed for several years with subcutaneous instrumentation without fusion. After reaching the age of 12, he underwent arthrodesis.

Surgical treatment is quite feasible for these children and should not be denied to them. At the same time, it is important to avoid fusing an excessive number of vertebrae, thereby reducing spinal mobility, which may be necessary for foot use. For this reason, the use of anterior instrumentation with Dwyer or Zielke devices may significantly lessen the number of lumbar vertebrae fused and maintain greater mobility of the spine than possible by conventional posterior surgery alone. This anterior surgery must usually be supplemented with additional posterior instrumentation incorporating levels proximal to the area of the Dwyer or Zielke device. With the use of combined anterior and posterior fixation using strong instrumentation and sublaminar wiring, it may be quite possible to manage the child without any external immobilization postoperatively. A much more active functional status is thereby maintained (Fig. 22–58).

References

1. Epps, C. H.: Upper extremity limb deficiency with concomitant infantile structural scoliosis. Inter-Clinic Information Bulletin, 5(2):1–9, Nov. 1965.
2. Lester, D. K., Painter, J. L., Berman, A. T., and Skinner, S.: Idiopathic scoliosis associated with congenital upper limb deficiency. Orthop. Trans., 9:113, 1985.
3. Makley, J. T., and Heiple, K. G.: Scoliosis associated with congenital deficiencies of the upper extremity. J. Bone Joint Surg., 52A:279–287, 1970.
4. Nell, G., and DuToit, G.: Congenital upper limb anomalies and scoliosis. S. Afr. Med. J., 63:893–895, 1983.
5. Powers, T. A., Haker, T. R., Derlin, V. J., et al.: Anomalies of the spine in relationship to congenital upper limb deficiencies. J. Pediatr. Orthop., 3:471–474, 1983.

Thoracic Cage Defects And Contractures With Scoliosis

Robert B. Winter, M.D.

INTRODUCTION

There are two basic types of thoracogenic scoliosis, those due to contractures secondary to empyema, and those due to the destabilizing effect of multiple rib resection. The removal of a single rib, as in a thoracotomy for tracheo-esophageal fistula repair or heart surgery such as a coarctation repair does not in itself result in scoliosis (see pp. 576–578 Congenital Heart Disease And Scoliosis).

CONTRACTURE SECONDARY TO EMPYEMA

Severe thoracic scoliosis was a common result of empyema. Pleural and lung scarring on one side inhibited the natural growth of that side and scoliosis resulted. These curvatures were often severe and the scoliosis, combined with the lung damage of the infection, often lead to major pulmonary function deficit and early death from cor pulmonale. This problem has almost totally disappeared with the widespread use of antibiotics and the prompt surgical drainage of intrapleural infection.

MULTIPLE RIB RESECTION

Thoracoplasty for Tuberculosis

In the early years of this century, thoracoplasty was a widely accepted procedure for the treatment of pulmonary tuberculosis. As a result of massive rib resections, the stabilizing effect of the intercostal muscles on the spine was destroyed and the spine would "buckle," always convex to the side of the rib resection.[1, 2, 4, 5] The more ribs that were removed, the worse the curvature. The closer to the spine the ribs were removed, the worse the curvature.[3] Multiple rib resection is almost the only way to make the adult spine scoliotic. It is for this reason that convex rib resection for the "treatment" of the rib hump of scoliosis is absolutely contraindicated except in conjunction with or subsequent to spinal fusion.

Rib Resection for Tumors

Currently, the most common cause of thoracogenic scoliosis is the resection of multiple ribs in the treatment of chest wall tumors, usually malignant. The early diagnosis, better surgical resection, chemotherapy, and advanced radiotherapy have combined to increase the survival of these children, and thus more will develop scoliosis.[3]

It is important that the pediatricians, surgeons, and oncologists caring for these children be aware that scoliosis can result from such treatment. At the earliest sign of scoliosis, the patient should be referred to a spine surgeon. Since these children all have periodic chest radiographs, a curve should readily be detected (Fig. 22–59).

Non-operative treatment does not appear to be feasible, since there are no lateral rib structures on which to apply the usual forces of a brace. Circumferential constrictive braces are contraindicated since these children already have diminished pulmonary function from lung resection, radiation, and altered chest wall dynamics.

If the child is of an adequate age for fusion (over age 10 in females and 12 in males), fusion is indicated. If possible, abundant internal fixation is desirable, since there is an inadequate chest wall against which to push with the postoperative cast or brace. Harrington instrumentation with a distraction rod, a long compression rod, and multiple cross-linkages is a good system for such patients. If the surgeon is familiar with the Luque system, it is ideal for these patients. Healing of the fusion may be delayed because tissues have been irradiated.[6]

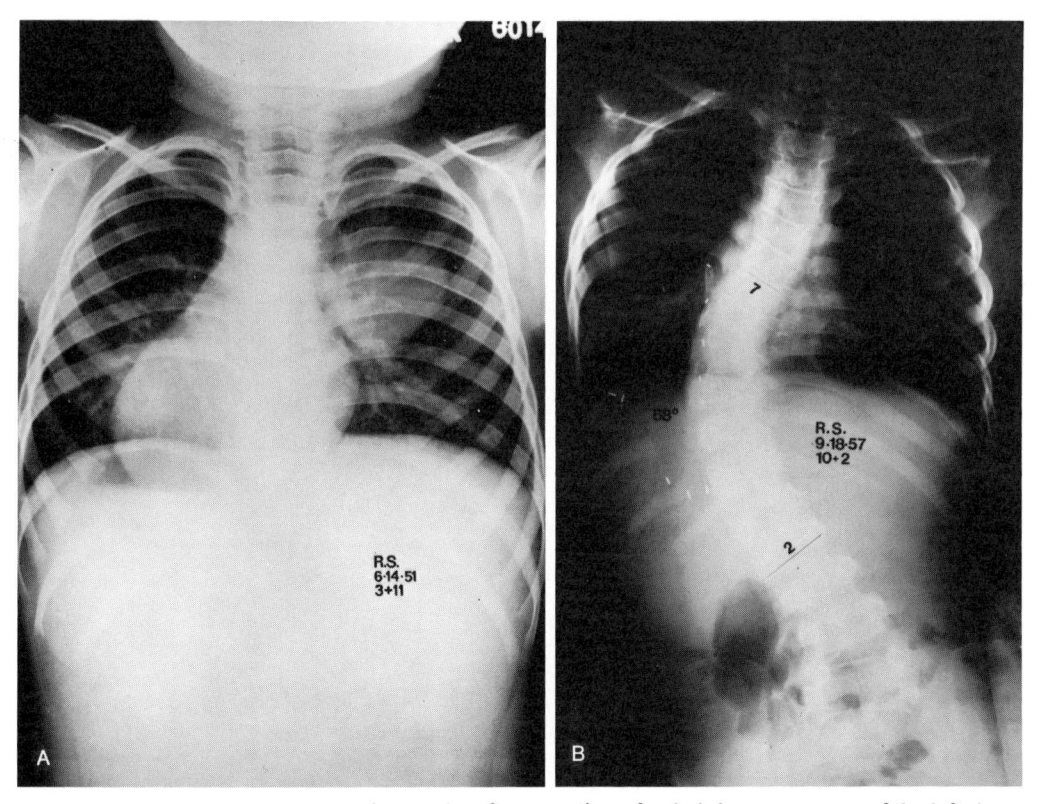

Figure 22–59. A, A 4 year old boy seen six months after resection of a rhabdomyosarcoma of the left chest wall. Note the large metastasis in the right lung. He had a local recurrence on the chest wall and had a second resection, radon seeds, resection of a left lung metastasis (not seen here), and resection of the right lung metastasis. B, When first seen by us in 1957 at age ten, he had no evidence of tumor, but had developed a scoliosis of 68 degrees. Fusion was done at this time. The patient was last contacted at age 32 and was alive and well.

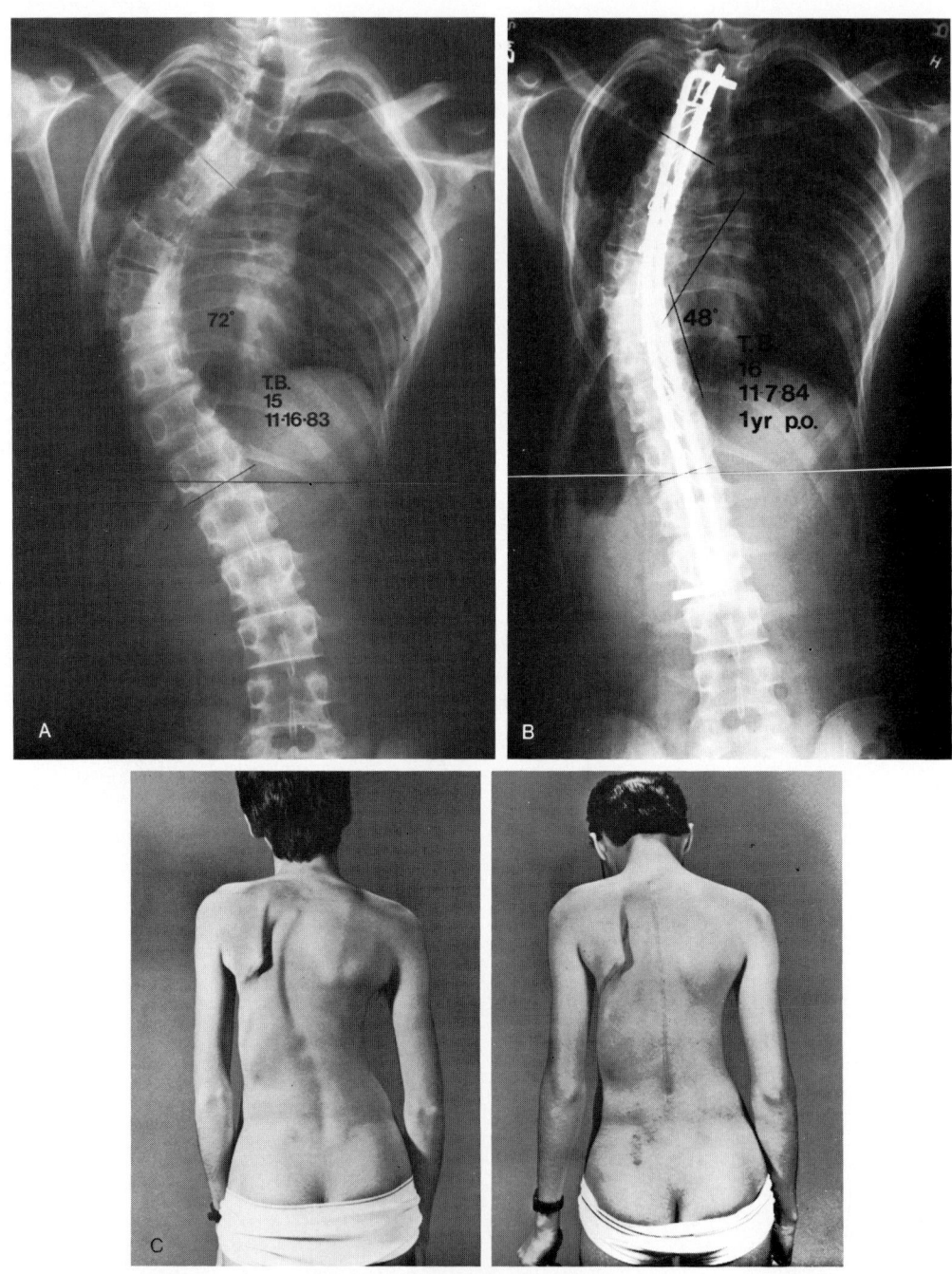

Figure 22–60. *A*, This 15 year old boy presented with a rapidly progressing 72 degree scoliosis. He had had five ribs resected for treatment of a Ewing's sarcoma of the chest wall. He also had extensive radiation. A radiograph in traction showed correction only to 52 degrees. His pulmonary function was only 38 per cent of normal. *B*, One year after fusion from T2 to L2, the curve is 48 degrees, the same as the day of surgery. No cast or brace was used after surgery. *C*, Pre- and postoperative photographs show the correction obtained.

For young patients in whom it would be highly advantageous to allow continued spinal growth and yet maintain control of the curve, instrumentation without fusion would appear to be the method of choice. The author has no personal experience with this technique in rib resection patients, but its proven benefits in juvenile idiopathic scoliosis and neuromuscular scoliosis would make it seem applicable (Fig. 22–60).

References

1. Alexandra, J.: Postoperative management of thoracoplastic patients. Am. Rev. Tuberc., 61:57, 1950.
2. Bisgard, J. D.: Thoracogenic scoliosis; influence of thoracic disease and thoracic operations of the spine. Arch. Surg., 29:417–445, 1934.
3. DeRosa, G. P.: Progressive scoliosis following chest wall resection. Spine 10:618–622, 1985.
4. Dwork, R. E., Dinken, H., and Hurst, A.: Post thoracoplasty scoliosis. Arch. Phys. Med., 32:722, 1951.
5. Stauffer, E. S., and Mankin, H. J.: Scoliosis after thoracoplasty; a study of thirty patients. J. Bone Joint Surg., 48A:339–348, 1966.
6. Winter, R. B., and Tongen, L. A.: A malignant chest wall sarcoma with bilateral pulmonary metastasis. A 15 year survival after multiple radial local excision and resection of bilateral pulmonary metastasis and a successful treatment of scoliosis secondary to tumor surgery. Surgery, 62:374–378, 1967.

Pulmonary Function Testing

Kathryn A. Hale, M.D. • *Fred L. Rasp, M.D.*

Preoperative pulmonary function testing in patients with spinal deformities allows one to better predict the risk of surgery as well as the possible need for postoperative mechanical ventilation. Pulmonary function tests in spinal deformities may be divided into three categories: lung mechanics, lung volumes, and arterial blood gases.

LUNG MECHANICS

Lung mechanics are measured with either a spirogram or a flow-volume curve. Both are accurate and helpful when assessing the operability of scoliosis patients. The basic maneuver for measuring mechanics is the same for both methods. The patient is asked to inhale to total lung capacity then exhale as hard and as fast as possible until the lungs are as empty as possible. This maneuver is called forced vital capacity (FVC). The spirometer plots volume versus time while the flow-volume curve displays instantaneous flow versus volume. The one second forced expiratory volume (FEV1), the ratio of FEV1 to FVC, and measures of midflow rates can be calculated from either curve. Normal values for these measurements are calculated using a regression equation based on sex, age, and body height.[41] There is a large variation of values among the normal population, so the tests are interpreted as abnormal if the results are outside of the 95 per cent confidence interval.[14] Patients with spinal deformities are screened initially with flow-volume curves. If the predicted FVC is less than 60 per cent or if pulmonary symptoms are present, lung volumes and arterial blood gases are tested.

Since predicted normal values are based on the patient's height, these values are often misleading in patients with spinal deformities whose height is frequently reduced. Alternate methods have been suggested to calculate the appropriate height of a scoliosis patient. The most accurate and easiest to use is the arm span method as described by Hepper and associates. The arm span/height ratio was calculated as 1.03/1 for men and 1.1/1 for women (SD ± 0.02). Johnson and Westgate found the differences among sex and age groups to be insignificant and arrived at a ratio of 1.03/1 (SD ± 0.02). The latter method is employed most widely.

LUNG VOLUMES

Lung volumes are measured indirectly because air remains in the lungs after complete exhalation. The volume of air that remains is the residual volume. The residual volume is measured by body plethysmography, nitrogen washout, or helium dilution. The relationship among lung volumes is shown in Figure 22–61. The effect of spinal deformities on pulmonary function is discussed below.

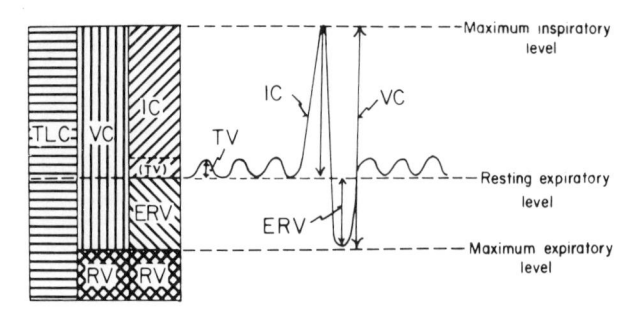

Figure 22–61. Pulmonary function. Relationship of the vital capacity (VC), residual volume (RV), tidal volume (TV), expiratory and inspiratory reserve volumes (ERV and IRV), and total lung capacity (TLC). (Adapted with permission from Comroe, J. H., Jr., et al. (eds.): The Lung. Clinical Physiology and Pulmonary Function Tests. Chicago, Year Book Medical Publishers, 1962, p. 8.)

ARTERIAL BLOOD GASES

Arterial blood gases are measured preoperatively when necessary in patients with scoliosis. Normal values for PaO_2 are dependent upon the barometric pressure, which varies with altitude. At sea level this value is 80 to 100 mm Hg. Normal value for $PaCO_2$ is 35 to 40 mm Hg.

PREOPERATIVE PULMONARY ASSESSMENT

Spirometry or flow-volume loops are measured in most patients who are being considered for surgical repair. Lung volumes and arterial blood gas examinations are performed only when the vital capacity is significantly diminished. It is difficult to establish a lower limit of pulmonary function that precludes surgery. Hypercarbia greater than 50 mm Hg and hypoxemia of less than 50 mm Hg are contraindications to surgery. Patients with severe impairment in their arterial blood gases or vital capacity may be placed on an intensive pulmonary training program consisting of inspiratory muscle strengthening, use of bronchodilators, and oxygen therapy. After six to twelve months, the individuals are retested, and if there has been significant improvement, surgery is considered. Occasionally, patients are placed in halo traction for several weeks with improvement in their pulmonary function to the extent that they become surgical candidates.

EFFECTS OF SCOLIOSIS ON PULMONARY FUNCTION

Pulmonary function may be impaired in patients with significant scoliosis. Abnormalities are found in lung mechanics and volumes, pulmonary gas exchange, and perhaps control of respiration. These abnormalities of pulmonary function, especially of vital capacity, are correlated with the severity of the curvature,[6, 19, 20, 23, 24, 32, 35, 36, 55] with consistent decrease being seen with curves over 60 degrees.[44, 57]

Lung volumes are impaired, and the impairment occurs in a pattern consistent with restrictive lung disease. The total lung capacity (TLC) in patients with scoliosis is often extremely small with characteristic decreases in components of the vital capacity (VC), the inspiratory capacity (IC) and the expiratory reserve volume (ERV). These volumes are frequently decreased to a greater degree than the residual volume (RV), which may be normal or only moderately decreased.[2] With neuromuscular disease, one may find further decreases in IC and ERV. In fact, patients with scoliosis secondary to poliomyelitis have lower values for TLC, FRC, and VC for a given angle of scoliosis than non-paralytic scoliotics.[17]

Several factors have been proposed to explain the alterations in lung volumes. Extensive studies have shown that the lungs themselves are not a major factor, except possibly in the case of early onset congenital scoliosis in which there seems to be failure of alveolar multiplication.[5] The compliance of the chest wall, however, is severely decreased as is the volume of the resting mid-position of the chest wall. The geometry of the thoracic cage deformity is suspected to be a major factor in decreasing chest wall compliance with resulting poor expansion of the lung parenchyma.

Similar chest wall compliance changes can be induced by simple strapping of the thorax. This has been shown to decrease maximum expiratory flow rate, maximum breathing capacity, and VC.[8] Makley and coworkers also demonstrated changes after application of a Risser localizer cast.[35] Thus, decreased compliance of the respiratory system is an important factor in impairment of lung volumes. Bergofsky also found the work of breathing increased and compliance decreased five times in patients with scoliosis compared with normal adults. These findings of decreased compliance and increased work of breathing have since been confirmed by other investigators.[18, 28, 49]

Impaired respiratory muscle performance has been shown to be an important factor in altering respiratory function in patients with scoliosis. As already noted, lung volumes are lower in patients with paralytic scoliosis compared with non-paralytic.[12] Cooper and associates found that the maximum inspiratory pressure (Pi max) was decreased in patients with idiopathic scoliosis, but the maximum expiratory pressure was normal. They argue that if the expiratory muscles are normal, then the inspiratory muscles are probably also normal. They hypothesize that the low Pi max occurs because the inspiratory muscles work at a mechanical disadvantage due to the chest deformity.

Thoracic lordosis may also play a role, as shown in a report by Winter, Lovell, and Moe, in which marked reduction in pulmonary function was seen.[56] Thoracic lordosis has a more profound effect on pulmonary functions than scoliosis or kyphosis.

Lung mechanics demonstrate pure restrictive ventilatory impairment in patients with scoliosis. The ratio of the FEV1 to the FEVC is usually preserved, indicating little or no obstructive component. Bjure and coworkers have demonstrated early closure of peripheral airways in lungs of patients with scoliosis,[3] but airway closure is suspected to be caused by lung compression rather than by airway obstruction per se. Dayman[15] and Fry and Hyatt[21] have shown that in normal subjects the gas flow rate changes proportionately with the degree of inflation of the lung. Since the vital capacity and thus the degree of inflation may be reduced in thoracic scoliosis, a decrease in maximum flow rates is found.

Impairment in pulmonary gas exchange occurs in patients with severe curves, as evidenced by arterial hypoxemia.[38, 51, 54] Three major mechanisms may contribute to the hypoxemia: ventilation-perfusion (V/Q) imbalance, limitation of diffusion, and alveolar hypoventilation. A progressive but modest worsening of V/Q imbalance occurs with increasing severity of scoliosis and with age.[30] Early airway closure and lung tissue adjacent to the convex portion of the curve that contains atelectatic areas[19] may create lung units with exceedingly low V/Q ratios and may result in hypoxemia. Riseborough and Shannon[42] and Westgate[53] found the lung on the convex side of the curve more affected, whereas Dollery and coworkers[16] and Littler and coworkers[34] found no significant difference in perfusion and ventilation between the two lungs. Such disparities in findings suggest that scoliosis can alter lung volume in one hemithorax with or without an alteration in ventilation and perfusion. The precise structural changes in the thoracic cage that produce altered regional ventilation and perfusion have not yet been delineated.

A decrease in pulmonary diffusion capacity beyond that associated with decrease in lung volume occurs in patients with advanced scoliosis, age, and cor pulmonale.[2] Alveolar hypoventilation may also contribute substantially to hypoxemia. These features of severe scoliosis can be accompanied by the previously mentioned severe V/Q imbalance and can also be associated with increased pulmonary artery pressure, hypercapnia, abnormal response to CO_2 stimulation, and increased work of breathing.[4]

Respiratory drive is probably normal in scoliosis patients with normal resting $PaCO_2$.[30] If resting $PaCO_2$ values are increased (averaging 55 mm Hg), the ventilatory response to inspired CO_2 becomes quite abnormal.[2] This would suggest that hypercapnia may effect ventilatory responses through tolerance to CO_2 or hydrogen ion. It is difficult to distinguish these factors from others affecting ventilatory response, such as compliance of the respiratory system or work of breathing.[49] Further studies have concluded that the effects of scoliosis on the ventilatory response to CO_2 resemble those of external resistance loading;[29] however, the influence of several other contributing factors, such as aging and muscle function, could not be distinguished. There is also a clear difference in ventilatory response between idiopathic and paralytic scoliosis. In the latter, no relationship between structured properties of the respiratory system and ventilatory response to CO_2 can be identified.[28]

Respiratory failure in scoliosis initially occurs at night and may occur in part because of alterations in sleep. Mezon and co-workers[40] and Guilleminault and co-workers[25] each evaluated five patients with severe kyphoscoliosis during sleep. Episodes of central apnea, obstructive apnea, and hypopnea were identified in addition to impaired oxygen saturation. Further study will be needed to define possible sleep disorders in patients with scoliosis but these findings suggest that altered breathing patterns during sleep may worsen nocturnal hypoxemia and contribute to development of right heart failure.

The cardiopulmonary response to exercise in patients with thoracic scoliosis (curves 20 to 130 degrees) has also been evaluated.[45] During a progressive exercise test, the maximum oxygen uptake was reduced, and this reduction was proportional to the FEV1 and maximum exercise ventilation. Exercise was limited by ventilatory factors in 80 per cent of patients with scoliosis in contrast to normal subjects whose exercise capacity is circulation-limited. The scoliosis patients also hyperventilated relative to their work rate. The extra work expended in hyperventilating with a poorly compliant deformed thorax decreased the amount of energy available for performing external work.[45]

EFFECTS OF SURGICAL CORRECTION ON PULMONARY FUNCTION

Numerous investigations have evaluated the effects of surgical correction of spinal curvature on pulmonary physiology with tests of pre- and post-fusion function. One would expect that correction of the spinal curvature would not only increase the size of the thoracic cavity, but improve its mechanical efficiency. This improvement could result either by improved mobility of the thoracic cage or by returning symmetry to the movement of the hemithoraces.[27] Excluding permanent alteration of lung parenchyma, these changes would result in increased lung volumes and perhaps mechanics. The actual results for post-fusion pulmonary function studies are varied and sometimes difficult to compare, as various methods for calculating predicted normal values are used, and varied patient groups with different etiologies, degrees of severity, and surgical methods are studied. However, some conclusions can be drawn from existing literature.

Immediate and Early Postoperative Periods

Immediately after surgery, lung volumes and flow rates may be reduced by 10 to 30 per cent for various reasons, including hypoventilation from analgesics or pain-induced splinting and postanesthetic changes. These transient reductions in postoperative pulmonary function will jeopardize any patient with severe reduction in preoperative pulmonary function. Patients with borderline pulmonary functions, therefore, require preoperative therapy as previously discussed.

A few investigators have evaluated pulmonary functions relatively early after surgical intervention for scoliosis. In a study by Kumano and Tsuyama[31] pulmonary functions were evaluated annually after surgical correction of scoliosis in 31 patients treated by either a posterior procedure with Harrington instrumentation or an anterior procedure with or without posterior instrumentation. At less than two years, there were no significant changes from preoperative values in the patients who had had a posterior procedure. The vital capacity of those treated with an anterior procedure was significantly lower than the preoperative value, ($p<0.05$). Banta and Park[1] evaluated pulmonary functions of 13 patients undergoing an anterior procedure before and ten months after surgery. They found that eight of ten patients demonstrated an increased peak flow, but other functions were mixed; vital capacity was increased in two, decreased in five, and unchanged in three patients.

Late Changes

Evaluating pulmonary functions after a longer postoperative period may provide more useful information about the efficacy of surgery for scoliosis. Numerous studies have demonstrated improvement in the vital capacity of patients with scoliosis after surgical intervention. Cotrel and associates[13] found an improvement of 30 to 40 per cent with the elongation derotation flexion method of casting and fusion, but this improvement was not calculated with a corrected height. Meznik and coworkers[39] showed a mean increase of 10 per cent, but provided no information on the method of predicting normal values. Similar results were found by Mazoyer[37] seven to eight years postoperatively. Kumano and Tsuyama[31] found improvement in the vital capacity in 20 patients treated with a posterior procedure, but not until two years after surgery.

Several studies have identified greater improvement in postoperative pulmonary functions in patients with more severe preoperative spinal curves. Boyer[9] evaluated lung volumes in severe adult idiopathic scoliosis (curves averaging 159 degrees). All cases showed improvement of 35 to 60 per cent, with greater increase being found in those with greater restriction of functions preoperatively. Similar large increases were found by Winter and coworkers[56] in cases of severe thoracic lordosis and moderate (30 to 47 degree) scoliosis. Lindh and Bjure[33] found a significant increase in pulmonary function in all cases, with a 10 per cent improvement in vital capacity, total lung capacity, functional reserve capacity, and residual volume. The height correction was calculated geometrically using a flexible rule to obtain spine length from the radiograph. However, a study by Gaziogler and coworkers[22] partially contradicts these findings. He identified a gain of 17 per cent vital capacity one year after surgery for scoliosis but did not find the results influenced by preoperative degree of curvature.

A few studies have demonstrated decreases in pulmonary function after surgical intervention for scoliosis. Some of these studies are within one or two years of surgery. Again, citing Kumano and Tsuyama,[31] pulmonary functions from 11 patients treated by an anterior procedure showed either no change or deterioration. Henche and coworkers[26] also showed a decrease in vital capacity one year after surgery for both idiopathic and paralytic scoliosis. Westgate and Moe[54] found a decrease in vital capacity up to five years postoperatively. However, the patients were kept recumbent and no chest window or routine pulmonary exercises were utilized.

Other investigators have reported no improvement in pulmonary function after surgery for scoliosis.[11, 24, 35] Master and Heine[38] and Vallbona and associates[50] both used corrected heights (preoperative and postoperative) for predicting vital capacity and reported no change in lung volumes one year after surgery. Shneerson and Edgar[46] reported no change in pulmonary functions after corrective surgery on ten females with adolescent idiopathic scoliosis. However, these patients had mild to moderate spinal curves (27.3 to 65.8 degrees) and none had abnormal functions before surgery.

Arterial oxygenation is one pulmonary function that is increased in all patients after surgical correction of scoliosis. The PaO_2 is consistently increased if it was reduced preoperatively. This improvement is undoubtedly associated with improved regional ventilation and perfusion but other factors such as improvement in diffusing capacity and decrease of dead space ventilation may play a role. Swank and associates[48] found good results in a group of patients with poliomyelitis and cor pulmonale with not only a substantial increase in the postoperative vital capacity, but also an increase in the mean PaO_2 from 55 to 64 mm Hg. One would expect this improvement in arterial oxygenation to have substantial impact on the cor pulmonale.

The preoperative and postoperative treatment routines probably influence the changes in pulmonary functions. Breathing exercises have been shown to be important for obtaining a prompt return to preoperative vital capacities.[33] However, no difference between the control and breathing exercise group was found when pulmonary functions were obtained at their long-term follow-up. Treatment with intermittent positive pressure breathing (IPPB) has been shown to cause early improvement in lung function after surgery on patients with kyphoscoliosis.[47] Because of extensive literature evaluating respiratory therapy modalities, IPPB has been replaced by incentive spirometry. Postoperative immobilization techniques that allow optimal thoracic cage movement are also thought to facilitate improvement in pulmonary functions.

In summary, the surgical correction of scoliosis improves lung volumes in most cases. This is especially true in patients with more severe preoperative restriction and with more severe spinal curvature. Some of the improvement may not be measured until over two years after surgery. Gas exchange seems to be uniformly improved if it was abnormal before surgery. These changes in pulmonary function may be enhanced by postoperative breathing exercises and casting techniques that limit physical restriction of thoracic cage movement. Further study is needed to evaluate the effect of surgical intervention on development of cor pulmonale, sleep and respiratory control, and longevity.

POSTOPERATIVE PULMONARY MANAGEMENT

The postoperative management of scoliosis patients requires a skilled, coordinated team consisting of orthopedic surgeons, anesthesiologists, experienced intensive care nurses, and pulmonary physicians. The decision to continue intubation and mechanical ventilation is made preoperatively and depends on the pulmonary function and arterial blood gas values. Those patients with normal or mild to moderate restrictive defects are usually extubated in the post-anesthesia recovery room (PAR) before being brought to the intensive care unit (ICU). Those with severe restrictive defects or preoperative carbon dioxide retention remain intubated and are brought directly to the ICU, bypassing the PAR. Patients in whom it is not possible to determine if they will need postoperative ventilation are monitored in the PAR and extubated if they can maintain adequate spontaneous ventilation.

Incentive spirometry is taught preoperatively to all patients and is started in the intensive care unit. Incentive spirometry has been shown to be effective in reducing postoperative pulmonary complications in a number of patient groups.[10] Intermittent positive pressure breathing is used infrequently and usually only when the patient is having difficulty with incentive spirometry. Bronchodilators are frequently administered to promote bronchodilatation and clearing of secretions. Beta agonists are usually administered by means of a hand-held nebulizer, but occasionally intermittent positive pressure breathing is used.

Patients who require mechanical ventilation are ventilated with a nasotracheal tube and a volume cycled ventilator in the assist-control mode. Ventilator settings are adjusted to maintain arterial blood gases at the preoperative level. If carbon dioxide retention was present preoperatively, then ventilator adjustments are made to maintain a similar postoperative PCO_2. These adjustments are made by changing the respiratory rate and tidal volume to achieve the desired level of PCO_2. The inspired oxygen concentration is reduced to the minimum that allows adequate oxygenation. The level of oxygenation is measured either by arterial blood gases or non-invasively by ear oximetry. Mechanical ventilation is continued overnight and weaning begins the first postoperative day. The ability to wean is initially assessed by weaning parameters.[43] This involves measuring tidal volume, respiratory rate, and minute ventilation with a Wright's spirometer while the patient is spontaneously ventilating. Negative inspiratory force is measured

TABLE 22–1. Weaning Parameters

Parameter	Acceptable Range
Minute Ventilation (MV)	<10 liters/minute
Maximum Voluntary Ventilation (MVV)	Double MV
Negative Inspiratory Force (NIF)	>-30 cm H_2O
Tidal Volume (TV)	3 cc/kg
Vital Capacity (VC)	10 cc/kg
Respiratory Rate (RR)	<35 breaths per min

by a manometer attached to the endotracheal tube. Values for weaning surgical patients from mechanical ventilation are shown in Table 22–1. Most spinal deformity patients are unable to reach this level of function so these values are used as a guideline rather than as absolutes for discontinuing mechanical ventilation. If the respiratory rate is less than 30 and tidal volume is 200 to 300 cc or if the negative inspiratory force is greater than -25 cm, weaning is started using a t-piece and wall oxygen.[43] Neither intermittent mechanical ventilation (IMV) nor continuous positive airway pressure (CPAP-0) is used. IMV is avoided for numerous reasons and CPAP-0 is avoided because most ventilators have inspiratory resistance, which increases the work of breathing.[52] If the patient remains comfortable on the t-piece and vital signs remain stable, arterial blood gases are obtained after one hour. If the patient is able to adequately oxygenate and maintain adequate minute ventilation without respiratory acidosis, the patient is extubated.

Weaning parameters are rechecked later during the first postoperative day if they are initially inadequate, and the protocol with t-tubing is repeated if the parameters are improved. Using this protocol, most patients are extubated on the first postoperative day. If the patient is unable to be extubated within two to three days, aminophylline, which not only bronchodilates but also may improve diaphragmatic contractility,[7] and inhaled beta agonists are administered. Careful attention to fluid balance and judicious use of narcotics also facilitate weaning. Patients rarely require mechanical ventilation for more than three to four days. Nasotracheal tubes are used for airway access for up to three to four weeks before tracheostomies are performed. The soft high compliance of nasotracheal tubes has been shown to be safe for this length of time. Using this protocol, tracheostomies are rarely required.

Pulmonary complications of atelectasis, extrapleural hematoma, hemothorax, and pneumonia are uncommon but do occur. Careful physical examination and chest roentgenograms when indicated allow early detection and treatment of these complications.

References

1. Banta, J. V., and Park, S. M.: Improvement in pulmonary function in patients having combined anterior and posterior spine fusion for myelomeningocele scoliosis. Spine, 8:765–70, 1983.
2. Bergofsky, E. H.: Respiratory failure in disorders of the thoracic cage. Am. Rev. Respir. Dis., 119:643–69, 1979.
3. Bjure, J., Grimby, G., Kasalicky, J., et al.: Respiratory impairment and airway closure in patients with untreated idiopathic scoliosis. Thorax, 25:451, 1970.
4. Blount, W., and Mellencamp, D.: Scoliosis treatment. Minn. Med., 56:382, 1973.
5. Boffa, P., Stovin, P., and Shneerson, J.: Lung developmental abnormalities in severe scoliosis. Thorax, 39:681–82, 1984.
6. Bohmer, D.: Lungenfunktion, Skoliose und Operation eine Statistische Analyse. Z. Orthop., 111:822, 1973.
7. Bukowsky, M., Nakatsu, K., and Munt, P. W.: Theophylline reassessed. Ann. Int. Med., 101:63–73, 1984.
8. Caro, C., and Dubois, A.: Pulmonary function in kyphoscoliosis. Thorax, 16:282, 1961.
9. Castex, M. R.: Insuficiencia Cardíaca en una Cifoescoliótica. La Prensa Med. Buenos Aires, Supp. 13, 1916.
10. Celli, B, R., Rodriquez, K. S., and Snider, G. L.: A controlled trial of intermittent positive pressure breathing, incentive spirometry, and deep breathing exercises in preventing pulmonary complications after abdominal surgery. Am. Rev. Respir. Dis., 130:12–15, 1984.
11. Cook, C. D., Barrie, H., Deforest, S. A., and Helliesen, P. J.: Pulmonary physiology in children. III, Lung volumes, mechanics of respiration and respiratory muscle strength in scoliosis. J. Pediatr., 25:766, 1960.
12. Cooper, D. M., Rojas, J. V., Mellins, R. B., et al.: Respiratory mechanics in adolescents with idiopathic scoliosis. Am. Rev. Respir. Dis., 130:16–22, 1984.
13. Cotrel, Y., Morel, G., and Rey, J. C.: La scoliose idiopathique. Acta. Orthop. Belg., 31:795, 1975.
14. Crapo, R. O., Morris, A. H., and Gardner, R. M.: Reference spirometric values using techniques and equipment that meets ATS recommendation. Am. Rev. Respir. Dis., 123:659–664, 1981.
15. Dayman, H.: The expiratory spirogram. Am. Rev. Respir. Dis., 83:842, 1961.
16. Dollery, C., Gillam, P. M. S., Hugh-Jones, P., and Zorab, P.: Regional lung function in kyphoscoliosis. Thorax, 20:175, 1965.
17. Editorial: Respiratory function in Scoliosis. Lancet: 84–85, 1985.
18. Fishman, A.: The syndrome of chronic alveolar hypoventilation. Bull. Physiopath. Respir., 8:971, 1972.
19. Flagstad, A., and Kollman, S.: Vital capacity and muscle study in one hundred cases of scoliosis. J. Bone Joint Surg., 10:724, 1928.
20. Freyschuss, U., Nilsonne, U., and Lundgren, K. D.: Idiopathic scoliosis in old age. Acta Med. Scand., 184:365, 1968.
21. Fry, D., and Hyatt, R.: Pulmonary mechanics, normal and diseased. Am. J. Med., 29:672, 1960.
22. Gazioglu, K., Goldstein, L. A., Femi-Pearse, D., and Yu, P. N.: Pulmonary function in idiopathic scoliosis. J. Bone Joint Surg., 50A:1391, 1968.
23. Godfrey, S.: Respiratory and cardiovascular consequences of scoliosis. Respiration, 27:67, 1970.
24. Gucker, T., III: Changes in vital capacity in scoliosis. J. Bone Joint Surg., 44A:469, 1962.
25. Guilleminault, C., Kurland, G., Winkle, R., and Miles, L. E.: Severe kyphoscoliosis, breathing, and sleep. Chest, 79:626–630, 1981.
26. Henche, H. R., Morscher, E., and Weisser, K.: The effects of the Harrington instrumentation on pulmonary functions in the treatment of scoliosis. In Operative Treatment of Scoliosis. Fourth International Symposium, Nymegen, Netherlands. Stuttgart, Georg Thieme, p. 89, 1973.
27. Jones, R. S., Kennedy, J. D., Hasham, F., et al.: Mechanical inefficiency of the thoracic cage in scoliosis. Thorax, 36:456–461, 1981.
28. Kafer, E.: Respiratory function in paralytic scoliosis. Am. Rev. Respir. Dis., 110:450, 1974.
29. Kafer, E.: Idiopathic scoliosis. Mechanical properties of the respiratory system and the ventilatory response to carbon dioxide. J. Clin. Invest., 55:1153, 1975.
30. Kafer, E.: Idiopathic scoliosis. Gas exchange and the age dependence of arterial blood gases. J. Clin. Invest., 58:825, 1976.
31. Kumano, K., and Tsuyama, N.: Pulmonary function before and after surgical correction of scoliosis. J. Bone Joint Surg., 64A:242–248, 1982.
32. Lamarre, A., Hall, J., Weng, T., et al.: Pulmonary functions in scoliosis one year after surgical correction. J. Bone Joint Surg., 53A:195, 1971.
33. Lindh, M., and Nachemson, A.: The effect of breathing exercises on the vital capacity in patients with scoliosis treated by surgical correction with the Harrington technique, Scand. Int. Rehab. Med., 2:1, 1970.
34. Littler, W., Brown, I. K., and Roaf, R.: Regional lung function in scoliosis. Thorax, 27:420, 1972.
35. Makley, J., Herndron, C. H., Inkley, S., et al.: Pulmonary function in paralytic and non-paralytic scoliosis before and after treatment. J. Bone Joint Surg., 50A:1379, 1968.
36. Mankin, H., Graham, J., and Schack, J.: Cardiopulmonary function in mild and moderate idiopathic scoliosis. J. Bone Joint Surg., 46A:53, 1964.
37. Mazoyer, D.: Seventy cases of scoliosis, late teenagers and adults, influence of treatment on breathing. Presented to the Scoliosis Research Society, Lyon, France, Sept., 1973.
38. Meister, R., and Heine, J.: Vergleichende Untersuchungen der Lungenfunktion bei jugendlichen Skoliosepatienten vor und nach der Operation nach Harrington. Z. Orthop., 111:749, 1973.
39. Meznik, F., Koller, H., and Kummer, F.: Die Enttwicklung der Lungenfunktion nach Skolioseoperationen. Z. Orthop., 110:542, 1972.

40. Mezon, B. L., West, P., Israels, J., and Kryger, M.: Sleep breathing abnormalities in kyphoscoliosis. Am. Rev. Respir. Dis., 122:617–621, 1980.
41. Morris, J. K., Koski, A., and Johnson, L. C.: Spirometric standards for healthy non-smoking adults. Am. Rev. Respir. Dis., 103:57–67, 1971.
42. Riseborough, E., and Shannon, D.: The effects of scoliosis on pulmonary function and changes occurring in the lungs following surgical correction of idiopathic scoliosis. In Keim, H. (ed.): Second Annual Postgraduate Course on Management and Care of the Scoliosis Patient. Warsaw, Ind., Zimmer, 1970.
43. Sahn, S. A., and Lakshminarayan, M. B.: Bedside criteria for discontinuation of mechanical ventilation. Chest, 63:1002–1005, 1973.
44. Shannon, D., Riseborough, E., and Kazemi, H.: Ventilation perfusion relationships following correction of kyphoscoliosis. JAMA, 217:579, 1971.
45. Shneerson, J. M.: The cardiorespiratory response to exercise in thoracic scoliosis. Thorax, 33:457–463, 1978.
46. Shneerson, J. M., and Edgar, M. A.: Cardiac and respiratory function before and after spinal fusion in adolescent idiopathic scoliosis. Thorax, 34:658–661, 1979.
47. Sinha, R., and Bergofsky, E.: Prolonged alteration of lung mechanics in kyphoscoliosis by positive pressure hyperinflation. Am. Rev. Respir. Dis., 106:47, 1972.
48. Swank, S. M., Winter, R. B., and Moe, J. H.: Scoliosis and cor pulmonale. Spine, 7:343–354, 1982.
49. Ting, E. Y., and Lyons, H. A.: The relation of pressure and volume of the total respiratory system and its components in kyphoscoliosis. Am. Rev. Respir. Dis., 89:379, 1964.
50. Vallbona, C., Harrington, P. R., Harrison, G. M., et al.: Pitfalls in the interpretation of pulmonary function studies in scoliotic patients. Arch. Phys. Med. Rehabil., 50:68, 1969.
51. Weber, B., Smith, J. P., Briscoe, W. A., et al.: Pulmonary function in asymptomatic adolescents with idiopathic scoliosis. Am. Rev. Respir. Dis., 111:389, 1975.
52. Weisom, I. M., Rinaldo, J. E., Rogers, R. M., and Sanders, M .H.: State of the art: Intermittent mandatory ventilation. Am. Rev. Respir. Dis., 127:641–647, 1983.
53. Westgate, H.: Hemi-lung ventilation and perfusion changes secondary to thoracic scoliosis. J. Bone Joint Surg., 50A:845, 1968.
54. Westgate, H., and Moe, J.: Pulmonary function in kyphoscoliosis before and after correction by the Harrington instrumentation method. J. Bone Joint Surg., 51A:935, 1969.
55. Westgate, H.: Pulmonary function in thoracic scoliosis, before and after currective surgery. Minn. Med., 53:839, 1970.
56. Winter, R., Lovell, W., and Moe, J.: Excessive thoracic lordosis and loss of pulmonary function in patients with idiopathic scoliosis. J. Bone Joint Surg., 57A:972, 1975.
57. Zorab, P. A.: Assessment of cardio-respiratory function. In Zorab, P. A. (ed.): Proceedings of a Symposium on Scoliosis. London, The National Fund for Research into Poliomyelitis and Other Crippling Diseases, Vincent House, p. 54, 1964.

Bone Transplantation, Bone Banking, And Establishing A Surgical Bone Bank

Nikki Jackson Jacobs, M.S., MT(ASCP)SBB
William E. Kline, M.S., MT(ASCP)SBB
J. Jeffrey McCullough, M.D.

Bone grafts are increasingly used in orthopaedic reconstructive surgery. In many cases the patient's own iliac cancellous bone is used for the bone graft. However, many patients do not have sufficient bone available for grafting owing to the size of the iliac crest or the size of the area to be grafted. In these patients, donor bone is often used. The use of donor bone in orthopaedic reconstructive surgery has led to the development of bone banks to procure, process, store, and distribute donor bone.

BONE TRANSPLANTATION

Bone Transplant Terminology

The terminology used to describe a bone graft is based on the immunologic relationship of the donor to the recipient. *Autografts* or *autogeneic grafts* are tissues taken from one site in the body and transplanted into another site in the same individual. The common donor sites for autogeneic bone grafts are the iliac crest for cancellous bone, and the midshaft of the fibula for cortical bone.[28]

Tissue transplanted between genetically identical individuals is termed an *isograft* or an *isogeneic* (or *syngeneic*) *graft*. An example of an isogeneic graft is the the transfer of tissues between human identical twins. This is rare. *Allografts* or *allogeneic grafts* are tissues obtained from one individual and transplanted into another individual that is of the same species, but is not genetically identical. Any graft between two humans who are not identical twins is an allogeneic graft. A *xenograft* or *xenogeneic graft* is the transfer of tissue between different species, such as a guinea pig to rabbit or cow to human. These terms are applicable to all tissue and organ transplants.

Source of Donor Bone

Allogeneic bone can be obtained from cadaver donors or from live donors having surgery during which a bone is removed. The bones that may be obtained from a cadaver donor include the long bones (humerus, radius, ulna, femur, tibia, fibula), ribs and the iliac crest.[14] Bones that may be obtained from a live donor include the femoral head, the femoral condyle, and ribs, which are removed during a total hip replacement, total knee replacement, or thoracotomy, respectively.

Autogeneic bone grafts have several advantages over allogeneic bone grafts.[5, 7] First, the autogeneic graft is histocompatible. Second, the chance of transmitting disease does not occur with autogeneic bone transplants. Third, the healing capacity (the osteogenic potential) is maximal with fresh autogeneic bone grafts. However, fresh autogeneic bone grafts have some disadvantages and cannot be used in all situations. As mentioned previously, autogeneic grafts may not be available in sufficient quantities. In addition, procuring autogeneic bone requires a second operative site and the temporary sacrifice of a normal bone structure elsewhere in the body. The second operative site may lead to infection, increased postoperative pain, increased anesthesia time, and increased blood loss. Bone procurement from a normal bone structure may result in a fatigue fracture, neuroma, or deformity at the donor site.

Use of Bone Grafts

Bone grafts are used to unite fractures, fuse joints, and repair skeletal defects resulting from injury, neoplasm, congenital malformation, and chronic infection.[5, 7, 28] Several varieties of bone can be used for transplantation purposes. Donor bone can be either cortical, cancellous, or a combination of the two and either crushed or shaped into dowels, wedges, strips, or blocks. The recipient's clinical situation will determine which type of bone is needed. In general, cancellous bone is used to fill small defects, whereas cortical bone segments are used as supportive struts.[6]

Bone grafts are used in a variety of skeletal reconstructive surgeries. Cortical bone strips are used in the fixation of long bone fractures, and cancellous bone chips are used in the arthrodesis of the spine and the replacement of excised bone tumors. Dowel- and wedge-shaped bone grafts are often used in the fusion of the spine anteriorly.[20]

Bone grafts function as internal splints or scaffolding upon which new bone can grow.[6, 7] They can provide some immediate support, such as in an anterior spinal fusion.[5] Eventually, the bone graft may be replaced by new bone of the recipient's own making.

Immunogenicity of Allogeneic Bone Transplants

The cellular components of a bone graft, which include osteocytes and hematopoietic cells, possess HLA and erythrocyte antigens. Therefore, fresh bone allografts, which contain these cells, are immunogenic.

The immunogenicity of matrix components has been studied with xenogeneic animal models. The matrix components that have been investigated include proteoglycan subunits, link protein, chondroitan sulfates, and keratin sulfate side chains.[13] Friedlaender and coworkers injected chondroitan sulfate A (of calf nasal cartilage origin), chondroitan sulfate C (of shark origin), and bovine proteoglycan subunits into the knee joints of rabbits to evaluate immunologic reactions to these matrix components. The chondroitan sulfate A and chondroitan sulfate C did not cause the production of humoral antibodies. However, histologic changes and rising titers of antiproteoglycan antibodies were detected after the injection of bovine proteoglycan subunits. Poole and colleagues, as reported by Friedlaender, demonstrated that purified proteoglycans and link proteins can be immunogenic in other xenogeneic animal models.[13] The immunologic effects of transplanting allogeneic matrix components have not been studied.

The current methods for storing allogeneic bone are freezing or freeze-drying. These methods reduce the immunogenicity of fresh bone allografts.[13] The immunogenicity of freeze-dried allogeneic bone is decreased the most. Frozen allogeneic bone has decreased immunogenicity intermediate between that of fresh allografts and freeze-dried allogeneic bone transplants. How freezing and freeze-drying effect the immunogenicity of allogeneic bone is not known, although the mechanism appears to be more complex than loss of cell viability.

Immune Response to Allogeneic Bone Transplants

A humoral response to transplanted allogeneic bone has been reported.[13] Cytotoxic antibodies against fibroblasts derived from donor tissue have been detected in the serum of recipients of fresh osteochondral allografts. Anti-HLA antibodies have also been demonstrated in serum from recipients of massive frozen bone allografts and freeze-dried bone allografts. The production of red cell antibodies following the transplantation of cancellous bone from frozen femoral heads has been reported.[18] Production of these antibodies appears to have no correlation with the clinical success of the transplant.

The cell-mediated immune response to allogeneic bone has been studied in animals, but not humans. The techniques used for these studies include the leukocyte migration test, the mixed lymphocyte culture, histologic assessment of the quantity and quality of cellular infiltrate surrounding the graft, second-set skin graft rejection following bone allograft transplantation, and changes in regional lymph nodes draining the site of graft implantation.[13] In general, the results show that a fresh allograft is capable of producing a cell-mediated response in the recipient, and reduced responses occur with the implantation of frozen or freeze-dried allografts.[13] Second-set skin graft assays also demonstrate that following transplantation of freeze-dried bone allograft, the rate of skin graft rejection is either the same or prolonged in comparison to first-set skin rejection. Some investigators have interpreted these results as evidence of the production of "blocking" antibody or induced tolerance.[13]

BONE BANKING

The function of a bone bank is to supply safe and efficacious donor bone for use in reconstructive surgery. Bone banking procedures have been developed for donor selection and bone procurement, processing, storage, and distribution.

Donor Selection

The donor selection process is designed to avoid the transfer of a potentially harmful disease, infection, or toxic substance from the graft to the recipient, and to provide a biologically suitable allograft.[2, 27] Selection of appropriate donors involves evaluating the donor's medical history, performing a physical examination or autopsy, and testing a donor blood sample for hepatitis B surface antigen (HBsAg), syphilis, and antibody to human T-lymphotrophic virus, type III (HTLVIII). Cadaver bone differs from live organ donation in that the donation of bone does not require intact cardiovascular function at the time of bone procurement. A dead-on-arrival (DOA) patient is an acceptable donor if the medical criteria are met. However, the procurement of bone must occur within 24 hours of death.[10]

The donor's medical history is evaluated to determine whether the donor meets the criteria for bone donation. The bone donor medical assessment criteria will differ from one bone bank to another, according to the bone bank's donor population, procurement technique, and the intended clinical application of the procured graft.

Cadaver donors must meet additional criteria relating to cause of death. Also, the donor criteria for infection are more stringent in a bone bank that procures bones with a sterile technique than in a bone bank that procures the bones in a non-sterile environment, then sterilizes the bones with ethylene oxide or irradiation. In addition, the medical criteria for bone structural integrity will be greater for the donor whose bone will be transplanted as a massive segmental allograft than for the donor whose bone will be crushed into chips or powder. The medical staff from each bone bank must determine which criteria are applicable to their bone bank program.

The most stringent medical criteria are established in bone banks that procure bones in a sterile environment and do not sterilize the bones prior to transplantation. Bone banks that collect sterilely procured surgical bone removed from live donors must be concerned with transmission of infection or disease from the donor graft to the recipient. Thus, the medical assessment criteria must defer donors from bone donation if the bones may be contaminated with microorganisms or the donor may have a transmissible disease or a condition that may cause a loss of bone structural integrity. The clinical application of the collected bone must also be considered. Patients who are undergoing total joint replacement surgeries are often older, and the donated bone may be osteoporotic; therefore, the donated bone is suitable only for crushing into cancellous or cortical bone chips and the structural integrity of the allograft is not often an important factor. In Tables 22–2, 22–3, and 22–4 are a compilation of criteria used by bone banks. The information in these tables is intended to include as many criteria as possible and does not imply that all of these criteria should be used.

Standards for donor acceptability must be determined by the local medical directors of each bone bank. In addition, not all of the criteria in this list are included among the suggested requirements and the standards of the American Association of Tissue banks (AATB).[2, 3]

Bone Donor Medical Criteria for Non-sterile Procurement of Bone with Subsequent Sterilization

Some bone banks have a cadaver program in which the bones are procured non-sterilely in a clean room, then sterilized after processing. The donor medical history assessment in these bone bank programs must be concerned with transmission of disease and the biologic suitability of the allograft material; however, the criteria relating to transmitting infection (see Table 22–2) are less important.

TABLE 22–2. Bone Donor Medical Criteria for Sterile Procurement of Bones Without Subsequent Sterilization to Avoid Transmitting Infection

In order to avoid transmitting infection, the presence of any of the following criteria may disqualify a donor.

Criterion	Reason
active systemic infection (septicemia, systemic mycosis, meningitis, encephalitis) or active infection involving tissue to be procured (osteomyelitis)	infection[4, 19]*
febrile hospital course	fever indicates possible infection[27]
on respirator for longer than 72 hours	high incidence of occult bacteria and septicemia detected by blood and tissue cultures[14]
died within 3 days of major surgery	frequently has positive blood cultures, thereby decreasing the possibility of obtaining sterile tissue[14]
severe superficial trauma (major burns or multiple puncture wounds) that would interfere with obtaining a sterile plane through which procurement of bones may be accomplished	risk of infection[12]
high-dose corticosteroids for longer than 1 week	high-dose corticosteroids may mask fever or infection, and the patient is more prone to bacteremia[14, 27]
no autopsy after bone procurement	an autopsy is required on all cadaver donors following bone procurement to minimize inadvertent transfer of infection or malignancy[14]
positive culture results from blood obtained at time of bone procurement	infection[14, 27]
positive culture results from any available body fluid (urine, pleural fluid) obtained at time of bone procurement	infection[27]
positive cultures of touch-swabs from sterilely prepared skin and all fluids that come into contact with procured bone	infection[14]

*See references.

TABLE 22-3. Bone Donor Medical Criteria for Sterile Procurement of Bones Without Subsequent Sterilization to Avoid Transmitting Disease

In order to avoid transmitting disease, the presence of any of the following criteria may disqualify a donor.

Criterion	Reason
history of or active hepatitis or unexplained jaundice	hepatitis has been transmitted through transfusion and transplantation[14, 25]
chronic parenteral drug abuse	high incidence of hepatitis virus carriers and bacteremia among drug abusers[14, 27]
positive HBsAg	hepatitis[14, 25]
serologic or clinical evidence of syphilis	transmission of spirochetes through donor graft (unlikely, since the graft is frozen or lyophilized). Syphilitic reagin can be transferred with donor bone and can theoretically cause temporary, positive serologic test in recipient[4, 14, 21]
tuberculosis, leprosy, or other granulomatous disease	theoretical possibility of inducing a serologic conversion following transplant from serologically positive donor. Tuberculosis has been documented to have been transmitted from donor to recipient through bone transplant[4, 14, 17]
malaria	malaria has been shown to be transmitted through transfused red cells of infected donors. However, plasma that has been frozen or dried has never been known to transmit malaria. The American Association of Blood Banks restricts the donation of red blood cell products from persons who have traveled in malaria endemic areas, taken antimalarial prophylactic drugs, or have had malaria. However, donations of blood products devoid of intact red blood cells are exempted from these restrictions[21, 26]
acquired immune deficiency syndrome (AIDS)	AIDS has been transmitted through blood transfusions[10]
history of or presence of active slow viral disease	fatal slow viral diseases (Creutzfeldt-Jakob disease and rabies) have been transmitted through corneal transplants[11, 14, 15]
malignant disease, except healed primary basal cell carcinoma	transmission of carcinoma, sarcoma, leukemia, and lymphoma are still not well enough understood to risk transplantation[14, 22, 30]
autoimmune disease, inflammatory disorder of unknown cause, or disease of unknown etiology, including rheumatoid arthritis, systemic lupus erythematosus, polyarthritis nodosa, sarcoidosis, and myasthenia gravis	present knowledge of these diseases is insufficient to determine the risks of transmitting these diseases through bone grafting[4, 14]
high-dose irradiation to tissues to be procured	concern over the possible induction of tumors in the years after exposure[14]
death from unknown causes	insufficient knowledge to assess donor suitability and the evaluation of risks to the allograft recipient[14]

*See references

TABLE 22–4. Bone Donor Medical Criteria for Sterile Procurement of Bones Without Subsequent Sterilization to Assure Biologically Suitable Allografts

In order to assure biologically suitable allografts, the presence of any of the following criteria may disqualify a donor.

Criterion	Reason
metabolic bone disease, diffuse connective tissue disorder, or serious systemic illness	these illnesses may potentially alter important biologic and biomechanical properties of the bone[14]
absorption of toxic substances in dosages sufficient to affect tissues to be procured	the pharmacologic nature of the toxic substance, its affinity for bone tissue, and the amount of bone to be procured for transplantation must be evaluated before victims of poisoning can be accepted as bone donors[14, 19]
maintenance dosages of steroids for greater than three months	bones are often too osteoporotic and brittle to provide structural integrity[14]
depending upon the intended clinical application of the graft, a donor under the age of 16 years	the long bones of children and growing adolescents have open epiphyseal plates, which should not be used in a massive segmental allograft procedure, since the plates may slip during the incorporation process. However, if the donor bone will be processed into chips, plugs, or powder, a lower age limit may not be significant[2, 14, 19]
an upper age limit may be established at the discretion of the medical director, depending upon the intended clinical application of the graft	aging is accompanied by physiologic osteopenia, which may compromise the intrinsic structural properties of the donor bone. However, if the structural integrity of the donor bone is of no consequence (i.e., bone is processed into chips or powder), an upper age limit may not be significant[2, 14, 19]

The bone to be used as the final product must be tested for sterility before it is released for transplantation.

Laboratory Testing of the Donor

The Musculoskeletal Council guidelines of the American Association of Tissue Banks recommend that a blood specimen be collected from cadaver and living bone donors for the detection of hepatitis B surface antigen (HBsAg) and syphilis.[2] The transmission of human T-lymphotrophic virus, type III (HTLVIII) through blood transfusion has led the American Red Cross to test all donor blood for antibody to the HTLVIII virus, and the American Association of Tissue Banks requires the detection of HTLVIII tissue donors.[24]

The detection of HBsAg should employ a commonly acceptable assay, such as radioimmunoassay (RIA), enzyme-linked immunosorbent assay (ELISA), or reversed passive hemagglutination (RPHA).[29] Syphilis testing should be performed using a serologic test for syphilis (STS), such as the venereal disease reference laboratory (VDRL) slide test or the rapid plasma reagin (RPR) test.[9]

Exposure to HTLVIII, the suspected etiologic agent of acquired immune deficiency syndrome (AIDS), is determined in the laboratory by the detection of anti–HTLVIII.[24] Tests for anti–HTLVIII, employing the ELISA technique, are commercially available. The donor's bone should be considered for allogeneic transplantation only if the tests for HBsAg, syphilis, and anti–HTLVIII are nonreactive. The Musculoskeletal Council guidelines also recommend that specimens are obtained from the donor for blood typing and HLA typing whenever possible. Although these typings are optional, the blood and HLA types may be used to further evaluate the significance of blood group and tissue antigens.

A case has been reported in which a patient was apparently sensitized by a cancellous bone transplant to produce Rh antibodies (anti-G and C).[18] The patient, who is Rh negative, received a bone graft consisting of cancellous bone chips mixed with donor marrow from two femoral heads obtained during total hip replacements. Both of the femoral head donors are Rh positive. Since the marrow elements were not removed, the patient was probably not sensitized by the cancellous bone itself, but rather by the marrow mixed in with the graft. This case has led the American Red Cross Bone Bank in St. Paul to Rh type all living bone donors and provide bones from Rh negative donors for transplantation to Rh negative recipients.

Bone Procurement

The bone bank medical directors at the Yale-New Haven Hospital and Massachusetts General Hospital prefer to procure bone aseptically, using standard operating room procedures.[14] Aseptic procurement of bones is also suggested in the Musculoskeletal Council guidelines of the American Association of Tissue Banks.[2] Thus, there is great emphasis on donor selection and bacteriologic testing of donor bone. For cadaver donors, bone procurement should be performed within 12 to 24 hours of death.[2] The bones are procured in an operating room, using standard operating room procedures. Prior to bone removal, samples of blood, urine, and pleural fluid are collected for culturing.[27] Culture samples for sterility testing are also collected from each procured bone. Following bone procurement, the cadaver frame is reconstructed by inserting wooden dowels in place of long bones.[19, 27]

In procuring surgical bone from live donors, the surgical bone is tested for sterility by culturing either a bone chip or a touch swab sample. After obtaining the culture specimens, the bone is placed in a sterile container for storage.[27]

Deferring donors with possible bacterial disease and testing each donor bone for sterility is necessary to avoid implantation of contaminated bone. Bone that is frozen or freeze-dried is non-viable and unvascular; however, many bacteria can survive freezing and freeze-drying. The transplantation of non-viable bone with viable bacteria can have devastating results. Since stored bone is unvascularized, intravenous antibiotics may not be capable of diffusing into the donor bone and eradicating the microorganisms within the donor tissue. Resection of the graft or amputation may be required following implantation of contaminated bone.[14, 27]

Sterilization of Donor Bone

Bones that are procured in a non-sterile environment are assumed to be contaminated and must be sterilized prior to transplantation. Several methods have been used to accomplish this. These include boiling, autoclaving, chemical sterilization with merthiolate (thimersol), ethylene oxide, polyvinylpyrrolidoneiodine, benzalkonium chloride, or beta-propiolactone, immersion into antibiotics (penicillin, streptomycin, tetracycline, bacitracin, neosporin), and irradiation with ionizing and high energy cathode rays.[8, 23, 27]

Most of the sterilization methods may have a detrimental effect on the bone or the bone graft recipient. Boiling, autoclaving, irradiation, and immersion into benzalkonium chloride, beta-propiolactone, and various antibiotics reduce the rate of graft incorporation.[23] Beta-propiolactone and merthiolate are toxic, and not recommended for use.[27] Ethylene oxide is an excellent sterilant, but ethylene oxide and its reactants, ethylene chlorohydrin and ethylene glycol, are toxic and must be removed from the bone before transplantation.[23] At higher doses, irradiation has been found to have a detrimental effect on bone, causing increased collagen and glycosaminoglycan solubility, destruction of the fibrillar network of the bone matrix, and production of mutagenic radicals.[23] The antibiotics used to sterilize bone may cause an allergic reaction in the recipient following transplantation.[27] The sterilization methods currently in use are irradiation and chemical sterilization by ethylene oxide.[4, 19, 23] However, because of the disadvantages of the sterilization methods, many bone banks prefer to procure bone under sterile conditions, and discard any bone that produces a positive bacteriologic culture.[27]

Storage of Donor Bone

STORAGE CONTAINERS

The bones are placed in sterile containers for storage. The containers currently in use for storage include glass jars, plastic jars, and sealed plastic bags. The critical features of any packaging system include durability and capacity to withstand sterilization by either ethylene oxide or steam autoclave. Materials from the container must not leach into the bone, and the container must withstand appropriate storage conditions, and must be air tight. All containers must be wrapped and sterilized according to the recommended practice of the American Association for the Advancement of Medical Instrumentation.[1] Since maintaining sterility during storage is so critical, a system with an outer container to protect the inner container from damage should be considered.

CONDITIONS

Freezing and freeze-drying are the two techniques currently used for long-term storage of bone. Both of these techniques result in non-viable bone with reduced immunogenicity, while the biologically useful properties of the bone are retained.[19]

Bones have been frozen at a variety of temperatures. Bones do not freeze at $-10°C$, so $-15°C$ or colder must be used for frozen storage.[2] Tissue enzymes are active at $-20°C$ or warmer, and at these temperatures, the enzymes will eventually destroy the tissue. For this reason, $-20°C$ or warmer is not recommended for bone storage for greater than a few months.[11] At $-80°C$ enzymatic destruction appears to be minimal. Mechanical freezers that reliably provide temperatures in the range of $-70°$ to $-85°C$ are available. These freezers should have a continuous temperature recorder and an alarm system. Storage in liquid nitrogen at $-179°C$ has also been used. At $-179°C$ molecular motion is minimal and there is little if any tissue destruction.[11] Clinical success has been achieved with bone frozen at $-20°C$, as well as $-179°C$, but the length of time bone can be stored at different temperatures is not well established.[14]

Freeze-drying is a three-step process in which the bone is first frozen to $-70°C$, then the water is removed from the tissue by direct sublimation of the ice. The dried tissue is sealed under vacuum and stored at room temperature. Storage at room temperature facilitates the shipment and handling of freeze-dried bone. In addition, the enzymatic destruction of the bone is virtually stopped because of the reduced moisture content and the low oxygen tension of vacuum-packed freeze-dried bone.[19] The disadvantages of freeze-drying include the mechanical changes due to dehydration, such as microfractures, the possibility of contamination during the procedure, and the expense of freeze-drying equipment.[6]

Sterility Testing of Donor Bone

The bacteriologic status of both the donor and donor bone must be established for sterilely procured bone that will not undergo subsequent sterilization. The bacteriologic status of the living donor is established through a complete medical history and a physical examination. The cadaver donor's bacteriologic status is determined by evaluating the donor's medical records and obtaining blood and any additional available body fluid (urine, pleural fluid) for routine culture.[14]

Sterility of the donor bone is determined by culturing either a touch swab sample of the bone surface or samples of bone obtained from the bone surface. The sterility testing is performed using routine microbiology protocols for detecting fastidious aerobic and anaerobic microorganisms.

In addition to evaluating the bacteriologic status of the donor and culturing a sample of donor bone, each fluid that comes into contact with the bone during the procurement (such as saline or glycerol) should be cultured for sterility. Also, a touch swab sample of the donor's prepared skin should be cultured aerobically to determine that the bone was obtained under aseptic conditions.[14]

Routine use of antibiotics during the tissue procurement process should be avoided.[14] The antibiotics would make interpretation of quality control cultures difficult and might preclude use of the graft in a patient sensitive to the drug. If antibiotics are used, the donor bone culture samples must be obtained before exposure of the bone to antibiotics.

Utilization of Bone for Grafting

Freeze-dried bone may require reconstitution with a sterile physiologic solution (saline, 0.9% w/v, 0.15 M NaCl) before usage. The time required for reconstitution depends upon the size and shape of the graft. Bone chips usually do not require any rehydration, whereas a massive segment of long bone may require eighteen hours of soaking for adequate reconstitution.[14]

Frozen bone may be cut and shaped while frozen. However, to thaw bone frozen at $-80°C$, the bone must be exposed to room temperature for one hour or immersed in warm physiologic solution for less than an hour. Generally, once thawed, bone should not be refrozen.

Quality Assurance

There are two major goals of the quality assurance program of any bone bank. The first is to insure as much as possible that there is no condition existing in the donor that would prove to be detrimental to the recipient's health. The second is to maximize the effectiveness of the bone graft's intended effect in the recipient.

Although there are several procedures that are exclusively performed to reassure and monitor the bone bank's compliance with the two major goals of the quality assurance program, in a general sense this is the real purpose of all of the operational procedures that are performed. Each procedure is specifically designed to eliminate as much risk to the recipient as possible while insuring that the bone graft can provide the maximum intended therapeutic effect.

Table 22–5 shows the procedures used in bone banking grouped as to whether they are designed to determine if the donor has a condition that may be hazardous to the health of the recipient, or to insure the efficacy of the graft.

Certain general principles apply to all of these procedures to insure that they have the maximum probability for fulfilling their intended function. First, all procedures are supplied in a comprehensive written form so that they can be easily followed by appropriately qualified individuals. All procedures are periodically reviewed by the medical staff of the bone bank and by the major users of bones to insure that they are still fulfilling their functions. Second, there is a program of orientation and instruction provided by the bone bank for personnel who will be actually performing the procedures. Third, there are qualified personnel available at the bone bank at all times to provide assistance and advice for anyone who is actually performing the procedures. Fourth, comprehensive written records are created to document that the procedure was performed correctly and who performed it. In addition, a complete system of records allows for the subsequent investigation of adverse reactions or ineffective graft performances and allows procedures to be modified as necessary. Thorough, accurate records are also critical from a medical-legal standpoint. Fifth, all records are reviewed by a second individual in the bone bank to act as a double check that all procedures were performed and that they were performed correctly. Sixth, there is medical monitoring of the recipients of bone grafts to insure that there are not adverse reactions or ineffective graft function.

An important concept is that quality assurance is not merely a set of separate and distinct procedures somehow separate from operational procedures, but rather it is an underlying principle that guides the development and execution of all activities of the bone bank.

ESTABLISHING A SURGICAL BONE BANK

A bone banking program that collects surgical bone from live donors is the easiest and least expensive way to begin a bone bank. The following section describes the operation of a surgical bone bank. A flow chart outlining the operational steps is presented in Figure 22–62.

Recognizing a Potential Donor

A potential donor is a patient scheduled for surgery during which bone is removed, such as, total hip replacement, total knee replacement, or thoracotomy. A system must be established to recognize these patients as potential donors. When a patient is admitted to the hospital for joint replacement surgery or a thoracotomy, the admitting or surgical staff can indicate that the patient is a potential donor during admission or by reviewing the next-day surgical schedule.

TABLE 22–5. The Major Procedures Performed in Bone Banking and Their Role in a Quality Assurance Program

Procedures to determine if the bone has any characteristics that may be harmful to the recipient.
  Medical History
  Laboratory Testing
    HBsAg
    STS
    Sterility Testing
    ABO/Rh
    Anti–HTLVIII

Procedures to insure that the bone graft will perform the expected therapeutic functions.
  Medical History
  Handling
    Packaging
    Storage
    Transportation
  Transplantation
    Thawing
    Follow-up of recipients

MISCELLANEOUS PROBLEMS

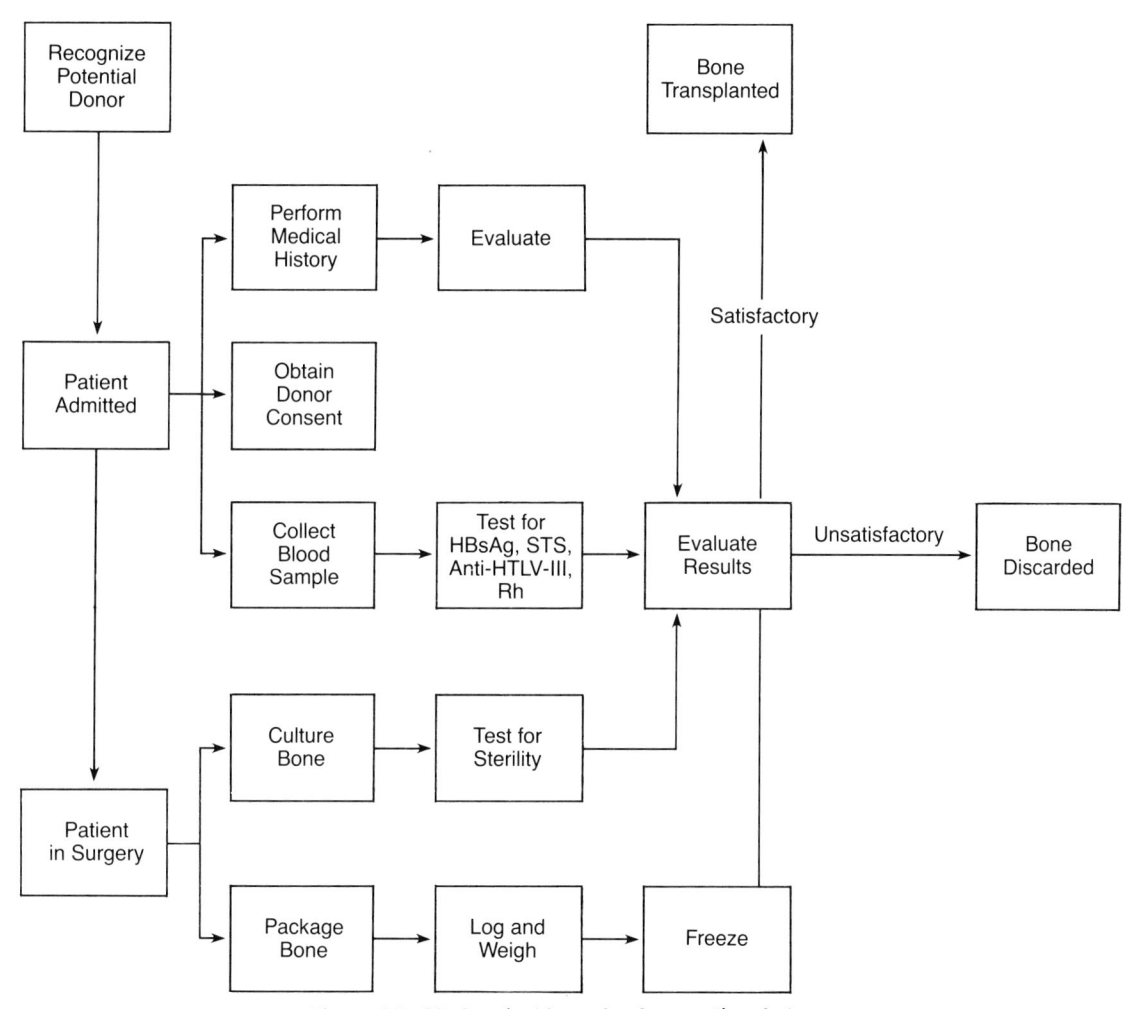

Figure 22–62. Surgical bone bank operational steps.

Assessing the Medical Suitability of the Donor

Prior to surgery, the potential donor's medical history must be evaluated by a registered nurse or physician to determine the existence of any condition that could be transmitted to the recipient through the bone graft or result in decreased efficacy of the bone graft. The patient's medical history assessment should consist of an interview with the patient and a review of the patient's chart. The American Red Cross Bone Bank in St. Paul has a medical history form containing ten questions to which the patient provides yes or no answers. Conditions precluding a patient from donating are listed in Table 22–6.

Obtaining Informed Consent for Donation

The consent of the potential donor should be obtained in writing after the donation procedure is explained in terms the donor can understand, and after the donor has had an opportunity to ask questions and to refuse consent. If the patient is not responsive or otherwise not able to understand and sign the consent form, the patient is deferred from donation.

TABLE 22–6. Conditions Precluding a Patient from Donating Bone

The presence of any of the following criteria disqualifies a patient from donating bone.
- A history of, or active viral hepatitis
- Acquired immune deficiency syndrome (AIDS)
- Symptoms or signs consistent with AIDS or pre-AIDS
- Close contact with a person with hepatitis or AIDS
- Recent history of any transmissible infectious disease or an active systemic infection
- Exposure to an infectious disease (must be evaluated individually for its risk of transmission)
- Parenteral drug users (high incidence of hepatitis)
- History of cancer, leukemia, or lymphoma
- Autoimmune disease
- Diffuse connective tissue disease
- Metabolic bone disease
- Granulomatous disease
- Serious systemic disorders of unknown etiology
- Heavy irradiation to the area of bone being collected
- A history of, or active tuberculosis, syphilis, malaria, or leprosy
- A history of, or an active slow viral disease, such as Creutzfeldt-Jakob disease or rabies

Obtaining Blood Specimen for HBsAg, STS, Anti–HTLVIII, and Rh Typing

If the patient is accepted as a bone donor, a blood sample is collected for HBsAg, STS, anti–HTLVIII testing, and Rh typing. One 7cc red-top (serum, clot) tube is needed for testing.

Packaging and Culturing Procured Donor Bone

BONE PROCUREMENT KIT

Bone storage jars and thioglycolate broth tubes for sterility testing of the procured bone are supplied in the operating room. Each donor bone will require one bone jar set and one thioglycolate broth tube. The bone storage jars are two glass jars (9 ounce and 17 ounce) with linerless plastic lids; the smaller jar fits inside the larger jar. The jars are cleaned, weighed, wrapped, and sterilized by steam autoclave. By weighing the empty jars, the amount of bone collected can be calculated by weighing the filled jars and subtracting the weight of the empty jars.

Thioglycolate broth tubes can be obtained commercially through a microbiology media supplier. However, since the tubes will be handled by a scrub nurse, the outside of the tubes must be sterile. The thioglycolate broth tubes are packaged in plastic envelopes with paper peel-back seals and sterilized by ethylene oxide. After sterilization, each batch of thioglycolate broth must be tested to assure the broth is sterile and that the broth will support the growth of aerobic and anaerobic microorganisms.

PROCURING AND CULTURING DONOR BONE (Fig. 22–63)

The scrub nurse is responsible for culturing and packaging the donor bone. The surgeon hands the procured bone to the scrub nurse. Using a rongeur, the scrub nurse obtains a few chips of bone from the bone surface for sterility testing and places the chips in the thioglycolate broth tube. Alternatively, the scrub nurse may use a touch swab to culture a large surface of bone. The swab is then used to inoculate the thioglycolate broth. The scrub nurse then places the donor bone into the smaller jar and the smaller jar into the

MISCELLANEOUS PROBLEMS 603

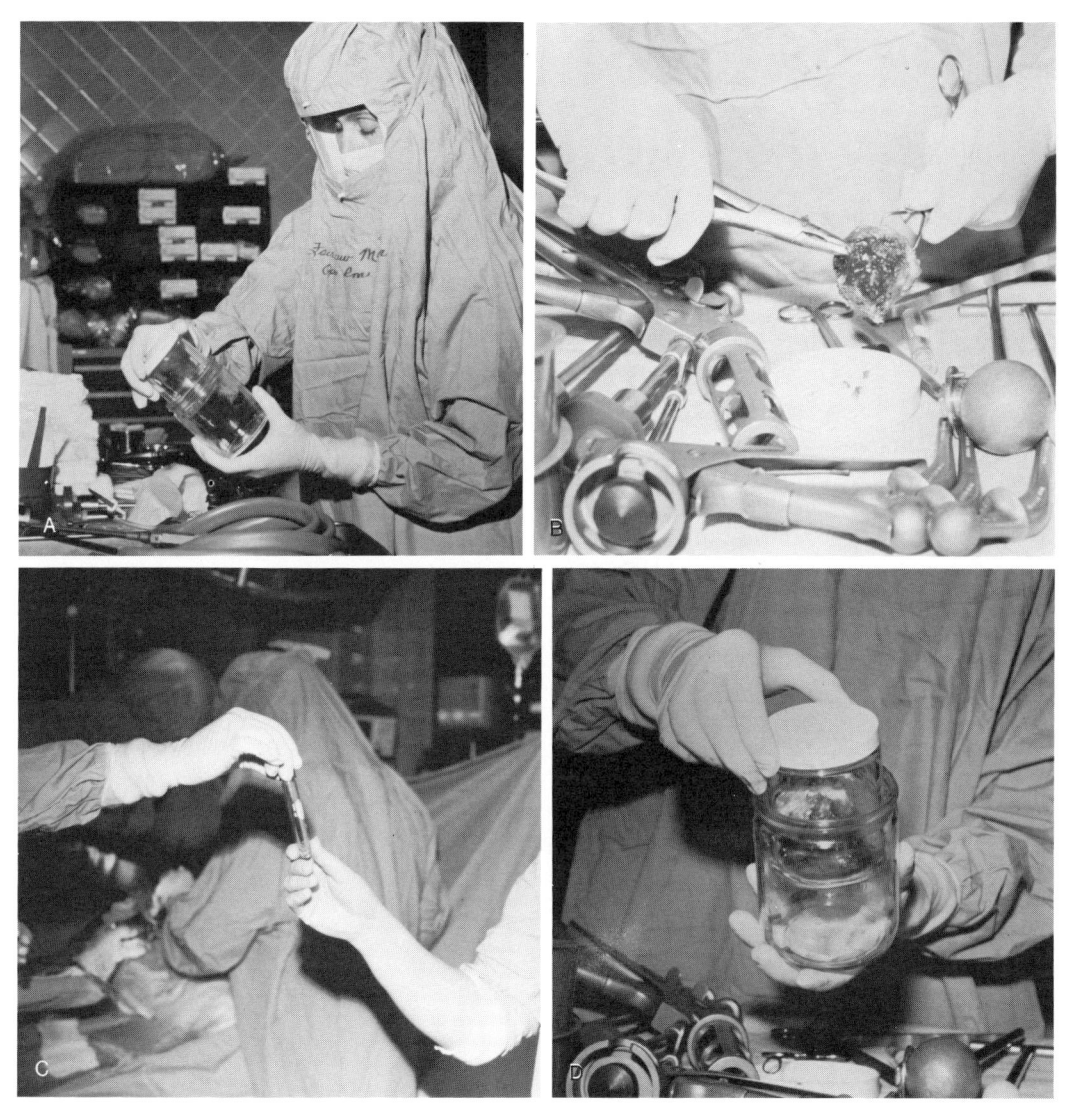

Figure 22–63. Collection of donor bone. *A*, After receiving the sterile bone jars from the circulating nurse, the scrub nurse removes the small inner jar from the outer jar. *B*, The scrub nurse receives the donor bone from the surgeon, then, using a rongeur, removes bits of bone from around the bone surface for sterility testing. *C*, The bone bits are placed in a culture tube and the tube is handed to the circulating nurse. *D*, The bone is placed in the smaller jar, then the smaller jar is placed in the larger jar.

larger jar. No antibiotics or preservative solutions are added. The thioglycolate broth tube and the bone jars are labeled with donor identification information and a description of the bone, e.g. femoral head. The thioglycolate broth tube is placed in the incubator soon after culture specimens are obtained to insure the growth of any contaminants. Likewise, the bone is placed in the freezer as soon as possible following procurement.

Storing Donor Bone

The donor bone is logged in, weighed, and frozen to $-20°C$ or colder. The American Red Cross Bone Bank in St. Paul stores donor bone at $-70°C$ in mechanical freezers. No expiration date is given to the bones. Bone which is accidentally thawed must be discarded.

Bone banking, much like blood banking, is much more effective and efficient when it is carried out on a community-wide coordinated basis, rather than with a fragmented approach in which each individual user institution has its own bone bank operating on its own policies and writing its own standards. This lack of uniformity makes communicating and sharing of resources difficult, if not impossible.

Several hospitals in the Minneapolis-St. Paul area have had in-house bone banks for over fifteen years. The surgical staff of these hospitals procured bone from their own patients undergoing total joint replacement surgery or thoracotomies, using their own procurement and processing techniques. Processing standards varied from one hospital to another. Laboratory testing of a donor blood sample for HBsAg, syphilis, and anti–HTLVIII usually was not done. Bones were shared between hospitals; however, the method for facilitating sharing was informal and, therefore, also unreliable and unpredictable. No one single individual in the community had a sense of the status of the community-wide supply of bones for transplantations. Each hospital kept a record of the bones collected and transplanted at their facility, but no centralized inventory was available.

In addition, when overseeing the operation of a bone bank is only a very small portion of what a person does (for example, when this is done by a surgical nurse), then the bone bank may not receive all of the attention that is required. Also, compliance with the standards of the AATB can be difficult for hospitals that are not involved in tissue banking on a regular basis. A centralized bone bank can provide information, education, and forms and can maintain records to help insure compliance with these standards. In addition, the central agency can insure that all bones in the system have been procured, processed, and stored according to certain minimum criteria. This facilitates sharing of bones among different institutions and can potentially increase the availability of bones to the total community.

The surgical staff from the hospitals with previous in-house bone banks have observed several changes since bone banking became a community-wide effort. First, a centralized system for monitoring bone inventory has been developed. With this system, bone can be transferred to the hospitals with the greatest bone usage. Second, a community-wide effort to generate bone has increased the availability of bone. Some of the hospitals participating in the bone bank program have more patients undergoing total joint replacement surgeries than spinal fusions. More bone is generated than transplanted at these hospitals, leading to a higher inventory. Third, criteria for a patient to be accepted for bone donations are more well-defined and stringent since the regional blood center became involved in bone banking. A medical history evaluation form with guidelines has been written, and bone donors are now being tested for HBsAg and syphilis. This uniformity of donor criteria has facilitated the interhospital sharing of donor bones. Fourth, a system for transferring bone from one institution to another by St. Paul Red Cross volunteer drivers has been incorporated.

Testing Donor Blood Specimen

The donor blood specimen is tested for HBsAg, syphilis, antibody to HTLVIII, and Rh type. The HBsAg, syphilis, and anti–HTLVIII test results must be nonreactive for the bone to be acceptable for transplantation. Recipients and bone for grafting are matched for Rh type. Recipients who are Rh negative receive bone from Rh negative donors only. Recipients who are Rh positive may receive bone from either Rh positive or Rh negative donors. However, since the supply of Rh negative bone is limited, Rh negative bone should be saved for Rh negative recipients.

Sterility Testing of Donor Bone

The bacteriologic status of both the donor and donor bone must be established. The bacteriologic status of the donor is established through a complete medical history and a physical examination.[14]

Sterility of the donor bone is determined by culturing either a touch swab sample of the bone surface or samples of bone obtained from the bone surface. The sterility testing is performed using routine microbiology protocols for detecting fastidious aerobic and anaerobic microorganisms. The AATB standard requires that the sterility testing procedure employed be that prescribed in section 610.12 of the Food and Drug Administration (FDA) Code of Federal Regulations.[3, 9]

Evaluating Test Results

The completed medical history evaluation and the test results are collected and evaluated. If all results are satisfactory, the donor bone is placed in the inventory and is available for transplantation. If the medical history evaluation or one of the test results is unsatisfactory, the bone is discarded or used for research.

Record Keeping

An inventory control system must be established that will allow the bone bank staff to identify the current location and status of each donor bone and to assess the probability of usage. Accurate records must be kept showing the disposition of each donor bone.

Requests for Donor Bone

Bone is selected for a grafting procedure according to source of bone needed (i.e., femoral head, rib, etc.) and quantity of bone required. The donor bone and recipient are matched for Rh type.

Frozen bone delivered from one institution to another should be transported on dry ice in a container that insulates the bone and ice from the outside environment.

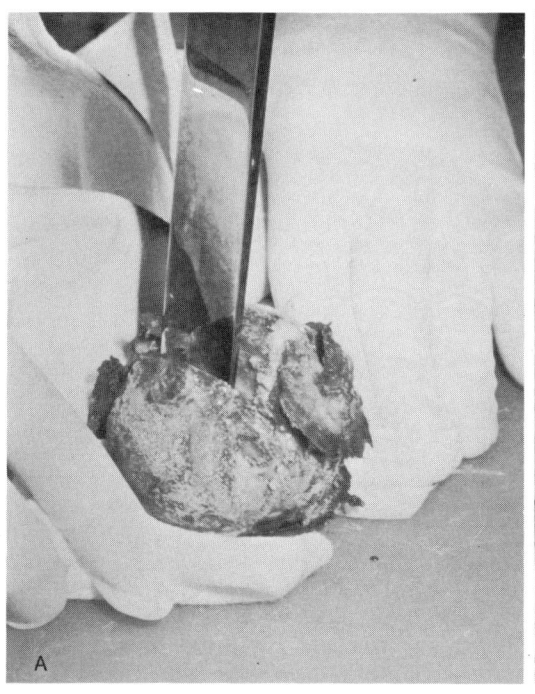

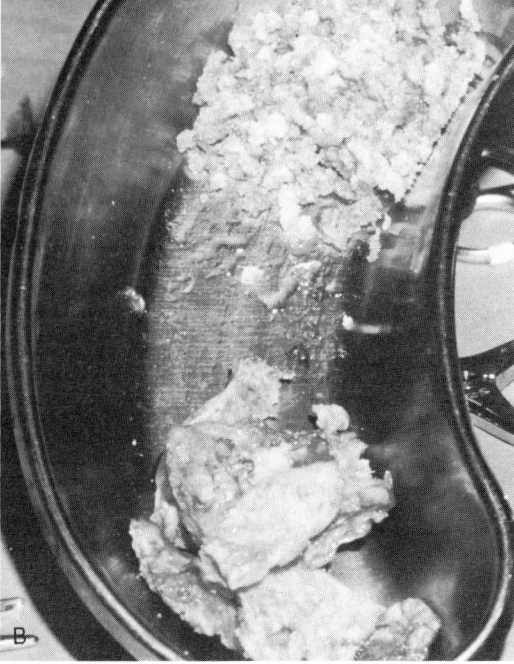

Figure 22–64. Preparing cancellous bone chips from a femoral head for grafting. *A,* Either after thawing or while still frozen, the femoral head is broken into four pieces with an osteotome and mallet. *B,* Using a rongeur, the cancellous bone and surrounding bone marrow are removed in small bits. The cancellous bone/marrow mixture (*upper portion*) is used for grafting and the cortical shell (*bottom portion*) is discarded.

Preparing Bone for Grafting

The donor bone may be cut and shaped either after thawing or while still frozen. To thaw the bone prior to shaping, the bone may be exposed to room temperature for one hour by placing the bone into a sterile pan, then covering the pan with a sterile drape to avoid contamination. If the bone must be thawed quickly, warm sterile saline may be poured into the sterile pan. Once thawed, the bone must be utilized or discarded.

The donor bone is selected and shaped according to the patient's need and the surgeon's specifications. For example, a femoral head is usually the bone of choice if cancellous bone chips are needed. The bone chips are prepared in the following manner: first, the frozen or thawed femoral head is cut into two halves with an osteotome and mallet; second, each half is again split into two pieces; third, the cancellous bone is removed in bits with a rongeur. Bone marrow is mixed with the cancellous bone chips. The cancellous bone/marrow mixture is used for grafting and the cortical shell is discarded (Fig. 22–64).

References

1. AAAMI Recommended Practice. American Association for the Advancement of Medical Instrumentation, Arlington, VA, 1980.
2. American Association of Tissue Banks: Musculoskeletal Council guidelines. Newsletter 4(Suppl): 32–33, 1980.
3. American Association of Tissue Banks: Standards for Tissue Banking. Arlington, VA, American Association of Tissue Banks, 1984.
4. Bright, R. W., Friedlaender, G. E., and Sell, K. W.: Tissue banking: The United States Navy Tissue Bank. Military Med., 142(7):503–510, 1977.
5. Brown, K. L. B., and Cruess, R. L.: Bone and cartilage transplantation in orthopaedic surgery. J. Bone Joint Surg., 64A(2):270–279, 1982.
6. Burchardt, H.: The biology of bone graft repair. Clin. Orthop. Rel. Res., 174:28–42, 1983.
7. Burchardt, H., and Enneking, W. F.: Transplantation of bone. Surg. Clin. North Am., 58(2):403–427, 1978.
8. Burwell, R. G.: The fate of freeze-dried bone allografts. Transplant Proc., 8(Suppl 1):95–111, 1976.
9. Code of Federal Regulations, Food and Drugs, 21, parts 600 to 799. Food and Drug Administration, Department of Health and Human Services. Washington, DC, U.S. Government Printing Office, p 114, 1984.
10. Curran, J. W., Lawrence, D. J., Jaffe, H. et al.: Acquired immunodeficiency syndrome (AIDS) associated with transfusion. New Engl. J. Med., 310(2):69–75, 1984.
11. Duffy, P., Wolf, J., and Collins, G.: Possible person-to-person transmission of Creutzfeldt-Jakob disease, letter. New Engl. J. Med., 290(12):692–693, 1974.
12. Friedlaender, G. E.: Personnel and equipment required for a "complete" tissue bank. Transplant Proc., 8(2)Suppl l:235–240, 1976.
13. Friedlaender, G. E.: Immune responses to osteochondral allografts. Clin. Orthop. Rel. Res., 174:58–68, 1983.
14. Friedlaender, G. E., and Mankin, H. J.: Bone banking: current methods and suggested guidelines. In Murray D. G. (ed.): Instructional Course Lectures, American Academy of Orthopedic Surgeons, Vol 30. St. Louis, CV Mosby Company, pp. 36–55, 1981.
15. Houff, S. A., Burton, R. C., Wilson, R. W., et al.: Human-to-human transmission of rabies virus by corneal transplant. New Engl. J. Med., 300(11): 603–604, 1979.
16. Jackson, N. L., Kline, W. E., Johnson, C., et al.: Sensitization of patient by cancellous bone transplant to produce Rh antibodies. Read before the Musculoskeletal Council Scientific Session during the American Association of Tissue Banks Annual Meeting, Arlington, VA, Sept 21, 1984.
17. James, J. I. P.: Tuberculosis transmitted by banked bone. J. Bone Joint Surg., 35B(4):578, 1953.
18. Johnson, C. A., Brown, B. A., and Lasky, L. C.: Rh immunization caused by osseous allograft. New Engl. J. Med., 312(2):121–122, 1985.
19. Kahn, R. A.: Establishing a tissue bank in a blood collection facility: an introduction to bone banking. In Glassman A. B., and Umlas J. (eds.): Cryopreservation of Tissue and Solid Organs for Transplantation. Arlington, VA, American Association of Blood Banks, pp. 13–28, 1983.
20. Malinin, T. I., and Brown, M. D.: Bone allografts in spinal surgery. Clin. Orthop. Rel. Res., 154:68–73, 1981.
21. Mollison, P. L.: Blood Transfusion in Clinical Medicine, 7th ed. Oxford, Blackwell Scientific Publications, pp. 768–780, 1983.
22. Penn, I.: The incidence of malignancies in transplant recipients. Transplant Proc., 8(2):323–326, 1975.
23. Prolo, D. J., Pedrotti, P. W., and White, D. H.: Ethylene oxide sterilization of bone, dura mater, and fascia lata for human transplantation. Neurosurgery, 6(5):529–539, 1980.
24. Schmitt, V., and Sandler, S. G.: HTLV-III Antibody testing. American Red Cross National Headquarters BSL No. 85–2, January 15, 1985.
25. Shutkin, N. M.: Homologous-serum hepatitis following the use of refrigerated bone-bank bone. J. Bone Joint Surg., 36A(1):160–162, 1954.
26. Standards for Blood Banks and Transfusion Services, 10 ed. Committee on Standards of the American Association of Blood Banks, Washington, DC, American Association of Blood Banks, p. 6, 1981.
27. Tomford, W. W., Doppelt, S. H., Mankin, H. J., and Friedlaender, G. E.: 1983 bone bank procedures. Clin. Orthop. Rel. Res., 174:15–21, 1983.
28. Urist, M. R.: Bone transplants and implants. In Urist, M. R. (ed): Fundamental and Clinical Bone Physiology. Philadelphia, JB Lippincott Company, pp. 331–368, 1980.
29. Widman, F. K. (ed): Technical Manual of the Amer-

Anesthesia for Surgery of the Spine

Bruce Ben-David, M.D.
Glenn S. Haller, M.D.
Peter D. Taylor, M.D.

The many advances in surgery of the spine have not only enabled surgeons to gain improved results but have led to intervention in cases previously believed to be inoperable. This, of course, has increasingly presented anesthesiologists with high risk patients who often must be brought through successive procedures each of which is of enormous magnitude.

The degree to which the anesthesiologist understands the patient's disorder and its physiologic ramifications clearly impacts on his ability to provide a high level of care. The degree to which he understands the surgeon's goals in any given case, the needs of the surgeon for optimal intraoperative manipulation, and the particulars of the surgical procedure can profoundly affect his handling of the case and thus his contribution toward a successful result. Likewise, it behooves the surgeon to gain some understanding of the anesthesiologist's concerns and the considerations that go into his decisions and management plan. In other words, good communication between services is instrumental in optimizing patient care. It is to this end that a chapter such as this is included in a surgical text.

PREOPERATIVE EVALUATION

The general thrust of the anesthesiologist's preoperative assessment of the patient differs somewhat from that of the surgeon. Beyond a general system review, our attention is directed with particular emphasis on the cardiovascular, neuromuscular, renal, and respiratory systems. The nature, degree, and etiology of the spine abnormality are vitally important both as they relate to the respiratory system and insofar as they may suggest abnormalities of these other organ systems.

The association of scoliosis and congenital heart lesions is well known.[68, 86, 118] Particularly in congenital scoliosis, in which the skeletal abnormality may be only one manifestation of an embryologic insult, one should suspect cardiovascular and renal anomalies.

A careful review of the patient's neurologic status is important. Existing deficits must be noted. Denervation, weakness, and spasticity all have implications both for response to anesthetic drugs and respiratory function. Evaluation of airway anatomy, a review of old anesthetic records, and the patient's account of any problems with previous anesthetics helps to anticipate problems. Special technical problems (e.g., the presence of pelvic traction pins, a halo, a body cast, an unstable spine, or limited shoulder or neck mobility) should be taken into account beforehand in order that a plan can be made to deal with them.

The preoperative evaluation must include those routine questions that we ask all our patients regarding their medical history: medications, allergies, prior illnesses, hospitalizations, surgery, and so on.[116] A history of prior spine surgery should alert the anesthesiologist to the possibility of unusually large blood loss. The preoperative visit should also be seen as one more component of the patient's psychological preparation for surgery. This is a process started by the surgeon and surgical team long before arrival at the hospital. For the occasional patient and family who are particularly anxious about anesthesia, it may be helpful to have a preliminary outpatient anesthesia consultation—one that is attuned to addressing any concerns, familiarizing the patient and family with what to expect, and relieving the fear that the anonymity of anesthesia seems to engender. Any preoperative visit should, of course, attempt to do these things. Specific mention should also be made about what the patient might experience: pre-operative medication, intraoperative wake-up tests, or postoperative assisted ventilation. Ideally, preoperative preparation should also include a visit from a representative from pulmonary therapy to at least acquaint the patient with this part of his/her postoperative care.

Necessary preoperative laboratory tests will vary greatly, depending on the patient's history and medical conditions. At one extreme is the young and healthy adolescent in whom only a test of hemoglobin is required. At the other extreme is the severely compromised patient with multiple system disease. This patient may require a complete blood count (CBC), coagulation profile, electrolyte level determination, urinalysis, arterial blood gases, chest x-ray, EKG, pulmonary function tests, and additional specialist consultation. For all patients blood should be typed and cross-matched in appropriate amounts if not already available by predisposition collection from the patient.

Of all the preoperative concerns, perhaps the most prominent is the potential for impaired pulmonary function. Relevant questions for the anesthesiologist include the level of the curve, the degree of curvature, its etiology and age of onset, any associated neuromuscular problems, the patient's exercise tolerance, smoking history, history of respiratory complications and management with previous surgery, history of past pulmonary infections, and the results of arterial blood gases and pulmonary function studies. Specific discussion of the associated respiratory problems—their assessment, nature, and management is found in Chapter 22.

While the end result of pulmonary impairment is respiratory failure,[10, 69] this deterioration is frequently parallelled by the development of pulmonary hypertension.[137] With pulmonary hypertension, there is potential for right ventricular failure (which on occasion may be curiously associated with left ventricular dysfunction) and a low output state, arrhythmias, and the increased possibility of coronary insufficiency particularly to a hypertrophied right ventricle.[21] Some feel that this warrants the use of a pulmonary artery catheter,[21, 84] especially in cases in which the magnitude of surgery suggests the likelihood of large volume replacement. Beyond optimizing fluid management, it can aid in distinguishing between right- and left-sided cardiac function, allows determinations of cardiac output and pulmonary vascular resistance, and permits measurement of the responses of those to therapeutic interventions with inotropes or vasodilators.

It has long been recognized that patients with severe scoliosis exhibit marked sensitivity to the respiratory depressant effects of narcotics.[74] This impairment in the central control of respiration is reflected in a sensitivity to CNS depressants in general, including general anesthetics and sedatives.[70] Kafer[70] therefore recommends controlled ventilation under anesthesia and until the effects of anesthetic drugs have diminished.

Malignant Hyperthermia

Certain specific diseases associated with scoliosis carry with them special concerns that are worthy of discussion. Possibly the most notorious of them is malignant hyperthermia (MH). Theory has it that MH is a disorder in which a triggering agent such as a potent inhalational anesthetic or succinylcholine leads to the decreased re-uptake of myoplasmic calcium by sarcoplasmic reticulum. The result of this is frequently a sustained muscle contracture and an abrupt increase in anaerobic and aerobic metabolism from cellular attempts to reverse increased calcium.[51] This translates into metabolic and respiratory acidosis, increased CO_2 production, and increased heat production.

A 1970 review of 89 cases of MH[19] revealed that six of the patients had idiopathic scoliosis. Despite this association, the incidence remains extremely small, one in 15,000 pediatric anesthetic patients and one in 50,000 adult anesthetic patients. The exact incidence among scoliosis patients is unknown.

Outside of the history of malignant hyperthermia's prior occurrence in the patient and actual muscle biopsy there is no reliable preoperative predictor of susceptibility. A previous uneventful use of an anesthetic does not rule out the possibility of MH. Nor does CPK screening have much predictive value.[5, 113] Therefore one must be alert intraoperatively for possible evidence of MH. This includes the absence of muscle relaxation, rigidity or a hypertonic contracture response to succinylcholine, tachycardia, ventricular arrythmias, cardiovascular instability, cyanosis, tachypnea and other evidence of increased CO_2 production, and a rising temperature.

The MH syndrome carries with it a significant mortality[51] and requires immediate intervention. This intervention includes the removal of all potential triggering agents, vigorous cooling, supportive maintenance of cardiovascular, respiratory, electrolyte, and acid-base status, maintenance of a high urine output with fluids and diuretics, and the administration of dantrolene. Late complications include disseminated intravascular coagulation, muscle necrosis with myoglobinemia, acute renal failure, hyperkalemia, pulmonary edema, inadvertent hypothermia, and the recrudescence of symptoms[37] following initially successful treatment. The latter point underscores the need to continue ICU observation and dantrolene administration for 24 to 48 hours after the initial episode.

For patients with known MH it is recommended that dantrolene be given preoperatively, and, of course, all triggering agents should be avoided. Flewellen and co-workers[39] suggest that an intravenous dose of 2.4 mg/kg of dantrolene 15 minutes preoperatively is optimal. Further discussion of MH and of anesthetic management of such cases is well reviewed by Gronert.[51]

Duchenne's Muscular Dystrophy

Duchenne's muscular dystrophy (DMD) is the most common and the most severe of the muscular dystrophies, all of which are characterized by a degeneration of muscle tissue. As with all the "neuromuscular scoliosis" patients, one is particularly concerned about pulmonary function and the potential for postoperative respiratory difficulties. Inkley and associates[62] described the problem as "a failure of muscle power to expand and compress the lung fully." This failure is superimposed on the restrictive defect of the scoliosis.

Another area of particular concern in DMD is cardiac involvement. Although interstitial fibrosis is present in a high percentage of cases, it is felt to be clinically significant in only 10 per cent of them,[94] and at that point it generally represents the terminal phase of the disease. The EKG has been reported to be abnormal in as many as 90 per cent of cases.[106] Echocardiography is a more discriminating measure of the degree of cardiac dysfunction in these patients.[61]

In two large series on anesthetics in DMD patients no particular problems beyond those of the disease process itself were reported.[26, 115] However, others have reported massive rhabdomyolysis and myoglobinuria,[15, 93] cardiac arrest (possibly due to rapid rise in extracellular potassium),[7, 13, 122, 126] and malignant hyperthermia.[7, 22, 117]

Myotonic Muscular Dystrophy

Myotonic muscular dystrophy (Steinert's disease) is characterized by sustained contracture of muscle after either voluntary or mechanical stimulation.[94] More precisely, there is a contracture of muscle that involves a lesion distal to the neuromuscular junction and is intrinsic to the muscle tissue itself. One of the anesthetic difficulties with myotonic muscular dystrophy patients is their response to neuromuscular blocking drugs. Succinylcholine can produce an unpredictable and generalized myotonic contracture[7] with several minutes of difficult to impossible ventilation[27, 101] because of involvement of the laryngeal muscles as well as rigidity of thoracic, abdominal, and presumably diaphragmatic musculature. Even with non-depolarizing blockade such patients may still present a problem of inadequate muscle relaxation and myotonic contractures. Percussion myotonia elicited by surgical manipulation and contractures in response to the use of electrocautery can severely hamper surgery. Neuromuscular blockers, spinal anesthesia, and peripheral nerve blocks are all ineffective against this problem because the site of the lesion is within the muscle itself. Therefore, one must attack the problem at the level of the muscle membrane. Various approaches have included quinine,[26, 110] procainamide,[26, 41, 83] steroids,[83] deep inhalation anesthesia,[97] and the direct injection of local anesthetic into the muscle.[7, 94] Deep general anesthesia, though usually effective, may cause unacceptable depression of these patients' potentially troublesome cardiovascular and respiratory systems.

The cardiac involvement encompasses both conduction and contractal dysfunction and need not parallel the severity of skeletal muscle involvement.[94] The most common EKG finding is a prolonged PR interval.[50] Stokes-Adams attacks have been reported in some.[7] The potential for pump failure seems to warrant aggressive cardiac evaluation and management.

Respiratory problems inherent in the disease compound those of the scoliosis. Here too, the process is restrictive in nature but is due to the abnormality of the muscles of respiration.[77] A CNS component to this respiratory dysfunction is reflected in somnolence, an attenuated response to CO_2,[76] and an extreme sensitivity to the respiratory depressent effect of medication.[96] In addition, oropharyngeal dysfunction with abnormal swallowing[108] makes these patients especially vulnerable to aspiration pneumonia.

Cerebral Palsy

Cerebral palsy is a heterogeneous group of non-progressive disorders with the commonality of upper motor neuron damage. Besides those problems presented by the degree, extent, and character of neuromuscular involvement, patients with cerebral palsy present several other potential problems. Mental retardation may make patient cooperation impossible and a wake-up test impractical. The presence of contractures and joint deformities should be taken into account prior to positioning. The prevalence of gastroesophageal reflux in combination with the possibility of dysfunctional laryngeal and pharyngeal reflexes is a significant concern especially since these patients already, even without intraoperative aspiration, have a high incidence of postoperative pulmonary complications. In addition, patients with cerebral palsy frequently have a seizure history and are on medication that may affect their response to anesthesia.

Neurofibromatosis

Neurofibromatosis (Von Recklinghausen's disease) presents several considerations. Neurofibromas in the upper airway can pose a difficult problem for laryngoscopy and intubation. The presence of fibromas compressing the larynx[24] or the neck or mediastinum may not only impair respiration but may cause obstruction upon induction of anesthesia. A primary involvement of lung parenchyma by a fibrosing alveolitis may further reduce pulmonary function and elevate pulmonary vascular pressures.[120] Pheochromocytoma occurs in approximately 1 per cent of cases[11] and can produce severe hypertension and cardiac arrhythmias. The possibility of a cervical spine abnormality as an associated defect should be considered.[145] Improper positioning of such a patient could result in a cervical cord injury. A small percentage of neurofibroma patients have associated intracranial tumors. A variable response to relaxants with reports of sensitivity to both depolarizing and non-depolarizing agents suggests caution in their use.[80, 144]

Marfan's Syndrome

Marfan's syndrome is a generalized disorder of connective tissue. The three particular areas of concern to the anesthesiologist are cardiovascular, respiratory, and muscoloskeletal. Cystic medial necrosis of arterial vessels leads to the formation of aneurysms. Most commonly it is the ascending aorta that is affected. This can culminate in aortic regurgitation by way of aneurysmal dilatation with stretching of the aortic ring or by actual dissection. The mitral valve too is affected, and mitral valve prolapse is common in these patients. Prophylactic antibiotics should be used as appropriate for any valvular problems. Anesthetic technique should be geared toward preventing any significant blood pressure elevations so as to avoid any increase in tension on the weakened arterial wall.

Respiratory function may be compromised not only by the restrictive aspects of the scoliosis but also by the emphysema occasionally seen in Marfan's patients.[14] The high incidence of spontaneous pneumothorax[14] suggests that caution is necessary in using high inflation pressures during controlled ventilation; a high index of suspicion for the development of a pneumothorax should be maintained. Pulmonary functions expressed as percentage of a calculated normal using arm span may be erroneous because such patients have disproportionately long arms. Joint laxity predisposes to joint injury and dislocations. Therefore, positioning should be meticulous, and undue traction on the temporomandibular joints should be avoided during laryngoscopy.

Trauma

The trauma patient often presents on this surgical service for decompression and stabilization of vertebral fractures. Anesthesia concerns are the same as for any trauma patient, for example, the nature of other associated injury, volume status, possibility of intracranial injury, possibility of an unstable neck, possibility of airway compromise or injury, full stomach, and prior medical status. Often these patients have associated pelvic and long bone fractures and thus the potential for fat embolism.[143]

The trauma patient who presents for spine surgery often has some degree of spinal cord injury. The unstable spine imposes restrictions on positioning and intubation. Since muscle spasm may bolster the area of instability, it may at times be desirable to accomplish intubation and positioning prior to putting the patient to sleep. (See Airway Management) If need be, laryngoscopy can be carried out and the patient can be intubated while axial traction is applied. Patients with low cervical spine injuries who are initially breathing well are still subject to further respiratory embarrassment. Their intercostal and abdominal muscles are unable to generate the pressures required to cough and clear secretions. Progressive spinal cord edema post-injury may envelope higher cervical cord, leading to ventilatory failure. Pulmonary edema, neurogenic or iatrogenic, can also compromise respiratory status. Acute gastric dilatation can restrict breathing as well. With the combination of poor muscle tone, immobility, venodilation, and stasis these patients are also at high risk for pulmonary embolism.

Cardiovascular problems can arise in the spinal cord injury patient because of spinal shock and loss of cardiac sympathetic tone. In spinal shock the loss of vasomotor tone causes tremendous peripheral venodilation requiring major fluid resuscitation (not necessarily pressors). Cardioaccelerator fibers (T_1-T_4), if lost, are unable to counter cardiac vagal innervation leaving the heart bradycardic. This combines with the loss of vascular tone to produce severe hypotension. Hypothermia can be a significant issue in these patients. Because of their inability to regulate cutaneous blood flow they lose a tremendous amount of body heat below the level of the injury. As the injury becomes chronic, other problems come into the picture, such as the mass reflex, autonomic dysreflexia, hyperkalemic response to succinylcholine, renal insufficiency secondary to amyloidosis and recurrent urinary tract infection, fluid and electrolyte disorders, malnutrition, and anemia of chronic disease.

MONITORING

One of the basic responsibilities of the anesthesiologist is that of intraoperative monitoring to continuously assess the anesthetized patient's vital organ function. For spinal surgery this includes the intraoperative monitoring of blood pressure, EKG, temperature, neuromuscular blockade, urine output, arterial blood gases as indicated, central pressures as indicated, and spinal cord function and auscultation of breath and heart sounds.

Blood pressure is monitored as an indirect indication of organ perfusion. Our most common indications for invasive arterial monitoring are for deliberate hypotension and for patients with major respiratory impairment in whom repeated arterial blood gas determination will be needed. Besides being an accurate indication of blood pressure, the shape and character of the arterial waveform is indicative of ventricular function, stroke volume, systemic vascular resistance, and intravascular volume. The importance of the *mean* blood pressure cannot be overemphasized as it and *not* the systolic pressure, correlates best with organ perfusion.

Central venous pressure monitoring is a useful adjunct for management of volume replacement in surgical procedures in which significant fluid shifts or blood loss is anticipated. In the presence of normal myocardial function, right atrial pressure is an adequate estimate of left ventricular filling pressure and volume. A pulmonary artery catheter rather than a central venous pressure line is indicated for patients with impaired ventricular function who require invasive monitoring for intraoperative assessment of volume status. However, in the vast majority of our cases we have not found either of these to be necessary.

Few complications of spinal surgery are more devastating than that of paraplegia. Schmitt's report from the Scoliosis Research Society Morbidity and Mortality Committee 1971–1979 quoted an incidence of 0.5 per cent spinal cord injuries.[123] Newer, more aggressive techniques such as the Luque procedure may increase this risk. Factors that predispose to neurologic injury include curves of greater severity, congenital scoliosis, kyphosis, postradiation curves, pre-existing neurologic deficit, neurofibromatosis, skeletal traction, Harrington instrumentation, spinal osteotomy, and possible induced hypotension.[55, 123] The critical issue with regard to monitoring is whether, given an abnormal result, a deficit or potential deficit can be reversed. In fact, the evidence indicates that this is so.[55, 99] One example is that of Hall and coworkers[58] who report three cases of reversible neurologic deficits that disappeared on release or reduction of the distraction force. Clearly, the evidence overwhelmingly supports the necessity of spinal cord monitoring. The two principal forms of spinal cord monitoring currently used are electrophysiologic (somatosensory evoked potentials) and clinical (wake-up test).

Somatosensory Evoked Potentials

Intraoperative electrophysiologic monitoring of spinal cord function using evoked potentials during spine surgery has become more common in the past few years, coincident with a reduction in cost and an improvement in technology. Systems for recording evoked potentials include: devices for providing sensory stimulation, filters and amplifiers to modify the signal, electrodes for detecting the neurphysiologic response to sensory stimulation, a computer to sum or average signals and to measure latencies and amplitudes, a device for storing and displaying averaged signals, and a printer for producing a permanent record of the averaged signals. Somatosensory evoked potentials are recorded from active electrodes placed in the scalp, the epidural space,[67] the interspinous ligament at a point proximal to the surgical procedure, or on spinous process of a cervical vertebra.[85] In each case, a reference and a ground electrode are required. A stimulating electrode is usually placed on the right or left posterior tibial nerve and occasionally on the right or left median nerve. For cortical recording the stimulus rate is usually set between 1 to 5 cycles per second. With an increasing stimulus rate the signal is increasingly damped;[49] this phenomenon is far more pronounced in cortical than in subcortical recording sites and is believed to be caused by physiologic fade of higher neurons or synapses.

The voltage generated by an evoked response is minute and must be amplified as well as filtered in preparation for further processing. Usually 100 to 500 successive responses are averaged, resulting in a tracing displayed on an oscilloscope. This tracing, the evoked potential, is a plot of microvolt versus milliseconds. A normal evoked potential consists of positive and negative deflections of various amplitudes occurring at various latencies, that is, the time interval between stimulation and the appearance of a deflection. That segment of the somatosensory evoked potential known as the primary specific complex usually occurs at latencies under 100 ms, whereas the non-specific complex occurs at longer latencies. It is this primary specific complex on which our attention is principally focused during an operation.

When interpreting somatosensory evoked potentials one must consider the potential effects of anesthetic agents on the evoked response. Inhalational anesthetic agents,[54] droperidol,[53] fentanyl,[103] thiopental,[3] morphine,[103] and diazepam,[54] may all cause a decrease in amplitudes and an increase in latencies of somatosensory evoked potentials. Meperidine, on the other hand, increases amplitudes of somatosensory evoked potentials.[52] These drug effects are generally more pronounced on late waves than on the primary specific complex. Furthermore, cortical potentials are more sensitive to effects of anesthetic agents than subcortical potentials.[102] Factors other than anesthetic agents, such as hemodilution,[98] hypotension,[56] and hypothermia,[133] including local hypothermia of the spinal cord from cold irrigating solutions, may also cause alterations in the evoked response.

Somatosensory evoked potentials assess the integrity of spinal cord sensory function. Halliday and associates,[15] studying cerebral evoked potentials in patients with dissociated sensory loss, concluded that the posterior columns were the major conductive pathways of the evoked response and that there was little to no contribution by the spinothalamic tracks. In a recent study Shufflebarger and coworkers,[130] evaluating somatosensory evoked potential changes during cordotomy, demonstrated the importance of the spinothalamic system as a second pathway for the evoked response.

Baseline measurements of evoked potentials are, in some institutions, recorded prior to anesthesia for both the baseline itself and to optimize electrode placement. However, unless there is a pre-existing neurologic abnormality we have not found this necessary. To maximize efficiency and minimize the cost of the monitoring, our practice is to institute monitoring in the operating room. Typically this is done with no appreciable delay of surgery. Baselines are run under anesthesia since we are not particularly interested in the effects of the anesthetic on the tracing. That is, the question being asked is "What are the effects of physiologic and surgical manipulations on spinal cord function and integrity?" Because these manipulations occur against a background of anesthesia, it seems reasonable to establish a stable anesthetic state and use this as the standard against which to compare future changes. Although the manipulation of greatest concern is that of spine distraction and its effect on cord blood flow,[32] it is recommended that monitoring be ongoing during the operation, since the possibility exists that other factors (for example, hypotension or passage of Luque wires) may also affect cord function.

Evoked potential wave forms are analyzed by measuring changes in specified peak to peak amplitudes and post-stimulus latencies of these peak deflections. One author considers amplitude decreases of 50 per cent or more and/or latency increases of 4 milliseconds or more from anesthesia steady state baselines to be significant.[56] There are, however, no studies in the literature clearly defining a range for changes in latencies and amplitudes that are consistently associated with the loss of neurologic function. Such a study would require a high number of patients as the incidence of this complication is relatively low. Despite the absence of hard data, there seems to be a concensus that severe prolongation, diminution, or obliteration of a wave form is an ominous sign and may portend a neurologic deficit.[57]

As with any other monitor, a marked change in the evoked potential signal requires further interpretation as to the possible causes and thus the significance of the change. Causes of a change may be technical errors (dislodged electrodes, altered settings on the machine, electrical interference), physiologic factors (whole body or localized hypothermia, hypotension, anemia, hypovolemia) pharmacologic factors (recent bolus of drugs), or surgical factors (direct injury by inadvertent blunt trauma, wire passage, ligation of feeding vessels, nerve root manipulation or retraction, rod insertion and distraction). In addition, one must establish the reproducibility of the change and whether changes have occurred at other stimulating and recording sites. The time course of the change (acute or gradual) may have great significance, particularly when considered in conjunction with these other factors. If a significant change in the somatosensory evoked potential is felt to be suggestive of neural injury, then further action is required. This may mean additional neurologic evaluation as by a wake-up test. Other interventions include raising the blood pressure, increasing the concentration of inspired oxygen, increasing the blood volume and hemoglobin, releasing retractors, and reducing the amount of distraction.

In general, the literature supports the reliability of somatosensory evoked potential monitoring both as a means of detecting deteriorating spinal cord function intraoperatively and predicting postoperative neurologic outcome following surgery involving the spine and spinal cord. McCallum and Bennet[89] evaluated electrophysiologic monitoring in 14 patients who had either spine or spinal cord surgery. Somatosensory evoked potential amplitudes decreased in all seven patients who had diminished cord function postoperatively. One patient who had improved neurologic function postoperatively demonstrated no significant change in the amplitude, whereas one patient who had no change in postoperative neurologic function demonstrated a decrease in amplitude intraoperatively. Engler and coworkers[35] monitored somatosensory evoked potentials in 55 patients undergoing Harrington rod instrumentation for correction of scoliosis. There were no significant changes in either latencies or amplitudes and no neurological deficits were detected postoperatively. Lueders and associates[85] observed significant changes in somatosensory evoked potential amplitudes during a spinal osteotomy when direct pressure was applied to the dura to stop bleeding. Fifteen to twenty minutes after direct pressure to the spinal cord was reduced, the amplitudes of the tracings returned to their original values. This patient had no neurologic complications postoperatively.

The reliance on electrophysiologic monitoring of spinal cord function during surgical procedures on the spine and spinal cord is based on the assumption that impairment of motor function is unlikely to occur in the absence of a significant and detectable change in sensory function. Theoretically a false negative result could occur if a lesion was produced that (1) spared only the fiber tracts that convey the evoked response or that (2) might ultimately affect those tracks but did not do so within the time that the patient was monitored in the operating room. Ginsberg and coworkers[45] reported a case of a posterior fusion with instrumentation during which somatosensory evoked potentials showed changes judged to be insignificant by experienced observers. The patient awoke paraplegic and demonstrated significant somatosensory evoked potential changes three hours later after re-exploration. Zaleske and associates[146] reported a case of partial spinal cord compression secondary to a mediastinal neuroblastoma treated with an anterior decompression. Somatosensory evoked potential amplitudes *increased* during the procedure, but the patient awoke paraplegic. These two cases illustrate the potential hazard of relying solely on electrophysiologic monitoring to assess spinal cord function during spine surgery.

Clinical Monitoring

The "clinical" form of spinal cord monitoring, the wake-up test, was first described in 1973 by Vauzelle and coworkers[138] and since then by others.[2, 58, 66] If done properly, it is simple, safe, and reliable. Although many authors cite potential hazards such as accidental extubation, air embolism, dislodgment of orthopedic instrumentation, and psychological trauma, we have not experienced a single complication during the thousands of wake-up tests performed in our institution. An ankle clonus test[60] is a viable option for mentally retarded patients who may not cooperate during a wake-up test. In spite of the growing body of literature on evoked potential monitoring, the improvements in equipment, and our own simultaneous use of evoked potential monitoring, our practice is to use the wake-up test for all patients undergoing spine surgery who are at risk of suffering a neurologic deficit intraoperatively. False negative results may occur if the test is done improperly or if further surgical manipulation of the implant occurs after the test. Also arterial spasm and cord ischemia could develop after a normal wake-up.

Because the complete reliability of both evoked potential monitoring and of the wake-up test have been questioned,[123] we are most comfortable with the overlap provided by the combined use of these techniques.

SURGICAL BLOOD LOSS AND INDUCED HYPOTENSION

Scoliosis surgery may be accompanied by major blood loss.[40, 46] This blood loss is related to both the duration and extent of the procedure, that is, the amount of muscle stripped away from the vertebrae and the area of exposed and oozing cancellous bone.[112] Although surgical technique clearly is a dominant factor, it is not the only factor. Proper positioning and good relaxation to minimize intraabdominal pressure (preventing diversion of venous blood to Batson's plexus) and attention to avoiding high mean airway pressures are of great help. Many surgeons also request induced hypotension for their patients to reduce blood loss, improve operative conditions, and shorten operating time. Clinical studies, in fact, support this practice and these conclusions.[75, 90]

To lower blood pressure one can use mechanical maneuvers such as head up tilt or positive end-expiratory pressure to increase mean airway pressure and reduce venous return. These are, however, neither applicable nor appropriate to spine surgery. Therefore, one must rely solely on pharmacologic intervention. A wide variety of pharmacologic agents can be used to induce hypotension. These include the inhalation anesthetic itself, vasodilators (e.g., nitroprusside, nitroglycerin, and hydralazine), ganglionic blockers (e.g., trimethaphan), calcium channel blockers (e.g., verapamil), alpha blockers (e.g., phentolamine), beta blockers (e.g., Inderal), ACE inhibitors (e.g., captopril), and various combinations of agents.

The use of induced hypotension necessitates the frequent and precise measurement of blood pressure. Profound hypotension requires an intraarterial catheter for continuous monitoring of arterial pressures, mean arterial pressure in particular, and analyses of arterial blood gasses. In addition to other basic monitoring, a Foley catheter is placed to assess urine output as an indirect indication of adequate renal perfusion.

Blood flow to any organ is usually constant over a wide range of pressures. However, the ability of an organ to autoregulate may be reduced in the setting of general anesthesia. Varying sensitivities of vascular beds to different hypotensive agents may redistribute blood flow to and within different organs considerably. The critical issue then is to define safe limits of induced hypotension wherein no organ is jeopardized by hypoperfusion.

There are many studies in both animals and humans on the effects of induced hypotension on regional blood flow and organ function. Unfortunately, there is a fair amount of disagreement among them, probably attributable to differences in technique (e.g., method of anesthesia, duration of hypotension, degree of hydration). For example, Colley and Sivarajan[28] studied the relation of both nitroglycerine (NTG) and nitroprusside (SNP) induced hypotension to mean arterial pressure (MAP) of 45 mm Hg in dogs. NTG maintained blood flow to brain, kidney, liver, gastrointestinal tract, and skeletal muscle and increased blood flow to the myocardium, whereas SNP caused a 14 to 18 per cent decrease in brain blood flow and a 44 per cent decrease in renal blood flow. In a similar study using a MAP of 50 mm Hg[29] these same researchers found SNP maintained blood flows at control levels to all major organs with the exception of the kidneys. However, Leighton and coworkers[82] using SNP-induced hypotension found that after an initial decrease, renal blood flow returned to normal after six minutes. Birch and Boyce[12] demonstrated the profound influence of hydration; SNP caused no change in renal blood flow when saline loading preceeded the induction of hypotension. This is not especially surprising, since ample evidence exists as to the effect of left atrial pressure on renal vascular tone and renal perfusion.[71] This may explain why Fan and associates[36] were able to decrease MAP's to 50 per cent of control values with no decrease in brain, kidney, liver, intestinal, or myocardial blood flow. Prior to inducing hypotension, Fan and associates infused lactated Ringer's solution until pulmonary artery wedge pressure was approximately 9 mm Hg, whereas Colley and Sivarajan[28] gave only maintenance fluids.

In line with these findings and those of others,[92] our practice is to avoid oligemia and limit hypotension (in non-hypertensive patients) to no lower than a MAP of 50 to 55 mm Hg. Such practice is supported not only by the laboratory data but by clinical data as well. Thompson and coworkers[135] studied the effects of hypotensive anesthesia on blood loss and organ function during total hip arthroplasty. Hypotension was induced to a mean blood pressure of 50 mm Hg with either high, inspired concentrations of halothane or a nitroprusside infusion. The control group MAP was maintained within 20 per cent of control. Blood loss was significantly reduced in the hypotensive groups and clinical and laboratory evaluation of cerebral, hepatic, renal, and myocardial function demonstrated no evidence of organ damage or dysfunction postoperatively.

What of the effects of induced hypotension on spinal cord blood flow and the combination of this with spine manipulation? Kling and associates[78] measured spinal cord blood flow in the dog model during halothane and nitroprusside-induced hypotension (mean arterial blood pressure was reduced to one half control). There was an initial significant fall in spinal cord blood flow, which returned to the control level within 30 minutes of induction of hypotension. Spine distraction during induced hypotension did not cause any further reduction in spinal cord blood flow. The authors concluded that the autoregulatory mechanism that controls spinal cord blood flow during induced hypotension is intact but its effect is delayed for approximately 30 minutes. In a similar study by Jacobs and coworkers,[63] no significant decrease in spinal cord blood flow was detected after 1 hour of hypotension to a mean of 60 mm Hg and after 30 minutes of hypotension to a mean of 50 mm Hg using nitroprusside in halothane anesthetized dogs. In addition, these authors established a linear relationship between spinal cord blood flow and PCO_2—blood flow decreased with decreasing PCO_2. It is therefore important to avoid hyperventilation and hypocarbia when using induced hypotension.

Some authors have suggested that hypotension predisposes to cord ischemia in scoliosis surgery. Brodkey and associates[20] studied the effects of direct pressure and hypotension on spinal cord function in the cat using evoked potentials. In this model, blood pressure was reduced by partial occlusion of the abdominal aorta. Neither the application of direct pressure nor the reduction of blood pressure alone resulted in any changes in the evoked potential tracings. Simultaneous application of direct pressure and reduction of blood pressure did result in significant changes in the evoked potential tracings. Although these data suggest a potential hazard of hypotension in the presence of spinal cord distraction, these results are difficult to extrapolate to the clinical setting of spinal cord surgery, since a reduction in blood pressure by partial occlusion of the abdominal aorta is by no means comparable to induced hypotension utilizing potent vasodilating agents. Likewise, Ponte's[107] report of paraplegia after hypercorrection of scoliosis and neurologic improvement with infusion of blood to correct *hemorrhagic* hypotension is not a comparable physiologic situation. These reports offer no insight into the relative safety or danger of induced hypotension as used in the operating room setting.

In conclusion, hypotension induced properly and maintained within established limits is a safe technique, not associated with any significant morbidity, which has been shown to reduce blood loss and operating time as well as improve operative conditions. This adjunct to anesthesia is not appropriate for all patients and should be limited to those who have no evidence of cerebrovascular, renal, hepatic, coronary artery, or certain cardiac disease.

INTRAOPERATIVE FLUID AND BLOOD MANAGEMENT

The elective surgical patient seldom has a major volume or electrolyte disturbance, but has incurred a fluid deficit (mostly water) by having been NPO since the previous evening. He also requires parenteral maintenance fluids for at least the duration of surgery. The use of crystalloid to replace deficit and for maintenance is relatively straightforward and non-controversial. A helpful formula applicable to patients of all ages is that they require 4 ml/kg/hr for the first 10 kg, 2 ml/kg/hr for the next 10 kg, and 1 ml/kg/hr for each kilogram over 20. Appropriate upward adjustment is made for fever and abnormal gastrointestinal losses. Deficit is simply the maintenance rate multiplied by the number of hours NPO and is generally replaced over the first two or three hours. Ideally hypotonic solutions are used to meet deficit and maintenance requirements, but in major surgery involving large replacement volumes, full strength salt solutions are used from the outset.

For procedures involving minimal tissue manipulation, maintenance fluids are all that is required. For more extensive operations, however, extra fluid is necessary to compensate for sequestration of edema in surgically traumatized tissue. The concept of third space losses is fairly recent, arising from work done by Shires in the early 1960's in which he showed that there is loss of functional extracellular fluid volume (ECF) during surgery which is independent of blood loss and proportional to the degree of retraction and surgical trauma.[127, 128] His studies indicated that ECF volume could be restored using balanced salt solutions such as Ringer's lactate and that the kidney could excrete the salt load postoperatively. This work has been challenged but nevertheless remains the theoretic mainstay of most intraoperative fluid regimens.

Surgical procedures and associated third space losses can be categorized according to the degree of tissue trauma involved.[42]

1. Operations involving *minimal* trauma require infusion of 2 to 4 ml/kg/hr of balanced salt solution over and above maintenance and deficit.

2. *Moderate* surgical trauma requires infusion of 4 to 6 ml/kg/hr of balanced salt solution.

3. *Extreme* surgical trauma requires infusion of 6 to 10 ml/kg/hr of balanced salt solution.

Most spine surgery falls somewhere near category 2, moderate surgical trauma. There are many different numerical schemes for calculating third space requirements but all have the common therapeutic goal of restoration of ECF volume and preservation of renal function. In patients with limited cardiopulmonary reserve it is safer to titrate fluid replacement to central venous or pulmonary artery pressure measurements rather than to rely on empiric formulas.

Surgical blood loss is measured by weighing sponges, recording volume in suction bottles, and surveying the field to estimate the amount on drapes, gowns, and so forth. Although studies have shown the inaccuracy of these techniques, it is important to keep a running estimate of blood loss.[23] Except in unusual circumstances (e.g., the preoperatively anemic patient) blood loss is seldom replaced red cell for red cell because most patients can tolerate moderate degrees of hemodilution without ill effect. A lower limit of hematocrit is set and a calculation is made to determine the amount of blood loss allowable before this limit is reached. The necessary parameters are baseline hematocrit and an estimate of the patient's blood volume.

The type of fluid used for volume resuscitation in hemorrhagic loss is a subject of debate. Some use crystalloid exclusively, and others argue that some form of colloid-containing solution must be used to maintain colloid osmotic pressure (COP) at near-normal values. Crystalloid is distributed through the entire extracellular space and therefore must be given in a volume exceeding blood loss in a ratio of approximately 3:1. Colloid, on the other hand, can be administered in a 1:1 ratio, and its proponents contend that volume replacement with pure crystalloid results in a reduction in COP and therefore predisposes the patient to edema formation. While it is true that COP does fall and edema does accumulate in peripheral tissues, the basic issue is whether or not fluid collects in the lung and adversely affects pulmonary oxygen exchange. In the absence of elevated left ventricular filling pressures, the weight of evidence suggests that it does not.[29, 139, 140] Whether or not peripheral edema is a serious disadvantage is a matter of opinion. Given that neither method is clearly superior, we opt for the more cost effective one and routinely use crystalloid for volume replacement up to the limit of allowable blood loss.

When blood replacement becomes necessary, many prefer whole blood because it supplies both volume and oxygen-carrying (red cell) requirements. If only packed cells are available, some compromise must be made. For losses exceeding ⅓ of blood volume (BV), packed cells are often supplemented with plasma protein fraction, albumin, or artificial colloid solution to provide the volume equivalent of whole blood. Fresh frozen plasma (FFP) should specifically *not* be used for this purpose.[30] If volume is replaced with crystalloid, care must be taken to match the plasma deficit with at least triple the volume of crystalloid to compensate for its redistribution.

Beyond 24 hours of storage, whole blood contains few viable platelets. Patients are at risk of bleeding secondary to dilutional thrombocytopenia when they have received a transfusion of more than one blood volume, and platelet concentrates should be given at that point. One unit of platelets raises the platelet count of a 70 kg adult by 5,000 to 10,000/µl, and it is recommended that 8 to 10 units be transfused at a time. Patients who have undergone losses greater than one blood volume should receive FFP to replace coagulation factors.

Since it is stored at 4° C, all blood is warmed before transfusion in the operating room. All blood products are administered through standard millipore (170 µm) filters that trap clots and other macroaggregates, which are invariably present. Micropore filters with pore sizes from 20 to 40 µm have been designed to remove the smaller fibrin-white cell-platelet microaggregates. The theoretical disadvantage of not filtering microaggregates is that they will lodge in the lung and cause deterioration of pulmonary function, perhaps contributing to adult respiratory distress syndrome (ARDS) in the massively transfused patient. There is no good evidence to support this claim, however.[95] Given the information at hand, a compromise is to use micropore filters for transfusions of greater than half a blood volume.

Autologous Transfusion Techniques

The surgical patient can serve as his own blood donor in three ways: (1) preoperative deposit and storage; (2) phlebotomy and hemodilution immediately preoperatively; (3) intraoperative salvage. The significant advantages of autologous transfusion are conservation of homologous banked blood and provision of blood with guaranteed compatibility and absence of infectious risk. Although hemolytic and other serious reactions are unusual, post-transfusion hepatitis is not. Despite HB_sAg screening and a trend away from paid donors, the overall incidence of hepatitis (icteric and non-icteric) is approximately 7 per cent of all recipients. Most cases are non-A, non-B of which a small percentage are fatal and another significant percentage progress to chronic active hepatitis.[1]

PREDEPOSIT

A healthy patient can donate blood preoperatively without increasing the risk of surgery.[51] An average adult male or postmenopausal female is able to donate four units in the three-week period preceding surgery with only a small change in hematocrit. Plasma is regenerated quickly; the rate-limiting process is erythropoesis, which can increase to three times its normal rate with the stimulus of phlebotomy if iron stores are adequate. The collected blood is usually stored under exactly the same conditions as for homologous donations, that is, as a liquid at 4°C in citrate phosphate dextrose (CPD) solution, which has a 21 day storage limit.

Recently approved CPD with adenine anticoagulant solution (CPDA-1) allows storage for 35 days and should expand predeposit capabilities. Storage of red cells in the frozen state greatly lengthens the time scale and permits collection of many more units, but it is an expensive process used mainly for patients' whose antibody status makes crossmatching of homologous blood difficult.

PREOPERATIVE HEMODILUTION AND AUTOTRANSFUSION

Hemodilution simply means the substitution of cell-free fluids for blood in the circulation, a procedure carried out on a limited basis in nearly every blood-losing surgery by allowing hematocrit to drop to a predetermined level before transfusing. Preoperative hemodilution extends this concept to controlled dilution by phlebotomy, aiming for a hematocrit in the range of 20 to 25 per cent. As well as lowering oxygen-carrying capacity, reduction of erythrocyte concentration causes a decrease in blood viscosity and therefore a decrease in total peripheral resistance.[47] The physiologic adaptation in patients with normal cardiac function is a reflex increase in cardiac output, almost entirely from augmented stroke volume. Heart rate and blood pressure remain unchanged. The increase in cardiac output is sufficient to offset the decrease in arterial oxygen carrying capacity and maintain tissue oxygenation.[64, 81, 91] Local tissue oxygenation has been studied using O_2 electrodes with the finding that microcirculatory flow becomes more homogeneous, a change attributed to the improved rheological properties of diluted blood. It should be emphasized that the increases in cardiac output can achieve full compensation for the reduction in oxygen content only under conditions of normovolemia and a hematocrit no less than 20 per cent.

Three major advantages are gained by hemodilution. First, the number of red cells lost through surgical bleeding is reduced, since what ends up on the sponges and in the suction bottle has a lower hematocrit from the outset. Second, it provides a source of fresh autologous blood with normal clotting factors, platelets, and oxyhemoglobin affinity. Third, if the phlebotomized blood is kept in continuity with the patient's circulation, the technique is acceptable to most Jehovah's Witnesses.[131]

Blood is withdrawn after induction of anesthesia. It is collected through venous or arterial catheters and stored in standard CPD donor bags at room temperature. The bag is continuously weighed during collection to monitor the rate of withdrawal and plasma substitute is infused simultaneously through another IV line. Both crystalloid and colloid have been used as diluents, with the same arguments for and against each as were raised in the preceding discussion on volume resuscitation during hemorrhage. Heart rate and blood pressure are monitored closely, and a rise in heart rate or fall in pressure demands re-evaluation of volume status. Dilution is usually carried out in two stages, checking hematocrit midway through the procedure. When surgical blood loss reaches approximately 300 ml (in an adult), reinfusion is begun with the last (most dilute) unit withdrawn and proceeds in reverse order of collection. Thus, the units with highest hematocrit and concentration of clotting factors are infused last.

An arterial catheter is advisable since it provides a sampling port for serial hematocrit and blood gas determinations as well as a better handle on volume status. A central venous or pulmonary artery catheter is useful for monitoring fluid replacement as well. Choice of anesthetic technique is not critical except that it should allow for high inspired oxygen concentration. Deliberate hypothermia (i.e., 30 to 31°C) is seldom employed with moderate hemodilution but is regularly used in conjunction with extreme (hct<20%) dilution to minimize tissue oxygen requirements. The concomitant use of hemodilution and profound hypotension is controversial, particularly during scoliosis surgery where the combination might increase the risk of spinal cord ischemia.

Acute normovolemic hemodilution is a safe and effective method of conserving blood in most surgical patients. Those with significant anemia or major organ system disease, particularly cardiac, should be excluded. Physicians responsible for ongoing care of the patient should be aware that the maximum benefit of this technique is dependent on the acceptance of postoperative hemodilution.

INTRAOPERATIVE SALVAGE

Intraoperative salvage involves collecting the patient's own blood from the operative field and reinfusing it instead of homologous transfusion. The technique has been in use since the mid 1960's; although it is a logical and appealing concept, its widespread application has been hindered by a series of problems. Adverse hematologic effects such as hemolysis, decreased erythrocyte survival time, platelet loss, coagulation disorders, fibrinogen loss, and development of fibrin degradation products and microemboli have all been reported.[38] Air embolism, sepsis, and spread of malignancy are further complications. Contamination of the blood with bacteria, usually from bowel contents, or tumor cells is a contraindication to the technique. The first commercial autotransfusion machine, the Bentley Autotransfusion System, was removed from the market after several incidents of fatal air embolism. The risk of embolism with more modern devices is minimal. Much of the hematologic damage has been eliminated by changes in suction design and by systems that automatically wash and concentrate red cells prior to reinfusion. Early machines required a technician to be present at all times, but the newer programmable models need minimal operator attention. Although the blood does not maintain continuity with the vascular tree, some Jehovah's Witness patients find use of intraoperative salvage acceptable.

AIRWAY MANAGEMENT

Airway management is another fundamental of anesthetic practice. A sizable percentage of anesthetic disasters derive specifically from some aspect of airway mismanagement.[33, 88] Spine surgery is one of the areas of anesthetic practice in which concern is especially great. Although the causes of difficult airways and intubations are many, those that pertain here generally have little to do with intrinsic airway pathology. Rather, the limitations of neck mobility[16] and the distortions of the cervical spine alone, or in combination, can create tremendous difficulty. Some examples that one sees with regularity on a spine service include Klippel-Feil syndrome, rheumatoid arthritis, ankylosing spondylitis, the unstable neck, and severe kyphoscoliosis. At times, external hardware or casting may be the limiting factor. At other times these devices may make access to the patient for standard laryngoscopy and intubation a problem.

Preoperative evaluation is critical in anticipating and averting airway problems. The patient's history (including prior anesthetic records) and physical examination results, the ability to flex and extend the neck, the size and mobility of the jaw, respiratory and cardiovascular status, AP and lateral neck films, flow-volume loop, and arterial blood gas determinations are all helpful pieces of information.

In general, it is difficult to argue with the safety of an awake intubation.[79, 134] The patient continues to breathe and protect his airway. With adequate explanation and reassurance, gentle and thorough anesthesia of the airway, and judicious sedation there are few patients who do not accept this well. Whether to use the oral or nasal route or to use a blind or visualized technique are strategies whose merit depend on both patient and the anesthesiologist. A direct visualized oral approach, utilizing a variety of blades and attachments at times in combination with rigid or flexible styletted tubes, has been used successfully on many occasions at this institution. Blind nasal intubation[6, 9] may prove easier than the oral approach and is further facilitated by having the patient hyperventilate, pulling the tongue forward or having the patient stick his own tongue out, and proper positioning of the head. If unsuccessful, intraoral manipulation of the tube with or without the additional use of a laryngoscope is possible.

Recent years have seen an eclipsing of these techniques by the fiberoptic bronchoscope applied to the difficult airway.[105, 142] This is especially true now with the newer pediatric fiberscopes[119] that allow the passage of smaller endotracheal tubes combined with suction capacity (or oxygen insufflation) and excellent optics. Either orally or nasally this technique is extremely well tolerated. Ovassapian and coworkers[100] using fiberoptic awake nasotracheal intubation on 200 patients demonstrated only small increases in blood pressure and heart rate, and only 4.5 per cent of patients considered the experience somewhat unpleasant. This technique is most efficient and successful when used early with a difficult intubation. As a last resort in an already traumatized airway, it is far more difficult and often impossible to use successfully. Furthermore, its skillful application in the difficult situation requires a facility gained by repeated use in less trying circumstances. For all these reasons one can make a strong argument for the regular use of awake fiberoptic intubations on patients suspected or known to have difficult airways.

There are advantages and disadvantages to oral versus nasal fiberoptic intubation. If one anticipates a need for postoperative mechanical ventilation, a nasal approach is preferable simply because the nasal tube is better tolerated postoperatively. Technical advantages of a nasal route include a more direct entry to the larynx and less interference from the tongue. Also the patient cannot bite down on the fiberscope. However, in practice an oral fiberoptic intubation does not seem any more difficult and does not have the same potential for tissue trauma and bleeding. Both techniques appear to elicit minimal cardiovascular response arising from pressure on or stimulation of pharyngeal tissues. In fact, for nasal fiberoptic intubation the only cardiovascular change has been associated with passing the endotracheal tube through the nostril.[100]

Certainly most patients do not present airway problems and do not require an awake intubation. Even when it is indicated, it is not always desirable or possible. In those cases an induction directed at maintaining spontaneous ventilation is indicated. Once induction is completed, fiberoptic intubation may be accomplished using either a Patel-Syracuse mask (a standard anesthesia mask with an additional endoscopic port) or using a nasal or binasal airway attached to the anesthesia circuit.[105] Hyperpnea to facilitate intubation, blind or otherwise, can be induced using doxapram. Should one repeatedly fail to intubate or have difficulty maintaining the airway, it is wise to stop before there is complete obstruction and consider either awakening the patient or performing a tracheostomy. The latter, though undesirable, is an option that rare times may be warranted as the initial management plan.

The establishment of an endotracheal tube raises the issue of how to then ventilate the patient. Positive-pressure ventilation increases mean airway pressure, which increases mean intrathoracic pressure and inhibits venous return. The resultant increase in venous pressure would be expected to increase flow to Batson's plexus and increase intraoperative venous bleeding.[112] Negative end-expiratory pressure reverses this effect,[112] but is not recommended because of the potential for air embolism and airway closure and atelectasis with resulting hypoxemia.[121] Controlled hyperventilation ($PaCO_2$ 25 to 30 mm Hg) may reduce blood loss by causing peripheral vasoconstriction,[112] but it would be countered in part by the increase in mean airway pressure from the controlled hyperventilation. Furthermore, spinal cord blood flow like cerebral blood flow, as noted earlier, is extremely responsive to $PaCO_2$ and will decrease with decreasing $PaCO_2$. There are already the potential effects of surgical manipulation, ligation of radicular arterial supply during anterior procedures, induced hypotension, and hemodilution on spinal cord blood flow, oxygen delivery, and ultimately spinal cord function. It seems unduly hazardous to add the additional risk of hypocarbia. Also, the combination of induced hypotension and hypocarbia may be a dangerous one with regard to cerebral perfusion. Therefore, it is recommended that along with zero end-expiratory pressure (ZEEP) the patient be ventilated to maintain normocarbia while minimizing inflation pressures as much as possible.

During anterior transthoracic procedures it may be desirable to improve operative exposure by selectively ventilating only the lung on the non-operative side. Today, double-lumen endotracheal tubes are generally the preferred method of providing one-lung anesthesia. The principal problem with one-lung anesthesia is the potential for hypoxemia due primarily to the shunt created by continued perfusion of the non-ventilated lung. The multiple factors at play and the optimum management of one-lung anesthesia are well detailed elsewhere.[4, 73] An arterial line and gas testing are necessary with this technique. Recently, the use of transcutaneous PO_2 monitoring[136] and pulse oximetry[124] have been described for use with one-lung ventilation. The latter, in particular, is extremely simple to use, requires no warm-up time, and provides a continuous and accurate accounting of arterial oxygen saturation.

POSITIONING

Proper positioning of the patient is of the utmost importance. Its significance relates to its role in optimizing surgical exposure and its physiologic impact on the anesthetized patient.

The Classic prone position, that is, the patient simply lying face down with his entire ventral surface in contact with the bed, has both respiratory and cardiovascular effects that make it unacceptable. The body's weight on the abdomen restricts diaphragmatic movement and thereby impairs ventilation. The abdominal compression is transmitted to the inferior vena cava, causing both hypotension secondary to decreased venous return and a shunting of blood to the valveless epidural venous plexus.[8] Engorgement of these veins obscures the surgical field and greatly increases operative blood loss. Because of the valveless nature of Batson's plexus and its communication with cranial venous drainage, this engorgement might also be expected to decrease cerebral perfusion pressure, a potentially critical issue when using induced hypotension.

To circumvent these problems Relton and Hall[114] devised a four-point positioning frame with padded supports angled inward to provide lateral stability while supporting the patient with the abdomen hanging free. Although some changes in functional residual capacity,[34, 111] intrapulmonary distribution of ventilation and perfusion,[72, 111] and the pattern of respiratory expansion[111] are seen, these are clinically of minimal significance. Even the most severe of the scoliotic pulmonary cases tolerate proper prone positioning quite well. In fact, prone positioning has been used to *improve* pulmonary function in the ICU setting both for adults[34] and neonates.[141] The use of this frame does alleviate the cardiovascular consequences of abdominal compression but it can create others. The dependent position of the legs in the anesthetized and fasted (therefore dehydrated) patient can itself produce significant hypotension. This is countered by the use of compressive stockings, additional fluid at the time of induction, and the use of light anesthesia or a technique less likely to cause vasodilation.

The frame itself is positioned so that the patient's anterior superior iliac spines lie in the middle of the lower supports. The upper supports underlie the anterolateral midchest. They should be low enough to avoid pressure in the axillae and high enough to avoid the lowermost ribs and abdomen. A local modification of Hall and Relton's original design uses four padded, wooden posts on a Velcro base. This affords both radiolucency for intraoperative x-rays and a set of easily movable and independently mobile posts that can rapidly and efficiently accommodate the most contorted of patients.

Turning the patient onto the frame is best accomplished from an adjacent litter. First, though, anesthesia is induced with the patient on the litter. The endotracheal tube, esophageal stethoscope, Foley catheter, eye tapes, and any additional intravenous or arterial lines are placed and fixed. Prior to turning, tubing lines and cables should be minimized as much as possible (e.g., temporarily disconnent endotracheal tube, arterial line, blood pressure cuff tubing, EKG cables) or placed in advance to avoid tangling during the turn. Positioning equipment must all be in place. The anesthetist should continue to auscult the esophageal stethoscope to avoid a total monitoring blackout during this time.

The turn requires four to six people, depending on the patient's size. After disconnecting the endotracheal tube, the anesthetist should grasp the head in such a manner as to stabilize and protect it through the move and prevent any sudden or extreme twisting of the neck. With one or two people on either side of the patient he is gently rolled into the arms of those "catching" who lift the patient onto the frame. The arms are swung down (to avoid shoulder dislocation) and forward and temporarily placed beside the head. The endotracheal tube is reattached, breath sounds verified bilaterally, and monitoring promptly re-established. The posts are positioned as indicated, and stability of the body mass atop the frame assured.

The head is turned to the side and positioned to avoid pressure on the eyes, ears, and nose. As much as possible the weight of the face should be evenly supported. Excessive extension or torsion of the neck is to be avoided (1) because of the potential for vertebral artery kinking or compression and jugular vein obstruction with resultant decrease in cerebral perfusion pressure, elevation of intracranial pressure, and superficial edema;[31] (2) because excessive extension could compress or disrupt the cervical cord, especially if there are spondylitic spurs; (3) because the combination may exert pressure on C2 as it emerges between the atlas and axis,[132] and (4) because it can so stretch the contralateral brachial plexus as to injure it.[17]

The brachial plexus is extremely vulnerable to positioning injury. Compression and stretching both play a role here. Again, supports must not extend cephalad into the axillae and abduction and anterior flexion of the arms greater than 90 degrees must be avoided.[18] To protect the ulnar nerve, arms should be positioned with sufficient padding and support beneath the upper arms to eliminate any weight bearing at the elbow.

Care should be taken that the female patient's weight does not rest on her breasts. Genitalia must be guarded against compression, abrasion (e.g., by the Velcro base), and encroachment by the electrocautery grounding plate. Patients whose abdomens protrude sufficiently to touch the Velcro base plate should be protected against abrasion there by placing a towel or sheet in between. Knees should be padded with small "donuts" underneath each one to prevent a small area of localized excessive pressure and skin ischemic injury.[43] Padding under the dorsum of each foot may protect both the toes and the anterior tibial nerve from injury, which can result from prolonged and excessive plantar flexion.[125]

Lastly, the relaxation of paraspinous muscles, the anesthetized patient's inability to guard himself, possibly combined with a prior anterior immobilizing procedure, may set the stage for a back or neck injury during turning[18] as a result of undue stretching of ligament, muscle, and nerve. Obviously a gentle, slow, and controlled turn is important. However, in cases in which there is particular concern, as with an unstable spine, the patient can be intubated awake and assist and participate in his own turning. Not only does this add an element of safety but it is very comforting to all involved to see the patient prone, positioned, and fixed into place moving all extremities normally prior to induction.

ANESTHETIC TECHNIQUE

Premedication choices vary, depending on the phychologic and physiologic status of the patient, intraoperative plans, and the anesthesiologist's style of practice. In our institution premedication is often a small dose of sedative, typically a benzodiazapine and a narcotic without an anticholinergic agent (in adults).

The choice of induction agent largely reflects the overall anesthetic plan, and it is difficult to discuss these separately. Anesthetic technique is generally based on either a narcotic or a potent inhalational agent. Because the narcotic-based techniques facilitate spinal cord monitoring (easier wake-up tests, less effect on evoked potentials) these are most often used for scoliosis surgery. The choice of narcotic and the particular means of administration—up front loading, loading plus additional small boluses, loading plus continuous infusions—are essentially all variations of the same theme. Fentanyl has become an extremely popular choice because of its rapid onset of action and the cardiovascular stability it affords.

Even fairly low doses of fentanyl have been shown to markedly blunt the cardiovascular response to laryngoscopy and intubation.[87] Sufentanyl, a new fentanyl analog, is extremely promising and is likely to see widespread use. With the methadone technique described by Gourley and coworkers[48] there is a slower onset of action, but one essentially administers the drug as a single front-end load. However, part of this dose can be given earlier in the premedication. Further titration of anesthetic depth can, as with any narcotic technique, be accomplished with low concentrations of inhalation agent. Pathak and associates[104] compared small loading doses plus continuous infusions of fentanyl and morphine (fentanyl 2.5 µg/kg plus 1.5 to 2.5 µg/kg/hour, morphine sulfate 250 µg/kg plus 150 to 250 µg/kg per hour) versus the same small loading doses plus additional boluses of drug as indicated. They concluded that the continuous infusion of either drug provided a smoother, easier, and more rapidly achievable wake-up test plus more stable and predictable suppression of the cortical somatosensory evoked potential.

The choice of sedative, beyond that given in the premedication, in this country almost always begins with thiopental 3 to 5 mg/kg. Some centers have taken to using thiopental infusions as a means of avoiding significant use of inhalational agents. The rationale here again is that of a lesser and a more stable suppression of somatosensory evoked response. Others prefer to use low concentrations of potent inhalational agents to achieve the same goal. It is worth noting that the narcotics, by themselves, are poor sedatives and should not be relied on to prevent intraoperative recall.

The choice of relaxant is less important than the point that relaxants should be used to decrease intraabdominal pressure and prevent straining. This should be advantageous in reducing blood loss. If one is applying evoked potential monitoring post-induction then obviously intubation with succinylcholine is preferable to a non-depolarizing agent because its effects are short-lived and allow localization of the nerve with a stimulator. In some patients the use of succinylcholine is contraindicated in which case one should accomplish nerve localization and afix the stimulator prior to induction. Intubation can then proceed using longer-acting non-depolarizing neuromuscular blockers. Paralysis is generally allowed to wear off as intraoperative wakeup is approached to facilitate its performance. Jones and coworkers[66] showed that this muscle tone mildly inhibits correction, and felt that it added an element of safety by preventing overdistraction.

Inhalational anesthetics include both nitrous oxide and the halogenated hydrocarbons. The former has for many years been a standard component of most anesthetics. Recently, some have suggested avoiding it because it has deleterious effects on the evoked potential response. On the other hand, its safety and reliability and the insolubility that provides us with the ability to rapidly reverse anesthesia still make it a highly desirable agent to use. Of the potent inhalational agents we prefer isoflurane or enflurane over halothane because they are less sensitizing to the myocardium of the arrhythmogenic effects of catecholamines.[61] The standard practice of infiltrating the operative site with a large volume of dilute epinephrine/saline solution makes this a significant consideration. Forane, because of its relative insolubility and thus rapidity of emergence, has become a favorite agent in our and many institutions.

Our technique in recent years has predominantly relied on fentanyl loading on induction with repeated small boluses through the operation, nitrous oxide 50 to 70 per cent, and low dose isoflurane as needed. Although a reliable technique that affords an easy intraoperative wake-up, the significant SCEP suppression from the inhalational agents does present a problem when relying on a cortical site for evoked potential recording. Achieving and maintaining high quality traces can be quite frustrating. Moreover the stimulus rate dependent degradation of the signal is pronounced, typically forcing the use of a 1 Hz rate.

Because of this we have turned to a Thiopental-fentanyl infusion (combined solution of a 2 mg/cc Pentothal, 2µg/cc fentanyl at 1 to 2cc/kg/hr) following initial loading doses of 10 to 12 µg/kg fentanyl and 3 to 4 mg/kg thiopental, oxygen, and low dose isoflurane ($<0.5\%$) for additional sedative, amnesia, and blood pressure control. Relaxants and hypotensive agents are otherwise used in standard fashion. Results with this approach have been outstanding. Besides high quality stable SCEPs that degrade little with stimulus rates up to 5 Hz, the intraoperative wake-ups have been prompt and without difficulty.

THE WAKE-UP TEST

Since we have not replaced the wake-up technique with the additional use of evoked potential monitoring, our anesthetic technique routinely plans for one (or possibly several) wake-up tests. To best accomplish a wake-up test, it is important to prepare the patient for what to expect (patients are very unlikely to remember and in any case will not experience pain) and for what will be expected (squeeze hand, move feet and wiggle toes), and to actually rehearse these movements with him. This last point not only gives the patient a clearer idea of what is expected of him but is a double check to pick up any neurologic deficits that might otherwise be interpreted as having arisen intraoperatively.

The wake-up test demands that the anesthetist pay close attention to the progress of the case to anticipate its timing and thus guide the conduct of the anesthetic. However, 20 to 30 minutes of advance warning by the surgeon is helpful. At this time the anesthesia is gradually lightened. Potent inhalational agents are decreased or are discontinued and no additional bolus of narcotic or relaxant is given. We have found no need to decrease or discontinue thiopental-fentanyl infusion until immediately prior to wake-up. Since induced hypotension appears to deepen anesthesia,[109] this is discontinued as well prior to wake-up. We differ from Hall[58] in that we do not routinely reverse relaxants or necessarily require spontaneous respirations to resume prior to wake-up if we believe neuromuscular blockade to have adequately worn off. If there is then a weak response, we titrate in small doses of Tensilon (a rapid acting anticholinesterase) until there is a strong hand grip.

At this point one is ready for wake-up. It is extremely important that the arms be strapped and held and the head held in place to avoid accidental extubation. All agents are discontinued and 100 per cent oxygen administered. After two minutes the patient is asked to squeeze his hands. If after several more minutes there is still no response, one can administer tiny doses of naloxone, 20 μg at a time, until the patient responds. Another approach is to use small doses of doxapram (20 mg, up to 1 to 1.5 mg/kg) for its analeptic effects. This is almost always effective and tends to provide a less abrupt and stormy wake-up. Once the patient is responding with hand movement he is asked to move his feet. If there is an absence of movement or weakness that persists, then distraction is decreased and the test repeated. In high risk cases one can prolong the wake-up and *increase* distraction during it to allow ongoing and simultaneous monitoring and the additional protection of the patient's muscle tone opposing the distraction thus preventing excessive distraction. On completing the test the patient is re-anesthetized with a small dose of thiopental. A small additional dose of benzodiazepine may be given for its amnesic effect. Along with the thiopental bolus and resumption of the thiopental-fentanyl infusion we often allow a brief period of "overpressure" with the inhalational agent to rapidly deepen anesthesia. Additional narcotic and/or relaxant may be given and controlled ventilation reinstituted.

EARLY POSTOPERATIVE CARE

At the conclusion of the operation the patient is ventilated with 100 per cent O_2 and neuromuscular blockade reversed. Patients are turned back onto the litter with the same caution used initially—lines and tubes, particularly the endotracheal tube, should be guarded against accidental dislodgment. Those without major respiratory impairment are extubated in standard fashion. For those borderline cases we tend toward a conservative approach of a short postoperative t-piece trial. In the most severe cases in which it is certain that postoperative ventilatory support is needed, no effort is made immediately postoperatively in this regard.

Another consideration in the recovery room is that of re-evaluating the patient's neurologic status. Pneumothorax is a recognized complication of anterior spinal surgery, and a chest x-ray is required postoperatively to rule this out. Vital signs and respiratory status should be followed closely. Supplemental O_2 should be administered routinely in the immediate postoperative period. Continuing blood loss and drains should be watched and fluid status reassessed. Blood gases should be checked as needed. Once awake, these patients are often in severe pain and analgesics should be titrated to the patient's needs. After one to two hours of stabilization patients are transferred to an intensive or semi-intensive care setting for further care. Here, too, the continued cooperation and communication among services (surgery, anesthesia, pulmonary, nursing) is of tremendous value in optimizing patient care.

References

1. Aach, R. D., and Kahn, R. A.: Post-transfusion hepatitis: current perspectives. Ann. Inter. Med., 92(4):539–546, 1980.
2. Abott, E. T., and Bentley, C. O.: Intraoperative awakening during scoliosis surgery. Anaesthesia, 35:298–302, 1980.
3. Abrahamian H. A., Allison, T., Goff, W. R., and Rosner, B. S.: Effects of thiopental of human cerebral evoked responses. Anesthesiology, 24:650, 1963.
4. Alfrey, D. D., and Benumof, J. L.: Anesthesia for thoracic surgery. In Miller, R. D. (ed.): Anesthesia. New York, Churchill-Livingstone, pp. 925–980, 1981.
5. Amaranath, L., Lavin, T. J., Trusso, R. A., et al.: Evaluation and creatine phosphokinase screening as a predictor of malignant hyperthermia: prospective study. Br. J. Anaesth., 55:531–533, 1983.
6. Ament, R.: A systemic approach to the difficult intubation. Anesthesiol. Rev., 5:12–16, 1978.
7. Azar, I.: The response of patients with neuromuscular disorders to muscle relaxants: a review. Anesthesiology, 61:173–187, 1984.
8. Batson, O. V.: The function of the vertebral veins and their role in the spread of metastases. Ann. Surg., 112:138–149, 1940.
9. Bennett, E. T., Grundy, E. M., and Patel, K. P.: Visual signs in blind nasal intubation. Anesthesiol. Rev., 5:18–20, 1978.
10. Bergofsky, E. H.: Respiratory failure in disorders of the thoracic cage. Am. Rev. Respir. Dis., 119:643–669, 1979.
11. Berryhill, R. E.: Skin and bone disorders. In Katz, J., Benumof, J., and Kodis, L. B. (eds.): Anesthesia and Uncommon Diseases. Philadelphia, W. B. Saunders Co., pp. 562–587, 1981.
12. Birch, A. A., and Boyce, W. H.: Renal blood flow autoregulation during anesthesia (abstract). Anesthesiology, 51:S123, 1979.
13. Boba, A.: Fatal post-anesthetic complications in two muscular dystrophy patients. J. Pediatr. Surg., 5:71–75, 1970.
14. Bolande, R. P., and Tucker, A. S.: Pulmonary emphysema and other cardiorespiratory lesions as part of the Marfan abiotrophy. Pediatrics, 33:356–366, 1964.
15. Boltshauser, E., Steinmann, B., Meyer, A., and Jerusalem, F.: Anesthesia induced rhabdomy-

olysis in Duchenne muscular dystrophy. Br. J. Anaesth., 52:559(letter), 1980.
16. Brechner, V. L.: Unusual problems in the management of airways: 1. Flexion-extension, mobility of the cervical vertebrae. Anesth. Analg., 47:362–373, 1968.
17. Britt, B. A., and Gordon, R. A.: Peripheral nerve injuries associated with anesthesia. Can. Anaesth. Soc. J., 11:514–536, 1964.
18. Britt, B. A., Joy, N., and Mackay, M. B.: Positioning trauma. In Orkin, F. K., and Cooperman, L. H. (eds.): Complications in Anesthesiology. Philadelphia, J. B. Lippincott Co., pp. 646–670, 1983.
19. Britt, B. A., and Kalow, W.: Malignant hyperthermia: a statistical review. Can. Anaesth. Soc. J., 17:293–315, 1970.
20. Brodkey, J. S., Richards, D. E., Blasingame, J. P., and Nulsen, F. E.: Reversible spinal cord trauma in cats. J. Neurosurg., 37:591, 1972.
21. Brooks, J. L., and Kaplan, J. A.: Cardiac diseases. In Katz, J., Benumof, J., and Kadis, L. B. (eds.): Anesthesia and Uncommon Diseases. Philadelphia, W. B. Saunders Co., pp. 268–312, 1981.
22. Brownell, A. K. W., Paasulke, R. J., Elash, A., et al.: Malignant hyperthermia in Duchenne muscular dystrophy. Anesthesiology, 58:180–182, 1983.
23. Cacares, E., and Whittembury, G.: Evaluation of blood losses during surgical operations, comparison of the gravimetric method with the blood volume determination. Surgery, 45:681, 1959.
24. Chang-lo, M.: Laryngeal involvement in Von Recklinghausen's disease: a case report and review of the literature. Laryngoscope, 87:435–442, 1977.
25. Clark, D. L., and Rosner, B. S.: Neurophysiologic effects of general anesthetics. Anesthesiology, 38:564, 1973.
26. Cobham, I. G., and Davis, H. S.: Anesthesia for muscular dystrophy patients. Anesth. Analg., 43:22–29, 1964.
27. Cody, J. R.: Muscle rigidity following administration of succinylocholine. Anesthesiology, 29:159–162, 1968.
28. Colley, P. S., and Sivarajan, M.: Regional blood flow in dogs during halothane anesthesia and controlled hypotension produced by nitroprusside and nitroglycerin. Anesth. Analg., 63:503, 1984.
29. Colley, P. S., and Sivarajan, M.: Regional blood flows during controlled hypotension. Anesthesiology, 53:588, 1980.
30. Consensus Conference: Fresh frozen plasma: inductions and risks. JAMA, 253:551–553, 1985.
31. Costley, D. O.: Peripheral nerve injury. Int. Anesthesiol. Clin., 10:189–200, 1972.
32. Dolan, E. J., Transfeldt, E. E., Tator, C. H., et al.: The effect of spinal distraction on regional spinal cord blood flow in cats. J. Neurosurg., 53:756–764, 1980.
33. Donlon, J. V., Jr.: Anesthetic management of patients with compromised airways. Anesthesiol. Rev., 7:22–31, 1980.
34. Douglas, W. W., Rehder, K., Beynen, F. M., et al.: Improved oxygenation in patients with acute respiratory failure: the prone position. Am. Rev. Respir. Dis., 115:559–566, 1977.
35. Engler, G. L., Speilholz, N. I., Bernhard, W. N., et al.: Somatosensory evoked potentials during Harrington rod instrumentation for scoliosis. J. Bone Joint Surg., 60A:528, 1978.
36. Fan, F. C., Kin, S., Simchan, S., et al.: Effects of sodium nitroprusside on systemic and regional hemodynamics and oxygen utilization in the dog. Anesthesiology, 53:113–120, 1980.
37. Fitzgibbons, D. C.: Malignant hyperthermia following preoperative oral administration of dantrolene. Anesthesiology, 54:73–75, 1981.
38. Fleming, A.: Intraoperative salvage. In Sandler, S. (ed.): Autologous Transfusion. Am. Assoc. Blood Banks, pp. 41–56, 1983.
39. Flewellen, E. H., Nelson, T. E., Jones, W. P., et al.: Dantrolene dose response in awake man: implications for management of malignant hyperthermia. Anesthesiology, 59:275–280, 1983.
40. Gardner, R. D.: Blood loss after spinal instrumentation and fusion in scoliosis (Harrington procedure). Clin. Orthop., 71:182–185, 1970.
41. Geschwind, N., Simpson, J. A.: Procainamide in the treatment of myotonia. Brain, 78:81–91, 1955.
42. Gieseck, A. H., Jr.: Perioperative fluid therapy—crystalloids. In Miller, R. D. (ed.): Anesthesia. Volume 2, New York, Churchill-Livingstone, pp. 865–875, 1981.
43. Gilbert, R. G. B., and Brindle, G. F.: Posture. Int. Anesthesiol. Clin., 4:815–817, 1966.
44. Gilcher, R. O., and Belcher, L.: Predeposit programs. In Sandler, S. (ed.): Autologous Transfusion. Am. Assoc. Blood Banks, pp. 11–22, 1983.
45. Ginsberg, H., Shetter, A., and Raudzens, P.: Postoperative paraplegia with preserved intraoperative somatosensory evoked potentials. Orthop. Trans., 8:161, 1984.
46. Goldstein, L. A.: Treatment of idiopathic scoliosis. J. Bone Joint Surg., 51A:209, 1969.
47. Gordon, R. J., and Ravin, M. B.: Rheology and anesthesiology. Anesth. Analg., 57:277–284, 1978.
48. Gourlay, G. K., Willis, R. J., and Wilson, P. R.: Postoperative pain control with methadone: influence of supplementary methadone doses and blood concentrate—response relationships. Anesthesiology, 61:19–26, 1984.
49. Gravenstein, M. A., Sasse, F., and Hogan, K.: Effect of stimulus rate and Halothane dose on canine far-field somatosensory evoked potentials. Anesthesiology, 61A:342, 1984.
50. Griggs, R. C., David, R. J., Anderson, D. C., and Dove, J. T.: Cardiac conduction in myotonic dystrophy. Am. J. Med., 59:37–42, 1975.
51. Gronert, G. A.: Malignant hyperthermia. Anesthesiology, 53:395–423, 1980.
52. Grundy, B. L., and Brown, R. H.: Meperidine enhances somatosensory cortical evoked potentials. Electroencephalogr. Clin. Neurophysiol., 50:177P, 1980.
53. Grundy, B. L., Brown, R. H., and Clifton, P. C.: Effect of Droperidol on somatosensory cortical evoked potentials. Electroencephalogr. Clin. Neurophysiol., 50:158P–159P, 1980.
54. Grundy, B. L., Brown, R. H., and Greenburg, P. S.: Diazepam alters cortical evoked potentials. Anesthesiology, 51:538, 1979.
55. Grundy, B. L., Nash, C. L., and Brown, R. H.: Arterial pressure manipulation alters spinal cord

function during correction of scoliosis. Anesthesiology, 54:249–253, 1981.
56. Grundy, B. L., Nash, C. L., and Brown, R. H.: Deliberate hypotension for spinal fusion: prospective randomized study with evoked potential monitoring. Can. Anaesth. Soc. J., 29:425, 1982.
57. Grundy, B. L., Nelson, P. B., Doyle, E., and Procopio, P. T.: Intraoperative loss of somatosensory evoked potentials predict loss of spinal cord function. Anesthesiology, 57:321, 1982.
58. Hall, J. E., Levine, C. R., and Sudhir, K. G.: Intraoperative awakening to monitor spinal cord function during Harrington instrumentation and spine fusion. J. Bone Joint Surg., 60A:533–536, 1978.
59. Halliday, A. M., and Wakefield, G. S.: Cerebral evoked potentials in patients with dissociated sensory loss. J. Neurol. Neurosurg. Psychiat., 26:211, 1963.
60. Hoppenfeld, S., Gross, A., and Andrews, C.: The ankle clonus test—an alternative to the Stagnara wake-up test and somatosensory evoked potentials in the assessment of spinal cord damage in the treatment of scoliosis with Harrington rod instrumentation. Presented at the meeting of the Scoliosis Research Society, 1984.
61. Hymsfield, S. B., McNish, T., Perkins, J. V., and Felner, J. M.: Sequence of cardiac changes in Duchenne muscular dystrophy. Am. Heart J., 95:283–294, 1978.
62. Inkley, S. R., Oldenburg, F. C., and Vignos, P. J.: Pulmonary function in Duchenne muscular dystrophy related to stage of disease. Am. J. Med., 56:297–306, 1974.
63. Jacobs, H. K., Lieponis, J. V., Bunch, W. H., et al.: The influence of halothane and nitroprusside on canine spinal cord hemodynamics. Spine, 7:35, 1982.
64. Jobes, D. R., and Gallagher, J.: Acute normovolemic hemodilution. Int. Anestheol. Clin., 20:77–95, 1982.
65. Johnston, R. R., Eger, E. I., and Wilson, C.: A comparative interaction of epinephrine with enflurane, isoflurane, and halothane in man. Anesth. Analg., 55:709–712, 1976.
66. Jones, E. T., Matthews, L. S., and Hensinger, R. N.: The wake-up technique as a dual protector of spinal cord function during spine fusion. Clin. Orthop., 168:113–118, 1982.
67. Jones, S. J., Edgar, M. A., Ransford, A. O., and Thomas, N. P.: A system for the electrophysiological monitoring of the spinal cord during operations for scoiosis. J. Bone Joint Surg., 65B:134–139, 1983.
68. Jordan, C. E., White, R. I., Fischer, K. C., et al.: The scoliosis of congenital heart disease. Am. Heart J., 84:463–469, 1972.
69. Kafer, E. R.: Respiratory and cardiovascular function in scoliosis. Bull. Eur. Physiopathol. Respir., 13:299–321, 1977.
70. Kafer, E. R.: Respiratory and cardiovascular functions in scoliosis and the principle of anesthetic management. Anesthesiology, 52:339–351, 1980.
71. Kahl, F. R., Flint, J. F., and Szidon, J. P.: Influence of left atrial distention on renal vasomotor tone. Am. J. Physiol., 226:240–246, 1974.
72. Kaneko, K., Milic-Emil, J., Dolovich, M. B., et al.: Regional distribution of ventilation and perfusion as a function of body position. J. Appl. Physiol. 21:767–777, 1966.
73. Kaplan, J. A.: Thoracic Anesthesia. New York, Churchill-Livingstone, 1983.
74. Katz, K. H., and Chandler, H. L.: Morphine hypersensitivity in kyphoscoliosis. New Engl. J. Med., 238:322–324, 1948.
75. Khambatta, H. J., Stone, J. G., Matteo, R. S., and Michelson, W. J.: Hypotensive anesthesia for spine fusion with sodium nitroprusside. Spine, 3:171, 1978.
76. Kilburn, K. H., Eagen, J. T., and Heyman, A.: Cardiopulmonary insufficiency associated with myotonic dystrophy. Am. J. Med., 26:929–935, 1959.
77. Kilburn, K. H., Eagen, J. T., Sicker, H. O., and Heyman, A.: Cardiopulmonary insufficiency in myotonic and progressive muscular dystrophy. New Engl. J. Med., 261:1089–1096, 1959.
78. Kling, T. F., Fergusson, N., Leach, A. W., et al.: The effect of induced hypotension and spine distraction on spinal cord blood flow in dogs. Orthop. Trans., 8:144, 1984.
79. Kopman, A. F., Wollman, S. B., Ross, K., and Surks, S. M.: Awake endotracheal intubation: a review of 267 cases. Anesth. Analg., 54:323–327, 1975.
80. Krishna, G., Haselby, K. A., Rao, C. C., et al.: The pediatric patient. In Stoelting, R. K., and Dierdorf, S. F. (eds.): Anesthesia and Co-existing Disease. New York, Churchill-Livingstone, pp. 741–810, 1983.
81. Laks, H., Pilon, R. N., Klovekorn, W. P., et al.: Acute hemodilution: its effects on hemodynamics and oxygen transport in anesthetized man. Ann. Surg., 180:103–109, 1974B.
82. Leighton, K. M., Bruce, C., and Macleod, B. A.: Sodium nitroprusside-induced hypotension and renal blood flow. Can. Anaesth. Soc. J., 24:637–640, 1977.
83. Leyburn, P., and Walton, J. A.: The treatment of myotonia: a controlled clinical trial. Brain, 82:81–91, 1959.
84. LoSasso, A. M.: Cor pulmonale. In Stoelting, R. K., and Dierdorf, S. F. (eds.): Anesthetics and Co-existing Disease. New York, Churchill-Livingstone, 1983.
85. Lueders, H., Gurd, A., Hahn, J., et al.: A new technique for intraoperative monitoring of spinal cord function. Spine, 7:110, 1982.
86. Luke, M. J., and McDonnell, E. J.: Congenital heart disease and scoliosis. J. Pediatr., 73:725–733, 1968.
87. Martin, D. E., Rosenberg, H., Aukburg, S. J., et al.: Low-dose fentanyl blunts circulatory responses to tracheal intubation. Anesth. Analg., 61:680–684, 1982.
88. Marx, G. F., Mateo, C. V., and Orkin, L. R.: Computer analysis of post anesthesia deaths. Anesthesiology, 39:54–58, 1973.
89. McCallum, J. E., and Bennett, M. H.: Electrophysiologic monitoring of spinal cord function during intraspinal surgery. Surg. Forum, 26:469, 1975.
90. McNeill, T. W., DeWald, R. L., Kuo, K. N., et al.: Controlled hypotensive anesthesia in scoliosis surgery. J. Bone Joint Surg., 56A:1167, 1974.
91. Messmer, K.: Hemodilution. Surg. Clin. North Am. 55(3):659–678, 1975.
92. Michenfelder, J. D., and Theye, R. A.: Canine

systemic and cerebral effects of hypotension induced by hemorrhage, trimethaphan, halothane, or nitroprusside. Anesthesiology, 46: 188–195, 1977.
93. Miller, E. D., Sanders, D. B., Rowlingson, J. C., et al.: Anesthesia induced rhabdomyolysis in a patient with Duchenne's muscular dystrophy. Anesthesiology, 48:146–148, 1978.
94. Miller, J., and Lee, C.: Muscle diseases. In Katz, J., Benumof, J., and Kadis, L. B. (eds.): Anesthesia and Uncommon Diseases. Philadelphia, W. B. Saunders, Co., pp. 531–562, 1981.
95. Miller, R. D., and Brzica, S.: Blood, blood component, colloid, and autotransfusion therapy. In Miller, R. D. (ed.): Anesthesia, Vol. 2. New York, Churchill-Livingstone, pp. 885–924, 1981.
96. Mudge, B. J., Taylor, P. B., and Vanderspek, A. F. L.: Perioperative hazards in mytonic dystrophy. Anaesthesia, 35:492–495, 1980.
97. Muller, J., and Suppan, P.: Case report: anesthesia in myotonic dystrophy. Anaesth. Inten. Care, 5:70–73, 1977.
98. Nagao, S., Rocaforte, P., and Moody, R. A.: The effects of isovolemic hemodilution and reinfusion of packed erythrocytes on somatosensory and visual evoked potentials. J. Surg. Res., 25:530, 1978.
99. Nordwell, A., Axelgaad, J., Harada, Y., et al.: Spinal cord monitoring using evoked potentials recorded from feline vertebral bone. Spine, 4:486–494, 1979.
100. Ovassapian, A., Yelich, S. J., Dykes, M. H. M., and Brummer, E. Z.: Blood pressure and heart rate changes during awake fiberoptic nasotracheal intubation. Anesth. Analg., 62:951–954, 1983.
101. Paterson, I. S.: Generalized myotonia following suxamethonium. Br. J. Anaesth., 34:340–342, 1962.
102. Pathak, K. S., Amaddio, M., Shaffer, J. W., and Scoles, P. V.: Effect of Halothane, nitrous oxide anesthesia on spinal versus cortical evoked potentials during spine surgery. Anesthesiology, 61:A346, 1984.
103. Pathak, K. S., Brown, R. H., Cascorbi, H. F., and Nash, C. L.: Effects of fentanyl and morphine on intraoperative somatosensory cortical evoked potentials. Anesth. Analg., 63:833, 1984.
104. Pathak, K. S., Brown, R. H., Nash, C. L., and Cascorbi, H. F.: Continuous opioid infusion for scoliosis fusion surgery. Anesth. Analg. 62:841–845, 1983.
105. Patil, V. U., Stehling, L. C., and Zauder, H. L.: Fiberoptic Endoscopy in Anesthesia. Chicago, Year Book Medical Publishers, 1983.
106. Perloff, J. K., deLeon, A. C., and O'Doherty, D.: The cardiomyopathy of progressive muscular dystrophy. Circulation, 33:625–648, 1966.
107. Ponte, A.: Postoperative paraplegia due to hypercorrection of scoliosis and drop of blood pressure. J. Bone Joint Surg., 56A:444, 1974.
108. Pruzanski, W., and Profis, A.: Pulmonary disease in myotonic dystrophy. Am. Rev. Respir. Dis., 91:874–879, 1965.
109. Rao, T. L. K., Jacobs, K., Salem, M. R., et al.: Deliberate hypotension and anesthetic requirements of halothane. Anesth. Analg., 60:513–516, 1981.
110. Ravin, M., Newmark, Z., and Saviello, G.: Myotonia dystrophica anesthetic hazard: two case reports. Anesth. Analg., 54:216–218, 1975.
111. Rehder, K., Knopp, T. K., and Sessler, A. D.: Regional intrapulmonary gas distribution in awake and anesthetized-paralyzed prone man. J. Appl. Physiol., 47:528–535, 1979.
112. Relton, J. E. S.: Anesthesia in the original correction of scoliosis. In Riseborough, E. J., and Herndon, J. H. (eds.): Scoliosis and other Deformities of the Axial Skeleton. Boston, Little Brown, pp. 309–316, 1975.
113. Relton, J. E. S., Britt, B. A., and Steward, D. J.: Malignant hyperpyrexia. Br. J. Anaesth., 45:269–275, 1973.
114. Relton, J. E. S., and Hall, J. E.: An operation frame for spinal fusion: a new apparatus designed to reduce hemorrhage during operation. J. Bone Joint Surg. (Am), 49B:327–332, 1967.
115. Richards, W. C.: Anaesthesia and serum creatinine phosphokinase levels in patients with Duchenne's pseudohypertrophic muscular dystrophy. Anaesth. Inten. Care, 1:150–153, 1972.
116. Roizen, M. F.: Routine preoperative evaluation in anesthesia. In Miller, R. D. (ed.): Anesthesia, Vol. 2. New York, Churchill-Livingstone, pp. 3–19, 1981.
117. Rosenberg, H., and Heiman-Patterson, T.: Duchenne's muscular dystrophy and malignant hyperthermia: another warning (letter). Anesthesiology, 59:362, 1983.
118. Roth, A., Rosenthal, A., Hall, J. E., and Mizel, M.: Scoliosis and congenital heart disease. Clin. Orthop., 93:95–102, 1973.
119. Rucker, R. W., Silva, W. J., and Worchester, C. C.: Fiberoptic bronchoscopic nasotracheal intubation in childen. Chest, 76(1)56–9, 1979.
120. Sagel, S. S., Forrest, J. V., and Askin, F. B.: Interstitial lung disease in neurofibromatosis. South. Med. J., 68:647–649, 1975.
121. Salem, M. R.: Anesthesia for orthopedic surgery. In Gregory, G. A. (ed.): Pediatric Anesthesia. New York, Churchill-Livingstone, pp. 851–898, 1983.
122. Schaer, H., Steinmann, B., Jerusalem, F., et al.: Rhabdomyolysis induced by anesthesia with intra-operative cardiac arrest. Br. J. Anaesth., 49:495–499, 1977.
123. Schmitt, E. W.: Neurological complications in the treatment of scoliosis. A sequential report of the Scoliosis Research Society 1971 through 1979. Reported at the 17th Annual Meeting of The Scoliosis Research Society, Denver Colorado, 1981.
124. Schulman, M. S., Brodsky, J. B., Mark, J. B. D., and Swan, M.: Non-invasive pulse oximetry during one-lung ventilation. Anesthesiology, 61:A98(abstract), 1984.
125. Schwartz, A. I., and Rosenblum, E.: Management of the anesthetized patient. Anesthesiology, 8:395–401, 1945.
126. Seay, A. R., Ziter, F. A., and Thompson, J. A.: Cardiac arrest during induction of anesthesia in Duchenne muscular dystrophy. J. Pediatr., 93:88–90, 1978.
127. Shires, T., Coln, D., and Corrico, J.: Fluid therapy in hemorrhagic shock. Arch. Surg., 88:688–693, 1964.
128. Shires, T., and Canizaro, P. C.: Fluid, electrolyte and nutritional management of the surgical patient. In Schwartz, S. I. (ed.): Principles of Surgery. New York, McGraw-Hill, pp. 65–96, 1974.

129. Shires, T., Peitzman, A. B., et al.: Response of extravascular lung water to intraoperative fluids. Ann. Surg., *197*:515–519, 1983.
130. Shufflebarger, H. L., Papazian, O., Morrison, G., and Corredor, C.: SSEP changes during cordotomy. Presented at the Scoliosis Research Society Meeting, Orlando, Florida, 1984.
131. Singler, R. C.: Special techniques: deliberate hypotension hypothermia, and acute normovolemic hemodilution. *In* Gregory, G. A. (ed.): Pediatric Anesthesia, New York, Churchill-Livingstone, pp. 553–577, 1983.
132. Smith, R. H.: The prone position. *In* Martin, J. T. (ed.): Positioning in Anesthesia and Surgery. Philadelphia, W. B. Saunders Co., pp. 32–43, 1978.
133. Stockard, J. J., Sharbrough, F. W., and Tinker, J. A.: Effects of hypothermia on the human brainstem auditory response. Ann. Neurol., 3:368, 1978.
134. Thomas, J. L.: Awake intubation: indications and techniques: a review. Anaethesia, 24:28–35, 1969.
135. Thompson, G. E., Miller, R. D., Stevens, W. C., and Murray, W. R.: Hypotensive anesthesia for total hip arthroplasty. Anesthesiology, *48*:91, 1978.
136. Tremper, K. K., Kapur, P. A., Thangathurai, C., et al.: Transcutaneous PO monitoring during one lung anesthesia. Anesth. Analg., 62:288 (abstract), 1983.
137. Turino, G. B., Goldring, R. M., and Fishman, A. P.: Cor pulmonale in musculoskeletal abnormalities of the thorax. Bull. N. Y. Acad. Med., *41*:959–980, 1965.
138. Vauzelle, L., Stagnara, P., and Jouvinroux, P.: Functional monitoring of spinal cord activity during spinal surgery. Clin. Orthop., *93*:173, 1973.
139. Virgilio, R. W., Rice, C. L., Smith, D. E., et al.: Crystalloid vs. colloid resuscitations: Is one better? Surgery, *85*:192–193, 1979.
140. Virgilio, R. W., Smith, D. E., and Zarins, C. K.: Balanced electrolyte solutions: experimental and clinical studies. Crit. Care Med., 7:98–106, 1979.
141. Wagaman, M. J., Shatack, J. G., Moomjian, A. S., et al.: Improved oxygenation and lung compliance with prone poisitioning of neonates. J. Pediatr., *94*:787–791, 1979.
142. Watson, C. B.: Fiberoptic bronchoscopy for anesthesia. Anesthesiol. Rev., 9:17–26, 1982.
143. Wilkins, K. E.: Fat embolism. *In* Zauder, H. L. (ed.): Anesthesia for Orthopaedic Surgery. Philadelphia, F. A. Davis Co, pp. 147–179, 1980.
144. Yamashita, M.: Anaesthetic considerations in Von Recklinghausen's disease (multiple neurofibromatosis). Abnormal response to muscle relaxants. Anaesthetist, 26:117–118, 1977.
145. Yong-Hing, K., Kalamchi, A., and MacEwen, G. D.: Cervical spine abnormalities in neurofibromatosis. J. Bone Joint Surg., *61*:695–699, 1979.
146. Zaleske, D. J., Hall, J. E., Vanter, G. H., et al.: Spinal deformity in a case of mediastinal neuroblastoma: its treatment including somatosensory evoked potentials during anterior decompression. J. Pediatr. Orthop., 2:416, 1982.

Ankylosing Spondylitis

David S. Bradford, M.D.

Ankylosing spondylitis is a systemic disease that primarily affects young men, producing progressive pain and stiffness of the spine. Kyphosis is a characteristic deformity. Roentgenograms show progressive sclerosis leading to ankylosis of the sacroiliac and facet joints along with ossification of the anulus fibrosus, the anterior longitudinal ligament, and the interlaminar and interspinous ligaments. Once the inflammatory component of the disease has run its course and interspinous ankylosis has occurred, spinal pain usually disappears. Patients, however, are left with a severe functional disability characterized by loss of normal lumbar lordosis and increased thoracic and cervical kyphosis. Bony ankylosis in this deformed position prevents the patient from standing upright even with knee flexion. This structural disability produces severe functional as well as psychological problems.[4, 20, 22, 28, 29]

REVIEW OF THE LITERATURE

Smith-Petersen, Larson, and Aufranc[32] in 1945 proposed surgical correction of the spinal deformity by lumbar osteotomy. Their procedure was carried out in six patients and consisted of resection of the spinous processes of L1 to L2 and L3 with removal of the edges of the lamina and portions of the superior and inferior articular facets and with correction by forceful manipulation and hyperextension. Local bone grafts were placed across the osteotomy sites, and the patient was immobilized in a postoperative cast for two months followed by a Taylor spinal brace for one year.

LaChapelle[14] recommended a two-stage osteotomy for correction of deformity, consisting of posterior neural arch resection under local anesthesia followed two weeks later by an anterior osteotomy, wedging open the lumbar spine, and filling in the disc space with bone plugs.

Briggs, Keats, and Schlesinger[4] presented their results on five cases of ankylosing spondylitis. Their procedure consisted of a posterior wedge osteotomy on the lumbar spine, pivoting the correction at the posterior margin of the intervertebral disc between the third and fourth lumbar vertebra. In two other cases the osteotomy site was fixed with metal plates after correction.

Herbert[10, 11] subsequently advocated either a one- or two-stage spinal osteotomy with the patient in the prone position. If the spine could be corrected after the first stage procedure, a second operation was not necessary.

Law has presented the largest series of cases reported to date.[15, 16] His total series consists of 120 patients of whom ten died and six developed neurologic complications following surgery.[17]

To prevent excessive lengthening of the anterior column, several authors have proposed modifications, which consist of shortening type procedures. Scudese and Calabro[27] have performed a similar posterior wedge resection between L2 and L3 but removed the back part of the upper surface of the body of L3 along with the disc. The most innovative procedure is that recently described by Thomasen,[31] which consists of a posterior vertebral body decancellation. During this procedure the lamina of L2 is removed along with the pedicles, and the spongy bone of the vertebral body is then removed through the base of the pedicle. A wedge fracture of L2 is created, producing lordosis and closing the wedge posteriorly. Other modifications of the original Smith-Petersen procedure have been described[12, 23] along with a technique for transpedicular fixation after osteotomy.[24] A more recent report by McMaster[21] supports the concept of stable internal fixation and controlled correction in preventing complications.

TECHNIQUES AND OPTIONS FOR CORRECTION

In assessing the patient for consideration of spinal osteotomy a careful evaluation of the magnitude of the deformity and its primary location (i.e., cervical, thoracic, or lumbar) should be determined. Of even greater importance is the determination of severe hip flexion contracture with or without associated hip joint disease. Soft tissue releases about the hips or, more commonly, total hip joint arthroplasty may be sufficient in itself to allow the patient to stand reasonably upright and see straight ahead irrespective of the spinal deformity.[2, 34]

In most cases the kyphosis originates in the lumbar region. The first manifestation is loss of lumbar lordosis and pelvic tilting; the sacrum becomes vertical in orientation. With relatively normal sagittal contour in the thoracic and cervical spine, lumbar osteotomy is the procedure of choice. The correction should be planned so that the plumbline from C7 falls within the body of S1. Even in cases in which the thoracic kyphosis is greater than normal, a compensatory lumbar osteotomy may correct sagittal plane malalignment and allow the patient to see ahead with the legs fully extended. In the presence of severe thoracic kyphosis where lumbar and cervical lordosis have been at least partially maintained but the patient is unable to see straight ahead, thoracic osteotomy would be indicated. If the primary deformity is at the cervical-thoracic junction where there is relatively normal thoracic kyphosis and lumbar lordosis, correction of the deformity by extension osteotomy of the cervical spine is indicated.

Techniques

Although satisfactory results have been reported using local anesthesia,[31] at our center we prefer endotracheal anesthesia. Extreme care must be taken in positioning the patient, and it may be necessary to use a fiberoptic laryngoscope during intubation. Once the patient has been anesthetized and intubated, the patient is positioned on a four-poster frame, which leaves the abdomen free and reduces intra-abdominal pressure. For details the reader is referred to the Techniques of Surgery section.

The technique of osteotomy is similar to that described by Smith-Petersen,[30] Adams,[1] Law,[15, 16] and McMaster.[21] We have generally preferred to perform one osteotomy only either at L2 and L3 or L3 and L4. This facilitates greater stability when the wedge is closed. It is also important to stress that the dura is frequently adherent to the posterior arch and may be easily torn during the osteotomy procedure. For maximum correction

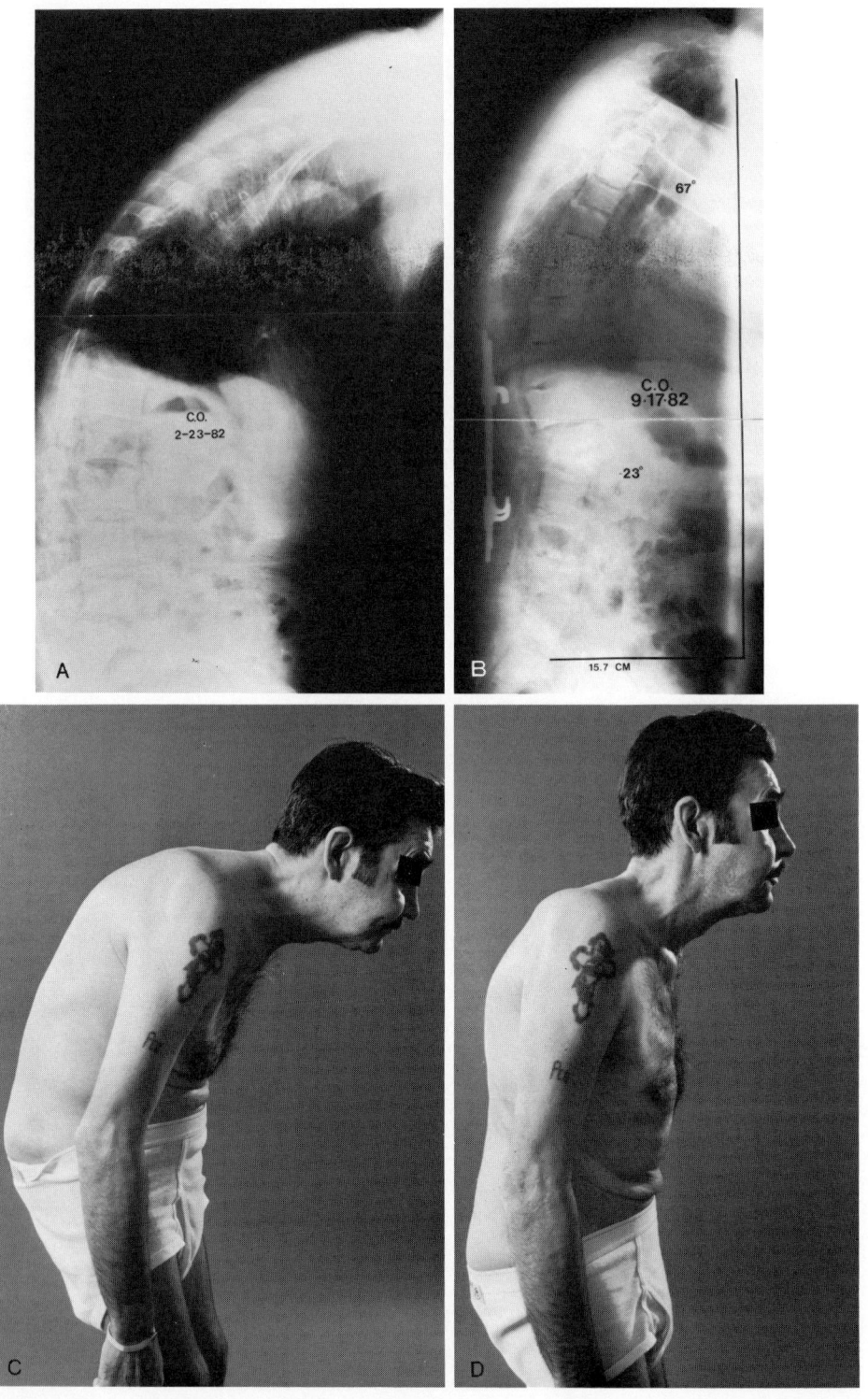

Figure 22–65. *A* and *B*, C.O. presented with severe thoracic lumbar kyphosis secondary to ankylosing spondylitis. Following posterior closing wedge osteotomy, significant correction was obtained. Although he can now see straight ahead with his knees fully extended, the correction was not optimal, and a larger posterior-based wedge would have been preferable. Preoperative clinical photograph (*C*) and postoperative photograph (*D*).

it may be necessary to remove at least 2 cm. of bone and a portion of each pedicle. The apex of the osteotomy must lie anterior to the neural tube, preferably at the junction of the posterior longitudinal ligament and intervertebral disc. If the apex of the cut lies posterior to the neural elements, anterior hinging and stretching of the neural elements may produce neurologic complications. After the osteotomy is completed, holes are made into the posterior fusion above and below the osteotomy to accept Harrington compression hooks (no. 1256). Compression rods are then applied and the table may be manipulated into gentle extension while compression is carried out through the implant. A routine wake-up test is performed to assure that the neural tissues have not been compromised. Local bone grafting is carried out along with the addition of cancellous iliac or bank bone allografts as felt necessary. Following surgery the patients are log-rolled for five to seven days, fitted for a molded TLSO brace, ambulated, and discharged. The brace is worn until the osteotomy is healed, which averages four to six months (Figs. 22–65 and 22–66).

THORACIC KYPHOSIS

When the primary deformity from ankylosing spondylitis is in the thoracic spine, the cervical and thoracic deformities are minimal, and correction or stabilization is felt desirable, we have favored a two-stage procedure consisting of a first stage anterior osteotomy with anterior interbody fusion followed one to two weeks later by posterior multiple level osteotomies with Harrington compression instrumentation. The approach is similar to that used for severe juvenile kyphosis (Fig. 22–67).[3] L-rod instrumentation may likewise be used, but may prove more difficult because of neural adhesions to the posterior arch. We have therefore generally favored the Harrington rod implant.

CERVICAL KYPHOSIS

Cervical osteotomy may occasionally be indicated in ankylosing spondylitis when the primary deformity is located at the cervical-thoracic junction. In 1953, Mason, Cozen, and Adelstein[19] reported successful correc-

Figure 22–66. A more optimal correction following lumbar osteotomy for ankylosing spondylitis. The seventh cervical vertebra is now positioned over the sacrum in the sagittal plane, and the patient's improvement, therefore, has been maximized. Preoperative (A) and postoperative (B) radiographs.

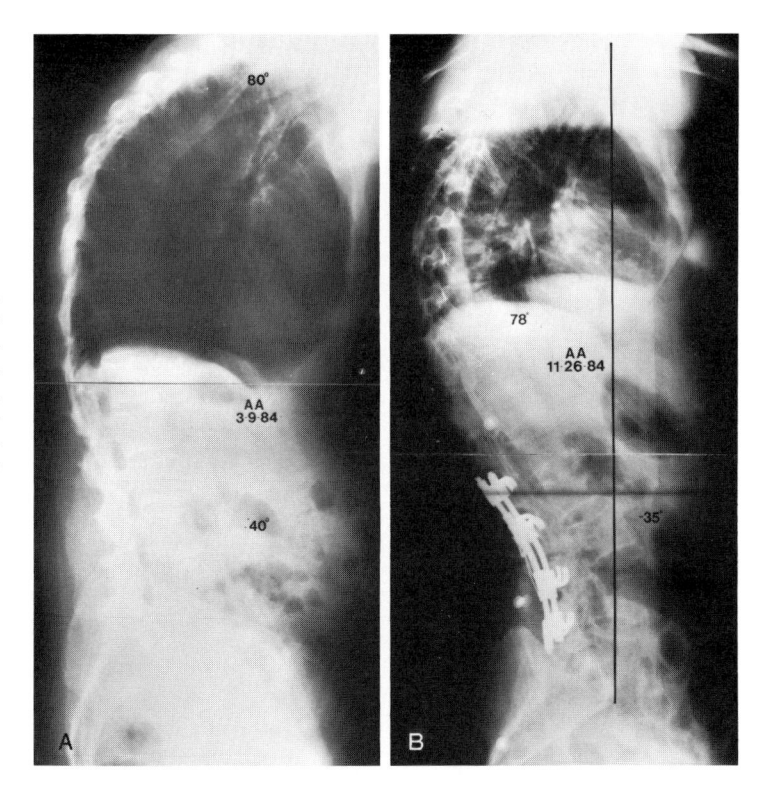

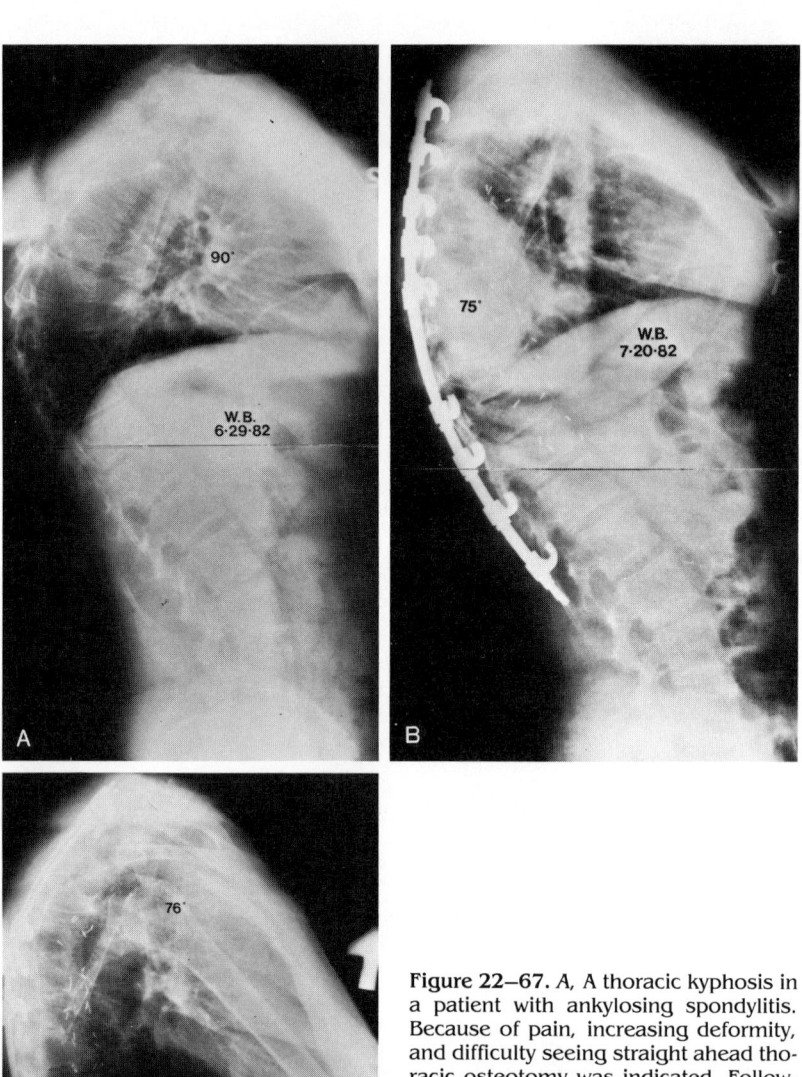

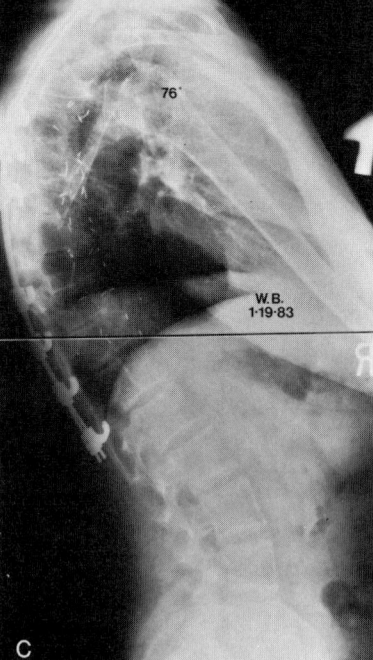

Figure 22–67. *A*, A thoracic kyphosis in a patient with ankylosing spondylitis. Because of pain, increasing deformity, and difficulty seeing straight ahead thoracic osteotomy was indicated. Following combined anterior and posterior surgery, satisfactory correction was maintained. However, the upper Harrington hook was noted to cut out (*B*). Reinstrumentation to a higher level resulted in a stable correction and solid arthrodesis (*C*).

tion of flexion deformity of the cervical-thoracic spine in a patient with ankylosing spondylitis. They carried out the osteotomy distal to C7 to avoid damage to the vertebral arteries. In 1958, Urist[33] reported a successful osteotomy at the cerivcal-thoracic junction in a patient awake under local anesthesia. Simmons[28] has reported experience in 11 patients (1972) consisting of a wide laminectomy from C6 to T2 with osteotomy at the C7 to T1 space. The procedure was done under local anesthesia with halo control. There was no mortality in his series and no major morbidity. Although our experience with cervical osteotomy is limited, the technique as outlined by Urist[33] and Simmons[28] has much to commend it. Performing the procedure under local anesthesia with controlled fixation by the use of a halo with careful controlled correction would, in our opinion, be the procedure of choice.

RESULTS AND COMPLICATIONS

In those series involving five or more cases in which kyphosis measurements have been calculated, the kyphosis correction has ranged from as low as 12 degrees to as high as 60 degrees.[8, 16, 21, 22, 29, 31] Recurrence of the deformity occurred in six of Herbert's series of 30 patients[10] and four of Law's series of 120 patients,[16] two of which were at the site of osteotomy and two in the thoracic kyphosis above the level of osteotomy. This problem has also been mentioned by Goel,[8] and it developed in one of his 15 cases.

It has been stated by review of several series[21, 29] that the mortality has varied from 8 per cent to 10 per cent, and neurologic complications have occurred in up to 30 per cent of patients. However, these quotes are misleading. If one analyzes the 12 large series, consisting of five or more cases, reported to date[4, 5, 8, 10, 11, 15–17, 20–22, 28–31] out of these combined 250 cases there was a 4 per cent incidence of neurologic complications and a 7 per cent mortality rate. However, more important is that in eight of these papers,[4, 5, 8, 17, 21, 29, 30, 32] consisting of 74 patients, there were no neurologic deficits and in nine of these papers,[4, 5, 8, 17, 21, 29–32] consisting of 85 patients, no mortality was reported. From careful review of published data and our own experience, it would appear that neurologic complications and mortality can be greatly lessened if not prevented all together by carefully avoiding compression of neurologic tissue, monitoring neurologic function during the osteotomy (wake-up test), use of internal fixation, and in avoiding translational displacement at the osteotomy site.

Postoperative ileus is common in these patients, and nasogastric drainage is essential. Although aortic rupture has been reported,[17] the case occurred following closed forceful osteoclasis of severe kyphosis in a patient who had previously been treated with radiation therapy for ankylosing spondylitis. The fear and likelihood of this complication, I feel, has been greatly overstated.

Fractures may occur in patients with ankylosing spondylitis and appear as focal spinal abnormalities on bone scans[25] or destructive lesions presenting as a nonspecific discitis.[13] These lesions appear to be an inflammatory process and may be referred to as a spondylodiscitis; however, they are secondary to stress fractures and are usually associated with significant pain and rarely a progressive neurologic deficit (Fig. 22–68).[5, 7] These lesions are more common in the cervical spine.[7, 26] As noted, progressive neurologic deterioration may occur with these stress fractures, but these patients may also develop cauda equina lesions with progressive neurologic deterioration in the presence of inactive disease. The etiology is not clear; it could be due to either arachnoiditis or local ischemia secondary to small vessel angiitis.[9] Laceration of the aorta with formation of an aortic spinal subarachnoid fistula has been reported in one case of a patient with ankylosing spondylitis who sustained a fracture dislocation of the spine after minor trauma.[6] As mentioned, although these stress fractures may heal with immobilization, more rapid pain relief and fracture union may be expected following internal fixation,[18] and we favor an operative approach in these situations.

We have now treated 21 patients with ankylosing spondylitis for pain and deformity, and eight patients with primary thoracic kyphosis have undergone combined anterior and posterior surgery with an average correction of 36 degrees. Eight patients have undergone lumbar osteotomy as a single stage procedure with Harrington compression instrumentation, with an average correction of 31 degrees. Five patients have presented with spondylodiscitis with evidence of pseudarthrosis. Four have under-

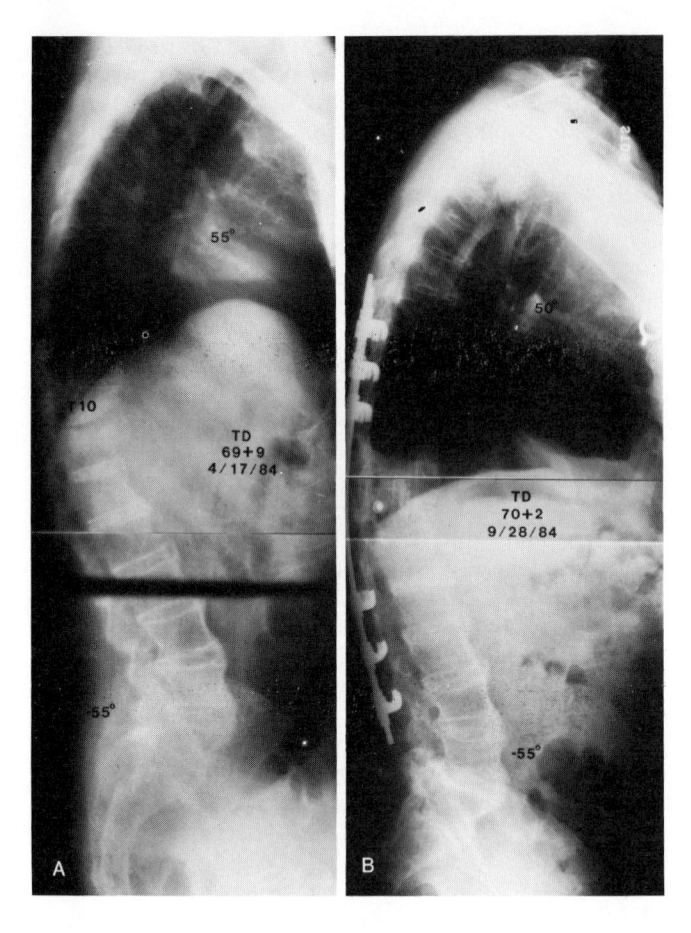

Figure 22–68. A, The lateral x-ray of a patient with spondylodiscitis secondary to a stress fracture. The patient presented with progressive pain and paraplegia. After anterior decompression with vascularized rib grafting followed by second stage posterior instrumentation and fusion, solid arthrodesis was achieved and complete neurologic recovery resulted.

gone combined surgery and one posterior surgery only. In these 21 cases, one developed a pseudarthrosis, which was successfully repaired, and one developed transient quadriceps weakness, which resolved spontaneously without consequence.

References

1. Adams, J. C.: Technique, dangers, and safeguards in osteotomy of the spine. J. Bone Joint Surg., 34B:226, 1952.
2. Biska, R. S., Ranawat, C. S., and Inglis, A. E.: Total hip replacement in patients with ankylosing spondylitis with involvement of the hip. J. Bone Joint Surg., 58A:233, 1976.
3. Bradford, D. S.: Kyphosis: Current Orthopaedic Management. W. J. Kane (Ed.) New York, Churchill-Livingstone, 1981.
4. Briggs, H., Keats, S., and Schlesinger, P.: Wedge osteotomy of the spine with bilateral intervertebral foraminotomy. J. Bone Joint Surg., 29:1075–1082, 1947.
5. Emneus, H.: Wedge osteotomy of spine in ankylosing spondylitis. Acta Orthop. Scand., 39:321–326, 1968.
6. Fazl, M., Bilbao, J. M., and Hudson, A. R.: Laceration of the aorta complicating spinal fracture in ankylosing spondylitis. Neurosurgery, 8:732–734, 1981.
7. Gelman, M. I., and Umber, J. S.: Fracture of the thoracolumbar spine in ankylosing spondylitis. Am. J. Roentenol., 130:485–491, 1978.
8. Goel, M. K.: Vertebral osteotomy for correction of fixed flexion deformity of the spine. J. Bone Joint Surg., 50A:287, 1968.
9. Gordon, A. L., and Yudell, A.: Cauda equina lesion associated with rheumatoid spondylitis. Ann. Intern. Med., 78:555–557, 1973.
10. Herbert, J. J.: Vertebral osteotomy for kyphosis, especially in Marie-Strumpell arthritis. J. Bone Joint Surg., 41A:291–320, 1959.
11. Herbert, J. J.: Vertebral osteotomy, technique, indications, and results. J. Bone Joint Surg., 30A:680, 1948.
12. Kallio, K. E.: Osteotomy of the spine in ankylosing spondylitis. Ann. Chir. Gynaec. Fenn., 52:615, 1963.
13. Kanefield, D. G., Mullins, B. P., Freehaffer, A. A., et al.: Destructive lesions of the spine in rheumatoid ankylosing spondylitis. J. Bone Joint Surg., 51A:1369, 1969.
14. LaChapelle, E. H.: Osteotomy of the lumbar spine for correction of kyphosis in a case of ankylosing spondyloarthritis. J. Bone Joint Surg., 28:851, 1946.

15. Law, W. A.: Lumbar spinal osteotomy. J. Bone Joint Surg., 41B:270, 1959.
16. Law, W. A.: Osteotomy of the spine. Clin. Orthop., 66:70, 1969.
17. Lichtblau, P. O., and Wilson, P. D.: Possible mechanism of aorta rupture in orthopaedic correction for ankylosing spondylitis. J. Bone Joint Surg., 38A:123, 1956.
18. Marsh, C. H.: Internal fixation for stress fractures of the ankylosed spine. J. R. Soc. Med., 78:377, 1985.
19. Mason, C., Cozen, L., and Adelstein, L.: Surgical correction of flexion deformity of the cervical spine. Calif. Med., 79:244, 1953.
20. McMaster, M. J.: Spinal osteotomy in ankylosing spondylitis: technique, complications, and long-term results. Mayo Clinic Proc., 48:476, 1973.
21. McMaster, M. J.: A technique for lumbar spinal osteotomy in ankylosing spondylitis. J. Bone Joint Surg., 67B:204, 1985.
22. McMaster, P. E.: Osteotomy of the spine for fixed flexion deformity. J. Bone Joint Surg., 44A:1207, 1962.
23. Nunziata, H.: Osteotomia de la columna. Operacion de Smith-Peterson. Prensa Med. Argent., 35:1536, 1948.
24. Puschel, J., and Zielke, K.: Transpedicular vertebral instrumentation using VDS-instruments in ankylosing spondylitis. Orthop. Trans., 9(1):130, 1985.
25. Resnick, D., Williamson, S., and Alazraki, N.: Focal spinal abnormalities on bone scans in ankylosing spondylitis: a clue to the presence of fracture or pseudarthrosis. Clin. Nucl. Med., 6:213, 1975.
26. Rosenberg, M., and Horowitz, I.: Fracture-dislocation of the cervical spine with rheumatoid spondylitis. J. Canad. Assn. Radiol., 16:241, 1965.
27. Scudese, V. A., and Calabro, J. J.: Vertebral wedge osteotomy: correction of rheumatoid (ankylosing) spondylitis. JAMA, 186:627, 1963.
28. Simmons, E.: The surgical correction of flexion deformity of the cervical spine of ankylosing spondylitis. Clin. Orthop., 86:132, 1972.
29. Simmons, E.: Kyphotic deformity of the spine in ankylosing spondylitis. Clin. Orthop., 128:65, 1977.
30. Smith-Petersen, M. N., Larson, C. B., and Aufranc, O. E.: Osteotomy of the spine for correction of flexion deformity in rheumatoid arthritis. J. Bone Joint Surg., 27:1, 1945.
31. Thomasen, E.: Vertebral osteotomy for correction of kyphosis in ankylosing spondylitis. Clin. Orthop., 194:142, 1985.
32. Thompson, W. A. L., and Ingersoll, R. E.: Osteotomy for correction of deformity in Marie-Strumpell arthritis. Surg. Gynecol. Obstet., 90:552, 1950.
33. Urist, M. R.: Osteotomy of the cervical spine. J. Bone Joint Surg., 40A:833, 1958.
34. Welch, R. B., and Charnley, C. B. E.: Law-friction arthroplasty of the hip in rheumatoid arthritis and ankylosing spondylitis. Clin. Orthop., 72:22, 1970.
35. Wilson, M. J., and Turkell, J. H.: Multiple spinal wedge osteotomy: its use in a case of Marie-Strumpell spondylitis. Am. J. Surg., 77:777, 1949.

Kyphosis in the Elderly

David S. Bradford, M.D.

It is well known that the incidence of spinal deformity, specifically scoliosis, may be correlated with age. Three peaks have been described: one in infancy, another in adolescence, and the last one after age 50 years.[9] Vanderpool, James, and Wynne-Davies have noted that the incidence of scoliosis in patients over 50 years of age is 6 per cent.[9] The incidence is six times greater in patients with osteoporosis and osteomalacia. The etiology appears to be directly related to the increased incidence of metabolic bone disease found in the elderly. On the other hand, Robin and co-workers[7] have stated that scoliosis can appear de novo in the elderly population and increase in severity. However, they feel that no direct relationship between the presence or progression of scoliosis and osteoporosis exists. Of less controversy is the known association of kyphosis with osteoporosis in the post-menopausal female. Cross-sectional data reported by Cowan,[2] Fon,[3] and Milne and Lauder[5] have reported kyphosis to be more severe in women and to increase with advancing age in both sexes. Recent longitudinal data reported by Milne and Williamson[6] demonstrate that kyphosis does increase with increasing age.

The management of patients presenting with increasing deformity, back pain, and progressive kyphosis has generally been relegated to the internist. Analgesics, anti-inflammatory medications, and underarm braces of flexible or rigid design, as well as extension exercises, are usually prescribed.[8]

Before initiating any type of treatment, however, careful thorough examination and medical evaluation and occasional bone biopsy are desirable. It is important to rule out other diseases that may mimic post-menopausal osteoporosis, such as primary or metastatic cancer, multiple myeloma, Cushing's disease, biliary cirrhosis, intestinal malabsorption, hyperparathyroidism, hyperthy-

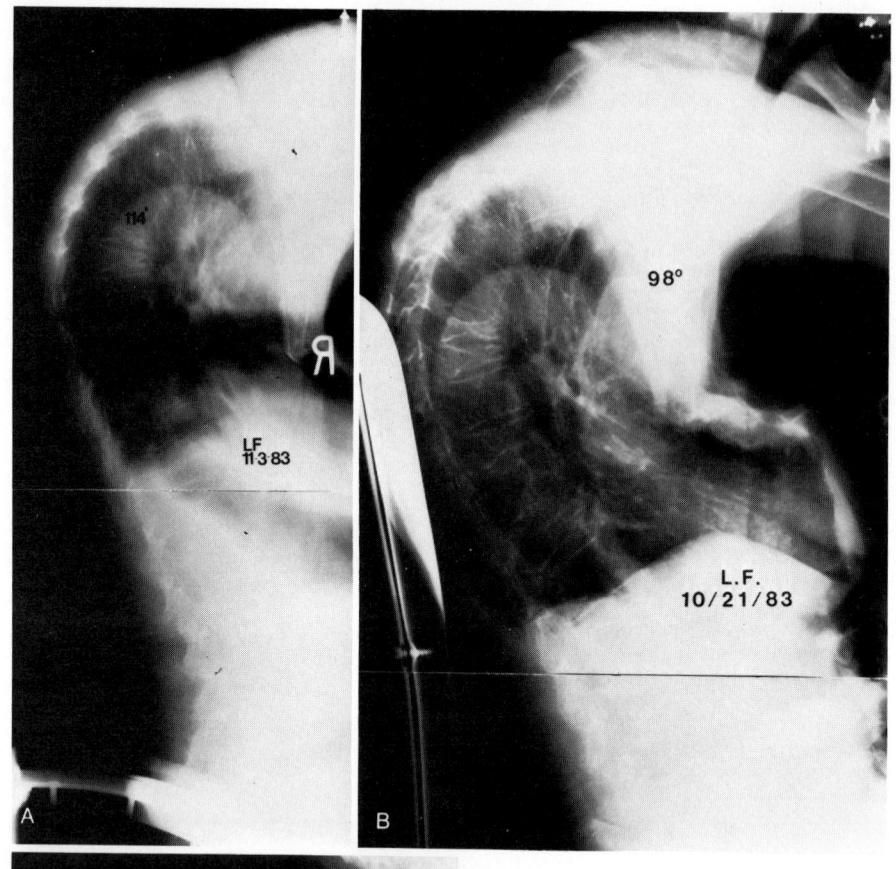

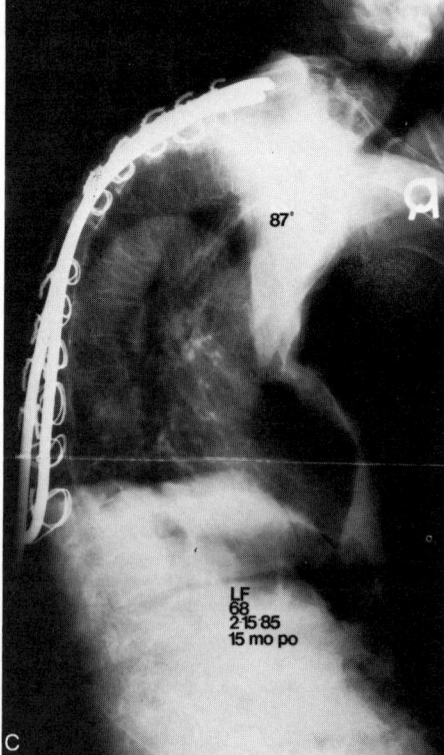

Figure 22–69. *A*, L.F. presented at age 67 with progressive kyphosis, intractable back pain, and difficulty feeding herself because of the fixed flexed position of her head, cervical spine, and upper thorax. Her sternum was markedly indented because of pressure from her mandible against her chest. *B*, She was placed in halo wheelchair traction for two weeks and then underwent posterior spinal fusion with L-rod instrumentation. *C*, Although the correction was less than optimal, the fixation is stable and she has shown no loss of correction over a year and a half since surgery.

roidism, and even osteogenesis imperfecta tarda.[4] To describe medical management of osteoporosis by fluoride calcium and estrogens with or without vitamin D, or of osteomalacia by vitamin D alone would be beyond the scope of this text, and the reader is referred elsewhere.[1]

Surgery may occasionally be indicated in this group of patients. As the elderly population becomes more healthier and lives longer, no doubt the spinal surgeon will be increasingly faced with the dilemma as to whether or not surgery should be undertaken in these patients. In the presence of progressive deformity, incapacitating pain unresponsive to conservative management, or the presence of neurologic impairment secondary to multiple compression fractures, we would consider surgery, providing the patient's health is satisfactory.

In the presence of neurologic deficit or neurologic deterioration secondary to compression fractures with retropulsed bone, we would recommend a first stage anterior transthoracic cord decompression followed by a second stage posterior L-rod instrumentation with fusion.

In those cases in which the patient primarily presents with progressive kyphosis and intractable back pain, we would recommend a single posterior approach with L-rod instrumentation and fusion. Some correction can be achieved by posterior transpedicular decancellation procedures along with the L-rod instrumentation (see Techniques of Surgery chapter)(Fig. 22-69).

References

1. American Academy of Orthopaedic Surgeons: Orthopaedic Knowledge Update Home Study Syllabus. Chicago, Illinois, 1984.
2. Cowan, N. R.: The frontal cardiac silhouette in older people. Br. Heart J., 27:231–235, 1965.
3. Fon, G. T., Pitt, M. J., and Thies, A. C.: Thoracic kyphosis: range in normal subjects. Am. J. Roentgenol., 134:979–983, 1980.
4. Gordon, G. S., Picchi, J., Roof, B. S., and Soika, C. V.: Postmenopausal osteoporosis. AFP 8, no. 6, pp. 74–83, 1973.
5. Milne, J. S., and Lauder, I. J.: Age effects in kyphosis and lordosis in adults. Ann. Hum. Biol., 1:327–337, 1974.
6. Milne, J. S., and Williamson, J.: A longitudinal study of kyphosis in older people. Age Ageing, 12:225–233, 1983.
7. Robin, G. C., Span, Y., Steinberg, R., et al.: Scoliosis in the elderly; a follow-up study. Spine, 7:355–359, 1982.
8. Sinaki, M.: Postmenopausal spinal osteoporosis: physical therapy and rehabilitation principles. Mayo Clin. Proc., 57:699–703, 1982.
9. Vanderpool, D. W., James, J. I. P., and Wynne-Davies, R.: Scoliosis in the elderly. J. Bone Joint Surg., 51A:446–455, 1969.

INDEX

Note: Page numbers in *italics* refer to illustrations; page numbers followed by the letter t refer to tables.

Abducens nerve, lesion of, from traction, 467
Achondroplasia, 522–528, *523–528*
   kyphosis in, 523, 525, *525–527*
     Milwaukee brace for, 523
   low back pain in, 525, 528
   scoliosis in, 525, *528*
Acquired immune deficiency syndrome, testing for, in bone banking, 597
Acute respiratory distress syndrome, postoperative, 475
Adolescent scoliosis, 203–228. See also *Scoliosis, adolescent*.
Adult scoliosis, 369–390. See also *Scoliosis, adult*.
Age, bone, definition of, 44
   skeletal, 44
   spinal growth and. See *Spine, growth of*.
AIDS. See *Acquired immune deficiency syndrome*.
Air embolism, 471
Airway management, intraoperative, 619–620
Alignment, body, definition of, 43
Allogeneic graft, 593
   bone source for, 593
   immune response to, 594
   immunogenicity of, 593–594
Allograft, 593
American Orthopaedic Association, 2
Amyotonia congenita. See *Spinal muscle atrophy*.
Anatomy, classification of spinal deformities by, 43
Anesthesia, 607–628
   inhalational, 623
   intraoperative monitoring of, 611–614
     clinical, 614
     somatosensory evoked potentials in, 612–614
   positioning for, 620–622
   postoperative care and, 624
   preoperative assessment for, 607–608
   techniques for, 622–623
   wake-up test for, 614, 623–624
Aneurysmal bone cyst, 494–495, *496*
Angiogram, in evaluation for spinal deformity, 85–86, *86*
Angle of thoracic inclination, definition of, 43
Ankylosing spondylitis. See *Spondylitis, ankylosing*.
Ankylosing spondylosis, treatment of, 629–631, *630*, *631*

Anterior column of spine, anatomy of, 8
Anterior strut fusion, *168–169*, 170–171
Antigravity cast, in juvenile kyphosis, 360
Anulus fibrosus, *8*, *9*
   anatomy of, *8*, *9*
Apical vertebra, definition of, 43
Apophyseal joints, anatomy of, 9
   asymmetry of, 10
Apophysis(es), iliac, definition of, 43
   vertebral ring, 44
     ossification of, 79, *79*
Arthrodesis, spinal. See *Spinal fusion*.
Arthrogryposis, *558*, *561*, 561–562
Astrocytoma, *508*, *509*, *510*, *519*
Asymmetry, facet, 10
Ataxia, Friedreich's, 298
Atlas, development of, 31
   ossification of, 32
Atrophy, of spinal muscles, 282–286, *285*, *287*
Autogeneic graft, 592
   bone source for, 593
Autograft, 592
Autotransfusion, 618
Axis, development of, 31
   ossification of, 32–33, *33*

Back, observation of, in evaluation for spinal deformity, 48, *49*
Balance, definition of, 43
Biomechanics, spinal, 7–23
Biopsy, vertebral, 491
Blood gases, arterial, 586
Blood loss, intraoperative, 474
   induced hypotension and, 614–616
   management of, 616–617
   surgical, in neuromuscular spinal deformity, 275
Blood transfusion, autologous, 617–618
Blood transfusion reaction, postoperative, 478
Body, vertebral. See *Vertebral body*.
Body alignment, definition of, 43
Body jacket. See *TLSO*.
Bone age, definition of, 44
   in evaluation for spinal deformity, 77
Bone bank. See also *Bone banking*.
   bone graft preparation at, *605*, 606
   bone procurement for, 602–604, *603*
   bone storage techniques in, *603*, 604
   bone testing for, 604–605

639

Bone bank (*Continued*)
  donor testing for, 602, 602(t)
  establishment of, 600–606, *601*, 602(t), *603*, *605*
    donor consent in, 602
    donor recognition for, 600
    donor suitability for, 602
Bone banking, 594–600, 595–597(t), 600(t). See also *Bone bank.*
  bone procurement for, 598
  bone sterilization for, 598
  donor selection for, 594–595, 596–597(t)
  donor testing for, 597–598
  freezing techniques for, 599
  medical criteria for, 595–597, 595–597(t)
  quality assurance for, 599–600, 600(t)
  sterility testing for, 599
  storage containers for, 598
  storage methods for, 598–599
Bone cyst, aneurysmal, 494–495, *496*
Bone transplantation, 592–594
  bone graft immunogenicity in, 593–594
  bone reconstitution for, 599
  bone source for, 593
  immune response to, 594
  mechanics of, 17–19, *18*
  technique of, 139
  terminology of, 592–593
  uses of, 593
Bone-in-bone appearance, 549, *549*
Brace, Milwaukee. See *Milwaukee brace.*
Brachial plexus, lesions of, from traction, 467
Bracing. See *Orthotics.*
Brackett and Bradford, horizontal distraction frame of, 4
Breast rating, in evaluation for spinal deformity, 55
Burst fracture, definition of, 448–449
  mechanism of, *450*
  neurologic deficit with, 454
  treatment of, 446, 448–454, *450–453*

Café-au-lait spots, definition of, 43
  in neurofibromatosis, 330, *331*
Calcium deficiency, juvenile kyphosis and, 349
Canal, neurenteric, 26, 27
Cardiac arrest, intraoperative, 471
Cardiovascular system, in spinal injury, 438
Cast(s), antigravity, in juvenile kyphosis, 360
  complications of, 468–470, *469*, *470*
  Cotrel E.D., 120, *120*
  femoral cutaneous nerve irritation from, 469
  halo, 110, *111*
    lo-profile supports in, *127–129*, 130
  hyperextension, application of, 126, *126*
  posterior fusion with, 251, *254*
  pressure sores from, 468–469, *469*
  reduction techniques with, for spondylolisthesis, 418, *419*, 420–422, *421*
  Risser localizer, *119*, 119–120
  Risser-Cotrel, 121, *122*
    application of, 121–125, *122–125*
  Stagnara (distraction and postoperative), 120, *121*
  techniques for application of, 119–133
  turnbuckle, 131–133, *132*

Cast(s) (*Continued*)
  underarm, application of, 126–129, *127*
  vascular compression of duodenum and, 469–470, *470*
  with leg extension, 130–131, *131*
Cast syndrome, 469–470, *470*
Centrum, vertebral, ossification of, 32
Cerebral palsy, 291, 293–298, *293–297*
  anesthetic considerations in, 610
  treatment of, approach to, 295
    non-operative, 293
    surgical, 293, 295
Cervical-thoracic-lumbar-sacral orthosis. See *Milwaukee brace.*
Charcot-Marie-Tooth disease, 298–299
Cholecystitis, acute, postoperative, 478
Chondrification, vertebral, 31, *32*
Chondrodystrophia calcificans congenita, 535, *537*
Chylothorax, postoperative, 475
Column failure, correction of, mechanics of, 15–17
  mechanics of, 12–15
Compensation, definition of, 43
Compensatory curve, definition of, 43
Compression, spinal. See *Spinal cord, compression of.*
Congenital dislocation of hip, infantile scoliosis and, 197
Congenital heart disease, scoliosis and, 576–578
  infantile, 197
Congenital kyphosis. See *Kyphosis, congenital.*
Congenital limb deficiency, scoliosis and, 578–582, *579–581*
  incidence of, 578, 580
  treatment of, *579*, 580, 581–582
Congenital lordosis, non-operative treatment of, 250
congenital.
Congenital scoliosis. See *Scoliosis, congenital.*
Congenital spine deformities, classification of, 233–235, *234–235*
  genetics of, 235–236
  natural history of, 237–239
  patient evaluation for, 236–237, *236–237*
  terminology for, 233–235
  treatment of, non-operative, 239–250
    operative, 250–269. See also names of specific procedures, e.g., *Spinal fusion.*
Contractures, of iliotibial band, treatment of, 279, *280*
Conversion scoliosis, 511–512, *512*
Cord, spinal. See *Spinal cord.*
Costal process of vertebra, 31, *31*
Costotransversectomy approach to spine, 166
Cotrel E.D. cast, 120, *120*
Cotrel-Dubousset instrumentation, in surgery for adolescent scoliosis, 225, *226*
  procedure for, 159
  technique of, 159–162
Cranial nerve(s), lesions of, from traction, 467
CT scanning, in spondylosis, 410
CTLSO (cervical-thoracic-lumbar-sacral orthosis). See *Milwaukee brace.*
Curve(s), compensatory, 43
  double thoracic, definition of, 43
  evaluation of, in patient evaluation for spinal deformity, 67–77, *70–77*
  fractional, definition of, 43

Curve(s) (*Continued*)
  full, 43
  lengthening of, postoperative problem of, 484
  measurement of, 71, 71–73, 72
    definition of, 43
  minor, 44
  nonstructural, 44
  patterns of. See *Curve patterns*.
  primary, definition of, 44
  progression of, 391–392
  structural, definition of, 44
Curve patterns, classification of, 194
  evaluation of, 71
  in cerebral palsy, *293*
  lumbar, single major, 195
  lumbosacral, 196
  multiple, 196
  thoracic, double major, 195
    and lumbar, 195
    and thoracolumbar, 195
  major, and minor lumbar, 195
  single major, 194
  single major high, 194
  thoracolumbar, single major, 195
Cyst(s). See also *Syringomyelia*.
  bone, aneurysmal, 494–495, *496*
  epidural, spinal, kyphosis and, *357*
Cystic fibrosis, juvenile kyphosis and, 349, *349*

Decompression, for degenerative spondylolisthesis, 427, *428*
  for fractures, 443–444
Decubital ulcers, in spinal cord injury patients, 438–439
Deformity, spinal. See *Spine, deformities of*, or name of specific deformity.
Diastrophic dwarfism, 528–529, *530–533*
Disc, intervertebral, anatomy of, 9
Discography, in evaluation for spinal deformity, 83–84
Displacement, tangential, in spondylolisthesis, 408–410
  translational, 408–410
Distraction injury, treatment of, 446, *447, 448*
Dorsal neural process, formation of, 30
Duchenne muscular dystrophy, 289–291, *292*
  scoliosis types in, 290
Duodenum, vascular compression of, from casts, 469–470, *470*
Dura, surgical trauma to, 473
Dural ectasia, in Marfan's syndrome, 555
  in neurofibromatosis, 332, *333*
Dwarfism, diastrophic, 528–529, *530–533*
  metatropic, 538
Dwarfs, 522–540. See also specific conditions, e.g., *Achondroplasia*.
Dysautonomia, familial, kyphoscoliosis in, 287, 289
Dysplasia, epiphyseal, multiple, 529
  spondyloepimetaphyseal, 538
  spondyloepiphyseal, 529, *534*
    Milwaukee brace for, 529
Dyspnea, 393
Dysraphism, spinal, treatment of, 265–269
Dystrophia myotonica, 291
Dystrophy, facioscapulohumeral, 291

Dystrophy (*Continued*)
  limb-girdle, 291
  muscular, Duchenne, 289–291, *292*
  myotonic, anesthetic considerations in, 609–610

Electric surface stimulation treatment, complications of, 215
  in juvenile scoliosis, 212–215, *214*
  mechanism of, 212–213
  methods in, 213
  patient selection for, 213
  results of, 215
Electrolytes, intraoperative management of, 616–617
Embolism, air, 471
Embryo, mesodermal differentiation in, 28, *29*
Embryology, 25–39
Empyema, contracture with, scoliosis and, 582
End vertebra, definition of, 43
Endodermal layer of notochord, 27, *27*
Endplate(s), vertebral, 44
  definition of, 44
Eosinophilic granuloma, 495, *498*
Ependymoma, *506–507*
Epiphyseal dysplasia, multiple, 529
Epiphysis(es), iliac, definition of, 43
  ossification of, 77–78, *78*
ERV (expiratory reserve volume), *586*
Evaluation, of patients, 47–88. See also *Patient(s), evaluation of*.
Examination, physical, in patient evaluation for spinal deformity, 48–58, *49–57*
Exercise, cardiopulmonary response to, scoliosis and, 588
  for adolescent scoliosis, 208
Expiratory reserve volume (ERV), *586*

Facet joints, anatomy of, 9
  asymmetry of, 10
  fusion of, 139–141, *140–141*
  in post-laminectomy spine deformity, 515, *516, 517*
Familial dysautonomia, kyphoscoliosis in, 287, 289
Family history, in evaluation of patient for spinal deformity, 48
Fascioscapulohumeral dystrophy, 291
Femoral cutaneous nerve, irritation of, from casts, 469
Femoral pins, complications of, 466
Fentanyl, 622
Ferguson view, in radiographic evaluation, 65, *68*
FEV1 (forced expiratory volume, one second), 585
Flexibility, of joints, in evaluation for spinal deformity, 53
  spinal, 48–53, *49–52*
Forced expiratory volume, one second (FEV1), 585
Forced vital capacity (FVC), 585
Formation defects, in congenital kyphosis, 262–265, *264*

Fracture(s), burst, *436*
  definition of, 448–449
  mechanism of, *450*
  neurologic deficit with, 454
  treatment of, 446, 448–454, *450–453*
 classification of, 439–440, *440*
 in ankylosing spondylitis, 633, *634*
 in children, 454, 459–460
 intraoperative, 474
 treatment of, decompression for, 443–444
  non-operative, 441–442
  operative, 442–460
  stabilization for, 442–443
 wedge compression, treatment of, 444–446, *445*
Fracture-dislocation, treatment of, 454, *455–459*
Frame, horizontal distraction, of Brackett and Bradford, *4*
Friedreich's ataxia, 298
Fusion, spinal. See *Spinal fusion.*
FVC (forced vital capacity), 585

Gastrointestinal tract, upper, radiographic evaluation of, 86, *86*
Genetics, of congenital spine deformities, 235–236
Giant cell tumor, 494, 495
Gibbus, definition of, 43
Gluteal artery, intraoperative laceration of, 474
Graft(s), bone. See *Bone transplantation.*
 isogeneic, 593
 rib, anterior vascularized, 179–181, *180–181*
 syngeneic, 593
 xenogeneic, 593
Granuloma, eosinophilic, 495, *498*
Growth, postoperative stunting of, 485
Growth plate, vertebral, 44

Halo cast, 110, *111*
 application of, *128–130*, 129–130
 lo-profile supports in, *127–129*, 130
Halo traction, application of, 113, *114–115*
 complications of, 465–466
 infected pins in, 465
 pin loosening in, 465–466
 slippage in, 466
Halofemoral traction, complications of, 115, *116*
Halohoop traction, complications of, 113–115
Halopelvic traction, complications of, 466
 in spondylolisthesis, 113
Harrington instrumentation, 143–148, *144–147*
 compression rod assembly in, 145–148, *146–147*
 for adolescent scoliosis, 217–225, *218, 221, 225*
 for juvenile scoliosis, 203
 hook placement in, 143, *144*
 outrigger in, 143–145
 paraplegia from, 472
 rod insertion in, 145, *145*
 sublaminar wires with, 157–158, *157–158*
 to lower lumbar spine and sacrum, 148

Harrington rod, postoperative dislodgement of, 478–479
 postoperative problems of, 481, *483*
Health, general, of patient with spinal deformity, 48
Heart disease, congenital, scoliosis and, 576–578
 infantile, 197
Hemangioma, 495
 cavernous, 494
Hemodilution, preoperative, 618
Hemothorax, intraoperative, 474
Hensen's node, *26, 27*
Hepatitis, postoperative, 478
 testing for, in bone banking, 597
Hip, congenital dislocation of, infantile scoliosis and, 197
Hippocrates, machine of, *2*
Histiocytosis-X, 495, *498*
History, of scoliosis, 1–5
 of spinal biomechanics, 7–23
 patient, in evaluation of spinal deformity, 47–48
Hooks, in Harrington instrumentation, placement of, 143, *144*
Horizontal distraction frame, of Brackett and Bradford, *4*
Hydrocephalus, postoperative, 475
Hydronephrosis, postoperative, 477
Hyperextension cast, application of, 126, *126*
 in juvenile kyphosis, 358
Hyperkyphosis, definition of, 43
Hyperthermia, malignant, anesthetic considerations in, 608–609
Hypochondroplasia, 528
Hypokyphosis, definition of, 43
Hypotension, induced, surgical blood loss and, 614–616
Hysterical scoliosis, 511–512, *512*
 definition of, 43

Idiopathic scoliosis. See *Scoliosis, idiopathic.*
Ileus, postoperative, 477
Iliac apophysis, definition of, 43
Iliac epiphysis, definition of, 43
Iliotibial band, contractures of, in poliomyelitis, 279, *280*
 treatment of, 279, *280*
Implant evaluation, 19–20
Incision, for spinal surgery, 135–139, *138*
Inclinometer, definition of, 43
Infantile scoliosis, 196–200. See also *Scoliosis, infantile.*
Infection, postoperative, 479
Injury(ies), seatbelt, treatment of, 446, 447–448
 spinal. See *Spinal injury.*
 translational, treatment of, 454, *455–459*
Inlay strut fusion, *167*, 170
Inspiratory reserve volume (IRV), *586*
Instability, spinal, 440–441
Instrumentation. See also names of specific types: *Cotrel-Dubousset; Harrington; L-rod; Zielke.*
 anterior, 174–177, *175–178*
 posterior fusion with, 253–258, *256–258*
 posterior spinal, 143–162. See also names of specific types, e.g., *Harrington; L-rod.*

Instrumentation (*Continued*)
   posterior spinal, without fusion, 177–179
   postoperative dislodgement and, 478–479, *480*
   postoperative problems with, 481–486, *482–485*
   segmental spinal, 149–157. See also *L-rod instrumentation.*
Interbody technique of spinal fusion, *166–167*, 167–170
Interspinous ligaments, 10
Intervertebral disc, anatomy of, 9
Intravenous pyelogram, in evaluation for spinal deformity, 84, *84*
Isogeneic graft, 593
Isograft, 593

Joint(s), apophyseal, 9
   anatomy of, 9
   asymmetry of, 10
   facet, anatomy of, 9
   asymmetry of, 10
   flexibility of, in evaluation for spinal deformity, 53
Juvenile kyphosis, 347–368. See also *Kyphosis, juvenile.*
Juvenile scoliosis, 200–203. See also *Scoliosis, juvenile.*

Kinematics, 10–12
   definition of, 10
Kniest syndrome, 538
Kugelberg-Welander disease. See *Spinal muscle atrophy.*
Kyphos, definition of, 43
Kyphoscoliosis, definition of, 44
   in Charcot-Marie-Tooth disease, 298–299
Kyphosing scoliosis, definition of, 44
Kyphosis, cervical, 631–632
   classification of, 42
   congenital, formation defects in, 262–265, *264*
     natural history of, 239, *248–249*
     non-operative treatment of, 250
     operative treatment of, 262–265, *263–264*
     segmentation defects in, 262, *263*
     vs. juvenile kyphosis, 354, *355*
   in achondroplasia, 523, 525, *525–527*
   in ankylosing spondylitis, 628–635, *630–632*, *634*
   in diastrophic dwarfism, 529, *531–533*
   in elderly, 635–637, *636*
   in neurofibromatosis, 334, 337–339, *338*
   in spinal muscle atrophy, 282–286, *285*, *287*
   in tuberculosis, 573, *574*, 574–575
   juvenile, 347–368
     atypical, 352–353, *354*
     complications of, 355–358, *356*, *357*
     cord angulation in, *357*
     cord compression in, 355
     cystic fibrosis and, 349, *349*
     diagnosis of, differential, 353–354, *355*
       radiographic, 352
     etiology of, 348–350, *349*, *350*
     histological studies of, 350, *350*
     normal, 347–348

Kyphosis (*Continued*)
   juvenile, pathogenesis of, 348–350, *349*, *350*
     physical examination in, 351, *352*
     prevalence of, 350
     radiographic findings in, 351–352
     spondylolisthesis in, 405
     spondylosis in, 355
     symptoms of, 351
     treatment of, electrical stimulation for, 361
       hyperextension case for, 358
       indications for, 358
       Milwaukee brace for, *359*, 359–360, *361*
       non-operative, 358–362, *359*, *361*, *362*
         patient management in, 360–361
       operative, 363–365, *364*, *365*
         patient management in, 365
       underarm brace for, 361, *362*
     Turner's syndrome and, 349, *349*
     vs. ankylosing spondylitis, 354
     vs. congenital kyphosis, 354, *355*
     vs. infectious spondylitis, 354
     vs. postural roundback, 352–353, *353*
     x-ray appearance of, *348*
   L-rod instrumentation for, 154
   post-laminectomy, 513
   radiation-induced, *549*
   spinal cord compression and, 540–547, *541–543*, *545*, *546*
     incidence of, 540
     pathogenesis of, 540–541, *541*, *542*
     presentation of, 541–543, *544*
     treatment of, 543–544, *545*, *546*
       anterior transthoracic approach for, 544
       plan for, 544–547, *546*
   spinal epidural cysts and, *357*
   thoracic, 631, *632*
     normal, 347–348
   thoracolumbar, in achondroplasia, Milwaukee brace for, 523
   vertebral rotation in, *76*, *77*

L-rod instrumentation, l49–157, *150–155*
   benefits of, 156
   complications of, 156–157
   convex technique with, 152–153, *153*
   determination of level of, 149–150, *150*
   disadvantages of, 156
   exposure for, 150–152, *151–152*
   for adolescent scoliosis, 217–225, *218*, *224*
   for arthrogryposis, *561*, 562
   for kyphosis, 154
   for lordosis, 154
   for pelvic obliquity, 154–156
   for spinal injury, 443
   general comments on, 156–156
   in myelomeningocele, 156, *156*
   neurologic complications of, 472
   pelvic fixation of, 153–154, *155*
   postoperative dislodgement of, 478–479
   technique of, concave, 153, *153*
     convex, 152–153, *153*
Laboratory tests, in evaluation for spinal deformity, 87
Laminectomy, deformities following, 513–522, *514–520*. See also *Post-laminectomy spine deformity.*

Laminectomy (*Continued*)
  deformities following, in neurofibromatosis, 339–340
  in spondylolisthesis, 415
Laminogram, in evaluation of patient for spinal deformity, 79–80, *80*
Leg extension cast, 130–131, *131*
Ligament(s), interspinous, 10
  of posterior column of spine, 10
  posterior longitudinal, 8, *8*
  supraspinous, 10
  yellow, anatomy of, 10
Ligamentum flavum, anatomy of, 10
Limb deficiency, congenital, scoliosis and, 578–582, *579–581*
Limb-girdle dystrophy, 291
Lisch nodules, in neurofibromatosis, 330, *331*, 332
Lo-profile supports, in halo casting, *127–129*, 130
Longitudinal ligament, posterior, 8, *8*
Lordoscoliosis, definition of, 44
  in neurofibromatosis, 339, *342*
Lordosis, classification of, 42
  congenital, non-operative treatment of, 250
  L-rod instrumentation for, 154
  lumbar, loss of, 392, *392*
    evaluation of, 393
    pain with, 393
    postoperative, 486
    symptoms of, 392–393
    treatment of, 395–396, *397*
  post-laminectomy, 513–514, *514*
  postoperative, 485–486
  thoracic, pulmonary function and, 587
    surgical management of, 181–184, *182–184*
Low back pain, in achondroplasia, 525, 528
Lung function. See *Pulmonary function*.
Lung volumes, 585–586, *586*
  impairment of, scoliosis and, 586
Luque instrumentation. See *L-rod instrumentation*.

Machine of Hippocrates, 2
Magnetic resonance imaging (MRI), 83
Malignant hyperthermia, anesthetic considerations in, 608–609
Marfan's syndrome, 554–560, *556–559*
  anesthetic considerations in, 610
  clinical manifestations of, 554
  patient evaluation in, 555–557, *556*
  treatment of, *557–559*, 557–560
    orthotic, 557
    periodic observation for, 557, *557*
    surgical, 557–560, *558*, *559*
Maturation, assessment of, Tanner system for, 55–57, *57*, 57t
  determination of, in adolescent idiopathic scoliosis, 207
Mechanical ventilation, postoperative, 590, 590(t)
Mental retardation, infantile scoliosis and, 197
Mesoderm, differentiation of, embryonic, 28, 29
Metatrophic dwarfism, 538

Milwaukee brace, for adolescent scoliosis, 208–210, *209*
  for adult scoliosis, 370
  for juvenile kyphosis, 359–360, *361*
  for postoperative immobilization in polio patients, 282
  for spondyloepiphyseal dysplasia, 529
  for thoracolumbar kyphosis in achondroplasia, 523
  history of, 97
Morquio's disease, 529, 535, *535*, *536*
Motor neuron disease, hereditary. See *Spinal muscle atrophy*.
MRI (magnetic resonance imaging), 83
Mucopolysaccharidoses, 529, 535, *535*, *536*
Multiple epiphyseal dysplasia, 529
Muscular dystrophy, Duchenne, 289–291, *292*
  anesthetic considerations in, 609
  myotonic, 609–610
Myelogram, in evaluation for spinal deformity, 80–83, *81*
  in evaluation for spondylosis, 410
Myelomeningocoele, 307–328
  congenital scoliosis in, operative treatment of, technique for, 318, *321*, 327
  kyphosis in, 322–326, 327
  L-rod instrumentation in, 156, *156*
  lordoscoliosis in, operative treatment of, technique for, 316, 318, *318–320*
  paralytic scoliosis in, 316, 318, *318–320*
  patient evaluation in, 308, 312, *313*
    history in, 308
    physical examination in, 308
    radiologic examination in, 312, *313*
  spinal deformity in, natural history of, 307–308, *309–311*
    operative treatment of, fusion area in, 316
      patient evaluation for, 316
      technique for, 316, *318–326*, 318–327
    treatment of, 312, *314*, 314–327, *315*, *317–326*
      non-operative, 312, 314, *314*, *315*
      operative, 316, *318–326*, 318–327
      rodding for, 316
      with braces, 314, *314*
  treatment of, bracing for, 314, *314*, *315*
Myotonic muscular dystrophy, anesthetic considerations in, 609–610

Neural folds, of notochord, 26, *27*
Neural plate, 26, *27*
Neural process, dorsal, formation of, 30
Neural tube, 26, *27*
  closure of, 27, *28*
  development of, 25–28, *26–28*
Neurenteric canal, 26, *27*
Neurofibromatosis, 329–346
  anesthetic considerations in, 610
  café-au-lait spots in, 330, *331*
  cervical spine deformity in, treatment of, 334, *336*, 337
  diagnosis of, 330–332, *331*, *332*
  dural ectasia in, 332, *333*
  dystrophic bony changes in, 332, *333*
  genetics of, 330
  incidence of, 329–330

Neurofibromatosis (*Continued*)
  intraspinal, 339, *344*
  kyphosis in, cervical, treatment of, 334, *336*, 337
  Lisch nodules in, 330, *331*, 332
  lordoscoliosis in, 339, *342*
  natural history of, 332, 334, *335*
  pathogenesis of, 330
  scoliosis in, 332
    cervical, treatment of, 334
    types of, 334, *335*, *336*
  spinal compression in, 339, 344, *344*
  spondylolisthesis in, treatment of, 339
  thoracic lordoscoliosis in, 339, *342*
  thoracic spine deformity in, 337–339, *338*, *340–343*
Neuromuscular spinal deformities, classification of, 271
  general principles of, 271–273, *272*
  patient evaluation in, 273–274
  pulmonary function in, 272, 273
  treatment of, 274–276, *275*
    observation in, 274
    orthoses for, 274, *275*
    surgery for, blood loss in, 275
Neuropraxia, Seddon's, 467
Node, Hensen's, 26, 27
Nodules, Lisch's, in neurofibromatosis, 330, *331*, 332
  Schmorl's, *348*
Notochord, development of, 25–28, *26–28*
  endodermal layer of, 27, *27*
  neural folds of, *26*, *27*

Obliquity, pelvic, definition of, 44
Occiput, development of, 31
Orthosis. See also *Orthotics*.
  cervical-thoracic-lumbar-sacral (CTLSO), history of, 97. See also *Milwaukee brace*.
  thoracolumbar sacral (TLSO), 98, *98*
Orthotics, 97–108
  biomechanics of, 98–102, *99–101*
  complications of, 106
  electrospinal treatment and, *102*, 102–103
  goals of, 97
  history of, 97–98, *98*
  in adolescent scoliosis, 208–212, *209*, *211*
  in Duchenne muscular dystrophy, 290
  in neuromuscular spinal deformities, 274, *275*
  prescription of, *102*, 102–103, 103–106, *104–106*
Ossification, of atlas, 32
  of axis, 32–33, *33*
  of sacrum, 33
  of vertebrae, 31, *32*
Osteoblastoma, 494
Osteogenesis imperfecta, 562–567, *564–566*
  incidence of, 562–563
  natural history of, 562–563
  treatment of, 563–567, *564–566*
Osteoma, osteoid, *492*, 492–494, *493*
  treatment of, *493*, 494
Osteomyelitis, 568–576, *569*, *570*, *573*, *574*
  non-tuberculous, 575
Osteotomy, anterior, technique of, 171, *172*
  combined anterior and posterior, with correction and fusion, 259–262, *261*

Osteotomy (*Continued*)
  lumbar, in ankylosing spondylitis, 629, *631*
  posterior spinal, 141–142, *142*
    of previously fused spine, 142, *143*

Pain, location of, in evaluation for spinal deformity, 50
Paralysis, due to spinal traction, 116
Paraplegia, 286–287, *288*
  fracture-dislocation and, 454, *455*
  from Harrington instrumentation, 472
  from spinal fusion, 472
  from traction, 466, *467*
  in children, 459
Pars interarticularis, stress to, spondylolisthesis and, 405
Patient(s), bone age of, 77
  effects of spinal deformity on, 91–93
  evaluation of, 47–88
    computerized tomography (CT scan) in, *82–83*, 83
    curve evaluation in, 67–77, *70–77*
    documentation in, 87
    family history in, 48
    for congenital spine deformity, 236–237, *236–237*
    general health in, 48
    history in, 47–48
    history of spinal deformity in, 47–48
    laboratory tests in, 87
    laminogram in, 79–80, *80*
    maturity assessment in, 48, 77–79
      Tanner system for, *55–57*, 57, 57t
    myelogram in, 80–83, *81*
    physical examination in, 48–58, *49–57*
    pulmonary function testing in, 87
    radiographic evaluation in, 58–67, *59–67*. See also *Spine, radiographic evaluation of*.
    special studies for, 79–86, *80–86*
    school screening in, 58
    spinogram in, 80–83, *81*
    upper gastrointestinal studies in, 86, *86*
  positioning of, for surgery, 135, *136*
Pedriolle method, for measuring vertebral rotation, 73, *75*
Pelvic obliquity, definition of, 44
  L-rod instrumentation for, 154–156
Peritoneum, intraoperative damage to, 474
Phalen-Dixon sign, 406, *408*
Physical examination, in evaluation for spinal deformity, 48–58, *49–57*
Pins, femoral, complications of, 466
  infected, in halo traction, 465
  loosening of, 465–466
Plagiocephaly, in infantile scoliosis, 197
Plan d'élection of Stagnara, in radiographic evaluation, 65–67, *69*
Plate, neural, *26*, *27*
Pneumothorax, intraoperative, *473*, 473–474
Poliomyelitis, Milwaukee brace for postoperative immobilization in, 282
  spinal deformity in, 276–282, *277*, *278*, *280*, *283*
    anterior fusion for, 281–282, *283*
    iliotibial band contractures in, 279, *280*
    posterior surgery for, 281
    postoperative immobilization for, 282

Poliomyelitis (*Continued*)
  spinal deformity in, preoperative traction for, 279
    pulmonary insufficiency and, 279, 281
    treatment of, non-operative, 276, *277*
      results of, 282
      surgical, 276–282, *278, 280*
Post-laminectomy spine deformity, incidence of, 513
  pathogenesis of, 514–516, *515–517*
  prevention of, 517
  treatment of, 517–521, *518–520*
  types of, 513–514, *514*
Posterior column of spine, anatomy of, 8, *8*
  ligamentous structures of, 10
Posterior ligament complex, in spinal injury, 439
Posterior longitudinal ligament, 8, *8*
Postural roundback, treatment of, 361
  vs. juvenile kyphosis, 352–353, *353*
Pressure sores, from casts, 468–469, *469*
  from traction, 468
Prominence, rotational, definition of, 44
Pseudarthrosis, 391
  evaluation of, 393
  following lumbosacral fusion, 416–417, *417*
  pain with, 392–393
  postoperative, 479, 481, *481*
  repair of, 394, *395*
  staged reconstruction of, 396
  symptoms of, 393
Pubertal stages, in boys and girls, 57t
Pulmonary function, evaluation of, 87
  in adult scoliosis, 372
  in Duchenne muscular dystrophy, 290
  in poliomyelitis, 279, 281
  in spinal injury, 437–438
  mechanics of, 585
  neuromuscular spinal deformities and, 272, 273
  postoperative, early, 588
    late, 588–589
    management of, 589–590, 590(t)
  postoperative complications of, 474–475, *475*
  preoperative assessment of, 586, 608
  scoliosis and, 586–588
  surgical curve correction and, 588–589
  testing of, 585–592, *586*, 590(t)

Quadriplegia, from traction, 466

Radiation, spine deformity following, 547–554, *548, 549, 551, 552*
  incidence of, 550
  treatment of, *551*, 551–553, *552*
Radiography, in evaluation of patient for spinal deformity, 58–67, *59–67*
  special studies in, 79–86, *80–86*
Reconstruction, anterior-posterior, 396, *399*
  posterior-posterior, 398, *401*
  staged, 396–402, *399–401*
    complications of, 400
    immobilization after, 400
Reduction, cast, for spondylolisthesis, *418*, *419*, 420–422, *421*

Reduction (*Continued*)
  for spondylolisthesis, *418–421*, 418–424, *423–425*
  posterior implant technique of, for spondylolisthesis, *419*, *422*, *423*
Residual volume (RV), 586
Respiratory drive, scoliosis and, 587
Respiratory failure, scoliosis and, 587
Retardation, mental, infantile scoliosis and, 197
Retroperitoneal approach to spine, 165
Rib(s), penciling of, in neurofibromatosis, 332
  resection of. See *Thoracoplasty.*
Rib deformity, tangential view of, 84–85, *85*
Rib grafting, anterior vascularized, 179–181, *180–181*
Rib hump view, in evaluation of spinal deformity, 84–85, *85*
Rib-vertebral angle (RVA), 197, *197*
Rib-vertebral angle difference (RVAD), in infantile scoliosis, 197, *197*
Risser localizer cast, *119*, 119–120
Risser sign, 78, *78*
Risser-Cotrel cast, 121, *122*
  application of, 121–125, *122–125*
Rod(s), Harrington. See *Harrington instrumentation.*
  L-. See *L-rod instrumentation.*
  Luque. See *L-rod instrumentation.*
Roentgen, Wilhelm Konrad, 2
Rotation, progressive, treatment of, 396
  vertebral, 73–77. See also *Vertebra(e), rotation of.*
Rotational prominence, definition of, 44
Roundback, postural, treatment of, 361
  vs. juvenile kyphosis, 352–353, *353*
Roy-Camille plates, 443
RV (residual volume), *586*
RVA (rib-vertebral angle), 197, *197*
RVAD (rib-vertebral angle difference), in infantile scoliosis, 197, *197*

Sacrum, ossification of, 33
Scapuloperoneal syndrome. See *Spinal muscle atrophy.*
Scheuermann's disease, 347–368. See also *Kyphosis, juvenile.*
Schmorl's nodules, *348*
School screening, in adolescent scoliosis, 207–208
  in patient evaluation for spinal deformity, 58
Sclerotome, differentiation of, 29, 30–32
Sclerotomic fissure of von Ebner, 30
Scoliosis. See also *Spine, deformities of.*
  adolescent, 203–228
    definition of, 43
    determination of maturation in, 207
    general findings in, 203–207
    Milwaukee brace for, 208–210, *209*
    school screening for, 207–208
    treatment of, 208–228
      non-operative, 208–215, *209, 211, 214*
      procedures associated with, 227–228
      surgical, 215–227, *218–227.* See also *Surgery, for adolescent scoliosis.*
  adult, 369–390
    cardiopulmonary decompensation in, 372

Scoliosis (*Continued*)
  adult, definition of, 43
    deformity of, 371, *371*
    functional loss in, 372
    natural history of, 369–370
    neurologic problems in, 372
    operative techniques for, 378–388, *379, 380, 381, 383–387*
      with double thoracic curves, 384–388, *385–388*
      with lumbar curve(s), 382, 384–388, *385–388*
      with nerve root compression, 382, 384, *384*
      with single thoracic curve, 378–379, *379–381*
      with single thoracolumbar curve, 382, *383*
    pain with, 370–372
    patient evaluation in, 372–373
      history in, 372–373
      radiographs for, 373
    presentation of, 370–372, *371*
      pain with, 370–372
    prevalence of, 369
    pulmonary function in, 372, 373
    treatment of, 373, 375–388
      evaluation for, 375, 377
      Milwaukee brace for, 370
      non-operative, 373, 375, *376*
      operative, 375, 377–388, *379–381, 383–387*
      orthosis for, 375, *376*
      principles of, 377–378
  congenital, classification of, 41–42
    definition of, 43
    natural history of, 237–239, *240–247*
    non-operative treatment of, 239–250, *250*
    operative treatment of, 250–262, *252–261*. See also names of specific procedures, e.g., *Spinal fusion*.
  congenital limb deficiency and, 578–582, *579–581*
  conversion, 511–512, *512*
  definition of, 1
  double major, definition of, 43
  effects on patient of, 91–93
  historical aspects of, 1–5
  hysterical, 511–512, *512*
    definition of, 43
  idiopathic, 191–232
    classification of, 41
    curve patterns in, 194–196
    definition of, 43
    etiology of, 191–193
    genetic aspects of, 191–193
    natural history of, 193–194
    preoperative skeletal traction in, 111, *112*
    types of, 196–228. See also specific types, e.g., *Scoliosis, adolescent*.
  in achondroplasia, 525, *528*
  in arthrogryposis, *558*, *561*, 561–562
  in congenital heart disease, 576–578
  in diastrophic dwarfism, 528–529
  in Friedreich's ataxia, 298
  in Marfan's syndrome, 554–560, *556–559*
  in neurofibromatosis, 332, *334*, *336*
  in osteogenesis imperfecta, 562–567, *564–566*
  in spinal muscle atrophy, 282–286, *285*, *287*
  in syringomyelia, 299–301, *300*, *301*

Scoliosis (*Continued*)
  infantile, 196–200
    defects associated with, 197
    definition of, 43
    rib-vertebral angle difference (RVAD) in, 197, *197*
    treatment of, 197–200, *198–199*
  juvenile, 200–203
    definition of, 43
    Harrington instrumentation for, 203
    treatment of, 200–201, *201–202*
      surgical, 201–203, *204–205*
  kyphosing, definition of, 44
  natural history of, 89–95
  neuromuscular, 271–305. See also *Neuromuscular spinal deformities*.
    classification of, 41
  nonstructural, 42
  osteoid osteoma and, 492
  paralytic, halogravity wheelchair traction in, 110, *111*
  post-laminectomy, 513
  prevalence of, 89–90
  pulmonary function and, 586–588
  radiation-induced, 548, *549*
  rib resection and, 582–585, *583*, 583–585, *584*
  spinal cord compression and, 540–547
  spondylolisthesis and, treatment of, 424–426, *425*
  structural, classification of, 41–42
  thoracic cage defects and, 582–585, *583*
  thoracoplasty and, 582–583
  traction in, 109–117, *110–116*. See also *Traction*.
  treatment of, orthotic, 97–108. See also *Orthotics*.
    surgical. See also *Surgery*.
    traction in, 109–117, *110–116*. See also *Traction*.
  untreated, studies of, 90–91, *91*, *92*
Scoliosis Research Society, 4
  classification and terminology used by, 41–45
Screening, school. See *School screening*.
Seatbelt injury, treatment of, 446, *447*, *448*
Seddon's neuropraxia, 467
Segmentation defects, in congenital kyphosis, 262, *263*
Shock lung syndrome, 471
Shoulders, levels of, in evaluation for spinal deformity, 48, *49*
Sign, Phalen-Dixon, 406, *408*
  Risser, 78, *78*
Skeletal age, definition of, 44
Skin, examination of, in evaluation for spinal deformity, 53, *53*
Somatosensory evoked potentials, anesthesia monitoring with, 612–614
Somites, formation of, 28–30, *29*
Spinal. See also *Spine*.
Spinal canal, cervical, in syringomyelia, 299, *300*
Spinal column, deformed, instrumental correction of, 15–17
  failure of, mechanics of, 12–15
Spinal cord, compression of, 540–547, *541–543*, *545*, *546*
  in juvenile kyphosis, 355
  in metastatic disease, 503

Spinal cord (*Continued*)
  compression of, in neurofibromatosis, 339, 344, *344*
  decompression of, anterior, 171–174, *173*
  injury to, 286–287, *288*
    decubital ulcers and, 438–439
  tumors of, 505–511, *506–508*, *510*
    classification of, 505
    diagnosis of, 505–509, *506–508*, *510*
    radiologic signs of, 509
    treatment of, 509, 511
Spinal deformity(ies). See *Spine, deformities of,* or name of specific deformity.
Spinal fusion, anterior, 166–169, 166–171
    inlay strut technique for, *167*, 170
    interbody technique for, 166–167, *167–170*
  anterior strut, *168–169*, 170–171
  convex, combined anterior and posterior, 258–259, *260*
  for neuromuscular spinal deformity, 275
  for poliomyelitis curvatures, 277
  for spondylolisthesis, 414–417, *415–417*
  in situ, 251, *252–253*
  paraplegia from, posterior, with cast correction, 251, *254*
    with traction, 251–253, *255*
  postoperative bending of, 484–485
  short, 392
    evaluation of, 393
    extension repair of, 394–395
    pain with, 393
    symptoms of, 392–393
  with combined anterior and posterior osteotomy, 259–262, *261*
  with instrumentation, 253–258, *256–258*
    after traction, 258, *259*
Spinal injury, 435–463. See also *Fracture(s).*
  complications of, cardiovascular, 438
    gastrointestinal, 438
    genitourinary, 438
    integumentary, 438–439
    pulmonary, 437–438
  decubital ulcers and, 438–439
  distraction, treatment of, 446, *447*, *448*
  evaluation of, 435–436
    computerized tomography in, 437
    myelography in, 437
    radiographic, *436*, 436–437
  in children, 454, 459–460
  mechanisms of, 439–440, *440*
  neurologic impairment in, 437–439
  posterior ligament complex in, 439
  pulmonary function in, 437–438
  spinal instability and, 440–441
  spinal stability and, 440–441
  stable, 439
  three column spine concept of, 439–440, *440*
  treatment of, anterior spinal implants for, 443
    Harrington distraction implants for, 442
    L-rod instrumentation for, 443
    non-operative, 441–442
    operative, 442–460. See also under *Fracture(s).*
    stabilization in, 442–443
    Roy-Camille plates for, 443
  unstable, 439
Spinal muscle atrophy, 282–286, *285*, *287*
  treatment for, 284–286, *285*, *287*

Spinal stenosis, in achondroplasia, 523, *524–527*
Spine, anatomy of, 8–10
  anterior approach to, surgical techniques for, 162–166, *163–165*
  anterior column of, anatomy of, 8
  anterior osteotomy of, technique of, 171, *172*
  biomechanics of, 7–23
    anatomy in, 8–10
    history of, 7
  column failure of, mechanics of, 12–15
  costotransversectomy approach to, 166
  curve of. See *Curve(s)* and *Curve patterns.*
  deformities of. See also specific deformities, e.g., *Scoliosis,* and associated conditions, e.g., *Myelomeningocoele.*
    classification of, 41-42
      by anatomic area, 43
    congenital, 233–269. See also *Congenital spine deformities.*
    effects on patient with, 91–93
    general health of patient with, 48
    history of, patient, 47–48
    in poliomyelitis. See *Poliomyelitis, spinal deformity in.*
    natural history of, 89–95
    neuromuscular, 271–305. See also *Neuromuscular spinal deformities.*
    patient evaluation for, 47–88. See also *Patient(s), evaluation of.*
    post-laminectomy, 513–522, *514–520*. See also *Post-laminectomy spine deformity.*
    radiation and, 547–554, *548*, *549*, *551*, *552*. See also *Radiation, spine deformity following.*
    traction in, 109–117, *110–116*. See also *Traction.*
  deformity of, natural history of, 89–95
  differentiation of, control of, 33
  dysraphism of, treatment of, 265–269, *268*
  embryonic development of, 25–39
  flexibility of, in evaluation for spinal deformity, 48–53, *50–52*
  fractures of, 435–463. See also *Fracture(s).*
  fusion of. See *Spinal fusion.*
  growth of, 34–39
    charting of, from birth to maturity, *34*
    sitting, *35*
    standing, *34*
    total thoracic and lumbar spines vs. segments, *36*
    velocity vs. angulation of curve in, *37*
  embryologic, 25–39
  percentage completed by age, 38t
  velocity of, 35t
    peak, vs. other parameters of development, *37*
  lumbar, injury to, 435–463. See also *Spinal injury.*
  lower, Harrington instrumentation to, 148
  posterior column of, anatomy of, 8, *8*
    ligamentous structures of, 10
  posterior osteotomy of. See *Osteotomy, posterior spinal.*
  radiographic evaluation of, 58–67, *59–63*
    derotated view in, 65–66, *69*
    evaluation of maturity by, 65
    Ferguson view in, 65, *68*
    flexibility views in, 63–65, *64*

INDEX649

Spine (*Continued*)
 radiographic evaluation of, hazards in, 58–60
  oblique views in, 65
  plan d'élection of Stagnara in, 65–66, 69
  radiation doses in, 60t
  routine, 58
  spot view in, 65
  supine evaluation in, 63
  upright examination in, 60–62, 60–63
 range of motion of, in evaluation for spinal deformity, 48–53, 50–52
 retroperitoneal approach to, 165
 thoracic, injury to, 435–463. See also *Spinal injury.*
 thoracoabdominal approach to, 164, 164–165
 transperitoneal approach to, 165–166
 transthoracic approach to, 162–164, 163
 tumors of, 491–511. See also *Tumor(s).*
Spinocerebellar degenerative diseases, 298–299
Spinogram, in evaluation of patient for spinal deformity, 80–83, 81
Spirometry, incentive, postoperative, 590
Spondylitis, ankylosing, 628–635, 630–632, 634
 fractures in, 633
 treatment of, 629–631, 630–631
 infectious, vs. juvenile kyphosis, 354
Spondylodiscitis, 635
Spondyloepimetaphyseal dysplasia, 538
Spondyloepiphyseal dysplasia, 529, 534
 Milwaukee brace for, 529
Spondylolisthesis, 403–434
 acquired, postoperative, 486
 asymptomatic, clinical risk factors and, 413
  radiographic risk factors and, 413
  slip angle and, 413
  slippage type and, 413
  stability and, 413
  treatment of, 413–414
 biomechanical considerations in, 404–405
 classification of, 403, 404
 clinical findings in, 406–407, 407, 408
 decompression for, 427, 428
 degenerative, radiographic evaluation of, 427
  symptoms of, 426–427
  treatment of, 427–430, 428, 429
   decompression for, 427, 428, 429
 etiology of, 403–404
 gait pattern in, 407
 growth and, 404
 hereditary factor in, 404
 in juvenile kyphosis, 405
 in neurofibromatosis, 339, 343
 in osteogenesis imperfecta, 567
 laminectomy in, 415
 neural arch failure and, 405
 radiographic findings in, 407–411, 409, 410
 sacral inclination of, measurement of, 409, 410
 sagittal rotation of, 409, 410
 scoliosis and, treatment of, 424–426, 425
 slip angle of, measurement of, 409, 410
 slippage percentage in, 408–410
 spinal fusion for, 414–417, 415–417
 stress x-rays for, 410–411
 trauma and, 404–405
 treatment of, 414–430, 415–421, 423–425, 428, 429

Spondylolisthesis (*Continued*)
 treatment of, anterior fusion for, 417
  lumbosacral fusion for, 414–416, 415
  spondyloptosis after, 416–417, 417
  posterolateral fusion for, 416, 416
  reduction for, 418–421, 418–424, 423–425
   anterior and posterior techniques in, 422, 424, 424, 425
   posterior implant technique in, 419, 422, 423
Spondylolysis, 403–434
 clinical findings in, 406–407, 407, 408
Spondyloptosis, 406, 407
 following lumbosacral fusion, 416–417, 417
Spondylosis, CT scanning in, 410
 in juvenile kyphosis, 355
 incidence of, 404
 myelographic evaluation in, 410
 stress x-rays for, 410
 treatment of, 411, 412
  cerclage wire fixation for, 411, 412
  fusion for, 411
  non-operative, 411
  operative, 411, 412
Stability, spinal, 440–441
Stabilization, spinal injury treatment with, 442–443
Stagnara, distraction cast of, 120, 121
 plan d'élection of, 65–67, 69
 postoperative cast of, 120, 121
Stenosis, spinal, in achondroplasia, 523, 524–527
Superior mesenteric artery syndrome, 469–470, 470
Supraspinous ligaments, 10
Surgery, airway management in, 619–620
 approaches to spine in. See under *Spine*, e.g., *Spine, anterior approach to.*
 blood loss during, induced hypotension and, 614–616
 blood salvage during, 618–619
 blood transfusion techniques for, 617–618
 bone grafting in, 139
 closure in, 141
 complications of, 471–488
  intraoperative, 471–474, 473
  postoperative, early, 474–479, 475, 477
   late, 478–485, 481–485
 facet joint fusion in, 139–141, 140–141
 fluid management during, 616–617
 for adolescent scoliosis, postoperative treatment in, 225–227
  preoperative distraction and casting in, 216
  selection of fusion area for, 216–217
  selection of instrumentation in, 217–225, 221–226
  two-stage anterior and posterior fusions in, 225
 for juvenile scoliosis, 201–203, 204–205
 for poliomyelitis, 276–282, 278, 280
 for thoracic lordosis, 181–184, 182–184
 incision in, 135–139, 138
 positioning for, 620–622
 positioning of patient for, 135, 136, 620–622
 reconstructive, 391–402. See also *Reconstruction, staged.*
 salvage, 391–402
 techniques of, 135–189. See also names of specific procedures, e.g., *Osteotomy.*

Surgery (*Continued*)
  techniques of, special, 177–185, *180–183*. See also names of specific procedures, e.g., *Thoracoplasty*.
  wake-up test after, 148–149, 614, 623–624
Syngeneic graft, 593
Syringomyelia, 299–301, *300, 301*

Tanner system, for assessment of maturity, 55–57, *57*, 57t
Test(s), forward bending, 50–53, *51–52*
  laboratory, in evaluation for spinal deformity, 87
  pulmonary function, 87
  wake-up, after spinal surgery, 148–149
Thiopental-fentanyl, 623
Thoracic cage, contractures of, scoliosis and, 582–585, *583*
  defects of, 582–585, *583*
Thoracic inclination, angle of, definition of, 43
Thoracoabdominal approach to spine, *164*, 164–165
Thoracolumbar sacral orthosis, history of, 98, *98*
Thoracoplasty, in treatment of idiopathic scoliosis, 227–228
  scoliosis due to, 582–585, *583–584*
  technique of, 184–185
Three column spine concept, in spinal injury, 439–440, *440*
Thrombophlebitis, from traction, 468
Tidal volume (TV), *586*
TLSO (thoracolumbar sacral orthosis), history of, 98, *98*
  in juvenile scoliosis, 210–212, *211*
Total lung capacity (TLC), *586*
Traction, 109–117, *110–116*. See also specific types of traction, e.g., *Halo traction*.
  clinical experience in, 110–113, *111–112*
  complications of, 113–116, *116*, 465–468, *467*
    neurologic, 466–467, *467*
      prevention of, 467
  followed by instrumentation at fusion, in congenital scoliosis, 258, *259*
  halo, 110, *111*
    application of, 113, *114–115*
    complications of, 465–466
    in poliomyelitis, 279
  halofemoral, complications of, 115, *116*
  halogravity wheelchair, in paralytic scoliosis, 110, *111*
  halohoop, complications of, 113–115
  halopelvic, 466
    in spondylolisthesis, 113
  mechanics of, 109–110
  paralysis due to, 116
  posterior fusion with, 251–253, *255*
  preoperative, in neuromuscular scoliosis, 279
  preoperative skeletal, in idiopathic scoliosis, 111, *112*
  pressure sores from, 468
  quadriplegia from, 466
  thrombophlebitis from, 468
Translational injury, treatment of, 454, *455–459*

Transperitoneal approach to spine, 165–166
Transthoracic approach to spine, 162–164, *163*
Trauma, anesthetic considerations in, 610–611
  spinal, 435–463. See also *Fracture(s)*.
  spondylolisthesis and, 404–405
Trophism, definition of, 10
Trunk, growth remaining in, at consecutive skeletal age levels, *39*
Tube, neural. See *Neural tube*.
Tuberculosis, 568–575, *569, 570, 573, 574*
  differential diagnosis of, 569–571, *570*
  history of, 568
  incidence of, 568
  pathogenesis of, 568–569, *569*
  spinal sites of, 568
  thoracoplasty for, scoliosis due to, 582–583
  treatment of, 571–575, *573, 574*
    current, 572–575, *573, 574*
    for late deformity, *573, 574*, 574–575
    for one vertebra, 572
    for two or more vertebrae, 572
    historical, 571–572
    with spinal cord involvement, 572, 574
Tumor(s), 491–511. See also specific types.
  benign, 491–495, *492, 493*
  biopsy of, 491
  malignant, metastatic, *499*, 500, *500–502*, 503
    spinal cord compression with, 503
  primary, 495, 500
  of spinal cord, 505–511, *506–508, 510*
  radiation treatment of, spine deformity following, *548*, 548–549, *549*
  rib resection for, scoliosis due to, *583–584*, 583–585
Turnbuckle cast, 131–133, *132*
Turner's syndrome, juvenile kyphosis and, 349, *349*
TV (tidal volume), *586*

Ulcers, decubital, in spinal cord injury patients, 438–439
Underarm cast, application of, 126–129, *127*
Urinary retention, postoperative, 476
Urogram, in evaluation for spinal deformity, 84

VC (vital capacity), *586*
Ventilation, mechanical, postoperative, 590, 590(t)
Ventrolateral costal element, formation of, 30
Vertebra(e), anatomy of, 8
  apical, definition of, 43
  chondrification of, 31, *32*
  costal process of, 31, *31*
  embryonic contributions to, *31*
  end, definition of, 43
  formation of, *29*
  ossification of, 31, *32*
  rotation of, 73–77
    evaluation of, 73, *74*
    grading of, 73
    measurement of, in kyphosis, *75, 76, 77*
      Pedriolle method for, 73, *75*

INDEX

Vertebral body, anatomy of, 8
  function of, 9
  resection of, 174
Vertebral centrum, ossification of, 32
Vertebral endplates, definition of, 44
Vertebral growth plate, definition of, 44
Vertebral ring apophyses, definition of, 44
  ossification of, 79, *79*
Viscera, intraoperative damage to, 474
Vital capacity (VC), *586*
von Ebner, sclerotomic fissure of, 30
von Recklinghausen's disease. See *Neurofibromatosis*.

Wake-up test, 148–149, 614, 623–624
Wedge compression fracture, treatment of, 444–446, *445*
Werdnig-Hoffmann disease, 282–286, *285, 287*

Werdnig-Hoffmann disease (*Continued*)
  treatment for, 284–286, *285, 287*
Wilms' tumor, radiation treatment of, spine deformity following, 549, *551, 552*
Wound, infection of, postoperative, 476, *477*

Xenogeneic graft, 593
Xenograft, 593

Yellow ligament, anatomy of, 10

Zielke instrumentation, in surgery for adolescent scoliosis, *223, 224, 225*
  technique of, 174–177, *175–178*